5.2 Chronic Liver Failure (CLIF) Organ Failure (OF) Score

Organ or System	Variable	Score = 1	Score = 2	Score = 3
Liver	Bilirubin (mg/dL)	<6	6 to ≤ 12	> 12
Kidney	Creatinine (mg/dL)	< 2	2 to < 3.5	≥ 3.5 or RRT
Brain	Grade of Hepatic encephalopathy (West-Haven)	0	1-2	3-4
Circulation	Mean arterial pressure (mm Hg)	≥ 70	< 70	Vasopressors
Coagulation	INR	< 2	2 to 2.5	≥ 2.5
Respiration	PaO_2/FiO_2 ratio, or SpO_2/FiC_2 ratio	> 300 > 357	200 – 300 215 - 357	≤ 200 ≤ 214

Grade of ACLF	Number of Organ Failures (OFs)	28-day mortality
1a	Single kidney failure	18.6%
1b	Single non-kidney organ failure with kidney or brain dysfunction	27.8%
2	Two OFs	32%
3a	Three OFs	68%
3b	Four or more OFs	88.9%

(Highlighted area shows defining criteria of each organ failure)

4.2 ALF Early Dynamic Model (ALFED)

Predictors of mortality based on dynamic assessment over 3 days		Score assigned
HE, persisting or progressed to ≥ grade 2		+2
IHR, persisting or progressed to ≥ 5		+1
Arterial ammonia, persisting or progressed to ≥ 123 μmol/L		+2
Serum bilirubin, persisting or increased to ≥ 15 mg/dL		+1
Risk Stratification	**Total Score**	**Mortality**
Low risk	0–1	0–5.6%
Moderate risk	2–3	19–21%
High risk	4	67%
	5	84%
	6	100%

42.5 Acute-on-Chronic Liver Failure (ACLF)

5.1 APASL-ACLF Research Consortium (AARC) score

Points Variable	1	2	3
Bilirubin (mg/dL)	<15	15–25	>25
Crade of HE	0	I–II	III–IV
INR	<1.8	1.8–2.5	>2.5
Serum Creatinine (mg/dL)	<0.7	0.7–1.5	>1.5
Lactate (mmol/L)	<1.5	1.5–2.5	>2.5
ACLF Grade I	**Score**	**28-day Mortality**	
Grade I	5–7	12.7%	
Grade II	8–10	44.5%	
Grade III	11–15	85.9%	

	Clinical or laboratory findings	Points
	0.1–0.2	1
	Normal (>0.2)	0
24-h Urinary Copper	>2x upper limit of normal	2
	1-2x upper limit of normal	1
	Normal	0
	Normal, but >5x upper limit of normal after D-penicillamine	2
Coombs-negative Hemolytic Anemia	Present	1
	Absent	0
Total Liver Copper Level (Micromol/g)	>5x upper limit of normal (>4)	2
	Increased (0.8–4)	1
	Normal (<0.8)	-1
	Rhodanine-positive granules present	1
Genetic Mutation	Present on both chromosomes	4
	Present on 1 chromosome	1
	Absent	0
Total Score	Diagnosed established	≥4
	Diagnosis possible	3
	Diagnosis unlikely	≤2

42.4 Acute Liver Failure (ALF) prognostic scores

4.1 Kings College Criteria

Acetaminophen induced ALF	**Non-Acetaminophen induced ALF**
List for Liver transplantation if –	List for Liver transplantation if –
1. Arterial pH < 7.3 after resuscitation and >24 hour after ingestion	1. INR > 6.5, or
2. Lactate >3mmol/L, or	2. **Three out of following 5 criteria** –
3. **All of the following** –	a. Aetiology – indeterminate hepatitis, drug induced liver injury
a. Prothrombin time > 100 sec (INR > 6.5)	b. Age < 10 or > 40 years
b. Serum creatinine > 3.4 mg/dL	c. Jaundice to encephalopathy interval > 7 days
c. Grade 3 or 4 hepatic encephalopathy	d. Bilirubin > 17.5 mg/dL
	e. INR > 3.5

Roussel UCLAF Causality Assessment Method (RUCAM) Score

Criteria	Explanation	Score
Time to onset of injury from initial exposure to the drug	Suggestive 2 Compatible 1 Inconclusive 0	0–2
Course of action	Highly suggestive 3 Suggestive 2 Compatible 1 Inconclusive 0 Against −2	−2 to 3
Known risk factors for DILI: alcohol exposure, age > 55Y	No risk factor 0 1 risk factor 1 2 and more: 2	0–2
Concomitant other drug exposure	No exposure 0 Drug exposure but not hepatotoxin-1 Hepatotoxin-2 Confirmed injury due to another drug −3	0 to −3
Alternative non-drug cause	Ruled out (HAV, HBV, HCV, HEV, alcohol, biliary pathology) 2 Some ruled out (based on number)1 to −2 Probable −3	2 to −3
Previous information on drug	None 0 Possible hepatotoxin1 Confirmed hepatotoxin 2	0–2
Response to rechallenge	Positive 3 Compatible 1 Not done 0 Negative −2	−2 to 3

Score	Interpretation
>8	High likely
6–7	Probable
3–5	Possible
<2	Unlikely

3.4 Wilson's Disease (Leipzig Score):

	Clinical or laboratory findings	Points
Kayser-Fleischer Rings	Present	2
	Absent	0
Neurological Symptoms or MRI Findings	Severe	2
	Mild	1
	Absent	0
Serum Ceruloplasmin Level (g/L)	<0.1	2

(continued)

Glasgow Alcoholic Hepatitis Score

Variable		Points
Age	<50	1
	≥50	2
White blood cell count	<15 × 10^9/L	1
	≥15 × 10^9/L	2
BUN (mg/dL)	<14	1
	≥14	2
Bilirubin (mg/dL)	<7.3	1
	7.3–14.6	2
	>14.6	3
PT ratio	<1.5	1
	1.5–2.0	2
	>2.0	3

A score of ≥9 is associated with 40% 28 days survival, compared with 80% survival in individuals with a score < 9.

3.2 Autoimmune liver diseases: Simplified scoring system for diagnosis of AIH

Category	Variable	Score
(1) AUTO ANTIBODIES		
ANA or SMA	1:40	+1
	>1:80	+2
Anti LKM-1	>1:40	+2
Anti SLA	Positive	+2
(2) IMMUNOGLOBULIN-G LEVEL	> Upper limit of normal	+1
	>1.1 Times upper limit of normal	+2
(3) HISTOLOGY	Compatible with AIH	+1
	Typical of AIH	−2
(4) VIRAL DISEASE	No viral markers	+2
DEFINITE DIAGNOSIS		≥7
PROBABLE DIAGNOSIS		6

3.3 Drug Induced Liver Injury: 'R-Score' = ALT/ALT (ULN) / ALP/ALP (ULN)

>5	Hepatocellular pattern
2–5	Mixed pattern
<2	Cholestatic pattern

2. **Medium/Large Varices**

Grouped together because management is the same.

- Nodular, tortuous, or beaded varices.
- Do **not** flatten with air insufflation.
- Typically **>5 mm**.
- Includes Grade II and Grade III from conventional grading.

AASLD: High-Risk Features
These determine whether prophylaxis is required:
High-risk stigmata

- **Red wale marks**
- **Cherry red spots**
- **Hematocystic spots**

2.7 **Ascites grading:**

International Ascites Club Grading system
Grade 1
Mild ascites detectable only by ultrasound examination
Grade 2
Moderate ascites manifested by moderate symmetrical distension of the abdomen
Grade 3
Large or gross ascites with marked abdominal distension

2.8 **Spontaneous Bacterial Peritonitis (SBP) Classification:**

Variants	Ascitic fluid culture	PMN/cumm
Spontaneous Bacterial Peritonitis	Positive	≥250
Culture negative neutrocytic ascitis	No growth	≥250
Monomicrobial non-neutrocytic bacterascites	Positive	<250
Polymicrobial bacterascites	Positive	<250

42.3 Etiology of Liver Diseases Related Scores and Grading

3.1 **Alcohol Related Hepatitis:**

$$\text{Maddrey Discriminant Function (mDF)} = 4.6\,(\text{patient prothrombin time} - \text{control prothrombin time}) + \text{total bilirubin (mg/dl)}$$

Poor prognosis mDF ≥32

Chapter 42
Hepatology Annexures

Vaibhav Patil, Karan Jain, Ruchi Rastogi, Dinesh Jothimani, and Sanjiv Saigal

42.1 Cirrhosis-Related Scores

1.1 Child Pugh score for severity of liver disease

Clinical and lab criteria	1	2	3
Encephalopathy	None	Mild to Moderate (grade 1or 2)	Severe (grade 3 or 4)
Ascites	None	Mild to Moderate (diuretic responsive)	Severe (Diuretic refractory)
Bilirubin (mg/dl)	<2	2 to 3	>3
Albumin (g/dl)	>3.5	2.8–3.5	<2.8
Prothrombin time			
Seconds prolonged	<4	4–6	>6
International Normalized Ratio	<1.7	1.7–2.3	>2.3
Class A: 5 to 6 points Class B: 7 to 9 Class C: 10 to 15			

V. Patil · K. Jain · D. Jothimani (✉)
Institute of Liver Disease and Transplantation, Dr Rela Institute and Medical Centre, Chennai, Tamil Nadu, India
e-mail: dinesh.jothimani@relainstitute.com

R. Rastogi
Department of Radiology, Max Super Speciality Hospital, Saket, New Delhi, India

S. Saigal
Hepatology and Liver Transplant Medicine, Max Institute of Liver and Gastrointestinal Sciences, Max Super Speciality Hospital, Saket, New Delhi, India

S. Saigal, D. Jothimani (eds.), *Fundamentals of Transplant Hepatology*,
https://doi.org/10.1007/978-981-95-2624-6_42

1.2. Model for End-Stage Liver Disease (MLED)

$$\text{MELD score} = 9.57 \times \log \text{Creatinine (mg/dl)} + 3.78 \times \log \text{Bilirubin (mg/dl)} + 11.20 \times \log \text{INR} + 6.43$$

$$\text{MELD} - \text{Na} = \text{MELD} + [1.32 \times (137 - \text{Na})] - [0.033 \times \text{MELD} \times (137 - \text{Na})]$$

$$\text{MELD 3.0} = 1.33 \times \text{if female} + 4.56 \times \log(\text{Bilirubin}) + [0.82 \times (137 - \text{Na}) - 0.24 \times (137 - \text{Na}) \times \log(\text{Bilirubin})] + 9.09 \times \log(\text{INR}) + 11.14 \times \log(\text{Creatinine}) + 1.85 \times (3.5 - \text{Albumin}) - 1.83 \times (3.5 - \text{Albumin}) \times \log(\text{Creatinine}) + 6$$

MELD Score	Mortality
≤9	1.9%
10–19	6.0%
20–29	19.6%
30–39	52.6%
≥40	71.3%

1.3 AST to Platelet Ratio Index (APRI)

Determines the likelihood of hepatic fibrosis and cirrhosis in patients with hepatitis C

$$\text{APRI} = [\text{AST(IU/L)} / \text{AST upper limit of normal (IU/L)}] \times [100 / \text{Platelets} (10^9/\text{L})]$$

Significant fibrosis: APRI threshold of 0.7 was 77% sensitive and 72% specific.
Severe fibrosis: APRI threshold of 1.0 was 61% sensitive and 64% specific.
Cirrhosis: APRI threshold of 1.0 was 76% sensitive and 72% specific.

1.4 Fibrosis-4 (FIB-4) Index for Liver Fibrosis

Non-invasive estimate of liver scarring in HCV and HBV patients, to assess the need for biopsy.

$$\text{FIB-4 Score} = [\text{Age (years)} \times \text{AST (IU/L)}] / [\text{platelet count} (10^9/\text{L}) \times \sqrt{\text{ALT (IU/L)}}]$$

Use with caution in patients <35 or >65 years old, as the score has been shown to be less reliable in these patients.

FIB-4 Score	Approximate fibrosis stage
<1.45	0–1
1.45–3.25	2–3
>3.25	4–6

42.2 Cirrhosis Complications-Related Scores

2.1 Hepatic encephalopathy:

West Haven criteria:

HE Grades	Description
Minimal	Objective tests like psychometric analysis suggestive of neurophysiological alterations without clinical evidence of mental change.
Grdae 1	Short attention span sleep reversal Euphoria, anxiety. Trivial lack of awareness.
Grade 2	Asterixis Lethargy, apathy Disorientation for time Obvious personality change Inappropriate behavior
Garde 3	Somnolence Gross disorientation Confusion Semi-stupor
Grade 4	Coma

2.2 Liver Frailty Index (LFI)*

Sex-adjusted Grip strength	Indicative of nutritional status
Number of chair stands	Muscle strength
Balance time	Neuromotor co-ordination

*LFI is calculated using an online calculator for above three components

Cutoffs of LFI:

<3.2	Robust
3.2–4.4	Prefrail
>4.5	Frail

2.3 Hepatorenal Syndrome (HRS)

HRS-AKI criteria

- ✓ ↑ in sCr ≥0.3 mg/dl (≥26.5µmol/L) in 48h; or ↑ ≥50% in 3 months
- ✓ No response after volume expansion with albumin 1g/kg/d x48H
- ✓ Cirrhosis with ascites
- ✓ Absence of shock
- ✓ No current or recent use of nephrotoxic drugs (diuretics, NSAIDs)
- ✓ Absence of parenchymal kidney disease
  - No Proteinuria (>500 mg/d)
  - No Hematuria (>50 RBC/HPF)
  - Normal kidney ultrasonography

Non-HRS AKI criteria

HRS-AKD

- ✓ ↑ in sCr < 50% in 3 months
- ✓ eGFR < 60 ml/min/1.73 m²
- ✓ No other cause of kidney disease
- ✓ Cirrhosis with ascites

HRS-CKD

- ✓ eGFR < 60 ml/min/1.73 m²
- ✓ No other cause of kidney disease
- ✓ Cirrhosis with ascites

2.4 Hepatopulmonary Syndrome Grading:

Stage	PaO_2 (Arterial Oxygen Tension)	A-aO_2 (Alveolar-arterial Gradient)
Mild	PaO_2 ≥80 mmHg	≥15 mmHg
Moderate	PaO_2 ≥60 and <80 mmHg	≥15 mmHg
Severe	PaO_2 ≥50 and <60 mmHg	≥15 mmHg
Very Severe	PaO_2 <50 mmHg (or <300 mmHg on 100% FiO_2)	≥15 mmHg

PaO_2 partial pressure of oxygen

2.5 Porto-Pulmonary Hypertension Grading:

Stage	Mean Pulmonary Arterial Pressure (mPAP)
Mild	mPAP: 25–35 mmHg
Moderate	mPAP: 35–45 mmHg
Severe	mPAP: >45 mmHg

2.6 AASLD Variceal Grading:

1. **Small Varices**

- Minimally elevated, straight.
- Flattens with air insufflation.
- Typically **<5 mm**.

17. Schütz E, Fischer A, Beck J, Harden M, Koch M, Wuensch T, et al. Graft-derived cell-free DNA, a noninvasive early rejection and graft damage marker in liver transplantation: A prospective, observational, multicenter cohort study. PLoS Med. 2017;14(4):e1002286.
18. Beck J, Bierau S, Balzer S, Andag R, Kanzow P, Schmitz J, et al. Digital droplet PCR for rapid quantification of donor DNA in the circulation of transplant recipients as a potential universal biomarker of graft injury. Clin Chem. 2013;59(12):1732–41.
19. Lagos-Quintana M, Rauhut R, Yalcin A, Meyer J, Lendeckel W, Tuschl T. Identification of tissue-specific micrornas from mouse. Curr Biol. 2002;12:735–9.
20. Wei L, Gong X, Martinez OM, Krams SM. Differential expression and functions of microRNAs in liver transplantation and potential use as non-invasive biomarkers. Transpl Immunol. 2013;29:123–9.

recommend that all physicians dealing with transplanted patients should acquaint themselves with the various drug interactions described above in the text (and tables).

References

1. Lim TY, Heneghan M. Biomarkers of immunosuppression. Clin Liver Dis. 2016;8(2):34.
2. Millán O, Rafael-Valdivia L, Torrademé E, López A, Fortuna V, Sánchez-Casbu S, et al. Intracellular IFN-γ and IL-2 expression monitoring as surrogate markers of the risk of acuterejection and personal drug response in de novo liver transplant recipients. Cytokine. 2013;61(2):556–64.
3. Kim N, Yoon Y-I, Yoo HJ, Tak E, Ahn C-S, Song G-W, et al. Combined detection of serum IL-10, IL-17, and CXCL10 predicts acute rejection following adult liver transplantation. Mol Cells. 2016;39(8):639–44.
4. Platz KP, Mueller AR, Haller GW, et al. Determination of alpha- and Pi-glutathione-S-transferase will improve monitoring after liver transplantation. Transplant Proc. 1997;29:2827–9.
5. Millán O, Rafael-Valdivia L, Torrademé E, et al. Intracellular IFN-γ and IL-2 expression monitoring as surrogate markers of the risk of acute rejection and personal drug response in de novo liver transplant recipients. Cytokine. 2013;61:556–64. https://doi.org/10.1016/j.cyto.2012.10.026.
6. He Q, Fan H, Li JQ, Qi HZ. Decreased circulating CD4+CD25highFoxp3+ T cells during acute rejection in liver transplant patients. Transplant Proc. 2011;43(5):1696–700.
7. Minguela A, Garcıa-Alonso AM, Marın L, Torio A, Sanchez-Bueno F, Bermejo J, et al. Evidence of CD28 upregulation in peripheral T cells before liver transplant acute rejection. Transplant Proc. 1997;29:499–500.
8. Rodrigo E, Lopez-Hoyos M, Corral M, Fabrega E, Fernandez-Fresnedo G, Segundo DS, et al. ImmuKnow as a diagnostic tool for predicting infection and acute rejection in adult liver transplant recipients: a systematic review and meta-analysis [Internet]. Database of Abstracts of Reviews of Effects (DARE): Quality-assessed Reviews [Internet]. Centre for Reviews and Dissemination (UK); 2012 [cited 2022 Mar 6]. Available from: https://www.ncbi.nlm.nih.gov/books/NBK115946
9. He Q, Fan H, Li JQ, et al. Decreased circulating CD4+CD25highFoxp3+ T cells during acute rejection in liver transplant patients. Transplant Proc. 2011;43:1696–700. https://doi.org/10.1016/j.transproceed.2011.03.084.
10. Lorho R, Turlin B, Aqodad N, et al. C4d: a marker for hepatic transplant rejection. Transplant Proc. 2006;38:2333–4.
11. Kaneku H. annual literature review of donor-specific HLA antibodies after organ transplantation. Clin Transpl. 2013;2013:63–75. PMID: 25095493.
12. O'Leary JG, Klintmalm GB. Impact of donor-specific antibodies on results of liver transplantation. Curr Opin Organ Transplant. 2013;18(3):279–84.
13. Martínez-Llordella M, Puig-Pey I, Orlando G, et al. Multiparameter immune profiling of operational tolerance in liver transplantation. Am J Transplant. 2007;7:309–19.
14. Li Y, Zhao X, Cheng D, et al. The presence of Foxp3 expressing T cells within grafts of tolerant human liver transplant recipients. Transplantation. 2008;86:1837–43.
15. Friedman BH, Wolf JH, Wang L, et al. Serum cytokine profiles associated with early allograft dysfunction in patients undergoing liver transplantation. Liver Transplant. 2012;18:166–76.
16. Beck J, Oellerich M, Schulz U, et al. Donor-derived cell-free DNA is a novel universal biomarker for allograft rejection in solid organ transplantation. Transplant Proc. 2015;47:2400–3.

Table 41.2 (continued)

Drugs	Interactions	Consequences
Prednisolone methylprednisolone	Ntifungals: ketoconazole, fluconazole, voriconazole, itraconazole	Increased blood levels of corticosteroids, inhibition of CYP3A4
	Antibiotics: rifampicin	CYP3A4 induction; enhanced metabolism of corticosteroids
	Antiviral agents: ritonavir	Irreversible inhibition of CYP3A4; increased blood levels of corticosteroids

Table 41.3 Drug interactions between various IMS medicines

Drugs	Interactions	Consequences
Cyclosporin Tacrolimus	Sirolimus, Everolimus	Increased blood levels of ciclosporin and mTOR inhibitors; increased risk of nephrotoxicity; ciclosporin decreases the clearance of sirolimus or everolimus
	Prednisolone	Decreased blood levels (induce the expression of the efflux pump transporter ABCB1 {P-glycoprotein} and CYP3A) due to enhanced metabolism of ciclosporin/tacrolimus, increased risk of rejection
Sirolimus Everolimus	Cyclosporin, Tacrolimus	Increased blood levels of ciclosporin and mTOR inhibitors; increased risk of nephrotoxicity
	Prednisolone	Decreased blood levels due to enhanced metabolism (induce the expression of the efflux pump transporter ABCB1 {P-glycoprotein} and CYP3A) due to enhanced metabolism of ciclosporin/tacrolimus, increased risk of rejection
Mycophenolate	Cyclosporin	Inhibition of enterohepatic circulation, a decrease in blood levels of mycophenolic acid

necessitating careful dose titration and therapeutic drug monitoring to maintain therapeutic levels (refer to Table 41.3 for guidance).

Additionally, CYP3A5 non-expressers (those with the **CYP3A5*3/*3 genotype) are more susceptible to glucocorticoid-induced enzyme induction compared to carriers of the CYP3A5*1 allele. Therefore, in these individuals, tacrolimus exposure may significantly increase after glucocorticoid withdrawal, and monitoring is essential to avoid toxicity.

41.7 Conclusion

Although imperfect, immunosuppression monitoring currently relies predominantly on therapeutic drug level monitoring of various immunosuppressants available. There are various techniques under evaluation which may help us better evaluate the net immunosuppression state of an individual patient. The liver transplant patients are going to be on these medications for life, thus necessitating the awareness of their drug interactions with commonly used medicines in clinical practice. We

Table 41.2 (continued)

Drugs	Interactions	Consequences
mTORi	Antifungals: Ketoconazole	CYP3A inhibition: Increase mTORi blood levels; sirolimus >11 fold, everolimus 15 fold. Advised to avoid the use of ketoconazole in post-transplant patients
	Fluconazole, voriconazole, and itraconazole	Inhibition of CYP3A4; dose reduction of sirolimus, everolimus is necessary. Voriconazole-sirolimus combination contradicts (increases sirolimus blood levels by seven-fold)
	Posaconazole	Increase sirolimus blood levels by nine-fold.
mTORi	Antibiotics: clarithromycin, erythromycin, azithromycin	Irreversible inhibition of CYP3A4; increased blood levels of sirolimus/ everolimus
	Rifampicin	CYP3A4 induction; enhanced metabolism of sirolimus/everolimus; increased risk of rejection
	Antiviral agents: ritonavir	Irreversible inhibition of CYP3A4; increased blood levels of sirolimus/ everolimus
mTORi	Antihypertensive agents: diltiazem, verapamil, amlodipine	Irreversible inhibition of CYP3A4, formation of metabolic intermediate complex; increased blood levels of sirolimus/everolimus; verapamil inhibits P-glycoprotein, increasing bioavailability of everolimus
	Antidiabetic agents: troglitazone, rosiglitazone	CYP3A4 induction; enhanced metabolism of sirolimus/everolimus; increased risk of rejection
	Psychopharmacants: carbamazepine, valproic acid	CYP3A4 induction; enhanced metabolism of sirolimus/everolimus; increased risk of rejection
Antimetabolites: Azathioprine	Allopurinol	Inhibition of xanthine oxidase; myelotoxicity
Mycophenolic acid	Antiviral agents: Ganciclovir, valganciclovir	Mycophenolate-glucuronide inhibits renal tubular secretion of ganciclovir; increased blood levels of ganciclovir and increased risk of toxicity (nephrotoxicity, neutropenia, leucopenia) Inhibits P-glycoprotein, caution!
	Antifungal: Posaconazole, ciprofloxacin	Decrease levels by interfering with enterohepatic circulation
	Bile acid sequestrants (e.g., cholestyramine)	Decrease levels by interfering with enterohepatic circulation

(continued)

Table 41.2 Drug interactions with post-transplant medications

Drugs	Interactions	Consequences
CNI	Antifungals: Ketoconazole	CYP3A inhibition: Increased blood levels of CNIs; Cyclosporin > 4 fold, tacrolimus > 2 fold. (73, 74) Advised to replace ketoconazole with other azole derivatives.
	Fluconazole, voriconazole, itraconazole	Alternative therapies to ketoconazole inhibit CYP3A to a lesser extent
	Posaconazole	Empiric dose reduction of CsA to 3/4th and TAC to 1/3rd of the normal dose
CNIs	Antibiotics: clarithromycin, erythromycin, azithromycin	Irreversible inhibition of CYP3A4; increased blood levels of ciclosporin/ tacrolimus
	Rifampicin	CYP3A4 induction; enhanced metabolism of ciclosporin, tacrolimus; increased risk of rejection
CNIs	Antihypertensive agents: diltiazem, verapamil, amlodipine	Irreversible inhibition of CYP3A4, formation of metabolic intermediate complex; increased blood levels of cyclosporin/tacrolimus
	Nifedipine	Reversible, competitive inhibition of CYP3A4
	Carvedilol	Inhibition of the ABCB1 transporter increases the absorption of oral cyclosporin
CNIs	Antidiabetic agents: troglitazone and rosiglitazone	CYP3A4 induction; enhanced metabolism of ciclosporin/tacrolimus; increased risk of rejection
	Anti-epileptics: carbamazepine, valproic acid Antiviral agents: Ritonavir	CYP3A4 induction; enhanced metabolism of ciclosporin/tacrolimus; increased risk of rejection
	Lipid-lowering agents: fluvastatin, simvastatin, atorvastatin	Irreversible inhibition of CYP3A4; increased blood levels of ciclosporin/ tacrolimus. Dose reduction of cyclosporine by 5–20% and tacrolimus by 1–3.5%. Increased statin exposure by ciclosporin; increased risk of myopathy and rhabdomyolysis

(continued)

5.3 Organ Failure Definition as per North American Consortium for Study of Liver Disease (NACSELD)

Organ failure	**Definition**
Renal	Need for renal replacement therapy
Brain	Grade 3 or 4 hepatic encephalopathy by West Haven classification
Circulation	Need for vasopressor support, mean arterial pressure <60 mm Hg or a reduction ≥40 mm Hg systolic blood pressure from baseline despite adequate volume resuscitation
Respiration	Need for positive pressure ventilation (BIPAP or mechanical ventilation)
Total Score	**Classification as per NACSELD criteria**
0–1 OFs	No ACLF
2–4 OFs	ACLF

42.6 Liver Transplant for Hepatocellular Carcinoma (HCC)

Milan Criteria:

- Single tumor ≤5 cm, or
- 2–3 tumors none exceeding 3 cms, and
- No vascular invasion and or extrahepatic spread

UCSF criteria:

- Single tumor ≤6.5 cms or
- 2–3 lesions, non exceeding 4.5 cms, with total tumor diameter ≤ 8 cms
- No vascular invasion and/or extrahepatic spread.

ALBI (Albumin-Bilirubin) Score for HCC
Predicts survival in HCC patients.

$$\text{ALBI} = \left(\log_{10} \text{bilirubin} \times 0.66\right) + \left(\text{albumin} \times -0.085\right)$$
$$\text{where bilirubin is in } \mu\text{mol / L and albumin in g / L.}$$

ALBI Score	**Grade**	**Median survival (months)**
≤ −2.60	1	18.5–85.6
> −2.60 to ≤ −1.39	2	5.3–46.5
> −1.39	3	2.3–15.5

42.7 Segmental, Sectoral, and Lobar Anatomy of the Liver

The liver is divided into right and left lobes by the plane extending through the midline of the gall bladder, portal bifurcation, and the IVC, corresponding to the plane of the middle hepatic vein, which further corresponds to Cantlie's line drawn during hepatic resection. The right and left lobes are divided vertically into right posterior, right anterior, left medial, and left lateral sectors by the three hepatic veins, and horizontally into superior and inferior segments of each sector by the portal vein branches (Table 42.1).

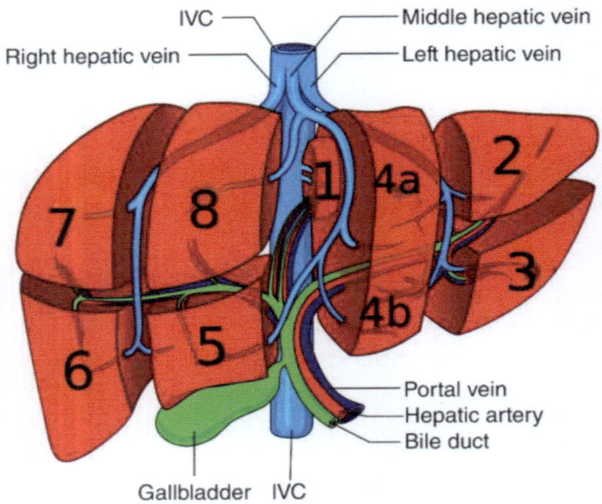

Table 42.1 The segmental, sectoral, and lobar divisions of the liver with segmental boundaries

Segment	Sector	Lobe	Landmark
I	–	Caudate	Anteriorly- Portal vein; Posteriorly- IVC
II	Left lateral (Posterosuperior)	Left	Medially-LHV; Inferiorly LPV
III	Left lateral (Anteroinferior)	Left	Medially-LHV; Superiorly-LPV
IV A	Left medial (Superior)	Left	Medially-LHV; Laterally-MHV; Inferiorly LPV
IV B	Left medial (Inferior)	Left	Medially-LHV; Laterally-MHV; Superiorly-LPV
V	Right anterior (Inferior)	Right	Medially-MHV; Laterally-RHV; Superiorly-RPV
VI	Right posterior (Inferior)	Right	Medially-RHV; Superiorly-RPV
VII	Right posterior (Superior)	Right	Medially-RHV; Inferiorly-RPV
VIII	Right anterior (Inferior)	Right	Medially-MHV; Laterally-RHV; Inferiorly-RPV

42.8 Hepatic Arterial Anatomical Variations

Typical hepatic arterial anatomy is described when celiac axis gives off common hepatic artery (CHA) which divides in gastroduodenal artery (GDA) and hepatic artery proper (HAP), which in turn divides in right hepatic artery (RHA) supplying the entire right lobe of liver (segments V, VI, VII & VIII) and left hepatic artery (LHA) supplying left lateral segments (II, III) with middle hepatic artery (MHA) supplying left medial segments (IVA, IVB) arising from RHA. Besides the conventional hepatic arterial anatomy in more than half of the population, different arterial anatomic variations are described by various authors, out of which Michels' classification is widely adopted, which is based on the origin of the three hepatic arteries along with identification of replaced and accessory arteries (Table 42.2).

Table 42.2 Michels' classification and variations in Hepatic arterial anatomy

Types	Population percentage (%)	Description
Type I	55	RHA, MHA, and LHA arising from the CHA.
Type II	10	RHA and MHA arising from the CHA; replaced LHA arising from the LGA.
Type III	11	RHA and MHA arising from the CHA; replaced RHA arising from the SMA.
Type IV	1	Replaced RHA and LHA arising from LGA and SMA, respectively.
Type V	8	RHA, MHA, and LHA arising from the CHA; accessory LHA arising from the LGA.
Type VI	7	RHA, MHA, and LHA arising from the CHA; accessory RHA arising from SMA.
Type VII	1	Accessory RHA and LHA.
Type VIII	2	Replaced RHA and accessory LHA or replaced LHA and accessory RHA.
Type IX	4.5	Entire hepatic trunk arising from the SMA.
Type X	0.5	Entire hepatic trunk arising from the LGA.

Michels NA. Blood Supply and Anatomy of the Upper Abdominal Organs with a Descriptive Atlas. Philadelphia: Lippincott, 1955

CHA common hepatic artery, *CT* Celiac trunk, *GDA* Gastroduodenal artery, *LGA* left gastric artery, *LHA* left hepatic artery, *MHA* middle hepatic artery, *PHA* Proper Hepatic artery, *RHA* right hepatic artery, *SMA* superior mesenteric artery, *SpA* Splenic artery

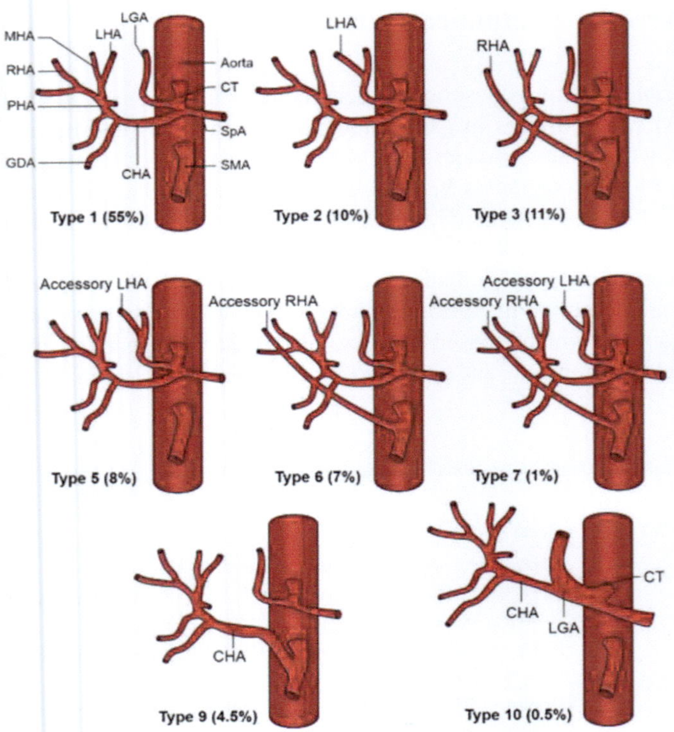

42.9 Portal Vein Anatomical Variations

Conventional portal vein anatomy, described as bifurcation of the main portal vein into right and left portal vein branches, which give supply to respective lobes, is present in the majority of the population, with few variations in the remaining people, primarily based on the separate origin of the right anterior portal vein branch. Nakamura et al. proposed a classification of portal vein anatomy in 2002, which is followed by many institutions due to its simplicity and easy adaptability (Table 42.3).

Table 42.3 Nakamura Classification of variations in Portal vein anatomy

Type	Population percentage (%)	Description
Type A	92.5	Bifurcation of MPV in RPV and LPV
Type B	2.5	Trifurcation pattern with separate origins of RAPV, LAPV, and LPV
Type C	2.5	Extrahepatic origin of RAPV from LPV
Type D	1.7	Intrahepatic origin of RAPV from LPV
Type E	<1	Undivided main portal vein trunk with individual segmental branches arising from the MPV

Nakamura T, Tanaka K, Kiuchi T, et al. Anatomical variations and surgical strategies in right lobe living donor liver transplantation: lessons from 120 cases. Transplantation. 2002; 73:1896–903
MPV Main portal vein, *RPV* Right portal vein, *LPV* Left portal vein, *RAPV* Right anterior portal vein branch, *RPPV* Right posterior portal vein branch

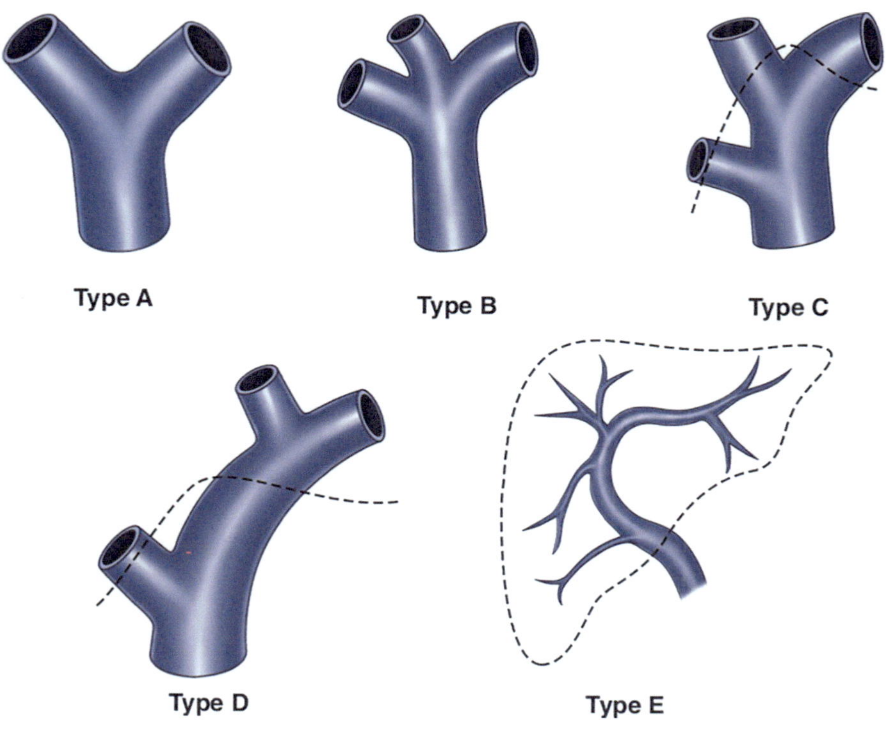

42.10 Hepatic Vein Anatomical Variations

The right, middle, and left hepatic veins form the basis of the sectoral division of the liver, with the right hepatic vein typically draining the right posterior sector, the middle hepatic vein draining the right anterior and the majority of the left medial sector, and the left hepatic vein draining the remaining left medial sector and left lateral sector, respectively. However, there can be considerable variations in the drainage patterns, especially pertaining to right hepatic venous drainage, with the presence of inferior right hepatic veins in many cases, as described by Varotti et al. (Table 42.4)

Table 42.4 Classification of the right liver hepatic venous anatomy

Types	Population percentage (%)	Description
Type Ia	13.8	Conventional anatomy with the right hepatic vein represents the main venous outflow of the right hemiliver.
Type Ib	7.7	Inferior right hepatic vein draining the right posterior segment of the liver to the IVC.
Type 2a	20	Segment 5 vein draining in MHV.
Type 2b	9.2	Inferior right hepatic vein draining the right posterior segment of the liver to the IVC, and the segment 5 vein draining into the MHV.
Type 3a	16.9	Segment 8 vein draining in MHV.
Type 3b	18.5	Inferior right hepatic vein draining the right posterior segment of the liver to IVC, and the segment 8 vein draining into the MHV.
Type 4a	10.8	Both segment 5 and 8 veins draining into MHV.
Type 4b	3.1	Inferior right hepatic vein draining the right posterior segment of the liver to IVC, and segment 5 and 8 veins draining into the MHV.

Varotti G, Gondolesi GE, Goldman J, et al. Anatomic variations in right liver living donors. J Am Coll Surg 2004;198:577–82

IRHV inferior right hepatic vein, *IVC* inferior vena cava, *LHV* left hepatic vein, *MHV* middle hepatic vein, *RHV* right hepatic vein

Types of Hepatic vein anatomical variations

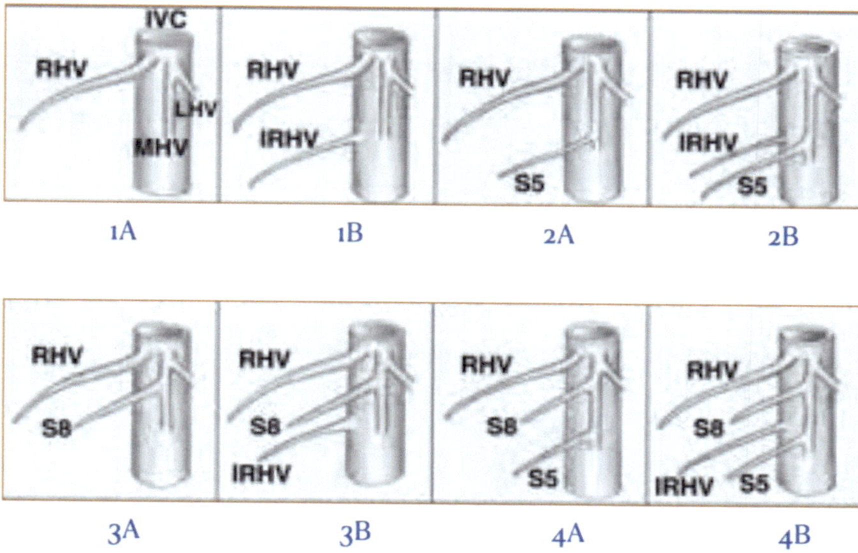

42.11 Biliary Anatomical Variations

Typically, the right anterior sectoral duct (RASD) and right posterior sectoral duct (RPSD) join to form the right hepatic duct (RHD) at the right secondary confluence, and the right and left hepatic ducts (LHD) join together to form the primary confluence, continuing as the common hepatic duct. Segment 4 duct opens in the left hepatic duct, forming the left secondary confluence. However, there are many variations in this biliary anatomy which have been described by various authors, out of which a commonly followed classification proposed by Choi et al. is described below (Table 42.5).

Table 42.5 Classification of Biliary anatomy variations

Type	Description
Type 1	RHD and LHD opening at the primary confluence
Type 2	Trifurcation pattern with RASD, RPSD, and LHD opening separately at the primary confluence
Type 3	RPSD draining anomalously in the left hepatic duct (Type 3A), common hepatic duct (Type 3 B), or cystic duct (Type 3C)
Type 4	The RHD draining into the cystic duct
Type 5	An accessory duct is present opening in CHD (Type 5A) or RHD (Type 5B)
Type 6	Segments II and III draining individually into the RHD or CHD
Type 7	Unclassified or complex variation

Choi JW, Kim TK, Kim KW, Kim AY, Kim PN, Ha HK, Lee MG. Anatomic Variation in Intrahepatic Bile Ducts: an Analysis of Intraoperative Cholangiograms in 300 Consecutive Donors for Living Donor Liver Transplantation. Korean J Radiol. 2003 Apr-Jun;4(2):85–90

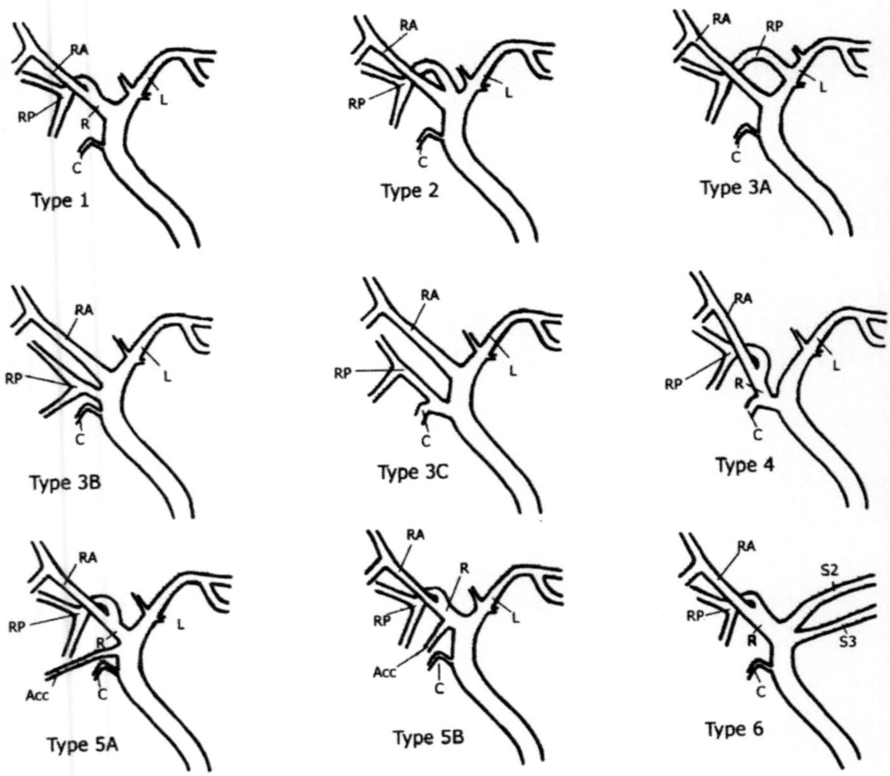

42.12 Liver Fat Quantification Based on MR-PDFF

MRI-based fat quantification by using Proton Density Fat fraction (PDFF) has been established as the most accurate non-invasive tool for liver fat quantification by various studies. The study by Tang et al. has established MR-PDFF thresholds for various grades of liver parenchymal steatosis vis-à-vis histopathological fat (Table 42.6).

Table 42.6 MR-PDFF thresholds of liver parenchymal steatosis in relation to histopathological grading

Steatosis Grade Classification	MR Imaging PDFF Threshold (%)
Grade 1	6.4
Grade 2	17.4
Grade 3	22.1

Tang A, Desai A, Hamilton G, Wolfson T, Gamst A, Lam J, Clark L, Hooker J, Chavez T, Ang BD, Middleton MS, Peterson M, Loomba R, Sirlin CB. Accuracy of MR imaging-estimated proton density fat fraction for classification of dichotomized histologic steatosis grades in nonalcoholic fatty liver disease. Radiology. 2015 Feb;274(2):416–25

42.13 Liver Imaging- Reporting & Data System (LI-RADS)

LI-RADS was created to standardize the reporting and data collection of CT and MR imaging for hepatocellular carcinoma (HCC). It is applicable in patients with cirrhosis, chronic hepatitis B infection, even in the absence of cirrhosis, or a personal history of HCC. It has also proposed post-treatment evaluation of proven or presumed HCC after locoregional therapy, with categorization of treated lesions as viable, nonviable, or equivocal (Figs. 42.1 and 42.2).

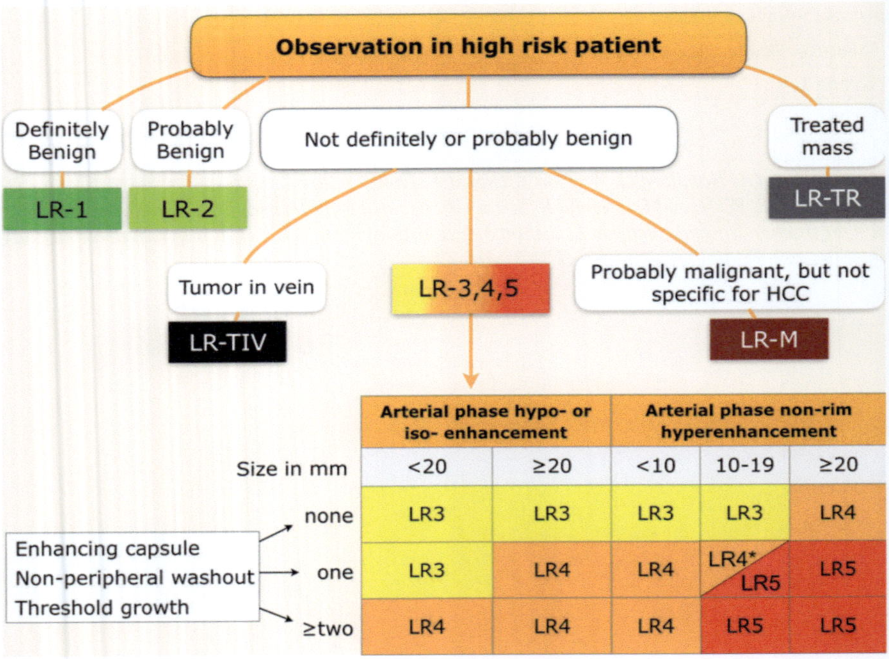

Fig. 42.1 CT and MRI LI-RADS diagnostic algorithm for untreated observations

Treatment Response Algorithm

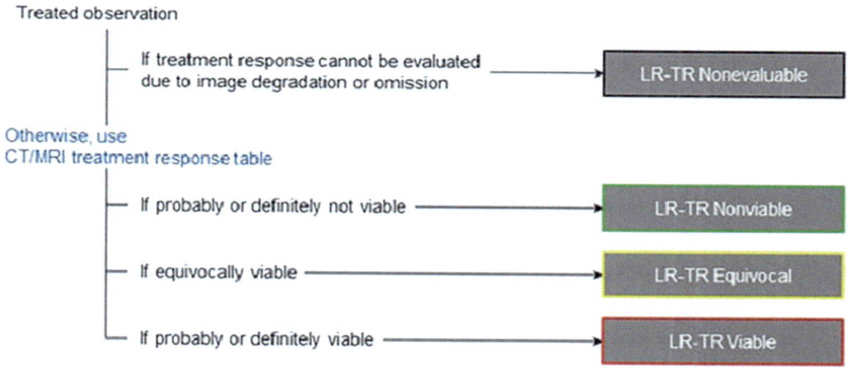

CT/MRI Treatment Response Table

Response Category	Criteria
LR-TR Nonviable	• No lesional enhancement **OR** • Treatment-specific expected enhancement pattern
LR-TR Equivocal	Enhancement atypical for treatment-specific expected enhancement pattern and not meeting criteria for probably or definitely viable
LR-TR Viable	Nodular, masslike, or thick irregular tissue in or along the treated lesion with any of the following: • Arterial phase hyperenhancement **OR** • Washout appearance **OR** • Enhancement similar to pretreatment

Fig. 42.2 LI-RADS Treatment Response (LR-TR) algorithm for assessing response to local-regional treatment of pathologically proven or imaging-presumed malignancies

Fundamentals of Transplant Hepatology

Sanjiv Saigal • Dinesh Jothimani
Editors

Fundamentals of Transplant Hepatology

Springer

Editors
Sanjiv Saigal, MD,DM,Inlaks Scholar, MRCP, FRCP
Vice Chairman and Head, Hepatology and Liver Transplant Medicine, Max Institute of Liver and Gastrointestinal Sciences
Max Super Speciality Hospital, Saket
New Delhi, India

Dinesh Jothimani, MBBS, MRCP, CCT, FRCP
Director of Hepatology and Medical Gastroenterology, Institute of Liver Disease and Transplantation
Dr Rela Institute and Medical Centre
Chennai, Tamil Nadu, India

ISBN 978-981-95-2623-9 ISBN 978-981-95-2624-6 (eBook)
https://doi.org/10.1007/978-981-95-2624-6

This Springer imprint is published by the registered company Springer Nature Singapore Pte Ltd.
The registered company address is: 152 Beach Road, #21-01/04 Gateway East, Singapore 189721, Singapore

Foreword

Liver transplantation now is a routine procedure that is available throughout many countries. A successful outcome for the patient is contingent on an effective teamwork involving a wide spectrum of healthcare practitioners including surgeons, physicians, anaesthetists and intensivists, microbiologists, radiologists, psychiatrists, histopathologists, immunologists, nurses, pharmacists, dieticians, physiotherapists and biomedical scientists. As the number of living transplant recipients continues to expand, more and more healthcare professionals are going to encounter transplant recipients, whether for problems relating to the graft, the treatment or unrelated problems.

Historically, assessment, transplant and follow-up of the patient lay with the local transplant unit. However, this model is becoming increasingly unsustainable due to the exponential increase in transplant recipients. Liver transplant units are developing their own patterns of referral, and good communication between the centre and the local practitioners remains essential. It is incumbent on all those healthcare professionals who care for those with liver disease to be aware of who and when to refer for consideration for transplant so that candidates can be assessed and where appropriate listed and grafted in a timely manner. Transplant units are also developing their own approaches of follow-up with many adopting devolved or shared care. Again, good communication between all parties remains a key to successful survival. Although liver transplantation leads to far better outcomes, both in terms of quality and quantity of life, neither reaches that of the normal population. The need, for the great majority of recipients at least, for lifelong immunosuppression and monitoring of complications relating to the graft, recurrent disease, donor transmitted disease and inherent consequences of immunosuppression, means that transplant recipients should remain under lifelong informed medical supervision. Thus, all healthcare practitioners need to be aware of knowing who and when to refer to a specialist unit, both before or after transplantation and when it is appropriate to manage the patient locally. Therefore, this book will be relevant not only for those working in transplant units but all those looking after patients with liver disease.

The tremendous advances already made in the management of liver disease and the ongoing and exciting research, especially in the fields of organ assessment and organ quality improvement, surgery, immunosuppression management and radiological interventions, should not ignore the fact that, for the physician at least, liver transplantation represents a failure to prevent end-stage disease; so it is important that research into transplantation should not detract resources and research into more effective prevention and treatment of liver disease so that transplantation becomes obsolete or, at best, reserved only for a small minority. I cannot see this happening in the near future at least.

While India was not in the vanguard of the development of liver transplantation, it is now very much at the forefront with several internationally renowned liver units, developing new surgical techniques, undertaking research and generating new paradigms for patient care. Data from the Global Observatory on Donation and Transplantation shows that in 2023 there were 41133 liver transplant procedures done worldwide in 436 centres; in that year India accounted for 4491 (11%) transplants which were done in 261 registered centres. Thus, India has rapidly become a major contributor to the worldwide experience.

While both the principles and practice for managing the liver transplant candidate and recipient are broadly similar around the world, variation in practice is not only necessary but desirable to tailor the care of the patient to their own personal, local and national environment. Transplantation is an expensive and resource-intensive procedure and is associated with legal, moral and ethical issues not often seen in other areas of clinical practice. The increasing burden of liver disease and the limited availability of organs in the context of ever increasing demands on the healthcare budget means that hard decisions have to be made regarding allocation of life-saving and life enhancing organs. It is for these reasons that this volume is so needed so that all those involved in liver transplantation, whether as donors or recipients and their families, healthcare professionals, managers, regulators and even politicians and law makers, need to understand and have confidence in the whole system.

Few, if any, ever read a textbook from cover to cover and many will dip in and out to find areas of relevance. The editors are to be congratulated in having brought together a comprehensive guide to all aspects of liver transplantation with contributions from clinicians with a wide spectrum of expertise. The focus on authors with knowledge of medical and social practice in the Asian subcontinent makes this especially relevant for those who practice in this location but, for those working elsewhere in the world, the book provides a useful guide to how medicine is practised in other jurisdictions with different pressures; we can all learn from the experience of others.

It has been said that the dangerous doctor is not the ignorant one but the lazy one: the lazy one will make assumptions whereas the ignorant one can easily find that knowledge. This volume provides a clear guide for those seeking clear and authoritative guidance on how to look after the patient with the care and quality they all deserve.

Finally, it is important to acknowledge the donors, whether living or deceased, without whose altruism and generosity transplantation could not take place. Both recipients and their healthcare professionals owe it to the donors and their families to ensure that the great gift is cherished.

Prof. James Neuberger, FRCP, DM

Professor of Medicine, Liver Unit,
Queen Elizabeth Hospital,
Associate Medical Director
(Organ Donation and Transplantation)
of NHS Blood and Transplant
University Hospitals of Birmingham
Birmingham, UK

Foreword

It gives me immense pleasure to write the Foreword for this book titled *Fundamentals of Transplant Hepatology* published by Springer.

Liver transplantation has seen a remarkable progress and acceptability over the last three decades. Surgical innovations in liver transplantation have considerably improved survival. It, however, remains a challenging field of modern medicine. Unlike other surgical procedures, the success of liver transplantation is dependent on a seamless coordination between several teams including hepatology, surgery, critical care, immunology, infectious diseases, and more. Moreover, there exists a significant disparity in policies and protocols across liver transplant centres. There is a need for comprehensive, practical, and authoritative resources that can guide the specialists involved in this field.

Increasing numbers of gastroenterology and hepatology trainees now undertake specialized training in 'transplant' hepatology as liver transplant centres are sprouting. Transplant hepatologists provide specialized pre- and post-transplant patient care, and co-ordinate decision-making strategies in liver transplantation. In recognition of the current need of transplant hepatologists, several countries including India offer a structured training in this discipline. This further endorses the need for a comprehensive textbook in the field of transplant hepatology.

I congratulate the editors—Dr Sanjiv Saigal and Dr Dinesh Jothimani, for creating this monumental work. It is a very timely addition to the field of transplant hepatology. The book has 42 elegantly written chapters which are divided into three sections: pre-transplant, perioperative, and post-transplant period. The contributors are nationally and internationally recognized experts from leading transplant centres. The chapters are lucidly written and thoughtfully structured with latest references, illustrative tables, diagrams, and practical algorithms wherever necessary. The editors have emphasized on evidence-based principles and practices, thus making it an invaluable resource for hepatologists, transplant surgeons, intensivists, fellows, and all members of the multidisciplinary transplant team.

I firmly believe that *Fundamentals of Transplant Hepatology* is a comprehensive treatise that encompasses the amazing progress in the field of liver transplantation and serves as a valuable resource for physicians and surgeons alike. I congratulate all the authors for their insightful contribution and wholeheartedly compliment Sanjiv and Dinesh for curating this book which I am confident will prove to be a 'must read' for the transplant community.

Prof. Shiv Kumar Sarin, MD, DM, DSc (Hons)

Senior Professor, Department of Hepatology, Chancellor and Director
Institute of Liver and Biliary Sciences (ILBS)
New Delhi, India

Preface

Liver transplantation is among the most challenging fields in medicine which involves a concerted multi-disciplinary teamwork for its success. Today, it is firmly established as a definitive treatment option for a large spectrum of liver diseases. Along with the remarkable success of liver transplantation, the field of transplant hepatology has evolved into a highly challenging speciality which serves as a backbone of any successful transplant programme. Despite this, there is a need of a comprehensive book that elaborates on the various issues involved in liver transplantation from a medical perspective.

This book titled *Fundamentals of Transplant Hepatology* has been conceived to serve as a comprehensive, reliable, evidence-based resource for ready reference for all those involved in the field of liver transplantation such as hepatologists, surgeons, intensivists, and various allied specialities.

This book has been elegantly edited by Dr Sanjiv Saigal and Dr Dinesh Jothimani, both being highly experienced hepatologists from leading transplant centres in India. The book truly reflects their deep understanding, commitment, and passion in dealing with liver transplant patients. The book comprises 42 chapters which have been divided into three major sections: pre-transplant, perioperative, and post-transplant care. All the chapters have been written by highly experienced national and international authors from leading transplant centres across the world, thus giving a flavour of both East and the West.

Each chapter is meticulously written in lucid manner, and includes key points. The chapters are further enriched with high-quality tables, algorithms, diagrams, and illustrations as and when necessary. In the end, there is an annexure that includes important grading and classification systems for quick reference for the readers. The book is intended to be a resource and a ready reference point, and help in clinical decision-making.

This book has been published by Springer, and every effort has been put to ensure high quality and authenticity of this book. We are confident that this book will be a much-needed addition for all those involved in liver transplantation, including the fellows and trainees.

We express our deep gratitude and appreciation for all those who have been involved in the creation of this book including the authors, the publisher Springer, and the transplant community which serves as a driving force for us to create this book.

Sincerely,

Sanjiv Saigal
Dinesh Jothimani

Acknowledgements

We would like to take this opportunity to look back, retrospect, and convey our deep gratitude to each and every individual who has been involved with us in the creation of this book, *Fundamentals of Transplant Hepatology*. This book involved numerous meetings, sacrosanct time, and our immense focus at all times despite several ups and downs in its journey. At each step, we were fortunate to have the right support from our well-wishers to whom we are extremely grateful.

The quality of any book of this magnitude entirely depends upon its content. In this regard, we would like to express our sincere thanks to all the distinguished national and international authors who took out time from their busy schedule and contributed such high-quality, evidence-based chapters. Our special thanks to Prof James Neuberger and Prof Shiv Kumar Sarin for graciously writing the Foreword for this book.

We extend our sincere thanks to Springer, the publisher, for doing a commendable job in publishing this book. Our special thanks to Raman Shukla, Senior Editor, for the guidance, and Stephanie, for handling the manuscripts, and all others from the Springer team for their invaluable support in the production of this textbook.

Patients are at the centre stage of any medical advancement. We owe huge respect for the patients who have to endure the burden of liver disease and show courage and determination at all stages of liver transplantation. In addition, we express our thanks to the care givers including all the paramedical staff who are involved in patient management. We would also like to thank our respective hospitals for providing the infrastructure and support to make liver transplantation a success story.

We deeply appreciate our supportive team members who have contributed directly or indirectly to this academic endeavour. In fact, our thanks reach out to each and every colleague of ours, individuals of the transplant community including the surgeons, hepatologists, anaesthesiologists, critical care physicians, intensivists, radiologists, pathologists, nurses, transplant co-ordinators, and other staff members.

We humbly pay respects to our parents for their blessings always. Lastly, this academic journey would not have been possible without the unwavering support of our families. A special thank you note from the bottom of our hearts for our wives, Jyoti and Nithya – without your understanding, patience, and support, this academic endeavour would not have been possible!

With gratitude,

Dr Sanjiv Saigal
Dr Dinesh Jothimani
Editors

Contents

Editors and Contributors

About the Editors

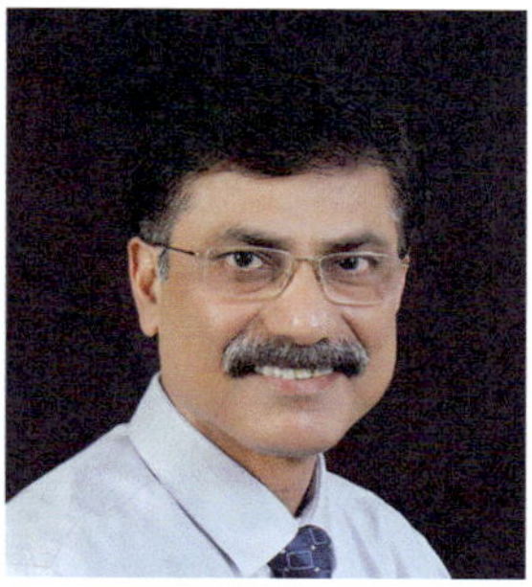

Dr. Sanjiv Saigal works as Vice Chairman and Head – Hepatology and Liver Transplant Medicine at Max Super Specialty Hospital, Saket, Delhi, India. As a skilled hepatologist, he has spearheaded the medical team of liver transplantation in India for over 24 years, with an experience in dealing with more than 5000 liver transplants, both living donor and cadaveric. He has over 175 peer-reviewed publications in reputed Journals, and has been the Editor of two books in Hepatology. He has received numerous awards, including the Calcutta University Gold Medal, National Pfizer Award and Human Care Award, and is an INLAKS Scholar trained at King's College Hospital, London. He is a member of the Royal College of Physicians (MRCP, Edinburgh) and a Fellow of the same (FRCP, Edinburgh). He is also the Fellow of the Indian National Association for Study of the Liver (Fellow-INASL), and the Master of the Indian Society of Gastroenterology (Master-ISG). He has been the Governing Council member of the Indian National Association for Study of the Liver (INASL). He has been a Member of several taskforces of INASL, such as Alcoholic Liver Disease, Hepatitis B, Hepatitis C, Acute Liver Failure & MASLD, and has regularly conducted Liver Transplant SIG meetings at the Annual INASL meetings.

He conducts Transplant Hepatology Fellowship program as the Course Director for over a decade now. He also conducts online certificate courses on management of various aspects of liver diseases. He is the Associate Editor of Journal of Clinical & Experimental Hepatology. He has been actively involved with the International Liver Transplant Society (ILTS) as its Education Committee Member (2017–2021), Member of Infectious disease SIG (2022–2025) and Membership & Communications Committee (2023–2026). He is currently the President of Liver Transplant Society of India (LTSI).

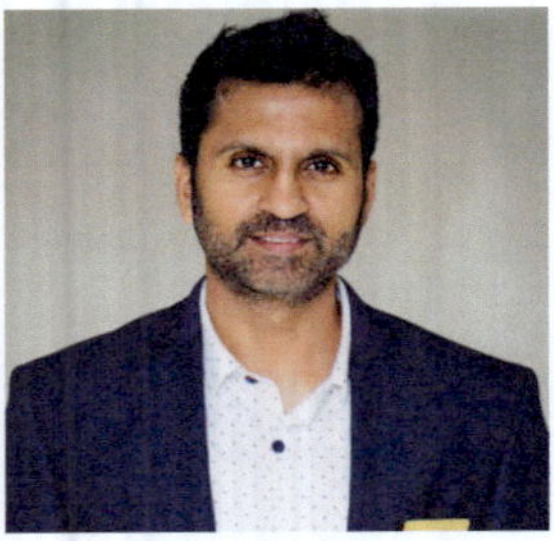

Dr. Dinesh Jothimani qualified from Madras Medical College and pursued his higher medical followed by higher specialist (Hepatology) training in Birmingham in the UK. He is a Member of the Royal College of Physicians, UK, and a Fellow of Royal college of Physicians and surgeons, Glasgow. He is a member of Indian Association for the Study of the Liver (INASL), Indian Society of Gastroenterology (ISG), International Liver Transplant Society (ILTS), and Liver Transplant Society of India (LTSI). He is the Director of Hepatology and Medical Gastroenterology at the Institute of Liver Disease and Transplantation, Dr Rela Institute and Medical Centre (RIMC), affiliated to Bharat Institute of Higher Education and Research, Chennai, India,

He loves sharing knowledge, spreading technical skills through simplified teaching.

He is the course director for Transplant Hepatology Fellowship programme at his institute, where he actively trains and guides gastroenterologists and hepatologists. He has several publications to his credit and actively collaborates with other centres nationally and internationally.

Contributors

Kalpana Acharya Department of Gastroenterology, Max Super Specialty Hospital, Saket, New Delhi, India

Subrat K. Acharya KIIT University, Bhubaneshwar, Odisha, India
Fortis Escorts Digestive & Liver Institute, New Delhi, India
Department of Gastroenterology, All India Institute of Medical Sciences, New Delhi, India

Jaya Agarwal Department of HPB Surgery and Solid Organ Transplant, Amrita School of Medicine, Amrita Vishwa Vidyapeetham, Faridabad, Haryana, India

Shaleen Agarwal Centre for Liver and Biliary Sciences (CLBS), Max Super Speciality Hospital, Saket, New Delhi, India

Dhiraj Agrawal Department of Gastroenterology and Hepatology, Continental Hospitals, Financial District, Hyderabad, India

Tanvir Ahmed Institute of Liver Disease and Transplantation, Dr Rela Institute and Medical Centre, Chennai, Tamil Nadu, India

Inbaraj Balradja Centre for Liver and Biliary Sciences (CLBS), Max Super Speciality Hospital, Saket, New Delhi, India

Shahnawaz Bashir Interventional Radiology, Max Super Speciality Hospital, Saket, New Delhi, India

Marina Berenguer Hepatology and Liver Transplantation Unit, Medical Research Institute (IISLaFe) La Fe University Hospital and University of Valencia, Valencia, Spain
CIBERehd (IISCarlosIII), Madrid, Spain

Naveen Bhagat Department of Hepatology, Postgraduate Institute of Medical Education and Research, Chandigarh, India

Prashant Bhangui Institute of Liver Transplantation and Regenerative Medicine, Medanta – The Medicity, Gurgaon, Delhi NCR, India

Ryan Chadha Departments of Anesthesiology and Peri-operative Medicine, Mayo Clinic, Jacksonville, FL, USA

Suchet Chaudhary Institute of Liver Transplantation and Regenerative Medicine, Medanta The Medicity, Gurugram, Delhi NCR, India

Yogesh K. Chawla Department of Gastroenterology and Hepatology, Kalinga Institute of Medical Sciences (KIMS), Bhubaneswar, Odisha, India

Arka De Department of Hepatology, Postgraduate Institute of Medical Education and Research, Chandigarh, India

Rajesh Dey Centre for Liver and Biliary Sciences, Max Saket and Vaishali Hospitals, New Delhi, India

Ajay Duseja Department of Hepatology, Postgraduate Institute of Medical Education and Research, Chandigarh, India

Maria A. Estevez Mayo Clinic, Jacksonville, FL, USA

James Fung Department of Medicine, The University of Hong Kong, Pok Fu Lam, Hong Kong SAR
The Liver Transplant Center, Queen Mary Hospital, Pok Fu Lam, Hong Kong SAR
State Key Laboratory Of Liver Research, The University of Hong Kong, Pok Fu Lam, Hong Kong SAR

Prasanna Gopal Star Institute of Comprehensive Liver Care & Transplantation, Star Hospitals, Hyderabad, India

Subhash Gupta Centre for Liver and Biliary Sciences (CLBS), Max Super Speciality Hospital, Saket, New Delhi, India

Amit Gupte Sir HN Reliance Foundation Hospital, Mumbai, India

Shekhar Singh Jadaun Hepatology and Liver Transplant Medicine, Max Institute of Liver and Gastrointestinal Sciences, Max Super Speciality Hospital, Saket, New Delhi, India

Karan Jain Institute of Liver Disease and Transplantation, Dr Rela Institute and Medical Centre, Chennai, Tamil Nadu, India

Dinesh Jothimani Institute of Liver Disease and Transplantation, Dr Rela Institute and Medical Centre, Chennai, Tamil Nadu, India

Patrick S. Kamath Division of Gastroenterology and Hepatology, Mayo Clinic College of Medicine and Science, Rochester, MN, USA

Jagdish Kanagaraj Nephrology and Renal Transplantation, Dr. Rela Institute and Medical Centre, Chennai, India

Akshay Kulkarni Department of Gastroenterology, Midas Multi-speciality Hospital, Nagpur, Maharashtra, India

Peeyush Kumar Liver and Digestive Institute, Fortis Escorts Hospital, New Delhi, India

Kaushal Madan Centre for Gastroenterology, Hepatology & Endoscopy, Max Super Specialty Hospital, Saket, New Delhi, India

Rakhi Maiwall Department of Hepatology, Institute of Liver and Biliary Sciences, New Delhi, India

Shweta Mallick Department of GI Surgery & Solid Organ Transplantation, Amrita Institute of Medical Sciences, Amrita Vishwavidyapeetham, Kochi, Kerala, India

Ameet Mandot Department of Hepatology and LICU, Gleneagles Hospital, Mumbai, India

Navin Marannan Institute of Liver Disease and Transplantation, Dr Rela Institute and Medical Centre, Chennai, Tamil Nadu, India

Rohit Mehtani Department of Hepatology, Amrita School of Medicine, Amrita Vishwa Vidyapeetham, Faridabad, Haryana, India

Krishnanunni Nair Department of GI Surgery & Solid Organ Transplantation, Amrita Institute of Medical Sciences, Amrita Vishwavidyapeetham, Kochi, Kerala, India

Gomathy Narasimhan Liver and Renal Transplant Surgery, Dr. Rela Institute and Medical Centre, Chennai, India

James Neuberger Liver Unit, Queen Elizabeth Hospital, Associate Medical Director (Organ Donation and Transplantation) of NHS Blood and Transplant, University Hospitals of Birmingham, Birmingham, UK

Laxmi Parsa University of Tennessee College of Medicine, Chattanooga, TN, USA

Vaibhav Patil Institute of Liver Disease and Transplantation, Dr Rela Institute and Medical Centre, Chennai, Tamil Nadu, India

Susan Paulin Liver anesthesia and Intensive Care, Institute of Liver Disease and Transplantation, Dr. Rela Institute and Medical Centre, Chennai, India

Anindita Phukan Institute of Digestive & Liver Diseases, BLK-Max Superspeciality Hospital, New Delhi, Delhi, India

Dibya Lochan Praharaj Department of Gastroenterology and Hepatology, Kalinga Institute of Medical Sciences (KIMS), Bhubaneswar, Odisha, India

Mithra Prasad VGM Hospital, Coimbatore, India

Akila Rajakumar Liver anesthesia and Intensive Care, Institute of Liver Disease and Transplantation, Dr. Rela Institute and Medical Centre, Chennai, India

Ashwin Rammohan Institute of Liver Disease & Transplantation, Rela Institute & Medical Centre, Chennai, India

Ruchi Rastogi Department of Radiology, Max Super Speciality Hospital, Saket, New Delhi, India

Mettu Srinivas Reddy Star Institute of Comprehensive Liver Care & Transplantation, Star Hospitals, Hyderabad, India
Rainbow Children's Hospitals, Hyderabad, India

Mohamed Rela Institute of Liver Disease & Transplantation, Rela Institute & Medical Centre, Chennai, India

Akash Roy Institute of Gastrosciences and Liver Transplantation, Apollo Multispeciality Hospitals, Kolkata, West Bengal, India

Omkar Rudra Department of Transplant Hepatology, Institute of Liver and Biliary Sciences, New Delhi, India

Sanjiv Saigal Hepatology and Liver Transplant Medicine, Max Institute of Liver and Gastrointestinal Sciences, Max Super Speciality Hospital, Saket, New Delhi, India

Shiv Kumar Sarin Department of Hepatology, Chancellor and Director, Institute of Liver and Biliary Sciences (ILBS), New Delhi, India

Sanjaya K. Satapathy Division of Hepatology, Department of Medicine, North Shore University Hospital/Northwell Health, Manhasset, NY, USA

Samir R. Shah Institute of Liver, Intestine and Pancreas Sciences, Liver Disease Unit, Nanavati Max Super Speciality Hospital, Mumbai, India

Sadhana Shankar Liver Transplant and Hepato-Pancreatico-Biliary Surgery Unit, Institute of Liver Studies, King's College Hospital NHS Foundation Trust, London, UK

Akash Shukla Sir HN Reliance Foundation Hospital, Mumbai, India
Seth GS Medical College & KEM Hospital, Mumbai, India

Ankita Singh Seth GS Medical College & KEM Hospital, Mumbai, India

Pankaj Singh Centre for Gastroenterology, Hepatology & Endoscopy, Max Super Specialty Hospital, Saket, New Delhi, India

Satender Pal Singh Department of Transplant Hepatology, Institute of Liver and Biliary Sciences, New Delhi, India

Shweta A. Singh Anesthesia & Critical Care, Centre for Liver and Biliary Sciences, Max Super Specialty Hospital, New Delhi, Delhi, India

Vikas Singla Department of Gastroenterology, Max Super Specialty Hospital, Saket, New Delhi, India

Arvinder Singh Soin Institute of Liver Transplantation and Regenerative Medicine, Medanta The Medicity, Gurugram, Delhi NCR, India

S Sreejith Centre for Liver and Biliary Sciences (CLBS), Max Super Speciality Hospital, Saket, New Delhi, India

Parthi Srinivasan Liver Transplant and Hepato-Pancreatico-Biliary Surgery Unit, Institute of Liver Studies, King's College Hospital NHS Foundation Trust, London, UK

S. Sudhindran Department of GI Surgery & Solid Organ Transplantation, Amrita Institute of Medical Sciences, Amrita Vishwavidyapeetham, Kochi, Kerala, India

Marta Tejedor Division of GI/Hepatology, University of Iowa Healthcare, Iowa City, United States

Shantan Venishetty AIG Hospitals, Hyderabad, India

Radhika Venugopal Institute of Liver Disease and Transplantation, Dr Rela Institute and Medical Centre, Chennai, Tamil Nadu, India

Mukul Vij Department of Pathology, Institute of Liver disease and Transplantation, Dr. Rela Institute and Medical Centre, Chennai, Tamil Nadu, India

Manav Wadhawan Institute of Digestive & Liver Diseases, BLK-Max Superspeciality Hospital, New Delhi, Delhi, India

Jyoti Wadhwa Department of Medical and Precision Oncology, Apollo Cancer Centres, Delhi, India

Julia Wendon Critical Care Division, Institute of Liver Diseases, King's College Hospital, Denmark Hill, London, UK

Sanjay Kumar Yadav Narayana Health, Gurugram, Haryana, India

Part I
Pre-transplantation

Chapter 1
Liver Transplantation: Historical Perspective and Evolution

James Neuberger

Abstract Successful human liver transplantation started, after a stuttering start, in 1967, led by the pioneering work of Thomas Starzl and others, such as Roy Calne, Rudolph Pichlmayr, Henri Bismuth, and Ruud Krom, supported by other health care professionals and scientists. The NIH Consensus Conference in 1983 marked the establishment of liver transplantation as a valid therapeutic option. Since that time, the number of liver transplants and transplant units has increased around the world, and outcomes have improved dramatically. Over the six subsequent decades, transplantation has evolved with many surgical advances, allowing donation from deceased and living donors, and use of liver segments and lobes and spliting livers to allow two recipients to receive a graft from one donor; Indications have evolved, and currently, alcohol-related liver disease and metabolic-dysfunction associated liver disease are the commonest indications. Immunosuppression has evolved from the early days using just prednisolone and azathioprine, sometimes with induction with anti-T cell induction, to triple therapy, most frequently using tacrolimus, mycophenolate, and prednisolone, although other drugs are also available to ensure optimal immunosuppression. As outcomes have improved, graft failure from acute or chronic (ductopenic) rejection, technical (often biliary) issues, and hemorrhage have become rare, and major causes of premature graft and patient loss are more related to recurrence of disease, cardiovascular and renal disease, and de novo malignancy.

To support liver transplantation, jurisdictions and international and national professional bodies have developed laws, regulations, policies, and procedures to ensure that organ donation and transplantation are carried out in a controlled way under clear ethical and legal frameworks.

J. Neuberger (✉)
Professor of Medicine, Liver Unit, Queen Elizabeth Hospital, Associate Medical Director (Organ Donation and Transplantation) of NHS Blood and Transplant, University Hospitals of Birmingham, Birmingham, UK
e-mail: jamesneuberger@hotmail.co.uk

S. Saigal, D. Jothimani (eds.), *Fundamentals of Transplant Hepatology*,
https://doi.org/10.1007/978-981-95-2624-6_1

Improvements in the outcomes after liver transplantation cannot be attributed to any one factor but occur as a result of the teamwork of many health care professionals and scientists. Issues still remain: relative organ shortage and potential shortage of skilled surgeons are of concern. In contrast, the use of machine perfusion is likely to improve outcomes and increase organ utilization. The place of xenotransplantation and other modalities is yet to be determined.

Keywords Liver transplantation · Indications · Outcomes · Immunosuppression · Ethics · Legal framework · Allocation

Key Highlights
- There has been a remarkable progress in the field of liver transplantation in the last six decades.
- Better patient selection, innovation in surgical techniques, and advancements in immunosuppression have improved graft and patient survival.
- Implementation of laws, regulations, and policies toward organ donation under a clear ethical and legal framework has contributed to the success of liver transplant programs globally.
- Teamwork is the cornerstone of a successful transplant program; however, organ shortage and universal accessibility to healthcare remain a concern.

1.1 Introduction

The earliest human liver transplants, performed in Denver, Boston, and Paris between 1963 and 1964, yielded extremely poor results—none of the patients survived beyond 23 days [1]. The youngest patient, a 3-year-old with biliary atresia, died during surgery due to uncontrollable hemorrhage. The remaining seven patients, most of whom were transplanted for cancer (including two with metastatic colon cancer), died mainly from sepsis, bleeding, or pulmonary embolism. These disappointing outcomes prompted a three-year suspension of the procedure. Liver transplantation resumed in 1967, led by Dr. Thomas Starzl in Denver, Colorado. A year later, a program commenced in Cambridge, UK, under the leadership of Sir Roy Calne in collaboration with Roger Williams in London.

In the initial years of the procedure, results remained poor. For instance, of the first 25 patients transplanted in Cambridge between 1968 and 1971, only six survived longer than 3 months, and just one survived more than a year—this patient had primary liver cell cancer [2]. Similar poor outcomes were reported across other European transplant centers, including those in Pittsburgh (Starzl), Groningen (Krom), Cambridge (Calne), and Hannover (Pichlmayr). The continued pursuit of liver transplantation, despite early failures, stands as a testament to the courage, insight, persistence, and commitment of these pioneering surgeons. They were supported by multidisciplinary teams—physicians, nurses, anesthetists, biomedical frameworks. Regulation has increased over time, sometimes in response to egregious misuse of responsibility. The WHO and the Transplantation Society have published a series of documents defining many legal and ethical aspects of donation and transplantation (see, for example, references [4–6]).

1.3 Surgical Techniques

The evolution of transplantation has been accelerated by the advances in anesthetic techniques, understanding of hemostasis, and control of infection. Surgical skills, supported by the understanding of the anatomy of the liver, have allowed the introduction and implementation of split, reduced liver, and segmental transplantation (Table 1.1). These advances have allowed not only greater use of organs but also ensured greater access to transplantation. The significant reduction in deaths of the pediatric waiting list is due in large part to the use of split livers, allowing two recipients (usually one adult and one child) to benefit. The introduction of living organ

Table 1.1 Some milestones in liver transplantation and the pioneers

Date	Event	Pioneers
1955	First article in literature about auxiliary liver transplant	Welch
1959	Models of canine total hepatectomy and replacement	Staudacher, Welch, Starzl, Cannon
1963	Introduction of corticosteroids/azathioprine	Starzl
1963	First attempt of a human liver transplant (survival up to 3 weeks)	Starzl
1967	1-year survival of human liver transplant recipients	Starzl
1969	Introduction of Collin's preservation solution	Collins
1979	Introduction of cyclosporine	Calne, White
1981	Reduced-size liver graft	Bismuth, Houssin
1983	Combined liver-kidney transplant	Margreiter
1984	Combined heart and liver transplant	Starzl
1987	Combined heart-lung liver transplant	Calne, Wallwork
1987	Introduction of the University of Wisconsin preservation solution	Belzer, Southard
1989	Combined liver-intestine transplant	Starzl
1989	Introduction of tacrolimus	Starzl
1989	First split liver transplant	Pichlmayr
1990	Living adult to child donor transplant	Raia, Strong
1993	Living adult-to-adult liver transplant	Shinshu
1993	Baboon to human liver transplant	Starzl
1994	Liver, kidney, stomach, intestine, and pancreas transplant	Calne
1995	Domino liver transplant	Furtado
1995	Introduction of mycophenolate	
1999	Introduction of sirolimus	

Legend: Some key dates in the field of liver transplantation

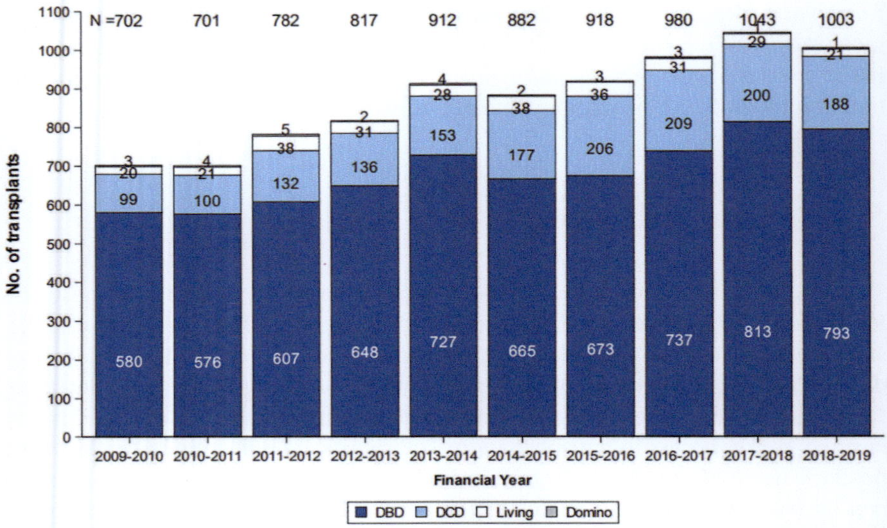

Fig. 1.3 Patterns of donor transplants in the UK. (From NHSBT Annual Report 2018/0 (www.odt.nhs.uk))

donation has evolved to allow organ donation to become accessible, especially in those areas of the world where deceased organ donation is very limited (Fig. 1.3).

1.4 Evolving Indications

In the early phase of liver transplantation, the primary indications included malignancy, cirrhosis, and acute liver failure. Between 1968 and 1985, the team at Cambridge and King's College Hospital performed 227 liver transplants, with approximately one-third conducted for malignant conditions—mainly hepatocellular carcinoma, though cases of cholangiocarcinoma, carcinoma of the hepatic ducts, and hepatic metastases were also represented [2]. Among patients with non-malignant liver disease, most suffered from end-stage cirrhosis, commonly due to primary biliary cholangitis, autoimmune hepatitis, cryptogenic cirrhosis, and alcohol-related liver disease. The series also included 13 cases of Budd-Chiari syndrome, six of acute liver failure, and 16 cases of biliary atresia and neonatal hepatitis. Over the following 40 years, the spectrum of indications has shifted (Table 1.2). Advances in therapies for liver cancer, effective control of hepatitis B, and curative treatments for hepatitis C have led to a decline in these indications. In their place, metabolic dysfunction-associated fatty liver disease (also referred to as non-alcoholic fatty liver disease, or NAFLD) and alcohol-related liver disease (ARLD) have emerged as increasingly prevalent indications.

Table 1.2 Indications for liver transplantation for adults on the US waiting list at the end of 2011 and 2021

Indications	2011	2021
Acute liver failure	31% (n = 4994)	10% (n = 1100)
Alcohol-related liver disease	23% (n = 3710)	34% (n = 3840)
Cholestatic disease	9% (n = 1502)	8% (n = 932)
Hepatocellular carcinoma	5% (n = 849)	11% (n = 2175)
Non-alcoholic fatty liver disease	8% (n = 1227)	19% (n = 2175)
Other/unknown	22% (n-3571)	17% (n = 1890)

Data from https://srtr.transplant.hrsa.gov/annual_reports/2021/Liver.aspx#tab:LIchar-adult-waiting-clin

1.4.1 Alcohol-Related Liver Disease and Alcoholic Hepatitis

ARLD has become one of the leading reasons for liver transplantation. In the early years, ARLD was not widely accepted as a suitable indication due to high infection risk and concerns about patients maintaining abstinence, which could affect graft function, medication adherence, and risk of extra-hepatic complications [7]. Starzl initially acknowledged ARLD as a valid indication but noted that very few patients could meet the abstinence criteria. However, within a decade, the same authors expressed greater support for liver transplantation in ARLD patients, citing favorable outcomes and low relapse rates [8].

Subsequently, ARLD became a subject of ethical debate in both the medical literature and popular media, particularly regarding the allocation of limited organs. Early public opinion opposed using donated organs for patients with ARLD [9], but perspectives have gradually shifted to become more supportive [10]. While concerns persist about alcohol relapse or non-adherence among these patients, studies indicate that graft loss due to resumed alcohol consumption is less frequent than previously feared and is lower than the graft loss from recurrent disease in other transplant indications.

Public perception remains vital to organ donation, as transplantation programs rely heavily on public trust. When that trust is compromised—as seen in Germany when patient data manipulation by clinicians was revealed—organ donation rates can sharply decline [11]. However, anecdotal reports and negative media attention surrounding alcohol misuse among transplant candidates have not been shown to significantly affect donation or consent rates [12].

The eligibility of patients with alcoholic hepatitis for transplantation has also evolved. Initially deemed an absolute contraindication, a landmark study by Mathurin demonstrated favorable outcomes in carefully selected patients [13]. Still, success rates remain lower than for many other indications, and around 25% of patients listed for transplant improved with medical therapy alone.

Today, transplant timing and eligibility for patients with ARLD and alcoholic hepatitis have become more standardized. Clinical guidelines now assist physicians in identifying suitable candidates and in providing structured post-transplant care and support [14].

1.4.2 Other Causes of Liver Disease

Metabolic dysfunction associated liver disease (or non-alcohol fatty liver disease: With rising global obesity rates and increasing prevalence of type 2 diabetes, NAFLD has emerged as a major indication for liver transplantation [15]. However, this condition brings unique challenges, particularly in evaluating patients for transplant due to associated comorbidities such as cardiovascular disease and diabetes and its associated microvascular complications, which complicate assessment and selection [15].

Acute on chronic liver failure: Acute-on-chronic failure (ACLF) is characterized by acute hepatic decompensation and often extra-hepatic organ failure. ACLF is often triggered by infection, alcohol consumption, or gastrointestinal bleeding and is associated with a high mortality [16]. More patients are now being considered for this indication.

Cholangiocarcinoma: Cholangiocarcinoma (CCA) was not an uncommon indication for liver transplant in the early years, but in the 1990s, this became a contraindication as outcomes were generally very poor, with 5-year survival rates around 30%, and death usually related to recurrent disease. Developments in understanding the natural history and classification of cholangiocarcinoma and the introduction of the "Mayo protocol" have resulted in some jurisdictions allowing the use of LT for this indication either when the Mayo protocol is followed (3-week course of external beam radiotherapy and continuous infusion of 5-Fluorouracil, followed by 2 weeks of brachytherapy, capecitabine, and abdominal laparotomy and staging to exclude spread). Patients with iCCA less than 2 cm on cross-sectional imaging seem to fare best, but outcomes remain poor. Treatments and protocols are evolving [17].

Colorectal metastases (CRM): Colorectal liver metastases were initially an indication for liver transplantation but soon became a contraindication. However, with a greater understanding of the natural history of CRM and the advent of newer technologies, it is becoming possible to select those with CRM who may benefit from liver transplant [18].

Neuroendocrine tumors: The role of LT in those with unresectable neuroendocrine liver metastases remains uncertain. Surgical resection is the best treatment when metastases are resectable, although liver transplantation shows good results for patients not eligible for surgery [19]. However, recurrence rates are relatively high (around 35%).

Budd-Chiari syndrome was initially considered a very good indication for LT. However, with greater understanding of the natural history and pathophysiology and the advent of improved radiological interventions such as thrombolysis and the use of transjugular intra-hepatic portal systemic stents (TIPS), Budd-Chiar is now an uncommon indication, offered to selected patients, mainly with acute liver failure [20].

HIV infections: The advent of highly effective anti-retroviral treatment has allowed those living with HIV with end-stage liver disease (often associated with HCV infection) to become suitable candidates for transplantation and can now be offered. Indications have been agreed upon, and outcomes are improving [21].

Hepatitis B and C infections: With the advent of successful treatments to treat or cure these viral infections, transplantation for end-stage disease with these indications is becoming much less common (Table 1.2).

1.5 Multiple Organ Transplants

Over time, the practice of multi-organ transplantation has become more widespread. The most frequently performed combination remains the liver-kidney transplant. In the United States, simultaneous liver-kidney transplants increased from 1.7% of all liver transplants to 9.9% by 2016 [22]. This rise is largely attributed to the MELD-based organ allocation system, which gives priority to patients with renal dysfunction or hepato-renal syndrome. Additional indications for combined liver-kidney transplants include conditions involving both organs, such as polycystic disease. Other less common combinations involve the liver transplanted alongside the heart alone, heart and lungs, pancreas, or small intestine (see Table 1.1).

1.6 Evolving Recipient Risk

As liver transplantation has progressed, the proportion of recipients presenting with risks beyond liver disease has increased [23]. Today's candidates tend to be older and are more likely to have associated comorbidities, including cardiovascular, respiratory, and cerebrovascular conditions, as well as malignancies.

It is now evident that transplant outcomes are influenced not only by recipient-specific factors and graft characteristics but also by the dynamic interaction between donor and recipient [24]. These evolving complexities present increasing challenges for transplant clinicians.

1.7 Organ Donation

1.7.1 Liver Transplantation and the Organ Shortage

In the early days of transplantation, liver transplants were done in an unplanned manner. There was no central or organized approach to obtaining donors. The process was very informal, and the retrieving surgical team was often the implanting team. Once liver transplantation became an accepted and successful form of therapy, the need to have an organized and regulated approach to organ donation became apparent, and countries set up their own systems for encouraging organ donation;

identifying, characterizing, and selecting organ donors; obtaining consent; and retrieving; transporting; and implanting organs. These processes are usually national and underpinned by a robust legislative framework.

One of the most significant ongoing challenges in solid organ transplantation is the mismatch between the number of patients who could benefit and the number of available, transplantable organs. This disparity necessitates rationing, prompting jurisdictions to establish transparent and ethically grounded policies that balance the sometimes-conflicting principles of utility, justice, equity, benefit, and fairness [25]. As a result, some patients who might derive some benefit from transplantation are not eligible because the projected benefit is not considered sufficient.

Establishing clear criteria to define futility is equally important, especially when the anticipated benefits of transplantation no longer justify allocating a scarce resource. In 1999, a working group proposed that liver transplantation should be considered only when there is greater than a 50% chance of the patient surviving 5 years post-transplant, with a quality of life deemed acceptable by the patient [26]. Although these criteria were somewhat arbitrary, they remain a helpful framework to avoid non-beneficial procedures. Most jurisdictions apply the same eligibility standards to recipients of both deceased and living donor organs, even though living donor transplantation does not directly impact the general organ supply. Whether this policy is appropriate remains a subject of debate beyond the scope of this article.

While clear and legally supported selection and allocation frameworks are essential, overly rigid criteria can hinder innovation and delay the acceptance of new indications. Advancing liver transplantation requires carefully reevaluating contraindications and exploring broader indications, which can enhance access for more patients. However, expanding eligibility must be matched by either increasing the supply of donor organs or discontinuing some current indications—otherwise, mortality among patients on the waiting list will increase. Because organ needs and availability vary across countries, so too do the transplant indications.

It is within this context of scarce, life-saving resources that new transplant indications must be considered. As many technical barriers to transplantation have been overcome, clinicians are increasingly exploring novel uses for this life-saving intervention.

One unfortunate result of the ongoing organ shortage is the emergence of unethical and sometimes illegal practices in organ procurement. The historical use of organs from executed prisoners has been discontinued due to concerns about coercion and lack of voluntary consent. Similarly, paying for organs is both unethical and illegal, as are organ trafficking and transplant tourism. Most jurisdictions explicitly prohibit these practices [26–29].

Organ donation is fundamental to transplantation, and several aspects surrounding donation—such as defining death, obtaining consent, and organ allocation—must be legally regulated. Legal frameworks vary across regions; several milestones have shaped the US system.

The Uniform Anatomical Gift Act (UAGA), introduced in 1968, marked a significant step forward by establishing the first Uniform Donor Card as a legally recognized consent document. The Act also outlined who could authorize organ donation on behalf of a deceased individual and permitted individuals aged 18 years or older to donate their organs posthumously. That same year also witnessed two other major developments: the first widely accepted definition of brain death and the establishment of the New England Organ Bank, the nation's first Organ Procurement Organization (OPO). These milestones paved the way for the first successful living donor liver transplant, also performed in 1968.

In 1981, the Uniform Determination of Death Act provided a legal definition of death as either the irreversible cessation of circulatory and respiratory function or the irreversible cessation of all brain activity.

The National Organ Transplant Act (NOTA) of 1986 further strengthened the ethical foundation of transplantation in the US by making it illegal to buy or sell human organs. It also created the Organ Procurement and Transplantation Network (OPTN) to ensure fair allocation of donated organs and established the Scientific Registry of Transplant Recipients to monitor and evaluate transplant outcomes.

The Required Request Law, also passed in 1986, mandated that hospitals must offer families of deceased patients the opportunity to consider organ donation. In 1988, this was reinforced when the Centers for Medicare & Medicaid Services (CMS) updated hospital participation requirements, compelling facilities enrolled in Medicare and Medicaid to report all deaths and imminent deaths to their regional OPO.

In 1999, the Institute of Medicine released the Organ Procurement and Transplantation report, which recommended that allocation of livers should be to those with the most urgent medical need—that is, those who are most likely to die. Since then, there have been further refinements to ensure the US has a transparent and equitable system of allocation that prioritizes the sickest first in an objective and transparent way. In 2000, the "Final Rule"established federal regulations on OPTN policies, including listing requirements, organ procurement, identification of an organ recipient, allocation of donated organs, designated transplant program requirements, reviews, evaluation, and enforcement of transplant programs.

Consent for organ donation is, of course, necessary. Consent for deceased donation may be explicit (opt-in), implied or assumed. With an opt-in process, the potential donor has either indicated their wishes by joining a national register or carrying a donor card or otherwise indicated their preference. Where the wishes have not been clear, the family is asked what the wishes of the donor would be, and these wishes are followed. In the UK, the organ donor card was introduced in 1971 and a national organ donor register established in 1994. After 10 years, there were 15 million registrants and currently over 25 million.

There has been much debate about whether an opt-in system is preferable to an opt-out system. In 2020, England followed the lead of Wales and some other jurisdictions changed the law on organ donation from one of opt-in to deemed consent; this was associated with a delayed but small increase in donation [30].

1.8 Development of Allocation Policies

Organs from deceased donors are considered a national resource. As liver transplantation has become a widely available routine procedure, the gap between the number of patients who need a liver transplant and the number of suitable organs available for transplant has increased and become more transparent. Despite a number of initiatives to increase organ donor availability, this gap remains a major problem, meaning that a resource that is life saving and life enhancing must be rationed, and therefore, jurisdictions have developed methodologies to provide an objective and transparent approach to organ allocation.

In the US, priority is given to those who have an acute onset of liver failure and are deemed not likely to survive more than a few days without an OLT (status 1A) and those who are very sick, chronically ill pediatric patients with cirrhosis who are younger than 18 years of age—pediatric population (status 1B). Other jurisdictions have developed other approaches to allocation.

1.8.1 Assessment of Disease Severity

Before 2002, the Child-Turcotte-Pugh (CTP) model was the standard for assessing liver disease severity. Initially developed to estimate surgical prognosis in patients with advanced cirrhosis, the model was largely empirical. Despite lacking rigorous validation, it became widely adopted, partly because it was created intuitively by clinicians, and rapidly became integrated into routine practice. However, criticism mounted over time due to both its limited statistical robustness and the inclusion of subjective factors such as the presence of ascites and hepatic encephalopathy.

In 2002, the Model for End-Stage Liver Disease (MELD) was introduced [31]. Developed by Kamath and colleagues, MELD was originally designed to predict outcomes in patients with advanced liver disease undergoing surgery for varices. It relied solely on objective laboratory values, enhancing its reliability, and was subsequently validated in various clinical settings. Although MELD proved to be a reasonably effective prognostic tool, several concerns and suggested revisions emerged over time.

One major revision involved incorporating serum sodium, leading to the adoption of the MELD-Na score in 2014, which was officially implemented in 2016. Critics also noted that using serum creatinine could disadvantage women due to differences in muscle mass and that non-hepatic factors—such as hemolysis—might skew results. Furthermore, MELD did not perform well in conditions where mortality was not primarily due to liver failure. For instance, patients with primary liver cancer often faced graft ineligibility due to extra-hepatic disease progression, despite having lower MELD scores. To address this, exception points were introduced to better align MELD-estimated prognosis with clinical reality.

Additional issues arose in specific conditions: MELD did not accurately represent the severity or outcomes for patients with hepatopulmonary syndrome, portopulmonary hypertension, or primary sclerosing cholangitis. Similarly, those experiencing debilitating symptoms such as severe pruritus or recurrent encephalopathy were not adequately prioritized. Pediatric patients are assessed using a separate tool—the Pediatric End-Stage Liver Disease (PELD) score—though it has not undergone validation as extensively as MELD.

1.8.2 Equity and Access

Concerns about equity in organ allocation persist, particularly in terms of geographic fairness. Ideally, patients with similar disease severity should have comparable access to donor livers regardless of where they live or which transplant center they attend. However, in practice, this goal is difficult to achieve because organ donor availability and recipient demand are unevenly distributed.

In an attempt to improve fairness, several sharing systems have been introduced in the United States:

- In 2005, the Regional Share 15 program began.
- In 2010, it was extended to include Status 1 patients.
- In 2013, the Regional Share 35 and the National Share 15 were implemented. Under the Share 35 rule, candidates with a MELD-Na score of 35 or higher would be prioritized for liver offers beyond their local Organ Procurement Organization (OPO) boundaries but within the same region.
- In 2020, the Acuity Circles model was adopted. This model aims to further reduce waiting list mortality by distributing organs more equitably, ensuring that geographic location does not unduly influence access.

Under the older donor service area system, some patients were listed at multiple transplant centers and/or traveled significant distances to increase their chances of receiving a transplant. This practice led to legal challenges, with critics arguing that it exacerbated inequities in access to transplantation.

In the UK, the approach is slightly different. The jurisdiction is small, both in terms of population and geography; for a population of around 66 million, there are only seven liver transplant centers, whereas New York (population 20 million) has 9 liver transplant centers, and California (population 39 million) has 21 active liver transplant centers. Furthermore, in the UK, with a primarily nationalized health care service, transplant units are not in financial competition with each other. In the UK, the current policy is that the success of any national donor offering scheme would be judged on the basis of survival from the point of registration on a national list for a liver transplant, rather than the point of transplant (although data are given for both). Allocation was initially center-based: there was a national priority for those with acute liver failure or primary graft failure. Thereafter, organs were allocated to the region allocated to the appropriate liver unit and, if the offer was declined, offered to other units in rotation. This system worked well but did not offer national equity of access. Hence, a national list was developed for non-urgent cases, with priority being given to the sickest (as evidenced by the UKELD score - this score is similar to MELD but validated for UK transplant-listed patients). In the last decade, NHS Blood and Transplant, which manages the allocation process, has introduced an allocation system based on survival benefit, with the liver being offered to the candidate with the greatest probability of survival, as estimated by the difference between estimated survival with and without transplant. Preliminary evidence suggests that this is a fair and equitable approach.

1.8.3 Allocation Based on Transplant Benefit

Different allocation models—based on medical need, utility, or transplant benefit (defined as net life years gained)—have been compared through simulation against the traditional unit-based allocation system. The transplant benefit model demonstrated superior performance, reducing waiting list mortality and maximizing overall life years in the population. As a result, since March 2018, donor livers from brain-dead donors in the UK have been allocated using a national list prioritized by transplant benefit, measured in net life years gained.

To support this system, the UK developed a specific scoring system, the United Kingdom Model for End-Stage Liver Disease (UKELD). The UKELD score was derived from survival data of patients listed for transplant in the UK and was found to be a more accurate predictor of outcomes than MELD or its variants. A UKELD score of 49 or higher currently serves as the threshold for listing, reflecting an estimated survival of one year or less without a transplant.

In addition to UKELD, specific minimum criteria have been established for listing patients with chronic liver disease, hepatocellular carcinoma, and certain less common syndromes where conventional scoring systems may not adequately capture the risk of death or symptom burden.

The UK and US systems reflect differing priorities. The US model focuses on minimizing waiting list mortality, while the UK approach seeks to maximize overall survival benefit. Both philosophies are ethically sound, yet they yield distinct methods for candidate selection and organ allocation. Notably, neither system currently incorporates quality of life assessments or provides a comprehensive definition of futility. It must be stressed that most allocation schemes are, in practice, offering schemes with the organ not transplanted into the first allocated recipient.

1.8.4 Equity of Access

Access to transplantation remains inequitable. A recent US review highlighted that racial and ethnic minorities, women, and individuals from lower socioeconomic groups are less likely to be referred for transplant evaluation or added to the waiting list. Other countries face similar disparities. In response, the US Congress tasked the National Institutes of Health with commissioning the National Academies of Sciences, Engineering, and Medicine to evaluate deceased donor organ procurement and allocation. Their report, *Realizing the Promise of Equity in the Organ Transplantation System* [32], outlined 14 recommendations across three strategic areas: improving equity, enhancing system performance, and increasing the effective use of donated organs.

1.9 Organ Preservation and Preservation Solutions

Organ preservation has evolved significantly since the introduction of the Collins solution in 1969, initially for kidney transplantation and later applied to liver grafts. This solution mimicked the intracellular electrolyte environment, characterized by low sodium, high potassium, a phosphate buffer, and high glucose content. The Euro-Collins solution, introduced in 1980 by the Eurotransplant Foundation, was a modified version of the original.

During the late 1970s, Marshall's solution (a hyperosmolar citrate, or HOC, solution) was developed by Ross and colleagues and remains in clinical use. Another major advancement was the HTK solution (histidine-tryptophan-ketoglutarate), introduced in the 1980s.

In 1987, the University of Wisconsin (UW) solution entered clinical practice and is now widely used. It shares similarities with Collins solution but replaces glucose with raffinose and lactobionic acid.

1.9.1 Machine Perfusion

Machine perfusion technology is now gaining traction in clinical transplantation [33]. Several devices are in use, and clinical trials have demonstrated clear benefits. While certain questions remain, machine perfusion is expected to become a central component of transplant practice. One notable advantage is the potential for scheduling transplants during daytime hours, which may reduce technical errors.

Two primary machine perfusion approaches exist:

- Hypothermic oxygenated perfusion, which perfuses the liver using an acellular solution at low temperatures (2–10 °C).
- Normothermic machine perfusion, which uses a red blood cell-based perfusate at body temperature to simulate physiological conditions.

Normothermic perfusion is believed to help reduce hyperfibrinolysis and inflammation after reperfusion, restore glycogen levels, and regenerate ATP [34]. Ongoing research aims to identify biomarkers that can predict organ quality and vulnerability to ischemia-reperfusion injury. Furthermore, machine perfusion provides opportunities for therapeutic interventions to enhance graft quality.

Preliminary data suggest that normothermic perfusion not only increases the number of usable donor livers but also leads to improved graft function, reduced ischemia-reperfusion injury, and fewer biliary complications. Normothermic regional perfusion (NRP), where organs are perfused in situ before retrieval, has also been shown to improve graft function and outcomes.

1.10 Surgical Techniques

In the early years, biliary problems were a major problem. Before the realization that bile was toxic to the ischemic biliary tree and the greater understanding of the arterial supply to the bile ducts, death from biliary leaks and biliary sepsis was common. Calne developed a technique known as the gall bladder conduit, in which the gall bladder is used as a pedicle graft between the donor and recipient common bile ducts. This technique helped resolve the issue [35], but with greater use of biliary washout and less dissection of the tissues around the biliary anastomosis, biliary issues became less of a problem, and the biliary conduit is hardly ever used. Biliary problems do remain an issue, affecting about one in 5 adult recipients, and have a significant impact on the risk of death and graft loss. Risk factors have changed and include donor type (living or deceased), recipient age, diagnosis, prior transplant, donor age, and donor cause of death (especially donations after circulatory death) [36].

Another major improvement was the introduction of the "piggyback" technique. The standard approach was to clamp the inferior vena cava to allow a section to be removed along with the diseased liver. However, this can decrease the blood returning to the heart and so may lead to a decreased cardiac output. In the piggyback method, developed by Calne and popularized by Tzakis, the recipient vein IVC is retained, and the donor IVC is then joined to the recipient vein. Although the data for a survival benefit is less clear, this offers another option for the surgeon [37]. Partial cardiopulmonary bypass was introduced in 1979 by Calne.

Other significant developments include the use of split livers, reduced-sized livers, and living donor livers. It is beyond the scope of this chapter to describe the heroic advances in detail [38].

1.11 Immunosuppression

Corticosteroids have been used since the development of immunosuppression. 6-mercaptopurine was one of the earliest drugs used to induce immunosuppression but was soon replaced by azathioprine as being more effective and less toxic; thus, corticosteroids and azathioprine became the mainstay of liver transplant immunosuppression in the early years. There was limited awareness of the side effects of steroids, and conditions such as osteoporosis became a major issue in longer term survivors, which was only partly later mitigated by the use of calcium supplements. The next major drug to be introduced was cyclosporine, which depresses both cellular and humoral immunity by inhibition of calcineurin. The early years following its introduction by the Cambridge team, led by Calne and White, were associated with better graft function and longer survival, but there were significant side effects such as neurological and pulmonary pathology. However, as assays became routinely available, their benefits became apparent, and cyclosporin was licenced for clinical use in 1984. The standard immunosuppression regimen became steroids, azathioprine, and cyclosporin. In several series, steroids were discontinued after 3 months. The initial formulation of Sandimmune was replaced by a microemulsion formulation (Neoral). A decade later, another calcineurin inhibitor (CNI), tacrolimus (initially known as FK506), was introduced into clinical practice, led by Starzl's team. Tacrolimus has gradually replaced cyclosporin, as many head-to-head studies have shown superiority in terms of liver function and a reduced spectrum of side effects. Both CNIs have significant side effects, notably renal impairment, although the profiles vary between the two agents. The next immunosuppressive agent to enter clinical practice was mycophenolate and its metabolite mycophenolic acid mofetil. This drug has gradually replaced azathioprine in most centers, although its superiority has yet to be convincingly shown. The most recent drug to enter routine clinical use is sirolimus, introduced in 1999.

In the early years of liver transplantation, induction was with anti-lymphocyte globulin and antibodies to the CD3 receptor on T-lymphocytes (OKT3). The first monoclonal antibody approved for clinical use was basiliximab, which has remained in clinical practice and is useful especially in those situations where delayed introduction of CNI is indicated.

The most commonly used immunosuppressive regimen is triple immunosuppression with tacrolimus, mycophenolate, and azathioprine. The increasing armamentarium of drugs is allowing tailored immunosuppression—a concept more actively discussed than implemented, but the widening range of agents allows for new combinations to allow good graft function with minimal side effects.

Tolerance and complete withdrawal of immunosuppression: it became clear in the early years of liver transplantation that a small number of recipients were able to stop immunosuppression without adverse effect. These operationally tolerant patients led to studies where some recipients are able to stop immunosuppression while under medical supervision. Early studies in the 1990s showed the potential of immunosuppression withdrawal, and some programs continue to establish withdrawal programs [39]. Development of tolerance remains a challenge nearly 3 decades later [40].

1.12 The Future

Liver transplantation has evolved over 6 decades from a very high-risk experimental procedure to a routine low-risk procedure. The future looks bright as access to transplant centers increases, outcomes improve (albeit slowly), and, with better immunosuppressive regimens, the adverse impact of medication will be reduced.

The place of machine perfusion needs to be established, but current data suggest that this technology will allow both improved outcomes from perfusion, allow implantation to be done in a timely way, allow techniques to assess the viability of the graft, and improve viability. The role of alternatives to solid organ transplants is developing, as is xenotransplantation. Of the risks facing transplantation, the shortage of organs and, more importantly, the possible shortage of surgeons and other skilled health care professionals and scientists will limit the application of this life-saving procedure. It must also be pointed out that transplantation is, for the physician, a mark of failure: research to advance transplantation should not therefore be at the expense of research to prevent and treat the consequences of liver disease.

References

1. Penn I, Halgrimson CG, Starzl TE. Liver transplantation in man. Ann N Y Acad Sci. 1970;170:251–8.
2. National Institutes of Health Consensus Development Conference Statement: liver transplantation—June 20–23, 1983. Hepatology 1984;4(1 Suppl):107s–110s.
3. Calne RY. Liver transplantation. New York/London: Grune and Stratton; 1983.
4. World Health Organisation. Human organ and tissue transplantation. https://apps.who.int/gb/ebwha/pdf_files/WHA75/A75_41-en.pdf#:~:text=In%20May%202010%2C%20the%20Sixty-third%20World%20Health%20Assembly,donors%20and%20ensuring%20the%20dignity%20of%20all%20involved.
5. The Transplantation Society. WHO Guiding Principles on human cell, tissue and organ transplantation. https://www.tts.org/education/tts-resources-and-guidelines/108-tts/about/tts-and-the-who/604-who-guiding-principles-on-human-cell-tissue-and-organ-transplantation.
6. The Declaration of Istanbul on Organ Trafficking and Transplant Tourism. https://declarationofistanbul.org/.
7. Starzl TE, Putnam CW, Ishikawa M, Picache R, Husberg B, Halgrimson CG, et al. Current policies in hepatic transplantation: candidacy of patients with alcoholic liver disease or preformed antidonor antibodies and a reappraisal of biliary duct reconstruction. Ann N Y Acad Sci. 1975;252:145–58.
8. Kumar S, Stauber RE, Gavaler JS, Basista MH, Dindzans VJ, Schade RR, et al. Orthotopic liver transplantation for alcoholic liver disease. Hepatology. 1990;11(2):159–64.
9. Neuberger J, Adams D, MacMaster P, Maidment A, Speed M. Assessing priorities for allocation of donor liver grafts: survey of public and clinicians. BMJ. 1998;317:172–5.
10. Tavabie OD, Srivastava A, Dillon A, Mirza D, Masson S, Smith PJ. Twitter debate: controversies in liver transplantation. Frontline Gastroenterol. 2022;13:262–5.
11. Schulte K, Borzikowsky C, Rahmel A, Kolibay F, Polze N, Fränkel P, Mikle S, Alders B, Kunzendorf U, Feldkamp T. Decline in organ donation in Germany. Dtsch Arztebl Int. 2018;115:463–8.
12. Madden S, Lucey MR, Neuberger J. Does publicity affect organ donation? Transpl Int. 2020;33(9):1146–8.
13. Mathurin P, Moreno C, Samuel D, Dumortier J, Salleron J, Durand F, et al. Early liver transplantation for severe alcoholic hepatitis. N Engl J Med. 2011;365(19):1790–800.
14. Crabb DW, Im GY, Szabo G, Mellinger JL, Lucey MR. Diagnosis and treatment of alcohol-associated liver diseases: 2019 practice guidance from the American Association for the Study of Liver Diseases. Hepatology. 2020;71:306–33.

15. Chalasani N, Younossi Z, Lavine JE, Charlton M, Cusi K, Rinella M, et al. The diagnosis and management of nonalcoholic fatty liver disease: practice guidance from the American Association for the Study of Liver Diseases. Hepatology. 2018;67:328–57.
16. Belli LS, Duvoux C, Artzner T, Bernal W, Conti S, Cortesi PA, et al. ELITA/EF-CLIF working group. Liver transplantation for patients with acute-on-chronic liver failure (ACLF) in Europe: results of the ELITA/EF-CLIF collaborative study (ECLIS). J Hepatol. 2021;75:610–22.
17. Sapisochin G, Ivanics T, Heimbach J. Liver transplantation for intrahepatic cholangiocarcinoma: ready for prime time? Hepatology. 2022;75(2):455–72.
18. Bonney GK, Chew CA, Lodge P, Hubbard J, Halazun KJ, Trunecka P, et al. Liver transplantation for non-resectable colorectal liver metastases: the International Hepato-Pancreato-Biliary Association consensus guidelines. Lancet Gastroenterol Hepatol. 2021;6(11):933–46.
19. Muttillo EM, Mazzarella G, Picardi B, Rossi S, Cinelli L, Diana M, et al. Treatment strategies for neuroendocrine liver metastases: a systematic review. HPB (Oxford). 2022;24:1832–43.
20. Gavriilidis P, Marangoni G, Ahmad J, Azoulay D. State of the art, current perspectives, and controversies of Budd-Chiari syndrome: a review. J Clin Med Res. 2022;14:147–57.
21. Zarinsefat A, Gulati A, Shui A, Braun H, Rogers R, Hirose R, et al. Long-term outcomes following kidney and liver transplant in recipients with HIV. JAMA Surg. 2022;157:240–7.
22. Nair G, Nair V. Simultaneous liver-kidney transplantation. Clin Liver Dis. 2022;26:313–22.
23. Durand F, Levitsky J, Cauchy F, Gilgenkrantz H, Soubrane O, Francoz C. Age and liver transplantation. J Hepatol. 2019;70(4):745–58.
24. Halldorson JB, Bakthavatsalam R, Fix O, Reyes JD, Perkins JD. D-MELD, a simple predictor of post liver transplant mortality for optimization of donor/recipient matching. Am J Transplant. 2009;9:318–26.
25. Neuberger J. Liver allocation. Minerva Gastroenterol Dietol. 2018;64(2):170–9.
26. Neuberger J, James O. Guidelines for selection of patients for liver transplantation in the era of donor-organ shortage. Lancet. 1999;354:1636–9.
27. Sahi MK, Shroff S, Navin S, Kumar P. Organ commercialism, trafficking and transplant tourism. Indian. J Med Ethics. 2022;VII:142–9.
28. Chapman JR, Stock P, Haberal M. Organs from executed people are not a source of scientific discovery. Transplantation. 2019;103:1534–5.
29. Halpern SD, Raz A, Kohn R, Rey M, Asch DA, Reese P. Regulated payments for living kidney donation: an empirical assessment of the ethical concerns. Ann Intern Med. 2010;152:358–65.
30. Madden S, Collett D, Walton P, Empson K, Forsythe J, Ingham A, et al. The effect on consent rates for deceased organ donation in Wales after the introduction of an opt-out system. Anaesthesia. 2020;75:1146–52.
31. Ruf A, Dirchwolf M, Freeman RB. From Child-Pugh to MELD score and beyond: taking a walk down memory lane. Ann Hepatol. 2022;27:100535.
32. National Academies of Sciences E, Medicine, Health, Medicine D, Board on Health Care S, Board on Health Sciences P, et al. The National Academies Collection: Reports funded by National Institutes of Health. In: Hackmann M, English RA, Kizer KW, editors. Realizing the Promise of Equity in the Organ Transplantation System. Washington (DC): National Academies Press (US) Copyright 2022 by the National Academy of Sciences. All rights reserved; 2022.
33. Ceresa CDL, Nasralla D, Pollok JM, Friend PJ. Machine perfusion of the liver: applications in transplantation and beyond. Nat Rev Gastroenterol Hepatol. 2022;19:199–209.
34. van Beekum CJ, Vilz TO, Glowka TR, von Websky MW, Kalff JC, Manekeller S. Normothermic machine perfusion (NMP) of the liver – current status and future perspectives. Ann Transplant. 2021;24(26):e931664.
35. Calne RY. A new technique for biliary drainage in orthotopic liver transplantation utilizing the gall bladder as a pedicle graft conduit between the donor and recipient common bile ducts. Ann Surg. 1976;184:605–9.
36. Many P, Seth A, Jackson K, Lentine K, Schnitzler M, Xiao H, et al. Biliary complications after liver transplantation in the United States: changing trends and economic implications. Transplantation. 2023;107:e127. https://doi.org/10.1097/TP0000000000004528.

37. Gurusamy KS, Pamecha V, Davidson BR. Piggy-back graft for liver transplantation. Cochrane Database Syst Rev. 2011;(1):CD008258. https://doi.org/10.1002/14651858.CD008258.pub2.
38. Petrowsky H, Busuttil RW. Evolving surgical approaches in liver transplantation. Semin Liver Dis. 2009;29:121–33.
39. Mazariegos GV, Reyes J, Marino IR, Demetris AJ, Flynn B, Irish W, et al. Weaning of immunosuppression in liver transplant recipients. Transplantation. 1997;63:243–9.
40. Takatsuki M, Eguchi S. Clinical liver transplant tolerance: recent topics. J Hepatobiliary Pancreat Sci. 2022;29:369–76.

Chapter 2
Indications and Patient Selection for Liver Transplantation

Akash Shukla, Amit Gupte, Ankita Singh, and Dinesh Jothimani

Abstract Liver transplantation (LT) is the only curative option for patients with end-stage liver disease, with a long-term survival exceeding 75%. Patients with decompensated cirrhosis of any etiology with no reversibility, hepatocellular carcinoma (HCC) within acceptable criteria and acute liver failure fulfilling poor prognostic score are standard indications for liver transplantation. With regard to the etiology of liver disease in patients for liver transplantation, hepatitis C was the most common indication. However, with exceptionally higher cure rates with directly acting antiviral, hepatitis C is no longer the most common indication. With increasing prevalence of obesity and associated metabolic syndrome, Metabolic associated steatotic liver disease (MASLD)-related liver disease has become the number one leading indications for liver transplantation. Alcohol-related liver disease continues to rise as a common indication for LT, particularly in the younger population. Acute-on-chronic liver failure (ACLF) is a recently defined disease entity with high short-term mortality. Selection of ACLF patients for liver transplantation can be a challenge.

Hepatocellular carcinoma is an important indication for liver transplantation. Availability of potent locoregional therapies and, in recent days, immunotherapy has changed the perspective of patient selection for LT. Tumor 'downstaging' with

A. Shukla
Sir HN Reliance Foundation Hospital, Mumbai, India

Seth GS Medical College & KEM Hospital, Mumbai, India

A. Gupte
Sir HN Reliance Foundation Hospital, Mumbai, India

A. Singh
Seth GS Medical College & KEM Hospital, Mumbai, India

D. Jothimani (✉)
Institute of Liver Disease and Transplantation, Dr Rela Institute and Medical Centre, Chennai, Tamil Nadu, India
e-mail: dinesh.Jothimani@relainstitute.com

S. Saigal, D. Jothimani (eds.), *Fundamentals of Transplant Hepatology*,
https://doi.org/10.1007/978-981-95-2624-6_2

above modalities has led to the expansion of liver transplant criteria in patients with HCC.

Less common indications for LT includes hepatopulmonary syndrome, portopulmonary hypertension, familial hypercholesterolemia, hepatic neuroendocrine tumor and other rarer conditions.

Careful patient selection and timing of liver transplantation are crucial for appropriate post-transplant outcomes. A multidisciplinary team approach is essential in the success of transplantation.

Keywords Liver transplantation · Model for end-stage liver disease · Acute-on-chronic liver failure · Variant syndromes · Hepatocellular carcinoma

Key Highlights

Patients with model for end-stage liver disease >15 should be considered for liver transplantation.

Comorbidities should be carefully evaluated in MASLD patients for liver transplantation.

Decision to transplant in patients with ACLF should be carefully made, considering the benefit and risks.

HCC patients with adequate response to 'downstaging' modalities should be offered liver transplantation.

2.1 Introduction

Liver transplantation (LT) has transformed lives of patients with liver cirrhosis. Since the first successful surgery in 1967 by Professor Thomas Starzl and subsequent pioneers over the years, the current long-term survival following liver transplantation exceeds 75%. The reason behind such improvement entails improvement in surgical techniques, refined postoperative care, optimization of immunosuppression and long-term follow-up with focus on lifestyle-related issues. Although, selection of patients has largely stratified over the years, there has been a considerable change in the spectrum of patients with chronic liver disease.

Over the last decade, a number of changes have occurred in the recognition and management of chronic liver disease. Introduction of directly acting antiviral (DAA) has been the game changer in patients with chronic hepatitis C infection. With closer to 100% cure rate, impacting its prevalence even in those with decompensated cirrhosis, Hepatitis C is no longer the most common indication for LT. On the other hand, with increasing prevalence of obesity and metabolic syndrome, MASH-related liver disease has shown enormous rise and with associated serious comorbidities.

Acute-on-chronic liver failure (ACLF) is relatively newer disease entity with lesser understanding of its pathogenesis and clinical course. Patients with ACLF encounter high short-term mortality in parallel with number of organ failures. Treating clinicians are challenged with selecting such patients for liver transplantation.

With improvement in critical care services, transplant-free survival of patients with acute liver failure (ALF) has improved significantly. Moreover, with disease heterogeneity across the world, the selection of patients for LT may vary including the timing.

Treatment of hepatocellular carcinoma (HCC) has evolved rapidly with the availability of locoregional therapy clearly impacting patient outcome following LT.

Thus, increasing complexity of patients with chronic liver disease compels the question on selection and timing of liver transplantation.

LT should be considered in patients in whom it is expected to improve the survival beyond what the natural history would predict or in whom LT would improve the quality of life [1]. Patients and their families should be counselled for a possible transplant when they develop one of the complications of liver cirrhosis.

The optimal timing of the transplant can be decided based on the prognostic scores.

Child-Turcotte-Pugh (CTP) score also helps to predict survival in patients with liver cirrhosis. The 1-year survival in CTP A, B and C is 95%, 80% and 45%, respectively, and the 2-year survival is 90%, 70% and 38%, respectively. A patient with CTP score >7 should be considered for LT [2].

Model for end-stage liver disease (MELD) score (MELD Score = 10 * {0.957 * ln[Creatinine]} + {0.378 * ln[Bilirubin]} + {1.12 * ln[INR]} + 6.43) was devised in 2000 for predicting the 3-month mortality of patients undergoing transjugular intrahepatic portosystemic shunt (TIPS) for variceal bleed [3] and then was used as a prognostic score for patients with cirrhosis [4]. In patients with MELD score less than or equal to 14, survival in the absence of liver transplantation was higher [5]. Hence, a MELD score of 15 or more has been a standard recommendation for LT. However, MELD score does not take into account ascites, hepatic encephalopathy (HE), development of hepatocellular carcinoma (HCC) and other complications like Hepatopulmonary syndrome (HPS) and portopulmonary hypertension (POPH). These patients should be given additional points—the MELD exception points in a MELD-based liver allocation system.

MELD-Na score and Delta MELD provide a better prognostic value than MELD score [1]. Recently, a new version of the MELD (the MELD 3.0) has been proposed for organ allocation. MELD 3.0 has additional variables: (a) female sex, albumin, (b) lowered ceiling for creatinine at 3 mg/dl and (c) inclusion of interaction between variables—sodium and bilirubin and bilirubin and albumin. MELD 3.0 offers a better mortality prediction than MELD-Na score [6]. Indications and selection of patient with ALF and ACLF are discussed later.

2.2 Indication and Patient Selection in ALF

In the pretransplant era for ALF, mortality exceeded 80%. With more widespread availability of liver transplant for this indication, mortality rates have reduced to around 33%, despite only approximately 25% of ALF patients undergoing transplantation [7, 8].

Prior to the era of LT, mortality of ALF patients was over 80% [9]. ALF as an indication for Liver transplantation was adopted in a consensus meeting by National Institute of Health in early 1980s, which has changed the outlook of these patients' survival [10].

In the initial era, liver transplantation was considered for patients with 'advanced' ALF. Unfortunately, the criteria for 'advanced' were not clearly defined and remained quite subjective with variations among different liver units.

Underlying etiology determines transplant-free survival and post-transplant outcomes [11]. Acetaminophen overdose is common in Western countries [12–14], while viral hepatitis, particularly hepatitis B in China and hepatitis E in India, dominates in Asia-Pacific [15–17]. Nonacetaminophen drugs, antitubercular therapy and alternative medicines are prevalent in Asia. An important cause of ALF in India is yellow phosphorus poisoning (rodenticide ingestion) which requires more aggressive therapeutic strategies like plasmapheresis and has low transplant-free survival [18]. Acetaminophen toxicity and hepatitis A virus (HAV)-related ALF have lower likelihoods of being listed for transplant, while Wilson's disease (WD) and seronegative ALF are more likely to be listed [12]. Common etiologic factors of ALF are summarized in Table 2.1.

Identification of patients for LT in ALF thus remained a challenge in the absence of a predictive model. An ideal criterion should be simple with higher sensitivity and specificity, applicable across all etiologies, and should be dynamic and reproducible with clinical and biochemical parameters.

Presence of accurate transplant criteria will on the one hand avoid false positive rates where patients may undergo potentially unnecessary liver transplantation and its relative complications, where otherwise improved with medical management. Similarly, false negative result may result in patients who would have benefitted by LT on time but not transplanted with jeopardized survival.

Table 2.1 Etiologic factors of ALF

Drug related
Acute viral hepatitis (HAV/hepatitis E virus)
Hepatitis B virus (HBV) reactivation
Toxin induced
Budd-Chiari Syndrome
Wilson disease
Autoimmune hepatitis flare
Ischemic hepatitis
Pregnancy related
Seronegative hepatitis

2.2.1 Clichy Criteria

Clichy criteria were introduced in 1986 and were one of the earliest model introduced in prognosticating ALF. Liver transplantation is recommended in ALF patients with grade III–IV HE and Factor V level less than 20% in patients under 30 years or <30% in over 30 years of age. The flip side of this criteria was the lack of wider availability of Factor V levels and that this model was studied in hepatitis B-related ALF [19].

King's College Hospital (KCH) criteria were introduced in 1987, based on a retrospective cohort of 588 ALF patients from King's liver unit from 1973 to 1985, and were validated in 1986 [20]. KCH criteria adopted slightly different parameters for paracetamol and non-paracetamol ALF. First time, etiology has been shown to determine clinical outcomes. Thus, patients with paracetamol ALF developed hyperacute ALF with higher chance of spontaneous recovery. KCH criteria are widely accepted and used worldwide. One of the major caveats of KCH criteria particularly in non-paracetamol ALF is its lower sensitivity (69%). This refers to 31% patients likely to improve with medical management despite fulfilling the criteria but may end up undergoing LT. On the other hand, KCH criteria have a higher specificity (92%), indicating the ability to pick up patients who do not benefit from LT in those who do not fulfil the criteria. Clinical performance of KCH criteria was slightly better for paracetamol ALF. A meta-analysis of KCH criteria in paracetamol ALF showed a sensitivity of 58–69% and specificity of 92–94% [21]. Addition of lactate following fluid resuscitation improved sensitivity of KCH criteria [22].

MELD score has been evaluated as a prognostic marker in patients with ALF. In a systematic comparative analysis of 23 studies involving 2153 ALF patients from 2001 to 2015 showed a diagnostic Odds ratio for KCH criteria 5.3 (95% CI 3.7–7.6) and MELD score 7.0 (95% CI 5.1–9.7) in predicting hospital mortality. In paracetamol ALF, the sensitivity and specificity of KCH criteria for predicting mortality were 58% (95% CI 51–65%) and 89% (95% CI 85–93%) and MELD score was 80% (95% CI 74–86%) and 53% (95% CI 47–59%). In non-paracetamol ALF, KCH sensitivity and specificity were 58% (95% CI 54–63%) and 74% (95% CI 69–78%). For MELD score, sensitivity and specificity were 76% (95% CI 72–80%) and 73% (95% CI 69–78%). Thus, KCH criteria had predictive value for paracetamol ALF, and MELD predicted better for non-paracetamol ALF [23].

2.2.2 Early Clinical Prognostic Indicators

A study from India on 144 ALF patients with viral hepatitis found a mortality of 63.9%. Presence of any three of the following six parameters was predictive of death: age ≥50 years, jaundice to HE >7 days, higher grade of HE, presence of cerebral edema, PT ≥35 and creatinine ≥1.5 mg/dl. This study was conducted in patients with ALF due to viral hepatitis and was found superior to MELD and KCH criteria [24].

ALF is a dynamic disease with variations in clinical findings. Using static criteria at baseline may be inappropriate. Kumar et al. developed and validated ALF early dynamic (ALFED) model score by prospectively studying 380 ALF patients [25]. The score consisted of arterial ammonia ≥123 umol/L, bilirubin ≥15 mg/dl, international normalised ratio (INR) ≥5 and HE >grade 2. Patients with score 1–3 had survival of 80%; whereas those with ≥4 had mortality of 80%. ALFED model demonstrated a better discriminant with AUROC 0.91. This study was conducted among patients with viral hepatitis. Table 2.1 illustrates predictive values of ALF prognostic scores.

Several other criteria were introduced predominantly based on intensive care unit (ICU) scores, such as acute physiology and chronic health evaluation (APACHE) and sequential organ failure assessment (SOFA) scores, but KCH criteria remain more reliable.

ALF related to yellow phosphorus poisoning, peculiar to south India, is discussed below [26]. In addition, ALF patients are much sicker in the intensive care unit with multiorgan support. Presence of multiorgan failure predicts transplant outcomes [27]. Availability of organ in a supraurgent situation has been a major drawback worldwide, particularly in Asian countries where organ donation rates remain considerably low per million population. Moreover, patients may not be suitable at the time of organ availability which may contraindicate LT.

Zinc phosphide (rodenticide)-induced ALF mandates special attention, as routinely used criteria have poor sensitivity in selecting patients for transplant. Associated extrahepatic organ failure, as a result of the direct effect of the toxin, leads to cardiomyopathy, rhabdomyolysis and acute renal failure, resulting in worse outcomes. MELD score more than 36 or a combination of INR over 6 and encephalopathy have been identified as excellent predictors for the need for liver transplantation [28].

Factors such as age >50 years, presence of multiorgan failure, requirement of vasopressor support and/or mechanical ventilation and high-grade HE are associated with post-transplant survival rates (<50%) and therefore such patients are less likely to get listed for LT [13].

Timing of LT is crucial for patient selection for the surgery. Timing of LT in ALF depends on disease etiology, time from jaundice to HE, donor–recipient age and presence of multiorgan failure.

In a study from King's College, 22% of ALF waitlisted patients either did not receive an organ or became too sick for transplantation and expired a median of 2 days from listing [29]. Waiting time more than 5 days from LT was associated with higher post-transplant mortality [30]. However, a subset of ALF patients do recover without LT and thereby avoid a major surgery and lifelong immunosuppression. The precise identification of such patients early in the course of disease is of prime importance. ALF presentation of autoimmune hepatitis, Wilson disease and Budd-Chiari syndrome should be considered for LT, despite their chronicity [31].

Optimal patient selection and time of transplant determine survival. ALF as an indication for liver transplantation (LT) was adopted in the 1980s by a consensus of the National Institutes of Health [10]. Currently, ALF represents about 8% of all liver transplants, based on data from the Scientific Registry of Transplant Recipients and the European Liver Transplant Registry [32, 33]. Significant progress has been achieved in this regard, with the development of multiple 'prognostic models' designed to guide clinicians in determining the appropriate timing for LT (Table 2.2).

Table 2.2 Prognostic models in ALF

Study	Year	Number of patients	Patient population	Parameters included in study or model	Comment
1. Bernuau et al.	1986	115	HBV	Age, Factor V levels	Clichy criteria
2. Bismuth et al.	1995	139	Mixed etiologies	Age, Factor V levels, HE Grade 3–4	
3. O'Grady et al.	1989	332	(a) Non-paracetamol	Age, etiology, serum bilirubin, jaundice to encephalopathy >7 days	KCH criteria
			(b) Paracetamol	Arterial pH, INR, serum creatinine, Grade 3–4 encephalopathy	
4. Hadem et al.	2008	102	Mixed etiologies	Etiology, serum bilirubin, lactate	BiLE score
5. Dhiman et al.	2007	144	Mixed etiologies	Age >50 year, prothrombin time >35 s, creatinine >1.5 mg/dl, jaundice to encephalopathy >7 days, HE grade 3–4, Cerebral edema	Any three of these six parameters Superior to KCH criteria and MELD
6. Bechmann et al.	2010	68	Mixed etiologies	Creatinine, INR, cytokeratin 18	Superior to KCH criteria and MELD
7. Rutherford et al.	2012	500	Mixed etiologies	INR, serum bilirubin, phosphate, M30, encephalopathy grade	ALFSG index; sensitivity 86%, superior to KCH criteria and MELD
8. Yantorne et al.	2007	120	Mixed etiologies	MELD score (INR, creatinine and bilirubin)	Similar to Clichy but superior to KCH criteria
9. Bernal et al.	2002	210	Paracetamol	Serum lactate (early 3.5 mmol/L, Postresuscitation 3.0 mmol/L)	
10. Schmidt and Dalhoff	2002	125	Paracetamol	Serum phosphate (1.2 mmol/L, 48–96 h after overdose)	Not superior to KCH criteria
11. Schmidt and Larsen	2007	460	Paracetamol	MELD score	Sensitivity 60%, not superior to KCH criteria
12. Taylor et al.	2006	29	HAV	ALT <2600 IU/L, creatinine >2.0 mg/dl, mechanical ventilation, requiring inotropes	Superior to KCH criteria and MELD

(continued)

Table 2.2 (continued)

Study	Year	Number of patients	Patient population	Parameters included in study or model	Comment
13. Ganzert et al.	2005	198	Amanita phalloides	Prothrombin index <25%, creatinine >106 μmol/L	Applicable from day 3, sensitivity 100%
14. Westbrook et al.	2010	54	Pregnancy related	Lactate >2.8 mg/dl, encephalopathy	90% sensitivity, 86% specificity, 98% specificity, 69%, specificity 65%

2.3 ACLF and Liver Transplantation

ACLF is an increasingly recognized condition defined by all major liver consortia (Table 2.3). Alcohol and sepsis lead the precipitating acute factors. ACLF is often seen in patients less than 60 years of age in contrast to decompensated cirrhosis. Patient selection for LT in ACLF is influenced by a number of clinical factors: age, acute event of the ACLF, sepsis, golden window period, number and type of organ failure(s). Interestingly, etiology of cirrhosis do not influence clinical outcome.

Unlike decompensated cirrhosis, MELD applicability is limited in patients with ACLF. Most patients with ACLF have acute precipitating factors which may not be fully reversible, leading to partial recovery but with organ failures. These are the patients who require liver transplantation.

Enhanced pretransplant intensive care has reduced mortality rates in ACLF, but a notable shift in patient outcomes emerged with increased transplantation listings. While various societies may differ in defining criteria and patient populations for ACLF, a unifying factor is the exceedingly high short-term mortality, prompting a recommendation for transplant listing in the earlier stages of the disease. ACLF patients benefit from rapid evaluation and listing. Even those who recover from the index ACLF event remain at risk of recurrent decompensation and more severe ACLF in the future [34]. Despite recovery, inherent 6-month mortality ranges from 40% to 50% [35, 36]. Development of infection portends a poor prognosis, and there is a narrow therapeutic window for these patients. Thus, patients with grade I and II ACLF should also be listed even if they are not transplanted.

ACLF grade 1: defined by single-organ failure either liver with bilirubin >12 mg/dl or creatinine >2 mg/dl.

MELD and CTP scores do not adequately reflect the high mortality in ACLF, necessitating the use of specific prognostic scores (Table 2.9). The CLIF-C ACLF score from CANONIC study [37], incorporating organ failures (CLIF-OF score), age and white blood cell count, outperforms other models, particularly in predicting

Table 2.3 Characteristics of definitions of ACLF developed by four different consortia

Characteristics	European Association for the Study of the Liver–Chronic Liver Failure (EASL-CLIF)	North American Consortium for the Study of End-stage Liver Disease (NACSELD)	Chinese Group on the Study of Severe Hepatitis B (COSSH)	Asian Pacific Association for the Study of the Liver (APASL) ACLF Research Consortium (AARC)
Population considered in definition	Acute decompensation of cirrhosis (patients with prior decompensation of cirrhosis are included)	Infection at admission or during hospital stay (patients with prior decompensation of cirrhosis are included)	Acute decompensation of HBV-related chronic liver disease with or without cirrhosis	Acute liver deterioration (see below) in patients with previously diagnosed or undiagnosed chronic liver disease (including cirrhosis) Both compensated cirrhosis and noncirrhotic chronic liver disease (nonalcoholic fatty liver disease, related chronic hepatic injury or chronic hepatitis with fibrosis or fibrosis due to other reasons) qualify as chronic liver disease
Population excluded from definition	Admission for scheduled procedure or treatment; Hepatocellular carcinoma outside Milan criteria; severe chronic extrahepatic diseases (HIV infection); ongoing immunosuppressive treatments	Outpatients with infection; HIV infection; prior organ transplant; disseminated malignancies	Other etiologies of chronic liver disease	Patients with bacterial infections; cirrhosis and known prior decompensation

(continued)

Table 2.3 (continued)

Characteristics	European Association for the Study of the Liver–Chronic Liver Failure (EASL-CLIF)	North American Consortium for the Study of End-stage Liver Disease (NACSELD)	Chinese Group on the Study of Severe Hepatitis B (COSSH)	Asian Pacific Association for the Study of the Liver (APASL) ACLF Research Consortium (AARC)
Definition	Presence of failure of 1 of the 6 major organ systems (CLIF-C Organ Failure [OF] scale)	≥2 OF (maximum 4)	≥1 OF (CLIF-C OF scale)	Acute hepatic insult manifesting as jaundice (total bilirubin levels of 5 mg/dl or more) and coagulopathy (INR of 1.5 or more, or prothrombin activity of less than 40%) complicated within 4 weeks by clinical ascites, encephalopathy or both.
Severity grading and risk stratification	Grading according to number of organ failures	Number of organ failures	Similar to EASL-CLIF	AARC score
Short-term mortality	By 28 days: Grade 1: 20% Grade 2: 30% Grade 3: 80%	By 30 days: 2 organ failures: 49% 3 organ failures: 64% 4 organ failures: 77%	By 28 days: Grade 1: 23% Grade 2: 61% Grade 3: 93%	By 28 days: Grade 1: 13% Grade 2: 45% Grade 3: 86%

short-term mortality [38, 39]. According to APASL, baseline criteria such as a MELD score >30, AARC Score >10 and advanced HE in the absence of overt sepsis or multiorgan failure may be considered for early liver transplantation [40]. These scores should be reassessed 3–7 days after diagnosis to predict patient outcomes. ACLF grade has the strongest correlation with post-transplant survival, and patients with grade 3 experience a higher rate of complications and a longer hospital stay [41]. Despite this, liver transplant remains the best therapeutic option for patients with grade 3 ACLF with 1 year survival of transplanted patients significantly higher than that of nontransplanted controls (83.9% vs. 7.9%) [42].

Scores at definite time intervals are used as threshold points to decide futility of care. EASL-CLIF score >64 points is commonly used to identify patients for whom rescue liver transplantation may not be a viable option [37]. APASL recommends that the presence of bilirubin level >22 mg/dL, HE grade 3 or 4, INR >2.5 with either creatinine level >1 mg/dL or lactate >1.5 mmol/L at baseline and persistent derangement at day 4 or 7 could indicate the futility of care [40]. Other factors like requirement of mechanical ventilation due to ARDS or brain-related conditions despite optimal therapy have also been suggested [43].

ACLF and organ failures define the grade and severity of ACLF. Presence of liver or renal failure with no improvement should be considered for liver transplantation [44]. Presence of progressive circulation failure and respiratory failure ($PiO_2/FiO_2 < 200$ mm Hg) is associated with poor post-transplant outcomes.

Improvement in ventilatory requirements and efforts to reduce lactate are associated with better post-transplant outcomes.

ACLF, being a dynamic condition, should be assessed for disease progression on a daily basis. Assessment of organ failure between day 3 and 7 has been shown to predict mortality [45]. APASL recommends early liver transplantation for patients with ACLF-grade 1 and grade 2 with AARC >8, MELD >28 and higher grades of HE in the absence of active sepsis or multiorgan failure [46].

Recent 'Kyoto' guidelines on ACLF strongly recommends to assess transplant benefit in ACLF patients based on the severity of acute liver injury, reversibility of underlying liver disease and the prognosis of associated extrahepatic organ failure. Given the similar transplant outcomes of ACLF patients compared to non-ACLF patients, liver transplant should be offered to appropriate ACLF patients [46].

2.4 Liver Transplantation for Decompensated Cirrhosis

Patients' survival following an episode of hepatic decompensation reduces to less than 2 years. Development of ascites, hepatic encephalopathy or liver synthetic dysfunction is associated with 20% 1-year mortality in contrary to 5.4% in patients with compensated cirrhosis [2]. In addition, these patients have increased risk of further decompensation resulting in hospitalization, septic complications and poor quality of life. In patients with decompensated cirrhosis, timely identification and referral for liver transplantation can significantly improve survival and quality of life. Therefore, patients with hepatic decompensation should be offered liver transplantation and perhaps constitute the most common indication. Given that the risk of liver transplant surgery is around 10%, patients with decompensated cirrhosis with an annual mortality of over 10% should be considered for liver transplantation.

As the global burden of chronic liver diseases continues to rise, the number of patients presenting with decompensation has increased, necessitating clear criteria for listing and prioritizing candidates.

Table 2.4 Indication for liver transplantation in chronic liver disease

Factors	Clinical significance for LT indication
Ascites	Especially if refractory or associated with spontaneous bacterial peritonitis (SBP)
Hepatic encephalopathy	Persistent or recurrent impacting quality of life
Jaundice and coagulopathy	Progressive hyperbilirubinemia and elevated INR
Hepatorenal syndrome (HRS)	Type 1 or 2 indicates severe portal hypertension

2.4.1 Indications for Liver Transplantation in Decompensated Cirrhosis

The decision to list a patient with decompensated cirrhosis for transplantation is based on a combination of clinical decompensation, biochemical markers and the survival benefit [1]. The factors necessitating consideration for LT in decompensated cirrhosis include ascites, hepatic encephalopathy and related complications (Table 2.4).

2.4.2 Refractory Ascites

Ascites is the most common complication in decompensated cirrhosis, developing in 5–10% of patients with compensated cirrhosis annually. Once ascites appears, the median survival drops to approximately 20 months [47]. Refractory ascites (RA) is diuretic-intractable in 93.3% cases and diuretic-resistant in 6.7%. RA was more frequent in patients who developed dilutional hyponatemia during the study (32.4% vs. 3.2%; $P < 0.0001$). The actuarial probability of RA after the first episode of ascites was 16.7% at 5 years of follow-up [48]. A key progression in its course is the development of refractory ascites. Once refractory ascites (RA) develops, the prognosis significantly worsens, with a mortality rate of approximately 50% within 6–12 months of diagnosis [49]. Liver transplantation (LT) remains the only definitive treatment. While transjugular intrahepatic portosystemic shunt (TIPS) may serve as a bridge to transplantation, in patients unsuitable for TIPS or with additional complications of cirrhosis, early liver transplantation is the preferred approach.

2.4.3 Spontaneous Bacterial Peritonitis

The occurrence of spontaneous bacterial peritonitis (SBP) among outpatient liver cirrhosis patients ranges from 1.5% to 3.5% and 10% in hospitalized cirrhotics [50]. Symptoms of SBP can often be mild and subtle, yet it may also trigger Acute

Chronic Liver Failure (ACLF), leading to septic shock, acute kidney injury (AKI) and multiorgan failure. The mortality rate for SBP episodes in liver cirrhosis patients could be 20% even with prompt diagnosis and intervention [51]. Following the resolution of SBP, it is crucial to consider the patient for an early liver transplantation. Ideally, a waiting period of 14 days after SBP resolution is recommended before proceeding with liver transplantation (LT). However, in instances that require immediate or urgent transplantation, LT can be performed as soon as SBP has been successfully resolved. The timing of LT for a patient who has recuperated from SBP should be determined on a case-by-case basis. Existing data on complications post-LT in individuals with a history of SBP vary. Patients who recently had SBP often experience more severe health challenges compared to those without SBP and may require preoperative mechanical ventilation or hemodialysis. In general, performing LT on a patient recovering from SBP can be technically difficult due to the formation of adhesions. One study reported a higher incidence of bile leaks in patients with a prior history of SBP undergoing LT. Furthermore, the rate of postoperative infections is elevated in those with a previous episode of SBP, although this does not seem to impact overall survival rates [52].

2.4.4 Hepatorenal Syndrome (HRS) (Table 2.5)

Hepatorenal syndrome is one of the most common causes of renal dysfunction in patients with liver cirrhosis, particularly in the setting of prerenal acute kidney injury (AKI). A key diagnostic indicator of HRS is the failure to respond to intravascular volume expansion with albumin, suggesting underlying pathophysiological mechanisms such as splanchnic vasodilatation, renal vasoconstriction and impaired cardiac function. If inadequately treated or if there is a poor response to therapy, HRS may progress to acute tubular necrosis (ATN), a more severe form of kidney injury. Types and definition of HRS are tabulated below [53].

Table 2.5 Definition of HRS

Cirrhosis; acute-on-chronic liver failure
Increase in serum creatinine ≥0.3 mg/dl within 48 h or ≥50% from baseline value and/or
Urinary output ≤0.5 ml/kg B.W. ≥6 h
No full or partial response after at least 2 days of diuretic withdrawal and volume expansion with albumin
Absence of shock
No current or recent treatment with nephrotoxic drugs
Absence of parenchymal disease as indicated by proteinuria >500 mg/day, microhematuria (>50 red blood cells per high power field), urinary injury biomarkers (if available) and/or abnormal renal ultrasonography
Suggestion of renal vasoconstriction with fraction excretion of sodium (FENa) of <0.2% (with levels <0.1% being highly predictive)

2.4.5 Hepatic Hydrothorax

Hepatic hydrothorax (HH) is the excessive (>500 mL) accumulation of transudate in the pleural cavity in patients with cirrhosis but without cardiopulmonary and pleural diseases. It is right sided in approximately 85% of cases and left sided in approximately 13% and bilateral in 2% [54]. The median survival in presence of HH is 8–12 months [55]. A significant event in the natural history of HH is development of Spontaneous Bacterial empyema, which carries a worse prognosis. Treatment of HH is parallel to management of ascites. Refractory HH not responding to standard management warrants a liver transplant especially with coexistence of other complications of liver cirrhosis. A study comparing outcomes of patients with HH undergoing LT with those of patients without HH did not show any difference in the 1-year survival rate, the duration of mechanical, the duration of ICU stay as well as the frequency of septic complications and early postoperative mortality [56].

2.4.6 Hepatic Encephalopathy

Hepatic encephalopathy (HE) is a potentially reversible neuropsychiatric syndrome in liver cirrhosis, ranging from subtle cognitive changes to coma. It is typically multifactorial and often triggered by identifiable precipitating factors. Prompt recognition and management of these factors are key to resolution and prevention of recurrence. Standard medical therapy includes lactulose, rifaximin and correction of contributing conditions. In cases where a large spontaneous portosystemic shunt is identified, interventional closure may effectively control symptoms. Recurrent or persistent HE, particularly when spontaneous, is considered an independent indication for liver transplantation [57].

2.4.7 Scoring Systems for Prioritization

Clinical scores may help determine patient selection for liver transplantation.

Child-Pugh score was formulated in 1972 mainly to identify patients with high risk of liver-related mortality in patients with decompensated cirrhosis. The score includes both clinical (ascites and hepatic encephalopathy grades) and biochemical variables (INR, bilirubin and albumin). The predictive value of this score for 28-day mortality is 68%, with a sensitivity and specificity of 77.3% and 52%, respectively [58]. It is still widely used for patient selection for liver transplantation. The advantage of this score is that it is simple, easy to use and extensively studied. However, presence of subjective variability in measuring ascites and challenges in grading hepatic encephalopathy may skew the score.

Model for end stage liver disease was developed in 2001 by Kamath et al., initially to identify patients for TIPS but subsequently found substantially beneficial in selecting patients for liver transplantation [4]. MELD score utilizes a logarithmic model of creatinine, bilirubin and INR values. The advantage of MELD is 'purely objective', easily reproducible with online calculators. Indeed, MELD-based organ allocation is the most common modality of patient selection for liver transplantation worldwide. A MELD score of 15 carries a 3-month mortality of 20% and is the minimal listing criteria for liver transplantation. However, MELD score may not identify cirrhotic patients with chronic hepatic encephalopathy, hepatopulmonary syndrome and importantly HCC. Thus, 'MELD exception' has been formulated for this specific cohort of patients with variant syndromes. Although MELD identifies liver-related complications, it may not be suitable for patients with predominant portal hypertension-related complications.

Hyponatremia in patients with liver cirrhosis is an important prognostic marker with significantly reduced 1-year survival. Addition of sodium to MELD (MELD-Na) appears better than the original score [59].

2.4.8 Child-Turcotte-Pugh (CTP) Score

The CTP score helps assess disease severity. One-year survival rates for classes A, B and C are approximately 95%, 80% and 45%, respectively. Patients with a CTP score >7 (Class B or C) should be evaluated for transplantation [47].

2.4.9 MELD and MELD-Na Score

The Model for End-Stage Liver Disease (MELD) score and its sodium-modified version (MELD-Na) predict short-term mortality and are used to allocate donor organs (Table 2.6). A MELD score ≥15 is generally recommended for transplant listing, as survival is better with LT beyond this threshold [59, 60]. MELD-Na further improves accuracy by incorporating serum sodium. Age have been proposed to enhance mortality prediction with improved prognostic accuracy over the original MELD [60].

Table 2.6 MELD score and 3-month mortality

MELD score range	3-month mortality risk (%)	Transplant recommendation
<10	<2	Monitor, no immediate listing
10–19	6–20	Consider evaluation
20–29	19–76	Listing generally appropriate
30–39	52–100	Urgent transplant required
≥40	~100	Highest priority

2.4.10 MELD 3.0 and Delta MELD

MELD 3.0, a newer model, includes additional factors such as female sex, albumin and refined creatinine limits, along with interaction terms among sodium, bilirubin and albumin. It offers superior mortality prediction compared to MELD-Na. Delta MELD (change in MELD over time) may also help identify patients with rapid disease progression and provide improved prognostic accuracy over the original MELD [6, 60].

2.4.11 Exceptions to MELD-Based Allocation

Several exceptions to the MELD score exist, including conditions like hepatic encephalopathy, pulmonary complications, amyloidosis and primary hyperoxaluria, where additional points may be granted to prioritize transplant candidates [61]. Hepatocellular carcinoma (HCC) is another exception, where extra points are awarded based on tumor characteristics, alpha-fetoprotein (AFP) levels and response to treatment.

2.5 Liver Transplantation Based on Disease Etiology

2.5.1 MASH

MASLD is the most common etiology of chronic liver disease, with increasing prevalence worldwide. MASH-related cirrhosis is the most common indication for LT across most centers worldwide. Presence of comorbidities may alter the timing of liver transplantation in patients with MASH. Obesity may delay postoperative recovery and delayed mobility. These patients must be urged to lose weight and more relevant in the setting of living donor liver transplantation (LDLT). Fluid overload may be responsible for increased weight in many patients, which requires optimal diuresis without compromising renal function.

A detailed cardiac evaluation with particular focus on coronary arteries is required in patients with MASH cirrhosis [62]. Presence of significant coronary artery disease (CAD) may warrant intervention prior to transplantation.

2.5.2 Alcohol

Patients with no improvement in hepatic decompensation despite abstinence. Although, 6 months abstinence is widely followed, the duration is a matter of debate. With increasing ACLF presentation, liver transplantation should be considered in selected patients.

LDLT offers an additional advantage in such scenarios where the decision to transplant can be expedited or withheld based on patient's clinical condition.

2.5.3 Hepatitis B

Patients with hepatitis B may present as decompensated cirrhosis, ACLF or ALF requiring liver transplantation. With the availability of potent drugs entecavir and tenofovir, use of hepatitis B immunoglobulin (HBIg) to prevent liver allograft reinfection is generally not required.

2.5.4 Hepatitis C

Hepatitis C cure (sustained virological response at 12 weeks after completion of therapy) can be achieved with currently available directly acting antiviral drugs. In sicker patients, 30 days of DAA achieving negative HCV RNA and considered for liver transplantation.

In case of limited time, patients can be transplanted and DAA can be initiated post-transplantation.

Contraindications to Liver Transplantation in Decompensated Cirrhosis (Table 2.7)

While liver transplantation offers substantial survival benefit in appropriately selected patients, certain absolute and relative contraindications must be considered to ensure optimal use of scarce donor organs and to protect patient safety [63]. Evaluation of contraindications is an essential part of transplant workup and often requires multidisciplinary assessment.

Selecting appropriate candidates for liver transplantation in decompensated cirrhosis is a dynamic and multifactorial process. It requires timely identification, careful risk-benefit analysis and collaboration among hepatologists, transplant surgeons and multidisciplinary teams. Early referral and individualized assessment are key to improving outcomes and maximizing the benefit of transplantation.

Table 2.7 Contraindications for liver transplantation

Absolute contraindications	Relative contraindications
Active alcohol or substance abuse	Age >70 years
Uncontrolled sepsis	Morbid obesity (BMI >40)
Advanced cardiopulmonary disease	Comorbidities affecting surgical outcomes
Metastatic malignancy	Limited psychosocial support or compliance
Severe extrahepatic infection	

2.6 Malignancies

2.6.1 Hepatocellular Carcinoma (HCC)

Indication for liver transplantation has evolved significantly in the last couple of decades. Initial poor long-term results of liver transplantation due to HCC recurrence was circumvented by improved patient selection based on size and number of lesions. Milan criteria, developed by Mazzoferro et al. [64], include a criteria of either a single lesion of maximal diameter of 5 cm or 3 lesions with largest not more than 3 cm. Application and patient selection based on this criteria has significantly improved long-term recurrence free post-transplant survival to over 75% [65]. Although this was widely accepted, Milan criteria were considered too restrictive for patient selection, and the initial study was based on radiological images from early 1990s [66].

University of California, San Francisco (UCSF) criteria were based on a retrospective analysis of liver explants following liver transplantation. Accordingly, a single lesion not more than 6.5 cm and up to 5 lesions with a combined diameter of not more than 8 cm in the absence of vascular invasion has been widely accepted for liver transplantation with a 5-year recurrence free survival of 80.9% [67].

Various other criteria based on size and number have been devised. A recent 'metro-ticket' criteria were published based on size and number, correlating with appropriate post-transplant recurrent free survival [68].

Barcelona clinic liver cancer (BCLC) staging system with recent modification based on HCC radiological characteristics, liver function and patient performance status recommends liver transplantation for BCLC-A and BCLC-B. Early stage (BCLC-A) is similar to Milan criteria and intermediate stage (BCLC-B) with higher tumor burden in the absence of vascular invasion [69].

The 2023 INASL Puri III recommendations introduced the INASL-BCLC staging system to better suit Indian patients. It allows liver transplantation in selected BCLC-B (intermediate) patients without vascular invasion after downstaging. BCLC-C and D stages are further subclassified (C1/C2, D1/D2) to guide therapy. Locoregional (e.g. Trans arterial radio embolization (TARE) and stereotactic brachyradiation therapy (SBRT)) and combination therapies are integrated. This system helps more patients qualify for transplant beyond the strict Milan criteria [70].

Downstaging of larger HCC allows better patient selection for liver transplantation. Downstaging involves application of locoregional therapies with transarterial chemo embolisation (TACE), TARE or SBRT followed by liver transplantation with improved survival.

2.6.2 Alpha-Fetoprotein (AFP)

AFP is the most validated tumor marker in diagnosis of HCC. Studies have evaluated its role in selection of patients for liver transplantation. Most centers follow an AFP >400 or >100 as an absolute contraindication for liver transplantation [71]. In the context of downstaging, patients with a significant reduction in AFP (<400) following locoregional therapy should be considered for liver transplantation.

Recent availability of immunotherapy may further expand the indication and selection of HCC patients for liver transplantation.

HCC stands out as the sixth most frequently diagnosed cancer globally and the third leading cause of cancer-related deaths [72]. Mazzaferro's seminal study in 1996 marked a turning point, making liver transplantation a curative treatment [64]. With advancements in surgical techniques, relaxation of inclusion criteria for transplant and 'downstaging' strategies for patients outside standard inclusion criteria, liver transplantation has become a standard of care for HCC [69]. HCC accounts for around 20–30% of all liver transplants done in Western countries [73, 74]. Due to a staggering disparity between available grafts and patients on wait-list, only patients with a significant survival advantage are usually selected for LT. Milan criteria were the first transplant selection criteria developed for HCC and continue to be widely used by organ procurement and transplant network for graft allocation. Since then, various criteria have been modelled and show favorable post-transplant survival (Table 2.8).

2.6.3 UCSF (University of California, San Francisco)

With these expanded criteria, greater number of patients can undergo transplant for HCC without significantly compromising on post-transplant survival and disease recurrence rate. Relying solely on tumor size and number is suboptimal, and incorporating parameters reflecting the expected evolutionary profile of the tumor is crucial. Several groups have integrated surrogates of this 'biological profile and behavior' into their selection criteria including tumor markers like AFP and DCP (des-gamma carboxyprothrombin) and histological features (microvascular invasion and tumor differentiation). This will further refine prediction of post-transplant recurrence and survival [82–84].

Table 2.8 Liver transplant criteria for HCC

Criteria (country)	Author	Donor setting	Inclusion criteria	Cases	Post-transplant survival
Milan (Milan, Italy)	Mazzaferro (1996) [64]	DD	Single tumor ≤5 cm OR	48	4-year survival rate: 85%
			Up to 3 tumors with diameter ≤3 cm		
UCSF (USA)	Yao [67, 75] (2001, 2007)	DD	Solitary tumor ≤6.5 cm OR	168	5-year survival rate: 80.9%
			< 3 nodules with the largest lesion ≤4.5 cm and total tumor diameter ≤8 cm		
Total tumor volume (TTV) (Alberta, Canada)	Toso [76] (2008)	DD	TTV ≤115 cm³ and AFP ≤400 ng/mL	228	Within Milan: 5-year survival rate: 82%
					Within TTV: 5-year survival rate: 80%
Up-to-7 (international multicenter)	Mazzaferro [77] (2009)	DD	Sum of the size of the largest tumor [in cm] and the number of tumors <7	1556	Within Milan: 5-year survival rate: 73.3%
					Beyond Milan: 5-year survival rate: 71.2%
Tokyo (Japan)	Sugawara [78] (2007)	LD	HCC diameter ≤5 cm, HCC number ≤5	78	5-year survival rate: 75%
Kyoto (Japan)	Kaido [79] (2013)	LD	≤10 tumors, ≤5 cm, DCP ≤400 mAU/mL	198	Beyond Milan 5-year survival rate: 65%
Asan (Korea)	Lee [80] (2008)	LD	HCC diameter 5 cm or less, HCC number 6 or less	229	5-year survival rate: 76%
Extended Toronto criteria (Canada)	Sapisochin [81] (2016)		No limit in size and number, no vascular invasion, no extrahepatic disease, no cancer-related symptoms Biopsy of largest tumor not poorly differentiated	605	Beyond Milan 5-year survival rate: 68%

2.6.4 Non-HCC Malignancies

Neuroendocrine tumor involving the liver, highly selected patients with intrahepatic cholangiocarcinoma (CCA) and stable colorectal metastasis may be considered for liver transplantation following a multidisciplinary approach.

2.7 Variant Syndromes

2.7.1 Refractory Ascites (RA) and Hepatic Hydrothorax (HH)

2.7.1.1 Hepatic Hydrothorax

Hepatic hydrothorax (HH) refers to the abnormal buildup of fluid (greater than 500 mL) in the pleural cavity among patients with cirrhosis, who do not have underlying cardiopulmonary or pleural conditions. This condition is typically found on the right side in about 85% of cases, while approximately 13% have it on the left side, and around 2% experience it bilaterally [54]. The median survival rate for individuals with HH is between 8 and 12 months [55]. A critical development in the course of HH is the onset of Spontaneous Bacterial Empyema, which is linked to a poorer prognosis. Managing HH aligns closely with treating ascites. When HH is resistant to standard treatments, liver transplantation becomes necessary, particularly if there are additional complications related to liver cirrhosis. A study that compared outcomes between patients with HH who underwent liver transplantation and those without it found no significant differences in 1-year survival rates, mechanical ventilation duration, ICU stay length or rates of septic complications and early postoperative deaths [56].

2.7.2 Hepatorenal Syndrome

Most common cause of renal dysfunction in patients with liver cirrhosis is prerenal AKI. Nonresponse to intravascular fluid volume expansion may indicate the presence of Hepatorenal syndrome (HRS) caused by splanchnic vasodilatation, renal vasoconstriction and cardiac dysfunction. Inadequate treatment and/or inadequate response of HRS to treatment can lead to development of Acute tubular Necrosis (ATN). The newer definition of HRS is shown in Tables 2.3 and 2.4 shows classification of subtypes of HRS.

The median survival of patients with HRS-AKI (HRS-1) is about 2 weeks and that of more chronic forms of HRS is about 6 months [85]. Hence, early recognition, initiation of therapy and consideration of early liver transplant are crucial for management of HRS. It is very important to rule out any structural or irreversible renal injury prior to liver transplant.

Biomarkers of renal injury may be of help in this situation. A urinary neutrophil gelatinase-associated lipocalin (NGAL) value of >194 mcg/gm of creatinine suggests presence of ATN [86]. Urinary Spot sodium and/or FENa <0.2% indicate presence of renal vasoconstriction and hence contribution from HRS pathophysiology.

Patients with liver cirrhosis who are candidate for liver transplant or patients presenting with Acute on chronic liver failure (ACLF) with Stage 3 AKI >4 weeks or on dialysis or eGFR <35 by MDRD-6 equation or evidence of structural renal disease should be considered for simultaneous liver–kidney transplant [86].

2.7.3 *Hepatopulmonary Syndrome (HPS)*

Hepatopulmonary Syndrome represents a progressive complication caused by liver cirrhosis and portal hypertension, characterized by the dilation of intrapulmonary precapillary and capillary vessels. This leads to a rapid flow of inadequately oxygenated blood entering the pulmonary veins while preserving alveolar ventilation, causing a mismatch between ventilation and perfusion [87]. The diagnostic criteria for HPS are outlined in Table 2.9.

HPS occurs in 10–17% of cirrhosis patients [88]. It is classified as mild when arterial oxygen partial pressure (PaO_2) exceeds 80 mm Hg, moderate when PaO_2 ranges from 60 to 80 mm Hg, severe when it falls between 50 and 60 mm Hg and very severe when PaO_2 drops below 50 mm Hg in room air. The presence of a significant intrapulmonary shunt that can be treated with endovascular intervention provides a non-liver transplant option. However, if no such shunt exists and there is no definitive medical therapy, liver transplantation remains the only solution to reverse HPS. Patients with severe HPS typically have a median survival of less than 12 months [89]. Therefore, evaluation for liver transplantation should be prioritized for patients with HPS, who also need close monitoring, especially as those with severe HPS face substantial perioperative risks [90]. In the absence of other indications, the best time for transplantation is when HPS reaches a moderate to severe level [57].

2.7.4 *Portopulmonary Hypertension (POPH)*

Portopulmonary hypertension is another complication affecting the pulmonary vasculature in cirrhosis and portal hypertension. It arises from increased resistance in pulmonary vessels due to endothelin-1-mediated vasoconstriction via ET-A receptors, reduced nitric oxide-mediated dilation and pulmonary vascular remodeling

Table 2.9 Diagnostic criteria for HPS

Impaired oxygenation (PaO_2 <80 mm Hg OR increased age corrected alveolar-arterial oxygen gradient while breathing on room air)
Intrapulmonary vasodilation (confirmed by bubble contrast echocardiography or brain shunt fraction >6% by 99 m Tc labelled macroaggregated albumin scan)
Liver disease (cirrhosis and/or portal hypertension)

[91]. A diagnosis is confirmed through right-heart catheterization, which reveals elevated mean pulmonary arterial pressure (MPAP >25 mm Hg), increased pulmonary vascular resistance and normal pulmonary capillary wedge pressure [91]. The severity of POPH is classified based on resting mPAP levels: mild (mPAP 25–35 mm Hg), moderate (mPAP 36–45 mm Hg) and severe (mPAP >45 mm Hg). Moderate or severe POPH cases exhibit poor survival rates following LT, making transplantation contraindicated when these conditions do not respond to medical treatments [57]. However, patients whose mPAP decreases to below 35 mm Hg with medical therapy are excellent candidates for LT [85] and should be given priority, even if no other conventional indications are present.

2.7.5 Hepatic Encephalopathy and Acquired Hepatocerebral Degeneration (AHCD)

Hepatic Encephalopathy (HE) refers to a potentially reversible brain dysfunction that encompasses a wide range of neuropsychiatric symptoms, from minor behavioral changes to coma. In cases of liver cirrhosis, HE is usually multifactorial and often linked to a precipitating factor. Identifying and treating this underlying cause can help resolve and prevent future HE episodes. Medical treatments include lactulose, rifaximin and addressing contributing factors. If a significant spontaneous portosystemic shunt is found, its closure through an interventional radiological approach may alleviate HE symptoms. Both spontaneous and recurrent or persistent HE can independently warrant consideration for LT [57].

Acquired Hepatocerebral Degeneration (AHCD) is a rare syndrome marked by ataxia, parkinsonism, various movement disorders, cognitive dysfunction and neuropsychiatric symptoms [92]. There is insufficient evidence regarding the reversibility of AHCD after LT, likely dependent on how long symptoms have been present. Although AHCD does not preclude LT for other reasons, there is inadequate support for recommending LT solely for AHCD. Some case reports indicate successful LT in AHCD patients, with symptom improvement noted within a period of up to 7 months [93].

2.8 Specific Disorders

2.8.1 Primary Sclerosing Cholangitis (PSC)

Primary sclerosing cholangitis (PSC) is a immune-mediated cholangiopathy with involvement of either extra hepatic or intrahepatic bile ducts or both, leading to inflammation, stricture formation, cirrhosis, portal hypertension, further decompensation and development of cholangiocarcinoma (CCA). Ursodeoxycholic (UDCA) acid is widely used for these patients, it improves liver biochemistry, and worsening of liver biochemistry, fatigue and pruritus have been seen on withdrawal of UDCA but there is no medical therapy shown to improve the histological lesions or alter natural progression of PSC [94]. Patients with PSC with classical indications of decompensation need LT as a definitive management. But, LT also need to be considered in patients with PSC with intractable pruritus and patients with recurrent cholangitis. MELD exceptions for LT are granted to patients with at least two admissions within a 1-year period for acute cholangitis with a documented bloodstream in infection or with evidence of sepsis requiring vasopressors for hemodynamic instability, as well as those with a diagnosis of CCA [95].

2.8.2 *Primary Biliary Cholangitis (PBC)*

PBC is an immune-mediated chronic progressive inflammatory liver disease resulting in chronic cholestasis, portal inflammation and fibrosis that can lead to cirrhosis and, ultimately, liver failure. The 10-year survival of asymptomatic patients ranged from 50% to 70%, whereas the median duration of survival for symptomatic patients ranged 5–8 years from the onset of symptoms [96]. The mainstay of therapy for PBC is UDCA, which has shown to improve liver biochemistry and slow down the disease progression and improve LT-free survival. In one third of the patients, the disease may not be sufficiently controlled and may need LT as an additional therapeutic option [96]. Apart from standard indications for LT for decompensated cirrhosis, intractable pruritus and profound fatigue may be considered for LT.

2.8.3 *Wilson Disease*

Wilson disease is a genetic disorder of copper metabolism resulting in liver disease and neuropsychiatric manifestations. Liver disease can present as decompensated cirrhosis and Acute liver failure for which LT is warranted. Whether patients with isolated neurological symptoms should be offered LT is debated. Studies have shown improvement of neurological symptoms in 58–78% of patients with WD [97]. Patients with long-standing neurological impairment from WD are unlikely to recover after LT contraindicating transplant in such cases [97].

Approach to patient selection for liver transplantation is illustrated in Fig. 2.1.

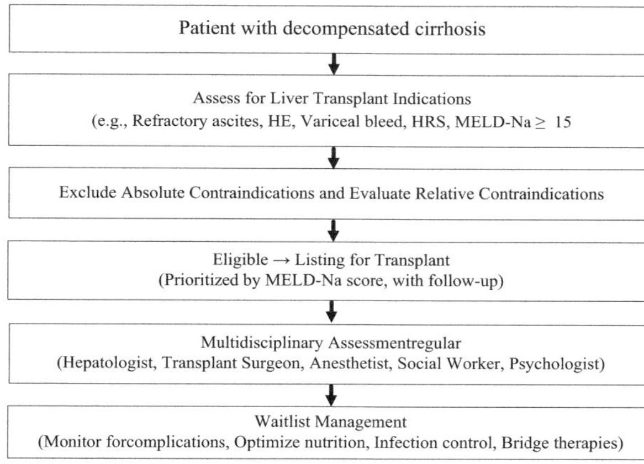

Fig. 2.1 Patient selection process for transplant in decompensated cirrhosis

2.9 Conclusion

Patient selection for liver transplantation is crucial to obtain optimal post-transplant outcomes.

Although clinical scores guide, individual patient selection should be carried out on a case-by- case basis. The complexities surrounding liver transplantation underscore the critical nature of appropriate patient selection. Successful outcomes hinge not only on the technical aspects of the surgery but also on the careful evaluation of candidate's overall health, disease severity and potential for post-transplant complications. By prioritizing comprehensive assessments and characterizing patient profiles, healthcare providers can streamline the selection process, thereby enhancing the effectiveness of liver transplantation and optimizing long-term patient outcomes.

References

1. European Association for The Study of the Liver. EASL clinical practice guidelines: liver transplantation. J Hepatol. 2016;64(2):433–85.
2. D'Amico G, Garcia-Tsao G, Pagliaro L. Natural history and prognostic indicators of survival in cirrhosis: a systematic review of 118 studies. J Hepatol. 2006;44(1):217–31.
3. Malinchoc M, Kamath PS, Gordon FD, et al. A model to predict poor survival in patients undergoing transjugular intrahepatic portosystemic shunts. Hepatology. 2000;31(4):864–71.
4. Kamath PS, Wiesner RH, Malinchoc M, et al. A model to predict survival in patients with end-stage liver disease. Hepatology. 2001;33(2):464–70.
5. Merion RM, Schaubel DE, Dykstra DM, et al. The survival benefit of liver transplantation. Am J Transplant. 2005;5(2):307–13.
6. Kim WR, Mannalithara A, Heimbach JK, et al. MELD 3.0: the model for end-stage liver disease updated for the modern era. Gastroenterology. 2021;161(6):1887–1895.e4.
7. Reuben A, Tillman H, Fontana RJ, et al. Outcomes in adults with acute liver failure between 1998 and 2013: an observational cohort study. Ann Intern Med. 2016;164:724–32.

8. Bernal W, Hyyrylainen A, Gera A, et al. Lessons from look-back in acute liver failure? A single centre experience of 3300 patients. J Hepatol. 2013;59:74–80.
9. Bernuau J, Rueff B, Benhamou JP. Fulminant and subfulminant liver failure: definitions and causes. Semin Liver Dis. 1986;6(2):97–106.
10. National Institutes of Health. Consensus development conference statement. Liver transplantation–June 20-23, 1983. Hepatology. 1984;4(1 Suppl):107S–10S.
11. Reddy KR, Ellerbe C, Schilsky M, et al. Determinants of outcome among patients with acute liver failure listed for liver transplantation in the United States. Liver Transpl. 2016;22:505–15.
12. Marudanayagam R, Shanmugam V, Gunson B, et al. Aetiology and outcome of acute liver failure. HPB (Oxford). 2009;11(5):429–34.
13. Karvellas CJ, Leventhal TM, Rakela JL, et al. Outcomes of patients with acute liver failure listed for liver transplantation: a multicenter prospective cohort analysis. Liver Transpl. 2023;29(3):318–30.
14. Stravitz RT, Lee WM. Acute liver failure. Lancet. 2019;394(10201):869–81.
15. Oketani M, Ido A, Nakayama N, et al. Intractable Hepato-Biliary Diseases Study Group of Japan. Etiology and prognosis of fulminant hepatitis and late-onset hepatic failure in Japan: summary of the annual nationwide survey between 2004 and 2009. Hepatol Res. 2013;43(2):97–105.
16. Zhao P, Wang C, Liu W, et al. Causes and outcomes of acute liver failure in China. PLoS One. 2013;8:e80991.
17. Khuroo MS, Kamili S. Aetiology and prognostic factors in acute liver failure in India. J Viral Hepat. 2003;10:224–31.
18. Eapen CE, Venkataraman J. Rodenticide (yellow phosphorus poison)-induced hepatotoxicity in India: constraints during management. J Clin Exp Hepatol. 2021;11(4):414–7.
19. Bernuau J, Goudeau A, Poynard T, et al. Multivariate analysis of prognostic factors in fulminant hepatitis B. Hepatology. 1986;6(4):648–51.
20. O'Grady JG, Alexander GJ, Hayllar KM, et al. Early indicators of prognosis in fulminant hepatic failure. Gastroenterology. 1989;97(2):439–45.
21. Craig DGN, Ford AC, Hayes PC, et al. Systematic review: prognostic tests of paracetamol-induced acute liver failure. Aliment Pharmacol Ther. 2010;31:1064–76.
22. Bernal W, Donaldson N, Wyncoll D, et al. Blood lactate as an early predictor of outcome in paracetamol-induced acute liver failure: a cohort study. Lancet. 2002;359(9306):558–63.
23. McPhail MJ, Farne H, Senvar N, et al. Ability of King's College criteria and model for end-stage liver disease scores to predict mortality of patients with acute liver failure: a meta-analysis. Clin Gastroenterol Hepatol. 2016;14(4):516–525.e5. quiz e43-e45.
24. Dhiman RK, Jain S, Maheshwari U, et al. Early indicators of prognosis in fulminant hepatic failure: an assessment of the Model for End-Stage Liver Disease (MELD) and King's College Hospital criteria. Liver Transpl. 2007;13(6):814.
25. Kumar R, Shalimar, Sharma H, et al. Prospective derivation and validation of early dynamic model for predicting outcome in patients with acute liver failure. Gut. 2012;61(7):1068–75.
26. Reddy MS, Rajakumar A, Mathew JS, et al. Liver Transplantation Society of India guidelines for the management of acute liver injury secondary to yellow phosphorus-containing rodenticide poisoning using the modified Delphi technique of consensus development. J Clin Exp Hepatol. 2021;11(4):475–83.
27. Devlin J, Wendon J, Heaton N, et al. Pretransplantation clinical status and outcome of emergency transplantation for acute liver failure. Hepatology. 1995;21(4):1018–24.
28. Saraf V, Pande S, Gopalakrishnan U, et al. Acute liver failure due to zinc phosphide containing rodenticide poisoning: clinical features and prognostic indicators of need for liver transplantation. Indian J Gastroenterol. 2015;34(4):325–9.
29. Bernal W, Cross TJ, Auzinger G, et al. Outcome after wait-listing for emergency liver transplantation in acute liver failure: a single centre experience. J Hepatol. 2009;50:306–13.
30. Yuan D, Liu F, Wei YG, et al. Adult-to-adult living donor liver transplantation for acute liver failure in China. World J Gastroenterol. 2012;18:7234–41.

31. European Association for the Study of The Liver. EASL Clinical Practical Guidelines on the management of acute (fulminant) liver failure. J Hepatol. 2017;66(5):1047–81.
32. Germani G, Theocharidou E, Adam R, et al. Liver transplantation for acute liver failure in Europe: outcomes over 20 years from the ELTR database. J Hepatol. 2012;57(2):288–96.
33. Freeman RB, Steffick DE, Guidinger MK, et al. Liver and intestine transplantation in the United States, 1997–2006. Am J Transplant. 2008;8(4 Pt 2):958–76.
34. Mahmud N, Sundaram V, Kaplan DE, et al. Grade 1 acute on chronic liver failure is a predictor for subsequent grade 3 failure. Hepatology. 2020;72(1):230–9.
35. Trebicka J, Sundaram V, Moreau R, et al. Liver transplantation for acute-on-chronic liver failure: science or fiction? Liver Transpl. 2020;26(7):906–15.
36. Gustot T, Fernandez J, Garcia E, et al., CANONIC Study Investigators of the EASL-CLIF Consortium. Clinical course of acute-on-chronic liver failure syndrome and effects on prognosis. Hepatology. 2015;62(1):243–52.
37. Jalan R, Saliba F, Pavesi M, et al., CANONIC study investigators of the EASL-CLIF Consortium. Development and validation of a prognostic score to predict mortality in patients with acute-on-chronic liver failure. J Hepatol. 2014;61(5):1038–47.
38. Barosa R, Roque Ramos L, et al. CLIF-C ACLF score is a better mortality predictor than MELD, MELD-Na and CTP in patients with acute on chronic liver failure admitted to the ward. Rev Esp Enferm Dig. 2017;109(6):399–405.
39. Engelmann C, Thomsen KL, Zakeri N, et al. Validation of CLIF-C ACLF score to define a threshold for futility of intensive care support for patients with acute-on-chronic liver failure. Crit Care. 2018;22(1):254.
40. Choudhury A, Jindal A, Maiwall R, et al., APASL ACLF Working Party. Liver failure determines the outcome in patients of acute-on-chronic liver failure (ACLF): comparison of APASL ACLF research consortium (AARC) and CLIF-SOFA models. Hepatol Int. 2017;11(5):461–471.
41. Choudhury A, Vijayaraghavan R, Maiwall R, et al., APASL ACLF Research Consortium (AARC) for APASL ACLF Working Party. 'First week' is the crucial period for deciding living donor liver transplantation in patients with acute-on-chronic liver failure. Hepatol Int. 2021;15(6):1376–1388.
42. Artru F, Louvet A, Ruiz I, et al. Liver transplantation in the most severely ill cirrhotic patients: a multicenter study in acute-on-chronic liver failure grade 3. J Hepatol. 2017;67(4):708–15.
43. Bajaj JS, O'Leary JG, Lai JC, Wong F, Long MD, Wong RJ, Kamath PS. Acute-on-chronic liver failure clinical guidelines. Am J Gastroenterol. 2022;117(2):225–52.
44. Xia L, Qiao ZY, Zhang ZJ, Lv ZC, Tong H, Tong Y, Wu HX, Chen XS, Sun HY, Zhang JJ, Thasler WE, Feng H, Xia Q. Transplantation for EASL-CLIF and APASL acute-on-chronic liver failure (ACLF) patients: the TEA cohort to evaluate long-term post-transplant outcomes. EClinicalMedicine. 2022;49:101476.
45. Gustot T, Fernandez J, Garcia E, Morando F, et al, CANONIC Study Investigators of the EASL-CLIF Consortium. Clinical course of acute-on-chronic liver failure syndrome and effects on prognosis. Hepatology. 2015;62(1):243–52.
46. Acute-on-chronic liver failure (ACLF): the 'Kyoto consensus'-steps from Asia. Hepatol Int. 2025;19(1):1–69.
47. Ginés P, Quintero E, Arroyo V, et al. Compensated cirrhosis: natural history and prognostic factors. Hepatology. 1987;7(1):122–8.
48. Planas R, Montoliu S, Ballesté B, et al. Natural history of patients hospitalized for management of cirrhotic ascites. Clin Gastroenterol Hepatol. 2006;4(11):1385–94.
49. Siqueira F, Kelly T, Saab S. Refractory ascites: pathogenesis, clinical impact, and management. Gastroenterol Hepatol (N Y). 2009;5(9):647–56.
50. Evans LT, Kim WR, Poterucha JJ, et al. Spontaneous bacterial peritonitis in asymptomatic outpatients with cirrhotic ascites. Hepatology. 2003;37(4):897–901.
51. Piano S, Fasolato S, Salinas F, et al. The empirical antibiotic treatment of nosocomial spontaneous bacterial peritonitis: results of a randomized, controlled clinical trial. Hepatology. 2016;63(4):1299–309.

52. Mounzer R, Malik SM, Nasr J, et al. Spontaneous bacterial peritonitis before liver transplantation does not affect patient survival. Clin Gastroenterol Hepatol. 2010;8(7):623–628.e1.
53. Angeli P, Garcia-Tsao G, Nadim MK, et al. News in pathophysiology, definition and classification of hepatorenal syndrome: a step beyond the International Club of Ascites (ICA) consensus document. J Hepatol. 2019;71(4):811–22.
54. Garbuzenko DV, Arefyev NO. Hepatic hydrothorax: an update and review of the literature. World J Hepatol. 2017;9(31):1197–204.
55. Abbasi A, Bhutto AR, Alam MT, et al. Frequency of hepatic hydrothorax and its association with child pugh class in liver cirrhosis patients. J Coll Physicians Surg Pak. 2016;26(7):566–9.
56. Sersté T, Moreno C, Francoz C, et al. The impact of preoperative hepatic hydrothorax on the outcome of adult liver transplantation. Eur J Gastroenterol Hepatol. 2010;22(2):207–12.
57. Siciliano M, Parlati L, Maldarelli F, et al. Liver transplantation in adults: choosing the appropriate timing. World J Gastrointest Pharmacol Ther. 2012;3(4):49–61.
58. Wan SZ, Nie Y, Zhang Y, Liu C, Zhu X. Assessing the prognostic performance of the child-Pugh, model for end-stage liver disease, and albumin-bilirubin scores in patients with decompensated cirrhosis: a large Asian cohort from gastroenterology department. Dis Markers. 2020;2020:5193028. https://doi.org/10.1155/2020/5193028. Retraction in: Dis Markers. 2023 Jul 12;2023:9831059.
59. Biggins SW, Kim WR, Terrault NA, et al. Evidence-based incorporation of serum sodium concentration into MELD. Gastroenterology. 2006;130(6):1652–60.
60. Huo TI, Wu JC, Lin HC, Lee FY, Hou MC, Lee PC, et al. Evaluation of the increase in model for end-stage liver disease (DeltaMELD) score over time as a prognostic predictor in patients with advanced cirrhosis: risk factor analysis and comparison with initial MELD and Child-Turcotte-Pugh score. J Hepatol. 2005;42:826–32.
61. Freeman RB Jr, Gish RG, Harper A, Davis GL, Vierling J, Lieblein L, et al. Model for end-stage liver disease (MELD) exception guidelines: results and recommendations from the MELD Exception Study Group and Conference (MESSAGE) for the approval of patients who need liver transplantation with diseases not considered by the standard MELD formula. Liver Transpl. 2006;12:S128–36.
62. Jothimani D, Marannan NK, Karan J, Aswin K, Mohamed R. Cardiac evaluation in liver transplant candidates. J Clin Exp Hepatol. 2025;15(5):102554.
63. Puri P, Malik S. Liver transplantation: contraindication and ineligibility. J Clin Exp Hepatol. 2023;13(6):1116–29.
64. Mazzaferro V, Regalia E, Doci R, et al. Liver transplantation for the treatment of small hepatocellular carcinomas in patients with cirrhosis. N Engl J Med. 1996;334(11):693–9.
65. Mazzola A, Costantino A, Petta S, Bartolotta TV, Raineri M, Sacco R, Brancatelli G, Cammà C, Cabibbo G. Recurrence of hepatocellular carcinoma after liver transplantation: an update. Future Oncol. 2015;11(21):2923–36. https://doi.org/10.2217/fon.15.239. Epub 2015 Sep 28.
66. Silva MF, Sherman M. Criteria for liver transplantation for HCC: what should the limits be? J Hepatol. 2011;55(5):1137–47. https://doi.org/10.1016/j.jhep.2011.05.012. Epub 2011 Jun 27.
67. Yao FY, Xiao L, Bass NM, Kerlan R, Ascher NL, Roberts JP. Liver transplantation for hepatocellular carcinoma: validation of the UCSF-expanded criteria based on preoperative imaging. Am J Transplant. 2007;7(11):2587–96.
68. Mazzaferro V, Sposito C, Zhou J, Pinna AD, De Carlis L, Fan J, Cescon M, Di Sandro S, Yi-Feng H, Lauterio A, Bongini M, Cucchetti A. Metroticket 2.0 model for analysis of competing risks of death after liver transplantation for hepatocellular carcinoma. Gastroenterology. 2018;154(1):128–39.
69. Reig M, Forner A, Rimola J, et al. BCLC strategy for prognosis prediction and treatment recommendation: the 2022 update. J Hepatol. 2022;76(3):681–93.
70. Kumar A, Acharya SK, Singh SP, et al. 2023 update of Indian national association for study of the liver consensus on management of intermediate and advanced hepatocellular carcinoma: the Puri III recommendations. J Clin Exp Hepatol. 2024;14(1):101269.
71. She WH, Chan ACY, Cheung TT, Lo CM, Chok KSH. Survival outcomes of liver transplantation for hepatocellular carcinoma in patients with normal, high and very high preoperative alpha-fetoprotein levels. World J Hepatol. 2018;10(2):308–18.

72. Sung H, Ferlay J, Siegel RL, et al. Global cancer statistics 2020: GLOBOCAN estimates of incidence and mortality worldwide for 36 cancers in 185 countries. CA Cancer J Clin. 2021;71(3):209–49.
73. Scientific Registry of Transplant Recipients. Annual data report: liver [Internet]. OPTN/SRTR. Available from https://srtr.transplant.hrsa.gov/annual_reports/2017/Liver.aspx. Accessed 22 Feb 2024.
74. Adam R, Karam V, Delvart V, et al., All contributing centers (www.eltr.org), European Liver and Intestine Transplant Association (ELITA). Evolution of indications and results of liver transplantation in Europe. A report from the European Liver Transplant Registry (ELTR). J Hepatol. 2012;57(3):675–887.
75. Yao FY, Ferrell L, Bass NM, et al. Liver transplantation for hepatocellular carcinoma: expansion of the tumor size limits does not adversely impact survival. Hepatology. 2001;33(6):1394–403.
76. Toso C, Trotter J, Wei A, et al. Total tumor volume predicts risk of recurrence following liver transplantation in patients with hepatocellular carcinoma. Liver Transpl. 2008;14(8):1107–15.
77. Mazzaferro V, Llovet JM, Miceli R, et al, Metroticket Investigator Study Group. Predicting survival after liver transplantation in patients with hepatocellular carcinoma beyond the Milan criteria: a retrospective, exploratory analysis. Lancet Oncol. 2009;10(1):35–43.
78. Sugawara Y, Tamura S, Makuuchi M. Living donor liver transplantation for hepatocellular carcinoma: Tokyo University series. Dig Dis. 2007;25(4):310–2.
79. Kaido T, Ogawa K, Mori A, et al. Usefulness of the Kyoto criteria as expanded selection criteria for liver transplantation for hepatocellular carcinoma. Surgery. 2013;154(5):1053–60.
80. Lee SG, Hwang S, Moon DB, et al. Expanded indication criteria of living donor liver transplantation for hepatocellular carcinoma at one large-volume center. Liver Transpl. 2008;14(7):935–45.
81. Sapisochin G, Goldaracena N, Laurence JM, et al. The extended Toronto criteria for liver transplantation in patients with hepatocellular carcinoma: a prospective validation study. Hepatology. 2016;64(6):2077–88.
82. Zheng SS, Xu X, Wu J, et al. Liver transplantation for hepatocellular carcinoma: Hangzhou experiences. Transplantation. 2008;85(12):1726–32.
83. Toso C, Meeberg G, Hernandez-Alejandro R, et al. Total tumor volume and alpha-fetoprotein for selection of transplant candidates with hepatocellular carcinoma: a prospective validation. Hepatology. 2015;62(1):158–65.
84. Mazzaferro V, Sposito C, Zhou J, et al. Metroticket 2.0 model for analysis of competing risks of death after liver transplantation for hepatocellular carcinoma. Gastroenterology. 2018;154(1):128–39.
85. Gupte A, Shukla A. Liver Transplantation - what the physician should know? J Assoc Physicians India. 2016;64(12):60–9.
86. Francoz C, Nadim MK, Durand F. Kidney biomarkers in cirrhosis. J Hepatol. 2016;65(4):809–24.
87. Koch DG, Fallon MB. Hepatopulmonary syndrome. Clin Liver Dis. 2014;18(2):407–20.
88. Rodríguez-Roisin R, Krowka MJ, Hervé P, et al, ERS Task Force Pulmonary-Hepatic Vascular Disorders (PHD) Scientific Committee. Pulmonary-hepatic vascular disorders (PHD). Eur Respir J. 2004; 24(5):861–80.
89. Krowka MJ, Porayko MK, Plevak DJ, et al. Hepatopulmonary syndrome with progressive hypoxemia as an indication for liver transplantation: case reports and literature review. Mayo Clin Proc. 1997;72(1):44–53.
90. Arguedas MR, Abrams GA, Krowka MJ, Fallon MB. Prospective evaluation of outcomes and predictors of mortality in patients with hepatopulmonary syndrome undergoing liver transplantation. Hepatology. 2003;37(1):192–7.
91. Cartin-Ceba R, Krowka MJ. Portopulmonary hypertension. Clin Liver Dis. 2014;18(2):421–38.
92. Listik C, Machado-Porto GCL, de Oliveira MO, et al. Acquired hepatocerebral degeneration: a case report. Dement Neuropsychol. 2012;6(1):59–63.
93. Domingos JP, et al. The role of liver transplant in the treatment of acquired hepatocerebral degeneration and hepatic encephalopathy (abstract). J Neurol Sci. 2013;e65–e108:e78.

94. Eaton JE, Talwalkar JA, Lazaridis KN, et al. Pathogenesis of primary sclerosing cholangitis and advances in diagnosis and management. Gastroenterology. 2013;145(3):521–36.
95. Update National Liver Review Board Guidance Documents and Policy Clarification-OPTN. Available from: https://optn.transplant.hrsa.gov/policies-bylaws/public-comment/update-national-liver-review-board-guidance-documents-and-policy-clarification/. Accessed 22 Feb 2024.
96. Akamatsu N, Sugawara Y. Primary biliary cirrhosis and liver transplantation. Intractable Rare Dis Res. 2012;1(2):66–80.
97. Catana AM, Medici V. Liver transplantation for Wilson disease. World J Hepatol. 2012;4(1):5–10.

Chapter 3
Contraindications for Liver Transplantation

Dinesh Jothimani, Mithra Prasad, and Patrick S. Kamath

Abstract Liver transplantation (LT) is the only curative option for most patients with decompensated cirrhosis. Indications for LT have been fairly well established over the years, but are no clear-cut guidelines on contraindications. The dynamic nature of complications in patients with liver disease in a given time point may influence the decision for LT, depending on disease severity in the recipient and on the expertise in the liver unit. Associated metabolic and cardiovascular comorbidities may also influence candidacy for liver transplantation in patients with Metabolic associated steatotic liver disease (MASH) cirrhosis. Likewise, duration of alcohol abstinence and severity of alcohol-related liver disease influence timing of liver transplantation. Severity of portopulmonary hypertension may be a contraindication for LT. Active sepsis and untreated acquired immunodeficiency syndrome are absolute contraindications for LT. Sarcopenia and frailty should be improved as much as possible, prior to the surgery. Acute-on-chronic liver failure (ACLF) is an increasing indication for LT. Patients with ACLF-3 should preferably be treated and the disease severity downgraded before being considered for LT. Despite expanding criteria for LT in hepatocellular carcinoma, patients with macrovascular invasion and extrahepatic disease are contraindicated from LT.

A multidisciplinary team approach should be carried out in the decision for LT. If contraindicated, and in case of relative contraindication, the reason should be clearly

D. Jothimani (✉)
Institute of Liver Disease and Transplantation, Dr Rela Institute and Medical Centre, Chennai, Tamil Nadu, India
e-mail: dinesh.jothimani@relainstitute.com

M. Prasad
VGM Hospital, Coimbatore, India

P. S. Kamath
Division of Gastroenterology and Hepatology, Mayo Clinic College of Medicine and Science, Rochester, MN, USA

S. Saigal, D. Jothimani (eds.), *Fundamentals of Transplant Hepatology*, https://doi.org/10.1007/978-981-95-2624-6_3

documented. Revisiting the case at a later date with discussion between the patient and their family members and members of the transplant team is encouraged.

Keywords Liver transplantation · Contraindication · Comorbidities

Key Highlights

Contraindications for liver transplantation can be absolute or relative.

Absolute contraindications for liver transplantation include severe cardiac or pulmonary disease, active sepsis, extra-hepatic malignancies, persistent substance abuse, untreated psychiatric conditions, irreversible neurological disease, severe systemic disease and lack of psychosocial support.

Relative contraindications are temporary, and decision to transplant requires multidisciplinary team approach and a detailed discussion with patient and their family members.

3.1 Introduction

Liver transplantation (LT) remains the most viable therapeutic option for patients with decompensated cirrhosis. With the increase in overall patient and graft survival, this procedure is increasingly carried out across several centres worldwide. Timing of LT in patients remains crucial for optimal clinical outcomes and is influenced by multiple clinical factors including comorbidities, some of which may be contraindications to LT. A multidisciplinary holistic approach involving hepatologists, liver surgeons, anaesthetists and allied specialists should be involved in meticulous planning and complex decisions in selecting patients for LT.

In the last decade, two major changes have been observed in the epidemiology of patients with chronic liver disease. Availability of high-efficacy antiviral drugs has improved the incidence and reduced the prevalence of chronic viral hepatitis. Introduction of directly acting antiviral drugs (DAA) in 2013 has significantly reduced the prevalence of hepatitis C infection; likewise, availability of the antiviral agents, entecavir and tenofovir, has greatly reduced the complications of chronic hepatitis B infection. On the contrary, there has been a dramatic increase in prevalence of alcohol-related and MASH-related cirrhosis. Alcohol remains the most common indication for LT across Europe [1]. With global increase in metabolic syndrome, obesity and diabetes, patients with MASH cirrhosis contribute significantly to chronic liver disease burden. This is clearly reflected in the increasing numbers of patients being selected for LT. MASH is the leading indication for LT in India surpassing viral hepatitis and increasing between 2009 and 2019 from 30.7% to 42% ($P = 0.001$) [2]. Patients with MASH-related end-stage liver disease (ESLD) have associated comorbidities which may influence the decision for LT. In patients with alcohol-related liver disease cirrhosis, 6 months abstinence policy was mandatory across several countries prior to consideration for LT. However, this policy has been challenged recently in several countries, particularly with increasing recognition of acute-on-chronic liver failure (ACLF) and more recently, alcohol-related hepatitis (AH) as indications for LT. Contraindications for liver transplantation are described according to the organ system.

3.2 Liver Related Contraindications

3.2.1 Acute Liver Failure (ALF)

Contraindication for LT in ALF is related to the potential for neurologic irreversibility despite liver transplantation. Acute liver failure with a sustained intracranial pressure >50 mmHg or a cerebral perfusion pressure <40 mmHg is a contraindication. Manifestations include severe brainstem dysfunction and, in particular, bilateral fixed and dilated pupils. Active sepsis, progressive escalation of inotropic requirements and acute pancreatitis are additional contraindications [3].

3.2.2 Acute on Chronic Liver Failure (ACLF)

Patients with acute on chronic liver failure (ACLF) are potential candidates for liver transplantation, and decisions regarding transplantation in these patients have to be made rapidly given their high risk of 28-day mortality. ACLF is characterised by extrahepatic organ dysfunction, at least in 40% of patients [4], with increasing risk of extrahepatic organ failure as disease severity increases. Most patients with ACLF have alcohol-related hepatitis with reactivation hepatitis B, drug-induced liver injury in patients with underlying metabolic associated steatotic liver disease (MASLD) and Wilson disease being some of the other causes. Since ACLF is associated with extrahepatic organ failure, the number and severity of extrahepatic organ failures determine whether patients should be excluded from transplantation or not. Acute kidney injury (AKI) is the most common organ failure in patients with ACLF [5] but is not a contraindication to liver transplantation. Active sepsis as a result of cholangitis or liver abscesses is not a contraindication to LT, but extrahepatic source of sepsis, especially if associated with the need of increasing pressor support is a contraindication. Similarly, requirement of ventilation for airway protection in patients with hepatic encephalopathy is not a contraindication, but not acute respiratory distress syndrome (ARDS).

APASL ACLF research consortium (AARC) prognostic model was derived using bilirubin, creatinine, international normalized ratio (INR), lactate and hepatic encephalopathy, and was found to predict 28-day mortality (AUROC 0.80) in patients with ACLF.

ACLF progressing with limited no response beyond a week may not be an ideal candidate for liver transplantation. AARC score study revealed that patients with a score 10 on admission had a survival of 89%, whereas at day 7 and 13, the survival was 54% and 45%, respectively, indicating rapid course after the first week of illness in ACLF patients. Extrapolation of this data suggests that the golden period for liver transplantation is probably a narrow window between the first and second week of presentation.

3.2.2.1 ACLF Grade 3

Grade 3 ACLF is defined by three or more organ failures with a 28-day mortality of 80%. In a study from United Network for Organ Sharing (UNOS) database among 5355 patients transplanted based on their model for end stage liver disease (MELD) score who on retrospective review had ACLF grade 3, the 1-year post-transplant survival was 81.8%, statistically poorer than other patient groups (88–91%, $P < 0.001$). Comparative analysis of ACLF grade 3 post-transplant survivors versus nonsurvivors showed that survivors were younger (51.7 vs. 52.9 years), required less mechanical ventilation pretransplant (33.1% vs. 49%, $P < 0.001$) and had less circulatory failure (49.8% vs. 60.6%, $P < 0.001$), higher coagulation failure (65.6% vs. 54.5%, $P < 0.001$) and lower four or more organ failure (42.3% vs. 50.3%, $P < 0.001$). Most important determinant of 1-year survival in ACLF grade 3 in a cox proportional hazard analysis was pretransplant mechanical ventilation (85.4% vs. 75.3%, HR 1.49, 95%CI: 1.22–1.49), predominantly related to respiratory failure. In addition, suboptimal donor (HR1.22, 95% CI 1.09–1.35) and duration on the transplant wait-list >30 days were associated with worse survival [6]. Patients on ventilatory support due to respiratory failure, particularly with PaO_2/FiO_2 <150, may be associated with poor survival following LT. Whereas ventilated ACLF-3 patients may not be ideal for liver transplantation; patients with improvement in ACLF grades following treatment may be considered for LT.

3.2.3 Risk Scores in Liver Transplantation

3.2.3.1 Model for End-Stage Liver Disease (MELD)

Patients are considered candidates for liver transplantation when they have liver disease severity to the extent that it impacts both quantity of life as well as quality of life. The MELD score and its iterations MELD-Na and MELD 3.0 accurately stratify patients at risk for 3-month mortality, thus identifying the ‘sickest’ patients among those listed for liver transplantation. Patients with a MELD score ≥15 have a transplant survival benefit, that is the likelihood of survival with liver transplantation at 1 year being higher with a liver transplant than without a liver transplant. With increasing MELD score, the transplant benefit increases, but at a risk of higher costs and morbidity is capped at 40 for maximal transplant benefit. It is uncertain what the upper limit of MELD score that is associated with transplant benefit is as in the liver allocation systems, the MELD score is capped at 40 [7]. That is, there is no upper limit of MELD score that can currently be used to define futility. Critical to determining transplant futility are donor characteristics and transplant centre experience.

3.2.3.2 Balance of Risk (BAR) Score

Multiple scores based on pretransplant variables have been identified to predict 3-month post-transplant mortality. Balance of risk (BAR) score was derived from 37,255 UNOS database patients using recipient and donor-derived variables: recipient age, MELD score, life-support and retransplantation, donor age and cold ischemic time (CIT). Predictability of 3-month mortality was 0.71 (c-statistic) [8] which is not high enough to make clinical decision regarding selection of patients for liver transplantation. European studies have compared various scores such as donor risk indices (DRI) and D-MELD on 4033 patients. A BAR score >18 was significantly associated with 3-month mortality [9] in high MELD (>30) patients.

3.2.3.3 Futility Risk Score

In a large Scientific Registry of Transplant Recipients database, analysis between 2002 and 2015 of liver transplant recipients to assess futility of the procedure was carried out. A multivariate analysis revealed that the presence of ventilatory support (HR 1.59 95% CI 1.47–1.72), recipient age >60 (HR 1.29 95% CI 1.23–1.36), haemodialysis (HR1.26 95% CI 1.16–1.37), diabetes (HR 1.20 95% CI 1.14–1.27) or creatinine ≥1/5 mg/dl (HR 1.15 95% CI 1.09–1.22) were the factors associated with liver allograft failure. These high-risk patients coupled with suboptimal donor led to poor 5-year patient and graft survival, irrespective of MELD score. Although not absolute contraindication, optimising such high-risk patients prior to liver transplantation may be advisable [10].

Given the difficulty in predicting post-transplant outcome based on risk scores alone, selection of patients for liver transplantation is as much art as science, taking into consideration factors such as sarcopenia, fragility, degree of portal hypertension (HT), previous abdominal surgery, donor risk indices, as well as transplant centre experience.

There are absolute and relative contraindications to liver transplantation. With increasing experience over the years, the absolute contraindications for LT have decreased significantly. Indeed, previously contraindications such as portopulmonary hypertension (PoPH) are now even considered possible indications for LT. In this chapter, we discuss contraindications for LT according to disease aetiology, severity of liver disease, complications of cirrhosis and comorbidities. In general, any comorbidity that cannot be corrected and is a prohibitive risk for surgery would be considered an absolute contraindication to liver transplantation.

3.2.4 Priority on Waitlist

Currently, in patients undergoing LT for ACLF, there are no specific formally accepted guidelines on 'prioritising' these patients. Most transplant centres prioritise them on case-to-case basis internally. Majority of these transplants are in the deceased donor setting. Living donor liver transplantation (LDLT) is commonly practised modality in Asia. LDLT may be a better option in ACLF patients because of uncertainties in the timing and narrow therapeutic window of opportunity. Studies have shown similar survival rates between deceased donor liver transplantation (DDLT) and LDLT in ACLF patients [11].

3.2.5 *Portal Vein Thrombosis (PVT)*

PVT occurs in 10–25% of patients, with higher prevalence in Child Pugh C disease [12]. Isolated portal vein thrombosis can be resolved at the time of liver transplantation and hence is not a contraindication for the surgery. However, complete porto-mesentric thrombosis with bowel compromise may be a surgical contraindication for LT even if a suitable collateral vessel is available for anastomosis to the donor portal vein.

3.2.6 *Malignant Tumours of the Liver*

When tumour is restricted to the liver, contraindications are related to the type of malignancy. Hepatocellular carcinoma (HCC) beyond Milan or UCSF criteria may be a contraindication; however, such patients may be considered candidates following downsizing of the tumour burden with loco-regional therapy. Criteria for transplant for cholangiocarcinoma are also defined in patients who are otherwise reasonable candidates for liver transplant. Contraindications include patients who have attempted prior resection with violation of tumour plane or have evidence of extrahepatic disease including positive lymph nodes. Vascular invasion is a contraindication for a transplant, although vascular encasement is not an exclusion criterion. When a mass is visible on imaging for patients with cholangiocarcinoma, the mass should be less than or equal to 3 cm in the radial diameter. In general, 'intrahepatic' cholangiocarcinoma is a contraindication, although the field is evolving. Liver failure due to diffuse infiltrative malignancy or lymphoma, even if the sole organ involved is the liver, is a contraindication for transplantation.

3.2.6.1 Hepatocellular Carcinoma (HCC)

Milan criteria are the gold standard in selecting patients for liver transplantation. Considering the 'too restrictive' nature of Milan criteria, there have been efforts at expanding criteria. Using UCSF criteria to select patients for liver transplantation is associated with an expected 5-year overall survival of 75%. Indeed, a total tumour volume of <115 cm^3 may be a better determinant of overall survival than Milan and UCSF (91%, 69% and 75%, $P < 0.001$). Thus, the upper limit of tumour diameter is not clearly established. In summary, HCC exceeding UCSF criteria would be a contraindication to transplantation in the absence of downsizing.

Rapidly increasing tumour size is likely associated with vascular invasion and poor differentiation. These features are relative contraindications for LT. Metastatic HCC is an absolute contraindication for LT. Studies that evaluated tumour size were retrospective, based on the explant, and highlighted the discordance between pathology and pretransplant radiology. With increasing 5-year post-transplant survival over 75%, expected survival that may be lower than this in the context of HCC should be considered as a relative contraindication for liver transplantation according to Indian National Association for the Study of the Liver guidelines [13].

Apart from metastatic disease, presence of radiological evidence of macrovascular invasion is associated with reduced post-transplant survival, due to higher rates of recurrence. Pathologically, in addition to tumour size and histological differentiation, microvascular invasion predicts HCC recurrence. Radiologically, presence of macrovascular invasion with involvement of main but not branched portal vein is a contraindication for LT.

Locoregional therapies have been used to downgrade the tumour size and activity, with tumour downstaging defined by a decrease in tumour diameter. A lack of response to downstaging modalities and reoccurrence of new lesions within 3 months of downstaging are contraindications for liver transplantation at present [14, 15].

3.3 Comorbidities

3.3.1 Age

The global increase in the overall age of the population has been associated with older patients being considered for liver transplantation. There is no fixed upper limit of biological age for liver transplantation, and selected patients ≥70 years of age have done well post-transplantation. Kurian et al. studied 20 elderly (age ≥70 years) liver transplant recipients: 1-year patient survival was 90.9% compared to 94.7% in the younger (<70 years) cohort ($P = 0.88$). There were no differences in complication rates. Interestingly, 67% of elderly patients referred for transplantation were declined due to comorbidities, and not due to age alone [16].

3.3.2 Obesity

Obesity and metabolic syndrome are growing epidemic worldwide and may complicate liver transplantation, but obesity is not an absolute contraindication to liver transplantation. Earlier studies revealed considerable differential clinical outcomes of obese patients undergoing liver transplantation. A study from 2002 comparing obese and nonobese patients revealed morbid obesity was associated with significantly higher primary graft function, and mortality 1 month and 1 year following liver transplantation. Patients with BMI >35 had higher 5-year mortality related to cardiovascular (CV) events [17]. In a study from UK, higher rates of septic complications (65.5%, $P < 0.01$) and longer hospital stay were noted in obese recipients without a difference in mortality [18]. Despite obesity and related comorbidities, survival benefit of liver transplantation was significantly ($P < 0.0001$) higher than waitlisted patients [19]. Additional procedures may be considered at the time of LT. Combining liver transplantation with sleeve gastrectomy resulted in effective weight loss and was associated with fewer post-LT metabolic complications in the DDLT setting [20]. Although not a contraindication, obese patients undergoing LDLT may pose a challenge due to the possibility of potential lower graft recipient weight ratio (GRWR).

3.3.3 Diabetes Mellitus (DM)

Diabetes mellitus is a common comorbidity in patients undergoing LT. Presence of DM increases cardiovascular risk and mortality post-transplant. A prospective study demonstrated the poor correlation of HbA1c and blood glucose in cirrhotics [21] (Bhattacharjee 2019 Diabetes). Thus, the level of glycemic control as a contraindication for LT is not established. In general, diabetes mellitus is not a contraindication to liver transplantation but the assistance of an endocrinologist to control the diabetes is recommended, especially in the immediate post-transplant when higher dose of steroids is being used.

3.4 Kidney related contraindications

3.4.1 Acute Kidney Injury (AKI)

AKI is the most common extrahepatic organ dysfunction in patients with end-stage liver disease. It is not uncommon for patients to undergo LT with some degree of renal impairment. Most patients recover renal function following liver transplantation with no long-term renal consequences. However, the cutoff level of creatinine or the degree of renal impairment is not established in deselecting patients for LT alone. Contraindications for LT from renal point of view remains fairly centre dependent. In a recent study with limited number of patients ($n = 62$), 40% 90-day mortality was observed in stage 3 ($n = 10$) AKI-hepatorenal syndrome (increase in serum creatinine > threefold from baseline, or Cr >4 mg/dl with an acute increase ≥0.3 mg/dl or initiation of continuous renal replacement therapy (CRRT)) patients [22]. In a study from UNOS database, 68% of patients on RRT initiated for AKI RRT, showed a complete renal recovery following liver transplant [23] (Northup 2010 Liver Transplantation). In chronic kidney disease patients, combined liver-kidney transplantation is necessary where reversibility is uncertain, when eGFR <30 ml/min and when patient has sustained an AKI necessitating haemodialysis in past 6 weeks. In summary, there is no actuarial renal contraindications for LT, and as per prevailing national policies, selected patients may require a simultaneous liver and kidney transplant, or a sequential kidney transplantation.

3.5 Cardiovascular Contraindications

With increase in MASH, selecting patients for liver transplantation who have coronary artery disease (CAD) can be challenging. Patients with severe CAD not amenable to revascularisation is a contraindication for Liver transplantation including patients with CAD and triple vessel disease, diffuse left anterior descending disease and heart failure with EF <40%. Patients with triple vessel disease with myocardial perfusion defect may have to undergo coronary artery bypass graft (CABG) surgery prior to, or uncommonly during liver transplantation. Combined liver transplantation and cardiac surgery procedures should be carried out only at centres with considerable expertise in both liver transplantation as well as coronary artery bypass graft surgery.

Nonobstructive coronary artery lesions and obstructive lesions that are treatable with intervention are not contraindication to liver transplantation.

3.5.1 Cardiovascular Risk in Orthotopic Liver Transplantation (CAR-OLT) Score

A risk score was developed based on 1024 consecutive patients who underwent assessment for LT and was developed using recipient age, sex, employment status, education, DM, HT, heart failure, atrial fibrillation (AF), pulmonary HT, respiratory failure and HCC. The score was developed to predict major cardiovascular complications defined as death from CV complications or hospitalization for a major CV event. The risk model scores range from <9 to >40. Scores of 10, 20, 30 and >40 predict absolute cardiovascular risk of 6%, 14%, 26% and 45%, respectively. A score >30 is considered high risk for cardiovascular mortality [24] and is an absolute contraindication to liver transplantation.

3.5.2 CAD-LT Score

A score to predict significant CAD (defined as CAD requiring percutaneous or surgical intervention) was developed by retrospective analysis of 1771 patients from a single centre in USA. The risk-adjusted predictors of significant CAD by multivariate analysis were older age (adjusted OR 1.05), male sex (1.69), diabetes (1.57), hypertension (1.61), tobacco use (1.01), family history (1.63) and personal history of CAD (6.55). The score termed ‘CAD LT score’ stratified the risk of significant

CAD as low (≤2%), intermediate (3–9%) and high (≥10%). The authors suggested an algorithm based on the above risks which would have identified 97% of all significant CAD and avoided unnecessary testing [25]. The study being retrospective and from a single centre in the West needs to be cautiously applied for Asian population.

3.5.3 *Cirrhotic Cardiomyopathy (CCM)*

CCM represents stiff ventricles with blunted response to stress, occurs in at least 40% patients with end-stage liver disease, irrespective of disease aetiology [26]. Hyperdynamic circulation associated with cirrhosis causes increased cardiac output, impaired diastolic response and prolongation of QT, indicative of defective ventricular depolarisation and repolarisation. As per the 2019 CCM consortium criteria, systolic dysfunction criteria involve any of LVEF ≤50% or absolute global longitudinal strain <18% or >22%. Advanced diastolic dysfunction with any 3 or more of the following: Septal e' velocity <7 cm/second, E/e' ratio ≥15, left ventricle (LV) volume index >34 mL/m^2 and tricuspid regurgitation (TR) velocity >2.8 m/s.
CCM may precipitate cardiac arrhythmias. Alterations in the cardiac haemodynamics following portal perfusion lead to increased LV filling during liver transplant surgery and this may precipitate heart failure in patients with CCM. Since liver transplantation reverses CCM, this entity is not a contraindication to LT.

3.5.4 *Cardiac Arrhythmias*

Atrial fibrillation is the most common arrhythmia reported in 10% of decompensated cirrhosis patients [27]. Pre-existent AF increases cardiovascular complications (OR 5.15, 95% CI 2.67–9.92) in the postoperative period. Similarly, new onset AF increases mortality (OR 2.34; 95%CI 1.10–5.0) in LT recipients [28]. Controlled AF and supraventricular tachycardia (SVT) are not contraindications for LT.

3.5.5 *Valvular Heart Disease (VHD)*

Presence of VHD may influence outcomes of noncardiac surgeries. Patients with structural VHD may develop perioperative cardiac dysfunction during noncardiac surgery. Severity of VHD, presence of myocardial damage and functional impairment of ventricles determine cardiac risk. With reduced prevalence of VHD, data in patients undergoing LT is limited.

3.5.5.1 Aortic Stenosis (AS)

Mild or moderate AS with no compromise in LV function can be considered for LT. However, severe or symptomatic aortic stenosis precludes liver transplantation due to severe haemodynamic instability and critically reduced myocardial perfusion.

Severe aortic stenosis increases the 10% risk of perioperative mortality and myocardial infarction following noncardiac surgery [29]. Moreover, intraoperative management of severe aortic stenosis is further difficult in the presence of low systemic vascular resistance and cardiomyopathy in cirrhosis and during acute decrease in venous return with cross-clamping of IVC.

Patients with severe AS (Valve area $\leq$1 cm^2 or jet velocity of >4 m/s), reduced left ventricular systolic function and symptomatic AS of moderate severity should undergo either surgical treatment or transcatheter aortic valve replacement (TAVR) prior to liver transplantation [30]. Postoperative mortality following open surgical AVR ranged from 17% to 26% in patients with cirrhosis, and the risk rises to 67% and low 1-year survival of 16% in Child C cirrhosis [31].

Recent data demonstrates comparable in-hospital (1.8% vs. 2%) and 30-day mortality (3.2% vs. 4.6%) among patients with cirrhosis undergoing surgical aortic valve repair (SAVR) and transcatheter aortic valve replacement (TAVR), respectively. However, in those with a MELD score less than 12, outcomes were superior with SAVR [32]. Valvular surgery prior to liver transplantation can be a viable option, and MELD score may help direct the treatment approach.
A meta-analysis of TAVR in chronic liver disease revealed a significant decrease in in-hospital mortality (OR 0.43) compared to SAVR. A propensity matched analysis showed that TAVR has similar mortality and 30-day readmission rates but shorter hospital stay [31]. However, TAVR requires dual antiplatelet therapy for a stipulated time thereby delaying LT. Valve replacement, preferably TAVR, followed by LT sequentially is a preferred modality in advanced liver disease. Aortic valvuloplasty as a bridge to LT has success rate from 26% to 74%. About 40% of the patients could avoid valve replacement surgery for 2 years [33].

3.5.5.2 Aortic Regurgitation

Severity of aortic regurgitation (AR) is measured by comparing the width of the LV outflow tract to the width of the AR jet across the valve. Severe AR is defined by the jet >2/3 of the LV outflow tract. These patients require valve replacement prior to LT. Unfortunately, patients with decompensated cirrhosis may not be suitable for the cardiac surgery.

3.5.5.3 Mitral Stenosis (MS)

Patients with symptomatic moderate MS with secondary pulmonary artery pressure (PASP >50 mmHg) or severe MS (valve area <1 cm^2 and mean valve gradient >10 mm Hg) require valvotomy or valve replacement, in case of unfavourable valve anatomy. Although, the data on patients undergoing liver transplantation is unavailable, aforementioned criteria can be extrapolated for these patients.

3.5.5.4 Mitral Regurgitation (MR)

MR severity is assessed by regurgitant orifice >0.40 cm^2, volume >60 mls, regurgitant fraction >50%, jet reaching posterior wall of LA and dilated left atrium (LV). However, these patients may not be suitable for noncardiac surgery, in particular liver transplantation [30].

MV repair or replacement is indicated in those with LVEF >30%. Patients with severe MR require edge-to-edge mitral repair prior to LT as they may not tolerate open surgery [31].

3.5.5.5 Tricuspid Regurgitation

Severe TR is a contraindication for LT, due to potential allograft congestion and high rates of failure. Patients with severe TR require valve repair, preferably minimally invasive, before the onset of severe right ventricle dysfunction.

3.5.6 Portopulmonary Hypertension

Portopulmonary hypertension (PoPH) occurs in 8.5% patients with end-stage liver disease; a mean pulmonary artery pressure (PAP) >35 mmHg and pulmonary vascular resistance (PVR) >250 dynes were associated with 36% perioperative mortality. However, with evolution of effective vasodilator therapy, medical management of PoPH can be implemented to reduce pulmonary arterial pressure. However, mPAP >45 mmHg or between 35 and 45 mm Hg with PVR <240 dyns.s.cm^{-5} (>3 Wood units) despite vasodilator therapy is an absolute contraindication for liver transplantation [34].

3.6 Pulmonary Contraindications

3.6.1 Interstitial Lung Disease (ILD)

Interstitial lung disease is a progressive fibrotic condition involving inter-alveolar tissue, resulting in reduced total lung capacity and forced vital capacity (functional lung volume (FVC)) with FEV1/FVC >70%. ILD rarely encountered in patients with chronic liver disease. Most patients with ESLD have reduced exercise tolerance due to liver disease and hence may not manifest ILD symptoms.

Most cases are identified during the evaluation for liver transplantation. Ley et al. developed gender, age and physiology (GAP) indices to evaluate the disease severity based on gender, age and lung physiology (FVD and Diffusing capacity of the lung for carbon monoxide (DLCo)). Those with score 4–5 have 1-year and 3-year mortality of 16.2% and 42.1% and with score 6–8 have 39.2% and 76.8% compared to score 0–3, where 1- and 3-year mortality was 5.6% and 16.3%. This extrapolates those with score 4 and above may be a high-risk candidate for liver transplantation.

3.6.2 Hepatopulmonary Syndrome (HPS)

HPS is an excellent indication for liver transplantation. However, the severity of HPS may vary depending on the degree of hypoxemia. Pretransplant hypoxemia influences post-transplant survival. Severe hypoxemia (PaO_2 <50 mmHg) was once considered an absolute contraindication for LT, studies showed higher mortality in HPS patients with PaO_2 <37 mmHg [35, 36]. Liver disease severity has no correlation with the severity of HPS. With improved ICU care, subsequent studies found that the severity of hypoxemia was associated with prolonged postoperative recovery but not mortality [37, 38]. As of now, there is no established degree of hypoxemia which is considered a contraindication to liver transplantation.

3.7 Neurological contraindications

Irreversible neurologic dysfunction or developmental defects preclude a transplantation in most individuals. However, certain conditions may improve following LT such as in some patients with Nieman pick's and neuro-Wilson disease.

Patients with new onset cerebrovascular event should wait for 4 weeks at least prior to LT. These patients should undergo investigations for thromboembolic event including carotid doppler for further stroke risk assessment.

3.7.1 Subdural Hematoma (SDH)

A large retrospective study from Taiwan reported SDH incidence 29.3 per 10,000 person-years compared to 10.9 per 10,000 person-years in patients with no cirrhosis. Patients with decompensated cirrhosis had a hazard ratio of 5.07 (95%CI 3.38–7.60) [39]. Chronic stable SDH is not a contraindication for LT. However, blood perioperative pressures should be maintained. Fluctuations in blood pressure may worsen intracranial bleed. Patients may require brain imaging (CT) in the post-operative period or in the presence of clinical symptoms.

3.7.2 Intracerebral Haemorrhage

Hypertension-related intracerebral bleed is not an absolute contraindication for LT. Transplant should be reconsidered once the acute episode subside. These patients should be evaluated in detail to identify the source of bleed.

3.8 Infection related contraindications

3.8.1 Sepsis

Active sepsis is a clear contraindication for LT. Timing of LT following sepsis may determine post-transplant outcomes. In a prospective study, Levesque et al. studied cirrhotic patients admitted to the ICU. From 2005 to 2009, 377 patients were admitted to the liver ICU with a mean MELD score of 24.9 (±10.8). Sepsis was observed in 44.8% of patients related to pneumonia (51%) followed by spontaneous bacterial peritonitis (21%). Sepsis was an independent predictor of ICU mortality (OR 3.51, 95%CI 1.35–9.15, $P = 0.01$). In addition, presence of infection was associated with poor 2-month survival (32% vs. 80.8%, $P < 0.001$) [40]. Among these critically ill cirrhotic patients, liver transplantation within a month of septic shock was associated with 2.4 times higher mortality in the postoperative period [41]. Petrowsky et al. showed a higher mortality in liver transplant patients with preop sepsis [42].

In general, presence of asymptomatic bacteriuria or candida in the urine is not contraindications for LT. Similarly, presence of urinary tract infection with negative blood cultures can be covered with perioperative antibiotics. Patients with SBP can be transplanted after 5 days of antibiotics; those with pneumonia requires a prolonged course of antibiotics with complete clinical resolution prior to LT. Similarly, blood stream infections, both bacteria and fungus, require longer course therapy with complete resolution.

3.8.2 Multidrug-Resistant (MDR) Bacteria

Infection with MDR bacteria is associated with poor clinical outcome. In a study by Eurotransplant, 9.26% patients were found to have MDR bacterial colonisation and post-transplant infection-related mortality was significantly higher in MDR colonised patients ($P < 0.001$) [43]. Timing of liver transplantation following MDR bacterial infection requires further clarity.

Active Mycobacterial tuberculosis infection is a relative contraindication for liver transplantation. LT is contraindicated with active viral infections such as influenza or COVID-19 [44]. Procedure should be postponed for a week or until recovery.

In summary, patients with active sepsis are a contraindication for LT. Following resolution, these patients deteriorate rapidly and LT should be considered in this critically ill cirrhotics. However, sepsis secondary to liver abscesses or cholangitis would not be considered a contraindication to liver transplantation as the risk of these infections is essentially removed following liver transplantation.

3.8.3 Sepsis (Including Fungal) and ACLF

Sepsis occurs in 30% of patients with ACLF as a precipitating factor. Active sepsis is an absolute contraindication for liver transplantation. Timing of liver transplantation is not established in ACLF patients with sepsis. Control of active sepsis with improvements in clinical and inflammatory markers may be a guide for the timing of liver transplantation, but this warrants further studies.

A European multicentre study found fungal infection in 2% of patients with ACLF, with associated higher mortality (78%) [45]. Timing of LT in patients following fungal sepsis is not established.

3.8.4 HIV/AIDS

In the past, HIV was considered an absolute contraindication for liver transplantation. With the advent of higher efficacy drugs, 1-year survival of liver transplant recipients with HIV was 79% which subsequently improved to 89% [46]. British Transplant Society issued a guideline in 2005 that liver transplantation in HIV patients can be safely carried out if CD >200 cells/ul or 100 cells/ul in the presence of portal hypertension, HIV RNA <50 copies/ml, no AIDS defining illness, absence of primary CNS lymphoma and the possibility of treatment in the post-transplant period [47]. These criteria, although arbitrary, are still valid. Thus, controlled HIV infection is no longer a contraindication for liver transplantation.

3.8.5 Viral Infections

Active viral infections such as Influenza, COVID-19, rhinovirus and adenovirus are contraindications for liver transplantation.

3.9 Sarcopenia and Frailty

Sarcopenia and frailty are associated with poor outcomes following liver transplantation in patients with decompensated cirrhosis. Data of sarcopenia in ACLF patients is scarce. In a study of 180 liver transplant waitlisted patients, sarcopenia was independently associated with the development of ACLF (OR 2.0, $p = 0.044$) [48]. The acceptable degree of sarcopenia, frailty and performance status in ACLF patients undergoing liver transplantation are not established. Large studies are required to clarify nutritional issues in these patients.

3.9.1 Sarcopenia

Sarcopenia, defined as loss of muscle mass, is an increasingly discussed yet an under-recognised complication of liver cirrhosis. Sarcopenia has been observed in 37.5% of patients with liver cirrhosis; 41.9% in men and 49.6% in alcohol-related liver cirrhosis. The degree of sarcopenia worsens with the increasing severity of liver disease, 28.7%, 37.9% and 46.7% in Child A, Child B and Child C cirrhosis, respectively. Presence of sarcopenia is associated with higher mortality (HR 2.61) in cirrhotic patients independent of MELD score [49]. Sarcopenia significantly influences survival with an inverse relationship before and after liver transplantation with impairment of quality of life.

Frailty is defined as the lack of functional physiological reserve to handle health issues. Up to 45% of patients with decompensated cirrhosis suffer from frailty related to muscle loss, encephalopathy, ascites and recurrent paracentesis. Frailty is an independent factor of poor prognosis in patients with decompensated cirrhosis [50].

In a study of 163 liver transplant recipients who underwent abdominal CT for other reasons, total psoas muscle area and density were measured. Total psoas muscle area was significantly ($P < 0.0001$, adjusted HR 0.27 per 1000 mm^2) associated with post-transplant mortality. HR increased from 0.07 to 6.65 with TPA ranging from 4.00 to 0.36 cm^2 [51]. Cutoff value of sarcopenia and associated frailty in patient selection for liver transplantation are not established.

Six-minute walk test as a performance marker have been tested and may be utilized in patient selection for LT. A 6-minute walk distance of less than 250 m is associated with poor outcome and may be taken as a cutoff to rule out liver transplantation. Various factors influence the test results and not specific to sarcopenia. Patients with extreme sarcopenia with Eastern cooperative oncology group (ECOG) performance status ≥ 3 are contraindications for LT.

3.10 Extra-Hepatic Malignancy

In general, active non-HCC malignancies are contraindications for liver transplantation.

Among patients who have been treated for cancer and are cancer free, the risk of cancer recurrence and worse outcome secondary to immunosuppression following transplantation must be weighed against the benefit the patient will receive from the transplant [52]. A minimum of 2 years between cancer treatment and transplant is recommended except for cancers with extremely low or zero risk of recurrence, such as ductal carcinoma in situ of the breast. For cancers at increased risk of recurrence, a wait time of 2–5 years or longer is advised.

3.10.1 Prostate Cancer

Diagnosis of prostate cancer is not a contraindication for liver transplantation. Presence of renal cell carcinoma at the time of liver transplantation is not a contraindication for the surgery provided an oncologic resection of the tumour carried out.

3.11 Psychosocial

Lack of family or social support: Presence of family and psychosocial support is a crucial element in patients undergoing liver transplantation. Lack of psychosocial support is a relative contraindication for LT.

Absolute (Fig. 3.1) and relative contraindications are illustrated in Tables 3.1 and 3.2, respectively.

3.12 Conclusion

Contraindication for liver transplantation can be absolute or relative. Organ-specific contraindications should be sought during the evaluation for liver transplantation.

Most contraindications are temporary and may require addressing prior to the surgery. The list of contraindications including absolute contraindications for liver transplantation has dwindled over the years. Careful patient selection is essential for successful clinical outcome. A multidisciplinary team approach is essential in the holistic management of these patients.

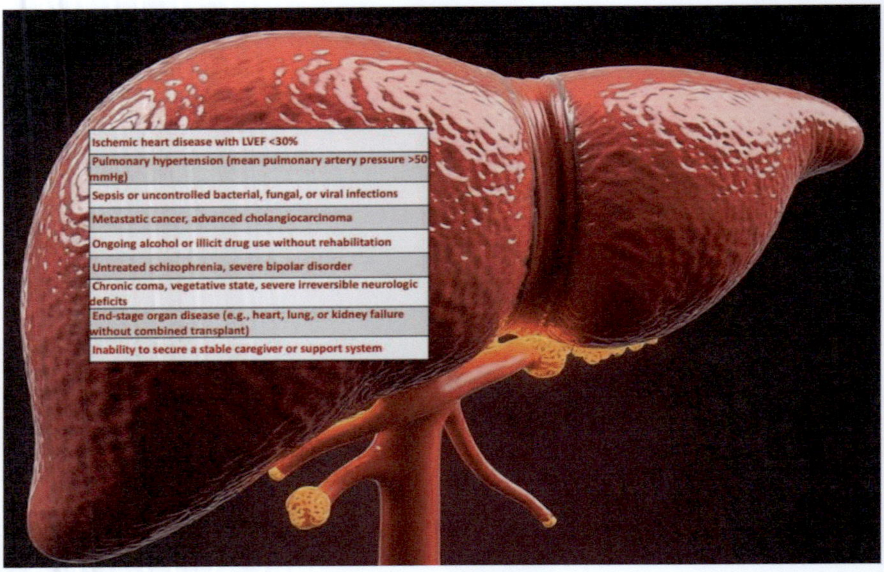

Fig. 3.1 Absolute contraindications for liver transplantation

Table 3.1 Absolute contraindications

Condition	
Severe cardiac or pulmonary disease	Ischemic heart disease with LVEF <30%
	Pulmonary hypertension (mean pulmonary artery pressure >50 mmHg)
Active systemic infection	Sepsis or uncontrolled bacterial, fungal or viral infections
Extrahepatic malignancies	Metastatic cancer and advanced cholangiocarcinoma
Persistent substance abuse	Ongoing alcohol or illicit drug use without rehabilitation
Untreated psychiatric conditions	Untreated schizophrenia and severe bipolar disorder
Irreversible neurologic disease	Chronic coma, vegetative state and severe irreversible neurologic deficits
Severe systemic disease	End-stage organ disease (e.g. heart, lung or kidney failure without combined transplant)
Lack of psychosocial support	Inability to secure a stable caregiver or support system

Table 3.2 Relative contraindications

Condition	
Age >70 years	Caution about coexistent comorbidities
Controlled systemic infections	Tuberculosis, cytomegalovirus or hepatitis B/C under control
Portal vein thrombosis	Complete or extensive thrombosis of the portal vein
Morbid obesity (BMI >40)	Increased surgical complications and graft dysfunction
Severe malnutrition	Muscle wasting and hypoalbuminemia
HIV infection	Active infection but controlled viral load
Recurrent substance use	History of uncontrolled alcohol/drug abuse
Untreated portal hypertension	Uncontrolled gastrointestinal bleeding or refractory ascites
Autoimmune disease	Coexisting autoimmune disorders (e.g. SLE)
Psychiatric instability	Severe depression or anxiety
Multiple abdominal surgeries	Complex surgical history, adhesions and bowel resections
Renal dysfunction	Chronic kidney disease with creatinine clearance <30 mL/min will need combined liver and kidney transplantation

References

1. Haldar D, Kern B, Hodson J, Armstrong MJ, Adam R, Berlakovich G, Fritz J, Feurstein B, Popp W, Karam V, Muiesan P, O'Grady J, Jamieson N, Wigmore SJ, Pirenne J, Malek-Hosseini SA, Hidalgo E, Tokat Y, Paul A, Pratschke J, Bartels M, Trunecka P, Settmacher U, Pinzani M, Duvoux C, Newsome PN, Schneeberger S, European Liver and Intestine Transplant Association (ELITA). Outcomes of liver transplantation for non-alcoholic steatohepatitis: a European Liver Transplant Registry study. J Hepatol. 2019;71(2):313–22. https://doi.org/10.1016/j.jhep.2019.04.011.
2. Jothimani D, Danielraj S, Narasimhan G, Kaliamoorthy I, Rajakumar A, Palaniappan K, Palanichamy S, Rammohan A, Ramachandran H, Rajalingam R, Rela M. Nonalcoholic steatohepatitis: a rapidly increasing indication for liver transplantation in India. J Clin Exp Hepatol. 2022;12(3):908–16. https://doi.org/10.1016/j.jceh.2021.09.017. Epub 2021 Sep 25. PMID: 35677507; PMCID: PMC9168702.
3. O'Grady J. Timing and benefit of liver transplantation in acute liver failure. J Hepatol. 2014;60(3):663–70. https://doi.org/10.1016/j.jhep.2013.10.024. Epub 2013 Nov 6.
4. Laleman W, Verbeke L, Meersseman P, Wauters J, van Pelt J, Cassiman D, Wilmer A, Verslype C, Nevens F. Acute-on-chronic liver failure: current concepts on definition, pathogenesis, clinical manifestations and potential therapeutic interventions. Expert Rev Gastroenterol Hepatol. 2011;5(4):523–37. https://doi.org/10.1586/egh.11.47.
5. Maiwall R, Chandel SS, Wani Z, Kumar S, Sarin SK. SIRS at admission is a predictor of AKI development and mortality in hospitalized patients with severe alcoholic hepatitis. Dig Dis Sci. 2016;61(3):920–9. https://doi.org/10.1007/s10620-015-3921-4. Epub 2015 Oct 15.
6. Sundaram V, Jalan R, Wu T, Volk ML, Asrani SK, Klein AS, Wong RJ. Factors associated with survival of patients with severe acute-on-chronic liver failure before and after liver transplantation. Gastroenterology. 2019;156(5):1381–1391.e3. https://doi.org/10.1053/j.gastro.2018.12.007. Epub 2018 Dec 18.

7. Kamath PS, Kim WR, Advanced Liver Disease Study Group. The model for end-stage liver disease (MELD). Hepatology. 2007;45(3):797–805. https://doi.org/10.1002/hep.21563.
8. Artru F, Samuel D. Approaches for patients with very high MELD scores. JHEP Rep. 2019;1(1):53–65. https://doi.org/10.1016/j.jhepr.2019.02.008. Erratum in: JHEP Rep 2019 Nov 09;1(5):414. doi: 10.1016/j.jhepr.2019.10.002. PMID: 32039352; PMCID: PMC7001538.
9. Schlegel A, Linecker M, Kron P, Györi G, De Oliveira ML, Müllhaupt B, Clavien PA, Dutkowski P. Risk assessment in high- and low-MELD liver transplantation. Am J Transplant. 2017;17(4):1050–63. https://doi.org/10.1111/ajt.14065. Epub 2016 Nov 14.
10. Asrani SK, Saracino G, O'Leary JG, Gonzalez S, Kim PT, McKenna GJ, Klintmalm G, Trotter J. Recipient characteristics and morbidity and mortality after liver transplantation. J Hepatol. 2018;69(1):43–50. https://doi.org/10.1016/j.jhep.2018.02.004.
11. Yadav SK, Saraf N, Choudhary NS, Sah JK, Sah SK, Rastogi A, Bhangui P, Saigal S, Soin AS. Living donor liver transplantation for acute-on-chronic liver failure. Liver Transpl. 2019;25(3):459–68. https://doi.org/10.1002/lt.25395.
12. Senzolo M, Garcia-Tsao G, García-Pagán JC. Current knowledge and management of portal vein thrombosis in cirrhosis. J Hepatol. 2021;75(2):442–53. https://doi.org/10.1016/j.jhep.2021.04.029. Epub 2021 Apr 27.
13. Kumar A, Acharya SK, Singh SP, Duseja A, Madan K, Shukla A, Arora A, Anand AC, Bahl A, Soin AS, Sirohi B, Dutta D, Jothimani D, Panda D, Saini G, Varghese J, Kumar K, Premkumar M, Panigrahi MK, Wadhawan M, Sahu MK, Rela M, Kalra N, Rao PN, Puri P, Bhangui P, Kar P, Shah SR, Baijal SS, Shalimar PSB, Gamanagatti S, Gupta S, Taneja S, Saraswat VA, Chawla YK. 2023 update of Indian national association for study of the liver consensus on management of intermediate and advanced hepatocellular carcinoma: the Puri III recommendations. J Clin Exp Hepatol. 2024;14(1):101269. https://doi.org/10.1016/j.jceh.2023.08.005. Epub 2023 Aug 19. PMID: 38107186; PMCID: PMC10724697.
14. Pomfret EA, Washburn K, Wald C, Nalesnik MA, Douglas D, Russo M, Roberts J, Reich DJ, Schwartz ME, Mieles L, Lee FT, Florman S, Yao F, Harper A, Edwards E, Freeman R, Lake J. Report of a national conference on liver allocation in patients with hepatocellular carcinoma in the United States. Liver Transpl. 2010;16(3):262–78. https://doi.org/10.1002/lt.21999.
15. Silva MF, Sherman M. Criteria for liver transplantation for HCC: what should the limits be? J Hepatol. 2011;55(5):1137–47. https://doi.org/10.1016/j.jhep.2011.05.012. Epub 2011 Jun 27.
16. Kurian J, Matevish LE, Feizpour C, Shah JA, Hwang C, Hanish SI, Mufti AR, Neill-Fogus S, Vagefi PA, Patel MS. Liver transplantation in elderly recipients: is age just a number? Am Surg. 2023;89(12):5737–43. https://doi.org/10.1177/00031348231173998. Epub 2023 May 4.
17. Nair S, Mason A, Eason J, Loss G, Perrillo RP. Is obesity an independent risk factor for hepatocellular carcinoma in cirrhosis? Hepatology. 2002;36(1):150–5. https://doi.org/10.1053/jhep.2002.33713. Erratum in: Hepatology 2002 Sep;36(3):774.
18. Hakeem AR, Cockbain AJ, Raza SS, Pollard SG, Toogood GJ, Attia MA, Ahmad N, Hidalgo EL, Prasad KR, Menon KV. Increased morbidity in overweight and obese liver transplant recipients: a single-center experience of 1325 patients from the United Kingdom. Liver Transpl. 2013;19(5):551–62. https://doi.org/10.1002/lt.23618. Epub 2013 Mar 17.
19. Pelletier SJ, Schaubel DE, Wei G, Englesbe MJ, Punch JD, Wolfe RA, Port FK, Merion RM. Effect of body mass index on the survival benefit of liver transplantation. Liver Transpl. 2007;13(12):1678–83. https://doi.org/10.1002/lt.21183.
20. Heimbach JK, Watt KD, Poterucha JJ, Ziller NF, Cecco SD, Charlton MR, Hay JE, Wiesner RH, Sanchez W, Rosen CB, Swain JM. Combined liver transplantation and gastric sleeve resection for patients with medically complicated obesity and end-stage liver disease. Am J Transplant. 2013;13(2):363–8. https://doi.org/10.1111/j.1600-6143.2012.04318.x. Epub 2012 Nov 8.
21. Bhattacharjee D, Vracar S, Round RA, Nightingale PG, Williams JA, Gkoutos GV, Stratton IM, Parker R, Luzio SD, Webber J, Manley SE, Roberts GA, Ghosh S. Utility of HbA_{1c} assessment in people with diabetes awaiting liver transplantation. Diabet Med. 2019;36(11):1444–52. https://doi.org/10.1111/dme.13870. Epub 2019 Apr 30. PMID: 30474191; PMCID: PMC6850030.

22. Li F, Wang T, Zhan L, Jia Z, Luo T, Chen S, Zhao Q, Guo Z, He X, Wang D. Clinical outcomes of liver transplantation in patients with hepatorenal syndrome: a single center study in China. Front Surg. 2022;8:781648. https://doi.org/10.3389/fsurg.2021.781648. PMID: 35155548; PMCID: PMC8831834.
23. Northup PG, Argo CK, Bakhru MR, Schmitt TM, Berg CL, Rosner MH. Pretransplant predictors of recovery of renal function after liver transplantation. Liver Transpl. 2010;16(4):440–6. https://doi.org/10.1002/lt.22008.
24. VanWagner LB, Harinstein ME, Runo JR, Darling C, Serper M, Hall S, Kobashigawa JA, Hammel LL. Multidisciplinary approach to cardiac and pulmonary vascular disease risk assessment in liver transplantation: an evaluation of the evidence and consensus recommendations. Am J Transplant. 2018;18(1):30–42. https://doi.org/10.1111/ajt.14531. Epub 2017 Nov 18. PMID: 28985025; PMCID: PMC5840800.
25. Rachwan RJ, Kutkut I, Timsina LR, Bou Chaaya RG, El-Am EA, Sabra M, Mshelbwala FS, Rahal MA, Lacerda MA, Kubal CA, Fridell JA, Ghabril MS, Bourdillon PD, Mangus RS. CAD-LT score effectively predicts risk of significant coronary artery disease in liver transplant candidates. J Hepatol. 2021;75(1):142–9. https://doi.org/10.1016/j.jhep.2021.01.008. Epub 2021 Jan 18.
26. Zardi EM, Abbate A, Zardi DM, et al. Cirrhotic cardiomyopathy. J Am Coll Cardiol. 2010;56(7):539–49. Erratum in: J Am Coll Cardiol. 2010 Sep 14;56(12):1000.
27. Han H, Qin Y, Yu Y, et al. Atrial fibrillation in hospitalized patients with end-stage liver disease: temporal trends in prevalence and outcomes. Liver Int. 2020;40(3):674–84.
28. Chokesuwattanaskul R, Thongprayoon C, Bathini T, Ungprasert P, Sharma K, Wijarnpreecha K, Pachariyanon P, Cheungpasitporn W. Liver transplantation and atrial fibrillation: a meta-analysis. World J Hepatol. 2018;10(10):761–71.
29. Kertai MD, Bountioukos M, Boersma E, et al. Aortic stenosis: an underestimated risk factor for perioperative complications in patients undergoing noncardiac surgery. Am J Med. 2004;116(1):8–13.
30. De Gasperi A, Spagnolin G, Ornaghi M, et al. Preoperative cardiac assessment in liver transplant candidates. Best Pract Res Clin Anaesthesiol. 2020;34(1):51–68.
31. Filsoufi F, Salzberg SP, Rahmanian PB, et al. Early and late outcome of cardiac surgery in patients with liver cirrhosis. Liver Transpl. 2007;13(7):990–5.
32. Peeraphatdit TB, Nkomo VT, Naksuk N, et al. Long-term outcomes after transcatheter and surgical aortic valve replacement in patients with cirrhosis: a guide for the hepatologist. Hepatology. 2020;72(5):1735–46.
33. Nwaejike N, Mills K, Stables R, et al. Balloon aortic valvuloplasty as a bridge to aortic valve surgery for severe aortic stenosis. Interact Cardiovasc Thorac Surg. 2015;20(3):429–35.
34. Bandara M, Gordon FD, Sarwar A, Knauft ME, Pomfret EA, Freeman RB, Wirth JA. Successful outcomes following living donor liver transplantation for portopulmonary hypertension. Liver Transpl. 2010;16(8):983–9. https://doi.org/10.1002/lt.22107.
35. Laberge JM, Brandt ML, Lebecque P, Moulin D, Veykemans F, Paradis K, Pelletier L, Lacroix J, Blanchard H, de Goyet JD, et al. Reversal of cirrhosis-related pulmonary shunting in two children by orthotopic liver transplantation. Transplantation. 1992;53(5):1135–8.
36. Krowka MJ. Hepatopulmonary syndrome and portopulmonary hypertension: the pulmonary vascular enigmas of liver disease. Clin Liver Dis (Hoboken). 2020;15(Suppl 1):S13–24. https://doi.org/10.1002/cld.846. PMID: 32140210; PMCID: PMC7050952.
37. Gupta S, Castel H, Rao RV, Picard M, Lilly L, Faughnan ME, Pomier-Layrargues G. Improved survival after liver transplantation in patients with hepatopulmonary syndrome. Am J Transplant. 2010;10(2):354–63. https://doi.org/10.1111/j.1600-6143.2009.02822.x. Epub 2009 Sep 22.
38. Iyer VN, Swanson KL, Cartin-Ceba R, Dierkhising RA, Rosen CB, Heimbach JK, Wiesner RH, Krowka MJ. Hepatopulmonary syndrome: favorable outcomes in the MELD exception era. Hepatology. 2013;57(6):2427–35. https://doi.org/10.1002/hep.26070. Epub 2013 Feb 15.

39. Lin Y-T, Cheng Y-K, Lin C-L, Wang I-K. Increased risk of subdural hematoma in patients with liver cirrhosis. QJM. 2017;110(12):815–20.
40. Levesque E, Hoti E, Azoulay D, Ichaï P, Habouchi H, Castaing D, Samuel D, Saliba F. Prospective evaluation of the prognostic scores for cirrhotic patients admitted to an intensive care unit. J Hepatol. 2012;56(1):95–102. https://doi.org/10.1016/j.jhep.2011.06.024. Epub 2011 Aug 9.
41. Levesque E, Winter A, Noorah Z, Daurès JP, Landais P, Feray C, Azoulay D. Impact of acute-on-chronic liver failure on 90-day mortality following a first liver transplantation. Liver Int. 2017;37(5):684–93. https://doi.org/10.1111/liv.13355. Epub 2017 Feb 27.
42. Petrowsky H, Rana A, Kaldas FM, Sharma A, Hong JC, Agopian VG, Durazo F, Honda H, Gornbein J, Wu V, Farmer DG, Hiatt JR, Busuttil RW. Liver transplantation in highest acuity recipients: identifying factors to avoid futility. Ann Surg. 2014;259(6):1186–94. https://doi.org/10.1097/SLA.0000000000000265.
43. Friedrich K, Krempl J, Schamoni S, Hippchen T, Pfeiffenberger J, Rupp C, Gotthardt DN, Houben P, Von Haken R, Heininger A, Brenner T, Mehrabi A, Weiss KH, Mieth M. Multidrug-resistant bacteria and disease progression in patients with end-stage liver disease and after liver transplantation. J Gastrointestin Liver Dis. 2019;28(3):303–10. https://doi.org/10.15403/jgld-212.
44. Jothimani D, Venugopal R, Abedin MF, Kaliamoorthy I, Rela M. COVID-19 and the liver. J Hepatol. 2020;73(5):1231–40. https://doi.org/10.1016/j.jhep.2020.06.006. Epub 2020 Jun 15. PMID: 32553666; PMCID: PMC7295524.
45. Fernández J, Acevedo J, Wiest R, Gustot T, Amoros A, Deulofeu C, Reverter E, Martínez J, Saliba F, Jalan R, Welzel T, Pavesi M, Hernández-Tejero M, Ginès P, Arroyo V, European Foundation for the Study of Chronic Liver Failure. Bacterial and fungal infections in acute-on-chronic liver failure: prevalence, characteristics and impact on prognosis. Gut. 2018;67(10):1870–80. https://doi.org/10.1136/gutjnl-2017-314240. Epub 2017 Aug 28.
46. Fung J, Eghtesad B, Patel-Tom K, DeVera M, Chapman H, Ragni M. Liver transplantation in patients with HIV infection. Liver Transpl. 2004;10(10 Suppl 2):S39–53. https://doi.org/10.1002/lt.20261.
47. O'Grady J, Taylor C. Guidelines for liver transplantation in patients with HIV infection, 2005. BTS.org.uk guidelines.
48. Mauro E, Crespo G, Martinez-Garmendia A, Gutierrez-Acevedo MN, Diaz JM, Saidman J, Bermudez C, Ortiz-Patron J, Garcia-Olveira L, Zalazar F, Narvaez A, Spina JC, Orta R, Savluk L, Piano S, Marciano S, Gadano A. Cystatin C and sarcopenia predict acute on chronic liver failure development and mortality in patients on the liver transplant waiting list. Transplantation. 2020;104(7):e188–98. https://doi.org/10.1097/TP.0000000000003222.
49. Tantai X, Liu Y, Yeo YH, Praktiknjo M, Mauro E, Hamaguchi Y, Engelmann C, Zhang P, Jeong JY, van Vugt JLA, Xiao H, Deng H, Gao X, Ye Q, Zhang J, Yang L, Cai Y, Liu Y, Liu N, Li Z, Han T, Kaido T, Sohn JH, Strassburg C, Berg T, Trebicka J, Hsu YC, IJzermans JNM, Wang J, Su GL, Ji F, Nguyen MH. Effect of sarcopenia on survival in patients with cirrhosis: a meta-analysis. J Hepatol. 2022;76(3):588–99. https://doi.org/10.1016/j.jhep.2021.11.006. Epub 2021 Nov 14.
50. Tandon P, Montano-Loza AJ, Lai JC, Dasarathy S, Merli M. Sarcopenia and frailty in decompensated cirrhosis. J Hepatol. 2021;75 Suppl 1(Suppl 1):S147–62. https://doi.org/10.1016/j.jhep.2021.01.025. PMID: 34039486; PMCID: PMC9125684.
51. Englesbe MJ, Patel SP, He K, Lynch RJ, Schaubel DE, Harbaugh C, Holcombe SA, Wang SC, Segev DL, Sonnenday CJ. Sarcopenia and mortality after liver transplantation. J Am Coll Surg. 2010;211(2):271–8. https://doi.org/10.1016/j.jamcollsurg.2010.03.039. Epub 2010 Jun 26. PMID: 20670867; PMCID: PMC2914324.
52. Al-Adra DP, Hammel L, Roberts J, Woodle ES, Levine D, Mandelbrot D, Verna E, Locke J, D'Cunha J, Farr M, Sawinski D, Agarwal PK, Plichta J, Pruthi S, Farr D, Carvajal R, Walker J, Zwald F, Habermann T, Gertz M, Bierman P, Dizon DS, Langstraat C, Al-Qaoud T, Eggener

S, Richgels JP, Chang GJ, Geltzeiler C, Sapisochin G, Ricciardi R, Krupnick AS, Kennedy C, Mohindra N, Foley DP, Watt KD. Pretransplant solid organ malignancy and organ transplant candidacy: a consensus expert opinion statement. Am J Transplant. 2021;21(2):460–74. https://doi.org/10.1111/ajt.16318. Epub 2020 Oct 23. PMID: 32969590; PMCID: PMC8576374.

Chapter 4
Pretransplant Assessment

Mettu Srinivas Reddy and Prasanna Gopal

Abstract All patients needing liver transplantation should undergo a detailed fitness evaluation to assess the benefit and risk of the procedure. Transplant evaluation should focus on conditions that may have the potential to derail intraoperative or postoperative course, enable a formal risk–benefit analysis and tailor intraoperative and postoperative management to a specific patient.

A protocolized assessment for liver transplantation should be followed. This includes a comprehensive medical history and physical examination, investigation for medical comorbidities and assessment of recipient's functional status along with preoperative imaging. Detailed preoperative cardiopulmonary evaluation is needed given the increasing prevalence of metabolic dysfunction-associated steatohepatitis and associated metabolic comorbidities. Upon completion of transplant evaluation, each patient should be discussed in a multidisciplinary transplant meeting to confirm suitability and document perioperative strategies. Living donor liver transplantation offers an advantage of better planning and timing of surgery following patient optimization.

Keywords Pretransplant assessment · Cardiopulmonary evaluation · Living donor liver transplantation · Surgical assessment

---

M. S. Reddy (✉)
Star Institute of Comprehensive Liver Care & Transplantation, Star Hospitals, Hyderabad, India

Rainbow Children's Hospitals, Hyderabad, India
e-mail: smettu.reddy@gmail.com

P. Gopal
Star Institute of Comprehensive Liver Care & Transplantation, Star Hospitals, Hyderabad, India

S. Saigal, D. Jothimani (eds.), *Fundamentals of Transplant Hepatology*, https://doi.org/10.1007/978-981-95-2624-6_4

Key Highlights

1. Patient assessment is the cornerstone of successful liver transplantation ensuring clear risk–benefit analysis and identifying factors that may complicate surgery or recovery.
2. A protocol-based approach is recommended for pretransplant evaluation, including detailed medical history, physical examination and advanced imaging.
3. Identifying and addressing medical conditions during pretransplant evaluation can mitigate postoperative complications and improve transplant outcomes.
4. Cardiovascular and pulmonary assessments are mandatory, given the high prevalence of metabolic comorbidities and the high impact of perioperative cardiorespiratory complications.
5. Multidisciplinary collaboration is essential for optimizing patients and ensuring successful transplantation.

4.1 Introduction

Liver transplantation (LT) is widely accepted as the treatment of choice for patients afflicted with end-stage liver disease. In recent years, there has been a significant improvement in the outcomes of LT recipients. At least, a part of this improvement is related to better risk assessment, risk stratification and preoperative optimization practices which have become part of LT practice.

The aims of preoperative LT assessment of a potential recipient are threefold.

1. To recognize the need for LT in a patient and ensure that the benefit–risk profile is clarified.
2. To identify medical and surgical factors in the recipient which may contraindicate LT or increase the risk of LT so that appropriate counselling of the patient is done.
3. To identify medical and surgical factors which can be optimized in the preoperative period so that the risk associated with these factors can be negated or mitigated.

It is increasingly recognized that a multidisciplinary assessment of the potential recipient lead by the LT team is essential to achieve all the above goals. Most LT centers now have a protocolized system of LT assessment, which includes a comprehensive medical history and physical examination, investigation for medical comorbidities, assessment of recipient's functional status along with a detailed assessment of preoperative imaging. While the specifics may vary between centers, the overall theme and principles of assessment are fairly standard and will be discussed in this chapter (Fig. 4.1). While this chapter primarily presents the assessment process for elective LT, it is not very different in the acute setting where LT is indicated for acute liver failure or acute-on-chronic liver failure (ACLF). Indications for liver transplantation and assessment of the pediatric recipient will be discussed elsewhere in this textbook.

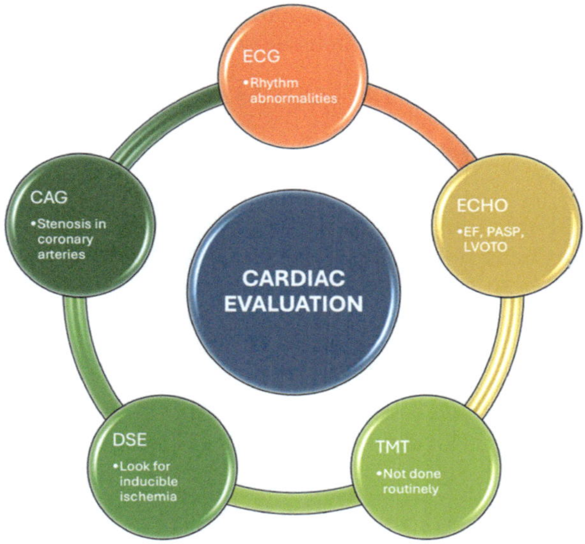

Fig. 4.1 Pretransplant Cardiac evaluation

4.2 History and Examination

An initial assessment by the LT team is essential before a potential recipient starts a formal evaluation for LT. This evaluation includes a detailed history centered on the duration, severity of liver disease, evaluation of the underlying etiologies, associated comorbidities such as diabetes, hypertension or coronary artery disease (CAD) and the presence of alcohol or substance abuse. This initial consultation will also help the clinician gain an understanding of the level of fitness of the patient and gives an opportunity to discuss the clinical pathway with the recipient and family. Clinical examination beyond the recognition of the standard features of liver disease also include a more objective assessment of recipient functional status.

4.3 Cardiovascular Assesment

Cardiovascular complications represent an important cause of perioperative and late mortality in patients undergoing LT. The increasing incidence of metabolic syndrome complicated by metabolic dysfunction-associated steatohepatitis (MASH) as an indication for LT along with the advancing age of transplant patients is increasing the likelihood of potential recipients presenting with coronary artery disease (CAD). It is notable that 13.3% of CAD patients are asymptomatic [1]. The classical symptoms of CAD, such as exertional dyspnea, may not be present in patients with decompensated liver disease due to restricted mobility caused by ascites and pedal edema. A rigorous preoperative cardiac evaluation is required to identify patients with cardiac disease. While CAD is an important factor to be evaluated, assessment should also include evaluation for arrythmias, valvular heart disease, cirrhotic cardiomyopathy and portopulmonary hypertension (PoPH).

4.3.1 Initial Cardiac Testing

The first line of cardiac testing involves an electrocardiogram (ECG) to identify rhythm abnormalities. A transthoracic echocardiogram (TTE) is then performed to assess the ejection fraction and right ventricular systolic pressure. An ejection fraction below 45% is considered abnormal and requires further evaluation by a cardiologist. Pulmonary artery systolic pressure (PASP) greater than 47 mmHg indicates pulmonary hypertension (PAH), which can be secondary to interstitial lung disease (ILD) or cardiac issues and needs detailed evaluation. TTE also helps in identifying significant valvular heart disease which needs further evaluation.

4.3.2 Coronary Artery Disease

Recognition of significant coronary artery disease and its risk stratification is an important goal of LT assessment. The precise protocol followed by individual centers varies; however, the aim is to obtain a detailed anatomical and physiological assessment of the cardiac effort tolerance of the patient. Patients are initially stratified for CAD based on risk factors recognized on history and examination. These risk factors include age greater than 50, diabetes mellitus, hypertension, hyperlipidemia, obesity, nonalcoholic steatohepatitis, smoking and family history of CAD. Recipients without these risk factors can undergo functional/noninvasive testing alone to assess cardiac fitness [2].

Noninvasive testing includes exercise stress testing (EST), dobutamine stress echo or stress thallium testing. Candidates for liver transplantation often present with ascites, sarcopenia and frailty which may prevent them from undergoing exercise stress testing. Dobutamine stress echocardiography (DSE) can be performed in younger patients where the pretest probability of CAD is low [3]. DSE is able to identify only those patients with CAD severe enough to impair cardiac muscle oxygenation. In order for DSE to be reliable, at least 85% of maximal heart rate must be achieved. However, many patients are beta-blocked and unable to achieve the target heart rate. Overall, DSE has a poor sensitivity for ruling out CAD but is reliable for predicting post-liver transplantation cardiovascular events. In cases where the pretest probability of CAD is high, angiography is necessary. Stress thallium is another noninvasive modality which is appropriate for patients who cannot undergo EST or DSE but have a low risk of CAD. It is also useful as an adjunct modality to assess the significance of mild to moderate CAD identified on angiography. Finally, computed tomography (CT) calcium score is being increasingly incorporated into LT assessment protocols due to its ease of performance and relatively low cost. It is primarily useful as an adjunct to noninvasive testing in patients deemed low risk for CAD. A calcium score of 0 in the absence of any other risk factors can rule out significant CAD in LT recipients.

Role of Coronary Angiography (CAG) The role of routine CAG in LT recipients is controversial. While CAG is an invasive procedure advances in technique such as radial access, low contrast usage have significantly reduced the risk of postprocedure hematomas, contrast-related renal injury and so on. CAG is indicated with recipients with past history or interventions of CAD, symptoms of CAD, risk factors (mentioned above) or positive findings on noninvasive testing. CAG helps in diagnosing significant CAD and also direct the need for pretransplant therapeutic interventions. Finally, the role of CT-CAG is still evolving, and its ability to replace conventional CAG is still unclear.

4.3.3 *Management of CAD in the Pre-LT Recipient*

Patients with CAD associated with physiological compromise of myocardial function during rest or exertion should be corrected in the pre-LT period. In patients with incidentally recognized CAD with no functional impairment, the decision to intervene is more complex and should be based on a multidisciplinary assessment and discussion among the cardiologist, anesthesiologist and the surgeon considering the extent of CAD, clinical urgency of LT and expected postoperative course of the patient.

Coronary artery stenting is the standard procedure to treat CAD in the pretransplant period. While bare metal stents were preferred previously due to the ability to de-escalate antiplatelet therapy earlier, drug-eluting stents are being increasingly preferred for their better long-term coronary outcomes. The decision regarding timing of LT and the risk/benefit of preoperative de-escalation of antiplatelet therapy is multifactorial and has to be taken after discussion in a multidisciplinary setting.

The role of preoperative coronary artery bypass grafting (CABG) is reducing as stent technology and coronary stenting techniques improve. However, in patients with multivessel disease or difficult to stent lesions, CABG may be indicated. In this scenario, an off-pump CABG is preferred to reduce the bleeding and renal risks [4]. The relative timing of CABG and LT is controversial, especially in the living donor liver transplantation (LDLT) setting, and should balance the risks of hepatic decompensation after CABG and the bleeding, hemodynamic and renal risks of combined procedures. Our strategy has been to complete the LD evaluation and formalities of LDLT before a planned sequential CABG-LDLT procedure with an interval of 24–72 h. This provides an opportunity for the assessment of post-CABG cardiac function and reduce bleeding risk while ensuring that the LT is performed before significant hepatic decompensation with its attendant risks.

Portopulmonary Hypertension (PoPH) poses a distinct challenge in liver transplant (LT) candidates. PoPH is caused by long-term injury, thrombosis and remodeling of the pulmonary vasculature in response to shear stress of the hyperdynamic circulation seen in cirrhosis. Patients with a pulmonary artery systolic pressure (PASP) greater than 47 mmHg on TTE should be subjected to right heart catheterization study to measure mean pulmonary arterial pressure (mPAP), pulmonary vascular resistance (PVR) and pulmonary capillary wedge pressure (PCWP). This differentiates POPH from fluid overload which is a much more common cause of increased PASP in cirrhotic patients. A diagnosis of PoPH is indicated by mPAP greater than 25 mmHg, PVR greater than 245 dyne/sec/cm^{-5} and PCWP less than 15 mmHg. In mild PoPH (mPAP <35 mmHg), LT can be considered and can reverse PoPH. The role of LT in patients with moderate and severe mPAP (>35 mmHg) is debatable as LT is associated with a 50% mortality and the reversal of POPH at this severity is unclear. An mPAP greater than 50 mmHg contraindicates LT. Patients with moderate PoPH should undergo medical therapy to reduce mPAP before being considered for LT. Response to medical therapy predicts good outcomes with LT.

4.4 Respiratory Assesment

Common respiratory issues in LT candidates are fluid overload, basal atelectasis, ascites reducing lung capacity, hepatic hydrothorax, hepatopulmonary syndrome (HPS) and rarely interstitial lung disease. Assessment of the respiratory assessment should start with history and examination to identify tachypnoea, dyspnea, abnormal breath sounds and signs of hypoxia such as cyanosis or clubbing. Pulse Oximetry is a simple bed-side test to assess oxygen saturation levels and should be performed in every LT recipient during assessment and at every out-patient visit. An SPO_2 less than 96% on room air should be evaluated.

Chest X-ray is useful for recognizing gross lung and pleural pathologies including tuberculosis (TB) sequelae and effusions. Further investigation of pulmonary symptoms should be performed only after large effusions or gross ascites is drained. CT scan of chest is now commonly performed along with CT abdomen in the post-COVID era to identify post-COVID lung pathology. CT can accurately assess pleural effusion, volume overload and ILD. Pleural effusion in CLD patients is more common in right side and an isolated or predominant left pleural effusion needs evaluation for tuberculosis.

Arterial blood gas (ABG) analysis should be performed in all potential recipients during evaluation. An arterial PaO_2 less than 80 mmHg in the absence of other contributing factors should trigger investigation for hepatopulmonary syndrome or interstitial lung disease. Further investigation is needed to rule out that ABG is done to look for arterial oxygen PaO_2 levels. If arterial oxygen levels are less than 80%, there is a need for bubble echo scan to look for HPS.

Pulmonary function test by spirometry should be performed to evaluate significant restrictive or obstructive lung disease. Restrictive pattern may be due to malnutrition causing muscle weakness and is defined by forced expiratory volume in one minute (FEV1)/forced expiratory capacity (FVC) ≥70 and total lung capacity (TLC) <80. Obstructive pattern may be secondary to due to chronic obstructive pulmonary disease (COPD) and defined as FEV1/FVC <70 and TLC ≥80 [5]. A mixed pattern (FEV1/FVC <70 and TLC <80) may also be noted. Investigations such as diffusion lung capacity for carbon mono oxide (DLCO) or high resolution chest computed tomography (HRCT) may be needed to clearly estimate the severity of lung dysfunction and prognosticate post-LT outcomes. Some of these patients may be candidates for combined liver and lung transplantation.

Table 4.1 Grading of HPS

HPS severity	PaO_2 in mm Hg on room air ABG
Mild	>80
Moderate	60–80
Severe	50–60
Very severe	<50

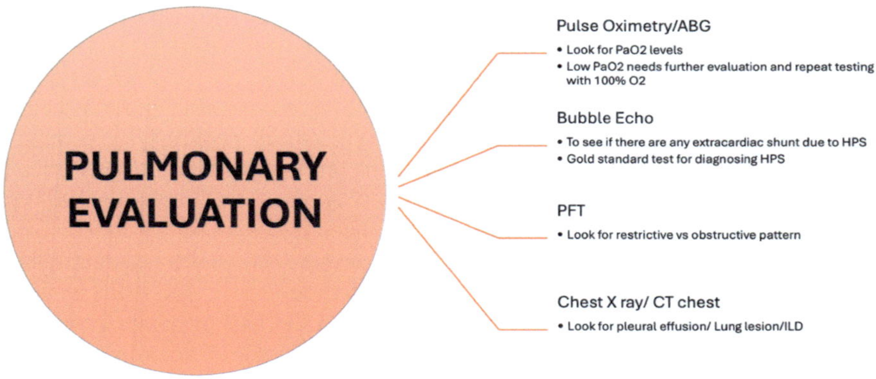

Fig. 4.2 Pulmonary evaluation, diagnostic tests and overview

4.4.1 Hepatopulmonary Syndrome (HPS)

HPS is caused due to abnormal intrapulmonary vasodilation and shunting, causing ventilation-perfusion mismatch resulting in low oxygen saturation. This is usually detected by hypoxia on pulse oximetry, which improves when the patient shifts from standing to supine position. Arterial hypoxemia on room air ABG which is completely corrected by 100% oxygen is also an indicator of HPS. Diagnosis of HPS is made by bubble, and appearance of contrast bubbles on the left side of the heart after the fourth cardiac cycle but before the tenth cycle is suggestive of intrapulmonary shunts. Macroaggregated albumin scan can also be used to diagnose and quantify the severity of shunting, although the shunt fraction has poor correlation with severity of symptoms or the likelihood of post-transplant reversibility.

Patients with HPS are grouped into four grades based on severity of arterial hypoxemia on room air ABG (Table 4.1). HPS with PaO_2 <60, that is, severe and very severe HPS are given model for end stage liver disease (MELD) exception points. Patients with very severe HPS and poor reversibility with 100% oxygen have poor outcomes post-transplant. Patients with moderate and severe HPS should be maintained on home oxygen therapy until LT. HPS recovers after liver transplantation, although patients with severe or very severe HPS may need prolonged home oxygen therapy in the post-LT period (Fig. 4.2).

4.5 Renal Assesment

Renal impairment is common in cirrhotic patients and affects both pretransplant and post-transplant outcomes such as intensive care unit stay, sepsis, need for dialysis and patient survival. It is important to assess renal function in LT candidates as it affects prognosis and to decide on liver alone/simultaneous liver kidney transplant and perioperative care including need for dialysis and post-op immnuosupression [6]. Both acute kidney injury (AKI) and chronic kidney disease (CKD) can affect cirrhotic patients. AKI is the most common presentation of cirrhotics with varied etiologies, and the prognosis each etiology carries also varies [7]. AKI is categorized as prerenal (hypovolemia, infection and use of vasodilators), intrarenal (glomerulopathy, acute tubular necrosis and acute interstitial nephritis) or postrenal causes (obstructive uropathy). Prerenal AKI is the predominant form resulting from reduced blood flow to kidneys. Advanced form of prerenal AKI is hepatorenal syndrome (HRS). These two disorders are differentiated by response to volume resuscitation, in which HRS does not respond to volume expansion. HRS is diagnosed by international club of ascites diagnostic criteria [8]. Prognosis of AKI-HRS is worse than other causes of AKI, and the development of AKI-HRS mandates early liver transplantation. Acute tubular necrosis is the most common differential for AKI-HRS, as both conditions are characterized by rapidly declining renal function. ATN has higher risk of developing into post-transplant CKD [9].

Renal assessment in LT candidates includes history, physical examination and review of patient drugs for nephrotoxicity. Laboratory assessment includes renal function tests such as urea, creatinine and electrolytes; urinalysis to look for casts/pus cells; spot urine tests for protein and creatinine; protein-to-creatinine ratio; renal ultrasound and kidney biopsy.

4.6 Surgical Assesment

Surgical assessment of the LT recipient is focused on anatomical factors which are likely to increase the complexity of the transplant procedure (Fig. 4.3). History of previous upper abdominal surgery, presence of scars and hernias on the anterior abdominal wall and groin areas should be recorded. Extensive abdominal wall edema and skin lesions can increase the risk of wound infections and should be treated, if possible, prior to surgery. Large abdominal wall collateral veins should be recognized so that excessive bleeding during laparotomy is avoided (Fig. 4.4).

Most centers perform a contrast CT or MRI scan of the abdomen as part of the LT assessment. Cross-sectional imaging provides a large amount of information regarding expected surgical complexity and should be reviewed in detail at the time of assessment and in the immediate preoperative period. Factors such as hepatomegaly, caval wrapping by enlarged caudate lobe, portal cavernoma formation and encapsulating peritonitis increase operating time, blood loss and transfusion requirement. Portal vein thrombosis (PVT) should be identified on preoperative imaging so

SURGICAL ASSESMENT	• Focus on anatomical factors which increase complexity
History of previous surgery	• Prior abdominal surgery can complicate explant hepatectomy due to adhesions • Examination to look for hernia, dilated veins • Hernial defect has to be closed at the time of surgery. Abdominal wall collaterals should be carefully addressed while opening abdominal wall
CT arterial phase	• SOL, artery branching pattern, Celiac axis stenosis
CT Portal phase	• PV patency, spleen size, Collaterals in abdominal wall, splenorenal collaterals, Left renal vein
CT hepatic venous phase	• Large caudate veins • Caudate wrap around IVC
Any phase	• Umbilical hernia/ inguinal hernia/ cocoon abdomen

Fig. 4.3 Surgical assessment and evaluation

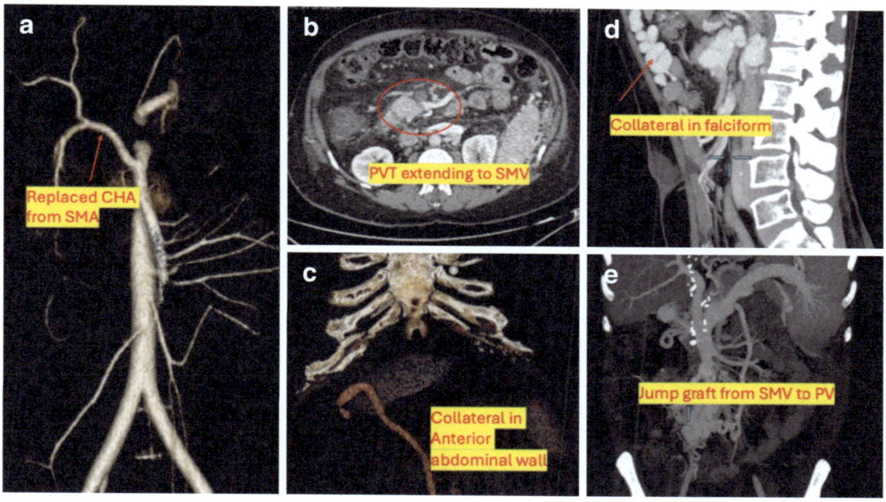

Fig. 4.4 CT scan findings (**a**) CT—arterial phase: showing common hepatic artery (CHA) arising from superior mesenteric artery (SMA). (**b**) CT—portal phase: showing grade 3 PVT involving superior mesenteric vein (SMV). (**c**) CT—portal phase: showing collaterals in anterior abdominal wall. (**d**) CT—portal phase: showing collaterals in falciform ligament. (**e**) CT—in post-transplant patient: showing jump graft from SMV to graft PV, done for grade 2 PVT

that arrangements are made for any vascular grafts. Similarly, coeliac artery stenosis, visceral artery aneurysms, presence of large portosystemic collaterals and presence of umbilical hernia should be recognized as they might impact intraoperative decisions. CT is now increasingly being used to estimate severity of sarcopenia which has been shown to have an impact on post-transplant recovery.

4.7 Functional Assessment—Frailty and Sarcopenia

Functional assessment is a key part of LT assessment as numerous studies have shown the strong link between preoperative functional status and postoperative morbidity and mortality. While end-of-bed assessment by experienced clinician is still valuable, more objective means are necessary. Generic instruments to assess performance status such as ECOG or Karnofsky score are being increasingly supplemented by objective scores assessing frailty in patients. Frailty in layman term means weakness and is a term derived from geriatric literature and is defined as a state of reduced physiological reserve associated with increased vulnerability to stressors which lead to adverse clinical outcomes [10]. General frailty is a multidimensional syndrome which includes physical, cognitive, emotional and psychosocial domains. In the context of CLD and LT, physical frailty and its association with LT outcomes have been the most extensively studied. Sarcopenia is a reduction in the quantity, quality and function of skeletal musculature and is associated with decompensated liver disease. Sarcopenia in cirrhosis is multifactorial. Multiple decompensation episodes, poor oral intake, repeated paracentesis with resultant protein loss, reduced mobility and cirrhosis-related inflammation can reduce muscle mass. Sarcopenia is closely related to frailty but the two are not always concordant. For example, patients with ACLF may be frail, although their muscle mass is still preserved due to the short duration of their disease. Frailty assessment may be more important in such patients than sarcometry alone.

Assessment of frailty and sarcopenia in LT candidates has to be multidimensional and objective to ensure valid estimation of its severity (Table 4.2). Sarcopenia and physical frailty are dynamic and progressive in nature with worsening liver disease. Measures to improve nutrition and activity levels can boost both these measures. A number of different measures are now available to estimate frailty in cirrhosis patients. However, very few of these measures have been validated in the Indian population. We have found the 6-minute walk test (6MWT) and hand grip strength to be the good indicators of functional status in elective LT recipients.

There is now increasing evidence that a preoperative regimen of exercise therapy reduces waiting list mortality and improves post-LT outcomes. All patients must be seen by a physiotherapist, and exercise program must be tailored to each patient based on disease severity and comorbidity (osteoarthritis and CAD). Exercise program should include a combination of aerobic (walking, jogging, cycling and swimming) and resistance training (wall squats, chair stands, leg raises, step-up and bridges) at least 2 days/week and be undertaken at level of moderate intensity [11].

Table 4.2 Methods of Frailty assessment

Methods			
Liver frailty index (LFI)	Composite metric of three performance-based measures	Hand grip strength Time to do five chair stands Time holding three balance positions (feet side by side, semitandem and tandem)	LFI <3.2, robust; 3.2–4.5, prefrail >4.5, frail
Short physical performance battery (SPPB)	Assess physical function	Three components: Time to complete five chair stands Time to walk 4 m Balance testing	Score ≤ 9/12 = higher wait-list mortality
6MWT	Assess physical function	Patient instructed to walk as far as possible in 6 min along set course	Reduced 6MWD (<250 m; HR = 2.1) predicts mortality among LT candidates
Hand grip strength	Assess physical function	Three consecutive measurements of static force (kg) produced by the nondominant hand around a dynamometer; mean value is used for analysis	Low HGS associated with hospitalization
L3SMI	Assess sarcopenia	Quantification of skeletal muscle is made using body-segmentation analysis software and then normalized to height to calculate the SMI	<50 cm^2/m^2 in men and <39 cm^2/m^2 in women

4.8 Nutritional Assessment

There is increasing evidence that malnutrition is an important contributor to pre-LT and post-LT morbidity. All LT recipients should have a consultation with an experienced clinical nutritionist to help guide dietary intake taking into consideration factors such as patients' current nutritional status, metabolic status and presence of complications such as encephalopathy. Daily energy intake of 35 kcal/kg/day in patients with a BMI of <30 kg/m^2 along with adequate protein intake is recommended [12]. Those who are not able to achieve energy requirements with oral intake alone needs enteral supplementation. Patients should be advised to reduce long fasting intervals and take frequent feeds every 3–4 h during day time along with a late evening snack to avoid muscle catabolism.

4.9 Psychological Assessment

LT is a life-changing event for a patient. All LT recipients should undergo a careful psychological evaluation to assess their mental capacity to undergo major surgery, adhere to medical advice and lifelong medications. In patients needing transplant for alcoholic liver disease, this is even more important as recidivism after LT significantly increases graft failure and death. In patients with CLD undergoing LT assessment, an abstinence period of at least 3 months should be considered as there is some evidence suggesting rates of recidivism in such patients. However, this may not always be possible in patients presenting with ACLF or severe alcoholic hepatitis resistant to medical management and being considered for early LDLT. In such patients, a detailed psychological assessment of the recipient is also not possible. Detailed discussion with family members will provide valuable insights to the psychologist and the transplant team regarding the patients' ability to maintain post-LT abstinence and his/her capacity for adherence to lifelong treatment and should be considered in the multidisciplinary discussion to assess the suitability of the patient for LT.

4.10 Anesthetic Assessment

In most centers, review by the transplant anesthesia team remains the key step in assessing fitness for transplantation. In addition to standard assessment for anesthesia, the 'liver anesthetic assessment' collates the varied medical opinions of the multidisciplinary team (MDT) to develop a comprehensive picture of a recipient's risk profile. This summative assessment along with the assessment of expected surgical complexity provides a final roadmap for preoperative optimization and perioperative management of LT recipients. It is recommended that the LT recipient is reviewed at least twice by the transplant anesthesia team—once at the beginning of evaluation and once after completion of the assessment process.

4.11 Management on the Waiting List

In patients who are on the waiting list for LT, regular monitoring is important. Assessment should include the status of liver disease and regular review of the cardiac and pulmonary function (Fig. 4.5) (Table 4.3). It is recommended that all recipients should be reviewed by the core transplant team (Hepatology, Surgery and Anesthesia) at least thrice monthly and more frequently if clinically necessary.

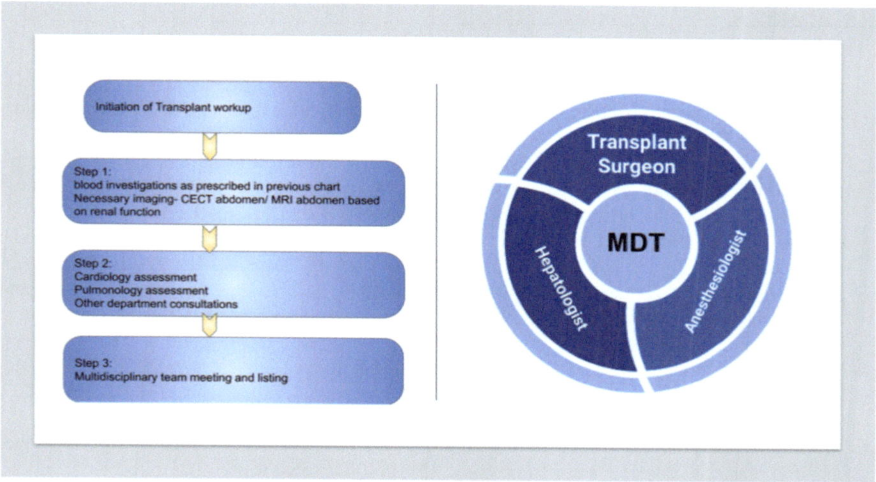

Fig. 4.5 Flow chart of assessment Process and MDT

Table 4.3 List of investigations and consultations

Complete hemogram	Blood group	Imaging
Renal function test	Coombs test—direct and indirect	CT, abdomen—contrast
Liver function test		CT, chest
PT/INR	AFP	X-ray, PNS
Lipid profile	Ca 19-9	DEXA scan—whole body
Thyroid profile	CEA	
HbA1C	PSA if male	Cardiology
HIV		Pulmonology
HBsAg	Reticulocyte count	Psychiatry
Anti HCV	G6PD assay	ENT
EBV VCA IgG	Bleeding time	Dental
EBNA IgG	S. Fibrinogen	Ophthalmology
CMV IgG	PTT	Infectious Disease
HSV 1 IgG	Factor V Leiden screen	Gynecology
HSV 2 IgG		Dermatology
VZV IgG		Nutritionist

4.12 Conclusion

Pretransplant assessment is the cornerstone in selecting and optimizing patients for liver transplantation. It involves a protocol based multidisciplinary team approach to address medical surgical, nutritional and psychological factors for successful post-transplant outcomes.

References

1. Carey WD, Dumot JA, Pimentel RR, Barnes DS, Hobbs RE, Henderson JM, et al. The prevalence of coronary artery disease in liver transplant candidates over age 50. Transplantation. 1995;59(6):859–64.
2. Tsochatzis EA, Watt KD, VanWagner LB, Verna EC, Berzigotti A. Evaluation of recipients with significant comorbidity – patients with cardiovascular disease. J Hepatol. 2023;78(6):1089–104. https://doi.org/10.1016/j.jhep.2023.03.023. PMID: 37208096.
3. Hogan BJ, Gonsalkorala E, Heneghan MA. Evaluation of coronary artery disease in potential liver transplant recipients. Liver Transpl. 2017;23(3):386–95. https://doi.org/10.1002/lt.24679.
4. Marui A, Kimura T, Tanaka S, Miwa S, Yamazaki K, Minakata K, for CREDO-Kyoto Investigators, et al. Coronary revascularization in patients with liver cirrhosis. Ann Thorac Surg. 2011;91(5):1393–9.
5. Bozbas SS, Eyuboglu F. Evaluation of liver transplant candidates: a pulmonary perspective. Ann Thorac Med. 2011;6(3):109–14. https://doi.org/10.4103/1817-1737.82436. PMID: 21760840; PMCID: PMC3131751.
6. Martin-Llahi M, Guevara M, Torre A, et al. Prognostic importance of the cause of renal failure in patients with cirrhosis. Gastroenterology. 2011;140(2):488–96.e4.
7. Cullaro G, Kanduri SR, Velez JCQ. Acute kidney injury in patients with liver disease. Clin J Am Soc Nephrol. 2022;17(11):1674–84. https://doi.org/10.2215/CJN.03040322.
8. Angeli P, Gines P, Wong F, Bernardi M, Boyer TD, Gerbes A, et al. Diagnosis and management of acute kidney injury in patients with cirrhosis: revised consensus recommendations of the International Club of Ascites. Gut. 2015;64(4):531–7.
9. Nadim MK, Genyk YS, Tokin C, Fieber J, Ananthapanyasut W, Ye W, et al. Impact of the etiology of acute kidney injury on outcomes following liver transplantation: acute tubular necrosis versus hepatorenal syndrome. Liver Transpl. 2012;18(5):539–48. https://doi.org/10.1002/lt.23384.
10. Williams FR, Milliken D, Lai JC, Armstrong MJ. Assessment of the frail patient with end-stage liver disease: a practical overview of sarcopenia, physical function, and disability. Hepatol Commun. 2021;5(6):923–37. https://doi.org/10.1002/hep4.1688.
11. Tandon P, Zanetto A, Piano S, Heimbach JK, Dasarathy S. Liver transplantation in the patient with physical frailty. J Hepatol. 2023;78(6):1105–17. https://doi.org/10.1016/j.jhep.2023.03.025. PMID: 37208097.
12. Bischoff SC, Bernal W, Dasarathy S, Merli M, Plank LD, Schütz T, et al. ESPEN practical guideline: clinical nutrition in liver disease. Clin Nutr. 2020;39(12):3533–62.

Chapter 5
Cardiac Issues in Liver transplantation

Dinesh Jothimani, Navin Marannan, and Karan Jain

Abstract With a rising prevalence of obesity and associated metabolic risk factors, cardiovascular disease in particular coronary artery disease, is increasingly recognized in patients for liver transplantation. Identification and management of these cardiovascular risk factors may influence post-transplant clinical outcomes. A detailed assessment of patients' cardiovascular status is therefore crucial in the decision-making of patients for liver transplantation (LT).

Patients with coronary artery disease (CAD) requires risk stratification around the perioperative and long-term postoperative periods. Advanced age, male sex, smoking, diabetes mellitus, hypertension, obesity, and non-alcoholic metabolic associated steatotic liver disease (MASLD) cirrhosis significantly increase the risk of CAD. Patients with these high-risk factors should undergo cardiac investigations with higher sensitivity to identify CAD and those with low-risk factors for CAD may undergo cardiac investigations with high specificity. Cirrhotic patients may suffer from conditions directly related to liver disease, such as cirrhotic cardiomyopathy and portopulmonary hypertension, and unrelated to liver disease, such as arrhythmias. Rarely, valvular heart disease may be identified during transplant evaluation. Clinicians managing patients for LT should carefully evaluate cardiovascular risk and treat appropriately prior to the surgery to minimize post-transplant complications. A multidisciplinary approach involving transplant physicians, anesthetists, cardiologists, and transplant surgeons is strongly recommended.

Keywords Liver transplantation · Cardiovascular system · Coronary artery disease · Valvular heart disease · Cirrhotic cardiomyopathy · Portopulmonary hypertension

---

D. Jothimani (✉) · N. Marannan · K. Jain
Institute of Liver Disease and Transplantation, Dr Rela Institute and Medical Centre, Chennai, Tamil Nadu, India
e-mail: dinesh.jothimani@relainstitute.com

S. Saigal, D. Jothimani (eds.), *Fundamentals of Transplant Hepatology*,
https://doi.org/10.1007/978-981-95-2624-6_5

Key Highlights

- Up to 40% of patients may encounter cardiovascular complications in the early post-transplant period.
- Advanced age, male sex, smoking, obesity, diabetes mellitus, hypertension, and MASLD is associated with coronary artery disease.
- Cardiac risk stratification is essential in patients for liver transplantation.
- Cirrhotic cardiomyopathy and portopulmonary hypertension should be evaluated preoperatively to reduce postoperative cardiac complications and allograft dysfunction.

5.1 Introduction

Liver transplantation (LT) is the therapeutic option for patients with end stage liver disease (ESLD). With the rising incidence of obesity and related metabolic disorders, cardiovascular disease (CVD) particularly coronary artery disease (CAD) is becoming increasingly prevalent among liver transplant candidates. The global burden of cardiovascular disease (CVD) is steadily increasing, particularly among older adults (age >50), smokers, and individuals with diabetes mellitus (DM), obesity, and other metabolic disorders. According to the CDC, approximately 523 million people worldwide are affected by CVD, especially CAD, and this number continues to grow annually [1]. In India, CAD is present in 21.4% of diabetics and 11% of non-diabetics [2].

Initially, CAD was considered less prevalent in patients with cirrhosis due to their vasodilated circulatory state, however subsequent studies have shown higher prevalence [3].

The prevalence of CAD among liver transplant candidates ranges from 2.5% to 27%, with higher rates observed in patients over 50 years old and those with diabetes [4]. Many individuals with ESLD remain unaware of their underlying cardiac conditions due to limited physical activity and reduced exercise tolerance, which often mask CAD symptoms. A retrospective study involving 1045 liver transplant candidates in South Korea revealed a greater prevalence of non-obstructive CAD among cirrhotic patients (30.6% vs. 23.4%, $P = 0.001$), emphasizing the silent nature of cardiac comorbidities in this population [5]. High-sensitivity C-reactive protein (hs-CRP), a marker commonly used to assess CAD risk, may not be elevated in cirrhotic patients due to impaired hepatic synthesis, further complicating diagnosis [6]. In addition, cirrhotic patients may present with other cardiac conditions, including cirrhotic cardiomyopathy, portopulmonary hypertension, and arrhythmias, which may be either related or unrelated to liver disease. Valvular heart disease, although less common, may also be identified during the transplant workup. Therefore, careful cardiovascular risk evaluation and timely intervention are critical to reduce post-transplant complications. A multidisciplinary team approach—involving transplant physicians, anesthesiologists, cardiologists, and transplant surgeons is highly recommended to optimize patient outcomes.

5.2 Liver Disease Etiology and CAD

Certain liver diseases appear to have a stronger association with CAD. Viral hepatitis and cholestatic disorders may not be an additional risk factor for CAD. However, the emergence of MASLD and possibly alcohol may cause additional risk. A Swedish study of 127 cirrhotic patients found that in comparison to the general population, alcohol (OR 9.5 95%CI 2.44-12.28) and age (OR 1.23 95%CI 1.06-1.43) were independent risk factors for CAD. This may be related to the sedentary lifestyle and behavioural pattern of these patients but also selection bias of the study population [7]. A meta-analysis reported a 44.6% prevalence of CAD among 67,070 patients with MASLD, particularly those with moderate to severe hepatic steatosis [8].

Interestingly, CAD prevalence in cirrhotic patients with MASLD varies by region: 70% in the USA, 34% in Japan, 21.6% in Italy, and 71.2% in Turkey [8–11]. In our study on liver transplant candidates, CAD was found in 11.9% of patients, with 57% of these cases occurring in those with MASLD [12]. Similarly, a U.S.-based transplant center identified CAD in 36.8% of 228 patients evaluated for LT, with a significantly higher prevalence (52.8%) among NASH patients [4]. These findings suggest that NASH-related cirrhosis poses the highest CAD risk compared to other liver disease etiologies.

5.3 Post-liver Transplantation Cardiac Complications

Pre-existing cardiovascular conditions can complicate outcomes following LT. A large study using logistic regression analysis on 54,697 transplant recipients reported that 2.9% of deaths occurred within 30 days post-transplant, with 42.1% due to cardiovascular causes and 27.9% due to sepsis [13]. Another study involving 5891 transplant recipients showed that 17.2% of deaths were related to CVD, nearly 40% of which happened within the first 30 days post-surgery. Overall, cardiovascular complications occur in approximately 8–40% of patients in the early post-transplant period [13, 14].

Cardiac arrhythmias such as atrial fibrillation also contributes to peri-operative cardiac events. The risk of cardiovascular events within the first year post-transplant ranges from 15% to 30%, primarily due to ischemic heart disease [15]. Long-term, liver transplant recipients are at increased risk of developing metabolic syndrome, which further aggravates their CAD risk. Among all solid organ transplant types, LT is associated with the highest incidence of metabolic syndrome, reaching up to 60% within the first year [16].

In a cohort of 455 post-transplant patients, cardiovascular events were observed in 10.6% at one year, 20.7% at 5 years, and 30.3% at 8 years post-transplant, majority of them presenting with acute coronary syndromes. MASLD (OR 3.22, 95% CI 0.97–10.63, $P = 0.055$) and post-transplant DM (OR 1.93, 95% CI 1.06–3.51, $P = 0.032$) were significantly associated with these events. Notably, elevated pre-transplant troponin levels (>0.07 ng/ml) and use of tacrolimus were also linked to CAD, even in patients without traditional risk factors [17]. A substantial number of candidates are disqualified from LT early in the evaluation process due to existing CAD.

5.4 Cardiac Risk Stratification

Patients being considered for LT should undergo cardiac risk stratification and be categorized into low- or high-risk categories. Non-modifiable risk factors for CAD include age and male gender, while modifiable ones comprise DM, hypertension (HT), obesity, MASLD, and chronic kidney disease. Additional high-risk indicators include a history of acute coronary syndrome, myocardial infarction (MI), left ventricular hypertrophy, prior coronary artery bypass grafting (CABG), and smoking. The absence of these risk factors generally places a patient in the low-risk category. Age-related CAD risk varies across studies, typically ranging from 45 to over 60 years [18]. Furthermore, individuals of South Asian ethnicity are at elevated risk of developing CAD. Experts from American college of cardiology developed atherosclerotic CVD score (ASCVD) to estimate 10 year risk of cardiovascular event or stroke. The formula is calculated using age, sex, race, cholesterol, blood pressure, diabetes and smoking. Risk score is represented in percentage 0-4.9% (low), 5-7.4% (borderline), 7.5-20% (intermediate), more than 20% (high). Treatment with statin in patients with intermediate and high scores to reduce the risk of cardiovascular events [19]. This score however may underestimate CVD risk in cirrhotics particularly at the stage when transplant is considered. Parameters such as blood pressure, blood sugar, cholesterol level are usually low due to hepatic dysfunction.

5.4.1 CAR-OLT Score

The CAR-OLT score was created using data from 1024 consecutive LT candidates to predict major cardiovascular events, defined as death from cardiovascular causes or hospitalization due to serious cardiac complications. The multivariate analysis identified significant predictors such as age, sex, employment status, education level, diabetes mellitus, hypertension, heart failure, atrial fibrillation (AF), pulmonary hypertension, respiratory failure, and hepatocellular carcinoma (HCC). Scores ranged from below 9 to over 40, correlating with an absolute cardiovascular risk of 6%, 14%, 26%, and 45% at scores of 10, 20, 30, and >40, respectively. A score exceeding 30 indicates a high risk for cardiovascular mortality [20].

5.4.2 *CAD-LT Score*

Another scoring system, the CAD-LT score, was developed from a retrospective analysis of 1771 patients at a single U.S. center. It aimed to predict significant CAD requiring surgical or percutaneous intervention. Independent predictors included older age (adjusted OR 1.05), male gender (1.69), DM (1.57), HT (1.61), tobacco use (1.01), family history of CAD (1.63), and a personal history of CAD (6.55). Risk levels were categorized as low ($\leq$2%), intermediate (3–9%), and high ($\geq$10%). The authors proposed an algorithm based on this scoring system, which identified 97% of clinically significant CAD cases while minimizing unnecessary testing. However, being a single-center, retrospective study from a Western population, the score's applicability to Asian patients requires cautious interpretation [21].

5.5 Cardiac Testing in Liver Transplant Evaluation

Cardiac assessment is a critical component of liver transplant evaluation. Testing must be tailored to each patient based on individual risk factors. Cardiac investigations are broadly divided into non-invasive and invasive types. There is considerable variability in cardiac testing protocols among transplant centers, partly due to differences in test availability and variations in sensitivity, specificity, positive predictive value (PPV), and negative predictive value (NPV). Moreover, many of these tests are inadequately validated in cirrhotic populations. Depending on the patient's risk profile, tests can be used to either rule out or detect significant CAD. Low-risk patients should undergo tests that exclude major CAD, whereas high-risk individuals should be evaluated with investigations aimed at detecting significant disease. Accurate history taking is crucial in evaluating cirrhotic patients for cardiovascular risk assessment. This involves history of chest discomfort, exertional dyspnoea including orthopnoea; although these symptoms can be observed in patients with decompensated cirrhosis particularly in the presence of ascites and hepatic hydrothorax. History of smoking along with packyears and alcohol should be elicited. History of type 2 DM and dyslipidemia should be obtained. Due to poor liver reserve most diabetic patients with advanced liver disease have normal blood sugar with significant reduction in the need for anti-diabetic drugs. History of palpitations, leg swelling syncopial episodes, history of sedentary lifestyle and occupation. Although uncommon, history of rheumatic fever during childhood as this may lead to valvular heart disease in the adulthood. History of cardiac arrhythmias, angina, myocardial infarction, coronary artery stenting and CABG may help assess baseline cardiac status of the potential liver transplant recipient. Family history of obesity, type 2 DM, hypertension dyslipidemia and coronary artery disease should be elicited as these patients have much higher risk of CVD.

Standard screening tests recommended for all LT candidates include electrocardiography (ECG) and a resting transthoracic echocardiogram. Treadmill testing (TMT), however, is generally not useful in patients with ESLD due to limited mobility, muscle wasting (sarcopenia), hepatic encephalopathy, ascites, and difficulty achieving target heart rates [22]. Younger patients (lesser than 35 years) with no risk factors for cardiovascular disease requiring liver transplantation basic investigations such as ECG, CXR and Echo may suffice and may not require stress test. This is particularly relevant in the setting of acute liver failure where the patient is considerably sicker in in the intensive care unit.

5.5.1 Dobutamine Stress Echocardiography (DSE)

DSE is a dynamic test that evaluates heart rate response, cardiac output, and overall myocardial performance under stress. It is a widely used, cost-effective, and generally safe tool for assessing LT candidates. In non-cirrhotic patients, DSE has a reported sensitivity of 85% and specificity of 77% for detecting CAD [23]. However, its diagnostic performance is diminished in ESLD patients. In one retrospective study of 105 LT candidates who underwent both DSE and coronary angiography, DSE demonstrated a sensitivity of only 13% and specificity of 85% [24], largely due to patients not achieving the target heart rate.

A meta-analysis reported pooled sensitivity and specificity of DSE for CAD diagnosis (with coronary angiography as the reference) at 28% and 82%, respectively. The estimated relative risk for major adverse cardiac events following a positive DSE was 30.2 (95% CI: 2.82–325.45), with moderate heterogeneity. For all-cause mortality, the relative risk was 4.71 (95% CI: 1.84–12.07) with low heterogeneity [25]. Another meta-analysis of seven studies involving DSE in LT candidates found sensitivity of 32%, specificity of 78%, PPV of 37%, and NPV of 75% [19]. Similar outcomes were noted in other clinical studies [26].

Several limitations reduce DSE utility in cirrhotic patients. Although it remains a valuable tool, ESLD-related pathophysiological changes can affect test accuracy. Many LT candidates are on beta-blockers, which dampen heart rate responses to dobutamine, preventing the achievement of target heart rates in 19–50% of patients. Additionally, cirrhosis-related vasodilation and elevated cardiac output hinder pharmacologic induction of myocardial ischemia. Patients' poor physical and cardiopulmonary condition further limits the effectiveness of DSE.

To improve the diagnostic yield of DSE, achieving at least 85% of the predicted maximum heart rate is essential—a challenging task in this population [27, 28]. Beta-blockers should be withheld before testing to enhance heart rate response. DSE may also be terminated early due to adverse events such as blood pressure changes, arrhythmias, or chest pain, which occur in up to 28% of patients [29, 30]. Therefore, while DSE can be a reliable screening tool to exclude CAD in low-risk patients, its predictive value in high-risk ESLD candidates is limited [31].

5.5.2 CT Coronary Artery Calcium Score (CACS)

CACS is a non-invasive tool that has demonstrated a 100% NPV for detecting clinically significant CAD [32]. The calcium score is also closely associated with the severity of arterial narrowing and plaque burden [33]. Initially developed for screening in the general population, a score above 400 Hounsfield Units (HU) has been linked to significant CAD.

In the context of LT, its utility has also been explored. For instance, Kong et al. retrospectively evaluated CACS in 443 LT candidates and found that a score >400 significantly predicted cardiovascular complications (e.g., MI and arrhythmias) within one month post-transplant (OR 4.62) [34]. Another study involving 227 adult LT recipients categorized patients into four calcium score groups: 0, 1–100, 101–400, and > 400 HU. Over a five-year follow-up, major adverse cardiac events occurred in 20.7% of patients, predominantly in those with scores >400 (HR 2.58; 95% CI 1.05–6.29) [35].

However, the reliability of CACS may be compromised by respiratory motion artifacts, the need for ECG gating, and the requirement for thin (3 mm) CT slices, especially in patients with ascites or respiratory difficulties [36]. Interestingly, calcium scores derived from standard chest CTs done for unrelated indications have also shown predictive value. In a study of 301 patients, event rates ranged from 7% to 27% depending on calcium score ($p = 0.007$) [37].

In conclusion, a CACS >400 is associated with significant CAD in LT candidates. Despite its cost-effectiveness, the exact placement of CACS within the transplant cardiac evaluation algorithm remains uncertain. It may be best suited for low-risk patients with a positive DSE or as an initial screening tool in high-risk individuals.

5.5.3 SPECT Myocardial Perfusion Imaging (SPECT-MPI)

SPECT evaluates myocardial perfusion and viability through uptake of radioactive tracers in response to adenosine-induced stress. In non-transplant populations, the test has high sensitivity (85%) and specificity (90%) [38]. However, its diagnostic accuracy is substantially reduced in liver transplant candidates.

In a study by Duvall et al., 2500 LT candidates underwent SPECT-MPI, of which 5.6% (142 patients) had abnormal findings. However, only 39% of these correlated with obstructive CAD, suggesting a high false-positive rate [39]. An earlier 2002 study with 83 patients showed a sensitivity of 37% and specificity of 63% [40]. A separate retrospective analysis of 473 LT candidates comparing adenosine SPECT to coronary angiography reported sensitivity of 62%, specificity of 82%, PPV of 30%, and NPV of 95% [41].

These findings suggest that while SPECT-MPI is not particularly effective for identifying CAD in high-risk patients, it may help exclude disease in low-risk candidates. Limitations in patients with cirrhosis include impaired coronary flow reserve, reduced microvascular circulation, chronic vasodilation, use of beta-blockers, and ascites, all of which may interfere with interpretation [42].

Emerging imaging technologies like cardiac PET are being explored for measuring coronary flow reserve in the general population, offering sensitivities of 81–89% [43]. While promising, cardiac PET has not yet been evaluated in ESLD patients.

5.5.4 Computed Tomography Coronary Angiography (CTCA)

CTCA is a non-invasive imaging modality with high sensitivity (95–99%) for diagnosing CAD in the general population [44]. Its role in liver transplant evaluations is also being recognized. In a retrospective analysis of 2118 LT candidates, CTCA detected obstructive CAD (>50% stenosis) in 21.7% of patients. Sensitivity, specificity, PPV, and NPV for post-transplant MI were 20%, 91.2%, 6.2%, and 97.5%, respectively [45].

The American Heart Association (AHA) now recommends CTCA combined with CT-derived fractional flow reserve (FFR) as a first-line, non-invasive test in high-risk LT candidates, such as those with abnormal ECGs, regional wall motion abnormalities on ECHO, or low ejection fraction. Detection of significant lesions on CTCA warrants invasive coronary angiography [46].

However, CTCA has notable limitations in ESLD patients, including ascites, renal dysfunction, and difficulties in performing FFR. It is also contraindicated in patients with contrast allergies, anaphylaxis, AF, or beta-blocker intolerance [47].

5.5.5 Invasive Coronary Angiography (CAG)

CAG is the gold standard for diagnosing CAD. The AHA recommends it for LT candidates at high cardiac risk, including those with:

Positive non-invasive stress tests indicating >10% myocardium at risk
Obstructive CAD on CTCA
Symptoms suggestive of CAD
Prior revascularization
Known CAD
Inability to undergo CTCA [46, 47]

The AASLD and EASL also support CAG in patients with suspected CAD or inconclusive non-invasive results [48, 49]. Though invasive, CAG is generally safe even in ESLD, with bleeding and contrast nephropathy risks around 2–3%. The need for dialysis post-CAG is rare (<1%) [50].

When obstructive CAD is found, further questions arise about the need for revascularization, stent type, duration of dual antiplatelet therapy, use of statins in Child-Pugh C cirrhosis, and timing of LT.

Patients with significant CAD (e.g., >70% LAD stenosis or multi-vessel disease) are often considered for revascularization prior to LT, although data on outcome benefits in asymptomatic individuals are limited [51]. One study compared 87 LT candidates who underwent CAG and coronary intervention to a matched group of 72 patients with CV risk factors but no CAG and 119 patients without CV risk. The survival rates of the revascularized group were comparable to those with non-obstructive CAD, irrespective of the number or severity of involved vessels [52]. This supports the idea that while obstructive CAD may warrant intervention, non-obstructive CAD can be managed medically [53].

5.6 Coronary Artery Stenting Prior to Liver Transplantation

Dual antiplatelet therapy (DAPT), typically comprising aspirin and a thienopyridine such as clopidogrel, is essential following coronary stent placement to prevent stent thrombosis. In cirrhotic patients, this therapy poses a significant bleeding risk due to underlying thrombocytopenia and coagulopathy. Historically, bare-metal stents (BMS) were favored, as drug-eluting stents (DES) required extended DAPT for up to 9 months.

In a study involving liver transplant patients who underwent coronary angiography, 96 had severe CAD and 55 had moderate disease. Those treated with angioplasty, stenting, or CABG prior to transplantation showed similar survival rates compared to those without CAD [54].

Recent multicenter trials involving Resolute Onyx and Xience-28 DES have shown promising results with only one month of DAPT, a significant development for patients with acute-on-chronic liver failure (ACLF) or those needing urgent transplantation [55]. In such cases, aspirin monotherapy may suffice, eliminating the need for clopidogrel.

Nevertheless, clinicians must not overlook the risks associated with PCI in cirrhotics. A meta-analysis of 28,100 cirrhotic patients undergoing PCI reported significantly higher rates of in-hospital mortality (OR 4.78), acute kidney injury (AKI, OR 3.66), stroke (OR 2.48), and gastrointestinal bleeding (OR 1.91) [56]. A multidisciplinary approach involving hepatologists, cardiologists, anesthetists, and liver surgeons is vital for safe management.

5.7 Use of Statins in Cirrhosis

Statins are well-established in both primary and secondary prevention of CAD. In cirrhotic patients, they can be used safely in Child-Pugh A and cautiously in Child-Pugh B stages. However, data are limited for their use in Child-Pugh C. Beyond lipid-lowering, statins also exhibit anti-fibrotic effects by inhibiting hepatic stellate cell activation, offering additional benefits in liver disease [57].

5.8 CABG and Liver Transplantation

The indications for CABG in LT candidates are similar to the general population. Patients with CAD unsuitable for PCI—such as those with >70% stenosis in three major vessels, double-vessel disease involving the proximal LAD, diffuse CAD, or reduced LVEF (30–50%)—should be considered for CABG.

However, in patients with advanced liver disease (Child-Turcotte-Pugh >7 or MELD >13), CABG carries a very high procedural risk and is contraindicated if done alone [58]. Although off-pump CABG has been proposed as safer, studies show no significant difference in outcomes compared to traditional on-pump surgery [59]. Combined CABG and LT has been successfully performed in select cases (off-pump CABG followed by living donor liver transplantation), but such cases are rare and not yet supported by formal guidelines [60]. This approach may be considered on a case-by-case basis depending on available expertise. Minimally invasive cardiac surgery (MICS) is an emerging option in selected patients.

5.9 Portopulmonary Hypertension (PoPH)

PoPH occurs in approximately 5–10% of patients with ESLD [61]. Elevated pulmonary artery pressure (PAP) is often due to volume overload, which typically responds well to diuretics. Symptoms like dyspnea, fatigue, and palpitations are common but nonspecific in cirrhosis.

Increased endothelin-1 levels have been implicated in PoPH pathogenesis. 2D-Echocardiography can detect elevated pulmonary artery systolic pressure (PASP) (>30 mmHg). Most commonly, high PASP in ESLD patients results from fluid overload but can also reflect true PoPH, or primary pulmonary hypertension. If PASP is elevated, right heart catheterization (RHC) is recommended to distinguish PoPH from volume overload.

Diagnostic criteria for PoPH using a right heart catheter (RHC) include:

Mean PAP >25 mmHg
Pulmonary vascular resistance ≥3 Wood units
Pulmonary capillary wedge pressure (PCWP) ≤15 mmHg
Elevated PCWP typically points to fluid overload rather than true PoPH [62].

Severity classification:

Mild: 25–<35 mmHg
Moderate: 35–<45 mmHg
Severe: ≥45 mmHg [63]

LT is safe in mild PoPH. Moderate cases require vasodilator therapy, and those responding (mPAP ≤35 mmHg) may proceed to transplant. Severe PoPH or non-responders should not be considered for LT due to poor outcomes [64].

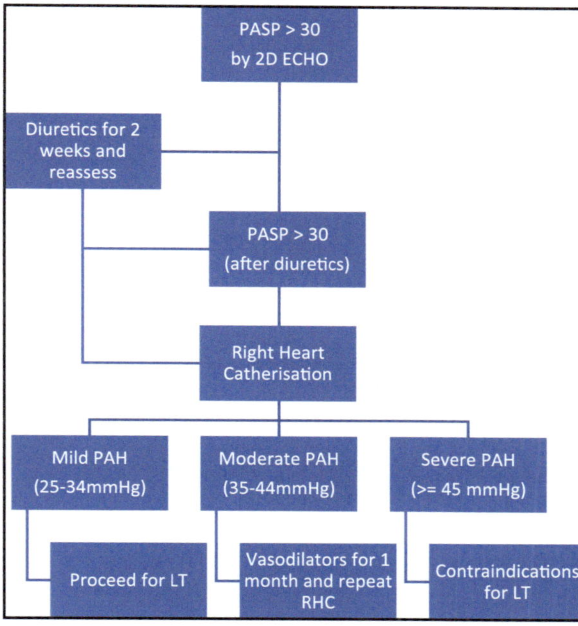

Fig. 5.1 Algorithmic approach to PoPH

Management involves collaboration with a cardiologist. Phosphodiesterase-5 (PDE5) inhibitors, such as sildenafil (20 mg TID) and tadalafil (once daily), are first-line treatments. Endothelin receptor antagonists like bosentan, ambrisentan, or macitentan serve as second-line options. Monitoring is essential, especially for bosentan, which may cause hepatotoxicity in \ ~5% of patients. A repeat RHC is necessary to confirm the reduction in PA pressure before proceeding to LT [65] (Fig. 5.1).

5.10 Cirrhotic Cardiomyopathy (CCM)

CCM is a chronic heart condition unique to cirrhosis, marked by impaired systolic and diastolic function and a blunted response to stress. It affects around 40% of ESLD patients, and its prevalence increases with disease progression, regardless of cause [63].

Patients exhibit hyperdynamic circulation, reduced myocardial contractility under stress, and often prolonged QT intervals—reflecting abnormal ventricular depolarization and repolarization. The underlying mechanism includes potassium channel dysfunction and autonomic dysregulation, leading to low systemic vascular resistance, elevated LV filling pressure, and reduced cardiac output.

Diagnostic criteria include:

Resting EF <55% or reduced response to stress
Diastolic dysfunction (E/A reversal <1, deceleration time >200 ms, IVRT >80 ms)
Prolonged QTc, elevated pro-BNP, or troponin [64]

CCM increases the risk of arrhythmias and heart failure during LT due to increased preload from portal reperfusion. While there is no definitive treatment, LT can reverse CCM over several months, though some patients may experience graft rejection or dysfunction postoperatively [66, 67]. Perioperative cardiac monitoring is essential.

5.11 Cardiac Arrhythmias

AF is the most frequent arrhythmia, observed in up to 10% of patients with ESLD [68]. Multiple factors contribute, including hemodynamic stress, CCM, sepsis, electrolyte imbalance, and systemic inflammation.

AF is associated with poor outcomes during and after LT. A meta-analysis of 38,586 patients found:

5.4% developed AF during LT
8.5% post-transplant
Pre-existing AF increased CV complications significantly (OR 5.15, 95% CI: 2.67–9.92)
New-onset AF raised mortality risk (OR 2.34, 95% CI: 1.10–5.0) [69]

5.12 Valvular Heart Disease

LT is classified as a high-risk surgical procedure, with a 6% risk of 30-day mortality, MI, or cardiac arrest, based on the Revised Cardiac Risk Index [70]. The presence of cardiovascular comorbidities, particularly valvular heart disease (VHD), further elevates this risk. For instance, severe aortic stenosis (AS) carries a 10% risk of perioperative mortality and MI in non-cardiac surgeries. Managing such patients intraoperatively becomes more complex due to the low systemic vascular resistance and cirrhotic cardiomyopathy, especially when venous return is reduced during inferior vena cava (IVC) cross-clamping [71].

Mild to moderate asymptomatic VHD is generally well tolerated in the perioperative period and does not typically contraindicate LT [72]. However, structural valvular disease may precipitate perioperative cardiac dysfunction depending on disease severity, ventricular function, and myocardial integrity.

Due to the lower prevalence of significant VHD in transplant candidates, data specific to this population remain limited. In general, mild VHD is not considered high-risk unless the patient is otherwise critically ill.

5.12.1 Aortic Stenosis (AS)

Patients with mild to moderate AS and preserved LV function may proceed to transplantation. However, individuals with severe AS (valve area $\leq$1 cm^2 or jet velocity >4 m/s), or those with symptomatic moderate AS, should undergo surgical aortic valve replacement (SAVR) or transcatheter aortic valve replacement (TAVR) before LT.

Open SAVR carries significant risk in cirrhotic patients, with postoperative mortality ranging from 17% to 26% and up to 67% mortality in Child-Pugh C patients, with a 1-year survival as low as 16% [73]. The transition to less invasive approaches like balloon valvuloplasty and TAVR has improved feasibility and outcomes. Valvuloplasty has been used successfully as a bridge to LT, with reported success rates between 26% and 74%, and 40% of patients avoiding valve replacement for up to 2 years [74].

A meta-analysis found lower in-hospital mortality with TAVR (OR 0.43) compared to SAVR in patients with chronic liver disease [75]. A propensity-matched study showed similar mortality and 30-day readmission rates between TAVR and SAVR, but TAVR was associated with shorter hospital stays [76]. However, DAPT following TAVR may delay LT. Thus, a sequential approach of valve replacement (preferably TAVR) followed by LT is currently favored [77]. Though there are reports of simultaneous AVR and LT, outcomes have been inconsistent [78, 79]. Additionally, coronary angiography is recommended in patients over 40 with AS to assess for coexisting CAD.

5.12.2 Mitral Stenosis (MS)

Patients with symptomatic moderate MS and PASP >50 mmHg, or severe MS (valve area <1 cm^2 with a mean gradient >10 mmHg), should undergo valvotomy or valve replacement, particularly when valve anatomy is unfavorable [80]. Although specific data on MS in liver transplant recipients is lacking, these general criteria are applicable.

5.12.3 Aortic Regurgitation (AR)

AR severity is assessed by comparing the AR jet width with the LV outflow tract. Severe AR, defined by a jet occupying >2/3 of the LVOT, typically warrants valve replacement. However, cardiac surgery may not be feasible in patients with decompensated cirrhosis [80].

5.12.4 Mitral Regurgitation (MR)

Significant MR is defined by:

Regurgitant orifice >0.40 cm^2
Regurgitant volume >60 mL
Regurgitant fraction >50%
Jet reaching the posterior left atrial wall
LV dilation

Mitral valve repair or replacement is advised in patients with LVEF >30%. However, these patients may not be ideal candidates for LT due to surgical risk [80].

5.12.5 Tricuspid Regurgitation (TR)

Severe TR is considered a contraindication to LT due to the risk of graft congestion and high failure rates. Treatment using minimally invasive techniques should be considered before proceeding to transplant [80].

Transthoracic echocardiography (TTE) is strongly recommended during LT evaluation to assess for VHD, supported by AHA/ACCF and AST guidelines (GRADE 1C). Mild to moderate VHD generally does not contraindicate LT [71]. However, severe AS remains a significant barrier due to poor hemodynamic stability and myocardial perfusion. Recent data indicate similar in-hospital (1.8% vs 2%) and 30-day mortality (3.2% vs 4.6%) between patients with cirrhosis undergoing SAVR and TAVR. In patients with MELD scores <12, outcomes were better with SAVR. Therefore, the MELD score may guide decision-making regarding valve surgery prior to LT [81, 82].

5.13 Congenital Heart Disease

Congenital defects like atrial or ventricular septal defects (ASD/VSD) are rare in adult LT candidates. These do not preclude transplantation unless associated with pulmonary hypertension and shunt reversal.

5.14 Heart Failure in Transplant Candidates

With increasing age among LT candidates, heart failure due to structural or valvular disease is more frequently encountered. Heart failure is categorized as:

HFrEF (Heart Failure with Reduced Ejection Fraction)
HFpEF (Heart Failure with Preserved Ejection Fraction)

5.14.1 *Systolic Heart Failure (HFrEF)*

Markedly reduced EF (<40%) is generally considered a contraindication to LT due to high perioperative mortality [83]. While no guideline specifies an EF threshold for LT candidacy, patients with severely impaired systolic function are typically excluded.

5.14.2 *Diastolic Heart Failure (HFpEF)*

Though it may not increase mortality, postoperative graft congestion is more common [83]. Current guidelines do not list diastolic dysfunction as a contraindication to LT.

The incidence of post-transplant heart failure ranges from 3% to 22%. Risk factors include:

Mean arterial pressure ≤65 mmHg
Pulmonary capillary wedge pressure ≥15 mmHg
Mean pulmonary artery pressure ≥32 mmHg [85]

In select cases, patients with advanced heart failure and cirrhosis may be considered for combined heart-LT (CHLT). CHLT is typically performed in conditions affecting both organs such as amyloidosis, hemochromatosis, familial hypercholesterolemia, and congenital heart disease with cardiac cirrhosis [86–88].

During liver graft reperfusion, cardiac output rises significantly. In patients with poor cardiac reserve, this can lead to acute heart failure or cardiac arrest, which occurs in \ ~1% of recipients. These cases have poor survival (mean 4.4 months), and interestingly, over 80% had no identifiable risk factors [89].

Here is the paraphrased version of your final section, covering cardiac contraindications, limitations of assessment, and conclusions—carefully reworded to maintain clarity, precision, and clinical integrity:

5.15 Cardiac Contraindications to Liver Transplantation

The cardiac risk associated with non-cardiac surgeries—including liver transplantation—depends on both the severity of existing cardiac conditions and the invasiveness of the procedure. Liver transplantation introduces substantial hemodynamic stress, particularly during the intraoperative period, which may exacerbate underlying cardiac conditions. Therefore, preoperative optimization of cardiovascular health is essential for improving surgical outcomes.

Absolute contraindications to LT include:

Portopulmonary hypertension (PoPH) with elevated mean pulmonary artery pressure (mPAP) that does not respond to vasodilator therapy
Uncontrolled heart failure, where cardiac function cannot be stabilized preoperatively

Relative contraindications include:

Severe CAD in patients who are not candidates for revascularization (e.g., percutaneous coronary intervention or CABG)
Symptomatic stenotic valvular lesions in individuals who cannot undergo surgical or percutaneous valve intervention
Severe regurgitant valve lesions where repair or replacement is not feasible

In such cases, proceeding with LT may present an unacceptably high perioperative risk.

5.16 Challenges in Cardiac Evaluation of Liver Transplant Candidates

Cardiac evaluation in patients with ESLD presents several unique challenges:

CAD prevalence and risk vary significantly across transplant populations
Non-invasive cardiac tests often show variable sensitivity and specificity, making interpretation difficult
ESLD patients frequently have sarcopenia, leading to attenuated test responses
Use of beta-blockers can blunt the chronotropic response during stress testing
There is no universally accepted standard for cardiac assessment in cirrhotic patients

Patients with acute liver failure (ALF) or severe ACLF are often critically ill and may be receiving multi-organ support, limiting their ability to undergo comprehensive cardiovascular testing. In these scenarios, individualized testing strategies should be employed, guided by patient-specific risk factors and determined through a multidisciplinary team approach.

5.17 Conclusion

Cardiac evaluation plays a central role in the pre-transplant workup, especially considering the high prevalence and impact of CAD in this population. However, clear guidelines for cardiac testing in ESLD patients remain lacking.

Low-risk patients should undergo tests with high specificity and NPV to rule out significant CAD.
High-risk individuals should be evaluated using tests with greater sensitivity, such as coronary angiography, to detect clinically relevant CAD.

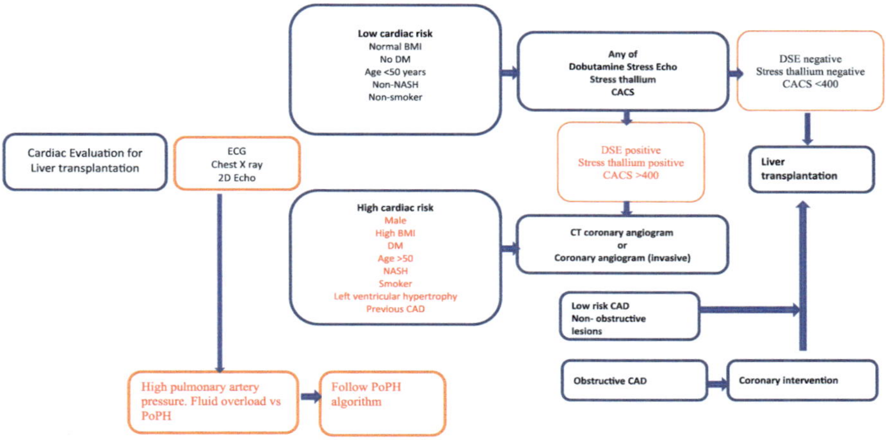

Fig. 5.2 Algorithmic approach for cardiac evaluation in liver transplant candidates

When present, obstructive CAD may benefit from revascularization. Clinicians should also be mindful of coexisting conditions such as PoPH and cirrhotic cardiomyopathy, which further complicate risk assessment.

Finally, candidates with ALF or ACLF may be too unstable for full cardiac evaluation. In such cases, decision-making should be guided by clinical judgment and team consensus, focusing on balancing urgency with patient safety.

An algorithm for cardiac evaluation in LT candidates is provided in Fig. 5.2 to guide clinical decision-making.

References

1. Roth GA, Mensah GA, Johnson CO, Addolorato G, Ammirati E, et al. Global burden of cardiovascular diseases and risk factors, 1990–2019: update from the GBD 2019 study. J Am Coll Cardiol. 2020;76:2982–3021.
2. Sreeniwas Kumar A, Sinha N. Cardiovascular disease in India: a 360 degree overview. Med J Armed Forces India. 2020;76(1):1–3.
3. Keeffe BG, Valantine H, Keeffe EB. Detection and treatment of coronary artery disease in liver transplant candidates. Liver Transpl. 2001;7(9):755–61.
4. Patel SS, Nabi E, Guzman L, Abbate A, Bhati C, et al. Coronary artery disease in decompensated patients undergoing liver transplantation evaluation. Liver Transpl. 2018;24(3):333–42.
5. An J, Shim JH, Kim S-O, Lee D, Kim KM, et al. Prevalence and prediction of coronary artery disease in patients with liver Cirrhosis. Circulation. 2014;130:1353–136.
6. An J, Shim JH, Kim SO, Lee D, Kim KM, Lim YS, Lee HC, Chung YH, Lee YS. Prevalence and prediction of coronary artery disease in patients with liver cirrhosis: a registry-based matched case-control study. Circulation. 2014;130(16):1353–62. https://doi.org/10.1161/CIRCULATIONAHA.114.009278. Epub 2014 Aug 5. PMID: 25095888.
7. Kalaitzakis E, Rosengren A, Skommevik T, Bjo¨rnsson E. Coronary artery disease in patients with liver cirrhosis. Dig Dis Sci. 2009;55:467.

8. Toh JZK, Pan X-H, Tay PWL, Ng CH, Yong JN, et al. A meta-analysis on the global prevalence, risk factors and screening of coronary heart disease in nonalcoholic fatty liver disease. Clin Gastroenterol Hepatol. 2022;20:2462.
9. Osawa K, Miyoshi T, Yamauchi K, Koyama Y, Nakamura K, et al. Nonalcoholic hepatic steatosis is a strong predictor of high-risk coronary-artery plaques as determined by multidetector CT. PLoS One. 2015;10(6):e0131138.
10. Fiorentino TV, Succurro E, Sciacqua A, Andreozzi F, Perticone F, Sesti G. Non-alcoholic fatty liver disease is associated with cardiovascular disease in subjects with different glucose tolerance. Diabetes Metab Res Rev. 2020;36(8):e3333.
11. Acikel M, Sunay S, Koplay M, Gündogdu F, Karakelleoglu S. Evaluation of ultrasonographic fatty liver and severity of coronary atherosclerosis, and obesity in patients undergoing coronary angiography. Anatol J Cardiol. 2009;9(4):273.
12. Jothimani D, Danielraj S, Narasimhan G, Kaliamoorthy I, Rajakumar A, Palaniappan K, Palanichamy S, Rammohan A, Ramachandran H, Rajalingam R, Rela M. Nonalcoholic Steatohepatitis: a rapidly increasing indication for liver transplantation in India. J Clin Exp Hepatol. 2022;12(3):908–16. https://doi.org/10.1016/j.jceh.2021.09.017. Epub 2021 Sep 25. PMID: 35677507; PMCID: PMC9168702.
13. Konerman MA, Fritze D, Weinberg RL, Sonnenday CJ, Sharma P. Incidence of and risk assessment for adverse cardiovascular outcomes after liver transplantation: a systematic review. Transplantation. 2017;101(7):1645–57. https://doi.org/10.1097/TP.0000000000001710. PMID: 28296809; PMCID: PMC5481461.
14. Koshy AN, Gow PJ, Han HC, Teh AW, Jones R, Testro A, Lim HS, McCaughan G, Jeffrey GP, Crawford M, Macdonald G, Fawcett J, Wigg A, Chen JWC, Gane EJ, Munn SR, Clark DJ, Yudi MB, Farouque O. Cardiovascular mortality following liver transplantation: predictors and temporal trends over 30 years. Eur Heart J Qual Care Clin Outcomes. 2020;6(4):243–53. https://doi.org/10.1093/ehjqcco/qcaa009. PMID: 32011663.
15. Barman PM, VanWagner LB. Cardiac risk assessment in liver transplant candidates: current controversies and future directions. Hepatology. 2021;73(6):2564–76. https://doi.org/10.1002/hep.31647. PMID: 33219576; PMCID: PMC8220582.
16. Watt KD, Charlton MR. Metabolic syndrome and liver transplantation: a review and guide to management. J Hepatol. 2010;53(1):199–206. https://doi.org/10.1016/j.jhep.2010.01.040. Epub 2010 Mar 31. PMID: 20451282.
17. Fussner LA, Heimbach JK, Fan C, Dierkhising R, Coss E, Leise MD, Watt KD. Cardiovascular disease after liver transplantation: when, what, and who is at risk. Liver Transpl. 2015;21(7):889–96. https://doi.org/10.1002/lt.24137. PMID: 25880971.
18. Tiukinhoy-Laing SD, Rossi JS, Bayram M, De Luca L, Gafoor S, Blei A, Flamm S, Davidson CJ, Gheorghiade M. Cardiac hemodynamic and coronary angiographic characteristics of patients being evaluated for liver transplantation. Am J Cardiol. 2006;98(2):178–81. https://doi.org/10.1016/j.amjcard.2006.01.089. Epub 2006 May 12. PMID: 16828588.
19. Nguyen P, Plotkin J, Fishbein TM, Laurin JM, Satoskar R, Shetty K, Taylor AJ. Dobutamine stress echocardiography in patients undergoing orthotopic liver transplantation: a pooled analysis of accuracy, perioperative and long term cardiovascular prognosis. Int J Cardiovasc Imaging. 2013;29(8):1741–8. https://doi.org/10.1007/s10554-013-0275-x. Epub 2013 Aug 23. PMID: 23974907.
20. VanWagner LB, Ning H, Whitsett M, Levitsky J, Uttal S, Wilkins JT, Abecassis MM, Ladner DP, Skaro AI, Lloyd-Jones DM. A point-based prediction model for cardiovascular risk in orthotopic liver transplantation: the CAR-OLT score. Hepatology. 2017;66(6):1968–79. https://doi.org/10.1002/hep.29329. Epub 2017 Nov 6. PMID: 28703300; PMCID: PMC5696007.
21. Rachwan RJ, Kutkut I, Timsina LR, Bou Chaaya RG, El-Am EA, Sabra M, Mshelbwala FS, Rahal MA, Lacerda MA, Kubal CA, Fridell JA, Ghabril MS, Bourdillon PD, Mangus RS. CAD-LT score effectively predicts risk of significant coronary artery disease in liver transplant candidates. J Hepatol. 2021;75(1):142–9. https://doi.org/10.1016/j.jhep.2021.01.008. Epub 2021 Jan 18. PMID: 33476745.

22. Murray KF, Carithers RL, AASLD. AASLD practice guidelines: evaluation of the patient for liver transplantation. Hepatology. 2005;41(6):1407–32. https://doi.org/10.1002/hep.20704. PMID: 15880505.
23. Fleischmann KE, Hunink MG, Kuntz KM, Douglas PS. Exercise echocardiography or exercise SPECT imaging? A meta-analysis of diagnostic test performance. JAMA. 1998;280(10):913–20. https://doi.org/10.1001/jama.280.10.913. PMID: 9739977.
24. Harinstein ME, Flaherty JD, Ansari AH, Robin J, Davidson CJ, Rossi JS, Flamm SL, Blei AT, Bonow RO, Abecassis M, Gheorghiade M. Predictive value of dobutamine stress echocardiography for coronary artery disease detection in liver transplant candidates. Am J Transplant. 2008;8(7):1523–8. https://doi.org/10.1111/j.1600-6143.2008.02276.x. PMID: 18510630.
25. Soldera J, Camazzola F, Rodríguez S, Brandão A. Cardiac stress testing and coronary artery disease in liver transplantation candidates: meta-analysis. World J Hepatol. 2018;10(11):877–86. https://doi.org/10.4254/wjh.v10.i11.877. PMID: 30533188; PMCID: PMC6280161.
26. Snipelisky D, Ray JC, Ung R, Duart M, Kauffman C, Kusumoto F. A comparison of bleeding complications between warfarin, dabigatran, and rivaroxaban in patients undergoing cryoballoon ablation. J Interv Card Electrophysiol. 2014;41(3):231–6. https://doi.org/10.1007/s10840-014-9948-1. Epub 2014 Nov 8. PMID: 25380703.
27. Snipelisky D, Levy M, Shapiro B. Utility of dobutamine stress echocardiography as part of the pre-liver transplant evaluation: an evaluation of its efficacy. Clin Cardiol. 2014;37(8):468–72. https://doi.org/10.1002/clc.22283. Epub 2014 Apr 9. PMID: 24719365; PMCID: PMC6649626.
28. Hogan BJ, Gonsalkorala E, Heneghan MA. Evaluation of coronary artery disease in potential liver transplant recipients. Liver Transpl. 2017;23(3):386–95. https://doi.org/10.1002/lt.24679. PMID: 27875636.
29. Su A, Almazan E, Sakulsaengprapha V, Shay J, Wittstein I, Hammami M, Pustavoitau A, Rizkalla N, Alqahtani S, Woreta T, Hamilton JP, Kohli R, Ottmann SE, Gurakar A, Chen PH. High coronary artery calcium score is associated with increased major adverse cardiac events after liver transplantation. Transplant Direct. 2023;9(2):e1426. https://doi.org/10.1097/TXD.0000000000001426. PMID: 36700067; PMCID: PMC9820787.
30. Gupta A, Bera K, Kikano E, Pierce JD, Gan J, Rajdev M, Ciancibello LM, Gupta A, Rajagopalan S, Gilkeson RC. Coronary artery calcium scoring: current status and future directions. Radiographics. 2022;42(4):947–67 https://doi.org/10.1148/rg.210122. Epub 2022 Jun 3. PMID: 35657766.
31. Gilstrap L, Bhatia RS, Weiner R, Dudzinski D. Dobutamine stress echocardiography: a review and update. Res Rep Clin Cardiol. 2014;5:69–81.
32. Bolick LE, Blankenhorn DH. A quantitative study of coronary arterial calcification. Am J Pathol. 1961;39(5):511–9. PMID: 13870788; PMCID: PMC1942427.
33. Breen JF, Sheedy PF 2nd, Schwartz RS, Stanson AW, Kaufmann RB, Moll PP, Rumberger JA. Coronary artery calcification detected with ultrafast CT as an indication of coronary artery disease. Radiology. 1992;185(2):435–9. https://doi.org/10.1148/radiology.185.2.1410350. PMID: 1410350.
34. Kong YG, Kang JW, Kim YK, Seo H, Lim TH, Hwang S, Hwang GS, Lee SG. Preoperative coronary calcium score is predictive of early postoperative cardiovascular complications in liver transplant recipients. Br J Anaesth. 2015;114(3):437–43. https://doi.org/10.1093/bja/aeu384. Epub 2014 Nov 21. Erratum in: Br J Anaesth. 2016;117(3):413. PMID: 25416273.
35. Zorzi A, Brunetti G, Cardaioli F, D'Arcangelo F, Fabris T, Gambato M, Iliceto S, Martini A, Mattesi G, Peluso C, Polacco M, Sartori C, Lorenzoni G, Feltracco P, Angeli P, Burra P, Cillo U, Pontisso P. Coronary artery calcium on standard chest computed tomography predicts cardiovascular events after liver transplantation. Int J Cardiol. 2021;339:219–24. https://doi.org/10.1016/j.ijcard.2021.06.046. Epub 2021 Jun 26. PMID: 34181996.
36. Parker MW, Iskandar A, Limone B, Perugini A, Kim H, Jones C, Calamari B, Coleman CI, Heller GV. Diagnostic accuracy of cardiac positron emission tomography versus single photon emission computed tomography for coronary artery disease: a bivariate meta-analysis. Circ

Cardiovasc Imaging. 2012;5(6):700–7. https://doi.org/10.1161/CIRCIMAGING.112.978270. Epub 2012 Oct 10. PMID: 23051888.
37. Duvall WL, Singhvi A, Tripathi N, Henzlova MJ. SPECT myocardial perfusion imaging in liver transplantation candidates. J Nucl Cardiol. 2020;27(1):254–65. https://doi.org/10.1007/s12350-018-1388-3. Epub 2018 Aug 23. PMID: 30141170.
38. Davidson CJ, Gheorghiade M, Flaherty JD, Elliot MD, Reddy SP, Wang NC, Sundaram SA, Flamm SL, Blei AT, Abecassis MI, Bonow RO. Predictive value of stress myocardial perfusion imaging in liver transplant candidates. Am J Cardiol. 2002;89(3):359–60. https://doi.org/10.1016/s0002-9149(01)02244-5. PMID: 11809445.
39. Bhutani S, Tobis J, Gevorgyan R, Sinha A, Suh W, Honda HM, Vorobiof G, Packard RR, Steadman R, Wray C, Busuttil R, Tseng CH. Accuracy of stress myocardial perfusion imaging to diagnose coronary artery disease in end stage liver disease patients. Am J Cardiol. 2013;111(7):1057–61. https://doi.org/10.1016/j.amjcard.2012.12.023. Epub 2013 Jan 18. PMID: 23337839.
40. Bonou M, Mavrogeni S, Kapelios CJ, Skouloudi M, Aggeli C, Cholongitas E, Papatheodoridis G, Barbetseas J. Preoperative evaluation of coronary artery disease in liver transplant candidates: many unanswered questions in clinical practice. Diagnostics (Basel). 2021;11(1):75. https://doi.org/10.3390/diagnostics11010075. PMID: 33466478; PMCID: PMC7824885.
41. Danad I, Raijmakers PG, Driessen RS, Leipsic J, Raju R, Naoum C, Knuuti J, Mäki M, Underwood RS, Min JK, Elmore K, Stuijfzand WJ, van Royen N, Tulevski II, Somsen AG, Huisman MC, van Lingen AA, Heymans MW, van de Ven PM, van Kuijk C, Lammertsma AA, van Rossum AC, Knaapen P. Comparison of coronary CT angiography, SPECT, PET, and hybrid imaging for diagnosis of ischemic heart disease determined by fractional flow reserve. JAMA Cardiol. 2017;2(10):1100–7. https://doi.org/10.1001/jamacardio.2017.2471. PMID: 28813561; PMCID: PMC5710451.
42. Deseive S, Pugliese F, Meave A, Alexanderson E, Martinoff S, Hadamitzky M, Massberg S, Hausleiter J. Image quality and radiation dose of a prospectively electrocardiography-triggered high-pitch data acquisition strategy for coronary CT angiography: the multicenter, randomized PROTECTION IV study. J Cardiovasc Comput Tomogr. 2015;9(4):278–85 https://doi.org/10.1016/j.jcct.2015.03.001. Epub 2015 Mar 12. PMID: 25926015.
43. Moon YJ, Kwon HM, Jung KW, Jeong HW, Park YS, Jun IG, Song JG, Hwang GS. Risk stratification of myocardial injury after liver transplantation in patients with computed tomographic coronary angiography-diagnosed coronary artery disease. Am J Transplant. 2019;19(7):2053–66. https://doi.org/10.1111/ajt.15263. Epub 2019 Feb 19. PMID: 30653845.
44. Cheng XS, VanWagner LB, Costa SP, Axelrod DA, Bangalore S, Norman SP, Herzog CA, Lentine KL, American Heart Association Council on the Kidney in Cardiovascular Disease and Council on Cardiovascular Radiology and Intervention. Emerging evidence on coronary heart disease screening in kidney and liver transplantation candidates: a scientific statement from the American Heart Association: endorsed by the American Society of Transplantation. Circulation. 2022;146(21):e299–324. https://doi.org/10.1161/CIR.0000000000001104. Epub 2022 Oct 17. PMID: 36252095; PMCID: PMC10124159.
45. Schönenberger E, Martus P, Bosserdt M, Zimmermann E, Tauber R, Laule M, Dewey M. Kidney injury after intravenous versus intra-arterial contrast agent in patients suspected of having coronary artery disease: a randomized trial. Radiology. 2019;292(3):664–72. https://doi.org/10.1148/radiol.2019182220. Epub 2019 Jul 2. PMID: 31264950.
46. Martin P, DiMartini A, Feng S, Brown R Jr, Fallon M. Evaluation for liver transplantation in adults: 2013 practice guideline by the American Association for the Study of Liver Diseases and the American Society of Transplantation. Hepatology. 2014;59(3):1144–65. https://doi.org/10.1002/hep.26972. PMID: 24716201.
47. European Association for the Study of the Liver. Electronic address: easloffice@easloffice.eu. EASL clinical practice guidelines: liver transplantation. J Hepatol. 2016;64(2):433–85. https://doi.org/10.1016/j.jhep.2015.10.006. Epub 2015 Nov 17. PMID: 26597456.

48. Maddur H, Bourdillon PD, Liangpunsakul S, Joseph Tector A, Fridell JA, Ghabril M, Lacerda MA, Bourdillon C, Shen C, Kwo PY. Role of cardiac catheterization and percutaneous coronary intervention in the preoperative assessment and management of patients before orthotopic liver transplantation. Liver Transpl. 2014;20(6):664–72. https://doi.org/10.1002/lt.23873. PMID: 24648247.
49. Patel SS, Lin FP, Rodriguez VA, Bhati C, John BV, Pence T, Siddiqui MB, Sima AP, Abbate A, Reichman T, Siddiqui MS. The relationship between coronary artery disease and cardiovascular events early after liver transplantation. Liver Int. 2019;39(7):1363–71. https://doi.org/10.1111/liv.14092. Epub 2019 Mar 26. PMID: 30848862; PMCID: PMC6620133.
50. Satapathy SK, Vanatta JM, Helmick RA, Flowers A, Kedia SK, Jiang Y, Ali B, Eason J, Nair SP, Ibebuogu UN. Outcome of liver transplant recipients with revascularized coronary artery disease: a comparative analysis with and without cardiovascular risk factors. Transplantation. 2017;101(4):793–803. https://doi.org/10.1097/TP.0000000000001647. PMID: 28099403; PMCID: PMC7228601.
51. Smith SC Jr, Feldman TE, Hirshfeld JW Jr, Jacobs AK, Kern MJ, King SB 3rd, Morrison DA, O'Neill WW, Schaff HV, Whitlow PL, Williams DO, Antman EM, Smith SC Jr, Adams CD, Anderson JL, Faxon DP, Fuster V, Halperin JL, Hiratzka LF, Hunt SA, Jacobs AK, Nishimura R, Ornato JP, Page RL, Riegel B, American College of Cardiology/American Heart Association Task Force on Practice Guidelines; ACC/AHA/SCAI Writing Committee to Update the 2001 Guidelines for Percutaneous Coronary Intervention. ACC/AHA/SCAI 2005 guideline update for percutaneous coronary intervention: a report of the American College of Cardiology/American Heart Association Task Force on practice guidelines (ACC/AHA/SCAI Writing Committee to update the 2001 guidelines for percutaneous coronary intervention). J Am Coll Cardiol. 2006;47(1):e1–121. https://doi.org/10.1016/j.jacc.2005.12.001. PMID: 16386656.
52. Valgimigli M, Cao D, Angiolillo DJ, Bangalore S, Bhatt DL, Ge J, Hermiller J, Makkar RR, Neumann FJ, Saito S, Picon H, Toelg R, Maksoud A, Chehab BM, Choi JW, Campo G, De la Torre Hernandez JM, Kunadian V, Sardella G, Thiele H, Varenne O, Vranckx P, Windecker S, Zhou Y, Krucoff MW, Ruster K, Zheng Y, Mehran R, XIENCE 90 and XIENCE 28 Investigators. Duration of dual antiplatelet therapy for patients at high bleeding risk undergoing PCI. J Am Coll Cardiol. 2021;78(21):2060–72. https://doi.org/10.1016/j.jacc.2021.08.074. PMID: 34794687.
53. Abraldes JG, Villanueva C, Aracil C, Turnes J, Hernandez-Guerra M, Genesca J, Rodriguez M, Castellote J, García-Pagán JC, Torres F, Calleja JL, Albillos A, Bosch J; BLEPS Study Group. Addition of Simvastatin to standard therapy for the prevention of variceal rebleeding does not reduce rebleeding but increases survival in patients with Cirrhosis. Gastroenterology. 2016;150(5):1160–1170.e3. https://doi.org/10.1053/j.gastro.2016.01.004. Epub 2016 Jan 14. PMID: 26774179.
54. Wray C, Scovotti JC, Tobis J, Niemann CU, Planinsic R, Walia A, Findlay J, Wagener G, Cywinski JB, Markovic D, Hughes C, Humar A, Olmos A, Sierra R, Busuttil R, Steadman RH. Liver transplantation outcome in patients with angiographically proven coronary artery disease: a multi-institutional study. Am J Transplant. 2013;13(1):184–91. https://doi.org/10.1111/j.1600-6143.2012.04293.x. Epub 2012 Nov 5. PMID: 23126562.
55. Simonneau G, Montani D, Celermajer DS, Denton CP, Gatzoulis MA, Krowka M, Williams PG, Souza R. Haemodynamic definitions and updated clinical classification of pulmonary hypertension. Eur Respir J. 2019;53(1):1801913. https://doi.org/10.1183/13993003.01913-2018. PMID: 30545968; PMCID: PMC6351336.
56. Khandait H, Jaiswal V, Hanif M, Shrestha AB, Iturburu A, Shah M, Ishak A, Garimella V, Ang SP, Mathew M. Percutaneous coronary intervention outcomes in patients with liver cirrhosis: a systematic review and meta-analysis. J Cardiovasc Dev Dis. 2023;10(3):92. https://doi.org/10.3390/jcdd10030092. PMID: 36975856; PMCID: PMC10059068.
57. Hoeper MM, Krowka MJ, Strassburg CP. Portopulmonary hypertension and hepatopulmonary syndrome. Lancet. 2004;363(9419):1461–8. https://doi.org/10.1016/S0140-6736(04)16107-2. PMID: 15121411.

58. Suman A, Barnes DS, Zein NN, Levinthal GN, Connor JT, Carey WD. Predicting outcome after cardiac surgery in patients with cirrhosis: a comparison of Child-Pugh and MELD scores. Clin Gastroenterol Hepatol. 2004;2:719–23. https://doi.org/10.1016/s1542-3565(04)00296-4.
59. Jiang SM, Liblik K, Baranchuk A, Payne D, El-Diasty M. CABG in patients with liver cirrhosis: to pump or not to pump? Expert Rev Cardiovasc Ther. 2022;20(2):95–9. https://doi.org/10.1080/14779072.2022.2045195. Epub 2022 Feb 23. PMID: 35188033.
60. Juneja R, Kumar A, Ranjan R, Hemantlal PM, Mehta Y, Wasir H, Vohra V, Trehan N. Combined off pump coronary artery bypass graft and liver transplant. Ann Card Anaesth. 2021;24(2):197–202 https://doi.org/10.4103/aca.ACA_194_19. PMID: 33884976; PMCID: PMC8253011.
61. Krowka MJ. Hepatopulmonary syndrome and Portopulmonary hypertension: the pulmonary vascular enigmas of liver disease. Clin Liver Dis (Hoboken). 2020;15(Suppl 1):S13–24. https://doi.org/10.1002/cld.846. PMID: 32140210; PMCID: PMC7050952.
62. European Association for the Study of the Liver. Electronic address: easloffice@easloffice.eu; European Association for the Study of the liver. EASL clinical practice guidelines for the management of patients with decompensated cirrhosis. J Hepatol. 2018;69(2):406–60. PMID: 29653741
63. Zardi EM, Abbate A, Zardi DM, Dobrina A, Margiotta D, Van Tassell BW, Afeltra A, Sanyal AJ. Cirrhotic cardiomyopathy. J Am Coll Cardiol. 2010;56(7):539–49. https://doi.org/10.1016/j.jacc.2009.12.075. Erratum in: J Am Coll Cardiol. 2010;56(12):1000. Van Tassel, Benjamin W [corrected to Van Tassell, Benjamin W]. PMID: 20688208.
64. Møller S, Henriksen JH. Cirrhotic cardiomyopathy. J Hepatol. 2010;53(1):179–90. https://doi.org/10.1016/j.jhep.2010.02.023. Epub 2010 Mar 31. PMID: 20462649.
65. Lau E, Giannoulatou E, Celermajer D, et al. Epidemiology and treatment of pulmonary arterial hypertension. Nat Rev Cardiol. 2017;14:603–14.
66. Torregrosa M, Aguadé S, Dos L, Segura R, Gónzalez A, Evangelista A, Castell J, Margarit C, Esteban R, Guardia J, Genescà J. Cardiac alterations in cirrhosis: reversibility after liver transplantation. J Hepatol. 2005;42(1):68–74.
67. Zardi EM, Zardi DM, Chin D, Sonnino C, Dobrina A, Abbate A. Cirrhotic cardiomyopathy in the pre- and post-liver transplantation phase. J Cardiol. 2016;67(2):125–30. https://doi.org/10.1016/j.jjcc.2015.04.016. Epub 2015 Jun 11. PMID: 26074443.
68. Han H, Qin Y, Yu Y, Wei X, Guo H, Ruan Y, Cao Y, He J. Atrial fibrillation in hospitalized patients with end-stage liver disease: temporal trends in prevalence and outcomes. Liver Int. 2020;40(3):674–84. https://doi.org/10.1111/liv.14291. Epub 2019 Dec 3. PMID: 31705572.
69. Chokesuwattanaskul R, Thongprayoon C, Bathini T, Ungprasert P, Sharma K, Wijarnpreecha K, Pachariyanon P, Cheungpasitporn W. Liver transplantation and atrial fibrillation: a meta-analysis. World J Hepatol. 2018;10(10):761–71. PMID: 30386469
70. Singh A. Cardiopulmonary resuscitation, Abernathy's surgical secrets. 6th ed. Mosby; 2009.
71. Kertai MD, Bountioukos M, Boersma E, et al. Aortic stenosis: an underestimated risk factor for perioperative complications in patients undergoing noncardiac surgery. Am J Med. 2004;116(1):8–13.
72. De Gasperi A, Spagnolin G, Ornaghi M, Petrò L, Biancofiore G. Preoperative cardiac assessment in liver transplant candidates. Best Pract Res Clin Anaesthesiol. 2020;34(1):51–68. https://doi.org/10.1016/j.bpa.2020.02.002. Epub 2020 Feb 18. PMID: 32334787.
73. Filsoufi F, Salzberg SP, Rahmanian PB, Schiano TD, Elsiesy H, Squire A, Adams DH. Early and late outcome of cardiac surgery in patients with liver cirrhosis. Liver Transpl. 2007;13(7):990–5. https://doi.org/10.1002/lt.21075. PMID: 17427174.
74. Nwaejike N, Mills K, Stables R, Field M. Balloon aortic valvuloplasty as a bridge to aortic valve surgery for severe aortic stenosis. Interact Cardiovasc Thorac Surg. 2015;20(3):429–35. https://doi.org/10.1093/icvts/ivu398. Epub 2014 Dec 8. PMID: 25487231.
75. Ma X, Zhao D, Li J, Wei D, Zhang J, Yuan P, Kong X, Ma J, Ma H, Sun L, Zhang Y, Jiao Q, Wang Z, Zhang H. Transcatheter aortic valve implantation in the patients with chronic liver

disease: a mini-review and meta-analysis. Medicine (Baltimore). 2020;99(16):e19766. https://doi.org/10.1097/MD.0000000000019766. PMID: 32311980; PMCID: PMC7220505.
76. Dhoble A, Chakravarty T, Nakamura M, Abramowitz Y, Tank R, Mihara H, Mangat G, Jilaihawi H, Shiota T, Makkar R. Outcome of paravalvular leak repair after transcatheter aortic valve replacement with a balloon-expandable prosthesis. Catheter Cardiovasc Interv. 2017;89(3):462–8.
77. Davari HR, Malek-Hosseini SA, Salahi H, Bahador A, Nikeghbalian S, Nemati MH, Sanjarian MA, Khosravi MB, Shahbazi S, Saberfiruzi M, Dehghani SM. Liver transplantation and aortic valve replacement. Int J Organ Transpl Med. 2011;2(1):32.
78. Giakoustidis A, Cherian TP, Antoniadis N, Giakoustidis D. Combined cardiac surgery and liver transplantation: three decades of worldwide results. J Gastrointest Liver Dis. 2011;20(4):415.
79. Lima B, Nowicki ER, Miller CM, Hashimoto K, Smedira NG, Gonzalez-Stawinski GV. Outcomes of simultaneous liver transplantation and elective cardiac surgical procedures. Ann Thorac Surg. 2011;92(5):1580–4.
80. Nishimura RA, Otto CM, Bonow RO, Carabello BA, Erwin JP 3rd, Guyton RA, O'Gara PT, Ruiz CE, Skubas NJ, Sorajja P, Sundt TM 3rd, Thomas JD, ACC/AHA Task Force Members. 2014 AHA/ACC guideline for the management of patients with valvular heart disease: executive summary: a report of the American College of Cardiology/American Heart Association Task Force on practice guidelines. Circulation. 2014;129(23):2440–92. https://doi.org/10.1161/CIR.0000000000000029. Epub 2014 Mar 3. Erratum in: Circulation. 2014;129(23):e650. PMID: 24589852.
81. Filsoufi F, Salzberg SP, Rahmanian PB, Schiano TD, Elsiesy H, Squire A, Adams DH. Early and late outcome of cardiac surgery in patients with liver cirrhosis. Liver Transpl. 2007;13(7):990–5. https://doi.org/10.1002/lt.21075. PMID: 17427174
82. Peeraphatdit TB, Nkomo VT, Naksuk N, Simonetto DA, Thakral N, Spears GM, Harmsen WS, Shah VH, Greason KL, Kamath PS. Long-term outcomes after Transcatheter and surgical aortic valve replacement in patients with cirrhosis: a guide for the hepatologist. Hepatology. 2020;72(5):1735–46. https://doi.org/10.1002/hep.31193. Epub 2020 Oct 15. PMID: 32080875.VHD.
83. Fatima I, Jahagirdar V, Kulkarni AV, Reddy R, Sharma M, Menon B, Reddy DN, Rao PN. Liver transplantation: protocol for recipient selection, evaluation, and assessment. J Clin Exp Hepatol. 2023;13(5):841–53. https://doi.org/10.1016/j.jceh.2023.04.002. Epub 2023 Apr 17. PMID: 37693258; PMCID: PMC10483012.
84. Xu ZD, Xu HT, Li WW, Zou Z, Shi XY. Influence of preoperative diastolic dysfunction on hemodynamics and outcomes of patients undergoing orthotopic liver transplantation. Int J Clin Exp Med. 2013;6(5):351–7.
85. Qureshi W, Mittal C, Ahmad U, et al. Clinical predictors of post-liver transplant new-onset heart failure. Liver Transpl. 2013;19(7):701–10.
86. Careddu L, Zanfi C, Pantaleo A, Loforte A, Ercolani G, Cescon M, Alvaro N, Pilato E, Marinelli G, Pinna AD. Combined heart-liver transplantation: a single-center experience. Transpl Int. 2015;28(7):828–34. https://doi.org/10.1111/tri.12549. Epub 2015 Mar 9. PMID: 25711771.
87. Gong T, Hall S. Considerations and experience driving expansion of combined heart-liver transplantation. Curr Opin Organ Transplant. 2020;25(5):496–500. https://doi.org/10.1097/MOT.0000000000000804. PMID: 32796180.
88. Rizvi SSA, Challapalli J, Maynes EJ, Weber MP, Choi JH, O'Malley TJ, Entwistle JW, Morris RJ, Samuels LE, Massey HT, Tchantchaleishvili V. Indications and outcomes of combined heart-liver transplant: a systematic review and met-analysis. Transplant Rev (Orlando). 2020;34(2):100517. https://doi.org/10.1016/j.trre.2019.100517. Epub 2019 Nov 22. PMID: 31831325.
89. Aufhauser DD Jr, Rose T, Levine M, Barnett R, Ochroch EA, Aukburg S, Greenblatt E, Olthoff K, Shaked A, Abt P. Cardiac arrest associated with reperfusion of the liver during transplantation: incidence and proposal for a management algorithm. Clin Transpl. 2013;27(2):185–92 https://doi.org/10.1111/ctr.12052. Epub 2012 Dec 27. PMID: 23278482.

Chapter 6
Monitoring and Preoperative Optimization of the Patient Awaiting Liver Transplantation

Akash Roy and Sanjiv Saigal

Abstract Liver transplantation (LT) is the ultimate therapeutic option for patients with life-limiting liver disease in the setting of advanced decompensated cirrhosis. While rapid strides have been made in LT surgery, adequate pre-operative optimization is one of the cornerstones for successful post-operative outcomes. Adequate pre-operative optimization entails managing conventional decompensation, nutritional rehabilitation, prevention of infections, and cardiopulmonary adequacy optimization. The optimization must be detailed and simultaneously spread across multiple axes, with a special focus on active surveillance for infection and risk stratification in the subgroup with acute on chronic liver failure (ACLF). In selected subgroups, transjugular intrahepatic portosystemic shunt (TIPSS) needs to be carefully considered in patients with recurrent portal hypertensive bleeding and refractory ascites. Renal failure has grave underpinnings in outcomes, and close attention to nephrotoxic stewardship needs to be paid. Evaluation and pragmatic strategies for transplant-listed patients' immunization need to be translated better into practice.

Keywords Liver transplant · Decompensation · Rehabilitation · Optimization · Nutrition · Cardiopulmonary

A. Roy
Institute of Gastrosciences and Liver Transplantation, Apollo Multispeciality Hospitals, Kolkata, West Bengal, India

S. Saigal (✉)
Hepatology and Liver Transplant Medicine, Max Institute of Liver and Gastrointestinal Sciences, Max Super Speciality Hospital, Saket, New Delhi, India
e-mail: sanjivsaigal@hotmail.com

S. Saigal, D. Jothimani (eds.), *Fundamentals of Transplant Hepatology*,
https://doi.org/10.1007/978-981-95-2624-6_6

Key Highlights

- Individuals with advanced cirrhosis are complex, and mandate optimization across multiple axes ranging from classical decompensations, nutrition, cardiopulmonary, and haemodynamic disturbances to active surveillance for infection and risk stratification in the subgroup with acute on chronic liver failure (ACLF).
- For classic decompensations (ascites, variceal haemorrhage, hepatic encephalopathy), close attention needs to be provided to medication adherence, dose optimization, and primary/secondary prophylaxis strategies.
- Transjugular intrahepatic portosystemic shunt (TIPSS) needs to be carefully considered in patients with recurrent portal hypertensive bleeding and refractory ascites.
- Hyponatraemia management has unique challenges and needs consideration of the acuity of need for correction as post-LT outcomes are impacted by the same.
- There is a global agreement to screen for malnutrition. A recommended total energy intake of 30–35 kcal/kg/d and a protein intake of 1.2–1.5 g/kg/d are desirable.
- Nephrotoxic stewardship needs to be carefully aimed at preserving renal function by stoppage of NSBB in advanced refractory ascites, avoidance of nephrotoxic drugs, avoiding overzealous diuresis, and excessive use of laxatives. Close monitoring for serial changes in creatinine clearance in patients with AKD.
- Cardiopulmonary optimization is a key determinant of better post-LT outcomes.
- Identification of infections early, aggressive approach to treating infections, and pragmatic immunization of LT candidates improve outcomes.

Liver transplantation (LT) is the ultimate therapeutic option for patients with life-limiting liver disease in the setting of advanced decompensated cirrhosis [1]. While rapid strides have been made in the domains of LT surgery, one of the cornerstones for successful post-operative outcome is adequate pre-operative optimization [2]. The complexity of a patient with advanced cirrhosis mandates optimization across multiple axes ranging from classical decompensations, nutrition, cardiopulmonary, and haemodynamic disturbances to active surveillance for infection and risk stratification in in the subgroup with acute on chronic liver failure (ACLF). Besides pre-operative optimization, patients listed for LT also need close monitoring as minor deviations from an optimized status lead to rapid downhill progress ultimately precluding LT and leading to enhanced morbi-mortality. In the following sections, we describe the principles of approaches towards pre-operative optimization and monitoring of patients awaiting LT specifically focused on *conventional decompensations, nutrition, cardiopulmonary stabilization, infection screen, and few special considerations.* Figure 6.1 provides an overview of key elements of care in monitoring and pre-optimization.

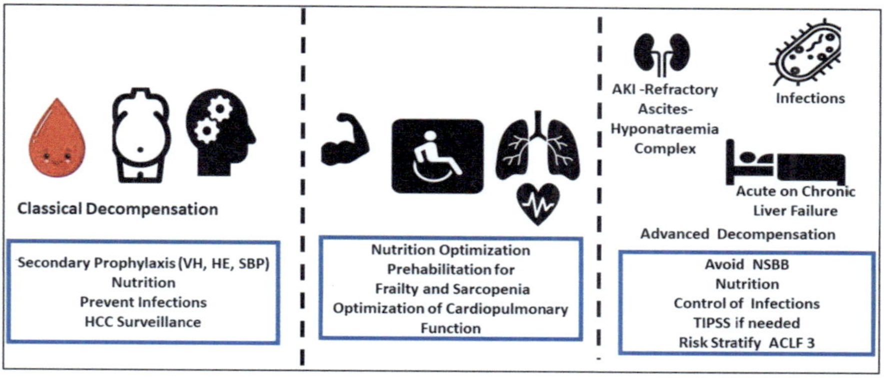

Fig. 6.1 Overview of elements in monitoring and pre-optimization of patients awaiting liver transplantation

6.1 Conventional Decompensations

Ascites, hepatic encephalopathy (HE), and variceal haemorrhage (VH) form the cornerstone of decompensation for any patient with cirrhosis. For any potential recipient awaiting LT, adequate optimization of each entity is essential.

Primary and secondary prophylaxis of HE using *lactulose alone or in combination with rifaximin* along with maintaining adequate nutrition form the standard strategy [3]. Assuring medication compliance and novel strategies like *Bristol stool chart* directed stool optimization and remote monitoring through *artificial intelligence aided smartphone* applications can aid in optimization and prevent frequent re-admissions [4, 5]. Those presenting with acute overt encephalopathy of higher grades (≥3 West Haven Scale) may benefit from *intravenous L-ornithine L-aspartate*, but the use of branched-chain amino acids and oral intravenous L-ornithine L-aspartate remains controversial [6, 7]. Patients with established HE or minimal HE are at *risk for falls* and should be educated about the implications while on wait-list with careful caregiver discussions [8].

Bleeding from oesophageal and gastric varices may prove catastrophic for LT recipients. Primary prophylaxis with *endoscopic therapy or non-selective beta blockers (NSBB)* and secondary prophylaxis using both endoscopic optimization and NSBB should be adequately achieved and monitored in check listed fashion while awaiting LT. For bleeding refractory to standard therapy, *emergency rescue transjugular intrahepatic portosystemic shunt (TIPSS)* is desirable [9]. Pre-LT TIPSS has been shown to be safe and is successfully used as a bridge to LT. The performance of TIPSS prior to LT is not a hindrance to LT and is associated with excellent outcomes [10].

Ascites and spontaneous bacterial peritonitis (SBP) management form one of the significant challenges in optimizing LT candidates. While uncomplicated ascites is relatively easily managed with *diuretic dose optimization*, recurrent and refractory ascites remain challenging, For recurrent ascites, besides diuretics, *long-term weekly intravenous albumin* administration has been shown to be beneficial [11]. The use of *midodrine* as an add-on agent to albumin has been shown to be controversial but is frequently used [12]. Use of simple tests like *urine sodium and potassium ratio* aids to assess diuretic responsiveness and may indicate progression to refractoriness with those having urine sodium <10 meQ/l frequently being diuretic refractory [13]. Once refractory ascites has set in, it is prudent to optimize patients on waitlist by *withholding further diuretics and avoiding non-selective beta blockers*, balancing the risk-benefit ratio. Long-term albumin on a weekly basis till transplant with or without midodrine may prove beneficial to be able to reach to LT. *Hyponatraemia* is a frequent complication in those having established refractory ascites. While free water restriction remains the first choice, it is often not completely therapeutic alone. Intravenous albumin and vaptans have shown to have some benefit [14]. Hyponatraemia in an imminent transplant candidate is detrimental and affects post-LT outcomes. LT awaiting patients with severe hyponatremia tended to have a longer stay in the ICU (median = 4.5 days) and hospital (17.0 days) compared to normo-natremic recipients (median ICU stay = 3.0 days, hospital stay = 14.0 days; $P = 0.02$ and 0.08, respectively) with an incidence of central pontine myelinolysis of 0.5% [15]. The challenges can be mitigated by measures to carefully increase the sodium levels pre-transplant with the use of water restriction, hypokalaemia correction, and administration of vaptans, albumin, or 3% saline [16]. While elective LTs allow time for the correction, emergency LT often pose a challenge. An approach to correction is shown in Fig. 6.2.

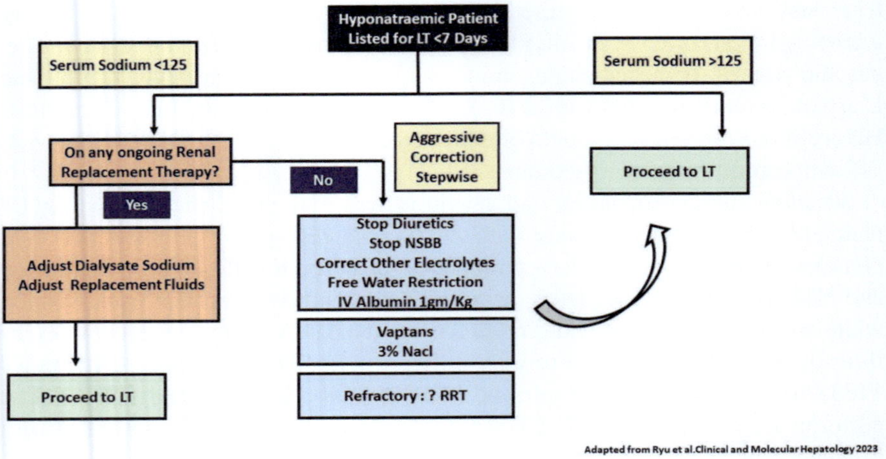

Fig. 6.2 Approach to patients with hyponatraemia and imminent LT

6.1.1 Nutrition

Malnutrition and sarcopenia are independent predictors of post-transplant infections, increased length of hospital stay, and 1-year post-transplant mortality [17]. The rates of complications further increase when severely sarcopenic patients receive suboptimal grafts [17]. Optimization of nutrition has long been an Achilles heel in LT candidates. *There is a global agreement to screen for malnutrition. A recommendation of total energy intake of 30–35 kcal/kg/d and a protein intake of 1.2–1.5 g/kg/d is desirable* [18, 19]. Standard nutrition regimens according to local dietary patterns are recommended. Specialized regimens (including BCAA-enriched, immune-enhancing diets) have not demonstrated superiority as opposed standard recommendations [20].

The challenges in nutritional optimization however are manifold. A granular analysis of available *literature has not shown robust evidence-based data on the impact of nutritional optimization.* A systematic review of seven studies including randomized trials showed no appreciable difference in mortality; post-transplant complication rate was noted across the studies [21]. Few studies have reported mortality outcomes. Plank and colleagues showed 98% 1-year survival in immunonutrition group in comparison to the 100% in the control groups, whereas Le Cornu et al. showed 95% survival in the supplementation group versus 82.5% survival in the control group, neither of which translate to statistical significance [22, 23]. Compared to mortality outcomes, literature is stronger for the impact of malnutrition on length of hospital stay. The analysis showed a trend towards reduced length of stay in those with lesser degrees of malnutrition. Based upon the available data, the panel of experts *suggests low-quality evidence* for short-term survival (within 90 days after transplant), post-operative complication, and moderate evidence for length of stay *for the impact of change in nutritional parameters pre-transplant* [21]. Based upon the available evidence, it would be prudent to *continue nutritional supplementation* according to available guidelines in all LT candidates, although *decision of undergoing transplant may not be only driven by the degree of malnutrition.*

Similar to sarcopenia, *frailty* before transplant has been shown to be an independent predictor of post-LT mortality even after adjusting for body mass index. Frail patients have higher odds of prolonged LT overall stay and ICU stay [24]. However, literature on pre-habilitation prior to LT is limited. In a recent two-arm pilot randomized trial, Serper and colleagues evaluated the feasibility and efficacy of a 14-week behavioural intervention to promote physical activity prior to LT in 30 (intervention, n = 20; control, N = 10). End-of-study step counts were nearly 1000 steps higher for intervention group, and on an average, the intervention group achieved daily step targets 51% of the time [25]. Similarly, another study showed that home-based nutritional and exercise recommendations improved both frailty and sarcopenia. However, it would be of interest to see in future studies to assess the impact of such pre-habilitation regimens on transplant outcome [26]. In line with continuation of nutritional improvement, physical activity and tailored exercise programs should be advocated in LT candidates for optimization.

6.1.2 Monitoring and Optimization of Renal Dysfunction

The impact of renal dysfunction on post-transplant outcomes has long been established supported by seminal works of Nair et al. who showed that renal failure was an independent predictor of 1-month and 2-year mortality after adjusting for multiple factors. A creatinine clearance of <40 mL/min significantly predicted lower short-term and long-term graft and patient survival rates [27]. While *hepatorenal syndrome* is often thought as being synonymous with renal dysfunction in cirrhosis, it is important to look for rule out *other causes like glomerular pathologies, acute tubular necrosis, and cholaemic nephropathy.* While vasoconstrictors provide the best solution in HRS, indiscriminate use of the same may be harmful in non-HRS AKI and is associated with cardiopulmonary risks [28]. It is key to optimize associated contributors like stoppage of NSBB in advanced refractory ascites, *avoidance of nephrotoxic drugs, avoiding overzealous diuresis, and excessive use of laxatives.* Close monitoring for *serial changes in creatinine clearance in patients with AKD* to understand regression or progression to CKD which may change transplant options towards combined liver kidney transplant is mandated. While on the waitlist, TIPSS have been attempted in HRS-AKI with debatable results. An ongoing multicentric randomized trial (Liver-HERO) should provide further evidence for the *role of TIPSS in HRS-AKI* [29].

Renal replacement therapy (RRT), in the form of continuous renal replacement therapy (CRRT) or haemodialysis (HD), is often resorted to in the peri-operative course of LT patients with renal dysfunction or chronic kidney disease. While for immediate optimization, pre-LT RRT is often unavoidable; a recent study demonstrates the importance of being able to take patients off RRT prior to post-LT. In a single centre experience, Fukumitsu et al. analysed 35 patients who were initiated on HD for AKI within 50 days before LDLT for acute renal failure, of which 29 (82.9%) successfully withdrew from HD after LDLT and demonstrated better prognosis (1-year OS, 69.0% vs. 16.7%) than those who continued HD [30]. Overall, RRT prior to LT, in patients without advanced CKD or ESRD, leads to longer IC stay, although the 180-day survival estimates are comparable to those not requiring RRT [31]. Therefore, in the appropriate setting, RRT is required to stabilize and optimize patients in selected cases although a close watch is required for SLKT candidacy.

6.1.3 Optimization of Porto Pulmonary Hypertension and Hepatopulmonary Syndrome

PoPH and HPS represent two unique challenges in a potential LT recipient. The screening for PoPH starts with non-invasive echocardiography surrogates indicated by *right ventricle systolic pressure* estimation. If echocardiography estimated pulmonary arterial pressures are >45 mmHg, cardiac catheterization and right heart studies are indicated. The diagnosis of PoPH is made based upon a *mean pulmonary artery pressure (m PAP) of >25 mmHg and pulmonary vascular resistance (PVR) >240 dyne/s/cm*$^{-5}$ *(>3 Wood Units)* [32]. However, it is important that this is established in the presence of a normal central venous pressure and pulmonary wedge pressure to exclude secondary causes like volume overload. It is important to classify PoPH as *mild (m PAP 25–35 mmHg), moderate (m PAP 35–45 mmHg), and severe (mPAP >45 mmHg)* as management approach and optimization varies. Patients with persistent severe PH with right ventricular failure are contraindicated for LT. Those with *moderate PoPH should first undergo a trial of pulmonary vasodilators* and taken for LT if responsive with sustained mPAP <35 [32, 33]. Moderate PoPH non-responsive to medical treatment constitutes a relative contraindication to LT [33].

HPS, on the other hand, should always be on the differential in patients with cirrhosis and hypoxia. The diagnosis, however, relies on carefully excluding other causes (hydrothorax, atelectasis, Syn pneumonic effusions). The diagnosis is established by *contrast-enhanced echocardiography* ('bubbling') to demonstrate *intrapulmonary shunting*. Unlike severe PoPH HPS is not a contraindication for LT and rather serves as MELD exception. However, therapy centres around oxygen supplementation. *High-inspiratory* O_2 *supplementation* is the first-line measure during LT in case of hypoxemia. Therefore, the response to high O_2 concentration should be evaluated before LT for ensuring intraoperative optimization [33].

6.1.4 Cardiovascular Optimization

Optimization of cardiac status prior to LT poses one of the key challenges for improved post-LT outcomes. Intraoperative challenges due to unique cardiovascular alterations in cirrhosis of high cardiac output and low systemic vascular resistance pose varied challenges. In addition to that multiple factors like acute blood loss, markedly reduced venous return, prolonged and resistant vasoplegia after graft reperfusion, massive transfusion, and acute right or left ventricular overload make pre-operative optimization a key goal [33]. Additionally, cardiac disease may have many shades in LT candidates ranging from *coronary artery disease, cirrhotic cardiomyopathy (CCM), arrhythmias and other structural heart disease.* Recently, important risk stratification scores including the *Framingham Risk Score (FRS) and coronary artery disease in LT score (CAD-LT)* have been validated to risk stratify LT candidates with excellent accuracy. When using FRS, scores ≥35% should be triaged towards cardiac catheterization as initial test of coronary artery disease, while those <35% can proceed towards stress testing [34]. Similarly, while using CAD-LT score, patients falling in high risk should directly proceed to cardiac catheterization and necessary intervention prior to LT for optimization. Recent data re-enforces the dictum that aggressive CAD screening with catheterization is associated with low rate of myocardial infarction and cardiac mortality [35]. For those at lower risk, spectrum although stress testing has been a commonly used test, the increasing use of *coronary artery calcium score* (CACS) and *coronary computed tomography angiography* (CCTA) have been shown to outperform nuclear tests [36]. Therefore, use risk stratification models, classifying into categories of risk and using strategies like CCTA and CACS first or direct catheterization may optimize post-LT outcomes.

Post-LT heart failure is influenced by multiple factors, including intraoperative transfusion of >11 units of packed red blood cells, presence of pre-transplant regional wall motion abnormalities, and those satisfying the updated diagnostic criteria for CCM being independent predictors. Moreover, as MASLD becomes the predominant aetiology and the median age of LT recipients increases, the incidence of HF is expected to increase. The management of patients with CCM remains a challenge. While *non-selective beta blockers* show benefit in the earlier stages, using NSBB in advanced cirrhosis in the setting of the vicious cycle of refractory ascites and hepatorenal syndrome may prove detrimental [37]. A recent study shows the use of *ivabradine in combination with carvedilol* to improve diastolic dysfunction [38]. However, further studies are mandates to establish efficacy. A specific challenge in cirrhosis is the restricted use if first-line cardiac remodelling drugs like angiotensin receptor blocker and angiotensin receptor/neprilysin inhibitor especially in the setting of established or impending renal dysfunction. Hence the optimization of patients awaiting LT with CCM primarily revolves around careful use of beta blocker in combination with ivabradine and haemodynamic stabilization. Regular involvement of cardiologist in the management of the complex physiology is mandated [33].

Arrhythmias especially atrial fibrillation have been shown to predict but worse perioperative outcomes [39]. *Appropriate anticoagulation strategies with warfarin or directly acting anticoagulants (DOACs)* need to be employed in those at risk of cerebrovascular events. DOACS have been shown to have lower risk than warfarin although the literature is sparse and emerges out of retrospective studies. A nationwide registry demonstrated that in comparison to warfarin, the risk of hospitalization for major bleeding is lower with DOACs as a class (HR, 0.69 [95% CI, 0.58–0.82]), apixaban (HR, 0.60 [95% CI, 0.46–0.78]), and rivaroxaban (HR, 0.79 [95% CI, 0.62–1.0], although this includes all-comers chronic liver disease and not those with advanced decompensated cirrhosis [40].

Lastly, cardiopulmonary endurance evaluation also helps to stratify patients prior to LT. *Cardiopulmonary exercise testing (CPET)* and the *6-min walk test* are reliable tests for cardiopulmonary endurance and to identify the degree of physical deconditioning. Additionally, assessment of metabolic equivalent of tasks through objective tools like *Duke Activity Status Index* may further aid in determining efforts for endurance optimization [33].

6.2 Identifying and Optimization of Sepsis

Pre-operative infections and sepsis are important determinants of post-transplant outcomes. Standard scores like SOFA, qSOFA, and presence of fever can predict microbiologically proven infections and should be treated aggressively [41]. Primary and secondary prophylaxis for SBP as per current guidelines should be instituted although debate remains about increased risk of MDRO and fungal infections in patients on prophylaxis [42]. Recent SBP when managed appropriately prior to LT does not seem to affect post-LT outcomes [43]. Similarly for overall infections, a recent large study highlights that although pre-LT infections increase the risk of post-LT infections, post-LT survival rates are excellent despite the risk [44]. The implications of such findings are not to delay LT because of concerns of pre-LT infections, but instead to actively monitor these patients pre- and post-LT [44].

6.3 Use of Liver Support Therapies

Unlike renal transplant, the Achilles heel of LT remains the lack of robust mechanisms to support a failing liver with artificial liver support devices. Previous trials with assist systems like Molecular Adsorbent Recirculating System have not gained popularity. *Plasma-exchange (PL-Ex)* has been shown to be helpful initially in ALF as a bridge to LT and recently for acute on chronic liver failure both as means to improve waitlist survival and act as a bridge [45–48]. While high volume PL-Ex was the initial norm, recent studies have demonstrated the safety of low and standard volume PL-Ex [49]. Questions and need for further data on timing of initiation to provide the maximum benefit, duration, and impact beyond the immediate short term, however, remain. *CRRT* has been shown to have good outcomes in ALF, and recent data also suggests its emerging role in patients with ACLF not meeting standard criteria like severe metabolic acidosis, uncorrectable dyselectrolytemia, and anuria. However, akin to PL-Ex, further data on timing of initiation to provide the maximum benefit, duration, and long-term impact is required to expand indications beyond conventional parameters. An emerging frontier looms with an upcoming system of liver dialysis known as *DIALIVE*, a novel extracorporeal liver support device to specifically address the pathophysiological derangements central to the development of ACLF by replacing dysfunctional albumin and removing pathogen- and damage-associated molecular patterns. In a pivotal phase II clinical trial, DIALIVE was safe and led to a faster time to the resolution of ACLF [50]. In the context of optimizing patients prior to LT, each of these entities may find a unique role especially in the sicker cohort of ACLF, thus expanding the eligible pool of ALF patients for LT.

6.4 Optimization and Monitoring of Acute on Chronic Liver Failure

Patients with ACLF pose a special challenge towards monitoring and optimization to LT. Inherently, the syndrome encompasses high mortality and selection of patients is of prime importance. Patients with ACLF Grade I and II are usually optimal for

LT but need close monitoring along all axes described above, as well as case-based use of liver support therapies while awaiting LT. ACLF Grade 3 forms the most challenging population with worse outcomes. Use of recently described scores like the *TAM score (age, lactate, mechanical ventilation, leucocytosis)* helps in stratifying this population into a *high-risk group (score >2) from a low-risk group (score ≤2)* with 1-year survival of 8.3% versus 83.9%, respectively. For high-risk groups, further optimization, downstaging of organ failures, control of infection, and inflammatory surges should be the foremost strategy [51].

6.5 Immunization

Patients with end-stage liver disease and LT recipients remain at high risk for vaccine-preventable infections in the pre- and post-LT period, and recommendations suggest inactivated vaccines to be given 2 weeks and live vaccines 4 weeks prior to LT to maximize response and safely proceed with immunosuppression.

6.6 Conclusion

Managing potential LT recipients requires close monitoring and goal-directed optimization. A collaborative and multidisciplinary effort of various transplant stakeholders is essential. A comprehensive assessment and individualized monitoring is essential to reach optimal LT outcomes.

References

1. Mahmud N. Selection for liver transplantation: indications and evaluation. Curr Hepatol Rep [Internet]. 2020 [cited 2024 Feb 19];19(3):203–12. Available from: https://link.springer.com/article/10.1007/s11901-020-00527-9.
2. Williams AM, Waits S, Englesbe MJ. The importance of prehabilitation in liver transplantation. Curr Transplant Rep [Internet]. 2015 [cited 2024 Feb 19];2(4):312–5. Available from: https://link.springer.com/article/10.1007/s40472-015-0080-7.
3. Bajaj JS, Lauridsen M, Tapper EB, Duarte-Rojo A, Rahimi RS, Tandon P, et al. Important unresolved questions in the management of hepatic encephalopathy: an ISHEN consensus. Am J Gastroenterol [Internet]. 2020 [cited 2024 Feb 19];115(7):989–1002. Available from: https://journals.lww.com/ajg/fulltext/2020/07000/important_unresolved_questions_in_the_management.10.aspx.
4. Duong NK, Shrestha S, Park D, Shahab O, Fagan A, Malpaya Z, et al. Bristol Stool Scale as a determinant of hepatic encephalopathy management in patients with cirrhosis. Am J Gastroenterol [Internet]. 2022 [cited 2024 Feb 19];117(2):295–300. Available from: https://journals.lww.com/ajg/fulltext/2022/02000/bristol_stool_scale_as_a_determinant_of_hepatic.21.aspx.

5. Fagan A, Gallagher ML, Mousel T, Davis BC, Fuchs M, Puri P, et al. AI evaluation of stool quality guides management of hepatic encephalopathy using a Smartphone App. Am J Gastroenterol [Internet]. 2023 [cited 2024 Feb 19]; Available from: https://journals.lww.com/ajg/fulltext/9900/artificial_intelligence_evaluation_of_stool.970.aspx.
6. Jain A, Sharma BC, Mahajan B, Srivastava S, Kumar A, Sachdeva S, et al. L-ornithine L-aspartate in acute treatment of severe hepatic encephalopathy: a double-blind randomized controlled trial. Hepatology [Internet]. 2022 [cited 2024 Feb 19];75(5):1194–203. Available from: https://pubmed.ncbi.nlm.nih.gov/34822189/.
7. Montagnese S, Rautou PE, Romero-Gómez M, Larsen FS, Shawcross DL, Thabut D, et al. EASL Clinical practice guidelines on the management of hepatic encephalopathy. J Hepatol [Internet]. 2022 [cited 2024 Feb 19];77(3):807–24. Available from: http://www.journal-of-hepatology.eu/article/S0168827822003464/fulltext.
8. Tapper EB, Nikirk S, Parikh ND, Zhao L. Falls are common, morbid, and predictable in patients with cirrhosis. J Hepatol [Internet]. 2021 [cited 2024 Feb 19];75(3):582–8. Available from: https://pubmed.ncbi.nlm.nih.gov/33887359/.
9. Garcia-Tsao G, Sanyal AJ, Grace ND, Carey WD. ACG & AASLD joint clinical guideline: prevention and management of gastroesophageal varices and variceal hemorrhage in cirrhosis. Am J Gastroenterol. 2007;102:2086–102.
10. Gonzales P, Dhanasekaran R, West J, Subramanian R, Parekh S, Spivey JR, et al. Influence of transjugular intrahepatic portosystemic shunt in patients awaiting orthotopic liver transplant on post-transplant outcome. Gastrointest Interv. 2012;1(1):69–73.
11. Caraceni P, Riggio O, Angeli P, Alessandria C, Neri S, Foschi FG, et al. Long-term albumin administration in decompensated cirrhosis (ANSWER): an open-label randomised trial. Lancet [Internet]. 2018 [cited 2024 Feb 19];391(10138):2417–29. Available from: http://www.thelancet.com/article/S0140673618308407/fulltext.
12. Kulkarni A V., Premkumar M, Reddy DN, Rao PN. The challenges of ascites management: an Indian perspective. Clin Liver Dis [Internet]. 2022 [cited 2024 Feb 19];19(6):234. Available from: /pmc/articles/PMC9248925/.
13. Lee JW, Hwang JS, Chung WJ, Lee HJ, Park JG, Lee CH, et al. Diagnostic usefulness of the spot urine sodium/potassium ratio in cirrhotic patients with ascites. PLoS One [Internet]. 2021 [cited 2024 Feb 19];16(6). Available from: /pmc/articles/PMC8224901/.
14. Praharaj DL, Anand AC. Clinical implications, evaluation, and management of hyponatremia in cirrhosis. J Clin Exp Hepatol [Internet]. 2022 [cited 2024 Feb 19];12(2):575–94. Available from: http://www.jcehepatology.com/article/S0973688321002449/fulltext.
15. Yun BC, Kim WR, Benson JT, Biggins SW, Therneau TM, Kremers WK, et al. Impact of Pretransplant Hyponatremia on Outcome Following Liver Transplantation. Hepatology [Internet]. 2009 [cited 2024 Feb 19];49(5):1610. Available from: /pmc/articles/PMC2902984/.
16. Ryu JY, Baek SH, Kim S. Evidence-based hyponatremia management in liver disease. Clin Mol Hepatol [Internet]. 2023 [cited 2024 Feb 19];29(4):924–44. Available from: https://pubmed.ncbi.nlm.nih.gov/37280091/.
17. Kalafateli M, Mantzoukis K, Choi Yau Y, Mohammad AO, Arora S, Rodrigues S, et al. Malnutrition and sarcopenia predict post-liver transplantation outcomes independently of the model for end-stage liver disease score. J Cachexia Sarcopenia Muscle [Internet]. 2017 [cited 2024 Jan 25];8(1):113–21. Available from: https://pubmed.ncbi.nlm.nih.gov/27239424/.
18. Merli M, Berzigotti A, Zelber-Sagi S, Dasarathy S, Montagnese S, Genton L, et al. EASL Clinical practice guidelines on nutrition in chronic liver disease. J Hepatol [Internet]. 2019 [cited 2024 Jan 25];70(1):172–93. Available from: https://pubmed.ncbi.nlm.nih.gov/30144956/.
19. Bischoff SC, Bernal W, Dasarathy S, Merli M, Plank LD, Schütz T, et al. ESPEN Guideline ESPEN practical guideline: clinical nutrition in liver disease. 2020 [cited 2024 Jan 25]; Available from: https://doi.org/10.1016/j.clnu.2020.09.001.
20. Trovato FM, Artru F. Nutritional optimization in liver transplant patients: from the pre-transplant setting to post-transplant outcome. Acta Gastro Enterologica Belgica. 2023;86:335.

21. Victor DW, Zanetto A, Montano-Loza AJ, Heimbach JK, Towey J, Spiro M, et al. The role of preoperative optimization of the nutritional status on the improvement of short-term outcomes after liver transplantation? A review of the literature and expert panel recommendations. Clin Transplant [Internet]. 2022 [cited 2024 Jan 25];36(10):e14647. Available from: https://onlinelibrary.wiley.com/doi/full/10.1111/ctr.14647.
22. Le Cornu KA, McKiernan FJ, Kapadia SA, Neuberger JM. A prospective randomized study of preoperative nutritional supplementation in patients awaiting elective orthotopic liver transplantation. Transplantation [Internet]. 2000 [cited 2024 Jan 25];69(7):1364–9. Available from: https://pubmed.ncbi.nlm.nih.gov/10798755/.
23. Plank LD, Mathur S, Gane EJ, Peng SL, Gillanders LK, Mcilroy K, et al. Perioperative immunonutrition in patients undergoing liver transplantation: a randomized double-blind trial. Hepatology [Internet]. 2015 [cited 2024 Jan 25];61(2):639–47. Available from: https://pubmed.ncbi.nlm.nih.gov/25212278/.
24. Lai JC, Shui AM, Duarte-Rojo A, Ganger DR, Rahimi RS, Huang CY, et al. Frailty, mortality, and health care utilization after liver transplantation: from the multicenter functional assessment in liver transplantation (FrAILT) study. Hepatology [Internet]. 2022 [cited 2024 Jan 25];75(6):1471–9. Available from: https://onlinelibrary.wiley.com/doi/full/10.1002/hep.32268.
25. Serper M, Jones LS, Clement T, Reddy RK, Reese PP. A randomized, controlled, prehabilitation intervention to maximize early recovery (PRIMER) in liver transplantation. Liver Transplant [Internet]. 2024 [cited 2024 Jan 25];30(1):10–9. Available from: https://journals.lww.com/lt/fulltext/2024/01000/a_randomized,_controlled,_prehabilitation.5.aspx.
26. Meena BL, Taneja S, Tandon P, Sahni N, Soundararajan R, Gorsi U, et al. Home-based intensive nutrition therapy improves frailty and sarcopenia in patients with decompensated cirrhosis: a randomized clinical trial. J Gastroenterol Hepatol [Internet]. 2023 [cited 2024 Jan 25];38(2):210–8. Available from: https://pubmed.ncbi.nlm.nih.gov/36268614/.
27. Nair S, Verma S, Thuluvath PJ. Pretransplant renal function predicts survival in patients undergoing orthotopic liver transplantation. Hepatology [Internet]. 2002 [cited 2024 Feb 5];35(5):1179–85. Available from: https://onlinelibrary.wiley.com/doi/full/10.1053/jhep.2002.33160.
28. Premkumar M, Kajal K, Reddy KR, Izzy M, Kulkarni AV, Duseja AK, et al. Evaluation of terlipressin-related patient outcomes in hepatorenal syndrome-acute kidney injury using point-of-care echocardiography. Hepatology [Internet]. 2023 [cited 2024 Feb 5]; Available from: https://journals.lww.com/hep/fulltext/9900/evaluation_of_terlipressin_related_patient.653.aspx.
29. Ripoll C, Platzer S, Franken P, Aschenbach R, Wienke A, Schuhmacher U, et al. Liver-HERO: hepatorenal syndrome-acute kidney injury (HRS-AKI) treatment with transjugular intrahepatic portosystemic shunt in patients with cirrhosis-a randomized controlled trial. Trials [Internet]. 2023 [cited 2024 Feb 7];24(1). Available from: https://pubmed.ncbi.nlm.nih.gov/37020315/.
30. Fukumitsu K, Kaido T, Matsumura Y, Ito T, Ogiso S, Ishii T, et al. Pretransplant renal dysfunction negatively affects prognosis after living donor liver transplantation: a single-center retrospective study. Transplant Proc. 2023;55(7):1623–30.
31. Ali H, Moond V, Lawson C, Budh D, Ohri R, Patel P, et al. Renal replacement therapy prior to liver transplant and inpatient mortality in patients without advanced kidney disease: a nationwide study. JGH Open [Internet]. 2024 [cited 2024 Feb 7];8(1):e13028. Available from: https://onlinelibrary.wiley.com/doi/full/10.1002/jgh3.13028.
32. Krowka MJ, Fallon MB, Kawut SM, Fuhrmann V, Heimbach JK, Ramsay MAE, et al. International liver transplant society practice guidelines: diagnosis and management of hepatopulmonary syndrome and portopulmonary hypertension. Transplantation [Internet]. 2016 [cited 2024 Feb 3];100(7):1440–52. Available from: https://pubmed.ncbi.nlm.nih.gov/27326810/.
33. De Gasperi A, Spagnolin G, Ornaghi M, Petrò L, Biancofiore G. Preoperative cardiac assessment in liver transplant candidates. Best Pract Res Clin Anaesthesiol. 2020;34(1):51–68.

34. Doctorian T, Nandkeolyar S, Fearon C, Nayak S, Tryon D, Sakr A, et al. Utility of Framingham score for optimizing preoperative evaluation among patients undergoing liver transplant evaluation. Transplant Proc. 2021;53(5):1616–21.
35. Kutkut I, Rachwan RJ, Timsina LR, Ghabril MS, Lacerda MA, Kubal CA, et al. Pre–liver transplant cardiac catheterization is associated with low rate of myocardial infarction and cardiac mortality. Hepatology [Internet]. 2020 [cited 2024 Feb 3];72(1):240–56. Available from: https://onlinelibrary.wiley.com/doi/full/10.1002/hep.31023.
36. Löffler AI, Gonzalez JA, Sundararaman SK, Mathew RC, Norton PT, Hagspiel KD, et al. Coronary computed tomography angiography demonstrates a high burden of coronary artery disease despite low-risk nuclear studies in pre-liver transplant evaluation. Liver Transpl [Internet]. 2020 [cited 2024 Feb 3];26(11):1398–408. Available from: https://pubmed.ncbi.nlm.nih.gov/32772465/.
37. Kaur H, Premkumar M. Diagnosis and management of cirrhotic cardiomyopathy. J Clin Exp Hepatol. 2022;12(1):186–99.
38. Premkumar M, Rangegowda D, Vyas T, Khumuckham JS, Shasthry SM, Thomas SS, et al. Carvedilol combined with Ivabradine improves left ventricular diastolic dysfunction, Clinical progression, and survival in cirrhosis. J Clin Gastroenterol [Internet]. 2020 [cited 2024 Feb 3];54(6):561–8. Available from: https://pubmed.ncbi.nlm.nih.gov/31305281/.
39. Dangl M, Grant JK, Vincent L, Ebner B, Maning J, Olorunfemi O, et al. The association of pretransplant atrial fibrillation with in-hospital outcomes in patients undergoing orthotopic liver transplantation: a propensity score matching analysis. J Card Surg [Internet]. 2022 [cited 2024 Feb 3];37(12):4762–73. Available from: https://onlinelibrary.wiley.com/doi/full/10.1111/jocs.17183.
40. Lawal OD, Aronow HD, Shobayo F, Hume AL, Taveira TH, Matson KL, et al. Comparative effectiveness and safety of direct oral anticoagulants and warfarin in patients with atrial fibrillation and chronic liver disease: a nationwide cohort study. Circulation [Internet]. 2023 [cited 2024 Feb 3];147(10):782–94. Available from: https://pubmed.ncbi.nlm.nih.gov/36762560/.
41. Kulkarni A, Rakam K, Avadhanam MVPY, Rachakonda C, Satyavadi A, et al. Predictors and outcomes of infections in ICU patients with cirrhosis: a single-center observational study. Cureus [Internet]. 2023 [cited 2024 Feb 7];15(10). Available from: /pmc/articles/PMC10652166/.
42. Kulkarni A V., Premkumar M, Arab JP, Kumar K, Sharma M, Reddy ND, et al. Early diagnosis and prevention of infections in cirrhosis. Semin Liver Dis [Internet]. 2022 [cited 2024 Feb 7];42(3):293–312. Available from: https://pubmed.ncbi.nlm.nih.gov/35672014/.
43. Nikam V, Srivastava M. The outcome of living donor liver transplant recipients with recent episodes of spontaneous bacterial peritonitis. Rev Esp enfermedades Dig [Internet]. 2021 [cited 2024 Feb 7];113(4). Available from: https://pubmed.ncbi.nlm.nih.gov/33207887/.
44. Incicco S, Tonon M, Zeni N, Gambino C, Gagliardi R, Calvino V, et al. Impact of bacterial infections prior to liver transplantation on post-transplant outcomes in patients with cirrhosis. JHEP Reports [Internet]. 2023 [cited 2024 Feb 7];5(9). Available from: http://www.jhep-reports.eu/article/S2589555923001398/fulltext.
45. Maiwall R, Bajpai M, Singh A, Agarwal T, Kumar G, Bharadwaj A, et al. Standard-volume plasma exchange improves outcomes in patients with acute liver failure: a randomized controlled trial. Clin Gastroenterol Hepatol [Internet]. 2022 [cited 2023 Jul 24];20(4):e831–54. Available from: http://www.cghjournal.org/article/S1542356521000860/fulltext.
46. Larsen FS, Schmidt LE, Bernsmeier C, Rasmussen A, Isoniemi H, Patel VC, et al. High-volume plasma exchange in patients with acute liver failure: an open randomised controlled trial. J Hepatol [Internet]. 2016 [cited 2024 Jan 14];64(1):69–78. Available from: https://pubmed.ncbi.nlm.nih.gov/26325537/.
47. Swaroop S, Arora U, Biswas S, Vaishnav M, Pathak P, Agarwal A, et al. Therapeutic plasma-exchange improves short-term, but not long-term, outcomes in patients with acute-on-chronic liver failure: A propensity score-matched analysis. J Clin Apher [Internet]. 2023 [cited 2024 Feb 7];38(4):376–89. Available from: https://pubmed.ncbi.nlm.nih.gov/36408827/.

48. Kumar SE, Goel A, Zachariah U, Nair SC, David VG, Varughese S, et al. Low volume plasma exchange and low dose steroid improve survival in patients with alcohol-related acute on chronic liver failure and severe alcoholic hepatitis—preliminary experience. J Clin Exp Hepatol. 2022;12(2):372–8.
49. Kulkarni AV, Venishetty S, Vora M, Naik P, Chouhan D, Iyengar S, et al. Standard-volume is as effective as high-volume plasma exchange for patients with acute liver failure. J Clin Exp Hepatol [Internet]. 2024 [cited 2024 Feb 7];0(0):101354. Available from: http://www.jcehepatology.com/article/S0973688324000112/fulltext.
50. Agarwal B, Cañizares RB, Saliba F, Ballester MP, Tomescu DR, Martin D, et al. Randomized, controlled clinical trial of the DIALIVE liver dialysis device versus standard of care in patients with acute-on-chronic liver failure. J Hepatol [Internet]. 2023 [cited 2024 Feb 7];79(1):79–92. Available from: http://www.journal-of-hepatology.eu/article/S0168827823001885/fulltext.
51. Artzner T, Michard B, Weiss E, Barbier L, Noorah Z, Merle JC, et al. Liver transplantation for critically ill cirrhotic patients: stratifying utility based on pretransplant factors. Am J Transplant [Internet]. 2020 [cited 2024 Feb 19];20(9):2437–48. Available from: https://pubmed.ncbi.nlm.nih.gov/32185866/.

Chapter 7
Muscle Health in Liver Disease and Transplant: The Sarcopenia Link

Subrat K. Acharya, Peeyush Kumar, and Dibya Lochan Praharaj

Abstract Loss of muscle mass (sarcopenia) and muscle function (frailty) is common in elderly patients. This is called primary sarcopenia. In contrast, patients may develop sarcopenia and frailty secondary to chronic diseases like decompensated cirrhosis. With worsening of underlying liver disease, the prevalence and severity of sarcopenia increase. Presence of ascites, repeated hospital admissions and prescription of low salt diet lead to significant reduction of dietary intake leading to malnutrition and sarcopenia. In addition, prolonged fasting in these patients leads to accelerated starvation, neo-glucogenesis and loss of muscle mass. Sarcopenia can be diagnosed by various clinical and radiological tests. Presence of sarcopenia has been associated with increased morbidity and short-term mortality. In addition, sarcopenia has been associated with increased morbidity and mortality in liver transplant recipients. The chapter aims to provide a brief overview regarding prevalence and etiopathogenesis of sarcopenia in patients with end-stage liver disease. In addition, diagnosis and management of sarcopenia will also be discussed. Management of sarcopenia will also be discussed briefly. Finally, clinical significance of sarcopenia and frailty in the setting of liver transplantation will also be discussed.

Keywords Sarcopenia · Frailty · Decompensated cirrhosis · Liver transplantation

S. K. Acharya
KIIT University, Bhubaneshwar, Odisha, India

Fortis Escorts Digestive & Liver Institute, New Delhi, India

Department of Gastroenterology, All India Institute of Medical Sciences, New Delhi, India

P. Kumar
Liver and Digestive Institute, Fortis Escorts Hospital, New Delhi, India

D. L. Praharaj (✉)
Department of Gastroenterology and Hepatology, Kalinga Institute of Medical Sciences (KIMS), Bhubaneswar, Odisha, India
e-mail: dibyalochanpraharaj@gmail.com

S. Saigal, D. Jothimani (eds.), *Fundamentals of Transplant Hepatology*,
https://doi.org/10.1007/978-981-95-2624-6_7

Key Highlights

- Sarcopenia and frailty are quite high in patients with cirrhosis ranging from 40% to 70% and 18% to 43%, respectively.
- Sarcopenia is strongly associated with higher risk of morbidity and mortality both pre- and post-liver transplantation.
- Incorporating the assessment and treatment of sarcopenia should be the standard of care in patients with cirrhosis.
- Simple, reliable, easily accessible tools with reproducibility are essential in the management of sarcopenia and frailty in cirrhotics.
- Aerobic exercise, muscle strengthening, balance enhancement and flexibility exercises along with small frequent meals, high-protein diet and late-evening snacks are strongly recommended in the management of sarcopenia in cirrhotics.

7.1 Sarcopenia Basics and Its Relevance

Sarcopenia is a progressive and generalized skeletal muscle disorder characterized by the loss of muscle mass and function. It is a complex syndrome that is rooted in adverse muscle changes that accrue across a lifetime. Sarcopenia is common among adults of older age, but it can also occur earlier in life [1].

Sarcopenia can be categorized broadly as ‘primary’, primarily linked to the ageing process, and ‘secondary’, which stems from an inherent disease process. In the management of secondary sarcopenia, it is crucial to identify and address the underlying cause. The prevalence of sarcopenia varies significantly due to differences in diagnostic methods, assessment criteria, study samples and ethnic backgrounds [2]. The updated consensus paper on sarcopenia, EWGSOP2, highlights low muscle strength as a central feature of this condition. The diagnosis of sarcopenia in older people is corroborated through the comprehensive evaluation of both quantity and quality of muscle, while its severity is further underscored by impaired physical performance, denoting an advanced stage of the condition [1] (Table 7.1).

Providing optimal care for individuals affected with sarcopenia is imperative, as the unaddressed condition imposes substantial personal, social and economic burdens. Aside from functional impairments, sarcopenia frequently leads to an increased risk of falls and subsequent injuries, exacerbating the constraints on one’s quality of life. In the Indian study, which involved 227 subjects aged over 60 years

Table 7.1 Operational definition of sarcopenia of EWGSOP2 2019

Sarcopenia	Criteria		
Probable	Low muscle strength		
Confirmed	Low muscle strength	Low muscle quantity or quality	
Severe	Low muscle strength	Low muscle quantity or quality	Low physical performance

attending the geriatric outpatient clinic, the prevalence of primary sarcopenia was found to be 39.2% [3].

7.2 Sarcopenia in the Setting of Chronic Liver Disease

Both sarcopenia and frailty are highly prevalent in patients with decompensated cirrhosis. The prevalence of both these conditions depends on the population that is being evaluated, and the method and definition that are used for assessment. Based on various studies, the prevalence of sarcopenia and frailty ranges from 40% to 70% and 18% to 43%, respectively [4–6]. While several definitions of both these apparently similar conditions exist in the field of hepatology, sarcopenia is defined as loss of muscle mass, while frailty is broadly defined as the phenotypic manifestation of loss of muscle function [7]. Standardized definitions or specific cut-off values for liver-related sarcopenia have not been established yet in patients with decompensated cirrhosis. This lack of standardization can be attributed to the considerable diversity in the assessment methods and definitions of sarcopenia utilized across different studies [1, 8–10] (Table 7.2).

Various methods exist for evaluating each aspect of sarcopenia (muscle mass, muscle function and muscle strength) (Table 7.3), but the field lacks a singular, dependable assessment tool that is both safe and consistent for accurately defining sarcopenia.

7.2.1 *Muscle Mass*

Various direct and indirect methods are routinely used to assess muscle mass. Anthropometry, bioelectrical impedance analysis (BIA), dual-energy X-ray absorptiometry (DXA), ultrasound, computed tomography (CT) scan and magnetic resonance imaging (MRI) have been widely used to assess muscle mass in patients with decompensated cirrhosis. Both BIA and DXA values are affected by the fluid status of the individual with decompensated cirrhosis which can be circumvented by using appendicular skeletal muscle [11, 12]. Similarly, anthropometric measurements may be subjective.

Cross-sectional imaging using either computed tomography (CT) or MRI scan is the most commonly used and validated method for assessing muscle mass, particularly in cirrhosis, where the focus lies on measuring the skeletal muscle index (SMI) at the level of the third lumbar vertebra [13, 14]. At this level, the thickness of the psoas and paraspinal muscles is measured. Moreover, CT scan is the only modality having an established sex-specific cut-off value, specifically <50 cm^2/m^2 in men and <39 cm^2/m^2 in women [9]. Previous research indicates that Asians, even after adjusting for height differences, typically have muscle mass approximately 15% lower than that of Western populations [15]. Sidhu et al. conducted a study involving

Table 7.2 Assessment of sarcopenia

Diagnostic parameter	Method of assessment	Sarcopenia cut-off INASL Consensus 2021	Japanese Society of Hepatology (2016)	Asian Working Group for Sarcopenia (2019)	North American Expert Opinion (2019)	EWGSOP2 (2019)
Muscle mass	DEXA	Male: 7.0 Kg/m^2 Female: 5.4 Kg/m^2	Male: 7.0 Kg/m^2 Female: 5.4 Kg/m^2	Male: 7.0 Kg/m^2 Female: 5.4 Kg/m^2	–	Male: 7.0 Kg/m^2 Female: 5.5 Kg/m^2
	BIA	Male: <7.0 kg/m^2 Female: <5.7 kg/m^2	Male: <7.0 kg/m^2 Female: <5.7 kg/m^2	Male: <7.0 kg/m^2 Female: <5.7 kg/m^2	–	–
	CT SMI Index: measure total muscle mass at the level of L3 divided by height squared	Men: <42 cm^2/m^2 Women: 38 cm^2/m^2	Men: <42 cm^2/m^2 Women: 38 cm^2/m^2	–	Men: <50 cm^2/m^2 Women: 39 cm^2/m^2	–
Muscle strength	Hand-grip strength	Male: <27 kg Female: <16 kg	Male: <26 kg Female: <18 kg	Male: <26 kg Female: <18 kg	–	Male: <27 kg Female: <16 kg
Muscle performance	Gait speed (4 m usual walking speed)	$\leq$0.8 m/s	$\leq$0.8 m/s	$\leq$1 m/s	–	$\leq$0.8 m/s

CT computed tomography, *BIA* bioelectrical impedance analysis, *DEXA* dual-energy X-ray absorptiometry, *SMI* skeletal muscle index

3,087 non-cirrhotic Indian patients, revealing that the mean CT SMI (skeletal

Table 7.3 Assessment modalities for sarcopenia: muscle mass, strength and function

Muscle mass	Muscle function	Muscle strength
CT L3 skeletal muscle index MRI Muscle ultrasound Dual-energy X-ray absorptiometry (DEXA) Bioelectrical impedance analysis (BIA) Mid-arm muscle circumference	Gait speed Short physical performance battery test (SPPB) Timed get-up-and-go test Liver frailty index (LFI) Aerobic exercise capacity 6-min walk distance (6MWD) Cardiopulmonary exercise testing (CPET)	Handgrip strength (HGS) Knee flexion/extension peak torque strength Liver frailty index (LFI)

CT computed tomography, *MRI* magnetic resonance imaging

muscle index) was 41.25 ± 4.42 in females and 44.33 ± 6.56 in males, significantly lower than values reported in Western populations [16]. Likewise, a study involving 149 Japanese individuals revealed reduced mean muscle mass, and the optimal cut-off values for CT L3 SMI to detect sarcopenia were determined as 42 cm^2/m^2 for men (AUC, 0.83; sensitivity, 89%; specificity, 57%) and 38 cm^2/m^2 for women [10]. The Indian National Association for the Study of the Liver (INASL) also suggests using cut-offs of 42 cm^2/m^2 for men and 38 cm^2/m^2 for women to diagnose sarcopenia [8] (Table 7.2).

However, there are challenges associated with using CT, such as its cost, potential for renal injury and the repeated exposure to radiation, which may limit its applicability in sarcopenia assessment to patients who already require CT imaging as part of their routine care (e.g. cancer screening or portal vein thrombosis evaluation). *Information pertaining to MRI is limited, and there is a lack of available reference values for normal measurements.*

Ultrasound has also been utilized for identifying sarcopenia. In a study by Tandon et al., thigh ultrasound was used to measure the thigh muscle index; they observed that utilizing a combination of body mass index and thigh muscle thickness could effectively detect sarcopenia in both male and female individuals, demonstrating nearly comparable accuracy to that of cross-sectional imaging (with area under the receiver operating characteristic curve values of 0.78 and 0.89, respectively). However, additional validation is required to confirm these results. Although muscle ultrasound is convenient and widely accessible, its utilization for diagnosing sarcopenia is still in its early stages of development [17].

7.2.1.1 Assessment of Body Composition

Multiple techniques are available to assess body composition, such as total body electrical conductivity, bioelectrical impedance, air displacement plethysmography, dual-energy X-ray absorptiometry (DEXA) and magnetic resonance spectroscopy. These methods enable the determination of total body weight, fat mass and lean body mass. DEXA is reproducible but involves low-dose X-rays, leading to radiation exposure. It may overestimate fat-free mass due to water retention. The Asian Working Group for Sarcopenia (AWGS) and INASL recommend height-adjusted skeletal muscle mass with cut-off values of 7.0 kg/m^2 in men and 5.4 kg/m^2 in women using DEXA [8, 18] (Table 7.2).

Bioelectrical impedance analysis (BIA) has emerged as an appealing method due to its portability, non-invasiveness, absence of radiation exposure and cost-effectiveness. Sarcopenia is defined as patients with skeletal muscle index (SMI) using BIA measurements of <7.0 kg/m^2 for males and <5.7 kg/m^2 for females [8] (Table 7.2). Nevertheless, both DEXA and BIA can be affected by hydration status and the presence of oedema and ascites in cirrhosis, posing significant limitations.

7.2.1.2 Assessment of Physical Performance and Muscle Strength

Assessments of physical performance, such as gait speed, and muscle strength, like handgrip strength (HGS), are indicative of the overall functional reserve and frailty. The term frailty (global frailty) was originally used to describe decreased physiological reserve along with increased vulnerability to stress [19]. In contrast to elderly patients, the frailty phenotype in patients with decompensated cirrhosis is the result of liver-specific factors (decreased protein synthesis, hyperammonemia-related muscle toxicity and hepatic encephalopathy-related immobility). Thus, physical frailty is the principal phenotype of muscular dysfunction in patients with decompensated cirrhosis. Gait speed is a widely used and reliable measure of physical performance in sarcopenia. It is a quick, safe and easy-to-perform test that can be done in a clinical setting. INASL recommends a <0.8 m/s threshold in a 6-meter walk test to indicate reduced physical performance. Hand grip strength (**HGS**) is a simple, inexpensive and effective method to assess muscle strength. It can be easily measured using a hand-held dynamometer. It is a good indicator of overall muscle strength and has been shown to be a reliable marker of sarcopenia in cirrhotic patients. INASL recommends using cut-off value <27 kg for males and <16 kg for females for low muscle strength [8]. Both HGS and gait speed are used as single-measure tests in patients with decompensated cirrhosis. Other methods to measure frailty include the liver frailty index, Fried frailty phenotype, short physical performance battery (SPPB), activity of daily living (ADL) and Karnofsky Performance Status (KPS). Though easy to measure, both HGS and gait speed tests need patient participation, which may not be always feasible in these sick patients (especially in patients with acute decompensation or acute on chronic liver failure). Thus, it remains to be seen in future studies whether all the above tests that were originally designed for patients with chronic generalized frailty in elderly can also be applied successfully to patients with decompensated cirrhosis and patients on LT waiting list.

7.3 Pathophysiology of Sarcopenia and Frailty in Cirrhosis

7.3.1 Sarcopenia

The presence of cirrhosis with portal hypertension in combination with its complications is the central mechanism in development of sarcopenia. The pathophysiological factors include hepatocellular necrosis with release of cytokines, host biomolecules like damage-associated molecular patterns (DAMPs), pathogen-associated molecular patterns (PAMPs), vascular changes associated with cirrhosis (portosystemic shunting), hyperammonemia and endotoxemia. Other factors like older age of patient, ethanol abuse, insulin resistance and cholestasis also contribute to development of sarcopenia in cirrhosis [20]. These physiological perturbations in decompensated cirrhosis produce a state of anabolic resistance characterized by lack of response to physiologic anabolic stimuli like increased nutrient intake and exercise (e.g. decreased proteolysis and increased protein synthesis) [21].

7.3.1.1 The Skeletal Muscle Protein Homeostasis

The skeletal muscle consists of both structural and contractile proteins. It is the largest storage site for protein in humans. A fine balance between protein synthesis and proteolysis is necessary to maintain the muscle homeostasis (involving ubiquitin proteasome pathway, lysosomal autophagy pathway and calcium-dependent calpain pathway) [22]. Metabolic tracer studies have shown decreased protein synthesis and increased proteolysis in patients with cirrhosis [23]. Similarly, myostatin, a transforming growth factor β superfamily member that is expressed primarily in skeletal muscles, prevents protein synthesis. Studies have demonstrated upregulation of myostatin in patients with cirrhosis, leading to decreased synthesis of muscle protein [24].

7.3.1.2 The Liver Muscle Axis

The mediators of liver muscle axis include endotoxemia, hyperammonemia and endocrine abnormalities like decreased testosterone levels and insulin-like growth factors. Of these, the role of hyperammonemia is strongly demonstrated as a mediator of sarcopenia in cirrhosis. Ammonia is a metabolic by-product of amino acid degradation, gut microbial metabolism and purine catabolism. Physiologically, disposal of ammonia occurs by ureagenesis. Impaired urea cycle, intestinal dysbiosis and porto-systemic shunting in cirrhosis lead to hyperammonemia. To compensate, muscle soaks up excess ammonia using glutamate, which ultimately leads to reduction of alpha-ketoglutarate, which is essential for ATP synthesis via Krebs cycle. The final result is reduced protein synthesis and sarcopenia. Hyperammonemia has also shown to upregulate myostatin in skeletal muscles further accentuating skeletal muscle protein synthesis and sarcopenia. Finally, gut dysbiosis, endotoxemia and increased inflammation shift the protein synthesis pathway towards an increased globulin synthesis at the cost of reduced synthesis of albumin leading to sarcopenia [20].

7.3.1.3 Metabolic and Hormonal Factors

Decreased testosterone levels along with an abnormal pattern of growth hormone secretion have been identified in patients with cirrhosis. Testosterone normally inhibits myostatin and promotes muscle growth. Low testosterone level in patients with cirrhosis thus promotes sarcopenia. Similarly, an abnormal growth hormone secretory pattern reduces muscle anabolism and promotes sarcopenia by acting on the myostatin receptor in muscles. Increased circulating angiotensin level in patients with non-alcoholic fatty liver disease-related cirrhosis binds to angiotensinogen receptors in the skeletal muscles, leading to proteolysis and skeletal muscle breakdown.

In line with increased glutamine and glutamate synthesis, patients with cirrhosis also have an alteration in substrate preferences. In the presence of hyperammonemia in cirrhosis, there occurs partitioning of L-leucine into mitochondria for oxidation instead of cytosol as a substrate for peptide chain elongation or translational regulation [25].

7.3.1.4 Endotoxemia/Gut Dysbiosis and Hyperinflammation

Altered gut microbiome and disrupted gut mucosal barrier lead to increased bacterial translocation. The endotoxin produced by these bacteria attaches to the toll-like receptors present in skeletal muscles leading to decreased protein synthesis and proteolysis. Various pro-inflammatory cytokines including IL-6 and TNF-α are produced in response to endotoxemia, leading to increased inflammation and muscle atrophy in cirrhosis [26, 27].

7.3.1.5 Systemic Hypermetabolism and Accelerated Starvation

Patients with cirrhosis often have significantly low hepatic glycogen reserve. In addition, these patients often have significantly decreased appetite due to zinc deficiency, ascites and prescription of salt-restricted diet. Patients are often kept on prolonged fasting, prior to various procedures and imaging. In view of decreased hepatic glycogen reserve, the pathway of neoglucogenesis is activated leading to loss of muscle protein and fatty acid. The final result is loss of muscle mass and development of sarcopenia [28, 29].

The pathophysiology of sarcopenia in cirrhosis has been summarized in Fig. 7.1.

7.3.2 Frailty

The development of frailty in elderly individuals occurs as a result of altered muscle protein homeostasis, progressively weakened immune system, chronic inflammation, neurologic changes and endocrine alteration. The mechanism of sarcopenia in patients with cirrhosis is not clear. However, a combination of sarcopenia, a pro-inflammatory state, low testosterone and gut dysbiosis may play an important role in the development of frailty even in young individuals with decompensated cirrhosis.

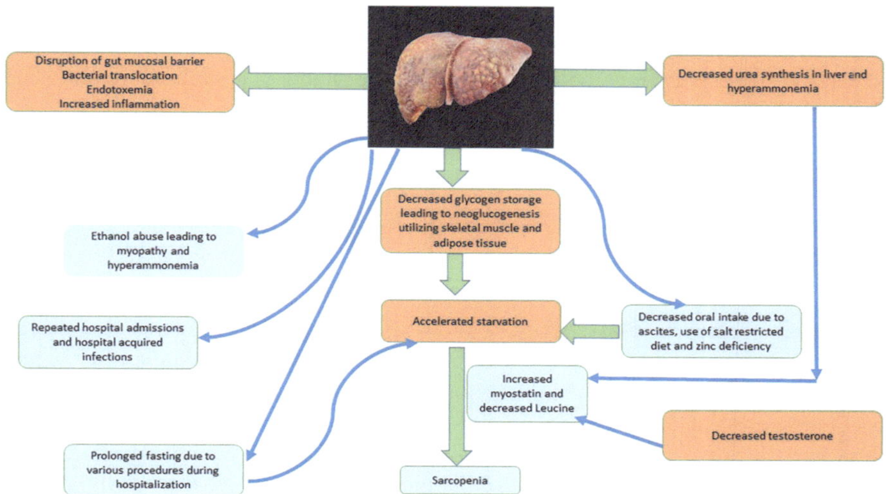

Fig. 7.1 Pathogenesis of sarcopenia in liver cirrhosis

7.4 Clinical Consequences of Sarcopenia and Frailty in Cirrhosis

The prevalence of sarcopenia and frailty increases with increased severity of decompensation in cirrhosis. Similarly, the presence of frailty and sarcopenia is independently associated with various adverse outcomes in patients with decompensated cirrhosis. Patients with decompensated cirrhosis and sarcopenia are at increased risk of developing newer decompensation, ACLF, poor health-related quality of life and increased mortality both pre-LT and post-LT. Similarly, duration of hospital stay, intensive care unit stay and risk of infection are increased in these patients. Similarly, risk of decompensation following transjugular intrahepatic portosystemic shunt (TIPS) is also higher in patients with concomitant sarcopenia. Episodes of hepatic encephalopathy (HE) are also higher in these patients, which is probably due to impaired extrahepatic ammonia metabolism and resulting hyperammonemia. Similarly, sarcopenia is a predictor of post-TIPS HE. Episodes of HE may gradually reduce over time with improvement in sarcopenia following TIPS.

Like sarcopenia, frailty (as defined by liver frailty index [LFI] >5) is associated with a high risk of morbidity and mortality. Similarly, 6-min walk test (6MWT) and gait speed are also associated with an increased morbidity and mortality [30, 31]. In hospitalized patients with cirrhosis, improvement in Karnofsky Performance Status (KPS) by 10 points was associated with a 30% reduction in odds of death at 30 days of discharge [32, 33].

While there may be a significant overlap between sarcopenia and frailty, combined studies (including both frailty) in patients being evaluated for LT have shown a poor correlation between these two with respect to increased morbidity and mortality [34–36]. While both these conditions may be interrelated in these patients, only physical frailty has been conclusively shown to be associated with an increased mortality. Thus, further studies are needed to establish a definite relationship between these two entities.

7.5 Sarcopenia-Frailty Interplay: Crucial Implication in Liver Transplantation

Frailty can be described as a unique biological condition characterized by reduced physiological capacity and heightened susceptibility to health challenges, which makes individuals more prone to negative health consequences. This state of frailty encompasses a variety of factors, involving multiple bodily systems such as organs (e.g. liver, kidney, heart), inflammatory and endocrine processes, cognitive function, musculoskeletal health and psychological aspects. It represents the final outcome of disturbances across these diverse physiological and psychosocial components. While sarcopenia is a central aspect of frailty, recent consensus from the American Society of Transplantation underscores that frailty encompasses more than just sarcopenia; it also involves muscle function and a patient's personal perception of their frailty state. Notably, physical frailty significantly predicts transplant waitlist and post-transplant mortality, as well as factors like mortality after hospitalization and length of hospital stay [37].

7.6 Point-of-Care Nutritional Assessment Tools

Physicians often gauge muscle wasting and physical capability based on a patient's appearance and activity level. However, these assessments can be subjective and vary among clinicians. Bedside muscle strength can be easily evaluated using HGS and physical ability with walking speed. HGS thresholds are <26 kg for men and <18 kg for women, while walking speed <0.8 m/s is considered a cut-off. Incorporating an objective measure like the liver frailty index (LFI) enhances frailty prediction accuracy. LFI combines grip strength (indicating nutritional status), balance testing (assessing neuro-muscular function) and chair stands (reflecting lower extremity weakness). This simple test can be conducted at the bedside or in outpatient settings. An LFI score of ≥4.5 indicates frailty, and detailed instructions are available at http://liverfrailtyindex.ucsf.edu.

7.7 Implications of Sarcopenia on Liver Transplantation in Cirrhosis

The presence of sarcopenia in end-stage liver disease (ESLD) is linked to poor prognosis. A mounting body of evidence shows marked increase in mortality among individuals with sarcopenia compared to those without it, particularly for patients awaiting liver transplant [38–40]. In a study by Lai et al., an analysis was conducted regarding the influence of compromised muscle functionality on the mortality rates of 309 individuals awaiting liver transplantation. Those with a SPPB score <10 had a 45% higher risk. Moreover, higher grip strength (1 kg), faster gait speed (0.1 m/s) and quicker chair stand (−1 s) each lowered mortality risk by 11%, 28% and 17%, respectively ($p < 0.01$) [38]. Wang et al. observed similar trends, associating waiting list mortality with grip strength (HR, 0.74; 95% CI, 0.59–0.92; $P = 0.008$), SPPB (HR, 0.89; 95% CI, 0.82–0.97; $P = 0.01$) and muscle quality indicated by skeletal muscle attenuation inversely linked to increased macroscopic fat infiltration (HR, 0.77; 95% CI, 0.63–0.95; $P = 0.02$) [35]. Studies demonstrated a more pronounced association between muscle function and waiting list mortality compared to muscle mass. This implies that evaluating muscle function holds greater clinical significance than assessing muscle mass for patients with ESLD who are awaiting liver transplantation [38, 40].

Remarkably, research indicates that the adverse effects of sarcopenia on the health outcomes of individuals with ESLD go beyond just liver transplantation. These effects encompass an extended ventilatory support, prolonged stays in the intensive care unit, increased overall hospital stay and a higher incidence of infections following transplantation [41].

A study from India showed that nearly half (47.8%) of the LT recipients had sarcopenia. Among individuals with sarcopenia, there was a significantly higher occurrence of postoperative sepsis (89% vs. 55%, $p = 0.001$), neurological complications (29.6% vs. 8.8%, $p = 0.040$), prolonged stay in the intensive care unit (median of 12 days [8–16] vs. 10 days [8–12], $p = 0.024$) and a need for ventilatory support (median of 1.5 days [1–3] vs. day [1–2], $p = 0.021$) [42].

A recent meta-analysis comprising 22 studies and 6965 cirrhosis patients revealed a notable association between sarcopenia and increased mortality risk. Patients diagnosed with sarcopenia faced approximately 2.3 times higher chances of mortality (adjusted hazard ratio [aHR] 2.30, 95% CI 2.01–2.63). This risk remained consistent across various patient subgroups, including those with low Model for End-Stage Liver Disease (MELD) scores [43].

The findings underscore the importance of including sarcopenia assessment in the initial evaluation of all cirrhosis patients and regular monitoring for sarcopenia in all cirrhosis patients, regardless of the degree of hepatic dysfunction.

7.8 Management of Sarcopenia in Cirrhosis

Treatment of sarcopenia involves integration of physical exercise and nutritional therapy.

7.8.1 *Physical Exercise*

It is strongly recommended to provide a diverse exercise program involving aerobic exercise, muscle strengthening, balance enhancement and flexibility exercises. It helps counteract sarcopenia and its impact on health.

Resistance training stands as prime approach to trigger muscle growth and enhance strength. It triggers anabolic signals for muscle protein synthesis, boosting muscle mass and overall physical performance, including balance [44, 45].

The World Health Organization (WHO) has formulated distinct guidelines regarding physical activity and sedentary behaviour for individuals with chronic conditions. The recommendations involve adopting consistent aerobic exercises (either 150 min or 75 min each week at moderate or vigorous intensity, respectively) and engaging in muscle strengthening routines (2–3 sessions every week) and ≥2–3 sessions per week of postural balance exercises [46].

Engaging in physical training can pose challenges for individuals with ESLD due to comorbidities, such as hepatic encephalopathy, cirrhotic cardiomyopathy, ascites, anaemia and porto-pulmonary hypertension. Customized training regimens should be developed for individual patient according to their physical capabilities. Prior to initiating exercise therapy, it is advisable to optimize the patient's overall medical condition, which includes addressing comorbidities. Additionally, it is recommended to start at low intensity and gradually advance to higher levels for individuals with chronic diseases [47, 48].

7.8.2 *Nutrition in Chronic Liver Disease with Sarcopenia*

Nutritional strategies for sarcopenia should focus on optimal caloric and protein intake to facilitate the growth of skeletal muscle mass and to hinder the deterioration of muscle mass. Optimal nutritional health plays a vital role in determining the outlook for cirrhosis patients and could potentially exert an influence on the overall survival. Cirrhosis patients experience continuous accelerated starvation, enhanced catabolism, alongside muscle anabolic resistance, which dampens metabolic reactions to nutrition. The European Association for the Study of the Liver (EASL) and the European Society for Parenteral and Enteral Nutrition (ESPEN) recommend tailored nutritional approaches for cirrhosis patients [49, 50].

For well-compensated patients, an ideal energy intake of 25–35 kcal/kg of dry body weight per day, along with 1.2–1.5 g/kg of body weight per day protein, is suggested. In contrast, for decompensated cirrhotic patients, a higher energy and protein intake is advised, targeting 35–40 kcal/kg and 1.5–2 g/kg, respectively [49, 50]. For patients retaining fluids, determining their optimal weight can be approximated through subjective evaluations using either [1] the weight measured after paracentesis or [2] by subtracting a proportion of weight based on the degree of fluid retention (mild, 5%; moderate, 10%; severe, 15%; with an additional 5% reduction if bilateral pedal oedema extends to the knees) [50].

Stable patients with obesity are advised to adopt a hypocaloric diet, creating a daily caloric deficit of 500–800 kcal, while ensuring sufficient protein intake. This strategy promotes simultaneous reduction of adipose tissue and preservation of muscle mass, complemented by an exercise regimen [50].

Optimal meal timing to prevent extended fasting is crucial, with beneficial options being early breakfast and late-evening snacks. Although specifics of snack composition need clarification, protein presence has shown to enhance nitrogen balance and muscle mass. Plank et al.'s study on cirrhosis patients revealed nocturnal supplementation significantly improved total body protein and fat-free mass [24, 51]. Similarly, systematic analysis highlighted late-evening snacks' potential to correct substrate utilization, elevate nitrogen retention, improve quality of life and reduce hepatic encephalopathy. Thus, cirrhosis patients should consume frequent, small meals (every 4–6 h), emphasizing high-protein breakfasts and energy-dense, complex-polysaccharide late-evening snacks (around 50 g) to avert detrimental early gluconeogenic state [51].

7.9 Conclusion

Sarcopenia has a strong clinical impact on health outcomes in chronic liver disease patients. It is a robust predictor of morbidity and mortality risk, with a considerable prevalence both prior and post-liver transplantation. However, the awareness of sarcopenia and its clinical implications in liver disease is limited. Incorporating the assessment and treatment of sarcopenia should be standard of care for individuals with cirrhosis. Detecting probable sarcopenia offers an opportunity for timely intervention to not only enhance muscle mass, strength and functionality but also holds potential to elevate patient outcomes.

The absence of consensus on sarcopenia diagnosis poses a substantial challenge, alongside it is equally vital to create simple screening tools that healthcare providers can utilize to identify this issue. At present, the cornerstone components of treating sarcopenia are physical exercise therapy and nutritional interventions. In order to advance treatment strategies and develop targeted therapeutic interventions, deeper comprehension of the intricate interplay between liver, muscle and adipose tissue is required.

References

1. Cruz-Jentoft AJ, Bahat G, Bauer J, Boirie Y, Bruyère O, Cederholm T, et al. Sarcopenia: revised European consensus on definition and diagnosis. Age Ageing. 2019;48(1):16–31.
2. Santilli V, Bernetti A, Mangone M, Paoloni M. Clinical definition of sarcopenia. Clin Cases Miner Bone Metab. 2014;11(3):177–80.
3. Rahman R, Wilson BP. Prevalence and factors contributing to primary sarcopenia in relatively healthy older Indians attending the outpatient department in a tertiary care hospital: a cross-sectional study. Aging Med. 2021;4(4):257–65.
4. Kim HY, Jang JW. Sarcopenia in the prognosis of cirrhosis: going beyond the MELD score. World J Gastroenterol. 2015;21(25):7637–47.
5. Montano-Loza AJ, Duarte-Rojo A, Meza-Junco J, Baracos VE, Sawyer MB, Pang JX, et al. Inclusion of sarcopenia within MELD (MELD-sarcopenia) and the prediction of mortality in patients with cirrhosis. Clin Transl Gastroenterol. 2015;6(7):e102.
6. Tandon P, Tangri N, Thomas L, Zenith L, Shaikh T, Carbonneau M, et al. A rapid bedside screen to predict unplanned hospitalization and death in outpatients with cirrhosis: a prospective evaluation of the clinical frailty scale. Am J Gastroenterol. 2016;111(12):1759–67.
7. Tandon P, Montano-Loza AJ, Lai JC, Dasarathy S, Merli M. Sarcopenia and frailty in decompensated cirrhosis. J Hepatol. 2021;75 Suppl 1(Suppl 1):S147–s62.
8. Puri P, Dhiman RK, Taneja S, Tandon P, Merli M, Anand AC, et al. Nutrition in chronic liver disease: consensus statement of the Indian National Association for study of the liver. J Clin Exp Hepatol. 2021;11(1):97–143.
9. Carey EJ, Lai JC. A North American expert opinion statement on sarcopenia in liver transplantation. Hepatology (Baltimore, Md.). 2019;70(5):1816–29.
10. Nishikawa H, Shiraki M, Hiramatsu A, Moriya K, Hino K, Nishiguchi S. Japan Society of Hepatology guidelines for sarcopenia in liver disease (1st edition): recommendation from the working group for creation of sarcopenia assessment criteria. Hepatol Res. 2016;46(10):951–63.
11. Lindqvist C, Brismar TB, Majeed A, Wahlin S. Assessment of muscle mass depletion in chronic liver disease: dual-energy x-ray absorptiometry compared with computed tomography. Nutrition (Burbank, Los Angeles County, Calif). 2019;61:93–8.
12. Sinclair M, Hoermann R, Peterson A, Testro A, Angus PW, Hey P. Use of dual X-ray absorptiometry in men with advanced cirrhosis to predict sarcopenia-associated mortality risk. Liver Int. 2019;39(6):1089–97.
13. Tandon P, Mourtzakis M, Low G, Zenith L, Ney M, Carbonneau M, et al. Comparing the variability between measurements for sarcopenia using magnetic resonance imaging and computed tomography imaging. Am J Transplant. 2016;16(9):2766–7.
14. Praktiknjo M, Book M, Luetkens J, Pohlmann A, Meyer C, Thomas D, et al. Fat-free muscle mass in magnetic resonance imaging predicts acute-on-chronic liver failure and survival in decompensated cirrhosis. Hepatology (Baltimore, Md.). 2018;67(3):1014–26.
15. Su H, Ruan J, Chen T, Lin E, Shi L. CT-assessed sarcopenia is a predictive factor for both long-term and short-term outcomes in gastrointestinal oncology patients: a systematic review and meta-analysis. Cancer Imaging. 2019;19(1):82.
16. Indian Society of Gastroenterology. Indian J Gastroenterol. 2018;37(1):1–137.
17. Tandon P, Low G, Mourtzakis M, Zenith L, Myers RP, Abraldes JG, et al. A model to identify sarcopenia in patients with cirrhosis. Clin Gastroenterol Hepatol. 2016;14(10):1473–80.e3.
18. Chen LK, Liu LK, Woo J, Assantachai P, Auyeung TW, Bahyah KS, et al. Sarcopenia in Asia: consensus report of the Asian working Group for Sarcopenia. J Am Med Dir Assoc. 2014;15(2):95–101.
19. Fried LP, Tangen CM, Walston J, Newman AB, Hirsch C, Gottdiener J, et al. Frailty in older adults: evidence for a phenotype. J Gerontol A Biol Sci Med Sci. 2001;56(3):M146–56.
20. Dasarathy S, Merli M. Sarcopenia from mechanism to diagnosis and treatment in liver disease. J Hepatol. 2016;65(6):1232–44.

21. Shalimar RG, Kumar R. Persistent or incident hyperammonemia is associated with poor outcomes in acute decompensation and acute-on-chronic liver failure. JGH Open. 2020;4(5):843–50.
22. Cohen S, Nathan JA, Goldberg AL. Muscle wasting in disease: molecular mechanisms and promising therapies. Nat Rev Drug Discov. 2015;14(1):58–74.
23. Periyalwar P, Dasarathy S. Malnutrition in cirrhosis: contribution and consequences of sarcopenia on metabolic and clinical responses. Clin Liver Dis. 2012;16(1):95–131.
24. Glass DJ. Skeletal muscle hypertrophy and atrophy signaling pathways. Int J Biochem Cell Biol. 2005;37(10):1974–84.
25. Dasarathy S. Myostatin and beyond in cirrhosis: all roads lead to sarcopenia. J Cachexia Sarcopenia Muscle. 2017;8(6):864–9.
26. Li H, Malhotra S, Kumar A. Nuclear factor-kappa B signaling in skeletal muscle atrophy. J Mol Med (Berl). 2008;86(10):1113–26.
27. Giusto M, Barberi L, Di Sario F, Rizzuto E, Nicoletti C, Ascenzi F, et al. Skeletal muscle myopenia in mice model of bile duct ligation and carbon tetrachloride-induced liver cirrhosis. Physiol Rep. 2017;5(7)
28. Glass C, Hipskind P, Tsien C, Malin SK, Kasumov T, Shah SN, et al. Sarcopenia and a physiologically low respiratory quotient in patients with cirrhosis: a prospective controlled study. J Appl Physiol (Bethesda, Md: 1985). 2013;114(5):559–65.
29. Tsien CD, McCullough AJ, Dasarathy S. Late evening snack: exploiting a period of anabolic opportunity in cirrhosis. J Gastroenterol Hepatol. 2012;27(3):430–41.
30. Carey EJ, Steidley DE, Aqel BA, Byrne TJ, Mekeel KL, Rakela J, et al. Six-minute walk distance predicts mortality in liver transplant candidates. Liver Transplant. 2010;16(12):1373–8.
31. Dunn MA, Josbeno DA, Tevar AD, Rachakonda V, Ganesh SR, Schmotzer AR, et al. Frailty as tested by gait speed is an independent risk factor for cirrhosis complications that require hospitalization. Am J Gastroenterol. 2016;111(12):1768–75.
32. Tapper EB, Finkelstein D, Mittleman MA, Piatkowski G, Lai M. Standard assessments of frailty are validated predictors of mortality in hospitalized patients with cirrhosis. Hepatology (Baltimore, Md). 2015;62(2):584–90.
33. Thuluvath PJ, Thuluvath AJ, Savva Y. Karnofsky performance status before and after liver transplantation predicts graft and patient survival. J Hepatol. 2018;69(4):818–25.
34. Yadav A, Chang Y-H, Carpenter S, Silva AC, Rakela J, Aqel BA, et al. Relationship between sarcopenia, six-minute walk distance and health-related quality of life in liver transplant candidates. Clin Transpl. 2015;29(2):134–41.
35. Wang CW, Feng S, Covinsky KE, Hayssen H, Zhou LQ, Yeh BM, et al. A comparison of muscle function, mass, and quality in liver transplant candidates: results from the functional assessment in liver transplantation study. Transplantation. 2016;100(8):1692–8.
36. Sinclair M, Chapman B, Hoermann R, Angus PW, Testro A, Scodellaro T, et al. Handgrip strength adds more prognostic value to the model for end-stage liver disease score than imaging-based measures of muscle mass in men with cirrhosis, Liver Transplant. 2019;25(10):1480–7.
37. Lai JC, Sonnenday CJ, Tapper EB, Duarte-Rojo A, Dunn MA, Bernal W, et al. Frailty in liver transplantation: an expert opinion statement from the American Society of Transplantation Liver and Intestinal Community of Practice. Am J Transplant. 2019;19(7):1896–906.
38. Lai JC, Dodge JL, Sen S, Covinsky K, Feng S. Functional decline in patients with cirrhosis awaiting liver transplantation: results from the functional assessment in liver transplantation (FrAILT) study. Hepatology (Baltimore, Md). 2016;63(2):574–80.
39. Hamaguchi Y, Kaido T, Okumura S, Fujimoto Y, Ogawa K, Mori A, et al. Impact of quality as well as quantity of skeletal muscle on outcomes after liver transplantation. Liver Transplant. 2014;20(11):1413–9.
40. Yadav A, Chang YH, Carpenter S, Silva AC, Rakela J, Aqel BA, et al. Relationship between sarcopenia, six-minute walk distance and health-related quality of life in liver transplant candidates. Clin Transpl. 2015;29(2):134–41.

41. Montano-Loza AJ, Meza-Junco J, Baracos VE, Prado CM, Ma M, Meeberg G, et al. Severe muscle depletion predicts postoperative length of stay but is not associated with survival after liver transplantation. Liver Transplant. 2014;20(6):640–8.
42. Kumar V, Benjamin J, Shasthry V, Subramanya Bharathy KG, Sinha PK, Kumar G, et al. Sarcopenia in cirrhosis: fallout on liver transplantation. J Clin Exp Hepatol. 2020;10(5):467–76.
43. Tantai X, Liu Y, Yeo YH, Praktiknjo M, Mauro E, Hamaguchi Y, et al. Effect of sarcopenia on survival in patients with cirrhosis: a meta-analysis. J Hepatol. 2022;76(3):588–99.
44. Aamann L, Dam G, Borre M, Drljevic-Nielsen A, Overgaard K, Andersen H, et al. Resistance training increases muscle strength and muscle size in patients with liver cirrhosis. Clin Gastroenterol Hepatol. 2020;18(5):1179–87.e6.
45. Agostini F, Bernetti A, Di Giacomo G, Viva MG, Paoloni M, Mangone M, et al. Rehabilitative good practices in the treatment of sarcopenia: a narrative review. Am J Phys Med Rehabil. 2021;100(3):280–7.
46. Bull FC, Al-Ansari SS, Biddle S, Borodulin K, Buman MP. World Health Organization 2020 guidelines on physical activity and sedentary behaviour. Br J Sports Med. 2020;54(24):1451–62.
47. Tandon P, Ismond KP, Riess K, Duarte-Rojo A, Al-Judaibi B, Dunn MA, et al. Exercise in cirrhosis: translating evidence and experience to practice. J Hepatol. 2018;69(5):1164–77.
48. Duarte-Rojo A, Ruiz-Margáin A, Montaño-Loza AJ, Macías-Rodríguez RU, Ferrando A, Kim WR. Exercise and physical activity for patients with end-stage liver disease: improving functional status and sarcopenia while on the transplant waiting list. Liver Transplant. 2018;24(1):122–39.
49. Plauth M, Bernal W, Dasarathy S, Merli M, Plank LD, Schütz T, et al. ESPEN guideline on clinical nutrition in liver disease. Clin Nutr (Edinburgh, Scotland). 2019;38(2):485–521.
50. EASL clinical practice guidelines on nutrition in chronic liver disease. J Hepatol. 2019;70(1):172–93.
51. Plank LD, Gane EJ, Peng S, Muthu C, Mathur S, Gillanders L, et al. Nocturnal nutritional supplementation improves total body protein status of patients with liver cirrhosis: a randomized 12-month trial. Hepatology (Baltimore, Md). 2008;48(2):557–66.

Chapter 8
Acute Liver Failure

Dinesh Jothimani, Navin Marannan, Tanvir Ahmed, and Julia Wendon

Abstract Acute liver failure (ALF) is characterized by a sudden and rapid decline in liver function, presenting with jaundice, coagulopathy, and hepatic encephalopathy (HE). The interval between the onset of jaundice and encephalopathy is used to classify ALF into hyperacute, acute, and subacute types, which also helps in predicting clinical outcomes.

There is notable geographic variation in the causes of ALF. In Western countries, paracetamol toxicity is the leading etiology, while in Asian countries, viral hepatitis is more common. In India, hepatitis A is the most frequent cause of ALF, while yellow phosphorus (YP) poisoning is frequently reported in the southern regions of the country.

Outcomes in ALF have improved markedly over the past three decades, primarily due to advancements in critical care, a better understanding of disease mechanisms, and the timely use of organ support therapies. Consequently, many ALF patients, particularly those with hyperacute presentations, recover with medical management alone. However, patients with seronegative hepatitis, non-paracetamol drug-induced liver injury (DILI), or subacute ALF are more likely to require liver transplantation (LT).

Management of ALF should take place at tertiary care centers with liver transplant capability. While emergency liver transplantation (LT) can be life-saving, determining the right candidates for LT remains challenging. Multiple prognostic scoring systems have been developed to assess mortality risk in the absence of LT. Among these, King's College Hospital (KCH) criteria are the most extensively

D. Jothimani (✉) · N. Marannan · T. Ahmed
Institute of Liver Disease and Transplantation, Dr Rela Institute and Medical Centre, Chennai, Tamil Nadu, India
e-mail: dinesh.jothimani@relainstitute.com

J. Wendon
Critical Care Division, Institute of Liver Diseases, King's College Hospital, Denmark Hill, London, UK

S. Saigal, D. Jothimani (eds.), *Fundamentals of Transplant Hepatology*,
https://doi.org/10.1007/978-981-95-2624-6_8

studied and widely used. However, due to its limited sensitivity, some patients who could benefit from LT may not meet its thresholds. The ALFED score, being dynamic, has shown better predictive accuracy but requires further validation.

A significant barrier to emergency LT in ALF patients in Asian populations is the limited availability of deceased donor organs, especially for those listed under "supra-urgent" categories. In response, countries like India have advanced the use of living donor liver transplantation (LDLT). Additionally, auxiliary partial orthotopic liver transplantation (APOLT) is a specialized surgical approach used in selected ALF cases. This technique supports native liver regeneration, potentially eliminating the need for lifelong immunosuppression.

Survival rates following LT in ALF have greatly improved, with current 1-year and 5-year survival rates around 80% and 70%, respectively—markedly better than in previous decades.

Keywords Acute liver failure · Ammonia · Cerebral edema · Organ dysfunction · Plasmapheresis · CRRT · Sepsis

Key Highlights

ALF is a rare but serious clinical condition characterized by the rapid onset of jaundice and coagulopathy, followed by the development of hepatic encephalopathy.

Treatment in ALF should be a goal-directed therapy toward hyperammonemia, metabolic acidosis, organ dysfunction, and sepsis.

Cerebral edema is a major complication in ALF; early detection and timely intervention improve overall survival.

King's College criteria are the most widely used prognostic markers in ALF, with higher specificity and lower sensitivity.

Living donor liver transplantation is a feasible option in ALF with good outcomes.

8.1 Introduction

Acute liver failure (ALF) is an uncommon yet serious clinical condition marked by a rapid decline in liver function, presenting with jaundice, coagulopathy, and hepatic encephalopathy (HE). It is associated with a high risk of mortality. The development of HE is a defining feature that distinguishes ALF from acute liver injury (ALI) in adults. This narrative review discusses the management of ALF, with an emphasis on the role of liver transplantation (LT).

8.2 Definition of ALF

Historically referred to as fulminant hepatitis, ALF was first described in the 1930s in patients who developed severe jaundice and liver cell failure, often resulting in death [1]. In the 1970s, Davidson et al. formally defined ALF as a syndrome involving severe yet potentially reversible liver injury, with the onset of hepatic encephalopathy within 8 weeks of symptom onset and no prior liver disease [2]. The Japanese criteria (1981) expanded on these characteristics by incorporating hepatic encephalopathy, prolonged prothrombin time, and histological evidence of liver inflammation within 8 weeks of injury.

Currently, there are approximately 40 different definitions of ALF, which vary based on the degree of liver dysfunction and the timing between jaundice and HE [3]. Among these, the most widely accepted is the O'Grady classification, which defines ALF as the sudden onset of jaundice, coagulopathy (INR $\geq$1.5), and subsequent encephalopathy within 8–28 days of jaundice onset. ALF is further subclassified by timing:

- Hyperacute: HE develops within 7 days of jaundice.
- Subacute: HE occurs more than 28 days later [4].

8.3 Limitations of Current Definitions

Despite an established definition, certain challenges persist. The interval between jaundice onset and encephalopathy varies significantly among patients. There is no standardized bilirubin threshold to quantify liver injury, unlike international normalized ratio (INR). Moreover, the diagnosis of hepatic encephalopathy, often based on the West Haven criteria, is subjective. Patients with subacute liver failure may not exhibit HE but may develop ascites due to transient portal hypertension, complicating diagnosis.

8.4 Epidemiology

Due to its rarity, the true incidence and prevalence of ALF are not well defined. Reported annual incidence ranges from 1 to 5 per million. A study conducted in Germany (2014–2018) reported an incidence of 1.13 per million [5], while a population-based study from Thailand noted a much higher prevalence of 62.9 per million, with indeterminate etiology being the most common (69.4%) [6]. In India, a lack of national data hampers accurate prevalence estimates.

There is considerable global variation in ALF etiology [7]. In the West, paracetamol toxicity accounts for the majority of cases (up to 57%), with the US ALF registry reporting it in 46% of cases [7]. In contrast, viral hepatitis is the dominant cause in Asia, particularly hepatitis B, which accounts for 20–22% of cases [8].

8.5 ALF in India

India has a distinct ALF profile. Single-center studies have reported acute viral hepatitis as the underlying cause in over 60% of patients. In some regions, hepatitis E accounts for up to 43% of ALF cases, followed by drug-induced liver injury (DILI), especially from anti-tubercular therapy (ATT) [9, 10]. Hepatitis A-induced ALF shows variability across centers (2–39%). However, a recent multi-center study indicated a shift, identifying hepatitis A as the most common cause (44.2%) [11].

ALF due to ATT has become increasingly common, contributing to 46.4% of DILI-related ALF cases. Complementary and Alternative Medicine (CAM)-related liver injury accounts for an additional 13.9%. In Southern India, yellow phosphorus (YP) poisoning (often from rodenticide ingestion) remains a common and notable cause [9, 11].

8.6 Clinical Implications

This etiological diversity likely explains variations in clinical presentation and prognosis across regions. For example, paracetamol-induced ALF typically presents as hyperacute and paradoxically has a favorable prognosis, even in the presence of multiple organ dysfunctions. Conversely, ALF caused by non-paracetamol drugs or viral hepatitis tends to have poorer spontaneous recovery rates.

Overall, ALF remains a high-mortality condition, with case fatality rates ranging from 60% to 80%, influenced by etiology, host factors, and disease severity.

8.6.1 Clinical Presentation

Jaundice followed by altered sensorium is the clinical hallmark of ALF. Clinical history is vital in assessing the cause and the severity of ALF. A history of travel, fever, and the presence of prodrome may favor viral hepatitis. A history of previous suicidal attempts, mental and psychosocial instability may provide a clue toward paracetamol or yellow phosphorus poisoning. Clinical examination is required to assess jaundice and the severity of hepatic encephalopathy. Once defined, patients should undergo basic investigations to identify the cause of ALF, which include an acute viral hepatitis panel, autoimmune hepatitis, and Wilson's disease screen. Serum samples should be sent for paracetamol levels whenever appropriate. Abdominal ultrasound may reveal a normal liver size, hepatomegaly, or, at times, a shrunken liver due to collapse of parenchyma.

Patients with ALF progress through four important clinical complications: cerebral dysfunction, acidosis, organ failure, and sepsis (Figs. 8.1 and 8.2).

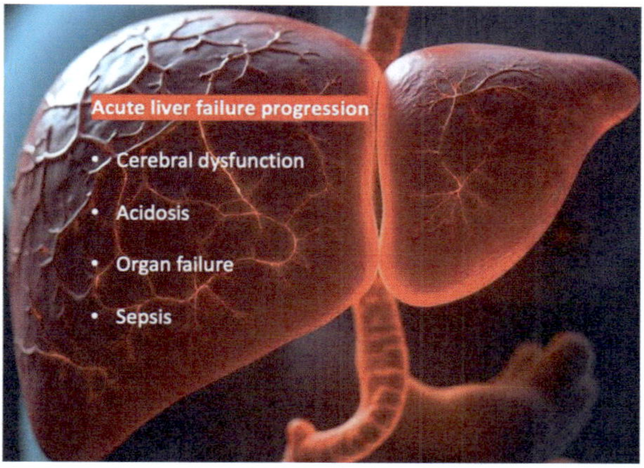

Fig. 8.1 Complications of acute liver failure

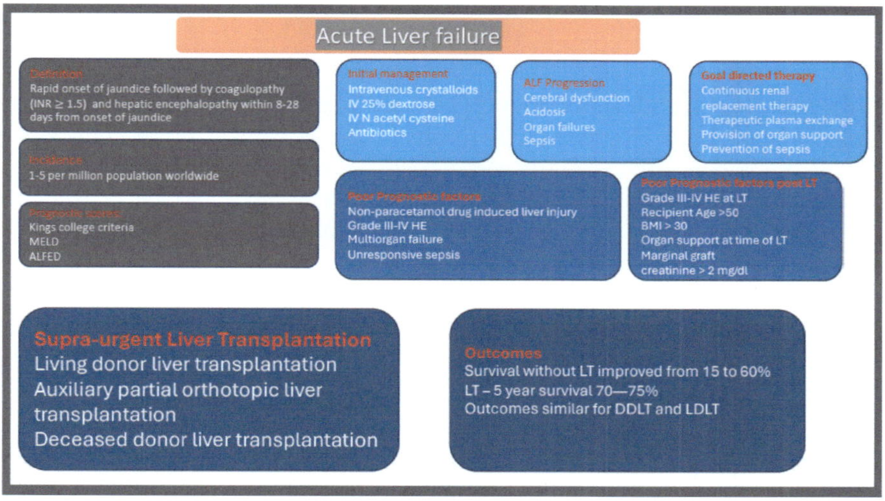

Fig. 8.2 Clinical approach to ALF

The unpredictable nature of ALF warrants management in specialized centers. ALF patients should be managed in a tertiary care liver unit with facilities for LT. Peripheral centers should liaise with the nearest liver unit for clinical support and safe transport for disease-directed therapies. These patients should be shifted at the earliest to centers equipped with an intensive care unit (ICU) managed by a team of critical care consultants and hepatologists, and preferably with the facility of liver transplantation. Effective communication between the unit aids safe patient transfer. The family should be counseled regarding the dynamicity of the situation and the need for specialized centers, even if LT is not feasible. Patients with grade III or IV encephalopathy should undergo elective endotracheal intubation prior to transfer. Whenever possible, patients should be accompanied by intensivists in an ambulance equipped with advanced life support. Hypoglycemia and acidosis should be corrected beforehand. Intravenous fluids should be used to maintain mean arterial pressure (MAP) to ensure adequate cerebral perfusion [12].

8.7 Medical Management of Acute Liver Failure (ALF)

Over recent years, the medical treatment of ALF has significantly advanced. Patients should be managed in intensive care units (ICUs) equipped for liver transplantation [13], with care ideally delivered through goal-directed protocols in specialized critical care settings. Key therapeutic objectives include reducing ammonia levels aggressively, managing cerebral edema, providing organ support, and preventing infections.

8.8 Initial Resuscitation and Supportive Measures

Early resuscitation with intravenous crystalloids is essential, as many ALF patients are volume-depleted. However, fluid overload must be avoided to prevent worsening cerebral edema. If hypotension persists despite adequate fluid resuscitation, noradrenaline should be initiated. Hyponatremia, often present and associated with worse outcomes, should be corrected using hypertonic saline. Blood glucose levels should be stabilized using intravenous dextrose.

Continuous renal replacement therapy (CRRT) is recommended to manage hyperammonemia, correct metabolic acidosis and hyponatremia, and remove lactate.

8.9 N-Acetylcysteine (NAC) Therapy

Intravenous NAC is the gold standard for treating paracetamol-induced ALF, particularly when administered within 8 hours of ingestion, improving transplant-free survival [14]. While also used in non-paracetamol ALF (NA-ALF), results have been mixed. A large randomized controlled trial (RCT) by the ALF Study Group showed improved transplant-free survival in early HE stages (HE grades I–II) with NAC (52% vs. 30%, *p* = 0.01), though overall survival was unaffected [15].

A meta-analysis involving 883 NA-ALF patients reported NAC significantly improved overall survival (OR 1.77), transplant-free survival (OR 2.85), and post-transplant survival (OR 2.44) [14].

The standard NAC dosing regimen involves:

- 150 mg/kg over 1 hour, followed by
- 12.5 mg/kg/h for 4 hours, then
- 6.25 mg/kg/h for 67 hours [16].

8.10 Fluid Management

ALF is characterized by a hyperdynamic circulation, leading to low mean arterial pressure (MAP), high cardiac output, and effective hypovolemia [4]. Although ideal fluids are not definitively established, balanced crystalloids are generally preferred. Colloids may be useful in cases with elevated intracranial pressure (ICP) or hypoalbuminemia [5, 6].

Fluid administration should be guided using pulse pressure variation, bedside ultrasound, and clinical markers [7].

If hypotension persists, vasopressors are necessary. Noradrenaline is first-line, with vasopressin added if needed [6].

Although optimal MAP is debated, a target of 60–75 mmHg is typically recommended to ensure organ and cerebral perfusion [8, 9].

In cases of vasopressor-resistant hypotension, stress-dose corticosteroids (e.g., hydrocortisone) may be beneficial due to relative adrenal insufficiency [10, 12].

Hypoglycemia should be corrected with dextrose to maintain levels between 150 and 180 mg/dL [14], while serum sodium should be maintained between 145 and 155 mEq/L using hypertonic saline or mannitol to mitigate cerebral edema [15].

Magnesium and phosphorus should be checked every 8–12 hours and replenished as needed [8].

Empirical antibiotics, such as ceftriaxone or piperacillin-tazobactam, are advised in patients with high-grade encephalopathy or systemic inflammatory response syndrome (SIRS), as these reduce infection-related complications [15].

Antifungal therapy should be considered in worsening encephalopathy or ongoing SIRS.

8.11 Neurological Monitoring and Cerebral Edema Management

ALF patients are at high risk of cerebral edema, necessitating frequent neurological assessments. Interventions include:

- Head elevation to 30°
- Minimal stimulation
- Therapeutic hypothermia (target 32 °C)
- Osmotic therapy with mannitol:
- 20% mannitol, 0.5–1 g/kg over 20 minutes, particularly in patients with raised ICP indicated by jugular bulb monitoring or optic nerve sheath diameter.

Hyponatremia (<130 mmol/L) is linked to elevated ICP. Maintaining serum sodium between 140 and 145 mmol/L improves outcomes. 30% saline can be infused at 5–20 mL/hour, avoiding rapid sodium shifts (>10 mmol/24 hours) [15].

Patients with grade 3–4 encephalopathy should be intubated to protect the airway and monitored closely for intracranial hypertension. Risk factors for cerebral edema include:

- HE grade 3–4
- Fever/SIRS
- Serum ammonia >150 μmol/L
- INR >5
- Acute kidney injury (AKI) [16]

CRRT: Treatment should be commenced promptly to reduce ammonia, the key pathogenic substance in ALF. Use of early (day 1) continuous renal replacement therapy (CRRT) has shown to reduce ammonia level reduced risk of cerebral edema and importantly improves patient survival [16]. CRRT should be initiated if ammonia more than 100 umol per decilitre. In addition to ammonia clearance; CRRT also improves lactic acidosis [17]. INASL recommends CRRT in the presence of uremia, acute kidney injury, fluid overload, oliguria and hyperkalemia [12]. A recent meta-analysis of 11 studies of 305 patients received CRRT for ALF showed an improved over all (RR 0.83, 95%CI 0.70-0.99, P = 0.002) and transplant free survival (RR = 0.65, 95%CI 0.49-0.85, P = 0.002) compared to patients (n = 1137) with no CRRT. The analysis also revealed a non-significant trend towards higher mortality (RR 1.24, P = 0.28) in ALF patients with no CRRT [18].

8.12 Plasma Exchange

Therapeutic plasma exchange (TPE) has shown benefit for ALF management. High-volume plasma exchange (HVPE) improves transplant-free survival, especially when used early, acting as a bridge to transplant or as a standalone therapy in ineligible candidates.

In a landmark RCT, Larsen et al. demonstrated that HVPE improved INR and bilirubin by day 2 and ammonia levels initially (120 → 113 μmol/L), though no significant change in lactate was seen [19]. HVPE involves large volumes of fresh-frozen plasma, which increases costs and fluid burden.

More recently, Maiwall et al. evaluated standard-volume plasma exchange (SVPE) using 1.5–2.0 plasma volumes per session in 20 ALF patients. SVPE improved transplant-free survival (75% vs. 45%) and significantly reduced bilirubin, INR, lactate, ammonia, SIRS, and cerebral edema [20]. SVPE offers cost-effectiveness with comparable outcomes to HVPE.

A retrospective study also found that low-volume plasma exchange combined with low-dose corticosteroids (prednisolone 10 mg/day) improved transplant-free survival (59%) in DILI-associated ALF [21]. Further prospective studies are needed to validate this combined approach.

8.13 Liver Transplantation in Acute Liver Failure (ALF)

Before the advent of liver transplantation (LT), mortality among patients with ALF exceeded 80% [22]. The significance of LT as a life-saving therapy for ALF was formally recognized during a National Institutes of Health consensus meeting in the early 1980s, transforming the outlook for these patients [23].

Initially, LT was considered for patients with what was termed "advanced" ALF. However, this designation was poorly defined, leading to subjective interpretations and variability in clinical decisions across transplant centers.

Selecting appropriate candidates for LT in the setting of ALF remains challenging due to the lack of a universally predictive model. An ideal prognostic criterion should be:

- Simple and easy to apply
- Highly sensitive and specific
- Applicable across etiologies
- Dynamic and reproducible, incorporating both clinical and biochemical variables

Effective transplant criteria are essential to avoid:

- False positives, which may lead to unnecessary transplantation and associated risks in patients who might otherwise recover
- False negatives, where timely transplantation is missed, compromising survival

8.14 Clichy Criteria

Introduced in 1986, the Clichy criteria were among the first models for predicting outcomes in ALF. According to this model, liver transplantation is advised for patients with:

- Grade III–IV hepatic encephalopathy
- Factor V level < 20% (in patients under 30 years) or < 30% (in those over 30 years)

However, this model had limited applicability due to:

- The need for Factor V testing, which is not widely available
- Development based primarily on patients with hepatitis B-related ALF [24]

8.15 King's College Hospital (KCH) Criteria

Introduced in 1987, the KCH criteria were based on a retrospective review of 588 ALF patients managed at King's Liver Unit between 1973 and 1985 and were validated in 1986 [25]. The KCH model was the first to distinguish between paracetamol and non-paracetamol ALF, recognizing that etiology affects prognosis.

- Paracetamol-induced ALF often presents as hyperacute, with a better likelihood of spontaneous recovery.
- The KCH criteria are widely adopted globally.

Limitations:

- Lower sensitivity (69%) in non-paracetamol ALF: 31% of patients who may improve with medical therapy alone might still meet criteria and undergo LT unnecessarily.
- High specificity (92%), suggesting good ability to identify those unlikely to benefit from LT when the criteria are not met.

In paracetamol-related ALF, a meta-analysis showed:

- Sensitivity: 58–69%
- Specificity: 92–94% [26]

The addition of serum lactate levels after fluid resuscitation has been shown to improve sensitivity [27].

8.16 Model for End-Stage Liver Disease (MELD) Score in ALF

The model for end-stage liver disease (MELD) score has also been evaluated for its ability to predict mortality in ALF patients. A meta analysis of 23 studies involving 2153 ALF patients (2001–2015) reported:

Diagnostic odds ratio for:

- KCH: 5.3 (95% CI: 3.7–7.6)
- MELD: 7.0 (95% CI: 5.1–9.7)

In paracetamol ALF:

- KCH sensitivity: 58% (95% CI: 51–65%), specificity: 89%
- MELD sensitivity: 80% (95% CI: 74–86%), specificity: 53%

In non-paracetamol ALF:

- KCH sensitivity: 58%, specificity: 74%

- MELD sensitivity: 76%, specificity: 73% [28]

These findings suggest that:

- KCH performs better for paracetamol-related ALF
- MELD may be more reliable in non-paracetamol cases

8.17 Early Clinical Prognostic Indicators

A study from India on 144 ALF patients due to viral hepatitis reported a mortality rate of 63.9%. The presence of any three of the following six criteria was predictive of poor outcomes:

1. Age ≥ 50 years
2. Interval from jaundice to HE >7 days
3. High-grade encephalopathy
4. Cerebral edema
5. PT ≥35 seconds
6. Serum creatinine ≥1.5 mg/dL

This model showed superior predictive ability compared to both KCH and MELD scores in viral hepatitis-related ALF [29].

8.18 ALF early dynamic (ALFED) Score

Recognizing the dynamic nature of ALF, Kumar et al. developed the ALFED score, validated through a prospective study of 380 patients with viral hepatitis-related ALF [30].

The score includes:

- Arterial ammonia ≥123 μmol/L
- Bilirubin ≥15 mg/dL
- INR ≥5
- HE >Grade 2

Outcomes:

- Score 1–3: 80% survival
- Score 4: 80% mortality

The ALFED model demonstrated excellent discrimination, with an area under receiver operating curve (AUROC) of 0.91 (Table 8.1).

Table 8.1 ALF prognostic scores and their predictive values

Prognostic Scores	Components	Sensitivity	Specificity	Remarks
King's College Criteria (Non-Paracetamol ALF)	INR Bilirubin Aetiology Age Jaundice to encephalopathy time	68–69%	82–92%	Most widely used, Poor sensitivity; Improves when advanced HE is a late event
Clichy Criteria	Hepatic EncephalopathyAge, Factor V levels	69%	50%	Factor V is not widely available
MELD	Bilirubin INR Creatinine	MELD >30 76%	MELD >30 73%	Cutoffs vary across studies
Arterial Ammonia	Baseline Ammonia > 124 mol/L	78.6%	76.3%	Accurate measurement is difficult, Varies with many factors—AKI, sepsis, bleeding, drugs
ALFED	Ammonia, INR, bilirubin, hepatic encephalopathy	73.5%	84.3%	AUC 0.91

8.19 Biomarkers and Prognostic Indicators in ALF

Among emerging biomarkers, von Willebrand factor (vWF) has been extensively studied in the context of acute liver failure (ALF). Secreted by vascular endothelial cells, vWF plays a crucial role in platelet adhesion and aggregation, and prolongs the half-life of Factor VIII, contributing significantly to hemostasis. Beyond its coagulative function, vWF is now recognized as a novel prognostic marker in liver disease. Studies have shown that elevated vWF levels are predictive of clinical decompensation and mortality in patients with cirrhosis, irrespective of disease stage or the severity of portal hypertension [31].

In acute-on-chronic liver failure (ACLF), vWF levels have also been found to correlate with disease severity and outcomes [32]. Similarly, patients with acute liver injury (ALI) and ALF demonstrate elevated vWF antigen levels. Conversely, reduced activity of ADAMTS13, the enzyme responsible for cleaving vWF, is associated with:

- Higher grades of hepatic encephalopathy
- Increased need for liver transplantation
- Worse survival outcomes [33]

Despite the emergence of ICU-based scoring systems such as acute physiology and chronic health evaluation (APACHE) and sequential organ failure asessment score (SOFA), the King's College Hospital (KCH) criteria continue to be regarded as more reliable for prognostication in ALF.

8.20 ALF from Yellow Phosphorus Poisoning

A unique form of ALF seen in Southern India involves yellow phosphorus poisoning, typically from rodenticides [34]. Patients presenting with this etiology often develop rapid hepatic failure and require intensive supportive care.

In general, ALF patients in the ICU tend to be critically ill, frequently requiring multi-organ support. The presence of multi-organ failure significantly influences post-transplant outcomes and is an important prognostic factor [35].

8.21 Challenges in Emergency Liver Transplantation

A major limitation in managing ALF worldwide—particularly in Asian countries—is the low rate of deceased organ donation, making supra-urgent liver transplantation (LT) challenging. Even when an organ becomes available, clinical deterioration in the recipient may render them unsuitable for surgery, excluding them from transplantation.

8.22 Timing of Liver Transplantation

Timely liver transplantation is critical to optimize outcomes in ALF. Factors influencing LT timing include:

- Etiology of liver failure
- Interval from jaundice to encephalopathy
- Age of donor and recipient
- Presence or progression of multi-organ dysfunction

A study from King's College Hospital reported that 22% of ALF patients listed for urgent LT either died or became unfit for transplantation, with a median survival of only 2 days post-listing [36]. Furthermore, waiting longer than 5 days for transplantation was associated with worse post-transplant survival [37].

However, it's important to recognize that some ALF patients recover spontaneously without requiring transplantation. Avoiding unnecessary LT in such cases spares patients from major surgery and lifelong immunosuppression. Therefore, the early and accurate identification of patients who are likely to recover without LT remains a critical priority in the management of ALF.

8.23 Survival Following Liver Transplantation in Acute Liver Failure (ALF)

The introduction of liver transplantation (LT) has significantly improved outcomes for patients with ALF. A large cohort study of 2095 ALF patients treated at King's College Hospital between 1973 and 2008 demonstrated a dramatic improvement in survival—from 16.7% to 62.2% ($P < 0.0001$)—attributed to advances in critical care and the timely availability of emergency LT. Transplant recipients also showed improved outcomes, with survival rising from 55.6% to 86% between 1984 and 2004. Survival among non-transplant patients also increased during this period (from 16.7% to 48.2%), especially among those with paracetamol toxicity, non-paracetamol drug-induced liver injury, and viral hepatitis. However, no survival gains were noted in patients with seronegative hepatitis and other rare causes of ALF [38]. One year survival of ALF liver transplant recipients has improved from 60% to 80% but much lesser compared to those transplanted for cirrhosis. In the largest ELTR database analysis, 4903 adult patients underwent LT for ALF between 1988 and 2009. Overall, 1-, 3-, 5- and 10-year survival was 74%, 70%, 68% and 63%, with graft survival of 63%, 59%, 57% and 50%, respectively. Patients transplanted in the later years had a better survival with 1-, 3- and 5-year survival of 79%, 75% and 72%, respectively compared to previous years ($P < 0.01$). Recipient age >50 years with deceased donor age more than 60 years were associated with higher mortality in the first year [39]. Similarly, experience from from King's college compared four time period (1984–93, 1994–98, 1999–2003 and 2004–08) of ALF and found improved overall survival from 66.3%, 67.6%, 78.8% to 86.4% ($P < 0.005$) respectively [40]. A Swedish study over 30 years studied transplant outcomes of 78 ALF patients. Five and 10-year survival was much better in patients transplanted after year 2000 (76% and 71%) than the previous era (63% and 52%), indicating improvement in critical care services [41]. A recent study from US ALF study group on 624 ALF waitlisted patients from 1998–2018, where 64% underwent liver transplantation with a 1 and 3-year survival of 91% and 90% [42].

Most of the above data come from Western countries, where deceased donor liver transplantation (DDLT) is the standard practice, supported by robust organ donation systems. Organs are often available within 72 hours, even though the timing of their availability remains a challenge. At times, marginal grafts are considered to overcome the major limiting factor with the risk of compromising post transplant graft and patient survival. Marginal grafts have one or more of the following: steatotic liver, elderly donor, long ischaemic times, donor on high inotropes and ABO-incompatible grafts. The system boasts to avoid unnecessary emotional pressure on the living donors to decide in limited time.

In Asia, including India, organ donation rates are extremely low (\~0.34 per million), prompting the widespread development of LDLT programs, which are more feasible and sustainable. Unlike DDLT, LDLT is center-driven and independent of organ availability. India now leads globally in LDLT volume, and the procedure is especially suited for ALF due to:

- Immediate access to a graft
- Avoidance of marginal organs
- Established surgical techniques
- Advancements like robotic-assisted donor hepatectomy

8.24 Auxiliary Partial Orthotopic Liver Transplantation (APOLT)

To address the limitations of both DDLT and LDLT, the technique of APOLT was introduced, with the first case reported in 1991 [43]. APOLT involves implanting a partial liver graft in the orthotopic position (natural liver location) while retaining part of the native liver. Over time, the native liver may regenerate, allowing graft removal and eliminating the need for lifelong immunosuppression.

Initial outcomes were poor, but with improved patient selection, surgical expertise, and critical care, 10-year survival rates have increased to 85–100%. Successful APOLT depends on several key factors:

1. Cause of ALF: Best suited for single-hit injuries like hepatitis A/E, acetaminophen overdose, or mushroom poisoning.
2. Recipient age: Children and adults under 40 have higher regenerative potential.
3. Clinical status: Patients with high inotrope requirements, severe SIRS, or elevated ICP are unsuitable due to the longer surgical time.
4. Graft volume: Adequate graft (e.g., right lobe in adults, left lobe in children) is essential to reverse encephalopathy and meet metabolic demands.
5. Graft quality: Non-marginal grafts are preferred.
6. Experienced surgical and ICU teams [44].

A French study involving 15 APOLT patients reported a 5-year survival of 59%. Carefully selected patients, especially those with hyperacute liver failure from toxins or hepatitis B, may eventually recover enough to permit graft explantation. In up to 70%, native liver regeneration occurs over 1–3 years [45].

8.25 ABO-Incompatible (ABOi) LDLT for ALF

Given the life-threatening nature of ALF and its high mortality without transplantation, the unavailability of timely matched grafts has prompted the use of ABO-incompatible (ABOi) liver transplantation in emergency settings. While still rare, most reports consist of single cases or small series [46, 47].

In a Japanese series, five patients with ALF underwent ABOi-LDLT from living donors. Pre-transplant desensitization involved rituximab administration 3–15 days before surgery, combined with perioperative plasma exchange and splenectomy. With a mean follow-up of 3.8 ± 3.7 years, patient survival was 80%.

Compared to decompensated cirrhosis, ALF poses unique challenges for ABOi-LT:

- Rituximab (300 mg/m^2), typically given 3 weeks before LT in cirrhosis, must be administered within days in ALF
- ALF patients are often too unstable to receive preoperative mycophenolate mofetil (MMF)
- Most require splenectomy and intravenous immunoglobulin G (IVIG) therapy [48]

A comparative Japanese study of ABOi-LT in ALF (n = 5) versus non-ALF (n = 33) found that ALF patients needed higher steroid doses, shorter rituximab-to-LT intervals (2 vs. 13 days, *P* <0.05), and more plasma exchanges. Notably, none developed antibody-mediated rejection, and 5-year survival was comparable (80% vs. 77.9%) [49].

8.26 Factors Influencing LT Survival in ALF

Despite improvements, 1-year survival after LT for ALF remains lower than in patients transplanted for chronic liver disease. The first 3 months post-LT carry the highest risk, primarily due to sepsis and multi-organ failure. A study from united network for organ sharing (UNOS) database on 1457 patients transplanted for ALF between 1988 and 2003 identified BMI >30, Cr >2, recipient age over 50 years and presence of organ support at the time of liver transplantation determined outcome. Patients fulfilling all 4 criteria had a 5-year survival of 42% as compared to those who filled none, the 5-year survival was 81% [50].

The severity of multi-organ failure and the quality of the liver graft remain major determinants of outcome. Recipients of marginal grafts, split grafts, or ABO-mismatched livers may have suboptimal outcomes [51].

Higher grades of hepatic encephalopathy (HE) are linked to poorer outcomes. A Taiwanese study of 11 ALF patients with grade 4 HE found that those transplanted within 48 hours of coma onset had a 3-year survival of 85%, compared to 50% for later transplants. This underscores the role of early LT in preventing irreversible cerebral edema [52].

Survival following DDLT vs LDLT for ALF was studied. Interestingly, they were not dissimilar; one year graft survival was 73%, 70% and 64% and patient survival 79%, 75% and 69% for DDLT, LDLT and ABO- I, respectively [53]. LDLT for ALF is less commonly performed in the West. Between 1998 and 2007, out of 1201 potential LDLT recipients in the ALF study group,10 patients [53].

In Western countries, LDLT for ALF remains a rare occurrence. From 1998 to 2007, only 10 of 1201 ALF patients in the US ALF Study Group (<1%) received LDLT, with 5-year survival of 70% for LDLT vs. 82% for DDLT [54].

An organ procurement and transplantation network (OPTN) database study by Urrunaga et al. (1987–2011) involving 2337 adults with ALF found 21 patients (0.9%) underwent LDLT. One- and five-year survival rates were: 71% and 79% for LDLT, and 71% and 71% for DDLT (P = 0.764) [55].

8.27 ALF Transplant Outcomes in India and Asia

A retrospective study from India (2007–2017) evaluated 69 ALF patients who underwent LDLT, reporting a mortality rate of 38%, primarily within 3 months. Sepsis was the leading cause of death (55.5%). Risk factors for higher postoperative mortality included:

- Seronegative ALF (OR 8.85, *P* = 0.053)
- Hepatitis A (OR 8.04, *P* = 0.072)
- Grade 4 HE (OR 8.81, *P* = 0.018)
- Creatinine >1.2 (OR 5.99, *P* = 0.051)

10-year survival was 60% in this cohort [56].

In another Indian study, 36 of 479 LT patients (7.5%) underwent LDLT for ALF (including 12 children). Viral hepatitis was the predominant cause. With a 4.5-year follow-up, survival was 80.5%. Five patients (13.6%) died postoperatively, mainly from cerebral edema and sepsis [57].

In a 10-year study from Japan 209 patients underwent LT for ALF, Hepatitis B was the most common cause of ALF (61%). One, five and 10-year patient survival rates were 79%, 74% and 73%, irrespective of the subtype of ALF (P = 0.48) and graft type (P = 0.21). Multivariate analysis revealed recipient age (HR 1.040, P = 0.002) and ABO-incompatibility (HR 4.169, P = 0.004) were associated with short term mortality (90 days) [58].

8.28 Pre-Transplant Factors Influence Post Transplant Outcomes

Pre-transplant factors that influence post-transplant survival for ALF was evaluated in a UNOS database analysis between 1998 and 2004. Out of 1457 patients transplanted for ALF, infection was the most common cause of mortality (23.6%), followed by brain death (13%) due to cerebral edema, brain stem herniation, followed by multi-organ failure (9.4%). A multi-variate model showed four risk factors, obesity (BMI $\geq$ 30) (HR 1.52, P = 0.008), serum creatinine > 2 mg/dl (HR 1.43,

P = 0.022), age >50 years (HR 1.39, P = 0.048) and presence of life support (HR 1.38, P = 0.056) determined post-transplant survival and a point based scoring system from 0-4 based on number of risk factors, accurately predicted post-transplant short and long term mortality with a HR 1.74 (score 1), 2.73 (score 2), 3.38 (score 3), and 6.22 (score 4) [50].

Overall, survival following liver transplantation for ALF has significantly improved, establishing LT as the most effective therapeutic strategy for this critical condition. However, outcomes remain heavily influenced by timing, pre-transplant patient status, organ quality, and center expertise. LDLT and ABOi-LT have expanded access in countries with low deceased organ donation rates, while innovations like APOLT provide hope for minimizing long-term immunosuppression.

8.29 Special Clinical Situations in Acute Liver Failure (ALF)

8.29.1 Autoimmune Hepatitis (AIH)

Severe AIH is characterized by INR >1.5, and the development of encephalopathy indicates progression to ALF. Due to the lack of prospective studies evaluating corticosteroid use or transplant timing in AIH-ALF, there are currently no standardized guidelines. However, based on available evidence, it is recommended that all AIH-ALF patients receive corticosteroids, along with empirical broad-spectrum antibiotics and antifungals.

Patients are more likely to respond to steroids if they have:

- MELD <27 [59]
- Lower grades of HE
- Declining bilirubin within one week
- Absence of submassive hepatic necrosis on biopsy [60, 61]

Poor steroid response is associated with elevated INR and thrombocytopenia at presentation [62]. Early liver transplantation should be considered in patients with higher MELD scores, advanced HE, or no bilirubin improvement by day 4 [60].

8.29.2 Wilson's Disease

Although typically a chronic liver condition, Wilson's disease-related ALF qualifies for supra-urgent transplant listing. As with AIH, prospective trials are lacking. The New Wilson's Index (NWI) is conventionally used to predict transplant need, with a score $\geq$ 11 indicating poor survival without LT (93% sensitivity, 98% specificity) [63]. Some studies suggest HE and bilirubin levels may more accurately predict the need for transplantation, though further validation is needed [64].

In regions where living donation is common (e.g., India), potential family donors—especially siblings or parents—may be heterozygous carriers of Wilson's disease (autosomal recessive inheritance). These individuals are safe to donate and not at risk for disease recurrence in recipients [65]. However, homozygous carriers are unsuitable as donors.

8.29.3 Budd-Chiari Syndrome (BCS)

BCS may present as acute liver failure. While angioplasty, TIPS, or DIPS are effective in chronic or subacute BCS, they are generally ineffective in ALF presentations [66]. This form of BCS progresses rapidly and carries a high in-hospital mortality (\~60%). Thus, BCS-related ALF is considered a valid indication for supra urgent liver transplantation [67, 68]. Liver transplantation can be challenging due to smaller caliber outflow tract and inferior vena cava (IVC) which may require complete reconstruction and thus requires an expert transplant team [69]. Patients with BCS requires etiology work up for underlying prothrombotic condition. BCS can recur in 7–11% of patients and hence requires lifelong anticoagulation following LT [70].

8.29.4 Acute Fatty Liver of Pregnancy (AFLP)

AFLP is a rare pregnancy-related liver disorder, typically occurring in the third trimester (35–37 weeks) due to fetal fatty acid oxidation defects, causing maternal microvesicular steatosis. Risk factors include nulliparous women, multiple gestation, low maternal BMI, male fetus, and fetal fatty acid oxidation defects are the commonly associated risk factors [71]

Common clinical features include:

- Nausea, vomiting, malaise, and jaundice
- Markedly elevated liver enzymes (300–10,000 IU/ml)
- Hypoglycemia, coagulopathy, and encephalopathy [72]

The Swansea criteria used for diagnosis of AFLP has 100% sensitivity, 57% specificity, 85% positive predictive value and 100% negative predictive value [76].

Liver biopsy is rarely needed, but when done, it reveals microvesicular fat [73].

Immediate fetal delivery is the cornerstone of treatment. Liver function generally improves postpartum and normalizes in 4–6 weeks [74, 75].

LT is indicated if the mother fails to recover post-delivery, showing persistent jaundice, coagulopathy, or encephalopathy. While consensus is lacking, Kushner et al. suggested transplantation should be pursued if no improvement occurs after delivery [76].

Recurrence in future pregnancies is possible, and multidisciplinary management is advised [77].

8.29.5 Yellow Phosphorus (YP) Poisoning

YP, a common rodenticide in India, is often ingested in suicide attempts via rat poison paste, though accidental exposure (e.g., through fireworks) also occurs. It contains zinc phosphide, which causes mitochondrial toxicity, impairing adenosine triphosphate (ATP) production and cellular respiration.

Initially asymptomatic, patients develop symptoms by day 3 (e.g., abdominal pain, vomiting) and marked liver dysfunction by day 5 [78]. Common findings include:

- Severe coagulopathy (INR unrecordable)
- High bilirubin
- Lactic acidosis
- Bone marrow suppression
- Occasional pancreatitis

The King's College criteria are not validated for YP-induced ALF. According to the Liver Transplant Society of India guidelines, LT should be considered if the patient has:

- INR >6.0
- MELD >36
- Persistent lactic acidosis
- Hepatic encephalopathy [34]

8.30 Futility of Liver Transplantation in ALF

The advent of liver transplantation (LT) has dramatically reduced ALF mortality from approximately 80% to 30% [79, 80]. However, not all ALF patients benefit from transplantation. A subset of patients presents at the end of illness severity, either being too unstable for surgery or having irreversible neurological injury, making LT unlikely to improve long-term quality of life.

In addition to clinical scores, significant medical or psychiatric comorbidities—such as poor likelihood of post-transplant adherence or survival—must be taken into account before recommending LT [81].

Absolute contraindications include:

- Irreversible brain damage or brain death
- More than three organ failures
- Refractory circulatory shock requiring multiple vasopressors
- Severe respiratory failure requiring high ventilatory settings (FiO_2 > 0.8, high positive end expiratory pressure (PEEP)) or ECMO [11]

Infections alone are not contraindications if responsive to therapy. However, persistent bacteremia, fungal sepsis, or failure to respond to antibiotics are reasons to delay or reconsider LT [12, 15].

Psychosocial considerations that may preclude LT include:

- Repeated acts of self-harm (>5 episodes)
- Severe, refractory psychiatric illness
- Ongoing intravenous drug use or chaotic alcohol consumption
- A clear and repeated wish to die without a diagnosable mental illness [12]
- Assessment in the context of hepatic encephalopathy and urgent timelines is challenging, further complicating decision-making.

8.31 Spontaneous Survival in ALF

Advancements in critical care, early organ support, and standardized management protocols have led to significant increases in transplant-free survival for many ALF patients.

Favorable predictors of spontaneous recovery include:

- Younger age (<40 years)
- Paracetamol-induced ALF
- Hyperacute presentations

Conversely, older age, indeterminate etiology, and subacute liver failure are associated with lower chances of survival without LT.

At King's College Hospital, analysis of 3300 ALF cases revealed an improvement in transplant-free survival from 15% to 60%. Outcomes improved significantly for ALF caused by:

- Paracetamol toxicity ($P < 0.001$)
- Non-paracetamol DILI ($P < 0.005$)
- Viral hepatitis ($P < 0.02$)

However, no significant survival gain was seen in cases of indeterminate or sero-negative hepatitis [34].

In an Indian study (Shalimar et al.), patients with hepatitis E-induced ALF ($n = 419$) had a 55.1% survival rate with medical therapy, while ATT-induced ALF had a 30.1% survival rate. Factors linked to poor outcomes included:

- Older age (OR 1.04)
- Female gender (OR 1.83)
- Cerebral edema (OR 2.48)
- Sepsis (OR 2.73)
- Elevated bilirubin (OR 1.04) [82]

The US ALF Study Group observed that 20% of 624 listed patients recovered without LT. Recovery was more likely in patients with:

- Paracetamol etiology (66% vs. 13%)
- Lower MELD scores (31 vs. 36)

- Less severe HE (33% vs. 55%)
- Lower rate of\ meeting KCH criteria (11% vs. 57%)

(*P* <0.002) [38]

8.32 Post-Transplant Complications in ALF

Unlike LT for cirrhosis, ALF recipients often face multi-organ complications and require extended ICU support.

Neurologic issues include:

- Persistent encephalopathy
- Seizures
- Posterior reversible encephalopathy syndrome (PRES)
- Intracranial hemorrhage

Cyclosporine may be favored over tacrolimus in those with delayed encephalopathy recovery.

Due to immune suppression, ALF patients are highly vulnerable to bacterial and fungal sepsis, which accounts for up to one-third of post-transplant deaths. Institutions often adopt prolonged antimicrobial protocols.

ALF recipients frequently present with renal dysfunction, prompting the use of basiliximab to delay calcineurin inhibitor initiation.

Psychological complications—such as anxiety, delirium, mood disorders, and PTSD—are common, necessitating early psychiatric intervention [12].

8.33 Unresolved Challenges in ALF

Several key questions in ALF management remain unanswered:

- Development of more sensitive and specific prognostic models
- Optimizing timing for both organ support initiation and transplantation
- Identifying patients who will recover without LT

Emerging technologies like machine learning (ML) and artificial intelligence (AI) hold promise for:

- Improving prognostic accuracy
- Enhancing donor-recipient matching
- Predicting post-transplant survival
- Identifying LT candidates more precisely [83]

8.34 Healthcare and Policy Gaps

While ALF patients should ideally be managed in tertiary liver centers, this is not always feasible in resource-limited settings. Capacity building through training local physicians and investing in extracorporeal support systems at secondary and tertiary care levels can bridge the gap.

Organ donation remains a significant challenge. For example, Spain leads globally with 48.9 donors per million population, while countries like India lag significantly. Public awareness campaigns, government support, and consideration of opt-out donation policies could help close the gap.

8.35 Conclusion

Acute liver failure is a rapidly progressive, life-threatening condition, typically presenting with sudden jaundice and encephalopathy. Early recognition and safe transfer to a transplant-capable tertiary center are crucial. Etiology and disease severity are the most important determinants of outcome, though causes vary by region.

The King's College criteria, despite limitations, remain the most widely accepted tool for LT candidacy. Advances in critical care, organ support, and plasma exchange therapy have significantly enhanced transplant-free survival, underscoring the importance of timely, multidisciplinary management.

References

1. Gaskell JF. The changes in the liver in a fatal case of epidemic "catarrhal" jaundice. J Pathol Bacteriol. 1933;36:008.
2. Trey C, Davidson CS. The management of fulminant hepatic failure. Prog Liver Dis. 1970;3:282–98.
3. Wlodzimirow KA, Eslami S, Abu-Hanna A, et al. Systematic review: acute liver failure—one disease, more than 40 definitions. Aliment Pharmacol Ther. 35:1245–56.
4. O'Grady JG, Schalm SW, Williams R. Acute liver failure: redefining the syndromes. Lancet. 1993;342(8866):273–5.
5. Weiler N, Schlotmann A, Schnitzbauer AA, et al. The epidemiology of acute liver failure. Dtsch Arztebl Int. 2020;117(4):43–50.
6. Thanapirom K, Treeprasertsuk S, Soonthornworasiri N, et al. The incidence, etiologies, outcomes, and predictors of mortality of acute liver failure in Thailand: a population-base study. BMC Gastroenterol. 2019;19(1):18.
7. Lee WM. Acetaminophen and the U.S. Acute Liver Failure Study Group: lowering the risks of hepatic failure. Hepatology. 2004;40(1):6–9.
8. Patterson J, Hussey HS, Silal S, et al. Systematic review of the global epidemiology of viral-induced acute liver failure. BMJ Open. 2020;10(7):e037473.
9. Anand AC, Nandi B, Acharya SK, et al. INASL Task-Force on Acute Liver Failure. Indian National Association for the study of the liver consensus statement on acute liver failure (part 1): epidemiology, pathogenesis, presentation and prognosis. J Clin Exp Hepatol. 2020;10(4):339–76.

10. Acharya SK. Acute liver failure: Indian perspective. Clin Liver Dis (Hoboken). 2021;18(3):143–9.
11. Roy A, Kumar K, Premkumar M, et al. HEPIN consortium. Current status of etiology and outcomes of acute liver failure in India-a multicentre study from tertiary centres. Indian J Gastroenterol. 2024;44(1):47–56.
12. Anand AC, Nandi B, Acharya SK, et al. Indian national association for the study of liver consensus statement on acute liver failure (Part-2): management of acute liver failure. J Clin Exp Hepatol. 2020;10(5):477–517.
13. Sehrawat SS, Premkumar M. Critical care management of acute liver failure. Indian J Gastroenterol. 2024;43(2):361–76. https://doi.org/10.1007/s12664-024-01556-8. Epub 2024 Apr 5.
14. Judith S-C, Sara T, Hao N, et al. N-acetylcysteine for the management of non-acetaminophen drug-induced liver injury in adults: a systematic review. Front Pharmacol. 2020;13:876868.
15. Wendon J, Cordoba J, Dhawan A, et al. EASL Clinical Practical Guidelines on the management of acute (fulminant) liver failure. J Hepatol. 2017;66(5):1047–81.
16. Bernal W, Wendon J. Acute liver failure. N Engl J Med. 2013;369:2525–34.
17. Cardoso FS, Gottfried M, Tujios S, et al. Continuous renal replacement therapy is associated with reduced serum ammonia levels and mortality in acute liver failure. Hepatology. 2018;67(2):711–20.
18. Dong V, Robinson AM, Dionne JC, et al. Continuous renal replacement therapy and survival in acute liver failure: a systematic review and meta-analysis. J Crit Care. 2024;81:154513.
19. Larsen FS, Schmidt LE, Bernsmeier C, et al. High-volume plasma exchange in patients with acute liver failure: an open randomised controlled trial. J Hepatol. 2016;64:69–78.
20. Maiwall R, Bajpai M, Singh A, et al. Standard-volume plasma exchange improves outcomes in patients with acute liver failure: a randomized controlled trial. Clin Gastroenterol Hepatol. 2022;20(4):e831–54.
21. Singh K, Kumar S, Zachariah U, Daniel D, David V, Subramani K, Pichamuthu K, Jacob E, Kodiatte TA, Eapen C, Goel A. Single-centre experience with low-volume plasma exchange and low-dose steroid to treat patients with idiosyncratic drug-induced acute liver failure. J Clin Exp Hepatol. 2024;14(2):101303.
22. Bernuau J, Rueff B, Benhamou JP. Fulminant and subfulminant liver failure: definitions and causes. Semin Liver Dis. 1986;6(2):97–106.
23. National Institutes of Health consensus development conference statement. Liver transplantation. Hepatology. 1984.
24. Bernuau J, Goudeau A, Poynard T, et al. Multivariate analysis of prognostic factors in fulminant hepatitis B. Hepatology. 1986;6(4):648–51.
25. O'Grady JG, Alexander GJ, Hayllar KM, et al. Early indicators of prognosis in fulminant hepatic failure. Gastroenterology. 1989;97(2):439–45.
26. Craig DGN, Ford AC, Hayes PC, et al. Systematic review: prognostic tests of paracetamol-induced acute liver failure. Aliment Pharmacol Therap. 2010;31:1064–76.
27. Bernal W, Donaldson N, Wyncoll D, et al. Blood lactate as an early predictor of outcome in paracetamol-induced acute liver failure: a cohort study. Lancet. 2002;359(9306):558–63.
28. McPhail MJ, Farne H, Senvar N, et al. Ability of King's College criteria and model for end-stage liver disease scores to predict mortality of patients with acute liver failure: a meta-analysis. Clin Gastroenterol Hepatol. 2016;14(4):516–525.e5; quiz e43–e45.
29. Dhiman RK, Jain S, Maheshwari U, et al. Early indicators of prognosis in fulminant hepatic failure: an assessment of the Model for End-Stage Liver Disease (MELD) and King's College Hospital criteria. Liver Transpl. 2007;13(6):814–21.
30. Kumar R, Shalimar, Sharma H, et al. Prospective derivation and validation of early dynamic model for predicting outcome in patients with acute liver failure. Gut. 2012;61(7):1068–75.
31. Ferlitsch M, Reiberger T, Hoke M, et al. von Willebrand factor as new noninvasive predictor of portal hypertension, decompensation and mortality in patients with liver cirrhosis. Hepatology. 2012;56(4):1439–47.

32. Prasanna KS, Goel A, Amirtharaj GJ, et al. Plasma von Willebrand factor levels predict in-hospital survival in patients with acute-on-chronic liver failure. Indian J Gastroenterol. 2016;35(6):432–40.
33. Hugenholtz GC, Adelmeijer J, Meijers JC, et al. An unbalance between von Willebrand factor and ADAMTS13 in acute liver failure: implications for hemostasis and clinical outcome. Hepatology. 2013;58(2):752–61.
34. Reddy MS, Rajakumar A, Mathew JS, et al. Liver transplantation society of India guidelines for the management of acute liver injury secondary to yellow phosphorus-containing rodenticide poisoning using the modified Delphi technique of consensus development. J Clin Exp Hepatol. 2021;11(4):475–83.
35. Devlin J, Wendon J, Heaton N, et al. Pretransplantation clinical status and outcome of emergency transplantation for acute liver failure. Hepatology. 1995;21(4):1018–24.
36. Bernal W, Cross TJ, Auzinger G, et al. Outcome after wait-listing for emergency liver transplantation in acute liver failure: a single centre experience. J Hepatol. 2009;50:306–13.
37. Yuan D, Liu F, Wei YG, et al. Adult-to-adult living donor liver transplantation for acute liver failure in China. World J Gastroenterol. 2012;18:7234–41.
38. Bernal W, Hyyrylainen A, Gera A, et al. Lessons from look-back in acute liver failure? A single centre experience of 3300 patients. J Hepatol. 2013;59(1):74–80.
39. Germani G, Theocharidou E, Adam R, et al. Liver transplantation for acute liver failure in Europe: outcomes over 20 years from the ELTR database. J Hepatol. 2012;57(2):288–96.
40. Bernal W, Auzinger G, Dhawan A, et al. Acute liver failure. Lancet. 2010;376(9736):190–201.
41. Sars C, Tranäng M, Ericzon BG, et al. Liver transplantation for acute liver failure - a 30-year single center experience. Scand J Gastroenterol. 2018;53(7):876–82.
42. Karvellas CJ, Leventhal TM, Rakela JL, et al. Outcomes of patients with acute liver failure listed for liver transplantation: a multicenter prospective cohort analysis. Liver Transpl. 2023;29(3):318–30.
43. Gubernatis G, Pichlmayr R, Kemnitz J, et al. Auxiliary partial orthotopic liver transplantation (APOLT) for fulminant hepatic failure: first successful case report. World J Surg. 1991;15:660–5.
44. Rela M, Kaliamoorthy I, Reddy MS. Current status of auxiliary partial orthotopic liver transplantation for acute liver failure. Liver Transpl. 2016;22(9):1265–74.
45. Jaeck D, Boudjema K, Audet M, et al. Auxiliary partial orthotopic liver transplantation (APOLT) in the treatment of acute liver failure. J Gastroenterol. 2002;37(Suppl 13):88–91.
46. Uribe M, Buckel E, Ferrario M, et al. ABO-incompatible liver transplantation: a new therapeutic option for patients with acute liver failure in Chile. In: Transplantation proceedings. 2005 Apr 1 (vol. 37, no. 3, pp. 1567–8). Elsevier.
47. Yasuda M, Ikegami T, Imai D, et al. The changes in treatment strategies in ABOi living donor liver transplantation for acute liver failure. J Med Investig. 2015;62(3.4):184–7.
48. Egawa H, Ohdan H, Saito K. Current status of ABO-incompatible liver transplantation. Transplantation. 2023;107(2):313–25.
49. Hirukawa K, Shinoda M, Hasegawa Y, et al. Long-term outcomes following ABO-incompatible living donor liver transplantation for acute liver failure: a single-center experience of over 20 years. Surg Today. 2023;53:1–3.
50. Barshes NR, Lee TC, Balkrishnan R, et al. Risk stratification of adult patients undergoing orthotopic liver transplantation for fulminant hepatic failure. Transplantation. 2006;81(2):195–201.
51. Bernal W, Wendon J, Rela M, et al. Use and outcome of liver transplantation in acetaminophen-induced acute liver failure. Hepatology. 1998;27(4):1050–5.
52. Yang HR, Thorat A, Jeng LB, et al. Living donor liver transplantation in acute liver failure patients with grade IV encephalopathy: is deep hepatic coma still an absolute contraindication? A successful single-center experience. Ann Transplant. 2018;23:176–81.
53. Mendizabal M, Silva MO. Liver transplantation in acute liver failure: a challenging scenario. World J Gastroenterol. 2016;22(4):1523.

54. Campsen J, Blei AT, Emond JC, et al. Adult-to-Adult Living Donor Liver Transplantation Cohort Study Group. Outcomes of living donor liver transplantation for acute liver failure: the adult-to-adult living donor liver transplantation cohort study. Liver Transpl. 2008;14(9):1273–80.
55. Urrunaga NH, Rachakonda VP, Magder LS, et al. Outcomes of living versus deceased donor liver transplantation for acute liver failure in the United States. In: Transplantation proceedings 2014 Jan 1 (vol. 46, no. 1, pp. 219–24). Elsevier.
56. Mallick S, Nair K, Johns SM, et al. Liver transplant in acute liver failure–looking back. J Clin Exp Hepatol. 2019;9(3):445.
57. Mehrotra S, Mehta N, Rao PS, et al. Live donor liver transplantation for acute liver failure: a single center experience. Indian J Gastroenterol. 2018;37:25–30.
58. Yamashiki N, Sugawara Y, Tamura S, et al. Outcomes after living donor liver transplantation for acute liver failure in Japan: results of a nationwide survey. Liver Transpl. 2012;18(9):1069–77.
59. Mendizabal M, Marciano S, Videla MG, et al. Fulminant presentation of autoimmune hepatitis: clinical features and early predictors of corticosteroid treatment failure. Eur J Gastroenterol Hepatol. 2015;27(6):644–8.
60. Verma S, Maheshwari A, Thuluvath P. Liver failure as initial presentation of autoimmune hepatitis: clinical characteristics, predictors of response to steroid therapy, and outcomes. Hepatology. 2009;49(4):1396–7.
61. Rahim MN, Liberal R, Miquel R, et al. Acute severe autoimmune hepatitis: corticosteroids or liver transplantation? Liver Transpl. 2019;25(6):946–59.
62. De Martin E, Coilly A, Chazouillères O, et al. FILFOIE consortium—France. Early liver transplantation for corticosteroid non-responders with acute severe autoimmune hepatitis: the SURFASA score. J Hepatol. 2021;74(6):1325–34.
63. Dhawan A, Taylor RM, Cheeseman P, et al. Wilson's disease in children: 37-year experience and revised King's score for liver transplantation. Liver Transpl. 2005;11(4):441–8.
64. Devarbhavi H, Singh R, Adarsh CK, et al. Factors that predict mortality in children with Wilson disease associated acute liver failure and comparison of Wilson disease specific prognostic indices. J Gastroenterol Hepatol. 2014;29(2):380–6.
65. Yoshitoshi EY, Takada Y, Oike F, et al. Long-term outcomes for 32 cases of Wilson's disease after living-donor liver transplantation. Transplantation. 2009;87(2):261–7.
66. Parekh J, Matei VM, Canas-Coto A, et al. Acute liver failure study group. Budd-Chiari syndrome causing acute liver failure: a multicenter case series. Liver Transpl. 2017;23(2):135–42.
67. O'Grady JG. Budd-chiari syndrome and acute liver failure: a complex condition requiring a rapid response. Liver Transpl. 2017;23(2):133–4.
68. Jayalakshmi VT, Bernal W. Update on the management of acute liver failure. Curr Opin Crit Care. 2020;26(2):163–70.
69. Ara C, Akbulut S, Ince V, et al. Living donor liver transplantation for Budd-Chiari syndrome: overcoming a troublesome situation. Medicine (Baltimore). 2016;95(43):e5136. https://doi.org/10.1097/MD.0000000000005136.
70. Ulrich F, Pratschke J, Neumann U, et al. Eighteen years of liver transplantation experience in patients with advanced Budd-Chiari syndrome. Liver Transpl. 2008;14(2):144–50.
71. Mentha G, Giostra E, Majno PE, et al. Liver transplantation for Budd–Chiari syndrome: a European study on 248 patients from 51 centres. J Hepatol. 2006;44(3):520–8.
72. Castro MA, Fassett MJ, Reynolds TB, et al. Reversible peripartum liver failure: a new perspective on the diagnosis, treatment, and cause of acute fatty liver of pregnancy, based on 28 consecutive cases. Am J Obstet Gynecol. 1999;181(2):389–95.
73. White M, Han H, Khungar V. Acute fatty liver disease of pregnancy. Clin Liver Dis (Hoboken). 2024;23(1):e0145.
74. Knight M, Nelson-Piercy C, Kurinczuk JJ, et al. UK Obstetric Surveillance System. A prospective national study of acute fatty liver of pregnancy in the UK. Gut. 2008;57(7):951–6.
75. Sheehan HL. The pathology of acute yellow atrophy and delayed chloroform poisoning. J Obstet Gynaecol Br Emp. 1940;47:49–62.

76. Ch'ng CL, Morgan M, Hainsworth I, et al. Prospective study of liver dysfunction in pregnancy in Southwest Wales. Gut. 2002;51(6):876–80. Erratum in: Gut. 2003 Feb;52(2):315.
77. Kushner T, Tholey D, Dodge J, et al. Outcomes of liver transplantation for acute fatty liver disease of pregnancy. Am J Transplant. 2019;19(7):2101–7.
78. Saraf V, Pande S, Gopalakrishnan U, et al. Acute liver failure due to zinc phosphide containing rodenticide poisoning: clinical features and prognostic indicators of need for liver transplantation. Indian J Gastroenterol. 2015;34(4):325–9.
79. Bismuth H, Samuel D, Gugenheim J, et al. Emergency liver transplantation for fulminant hepatitis. Ann Intern Med. 1987;107:337–41.
80. Donnelly MC, Hayes PC, Simpson KJ. The changing face of liver transplantation for acute liver failure: assessment of current status and implications for future practice. Liver Transplant. 2016;22:527–35.
81. Kumar SS, Mashour GA, Picton P. Neurologic considerations and complications related to liver transplantation. Anesthesiology. 2018;128:1008–14.
82. Shalimar, Kedia S, Gunjan D, et al. Acute liver failure due to hepatitis E virus infection is associated with better survival than other etiologies in Indian patients. Dig Dis Sci. 2017;62(4):1058–66.
83. Bhat M, Rabindranath M, Chara BS, et al. Artificial intelligence, machine learning, and deep learning in liver transplantation. J Hepatol. 2023;78(6):1216–33.

Chapter 9
Liver Transplant in Acute-on-Chronic Liver Failure: Selection and Outcomes

Shantan Venishetty and Shiv Kumar Sarin

Abstract Acute-on-chronic liver failure (ACLF) involves failure of organs outside the liver and carries a high risk of mortality. It represents a sudden decline in liver function in individuals with pre-existing chronic liver disease. Liver transplantation (LT) is the definitive treatment for ACLF. However, patients with ACLF tend to experience greater complications after LT compared to matched individuals with decompensated cirrhosis. Early identification of ACLF patients who would benefit from transplantation within 30 days is essential. Those with advanced ACLF grades or multiple organ failures (OF) are unlikely to benefit from LT, making it crucial to recognize patients for whom LT would be ineffective. Long-term outcomes are excellent for patients who survive the first year following transplantation. Donors with a risk index of 1.7 or higher and those with hepatic macrosteatosis exceeding 15% are generally unsuitable for organ donation.

Keywords Liver transplantation · ACLF · TAM score · Share 35 · Golden window · Futility

Key Highlights

- Acute-on-chronic liver failure (ACLF), as defined by the Asian Pacific Association for the Study of the Liver (APASL), is an acute hepatic insult manifesting as jaundice and coagulopathy complicated within 4 weeks by clinical ascites and/or

S. Venishetty
AIG Hospitals, Hyderabad, India

S. K. Sarin (✉)
Department of Hepatology, Chancellor and Director,
Institute of Liver and Biliary Sciences (ILBS), New Delhi, India
e-mail: sksarin@ilbs.in

S. Saigal, D. Jothimani (eds.), *Fundamentals of Transplant Hepatology*,
https://doi.org/10.1007/978-981-95-2624-6_9

encephalopathy in a patient with previously diagnosed or undiagnosed chronic liver disease/cirrhosis and is associated with a high 28-day mortality.
- Liver transplantation (LT) should be cautiously considered in patients with higher grades of ACLF with organ failures to avoid futility.
- Timely Liver transplantation in ACLF patients is associated with a comparable survival to that of non-ACLF patients.

9.1 Introduction

Acute-on-chronic liver failure (ACLF) is characterized by a sudden liver injury presenting with jaundice and coagulopathy, followed within 4 weeks by the development of clinical ascites and/or encephalopathy in individuals with either diagnosed or previously undiagnosed chronic liver disease or cirrhosis. This condition is linked to a high 28-day mortality rate [1]. Despite differences in their specific criteria, the three major definitions of ACLF—from the European Association for the Study of the Liver, the Asian Pacific Association for the Study of the Liver (APASL), and the North American Consortium for the Study of End-Stage Liver Disease (NACSELD)—consistently recognize its association with significant short-term mortality (see Table 9.1).

Recent evidence indicates that liver transplantation (LT) can lead to highly favorable outcomes in patients with ACLF. The risk of death increases with higher ACLF grades, and the overall incidence of ACLF has risen markedly in recent years [2]. Without LT, prognosis remains poor despite advances in supportive care. However, timely LT is often hindered by organ shortages, the presence of sepsis, and the extent of extrahepatic organ dysfunction. In Asian countries, additional barriers such as limited healthcare infrastructure, fewer experienced centers, and inadequate financial support further delay LT. The ideal timing and criteria for transplantation following the onset of organ failure remain subjects of ongoing debate. Nonetheless, early LT—within 30 days—may improve survival in selected patients.

This article highlights the challenges, selection of ideal patients, predictors of survival, and outcomes of LT, along with its futility in patients with ACLF.

9.2 Is Liver Transplantation Always Necessary in ACLF?

In the absence of liver transplantation, mortality rates in patients with ACLF are significantly high. The 28-day transplant-free mortality rates are reported as 23%, 32%, and 75% for ACLF grades 1, 2, and 3, respectively [3]. Despite this, due to the liver's regenerative capacity and the dynamic nature of ACLF, spontaneous resolution may occur in 55% of patients with ACLF-1, 35% with ACLF-2, and 15% with ACLF-3 [4]. Outcomes are strongly influenced by the ACLF grade assessed between days 3 and 7, with those in advanced stages requiring early transplant evaluation and listing. Without a transplant, the 1-year survival drops to just 8%, compared to 80% in those who undergo liver transplantation [5]. While LT is the preferred treatment, early listing—within the first 7 days—remains challenging in settings with limited resources.

Table 9.1 Acute on chronic liver failure—three major definitions

	APASL	NACSELD	EASL-CLIF
Definition	Jaundice (>5 mg/dL) and coagulopathy (INR >1.5) followed by ascites and/or hepatic encephalopathy within 4 wk. in a patient with known or unknown liver disease	Often infection-related extrahepatic organ failure in a patient with cirrhosis	Acute decompensation presenting with extrahepatic organ failure in a patient with cirrhosis
Liver involvement	Bilirubin >5 mg/dL	Not required	Not required (bilirubin >12 mg/dL is considered as organ failure)
Coagulopathy	INR >1.5 is must	Not required	Not required (INR >2.5 is considered as organ failure)
Infection	Considered as a consequence	Most often is a precipitant	Most often is a precipitant
Renal involvement	Not required	Renal replacement therapy is required	Must (serum creatinine level should be >1.5 mg/dL to identify ACLF and >2 to define organ failure)
Reversibility	Possible	Unlikely	Unlikely
Severity scores	AARC	–	CLIF-C ACLF; CLIF-C OF
Validation of the TAM score to predict post-LT outcomes	No	No	Yes

Abbreviations: *APASL* Asian Pacific Association for Study of the Liver, *EASL-CLIF* European Association for Study of Liver-Consortium for Liver Failure, *NACSELD* North American Consortium for Study of End-Stage Liver Disease, *CLIF-C OF* chronic liver failure-consortium organ failure, *CLIF-C ACLF* chronic liver failure-consortium ACLF, *INR* international normalized ratio, *AARC* APASL ACLF research consortium, *TAM* transplantation for ACLF-3 model

9.3 Identifying the Ideal Liver Transplant Candidate

Multiple scoring systems have been designed to estimate transplant-free survival in ACLF patients [6, 7], including the Model for End-Stage Liver Disease (MELD), CLIF-C ACLF, CLIF-C OF, and AARC scores. However, these tools do not reliably predict post-transplant outcomes, which are more dependent on recipient and donor characteristics [8–11].

Several models have been proposed for predicting post-LT survival:

Levesque et al. [12] introduced a model predicting 90-day mortality based on recipient and donor gender, age, the LT indication (hepatocellular carcinoma vs. end-stage cirrhosis), recent infections, and the presence of ACLF at transplantation.

End-stage cirrhosis in male recipients was associated with reduced mortality risk, while infections, ACLF at transplant, and donor-recipient age and sex factors increased risk.

Huebener et al. [13] proposed the orthotopic liver Transplantation (OLT)-Survival Score, derived from the CLIF-C ACLF score at transplant and whether there was clinical improvement (defined as the recovery of at least one previously failed organ). The score is calculated as:

0.03 × CLIF-C Score—Clinical improvement (yes: 1; no: 0)
This tool effectively predicted 90-day survival post-transplant.

Artzner et al. [14] developed a model for ACLF grade 3 patients, using four pre-transplant risk factors: age ≥53, arterial lactate ≥4 mmol/L, mechanical ventilation with P/F ratio ≤200 mm Hg, and leukocyte count ≤10 G/L. These were incorporated into the Transplantation for ACLF-3 Model (TAM) score, assigning 1 point per factor. Patients with a TAM score >2 had a 1-year survival rate of 8%, compared to 84% in those with a score ≤2. This score performed better when calculated within 48 h before LT, and patient optimization (i.e., lowering the score) prior to LT improved outcomes.

Chen et al. [15] created a nomogram to predict 1-year survival in HBV-related ACLF patients undergoing LT, incorporating white blood cell count, alanine aminotransferase (ALT)/aspartate aminotransferase (AST) ratio, and the number of organ failures.

Singal et al., [16] using United Network for Organ Sharing (UNOS) data, devised a model for ACLF-3 patients based on recipient age, alcohol-related liver disease, and failures in pulmonary, neurological, and cardiovascular systems. Patients were grouped by risk:

Low risk (score <7.55): 1-year survival 89%
Medium risk (score 7.55–11.57): survival 82%
High risk (score >11.57): survival 80%

Notably, high-risk patients receiving high-quality grafts (donor risk index (DRI) <1.5) had better 1-year survival (83%) than those with lower-quality grafts (DRI ≥1.5; survival 78%).

Wackenthaler et al. [17] used pre-transplant CT imaging to predict 1-year survival post-LT. Their score included three factors: splenomegaly (>500 cm^3), liver atrophy (>20% smaller than expected), and inferior vena cava diameter ratio (VCR ≤0.2). The VCR was calculated based on measurements 1 cm above and below the left renal vein. A score above 10 was linked to poorer outcomes.

All these models require additional validation through prospective studies (Table 9.2).

Table 9.2 Models predicting post-LT outcomes in ACLF

Score	Author	Year	Components of score	Highlights
Model by Levesque et al	Levesque et al. [12]	2017	Recipient age (>57.2 year) and gender (male) Male donor Indication for LT (ESLD or HCC) Infection Presence of ACLF	90-day post-LT mortality
OLT-survival score	Huebener et al. [13]	2018	CLIF-C score Clinical improvement	90-day post-LT survival Applicable for all grades of ACLF
Transplantation for ACLF-3 model (TAM score)	Artzner et al. [14]	2020	Recipient age ≥53 year Pre-LT arterial lactate level ≥4 mmol/L PaO_2/FIO_2 ≤200 mm Hg Pre-LT leukocyte count ≤10 G/L	Predicts 1 year survival post-LT (Score ≤2: 84% survival Score >2: 8.3% survival)
Nomogram	Chen et al. [15]	2021	White cell counts ALT/AST ratio Number of organ failures	Predicts 1-year post-LT survival Applicable for HBV-related ACLF diagnosed by either APASL or European Association for the Study of the Liver (EASL) criteria
Model by Singal	Singal et al. [16]	2022	Recipient age Pulmonary failure Brain failure Cardiovascular failure Alcohol etiology	1-year post-LT survival Applicable for ACLF grade 3 Score >9.7 is inversely related to survival
Computed tomography-based score	Wackenthaler et al. [17]	2022	Splenomegaly (>500 cm^3): 5 points Liver atrophy (>20% smaller than the expected liver volume): 5 points Inferior vena cava diameter ratio (VCR ≤0.2): 12 points	Applicable for patients with ACLF-3 Score >10—poor survival post-LT

Abbreviations: *ALT* alanine transaminase, *AST* aspartate transaminase, *CLIF-C ACLF* chronic liver failure-consortium ACLF, *ESLD* end-stage liver disease, *FiO_2* fraction of inspired oxygen, *HCC* hepatocellular carcinoma, *OLT* orthotopic liver transplantation, *TAM* Transplantation for ACLF-3 model

9.4 Futility of Liver Transplantation in Acute-on-Chronic Liver Failure

In patients with ACLF, identifying an appropriate candidate and determining the timing of LT have a significant impact on outcomes. In advanced grades of ACLF, the futility of transplant, considering the low survival post-LT, has to be recognized [18]. A "potentially inappropriate candidate" is a patient with ACLF who has a high probability of mortality early after LT or has an unacceptable quality of life (QoL) and/or multiple complications post-LT [11]. A post-LT survival of less than 3 months (or in-hospital mortality) is considered a futile LT [10].

Preallocation survival outcomes following liver transplantation (SOFT) score [19], balance of risk (BAR) score [20], liver transplant risk score (LTRS) [21], and University of California, Los Angeles (UCLA) score [22] are some of the scores for the prediction of survival post-LT. However, Artru et al. [5] reported that none of the scores could identify survival accurately. However, the UCLA score was a better predictor of post-LT survival in comparison to other scores. A few indicators of futility are as follows:

- MELD-Na greater than 30 with advanced hepatic encephalopathy (HE) at baseline [23].
- Persistently high lactate levels [24–27].
- Greater than or equal to four organ failures [4].
- Futility risk score greater than 8 [28, 29]—Futility risk score is based on ventilator support (5 points), recipient age greater than 60 years (3 points), preoperative dialysis (3 points), preoperative diabetes (2 points), and preoperative creatinine levels greater than or equal to 1.5 mg/dL but no dialysis (2 points). A score greater than 8 is associated with poor graft survival.
- CLIF-C score greater than 64 at day 3–7 [4].
- Respiratory failure and/or requiring mechanical ventilation [9, 25, 26, 30].
- Patients with ACLF grade 2/3, with either active gastrointestinal bleed, controlled sepsis for less than 24 h, high vasopressor support, and/or P/F ratio less than 150 [5].
- Active drug abuse, infections by multidrug-resistant organism (MDROs) or invasive fungal infections, high cardiac risk, significant comorbidities [10, 31].
- Clinical frailty score greater than or equal to 7 [24] (Table 9.3).

Table 9.3 Factors associated with poor outcomes post-LT

Recipient factors	Donor-related factors
Transplantation from ICU [13]	DRI ≥1.7 [28, 30, 32]
Portal vein thrombosis [31]	Male donor [12]
Mechanical ventilation at LT	Donor BMI
Cerebral failure [9, 15]	Hepatic macrosteatosis >15% [16]
CLIF-C ACLF score >64 >3 OF [15]	
Need for RRT [33]	
Arterial lactate >4 mmol/L	
MDROs [33]	
Pre-transplant ICU care (shorter stay, better outcomes) [32, 34]	
TAM score >2	
Futility risk score >8 [28, 35]	
Clinical frailty score ≥7 [24]	
Cold ischemia time >8.5 h [11]	

Abbreviations: *BMI* body mass index, *DRI* donor risk index, *FiO_2* fraction of inspired oxygen, *ICU* intensive care unit, *OFs* organ failures, *RRT* renal replacement therapy, *TAM* transplantation for ACLF-3 model

9.5 MELD Score-Based Early Liver Transplantation and Challenges in ACLF

9.5.1 Limitations of MELD Scoring in ACLF Patients

The Model for End-Stage Liver Disease score, the current standard for organ allocation, does not adequately reflect the extrahepatic organ failures that are central to the diagnosis of ACLF. This limits the score's effectiveness in accurately prioritizing ACLF patients for liver transplantation. However, MELD may have more predictive value in ACLF cases defined by the APASL criteria, which focus primarily on liver dysfunction [36, 37].

In a retrospective study involving 18,979 hospitalized ACLF patients, 48.5% had grade 1, 38.2% had grade 2, and 13.3% had grade 3 ACLF. The median MELD-Na scores were 24, 27, and 32 for grades 1, 2, and 3, respectively. Notably, 90-day mortality in ACLF patients was higher than expected based on MELD-Na, particularly among those with scores between 10 and 30. The lower the MELD-Na score, the greater the underestimation of mortality risk. This pattern was consistent across definitions from Chronic Liver Failure–Acute-on-Chronic Liver Failure in Cirrhosis (European CANONIC Study by EASL-CLIF Consortium) (CANONIC), NACSELD, and APASL [38]. As a result, many ACLF patients were not listed for LT, despite being at high risk. Another study reported a 33–40% waitlist mortality in ACLF patients with MELD scores under 25, compared to less than 10% in non-ACLF patients with similar MELD scores [39].

9.5.2 *Impact of "Share 35" and MELD-Based Allocation*

Implemented in 2013, the "Share 35" policy was intended to prioritize severely ill patients for liver transplantation and reduce waitlist mortality, especially those with MELD-Na scores ≥35 [40]. While this policy has lowered mortality in some ACLF patients, [41] most ACLF patients tend to have MELD-Na scores in the 30–35 range, often falling just short of meeting the "Share 35" threshold. This phenomenon contributes to inequities in access to timely transplantation. As such, MELD-based allocation may disadvantage ACLF patients [41].

9.6 Timing of Liver Transplantation in ACLF

Accurate identification of ACLF patients who require transplantation is crucial to improving survival. A study by the APASL ACLF research consortium (AARC) found that transplant eligibility increased from 35% to 60% within 7 days after stabilization of sepsis and organ dysfunction [23]. However, delaying LT beyond 7 days led to higher rates of multiorgan failure and increased mortality—23% of deaths occurred within the first week and 55% within 28 days. Yet, only 4% of 1021 patients assessed in this multicenter study ultimately underwent transplantation.

The development of hepatic encephalopathy, rising white blood cell counts, and elevated creatinine within the first week were all predictors of 28-day mortality. Importantly, LT performed within 30 days of listing significantly improved both performance status and survival outcomes.

The CANONIC study from the EASL-CLIF Consortium [4] reported that 81% of patients reached their final ACLF grade by day 7, making this time frame critical for outcome prediction. Among those who received early LT (within 28 days), 75% survived at least one year. The ACLF grade largely determined outcomes between days 3 and 7. For instance, 6-month survival for ACLF grade 2 and 3 patients who underwent LT within 28 days was 81%, compared to just 10% in those who were not transplanted. Mortality was 100% at 90 days for patients with four or more organ failures or a CLIF-C score >64 who did not undergo LT [30].

9.7 Predictive Models and Waitlist Mortality

Goudsmit et al. [42] introduced the ACLF Joint Model (ACLF-JM) to help assess the urgency for LT. The model incorporates age, ACLF grade, sex, life support requirement, presence of spontaneous bacterial peritonitis, MELD-Na score, and changes in MELD-Na over 2, 7, and 14 days. It was effective in predicting 28-day and 90-day mortality on the waitlist.

Waitlist outcomes are closely tied to the number of organ failures [30, 43]. Within 30 days:

10% of patients without organ failure are delisted.
80% of those with two organ failures are delisted.
98% of those with three or more organ failures are delisted.

Improvement in a patient's condition before transplantation is strongly associated with better outcomes [44]. Specifically, recovery in circulatory and cerebral functions, respiratory improvement, and weaning from mechanical ventilation reduce post-transplant mortality. Thus, supportive interventions aimed at stabilizing failing organs and bridging patients to LT are essential [45–47]. A multidisciplinary approach to care is critical in achieving optimal outcomes for ACLF patients.

9.8 Outcomes of Liver Transplantation in ACLF

The post-transplant survival depends on the grade of ACLF. Survival post-LT for ACLF grade 1 is 90% compared with 70–80% in patients with ACLF grades 2 and 3 at 1 year [4]. The long-term survival of patients with ACLF undergoing LT is greater than 80% compared with less than 40% in non-transplant patients with ACLF [5, 48]. Initial studies reported poorer outcomes in patients with ACLF and multiorgan failures [12]. However, several retrospective and national database-based studies have demonstrated excellent outcomes with LT in ACLF.

Based on the ACLF defined by APASL, Finkenstedt et al. [49] compared 33 ACLF patients (mean MELD-Na-30) with 356 non-ACLF patients (mean MELD-Na-18) who underwent transplant and found similar survival rates (85% vs. 84%) at 29 months. However, the waitlist mortality was 54%. Chen et al. [15] studied 290 patients with HBV ACLF who underwent transplant, out of which 35.5% had more than three organ failures at the time of LT. The mean survival was 77% at 1 year. However, patients with circulatory, cerebral, and respiratory failure had high post-LT mortality. Chen et al. [48] in 2022 compared 29 ACLF patients who underwent transplant with 110 ACLF patients who were non-transplant. The 1-year survival was 87% in the transplanted group, compared to 42.7% in the non-transplanted group. However, the transplanted ACLF patients had higher morbidity and risk of pulmonary infections when compared to a matched cohort of decompensated cirrhosis patients who underwent transplantation. Wang et al. [50] demonstrated 95.5% survival at 3 years and 93% survival at 5 years in ACLF patients who underwent transplantation. They had frequent portal vein complications post-LT. Kulkarni et al. [51] retrospectively studied 73 ACLF patients who underwent living donor liver transplantation (LDLT), out of which 18 patients died within 30 days. Most were in grade II ACLF (87.3%) at the time of LDLT (APASL ACLF Research Consortium [AARC] score: 9.05 ± 1; MELD NA: 28.15 ± 4.13). The survival rate was 72.73%, with a mean follow-up period of 925.21 days; 58.2% (32/55) developed complications during the first year post-LT, and 45% (25/55) and 12.7% (7/55) developed infections within and after 3 months.

Toshima et al. [35], based on newly proposed Japanese criteria, showed 80–100% survival at 5 years in the ACLF grade 0–2 group, while the survival was only 33.3% in the grade 3 ACLF, demonstrating that ACLF-3 had a poor outcome post-LDLT.

Based on the CANONIC definition and the European Association for the Study of the Liver–Chronic Liver Failure (EASL-CLIF) criteria, Gustot et al. [4] prospectively evaluated 388 patients with acute-on-chronic liver failure (ACLF), among whom 35 underwent early liver transplantation. At the time of transplant, 10 patients had no ACLF, 5 patients had grade 1 ACLF, and 11 patients had grade 2 ACLF. The 1-year survival was 90% in the no ACLF group, while it was 80% in the ACLF-1 group and 71.6% in the ACLF-2 group. The grade of ACLF at day 3–7 determined the outcome. Levesque et al. [12] showed that the survival rates at 3 and 12 months among patients with ACLF compared to those without ACLF were 79.3% vs. 96.2% and 70% vs. 91.4%, respectively. Compared to patients without ACLF, those with ACLF experienced a significantly longer stay in the intensive care unit (ICU) (11.5 ± 16.5 vs. 17.5 ± 19 days). The 90-day and one-year survival probabilities in patients with ACLF grade 1 or 2 were 84.5% and 77.2%, respectively, while they were 60% and 43.3% in patients with ACLF grade 3. Huebener P et al. [13] retrospectively analyzed 250 cirrhotic liver transplant recipients, of whom 98 patients fulfilled diagnostic criteria for ACLF. Compared to non-ACLF patients, ACLF was associated with significantly higher short-term morbidity and mortality after liver transplantation (90-day patient survival: 96.1% non-ACLF vs. 72.4% ACLF patients). ACLF patients required approximately twice as many transfusions as non-ACLF recipients during OLT. ACLF recipients had to undergo significantly more surgical interventions as well as invasive procedures (i.e., thoracocentesis, chest tube insertions, tracheotomies, and endoscopic interventions) before discharge from the hospital and required longer hospitalization in the intensive care unit (median 16.0 vs. 4.0 days). Following the 90-day post-transplant period, patient survival and long-term graft functions were comparable between ACLF and non-ACLF liver transplant recipients for up to 5 years. Another retrospective analysis of a single-center study by Agbim et al. [52] showed that patients with ACLF experienced prolonged hospitalization and ICU care. Early surgical re-explorations occurred in 26.7% of the ACLF group compared to 14.6% of the non-ACLF group; graft loss depended on ACLF grade, with rates of 6%, 19%, and 21%, respectively; and there was a higher need for renal replacement therapy (RRT) post-LT in the ACLF group. Sundaram et al. [27] retrospectively reviewed data from 318 patients who underwent LT. The length of stay post-LT was correlated with the grade of ACLF. Higher acute cellular rejection (ACR) post-LT was seen in patients with grade 3 ACLF (13%). There were more infections in patients with ACLF grades 2 and 3. PVT increased the risk of post-LT mortality within 1 year. Comparable outcomes were seen between those with and without circulatory failure. There was a high utilization of resources in ACLF grades 2 and 3 [53].

In short, LT in ACLF patients shows frequent complications in the early post-LT period (initial 6–12 months), and patients surviving the early period have excellent long-term outcomes [54, 55]. Patients with ACLF have higher morbidity post-LT, requiring higher health care utilization due to prolonged hospitalization, ICU care, renal replacement therapy, and recurrent readmissions for infections [33, 51, 52]. Post-transplant vascular and biliary complications, re-explorations, and pulmonary, neurologic, and cardiovascular complications are significantly higher in patients with ACLF grade 3 who undergo LT [5, 52].

The prevalence of infections post-LT increases with the grade of ACLF at LT. Common sites of infection include the urinary tract, lung, and spontaneous bacteremia. Patients with ACLF grade 3 are prone to develop multisite infections [53]. Kidney dysfunction is frequent in patients with ACLF. The incidence of chronic kidney disease post-LT is slightly higher in patients with ACLF than in non-ACLF, although renal recovery is similar [54, 56, 57]. However, the development of other comorbidities, including diabetes mellitus, dyslipidemia, systemic hypertension, and obesity, is similar among patients with ACLF and those without ACLF post-LT.

Goosmann and colleagues [54] compared the quality of life post-LT among patients with ACLF and non-ACLF. The median follow-up in the whole cohort was 8.7 years. Patients with ACLF reported an inability to perform usual activities and had a higher incidence of anxiety/depression, and less than 50% of patients reported "optimal" health. Patients with ACLF reported poorer physical and psychological health. The QoL was inversely related to the duration of ICU hospitalization following LT, indicating a measurable and significant impact of liver disease severity on long-term outcomes.

9.9 Conclusion

Liver transplantation (LT) is a viable option for patients with ACLF, provided they are carefully selected and a suitable donor organ is available in a timely manner. However, in cases where the prognosis is poor, it is essential to consider the futility of proceeding with LT. Decisions regarding transplant listing should ideally be made within the first week of diagnosis. There is a need for prospective studies in living donor liver transplantation (LDLT) settings to evaluate both the practicality and limitations of early LDLT in ACLF, as most current evidence is derived from retrospective or registry-based studies.

Early identification of ACLF patients who could benefit from LT—preferably within 30 days—is a cornerstone of effective management. Patients with ACLF grade 3, an APASL score ≥13, or more than three organ failures as defined by EASL-CLIF may already be beyond the window of benefit, indicating that LT may be futile in these cases. One-year post-transplant survival is around 90% for patients with ACLF grade 1, compared to 70–80% for those with grades 2 and 3. Therefore, early referral is advantageous. Additionally, bridging therapies may help downgrade ACLF severity or improve organ function, allowing for relisting and improving the chances of successful transplantation.

References

1. Sarin SK, Choudhury A, Sharma MK. Acute-on-chronic liver failure:consensus recommendations of the Asian Pacific association for the study of the liver (APASL): an update. Hepatol Int. 2019;13(4):353–90.
2. Allen AM, Kim WR, Moriarty JP. Time trends in the health care burden and mortality of acute on chronic liver failure in the United States. Hepatology. 2016;64(6):2165–72.
3. Moreau R, Jalan R, Gines P. Acute-on-chronic liver failure is a distinct syndrome that develops in patients with acute decompensation of cirrhosis. Gastroenterology. 2013;144(7):1–1437.
4. Gustot T, Fernandez J, Garcia E. Clinical course of acute-on-chronic liver failure syndrome and effects on prognosis. Hepatology. 2015;62(1):243–52.
5. Artru F, Louvet A, Ruiz I. Liver transplantation in the most severely ill cirrhotic patients: a multicenter study in acute-on-chronic liver failure grade 3. J Hepatol. 2017;67(4):708–15.
6. Zheng YX, Zhong X, Li YJ. Performance of scoring systems to predict mortality of patients with acute-on-chronic liver failure: a systematic review and meta-analysis. J Gastroenterol Hepatol. 2017;32(10):1668–78.
7. Vipani A, Lindenmeyer CC, Sundaram V. Treatment of severe acute on chronic liver failure: management of organ failures, investigational therapeutics, and the role of liver transplantation. J Clin Gastroenterol. 2021;55(8):667–76.
8. Zhou Z, Yi J, Li Q. Factors prognostic of survival in liver transplant recipients with hepatitis B virus related acute-on-chronic liver failure. Can J Gastroenterol Hepatol. 2022;2022(6390809)
9. Xia L, Qiao ZY, Zhang ZJ. Transplantation for EASL-CLIF and APASL acuteon- chronic liver failure (ACLF) patients: the TEA cohort to evaluate long-term post-transplant outcomes. EClinicalMedicine. 2022;49(101476):101476.
10. Petrowsky H, Rana A, Kaldas FM. Liver transplantation in highest acuity recipients: identifying factors to avoid futility. Ann Surg. 2014;259(6):1186–94.
11. Linecker M, Krones T, Berg T. Potentially inappropriate liver transplantation in the era of the "sickest first" policy – a search for the upper limits. J Hepatol. 2018;68(4):798–813.
12. Levesque E, Winter A, Noorah Z. Impact of acute-on-chronic liver failure on 90-day mortality following a first liver transplantation. Liver Int. 2017;37(5):684–93.
13. Huebener P, Sterneck MR, Bangert K. Stabilisation of acute-on-chronic liver failure patients before liver transplantation predicts post-transplant survival. Aliment Pharmacol Ther. 2018;47(11):1502–10.
14. Michard B, Artzner T, Deridder M. Pretransplant intensive care unit management and selection of grade 3 acute-on-chronic liver failure transplant candidates. Liver Transpl. 2022;28(1):17–26.
15. Chen L, Zhang J, Lu T. A nomogram to predict survival in patients with acute-on-chronic hepatitis B liver failure after liver transplantation. Ann Transl Med. 2021;9(7):555.
16. Singal AK, Kuo YF, Waleed M. High-risk liver transplant recipients with grade 3 acute on chronic liver failure should receive the good quality graft. Liver Int. 2022;42(7):1629–37.
17. Wackenthaler A, Molie're S, Artzner T. Pre-operative CT scan helps predict outcome after liver transplantation for acute-on-chronic grade 3 liver failure. Eur Radiol. 2022;32(1):12–21.
18. Ferna´ndez JSF. Liver transplantation in patients with ACLF and multiple organ failure: time for priority after initial stabilization. J Hepatol. 2018;69(5):1004–6.
19. Rana A, Hardy MA, Halazun KJ, Woodland DC, Ratner LE, Samstein B, et al. Survival outcomes following liver transplantation (SOFT) score: a novel method to predict patient survival following liver transplantation. Am J Transplant. 2008;8(12):2537–46.
20. Martínez JA, Pacheco S, Bachler JP, Jarufe N, Briceño E, Guerra JF, et al. Accuracy of the BAR score in the prediction of survival after liver transplantation. Ann Hepatol. 2019;18(2):386–92.

21. Kaltenmeier C, Jorgensen D, Dharmayan S, Ayloo S, Rachakonda V, Geller DA, et al. The liver transplant risk score prognosticates the outcomes of liver transplant recipients at listing. HPB. 2021;23(6):927–36.
22. Ghobrial RM, Gornbein J, Steadman R, Danino N, Markmann JF, Holt C, et al. Pretransplant model to predict posttransplant survival in liver transplant patients. Ann Surg. 2002;236(3):315–23.
23. Choudhury A, Vijayaraghavan R, Maiwall R. First week' is the crucial period for deciding living donor liver transplantation in patients with acute-on-chronic liver failure. Hepatol Int. 2021;15(6):1376–88.
24. Weiss E, Saner F, Asrani SK. When is a critically ill cirrhotic patient too sick to transplant? Development of consensus criteria by a multidisciplinary panel of 35 international experts. Transplantation. 2021;105(3):561–8.
25. Michard B, Artzner T, Lebas B. Liver transplantation in critically ill patients: preoperative predictive factors of post-transplant mortality to avoid futility. Clin Transpl [Internet]. 2017;31(12) Available from: https://doi.org/10.1111/ctr.13115.
26. Laici C, Guizzardi C, Morelli MC. Predictive factors of inhospital mortality for ICU patients with acute-on-chronic liver failure undergoing liver transplantation. Eur J Gastroenterol Hepatol. 2022;34(9):967–74.
27. Sundaram V, Patel S, Shetty K. Risk factors for posttransplantation mortality in recipients with grade 3 acute-on-chronic liver failure: analysis of a north American consortium. Liver Transpl. 2022;28(6):1078–89.
28. Sundaram V, Jalan R, Wu T. Factors associated with survival of patients with severe acute-on-chronic liver failure before and after liver transplantation. Gastroenterology. 2019;156(5):1381–91.
29. Asrani SK, Saracino G, O'Leary JG. Recipient characteristics and morbidity and mortality after liver transplantation. J Hepatol. 2018;69(1):43–50.
30. Thuluvath PJ, Thuluvath AJ, Hanish S. Liver transplantation in patients with multiple organ failures: feasibility and outcomes. J Hepatol. 2018;69(5):1047–56.
31. Artzner T, Bernal W, Belli LS. Location and allocation: inequity of access to liver transplantation for patients with severe acute-on-chronic liver failure in Europe. Liver Transpl. 2022;28(9):1429–40.
32. Sundaram V, Kogachi S, Wong RJ. Effect of the clinical course of acute-onchronic liver failure prior to liver transplantation on post-transplant survival. J Hepatol. 2020;72(3):481–8.
33. Belli LS, Duvoux C, Artzner T. Liver transplantation for patients with acuteon- chronic liver failure (ACLF) in Europe: results of the ELITA/EF-CLIF collaborative study (ECLIS). J Hepatol. 2021;75(3):610–22.
34. Thuluvath PJ, Thuluvath AJ, Savva Y. Karnofsky performance status following liver transplantation in patients with multiple organ failures and probable acute-on-chronic liver failure. Clin Gastroenterol Hepatol. 2020;18(1):234–41.
35. Toshima T, Harada N, Itoh S. Outcomes of living-donor liver transplantation for acute-on-chronic liver failure based on newly proposed criteria in Japan. Clin Transpl. 2022;36(8)
36. Laique SN, Zhang N, Hewitt WR. Increased access to liver transplantation for patients with acute on chronic liver failure after implementation of Share 35 Rule: an analysis from the UNOS database. Ann Hepatol. 2021;23(100288):100288.
37. Kumar R, Krishnamoorthy TL, Tan HK. Change in model for end-stage liver disease score at two weeks, as an indicator of mortality or liver transplantation at 60 days in acute-on-chronic liver failure. Gastroenterol Rep Oxf. 2015;3(2):122–7.
38. Hernaez R, Liu Y, Kramer J. Model for end-stage liver disease-sodium underestimates 90-day mortality risk in patients with acute-on-chronic liver failure. J Hepatol. 2020;73(6):1425–33.
39. Chang J, Matheja A, Krzycki S. Model for end-stage liver disease underestimates mortality of patients with acute-on-chronic liver failure waiting for liver transplantation. Dig Liver Dis. 2022;54(6):784–90.

40. Sharma P, Schaubel DE, Gong Q. End-stage liver disease candidates at the highest model for end-stage liver disease scores have higher wait-list mortality than status-1A candidates. Hepatology. 2012;55(1):192–8.
41. Sundaram V, Shah P, Mahmud N. Patients with severe acute-on-chronic liver failure are disadvantaged by model for end-stage liver disease-based organ allocation policy. Aliment Pharmacol Ther. 2020;52(7):1204–13.
42. Goudsmit BFJ, Braat AE, Tushuizen ME. Development and validation of a dynamic survival prediction model for patients with acute-on-chronic liver failure. JHEP Rep. 2021;3(6)
43. Reddy KR, O'Leary JG, Kamath PS. High risk of delisting or death in liver transplant candidates following infections: results from the North American consortium for the study of end-stage liver disease. Liver Transpl. 2015;21(7):881–8.
44. Kim JE, Sinn DH, Choi GS. Predictors and outcome of emergent liver transplantation for patients with acute-on-chronic liver failure. Dig Liver Dis. 2021;53(8):1004–10.
45. Wong F, Pappas SC, Reddy KR. Terlipressin use and respiratory failure in patients with hepatorenal syndrome type 1 and severe acute-on-chronic liver failure. Aliment Pharmacol Ther. 2022;56(8):1284–93.
46. Abbas N, Rajoriya N, Elsharkawy AM. Acute-on-chronic liver failure (ACLF) in 2022: have novel treatment paradigms already arrived? Expert Rev Gastroenterol Hepatol. 2022;16(7):639–52.
47. Larsen FS. Artificial liver support in acute and acute-on-chronic liver failure. Curr Opin Crit Care. 2019;25(2):187–91.
48. Chen GH, Wu RL, Huang F. Liver transplantation in acute-on-chronic liver failure: excellent outcome and difficult posttransplant course. Front Surg. 2022;9(914611)
49. Finkenstedt A, Nachbaur K, Zoller H. Acute-on-chronic liver failure: excellent outcomes after liver transplantation but high mortality on the wait list. Liver Transpl. 2013;19(8):879–86.
50. Wang YC, Yong CC, Lin CC. Excellent outcome in living donor liver transplantation: treating patients with acute-on-chronic liver failure. Liver Transpl. 2021;27(11):1633–43.
51. Kulkarni AV, Reddy R, Sharma M, Iyengar S, Rambhatla A, Gv P, et al. Healthcare utilization and outcomes of living donor liver transplantation for patients with APASL-defined acute-on-chronic liver failure. Hepatol Int. 2023;17:1233.
52. Agbim U, Sharma A, Maliakkal B. Outcomes of liver transplant recipients with acute-on-chronic liver failure based on EASL-CLIF consortium definition: a single-center study. Transpl Direct. 2020;6(4)
53. Sundaram V, Lindenmeyer CC, Shetty K. Patients with acute-on-chronic liver failure have greater healthcare resource utilization after liver transplantation. Clin Gastroenterol Hepatol. 2023;21(3):704–12.
54. Goosmann L, Buchholz A, Bangert K. Liver transplantation for acute-onchronic liver failure predicts post-transplant mortality and impaired long-term quality of life. Liver Int. 2021;41(3):574–84.
55. Sundaram V, Mahmud N, Perricone G. Longterm outcomes of patients undergoing liver transplantation for acute-on-chronic liver failure. Liver Transpl. 2020;26(12):1594–602.
56. O'Leary JG, Bajaj JS, Tandon P. Outcomes after listing for liver transplant in patients with acute-on-chronic liver failure: the multicenter North American consortium for the study of end-stage liver disease experience. Liver Transpl. 2019;25(4):571–9.
57. Marciano S, Mauro E, Giunta D. Impact of acute-on-chronic liver failure on post-transplant survival and on kidney outcomes. Eur J Gastroenterol Hepatol. 2019;31(9):1157–64.

Chapter 10
Chronic Hepatitis B and C Infection

Yogesh K. Chawla and Dibya Lochan Praharaj

Abstract Infection with hepatitis B and C virus are the two most common cause of chronic hepatitis, cirrhosis, and hepatocellular carcinoma worldwide. Hepatitis B virus (HBV) is a DNA virus and possesses remarkable ability to integrate in to host genome using its covalently closed circular DNA. This constitutes the major barrier in cure from HBV infection. Immune response to HBV infection is dynamic and differs with respect to age of acquisition of infection, mode of transmission of infection, and viral genotype. Nucleotide analogues are commonly used to treat HBV infection in a few selected group of patients though complete cure from the infection using these agents is unlikely. In contrast, hepatitis C virus is an RNA virus. With advent of directly acting antivirals (DAAs) management of HCV infection has been simplified and complete elimination of the virus may be achieved in near future. The aim of the chapter is to provide a brief outline of pathogenesis, clinical manifestations, and current management and prevention of HBV and HCV infection.

Keywords Hepatitis B virus · Hepatitis C virus · Directly acting antiviral agents · Extrahepatic manifestations

Y. K. Chawla · D. L. Praharaj (✉)
Department of Gastroenterology and Hepatology, Kalinga Institute of Medical Sciences (KIMS), Bhubaneswar, Odisha, India
e-mail: dibyalochanpraharaj@gmail.com

S. Saigal, D. Jothimani (eds.), *Fundamentals of Transplant Hepatology*,
https://doi.org/10.1007/978-981-95-2624-6_10

Abbreviations

AFP	Alfa-fetoprotein
ALF	Acute liver failure
ALT	Alanine transaminase
DAA	Directly acting antivirals
HBIG	Hepatitis B immunoglobulin
HBV	Hepatitis B virus
HCV	Hepatitis C virus
HCV	Hepatocellular carcinoma
LT	Liver transplantation
NANBH	Non A Non B hepatitis
ULN	Upper limit of normal

Key Highlights

- Hepatitis B virus and hepatitis C virus are the two most common causes of chronic hepatitis, liver cirrhosis, and hepatocellular carcinoma worldwide
- Hepatitis B virus integrates into host genome using covalently circular DNA, enabling the virus to evade immune system and preventing its elimination
- In contrast, hepatitis C virus is an RNA virus and can now be easily cured using directly acting antivirals (DAAs)
- The natural history of HBV infection in humans is dynamic and depends on various host and viral factors
- In addition to chronic hepatitis, both these viruses are associated with various extrahepatic manifestations
- A highly efficacious vaccine is available to prevent transmission of HBV infection, which, along with DAAs are likely to play a pivotal role in achieving the WHO goal of eliminating viral hepatitis by 2030

10.1 Introduction

Hepatitis B virus (HBV) and hepatitis C virus (HCV) are the two most common hepatotropic viruses that cause chronic hepatitis, cirrhosis, and hepatocellular carcinoma (HCC). Despite significant advances in understanding of pathogenesis and treatment in the last two decades, both these viruses constitute major cause of cirrhosis, HCC, and death worldwide. The capability of HBV to incorporate its covalently closed circular DNA into the host hepatocyte genome constitutes a major barrier in eradication of the virus in chronic stage. Nonetheless, few of these patients are able to eradicate the virus which depends on an extremely complex interaction between host immunity, virus, and treatment regimen commonly used. One important advance in HBV infection is the widespread availability of a highly effective vaccine, which has made prevention of HBV infection a reality. In contrast, with recent advent of directly acting antivirals (DAAs), the treatment of HCV infection has been simplified and has been proven to be extremely effective, with about 85–99% of patients being able to achieve virological response. However, due to high mutagenicity and heterogeneity of the HCV virus, an effective vaccine has not been developed till now. Moreover, some of these patients fail to clear the virus even with DAA therapy. The chapter aims to provide a brief overview regarding epidemiology and microbiological properties of both these viruses. Recent advances in pathogenesis and management of HBV and HCV infection will also be briefly described.

10.2 History

10.2.1 Hepatitis B Virus

Hepatitis B-related liver diseases were recognized since ancient times but the etiologic agent was identified only recently. The first clue in unraveling the mystery was the discovery of an enigmatic protein initially named as the Australian antigen (as it was discovered in sera of an Australian aborigine) by Baruch Blumberg. Later on, this protein was identified as the HBV surface antigen (HBsAg) [1]. Discovery of this antigen laid down the basis for the first-time screening of apparently infected blood donors for a dangerous pathogen. The HBsAg became the first virological marker to be identified by radioimmunoassay. The phenomenon of seroconversion was first noted in a patient with Down's syndrome who was initially negative for the Australian antigen (Au) but later turned positive. Simultaneously, liver functions were also found to be deranged in these patients. This led open to a possible association between the Australian antigen and chronic hepatitis. Blumberg and colleagues reported that most of the disease association can be explained by possible association of the antigen with a virus. The fact that the Australian antigen can be transmitted by transfusion was first noted by Dr. Kazuo Okochi of the University of Tokyo. He also noted that some of these patients developed hepatitis while others developed anti-Au antibodies [2, 3]. In addition, it was also noted that patients receiving blood from the donors having Au antigen are more likely to transmit hepatitis than the donors who don't have this antigen. This formed the basis for universal screening of donor sera for presence of the Au antigen [4]. Following this, senior and colleagues observed a dramatic reduction in transfusion hepatitis from 18% to 6%.

10.2.2 *Hepatitis C Virus*

Following the discovery of hepatitis A virus and HBV, it was presumed that by universal screening, transfusion-transmitted hepatitis can be entirely prevented. However, very soon it was noted that about 10% of patients developed hepatitis even after exclusion of HAV and HBV infections [5]. It was also noted that about half of these patients developed chronic hepatitis out of which about 20% patients developed cirrhosis [6]. This led to a hypothesis that there may exist another virus that is transmissible by blood transfusion. It was named as posttransfusion non-A non-B hepatitis (PT-NANBH) virus. Studies in chimpanzees infected with the virus served as the basis for further characterization of the virus. Double-walled tubular structures were seen in cytoplasm of hepatic cells, and intranuclear particles were seen in hepatocytes from chimpanzee [7]. These were called tubule-forming agent and thought to be related to NANBH. As these agents were easily rendered noninfectious by treatment with chloroform or formalin thus indicating the NANBH may be lipid-containing enveloped virus rather than prions or virioids [8]. Finally, this virus was discovered after the pioneering work done by Harvey J Alter, Michael Hougton, and Charles M Rice. For the path-breaking discovery, the trio were awarded Nobel Prize in 2020 [9].

10.3 Epidemiology of Viral Hepatitis B and C

Hepatitis B is globally one of the most common and lethal infectious disease which is responsible for significant morbidity and mortality [10]. Around 3% of the world population (292 million individuals) is infected by the virus out of which about 5% are chronic carriers. About 25% of these chronic carriers develop chronic hepatitis, cirrhosis, and hepatocellular carcinoma [11]. Worldwide, about eight lakh patients die due to HBV infection-related causes [11]. About 3.5% of all HBV infections are in the high-income countries while the remaining occur in middle- and low-socioeconomic countries [12]. The majority of population with HBV infection is concentrated in sub-Saharan Africa and Asia. The majority of immigrant population from these countries constitutes the majority of population in the West. About half of the hepatitis B population all over the world is contributed by the four countries (China, India, Nigeria, and Indonesia) [12]. According to the prevalence of HBV infection, the world can be divided into three regions (high endemicity zone, intermediate zone, and the low endemic zone). India falls into the intermediate endemicity zone with a prevalence of 1.1–2.5% [13]. In sub-Saharan Africa and the Asian countries, the perinatal mode of transmission predominates over horizontal mode (sexual/intravenous drug abuse) that is more common in the western countries [14].

As the risk of acquiring chronic infection is inversely related to the age of individual, perinatal mode of transmission promotes chronic infection in Asian and African countries. Use of a birth dose of vaccine along with use of immunoglobulin and antivirals in infected mothers is helpful to curb down perinatal transmission which has led to significant reduction of prevalence of HBV in individuals less than 5 years of age [12]. However, HBV remains the greatest public health failure in late twentieth century despite availability of a very highly effective vaccine which has significantly cut down the incidence of new infections [15, 16]. Effect of vaccine on disease burden (liver cirrhosis and hepatocellular carcinoma) has remained minimal. In 2015, about nine lakh individuals succumbed to HBV-related illness corresponding to about one death every 36 seconds [17]. Currently used treatment is highly effective in reducing the progression of illness but globally only 10% of all infected individuals are diagnosed and only 5% of the eligible population are treated [12]. Thus, diagnosis of individuals who are already infected is vital to achieve the WHO target of elimination of viral hepatitis by 2030 [18].

With advent of highly effective oral directly acting antivirals (DAAs), prevalence of HCV infection has significantly reduced (80 million individuals in 2013 to 71 million individuals in 2015) [19]. Death of ageing population has also significantly contributed to this. However, this decrease in prevalence has been offset by an increased prevalence of intravenous drug abuse in western countries [20]. Six countries (China, Pakistan, India, Egypt, Russia, and the United States) contribute to almost 50% of all HCV infection all over the world [21]. Most common genotype to cause the HCV infection worldwide is genotype 1 (44%). About a quarter of infection were caused by genotype 3 while 15% were due to genotype 4 [4]. In India, genotype 3 is the predominant cause of most infections [21, 22].

10.4 Clinical Manifestations and Natural History

10.4.1 Hepatitis B Virus

The spectrum of clinical manifestations of hepatitis B virus can be divided into acute hepatitis or chronic hepatitis. The spectrum of illness in acute hepatitis varies from subclinical or anicteric hepatitis to icteric hepatitis. Rarely, patients may develop acute liver failure. Similarly, in the chronic phase, the manifestations range from asymptomatic carrier state to chronic hepatitis, cirrhosis, or hepatocellular carcinoma. Along with the hepatitis illness, some of these patients may also develop extrahepatic manifestations related to HBV infection. As mentioned before, earlier age of acquisition of the HBV infection is associated with a higher risk of chronicity.

- *Acute hepatitis*: Most of the patients (about 70%) with acute hepatitis B have anicteric hepatitis while about 30% develop icteric hepatitis. Patients with underlying liver disease or coinfection tend to have more severe infection [23]. Fulminant hepatic failure is extremely rare with HBV infection (0.1–0.5% of patients). The cause of the fulminant presentation is unclear. However, patients with history of ethanol abuse/acetaminophen intake and infection with genotype D have been shown to be associated with fulminant hepatic failure in a retrospective study. The pathogenesis of fulminant hepatitis involves massive immune-mediated destruction of infected hepatocytes which may explain paucity of viral replication in these patients [24].
  The incubation period for HBV infection lasts 1–4 months. A serum sickness-like syndrome may develop during the prodromal period, which is characterized by constitutional symptoms, anorexia, nausea, jaundice, and right upper quadrant pain. These symptoms usually resolve by 1–3 months though some patients may experience prolonged jaundice and fatigue.
  Laboratory findings in the patients with acute hepatitis include elevated transaminases (in thousands). Serum bilirubin may also be elevated though it remains normal in patients with anicteric hepatitis. Patients with acute liver failure (ALF) also have encephalopathy and coagulopathy. Recovery from ALF is characterized by improvement in encephalopathy and coagulopathy. Patients with acute hepatitis often recover within 2–4 months. Persistence of elevated transaminases even after 6 months of illness indicates development of chronic hepatitis.
  Overall outcome of acute viral hepatitis related to HBV is usually good. However, despite presence of anti-HBsAg antibodies in serum, these patients continue to have detectable HBV-DNA by polymerase chain reaction for many years. Similarly, HBV-specific cytotoxic T cells may also be detected for a prolonged time period [25–27]. However, the more worrisome figure is despite complete serological recovery, persistent histological abnormalities (inflammation and fibrosis) may be seen up to 10 years following clinical and serological recovery [28].
  The rate of progression from acute to chronic viral hepatitis in immunocompetent individuals is primarily determined by the age of acquisition of the infection. About 90% of perinatally acquired infection, 20–50% of infection acquired between 2 and 5 years, and less than 5% infection acquired in adulthood become chronic [29].
- *Chronic Hepatitis*: Patients with chronic hepatitis are usually asymptomatic and most of the time, they are incidentally detected during voluntary blood donation or during routine virus screening prior to surgery. About 30–50% of patients who have acquired infection during adulthood may have prior episodes of hepatitis. In contrast, prenatally acquired infections as seen in most patients in high prevalent countries, history of acute hepatitis is usually absent. Some of these patients experience nonspecific symptoms like fatigue. Few patients experience exacerbations of underlying viral infection, which may be asymptomatic or mimic an episode of acute hepatitis. Some of the patients may develop ALF.

Physical examination in the patients with chronic hepatitis is usually unrevealing. Patients with decompensated cirrhosis may have peripheral stigmata like spider angioma, palmar erythema, and gynecomastia along with ascites and/or splenomegaly. Laboratory parameters may show elevated transaminases and cytopenia (especially in advanced cirrhosis with portal hypertension). Liver functions may be normal but there may be elevation of transaminases. Uncommonly, these patients may develop episodes of acute exacerbation which is characterized by a marked elevations of transaminases (50 times upper limit of normal) and serum alfa-fetoprotein (AFP) levels [30]. With progression of cirrhosis and as the patient develops features of hepatic decompensation, patients develop thrombocytopenia, hypoalbuminemia, raised international normalized ratio (INR), and hyperbilirubinemia.

- *Extrahepatic Manifestations* (Table 10.1): Along with the hepatitis illness, patients infected with HBV may also have extrahepatic organ involvement [31]. Patients with both acute and chronic hepatitis may have extrahepatic manifestations. Acute hepatitis occurs as serum sickness like illness and characterized by fever, arthralgia, arthritis which subsides with development of jaundice. Two of the classical extrahepatic manifestations of chronic viral hepatitis B are polyarteritis nodosa and glomerulopathy.
- *Natural history of chronic HBV infection* (Table 10.2): The natural course of chronic HBV infection is determined by the interplay between host immune response and viral replication. Other factors that play important role in progression of the liver disease include gender, ethanol abuse, and concomitant infection with other hepatotropic viruses. Presence of obesity and fatty liver disease has also shown to accelerate the progression of liver disease in patients with HBV infection [32–34].

  Though chronic HBV infection generally consists of four phases (Table 10.2), not all patients pass through all these phases. Similarly, while most patients move from one phase to next phase of illness, rarely reversal to an earlier phase can also occur.

  (a) *Immune-tolerant phase*

    This phase is particularly prominent in patients with perinatally acquired infection. The phase is characterized by HBeAg positivity, very high HBV-DNA level with normal serum ALT level. Liver biopsy reveals only minimal change. However, studies have shown that about 50–70% of these patients may have stage I fibrosis [35]. More importantly, the stage of fibro-

Table 10.1 Extrahepatic manifestations of viral hepatitis B

Acute hepatitis	Chronic hepatitis
1. Serum sickness	1. Polyarthritis nodosa
2. Arthralgia	2. Glomerular disease
3. Arthritis	Membranous glomerulonephritis
4. Skin rashes	Membranoproliferative glomerulonephritis
5. Fever	3. Aplastic anemia

Table 10.2 Phases in the natural history of chronic HBV infection

Immune-tolerant phase	Immune active HBeAg-positive phase	Inactive carrier phase	Immune active HBeAg –ve phase
Classically seen in prenatally acquired infections HBeAg-positive and very high HBV-DNA levels Patients are asymptomatic with normal enzymes and near-normal liver biopsy Transplacental transfer of HBeAg plays important role in immune tolerance This phase lasts for 10–30 years Responsible for high rates of MTCT	Occurs in second to third decade in perinatally acquired infections Annual seroconversion (disappearance of HBeAg with appearance of anti-HBeAg) rate 10–20% Seroconversion earlier with genotype B Abrupt elevation of ALT levels is frequent due to immune-mediated lysis of hepatocytes Elevated HBV-DNA levels	HBeAg-negative and anti-HBeAg-positive HBV-DNA levels are low Normal ALT level	HBeAg-negative due to pre-core or core mutations ALT level fluctuating HBV-DNA levels also fluctuate

sis in these patients remains unchanged if the patients remain in immune-tolerant phase for 5 years [35].

The relative lack of hepatic inflammation despite very-high HBV-DNA levels is suggestive of inability to mount an adequate immune response. This may be explained by presence of HBeAg in patient which promotes immune tolerance. Presence of HBeAg was classically thought to prevent development of an adequate immune response against the virus. The immune tolerance is also believed to be the major reason for poor response to interferon therapy. However, more recent studies have shown that T-cell immune response in immune-tolerant phase is similar to other phases of chronic HBV infection [36]. This period lasts for 10–30 years and is associated with very low rate of spontaneous clearance of HBeAg. This low rate of HBeAg clearance promotes perinatal transmission of HBV infection.

(b) *Immune active, HBeAg-positive phase*

The transition from immune tolerance to immune active or clearance occurs during second to third decade of life in perinatally acquired infections. The rate of spontaneous HBeAg clearance ranges from 10% to 20% annually [37]. The HBeAg seroconversion is frequently but not always accompanied by a biochemical exacerbation (as defined by rise in serum alanine transaminase [ALT] level > 10 times of normal). This exacerbation is usually immune mediated and rise in transaminases occurs due to immune-mediated lysis of the hepatocytes. The episodes of exacerbation are often preceded by an increase in HBV-DNA level in serum. These exacerbations are more commonly seen in men than women. Though the exact cause of this gender predilection is unknown, an increased frequency of exacerbation may explain higher incidence of cirrhosis and HCC in males. Although the majority of episodes of exacerbations are asymptomatic, a fraction of individuals may develop decompensation or liver failure and may require liver transplantation. High HBV-DNA levels (>8 log IU/ml) have been shown to be a predictor of decompensation in HBeAg-positive patients without cirrhosis [38].

Another important point to note is that not all episodes of exacerbation result in HBV clearance. Rather, these individuals experience repeated exacerbations and ultimately develop cirrhosis or HCC. Early HBeAg seroconversion has been noted in individuals who have acquired the infection after perinatal period and have low HBV-DNA levels (<6 log IU/ml) [39].

(c) *Inactive chronic HBV*

These patients are in low nonreplicative phase or inactive carrier phase. This phase is characterized by absence of HBeAg, presence of Anti-HBeAg, low HBV-DNA level along with normal liver enzymes. Liver biopsy usually reveals resolution of necro-inflammation and absence of significant fibrosis especially in individuals with persistently normal ALT and low DNA levels [40]. In view of fluctuating nature of chronic HBV infection, a patient should never declared as inactive carrier unless three ALT levels over a span of 12 months is consistently normal and HBV-DNA levels are persistently less than 2000 IU/mL. In such a crucial scenario, quantitative estimation of HBsAg and HBV-DNA may be useful to distinguish between inactive carriers and HBeAg-negative chronic active hepatitis patients. In a HBeAg-negative patient, presence of quantitative HBsAg (<1000 IU/mL) and HBV-DNA (<2000 IU/mL) can identify patients of inactive carrier state with accuracy of 94% [41].

(d) *Immune active HBeAg-negative*

Despite being HBeAg-negative, some patients with chronic hepatitis B infection continue to have persistent HBV replication, elevated liver enzymes, and necro-inflammation on liver biopsies. Negative HBeAg in these patients is the result of core or pre-core genetic mutations. Patients in HBeAg-negative immune-active phase are usually older and have more advanced liver disease. Spontaneous ALT flares (ALT level more than 2 times the baseline) are common in these patients. The cumulative probability of developing flares is about 11% and 47% at 5 years and 10 years, respectively. Age more than 30 years, male sex, and presence of pre-core mutation were shown to be associated with flares [42]. Following seroconversion, patients with persistently elevated ALT and HBV-DNA levels are shown to be at increased risk of developing cirrhosis and HCC in contrast to patients with normal liver enzymes.

(e) *Resolution of chronic infection*

Few patients with chronic HBV infection are able to completely clear the infection and become HBsAg-negative. The rate of HBsAg clearance is higher in western patients (0.5–2%) compared to the Asian counterparts (0.2–0.8%) [43]. In a Taiwanese study, the rate of HBsAg seroclearance was 8% at 10 years which increased to 25% at 25 years [44]. HBsAg clearance may be preceded by decrease in HBV-DNA and HBsAg levels [45]. Following HBsAg clearance, patients without underlying cirrhosis have overall good long-term outcomes. However, the risk of development of HCC still remains especially in patients who achieve HBsAg seroclearance at old age (>50 years) or have coinfection (HCV/hepatitis D virus) [46].

Despite disappearance of HBsAg, vast majority of patients have detectable HBV-DNA in liver biopsy samples though it may not be detected in serum. These patients are anti-HBc-positive and over time may develop anti-HBs antibodies. The patients with anti-HBc-positive, HBsAg-negative with detectable HBV-DNA in serum/liver biopsy samples are termed occult HBV infection [47].

10.4.2 Hepatitis C Virus

10.4.2.1 Acute HCV Infection

Introduction By convention, acute HCV infection refers to the first 6 months of infection following presumed exposure to the virus. In contrast to acute viral hepatitis due to HBV or other hepatotropic viruses, most of these patients are asymptomatic [48]. Despite the use of highly effective DAAs, the incidence of acute HCV infection continues to rise due to IV drug abuse.

Clinical Features The incubation period of HCV infection is 2–26 weeks after exposure to HCV with a mean onset of symptoms at 7–8 weeks. The illness usually lasts for 2–12 weeks. Most of the patients with acute HCV infection are asymptomatic. However, some patients may experience jaundice, right upper quadrant pain, and nausea. In symptomatic patients, jaundice is seen in almost 70% of patients. In contrast, abdominal pain and nausea are relatively uncommon (20–30%). Other less-reported symptoms include fatigue, joint pain, pruritus, myalgia, and dyspepsia [49]. Development of ALF is still rare in patients with acute HCV infection. However, it may be common in patients with HBV coinfection. This subset of patients may also clear HCV spontaneously [50].

Laboratory findings In patients with symptomatic acute HCV infection, elevated transaminases are seen, which may be up to 20 times the upper limit normal, though at most of the times the level of elevation is only moderate [51]. Elevation of transaminases usually occurs just prior to onset of the symptoms and well before the development of antibodies. About 50% patients may have elevated serum bilirubin levels [52]. Detection of HCV-RNA in absence of Anti-HCV antibodies that becomes detectable at about 12 weeks of onset of symptoms is usually diagnostic of acute HCV infection.

10.4.2.2 Chronic HCV Infection

Introduction

Following infection with HCV, about 50–85% patients develop chronic hepatitis. However, the natural progression of HCV infection is usually very slow. There may not be any clinically apparent liver disease in most of the patients for a long period of time. Over a period of 20–30 years, only 5–30% chronically infected individuals may develop cirrhosis.

Clinical Features

Most of the symptoms in patients with chronic HCV infection are nonspecific and include lethargy, abdominal discomfort, pruritus, myalgia, arthralgia, and nausea [53]. Neuropsychiatric symptoms (depression and anxiety) are also commonly seen. Despite this, there is often a decrease in quality of life in these patients which may be due to increased awareness regarding the infection and can be improved following successful treatment [54]. Cognitive impairment is also common in patients with chronic HCV infection. The mechanism of cognitive impairment, though unknown, improves with successful treatment [55].

Extrahepatic Manifestations

Quite a number of extrahepatic manifestations are described with chronic HCV infection. In contrast to the nonspecific clinical features, these extrahepatic manifestations are relatively specific to chronic HCV infection. Various hematological, renal, autoimmune, dermatologic, and endocrine diseases have been shown to be associated with chronic HCV infection (Table 10.3). The frequency of these manifestations is uncertain though not uncommon. In one series of 321 patients, HCV infection was seen in 38% patients [56].

Laboratory Findings

There is a wide variation in the level of transaminases in patients with chronic HCV infection. About a third of patients have normal serum aminotransferases. A quarter of these patients have elevated liver enzymes by twice the upper limit of normal. In contrast to chronic HCV infection, raised liver enzymes rarely correlate with the histopathology of liver. Similar to elevated transaminases, level of HCV-RNA also widely fluctuates and doesn't correlate with transaminases and severity of liver disease [57]. Coinfection with other viruses has also been shown to influence HCV-RNA level. While infection with Human Immunodeficiency Virus generally increases HCV-RNA level, HBV coinfection reduces HCV proliferation. However,

Table 10.3 Extrahepatic manifestations of viral hepatitis C in decreased order of prevalence

Organ system involved	Specific disease
Dermatological	1. Purpura 2. Raynaud's phenomenon 3. Cutaneous vasculitis 4. Pruritus 5. Psoriasis 6. Porphyria cutanea tarda 7. Lichen planus
Rheumatological	1. Arthralgia 2. Arthritis 3. Myalgia
Neurologic	1. Sensory neuropathy 2. Motor neuropathy
Miscellaneous	1. Sicca syndrome 2. Hypertension 3. Uveitis
Endocrinological	Diabetes mellitus

Coinfection with both these viruses has conclusively shown to reduce hepatic fibrosis. Other laboratory abnormalities may be seen as part of extrahepatic manifestations (e.g., hematuria/proteinuria as part of glomerulonephritis, raised rheumatoid factors in arthritis). Patients with cirrhosis may present with features of portal hypertension (splenomegaly, ascites, and variceal bleed). Laboratory abnormalities may include coagulopathy, thrombocytopenia, and hypoalbuminemia. Some of these patients may have elevated AFP level even without HCC, though dynamic cross-sectional imaging should be done in all these patients to rule out HCC.

Natural History of Chronic HCV Infection

The natural history of HCV infection is difficult to define because of long course of illness, difficulty in measuring the duration of infection, and various factors that affect the course of illness. A systemic review including 111 studies analyzed the natural history of HCV infection. It was noted that the prevalence of cirrhosis at 20 years of HCV infection is about 16% (95% CI; 14–19%) [58]. The overall estimated time to develop cirrhosis is 39 years [58]. Though the rate of progression of liver disease is slow, once the patient develops fibrosis, the rate of progression to cirrhosis and HCC is fast [59]. A vast majority of patients who acquire HCV don't clear the virus spontaneously and develop chronic infection which ultimately leads to fibrosis and cirrhosis. Finally, if untreated, some of these patients develop ascites, variceal bleed, and hepatic encephalopathy (HE). Increased risk of chronic infection can be due to both host and viral factors. Rapid mutation and extensive virus diversity enable it to escape from the host immunity. Similarly, polymorphism of a chromosomal locus close to Interleukin-28 (IL-28) gene has been shown to promote chronicity of HCV. The presence of CC locus is associated with spontaneous viral clearance of 50–55% compared to only 15–20% clearance in presence of TT locus. During interferon and ribavirin era, these mutations were also shown to predict treatment response [60]. Other host factors that have been shown to be associated with spontaneous clearance of viruses include specific human leukocyte antigen (HLA) alleles, female sex, high titer neutralizing antibodies against HCV structural proteins, the persistence of HCV-specific T cell response, low peak viremia during acute phase, infection acquired during childhood, and symptomatic acute infection (Up to date, 2023). Acute exacerbations of chronic HCV infection as can be suspected by elevated transaminases have been described especially in genotype-2 infections, immunosuppressed individuals, and patients on chemotherapy. Most of these patients achieve sustained viral response (SVR) with treatment [61]. These episodes of exacerbations have also been shown to be associated with rapid progression of the underlying liver disease [61].

One patient has developed cirrhosis; the rate of developing decompensation has been shown to be about 18% at 5 years in the IFN+ Ribavirin era [62]. Even now in the era of DAAs, the yearly rate of decompensation has significantly improved. A prospective cohort study from Egypt included 1789 HCV-positive patients with cirrhosis who have completed treatment with DAAs. They were followed up for 2 years. At the end of 2 years, about 10% patients developed decompensation, with ascites being the most common decompensating event [63].

In the large prospective hepatitis C antiviral long-term treatment against cirrhosis (HALT-C) trial, 1050 patients were included. These had either advanced fibrosis or cirrhosis. All of them were nonresponders to IFN treatment. Over 8 years, there were 679 liver-related outcomes with most common outcomes being Child-Turcotte-Pugh (CTP) ≥ 7 and development of HCC. Other outcomes included development of ascites, HE, and variceal bleed. Liver-related complications were more common in patients with cirrhosis compared to advanced fibrosis (7.5% vs. 3.3%). Once a patient developed CTP ≥ 7, the rate of subsequent clinical events increased to 12% with annual mortality of 10% [59]. However, in the current era of DAAs, nonresponse to treatment is very rare, and overall outcome may be better. Once a patient develops various complications of HCV infection LT remains the only curative treatment. In the IFN era, recurrent HCV infection of graft was universal. However, with advent of highly effective DAAs, the incidence of recurrent HCV infection has significantly reduced [64].

HCV infection accounts for about one-third of all cases of HCC. The risk of developing HCC is higher with genotype-1 compared to genotype-2. Obesity is also a predisposing factor for developing HCC [65, 66].

10.5 Management

10.5.1 Hepatitis B

1. *Acute HBV infection*: The diagnosis of acute HBV infection is based on serological detection of HBsAg and IgM anti-HBc. Treatment is purely based on the clinical scenario. Appropriate measures should be taken to prevent infection following exposure (e.g., sexual exposure or needle stick injury) in nonimmunized individuals. Timely administration of hepatitis B immunoglobulin following high-risk exposure to unvaccinated individuals has been shown to prevent acute viral hepatitis [67]. Management of patients after high-risk exposure to HBV has been described later.

   Treatment of patients with acute viral hepatitis related to HBV is usually supportive. Use of antivirals is usually not recommended in immunocompetent adults as rate of progression to ALF and chronic hepatitis is only 1% and 5% respectively [68]. In contrast, in immunocompromised individuals, patients with underlying liver disease or coinfection with HCV/HIV the role of antivirals in uncomplicated acute hepatitis is uncertain in absence of high-quality literature.

   In contrast, patients with prolonged jaundice (serum bilirubin ≥3 mg/dL) along with coagulopathy for more than 4 weeks should be started on antivirals. Similarly, patients with HBV-related ALF should also be started on antiviral agents [69]. These patients should receive antivirals with high barrier to resistance (e.g., tenofovir and entecavir). These agents can be stopped once HBsAg has become negative as confirmed by two reports at an interval of 4 weeks. The distinction between acute hepatitis B and the reactivation of underlying chronic disease is often difficult. In such a scenario, starting antivirals becomes necessary.
2. *Chronic hepatitis B infection*

   The management of these patients is not straightforward and depends on host and viral factors along with clinical variables. The host factors include the immunologic response of host to the viral infection (HBeAg status) and degree of hepatic injury (hepatic necro-inflammation or cirrhosis). The viral factors include viral load and genotype. Few host factors that are associated with an aggressive clinical outcome (e.g., age more than 40 years along with family history of HCC) are also considered prior to initiating treatment. Treatment of patients with chronic hepatitis can be divided into two categories (patients without cirrhosis and patients with cirrhosis).

10.5.2 Treatment of Patients with Chronic Hepatitis B Without Cirrhosis

Patients with CHB and HBeAg-positive should be treated if ALT level is twice the upper limit of normal (ULN) and HBV-DNA levels are more than 20,000 IU/mL. In contrast, patients with normal ALT level with HBV-DNA level less than 20,000 IU/mL should be monitored every 3–6 months with ALT and HBV-DNA levels. These patients should also be monitored for HBeAg seroconversion every 6–12 months. Patients with HBV-DNA level more than 20,000 with elevated ALT level (<2 ULN) should be evaluated thoroughly to rule out other possible etiology of elevated transaminases. Liver biopsy may be done if there is persistence of elevated transaminases. Presence of >F2 fibrosis or moderate to severe necro-inflammation without any other explainable etiology mandates initiating treatment with antivirals (Especially patients with age > 40 years) [69]. Instead of liver biopsy, noninvasive tests may also be used to estimate degree of fibrosis and/or inflammation. Liver stiffness measurement (elastography of liver) is more accurate than the serum markers (e.g., AST to platelet ratio index [APRI] and FIB-4) [70].

All patients with CHB but HBeAg-negative should be treated when HBV DNA level is more than 2000 IU/mL and ALT is elevated more than twice ULN, while patients with HBV-DNA less than 2000 IU/mL with normal ALT level should not be started on medications. In contrast, patients with intermediate level of HBV-DNA and ALT level should be followed up regularly [70].

10.5.3 Treatment of Patients with CHB with Cirrhosis

All HBsAg-positive patients with cirrhosis (Decompensated or compensated) should be started on antivirals with high barrier to resistance irrespective of HBV-DNA levels. In addition, all patients with decompensated cirrhosis should be put on LT waiting list. Early initiation of treatment has been shown to improve survival in patients with decompensated cirrhosis. Moreover, some of the patients can be recompensated and removed from the LT waiting list [71]. Despite all these benefits provided by the use of antivirals, the risk of HCC remains, though lower in patients on antivirals. For the same reason, these patients need to be screened regularly for the same [72]. While Peg-Interferon is contraindicated in patients with decompensated cirrhosis, both entecavir and tenofovir can be used safely.

10.5.4 Treatment of CHB in Special Populations

Management of patients who are coinfected with HBV and HCV has to be individualized. Patients with detectable HCV-RNA must be started on DAAs. Treatment of HBV infection in these patients is determined by status of underlying liver disease, serum ALT level, and HBV-DNA levels as described before. Treatment of one infection may lead to changes in activity of the other virus which mandates frequent monitoring of viral activity during and after treatment [73].

Patients who are coinfected with HIV and HBV constitute another special category. Three Nucleotide Analogues (NAs) with activity against both HBV and HIV include tenofovir, lamivudine, and emtricitabine. Patients having HIV coinfection should receive a combination of two drugs with activity against HBV. Ideal treatment combination includes tenofovir disoproxil fumarate (TDF)/tenofovir alefnamide (TAF) with lamivudine/emtricitabine. In general, TAF is preferred over TDF in view of its better safety profile [74]. Alternately, entecavir can also be used, especially in patients who are on a fully suppressive antiretroviral regimen [75]. Modification of dose of TDF is needed if creatinine clearance is less than 50 ml/min while patients with creatinine clearance less than 30 ml/min should not be prescribed TAF. Initiation of antiviral therapy may be associated with HBV flares following a few weeks of initiation of therapy due to immune reconstitution or HBV medications are discontinued without HBeAg seroconversion [76]. Ideally, treatment should be continued indefinitely.

Patients with CHB and on immunosuppressive agents/chemotherapy constitute another special group. These patients run the risk of developing reactivation/flares of hepatitis B. The risk of having HBV reactivation depends on the nature of treatment used and the serological status of host. Previous studies have shown that in patients on anti-cancer therapy, the risk varies from 41% to 53% in patients positive for both HBsAg and total anti-HBc while the risk reduces to 8–18% in patients who are positive for only total anti-HBc [77]. Thus, all the patients (especially in moderate to high prevalence areas) should be screened for HBsAg and total anti-HBc prior to starting treatment with these agents [78, 79]. Ideally, these patients should be started on highly potent nucleic acid analogue 7 days before initiation of chemotherapy. As life-threatening flares have been documented even in patients after completion of chemotherapy/immunosuppression, it is often indicated to prolong the duration of HBV treatment by at least 6–12 months following completion of therapy [69, 79]. However, the duration of therapy is unclear in patients on chronic or lifelong immunosuppression, e.g., organ transplant recipients and patients on biologics [80, 81].

Finally, patients on liver transplant waiting list should be started on antivirals and continued in the posttransplant period. These patients should be started on antivirals having high barrier to resistance, e.g., entecavir, TDF/TAF. In patients with decompensated cirrhosis with a prior history of lamivudine resistance, TAF may be preferred over TDF to mitigate risk of development of bone/renal disease with the later. Irrespective of HBeAg/HBV-DNA status, all the liver transplant recipients should be continued on the antivirals indefinitely. Use of entecavir alone post-LT was shown to be sufficient to prevent HBV recurrence in a study conducted in Hong Kong. In this study, 265 patients after giving entecavir monotherapy, 85%, 88%, 87%, and 92% patients were HBsAg-negative at 1, 3, 5, and 8 years of follow-up, respectively. All 100% patients had undetectable HBV-DNA levels [82].

10.5.5 Hepatitis C

10.5.5.1 Evaluation of Infected Patients

All patients with chronic HCV infection with detectable viral load should be treated irrespective of stage of the underlying liver disease. Moreover, with advent of DAAs, the management of the infection has been simplified, and the WHO goal of eliminating viral hepatitis B can be a reality. To achieve this goal, all the individuals at high risk of acquiring infection must be screened once, annually, or periodically [83] (Table 10.4). Male patients with HIV coinfection who have unprotected sex with males and injection drug abusers should be annually screened for HCV infection [83]. Prior to starting treatment, all patients should be evaluated for the stage of underlying liver disease (e.g., stage of fibrosis or cirrhosis), viral load, genotype, and renal functions.

Various extrahepatic manifestations of chronic HCV infection including cryoglobulinemia, HCV-associated renal diseases, and porphyria cutanea tarda must be identified and should be treated in these patients. Finally, all patients with chronic HCV infection must be screened for HBV and HIV infection because of common mode of transmission and a rapid disease progression associated with the coinfection. In a worst-case scenario, HBV reactivation may occur after initiating DAA therapy and can precipitate liver failure.

Table 10.4 Selected high-risk behaviors, conditions, and circumstances associated with an increased risk of acquiring HCV infection

Behavioral risk	1. Injection drug use 2. Intranasal illicit drug use 3. Men having sex with men (MSM)
Risk exposures	1. Persons on long-term hemodialysis 2. Needle stick/sharp/mucosal exposure to HCV-infected blood especially in health care setting 3. Children born to HCV-infected women 4. Persons receiving blood products from HCV-infected individuals
Risk conditions and circumstances	1. HIV-infected individuals 2. Sexually active individuals who have not started pre-exposure prophylaxis for HIV 3. Unexplained chronic liver disease/chronic hepatitis including elevated ALT levels 4. Solid organ donors and transplant recipients

HCV hepatitis C virus, *ALT* alanine aminotransferase

10.5.5.2 General Management

The psychosocial issues (e.g., depression, intravenous drug abuse) are common in HCV-infected individuals and must be addressed. Psychiatric evaluation and opioid substitution therapy may be provided to the patient. All the infected patients should also be counselled regarding the various routes of transmission of HCV infection and ways to prevent transmission (e.g., sharing of tooth brushes/shaving equipment, avoiding blood donation, and covering bleeding areas so as to prevent others from coming in contact with blood). Sexual transmission of HCV is uncommon, and use of barrier contraception is usually not warranted in patients with isolated HCV infection. However, patients who are coinfected with HIV or having multiple sexual partners should be advised to use barrier contraception. Similarly, vertical transmission of HCV is fairly low though incidence may be higher (About 12%) in pregnant women who are coinfected with HIV [84]. The natural history of chronic HCV infection and factors associated with an aggressive clinical course (obesity, smoking, and ethanol abuse) must be explained to patients. They should be advised to shed weight, abstain from ethanol abuse, and stop smoking.

10.5.5.3 Specific Treatment for HCV Infection (Table 10.5)

With advent of DAAs, the treatment of HCV infection has been simplified. In contrast to interferon, DAAs can be prescribed by general physicians (Especially to patients without cirrhosis) without significant concerns of adverse events [85]. Prior to initiation of treatment, all the patients should be categorized as per status of underlying liver disease. All patients should undergo a battery of preliminary tests like blood counts, liver functions, and calculated glomerular filtration rates (eGFR). HCV-RNA levels must be determined in all the patients as only patients with detectable HCV-RNA levels need treatment. As both hepatitis B and hepatitis C viruses share similar modes of transmission, all patients with HCV seropositivity must be screened for HBsAg and HIV. Similarly, pregnancy must be ruled out in all the women of childbearing age. Risk associated with various HCV medications when given during pregnancy should also be explained to all HCV-positive women of childbearing age. Severity of underlying liver diseases can be predicted by using various noninvasive scores like APRI, FIB-4, or fibroscan. Similarly, patients with prior comorbidities may on other medications. Prior to starting DAAs, a thorough review of all possible drug interactions should be done. Following this, the patients may be categorized in to following three groups.

Table 10.5 Comparison of various classes of directly acting antiviral (DAA) agents

Class of DAAs	NS3/4A protease inhibitors	NS5A protein inhibitor	NS5B polymerase inhibitors
Mechanism of action	NS3/4A is a serine protease involved in posttranslational processing and replication of HCV	Involved in viral replication and assembly of HCV	NS5B is an RNA-dependent RNA polymerase involved in posttranslational processing necessary for replication of HCV Nucleotide/nucleoside analogues attach to catalytic site of NS5B resulting in chain termination Non-nucleoside agents act as allosteric inhibitors
Spectrum of action	Usually effective only against genotype-1	Usually effective against genotype-1. However, newer agents have pan-genotypic activity.	Usually have pan-genotypic activity and equal activity against both genotype 1a and 1b
Barrier to resistance	Low	Low	High
Potential for drug interactions	High	Low to moderate	Low
Adverse events	Rash, anemia, and high bilirubin levels	Mild variable toxicity like headache, nausea, myalgia	Mitochondrial toxicity Potential interaction of nucleotide/nucleoside agents with anti-retroviral agents and ribavirin
Antiviral agents	*First-generation protease inhibitors*—Telepravir and bocepravir *Newer protease inhibitors*—Glecaprevir/Gazoprevir/Paritaprevir/simeprevir/Voxilaprevir	Daclatasvir/Ledipasvir/Elbasvir/Ombitasvir/Pibrentasvir/Velpatasvir	Nucleot(s)ide analogues—Sofosbuvir Non-nucleot(s) ide polymerase inhibitors—Dasabuvir
Special comments	Newer protease inhibitors tend to have high barrier to resistance and tend to be effective across genotypes	They have multiple mechanisms of action	None

NS nonstructural, *HCV* hepatitis C virus, *RNA* ribose-nucleic acid

10.5.6 HCV-Positive Treatment-Naïve Patients Without Cirrhosis

Patients who are HCV-positive and don't have cirrhosis, can be started on either sofobuvir (NS5B inhibitor) + velpatasvir (NS5A inhibitor) for 12 weeks or glecaprevir + pibrentasvir for 8 weeks. Regardless of the genotype, this regimen results in a Sustained Virological Response (SVR) in about 95% of patients. In India, glecaprevir + pibrentasvir combination is not available at present. A single tablet, combining both sofosbuvir (400 mg) and velpatasvir (100 mg), is often the initial agent of choice for treatment-naïve patients (without cirrhosis or with compensated cirrhosis) with HCV infection. It has to be administered once daily with or without food at same dose irrespective of hepatic or renal functional status. Several trials have demonstrated very high efficacy of the combination for management of HCV in patients without cirrhosis or only compensated cirrhosis [86–88]. This regimen holds good even for noncirrhotic patients having infection with genotype-3 (>97%) [89]. However, certain subtypes of genotype-3 (genotype 3b) especially in patients with cirrhosis may be less susceptible to the sofosbuvir-velpatasvir regimen as reported in an Asian study [90].

Some drugs may have interaction with the sofosbuvir + velpatasvir combination. Coadministration of drugs like amiodarone, certain anti-convulsants (phenytoin, carbamazepine, and oxcarbamazepine), and rifamycins should be avoided while the patient is on the combination therapy. More importantly, elevated gastric p^H reduces absorption of sofosbuvir-velpatasvir. To avoid this, adequate gap should be kept between the two medications.

The combination is generally well tolerated and serious adverse events requiring dose modification/drug withdrawal are uncommon. Most commonly reported adverse events are fatigue, headache, nausea, nasopharyngitis, and insomnia [91].

Various alternative regimes have also been used in individuals who can't assess the preferred regimen because of pricing issues or sole availability of alternate regimen. The commonly used alternate regimen include sofosbuvir-daclatasvir/sofosbuvir-ledipasvir and elbasvir-grazoprevir [92–95]. However, with availability of highly effective DAAs against all the genotypes, use of sofosbuvir/velpatasvir for HCV-infected patients has completely obviated doing routine genotyping, treatment monitoring or regular follow-up visits. In resource-constraint countries, the regimen can be dispensed at one time at initiation of treatment and has shown to provide SVR in about 95% of patients [96].

10.5.7 HCV-Positive Patients with Cirrhosis

10.5.7.1 Compensated Cirrhosis

For patients with compensated cirrhosis, pan-genotypic regimen is quite effective and routine determination of HCV genotype is not essential. However, genotype-3 is hardest to treat in this subset of patients, and determining genotype may result in improved SVR by few points (especially genotype-3). In patients infected with genotype-3 the preferred treatment regimen is either glecaprevir/pibrentasvir for 8 weeks or sofosbuvir/velpatasvir for 12 weeks. Because of shorter duration of treatment, the former regimen is often preferred for genotype-3 infection. Use of glecapravir/pibrentasvir leads to about 95% SVR in patients with HCV-related compensated cirrhosis [97]. However, in case glecaprevir/pibrentasvir is not available or can't be given due to interaction with other drugs then sofosbuvir + velpatasvir regimen for 12 weeks may be given.

However, regimen containing sofosbuvir + velpatasvir is associated with inferior SVR in patients with compensated cirrhosis related to genotype-3 infection. Prior to initiation of therapy, testing for NS5A resistance-associated substitutions should be performed for Y93H variant. Presence of Y93H substitution results in treatment failure. In contrast, in absence of this mutation, SVR of 97% can be achieved with sofosbuvir + velpatasvir regimen for 12 weeks [89]. In presence of Y93H substitution sofosbuvir + velpatasvir + voxilaprevir regimen for a duration of 12 weeks is recommended [98]. In this scenario, in countries where voxilaprevir is not available, ribavirin may be added to improve overall SVR. Another less preferred alternative is the use of the sofosbuvir + daclatasvir combination for 24 weeks [99].

10.5.7.2 Decompensated Cirrhosis

In patients with decompensated cirrhosis, the patients should be stratified based on their need of LT in near future. Patients who are quite sick and require urgent LT may not be able to complete the full course of treatment by transplant. Similarly, treatment of HCV infection in these patients may not necessarily improve their overall liver function so that they can be put off from the transplant waiting list. Generally speaking, patients with low baseline MELD score (<16), CTP score, and absence of significant complications of portal hypertension may have significant improvement with antiviral therapy [100, 101]. Similarly, in patients with advanced decompensated cirrhosis (MELD >27), the response to DAAs has been shown to be inferior to patients having normal liver function. Moreover, this subset of patients may actually be disadvantaged by use of DAAs as mild improvement in MELD score can actually prolong the waiting time for LT [102]. The preferred treatment regimen is use of sofosbuvir + velpatasvir along with weight-based ribavirin (1200 mg for body weight more than 75 kg and 1000 mg for body weight < 75 kg). The duration of treatment is usually 12 weeks. The rate of SVR with this regimen is

100% for all genotypes except for genotype-1a (94%) and genotype-3 (85%) [103]. Patients who can't tolerate ribavirin, use of sofosbuvir and velpatasvir may be extended for 24 weeks which results in a comparable SVR irrespective of genotype [104]. Alternately, these patients may be started on a low dose of ribavirin (400–600 mg/day) which can be increased later based on tolerance of the patient. The alternative DAA regimen in patients with genotype 1, 4, 5, and 6 includes use of sofosbuvir and ledipasvir for 12 weeks or sofosbuvir, ledipasvir with ribavirin for 12 weeks [105]. In a trial of patients with genotype 1 and 4 infection, ledipasvir + sofosbuvir for 24 weeks or ledipasvir + sovosbuvir + ribavirin for 12 weeks results in similar high SVR rates [106]. Other antiviral combinations like glecaprevir-pibrentasvir, elbasvir-grazoprevir, sofusbuvir-velpatasvir-voxilaprevir, and simeprevir are contraindicated in patients with child B/C cirrhosis.

10.5.8 HCV Treatment in Special Population Groups

Treatment of HCV infection in patients with renal impairment is often similar to patients without renal disease. However, dose modification of patients with chronic kidney disease on maintenance hemodialysis may be needed. Similarly, patients with HIV coinfection special consideration must be given regarding potential interactions with antiretroviral agents. Finally, in post-LT settings, all recipients (without cirrhosis or compensated cirrhosis) should be treated with glecaprevir-pibrentasvir/sofosbuvir-velpatasvir for 12 weeks. Alternative regimen includes sofosbuvir-ledipasvir-ribavirin for 12 weeks. All the three regimens result in very-high SVR rates in patients post-LT [105, 107].

10.6 Prevention

Both HBV and HCV infection are transmitted by percutaneous or mucosal exposure of body fluids. In addition, mother-to-child transmission of HBV is also common in mothers with high viral load and HBeAg-positive status. All pregnant women should be screened for HBV/HCV/HIV infection during prenatal checkup. Similarly, during blood donation, all the blood samples must be screened for presence of HBV/HCV/HIV infection.

10.6.1 Prevention of HBV Infection (Table 10.6)

All HBV-positive individuals should refrain from voluntary blood donation and unprotected sexual intercourse. Similarly, they should use separate combs, toothbrushes, and shaving kit. All pregnant women who are HBsAg-positive should be

Table 10.6 Post-exposure prophylaxis for hepatitis B virus (HBV) (to be given within 72 hours of exposure)

Exposed individual vaccination status	Source HBsAg-positive	Source HBsAg-negative or not available	Source not known; known high risk
Unvaccinated/nonimmune	HBIg-0.06 ml/kg IM Initiate HBV vaccine series	Initiate the vaccine series	Treat as if the source is HBsAg-positive
Previously vaccinated and known responder	No treatment needed	No treatment needed	No treatment needed
Previously vaccinated and known nonresponder	HBIg-0.06 ml/kg IM Initiate HBV vaccine series	No treatment needed	Treat as if the source is HBsAg-positive
Previously vaccinated but antibody response is not known	Administer single dose of vaccine and check titer If titer is low, complete three vaccine series	No treatment needed	Treat as if the source is HBsAg-positive
Undergoing vaccination at the time of exposure	HBIg-0.06 ml/kg IM Initiate HBV vaccine series	Complete vaccine series	Complete vaccine series

IM intramuscular, *HBV* hepatitis B virus, *HBIg* hepatitis B immunoglobulin

evaluated for viral load, HBeAg positivity, and underlying liver disease. Pregnant women with HBV-DNA level more than 200,000 IU/Ml, HBsAg level of more than 4–4.5 log10 IU/mL, and HBeAg positivity are associated with a high risk of MTCT. These women should be started on antivirals at 28–32 weeeks of gestational age and should be continued till about 12 weeks' postpartum. The preferred antivirals in this scenario are usually TDF, the use of which has been shown to reduce transmission of HBV from 7% to 0% [108]. In addition, the newborn should receive hepatitis B immunoglobulin (HBIG) and vaccination given within 12 hours of birth is also recommended to further reduce the risk of perinatal transmission. The combined use of active and passive immunization leads to reduction of perinatal transmission from 90% to 10% [78, 109]. Mandatory vaccination of all neonates and high-risk individuals (before chemotherapy and organ transplantation) can significantly reduce risk of horizontal transmission. Similarly, HBsAg-positive LT recipients who receive anti-HBc-positive liver graft should receive HBIG and nucleoside analogues to prevent graft infection [110].

10.6.2 Prevention of HCV Infection

In contrast to HBV infection, no specific vaccine against HCV is available at present. Perinatal transmission of HCV occurs in 3–10% of cases [111, 112]. Risk factors for transmission of HCV from mother to child include high HCV RNA levels in mother, concomitant HIV infection, prolonged or difficult delivery, and invasive fetal monitoring during delivery [113]. Similarly, breastfeeding has not shown to increase risk of transmission to the neonate. However, feeding from cracked and bleeding nipple may be associated with increased risk of transmission to the baby [114]. At present, the use of DAAs is not recommended in pregnant women and children younger than 3 years of age. All neonates born to HCV-positive mother should be tested for anti-HCV positivity at 18 months of age. Anti-HCV positivity at this age usually suggests prenatally acquired infection and HCV-RNA quantification must be done. Treatment with DAAs may be initiated once the child turns 3 [115].

10.7 Conclusion

Both the chronic HBV and HCV infection are associated with increased risk of developing cirrhosis and HCC thus increasing morbidity, mortality and health care expenditure. With advent of DAAs the treatment of HCV infection has been simplified. Availability of an effective vaccine and highly potent nucleoside analogues have significantly reduced prevalence, morbidity, and mortality associated with HBV infection. However, few concerns still remain. Genotype-3 remains the most difficult HCV variant to treat with currently available DAAs. In presence of resistance-associated substitutions, this genotype may be difficult to treat. Similarly, optimal timing and duration of treatment of DAAs in patients with decompensated cirrhosis (especially in patients in LT waiting list) needs further studies. Finally, even with use of highly effective nucleoside analogues, functional cure of HBV has been a distant dream. Use combination therapies (interferon and nucleoside analogues) in achieving functional cure needs to be studied further [116].

References

1. Blumberg BS. Hepatitis B: the hunt for a killer virus. Princeton: Princeton University Press; 2002.
2. Okochi K, Murakami S. Observations on Australia antigen in Japanese. Vox Sang. 1968;15(5):374–85.
3. Okochi K, Murakami S, Ninomiya K, Kaneko M. Australia antigen, transfusion and hepatitis. Vox Sang. 2017;18(4):289–300.
4. Gocke DJ, Kavey NB. Hepatitis antigen. Correlation with disease and infectivity of blood-donors. Lancet (London, England). 1969;1(7605):1055–9.
5. Feinstone SM, Kapikian AZ, Purcell RH, Alter HJ, Holland PV. Transfusion-associated hepatitis not due to viral hepatitis type A or B. N Engl J Med. 1975;292(15):767–70.
6. Pawlotsky J-M. Hepatitis C virus: from laboratory to clinic. By Mark A. Feitelson. 256 pp. $48.00. Cambridge University Press, New York, New York, 2002. ISBN 0-521-79959-7. Web address for ordering: https://www.cambridge.org. Gastroenterology. 2003;124(7):1996.

7. Bradley DW, Maynard JE, Cook EH, Ebert JW, Gravelle CR, Tsiquaye KN, et al. Non-A/non-B hepatitis in experimentally infected chimpanzees: cross-challenge and electron microscopic studies. J Med Virol. 1980;6(3):185–201.
8. Merz PA, Somerville RA, Wisniewski HM, Manuelidis L, Manuelidis EE. Scrapie-associated fibrils in Creutzfeldt-Jakob disease. Nature. 1983;306(5942):474–6.
9. Ghany MG, Lok ASF, Dienstag JL. The 2020 nobel prize for medicine or physiology for the discovery of Hepatitis C virus: a triumph of curiosity and persistence. Hepatology. 2021;74(5):2813–23.
10. Franco E, Bagnato B, Marino MG, Meleleo C, Serino L, Zaratti L. Hepatitis B: epidemiology and prevention in developing countries. World J Hepatol. 2012;4(3):74–80.
11. Sharma SK, Saini N, Chwla Y. Hepatitis B virus: inactive carriers. Virol J. 2005;2:82.
12. Polaris Observatory Collaborators. Global prevalence, treatment, and prevention of hepatitis B virus infection in 2016: a modelling study. Lancet Gastroenterol Hepatol. 2018;3(6):383–403.
13. Razavi H. Global epidemiology of viral hepatitis. Gastroenterol Clin N Am. 2020;49(2):179–89.
14. Schweitzer A, Horn J, Mikolajczyk RT, Krause G, Ott JJ. Estimations of worldwide prevalence of chronic hepatitis B virus infection: a systematic review of data published between 1965 and 2013. Lancet (London, England). 2015;386(10003):1546–55.
15. Cui F, Shen L, Li L, Wang H, Wang F, Bi S, et al. Prevention of chronic hepatitis B after 3 decades of escalating vaccination policy, China. Emerg Infect Dis. 2017;23(5):765–72.
16. Liang X, Bi S, Yang W, Wang L, Cui G, Cui F, et al. Reprint of: epidemiological serosurvey of Hepatitis B in China--declining HBV prevalence due to Hepatitis B vaccination. Vaccine. 2013;31(Suppl 9):J21–8.
17. World Health O. Global hepatitis report 2017. Geneva: World Health Organization; 2017.
18. World Health O. Combating hepatitis B and C to reach elimination by 2030: advocacy brief. Geneva: World Health Organization; 2016. Report No.: Contract No.: WHO/HIV/2016.04.
19. Polaris Observatory HCV Collaborators. Global prevalence and genotype distribution of hepatitis C virus infection in 2015: a modelling study. Lancet Gastroenterol Hepatol. 2017;2(3):161–76.
20. Gower E, Estes C, Blach S, Razavi-Shearer K, Razavi H. Global epidemiology and genotype distribution of the hepatitis C virus infection. J Hepatol. 2014;61(1 Suppl):S45–57.
21. Blach S, Zeuzem S, Manns M, Altraif I, Duberg A-S, Muljono DH, et al. Global prevalence and genotype distribution of hepatitis C virus infection in 2015: a modelling study. Lancet Gastroenterol Hepatol. 2017;2(3):161–76.
22. Anand A, Shalimar. Hepatitis C virus in India: challenges and successes. Clin Liver Dis. 2021;18(3):150–4.
23. Liaw YF, Tsai SL, Sheen IS, Chao M, Yeh CT, Hsieh SY, et al. Clinical and virological course of chronic hepatitis B virus infection with hepatitis C and D virus markers. Am J Gastroenterol. 1998;93(3):354–9.
24. Wright TL, Mamish D, Combs C, Kim M, Wright TL, Mamish D, et al. Hepatitis B virus and apparent fulminant non-A, non-B hepatitis. Lancet. 1992;339(8799):952–5.
25. Rehermann B, Ferrari C, Pasquinelli C, Chisari FV. The hepatitis B virus persists for decades after patients' recovery from acute viral hepatitis despite active maintenance of a cytotoxic T-lymphocyte response. Nat Med. 1996;2(10):1104–8.
26. Yotsuyanagi H, Yasuda K, Iino S, Moriya K, Shintani Y, Fujie H, et al. Persistent viremia after recovery from self-limited acute hepatitis B. Hepatology (Baltimore, Md). 1998;27(5):1377–82.
27. Marusawa H, Uemoto S, Hijikata M, Ueda Y, Tanaka K, Shimotohno K, et al. Latent hepatitis B virus infection in healthy individuals with antibodies to hepatitis B core antigen. Hepatology (Baltimore, Md). 2000;31(2):488–95.
28. Yuki N, Nagaoka T, Yamashiro M, Mochizuki K, Kaneko A, Yamamoto K, et al. Long-term histologic and virologic outcomes of acute self-limited hepatitis B. Hepatology (Baltimore, Md). 2003;37(5):1172–9.

29. Coursaget P, Yvonnet B, Chotard J, Vincelot P, Sarr M, Diouf C, et al. Age- and sex-related study of hepatitis B virus chronic carrier state in infants from an endemic area (Senegal). J Med Virol. 1987;22(1):1–5.
30. Lok AS, Lai CL. Alpha-fetoprotein monitoring in Chinese patients with chronic hepatitis B virus infection: role in the early detection of hepatocellular carcinoma. Hepatology (Baltimore, Md). 1989;9(1):110–5.
31. Cacoub P, Asselah T. Hepatitis B virus infection and extra-hepatic manifestations: a systemic disease. Am J Gastroenterol. 2022;117(2):253–63.
32. Chan AW, Wong GL, Chan HY, Tong JH, Yu YH, Choi PC, et al. Concurrent fatty liver increases risk of hepatocellular carcinoma among patients with chronic hepatitis B. J Gastroenterol Hepatol. 2017;32(3):667–76.
33. Yan LB, Liao J, Han N, Zhou LY, Wang XE, Wang YJ, et al. Association between hepatitis B virus infection and metabolic syndrome in Southwest China: a cross-sectional study. Sci Rep. 2020;10(1):6738.
34. Chan TT, Chan WK, Wong GL, Chan AW, Nik Mustapha NR, Chan SL, et al. Positive Hepatitis B core antibody is associated with cirrhosis and hepatocellular carcinoma in nonalcoholic fatty liver disease. Am J Gastroenterol. 2020;115(6):867–75.
35. Hui CK, Leung N, Yuen ST, Zhang HY, Leung KW, Lu L, et al. Natural history and disease progression in Chinese chronic hepatitis B patients in immune-tolerant phase. Hepatology (Baltimore, Md). 2007;46(2):395–401.
36. Bertoletti A, Kennedy PT. The immune tolerant phase of chronic HBV infection: new perspectives on an old concept. Cell Mol Immunol. 2015;12(3):258–63.
37. McMahon BJ, Holck P, Bulkow L, Snowball M. Serologic and clinical outcomes of 1536 Alaska Natives chronically infected with hepatitis B virus. Ann Intern Med. 2001;135(9):759–68.
38. Jeng WJ, Sheen IS, Liaw YF. Hepatitis B virus DNA level predicts hepatic decompensation in patients with acute exacerbation of chronic hepatitis B. Clin Gastroenterol Hepatol. 2010;8(6):541–5.
39. Kim HS, Kim HJ, Shin WG, Kim KH, Lee JH, Kim HY, et al. Predictive factors for early HBeAg seroconversion in acute exacerbation of patients with HBeAg-positive chronic hepatitis B. Gastroenterology. 2009;136(2):505–12.
40. Papatheodoridis GV, Manolakopoulos S, Liaw YF, Lok A. Follow-up and indications for liver biopsy in HBeAg-negative chronic hepatitis B virus infection with persistently normal ALT: a systematic review. J Hepatol. 2012;57(1):196–202.
41. Brunetto MR, Oliveri F, Colombatto P, Moriconi F, Ciccorossi P, Coco B, et al. Hepatitis B surface antigen serum levels help to distinguish active from inactive hepatitis B virus genotype D carriers. Gastroenterology. 2010;139(2):483–90.
42. Kumar M, Chauhan R, Gupta N, Hissar S, Sakhuja P, Sarin SK. Spontaneous increases in alanine aminotransferase levels in asymptomatic chronic hepatitis B virus-infected patients. Gastroenterology. 2009;136(4):1272–80.
43. Liu J, Yang HI, Lee MH, Lu SN, Jen CL, Wang LY, et al. Incidence and determinants of spontaneous hepatitis B surface antigen seroclearance: a community-based follow-up study. Gastroenterology. 2010;139(2):474–82.
44. Chu C-M, Liaw Y-F. HBsAg seroclearance in asymptomatic carriers of high endemic areas: appreciably high rates during a long-term follow-up. Hepatology (Baltimore, Md). 2007;45(5):1187–92.
45. Chen YC, Jeng WJ, Chu CM, Liaw YF. Decreasing levels of HBsAg predict HBsAg seroclearance in patients with inactive chronic hepatitis B virus infection. Clin Gastroenterol Hepatol. 2012;10(3):297–302.
46. Yuen MF, Wong DK, Fung J, Ip P, But D, Hung I, et al. HBsAg Seroclearance in chronic hepatitis B in Asian patients: replicative level and risk of hepatocellular carcinoma. Gastroenterology. 2008;135(4):1192–9.

47. Raimondo G, Locarnini S, Pollicino T, Levrero M, Zoulim F, Lok AS. Update of the statements on biology and clinical impact of occult hepatitis B virus infection. J Hepatol. 2019;71(2):397–408.
48. Blackard JT, Shata MT, Shire NJ, Sherman KE. Acute hepatitis C virus infection: a chronic problem. Hepatology (Baltimore, Md). 2008;47(1):321–31.
49. Loomba R, Rivera MM, McBurney R, Park Y, Haynes-Williams V, Rehermann B, et al. The natural history of acute hepatitis C: clinical presentation, laboratory findings and treatment outcomes. Aliment Pharmacol Ther. 2011;33(5):559–65.
50. Wietzke-Braun P, Manhardt LB, Rosenberger A, Uy A, Ramadori G, Mihm S. Spontaneous elimination of hepatitis C virus infection: a retrospective study on demographic, clinical, and serological correlates. World J Gastroenterol. 2007;13(31):4224–9.
51. Maheshwari A, Ray S, Thuluvath PJ. Acute hepatitis C. Lancet (London, England). 2008;372(9635):321–32.
52. Maheshwari A, Thuluvath PJ. Management of acute hepatitis C. Clin Liver Dis. 2010;14(1):169–76. x
53. Evon DM, Stewart PW. A comprehensive assessment of patient reported symptom burden, medical comorbidities, and functional well being in patients initiating direct acting antiviral therapy for chronic hepatitis C: results from a large US multi-center observational study. PLoS One. 2018;13(8):e0196908.
54. Spiegel BMR, Younossi ZM, Hays RD, Revicki D, Robbins S, Kanwal F. Impact of hepatitis C on health related quality of life: a systematic review and quantitative assessment. Hepatology (Baltimore, Md). 2005;41(4):790–800.
55. Forton DM, Thomas HC, Murphy CA, Allsop JM, Foster GR, Main J, et al. Hepatitis C and cognitive impairment in a cohort of patients with mild liver disease. Hepatology (Baltimore, Md). 2002;35(2):433–9.
56. Cacoub P, Renou C, Rosenthal E, Cohen P, Loury I, Loustaud-Ratti V, et al. Extrahepatic manifestations associated with hepatitis C virus infection. A prospective multicenter study of 321 patients. The GERMIVIC. Groupe d'Etude et de Recherche en Medecine Interne et Maladies Infectieuses sur le Virus de l'Hepatite C. Medicine. 2000;79(1):47–56.
57. Anand BS, Velez M. Assessment of correlation between serum titers of hepatitis C virus and severity of liver disease. World J Gastroenterol. 2004;10(16):2409–11.
58. Erman A, Krahn MD, Hansen T, Wong J, Bielecki JM, Feld JJ, et al. Estimation of fibrosis progression rates for chronic hepatitis C: a systematic review and meta-analysis update. BMJ Open. 2019;9(11):e027491.
59. Dienstag JL, Ghany MG, Morgan TR, Di Bisceglie AM, Bonkovsky HL, Kim HY, et al. A prospective study of the rate of progression in compensated, histologically advanced chronic hepatitis C. Hepatology (Baltimore, Md). 2011;54(2):396–405.
60. Thomas DL, Thio CL, Martin MP, Qi Y, Ge D, O'Huigin C, et al. Genetic variation in IL28B and spontaneous clearance of hepatitis C virus. Nature. 2009;461(7265):798–801.
61. Sagnelli E, Pisaturo M, Stanzione M, Messina V, Alessio L, Sagnelli C, et al. Clinical presentation, outcome, and response to therapy among patients with acute exacerbation of chronic hepatitis C. Clin Gastroenterol Hepatol. 2013;11(9):1174–80.e11.
62. Fattovich G, Giustina G, Degos F, Tremolada F, Diodati G, Almasio P, et al. Morbidity and mortality in compensated cirrhosis type C: a retrospective follow-up study of 384 patients. Gastroenterology. 1997;112(2):463–72.
63. Marie MS, Shousha HI, Abdelrazek W, Hassany M, Dabees H, Abdelghafour R, et al. Prediction of hepatic decompensation and hepatocellular carcinoma after direct-acting antiviral therapy in patients with hepatitis C-related liver cirrhosis: a cohort study. Egypt Liver J. 2023;13(1):12.
64. Young K, Liu B, Bhuket T, Wong RJ. Lower likelihood of post-transplant graft failure, death, and retransplantation in the era of direct-acting antivirals. J Clin Exp Hepatol. 2020;10(6):581–9.

65. Bruno S, Crosignani A, Maisonneuve P, Rossi S, Silini E, Mondelli MU. Hepatitis C virus genotype 1b as a major risk factor associated with hepatocellular carcinoma in patients with cirrhosis: a seventeen-year prospective cohort study. Hepatology (Baltimore, Md). 2007;46(5):1350–6.
66. Ohki T, Tateishi R, Sato T, Masuzaki R, Imamura J, Goto T, et al. Obesity is an independent risk factor for hepatocellular carcinoma development in chronic hepatitis C patients. Clin Gastroenterol Hepatol. 2008;6(4):459–64.
67. Schillie SVC, Reingold A. Prevention of hepatitis B virus infection in the United States: recommendations of the advisory committee on immunization practices. MMWR Recomm Rep. 2018;67:1–31.
68. Kumar M, Satapathy S, Monga R, Das K, Hissar S, Pande C, et al. A randomized controlled trial of lamivudine to treat acute hepatitis B. Hepatology (Baltimore, Md). 2007;45(1):97–101.
69. Terrault NA, Lok ASF, McMahon BJ, Chang K-M, Hwang JP, Jonas MM, et al. Update on prevention, diagnosis, and treatment of chronic hepatitis B: AASLD 2018 hepatitis B guidance. Hepatology. 2018;67(4):1560–99.
70. Xiao G, Yang J, Yan L. Comparison of diagnostic accuracy of aspartate aminotransferase to platelet ratio index and fibrosis-4 index for detecting liver fibrosis in adult patients with chronic hepatitis B virus infection: a systemic review and meta-analysis. Hepatology. 2015;61(1):292–302.
71. Jang JW, Choi JY, Kim YS, Woo HY, Choi SK, Lee CH, et al. Long-term effect of antiviral therapy on disease course after decompensation in patients with hepatitis B virus-related cirrhosis. Hepatology (Baltimore, Md). 2015;61(6):1809–20.
72. Singal AK, Salameh H, Kuo YF, Fontana RJ. Meta-analysis: the impact of oral antiviral agents on the incidence of hepatocellular carcinoma in chronic hepatitis B. Aliment Pharmacol Ther. 2013;38(2):98–106.
73. Terrault NA, Bzowej NH, Chang KM, Hwang JP, Jonas MM, Murad MH. AASLD guidelines for treatment of chronic hepatitis B. Hepatology. 2016;63(1):261–83.
74. Huhn GD, Tebas P, Gallant J, Wilkin T, Cheng A, Yan M, et al. A randomized, open-label trial to evaluate switching to Elvitegravir/Cobicistat/Emtricitabine/Tenofovir Alafenamide plus Darunavir in treatment-experienced HIV-1-infected adults. J Acquir Immune Defic Syndr (1999). 2017;74(2):193–200.
75. Dybul M, Fauci AS, Bartlett JG, Kaplan JE, Pau AK. Guidelines for using antiretroviral agents among HIV-infected adults and adolescents. Recommendations of the Panel on Clinical Practices for Treatment of HIV. MMWR Recomm Rep. 2002;51(Rr-7):1–55.
76. Manegold C, Hannoun C, Wywiol A, Dietrich M, Polywka S, Chiwakata CB, et al. Reactivation of hepatitis B virus replication accompanied by acute hepatitis in patients receiving highly active antiretroviral therapy. Clin Infect Dis. 2001;32(1):144–8.
77. Lau GK, Yiu HH, Fong DY, Cheng HC, Au WY, Lai LS, et al. Early is superior to deferred preemptive lamivudine therapy for hepatitis B patients undergoing chemotherapy. Gastroenterology. 2003;125(6):1742–9.
78. EASL. 2017 Clinical Practice Guidelines on the management of hepatitis B virus infection. J Hepatol. 2017;67(2):370–98.
79. Lau G, Yu M-L, Wong G, Thompson A, Ghazinian H, Hou J-L, et al. APASL clinical practice guideline on hepatitis B reactivation related to the use of immunosuppressive therapy. Hepatol Int. 2021;15(5):1031–48.
80. Morisco F, Castiglione F, Rispo A, Stroffolini T, Vitale R, Sansone S, et al. Hepatitis B virus infection and immunosuppressive therapy in patients with inflammatory bowel disease. Dig Liver Dis. 2011;43:S40–S8.
81. Hwang JP, Lok AS. Management of patients with hepatitis B who require immunosuppressive therapy. Nat Rev Gastroenterol Hepatol. 2014;11(4):209–19.
82. Fung J, Wong T, Chok K, Chan A, Cheung T-T, Dai JW-C, et al. Long-term outcomes of entecavir monotherapy for chronic hepatitis B after liver transplantation: results up to 8 years. Hepatology. 2017;66(4):1036–44.

83. Ghany MG, Morgan TR, Panel A-IHCG. Hepatitis C Guidance 2019 update: American Association for the Study of Liver Diseases–Infectious Diseases Society of America recommendations for testing, managing, and treating hepatitis C virus infection. Hepatology. 2020;71(2):686–721.
84. Ades AE, Gordon F, Scott K, Collins IJ, Claire T, Pembrey L, et al. Overall vertical transmission of hepatitis C virus, transmission net of clearance, and timing of transmission. Clin Infect Dis. 2022;76(5):905–12.
85. Singla K, Boeke CE. Progress toward hepatitis C elimination in Punjab, India. Clin Liver Dis. 2023;21(1):36–40.
86. Feld JJ, Jacobson IM, Hézode C, Asselah T, Ruane PJ, Gruener N, et al. Sofosbuvir and Velpatasvir for HCV genotype 1, 2, 4, 5, and 6 infection. N Engl J Med. 2015;373(27):2599–607.
87. Everson GT, Towner WJ, Davis MN, Wyles DL, Nahass RG, Thuluvath PJ, et al. Sofosbuvir with Velpatasvir in treatment-naive noncirrhotic patients with genotype 1 to 6 hepatitis C virus infection: a randomized trial. Ann Intern Med. 2015;163(11):818–26.
88. Pianko S, Flamm SL, Shiffman ML, Kumar S, Strasser SI, Dore GJ, et al. Sofosbuvir plus Velpatasvir combination therapy for treatment-experienced patients with genotype 1 or 3 hepatitis C virus infection: a randomized trial. Ann Intern Med. 2015;163(11):809–17.
89. Foster GR, Afdhal N, Roberts SK, Bräu N, Gane EJ, Pianko S, et al. Sofosbuvir and Velpatasvir for HCV genotype 2 and 3 infection. N Engl J Med. 2015;373(27):2608–17.
90. Wei L, Lim SG, Xie Q, Văn KN, Piratvisuth T, Huang Y, et al. Sofosbuvir-velpatasvir for treatment of chronic hepatitis C virus infection in Asia: a single-arm, open-label, phase 3 trial. Lancet Gastroenterol Hepatol. 2019;4(2):127–34.
91. Jacobson IM, Bourgeois S, Mathurin P, Thuluvath P, Ryder SD, Gerken G, et al. The tolerability of sofosbuvir/velpatasvir for 12 weeks in patients treated in the ASTRAL 1, 2 and 3 studies: a pooled safety analysis. J Viral Hepat. 2023;30(5):448–54.
92. Sulkowski MS, Gardiner DF, Rodriguez-Torres M, Reddy KR, Hassanein T, Jacobson I, et al. Daclatasvir plus Sofosbuvir for previously treated or untreated chronic HCV infection. N Engl J Med. 2014;370(3):211–21.
93. Nelson DR, Cooper JN, Lalezari JP, Lawitz E, Pockros PJ, Gitlin N, et al. All-oral 12-week treatment with daclatasvir plus sofosbuvir in patients with hepatitis C virus genotype 3 infection: ALLY-3 phase III study. Hepatology (Baltimore, Md). 2015;61(4):1127–35.
94. Surendra M, Raju SB, Sridhar N, Vijay Kiran B, Rajesh G, Anvesh G, et al. Ledipasvir and Sofosbuvir for untreated HCV genotype 1 infection in end stage renal disease patients: a prospective observational study. Hemodial Int. 2018;22(2):217–21.
95. Buggisch P, Vermehren J, Mauss S, Günther R, Schott E, Pathil A, et al. Real-world effectiveness of 8-week treatment with ledipasvir/sofosbuvir in chronic hepatitis C. J Hepatol. 2018;68(4):663–71.
96. Solomon SS, Wagner-Cardoso S, Smeaton L, Sowah LA, Wimbish C, Robbins G, et al. A minimal monitoring approach for the treatment of hepatitis C virus infection (ACTG A5360 [MINMON]): a phase 4, open-label, single-arm trial. Lancet Gastroenterol Hepatol. 2022;7(4):307–17.
97. Brown RS Jr, Buti M, Rodrigues L, Chulanov V, Chuang WL, Aguilar H, et al. Glecaprevir/pibrentasvir for 8 weeks in treatment-naïve patients with chronic HCV genotypes 1-6 and compensated cirrhosis: the EXPEDITION-8 trial. J Hepatol. 2020;72(3):441–9.
98. European Association for the Study of the Liver. EASL recommendations on treatment of hepatitis C 2018. J Hepatol. 2018;69(2):461–511.
99. Hézode C, Lebray P, De Ledinghen V, Zoulim F, Di Martino V, Boyer N, et al. Daclatasvir plus sofosbuvir, with or without ribavirin, for hepatitis C virus genotype 3 in a French early access programme. Liver Int. 2017;37(9):1314–24.
100. Belli LS, Berenguer M, Cortesi PA, Strazzabosco M, Rockenschaub SR, Martini S, et al. Delisting of liver transplant candidates with chronic hepatitis C after viral eradication: a European study. J Hepatol. 2016;65(3):524–31.

101. Martini S, Sacco M, Strona S, Arese D, Tandoi F, Dell Olio D, et al. Impact of viral eradication with sofosbuvir-based therapy on the outcome of post-transplant hepatitis C with severe fibrosis. Liver Int. 2017;37(1):62–70.
102. Terrault NA, McCaughan GW, Curry MP, Gane E, Fagiuoli S, Fung JYY, et al. International liver transplantation society consensus statement on hepatitis C management in liver transplant candidates. Transplantation. 2017;101(5):945–55.
103. Liu CH, Chen CY, Su WW, Liu CJ, Lo CC, Huang KJ, et al. Sofosbuvir/velpatasvir plus ribavirin for Child-Pugh B and Child-Pugh C hepatitis C virus-related cirrhosis. Clin Mol Hepatol. 2021;27(4):575–88.
104. Curry MP, O'Leary JG, Bzowej N, Muir AJ, Korenblat KM, Fenkel JM, et al. Sofosbuvir and Velpatasvir for HCV in patients with decompensated cirrhosis. N Engl J Med. 2015;373(27):2618–28.
105. Charlton M, Everson GT, Flamm SL, Kumar P, Landis C, Brown RS Jr, et al. Ledipasvir and Sofosbuvir plus Ribavirin for treatment of HCV infection in patients with advanced liver disease. Gastroenterology. 2015;149(3):649–59.
106. Bourlière M, Bronowicki JP, de Ledinghen V, Hézode C, Zoulim F, Mathurin P, et al. Ledipasvir-sofosbuvir with or without ribavirin to treat patients with HCV genotype 1 infection and cirrhosis non-responsive to previous protease-inhibitor therapy: a randomised, double-blind, phase 2 trial (SIRIUS). Lancet Infect Dis. 2015;15(4):397–404.
107. Manns M, Samuel D, Gane EJ, Mutimer D, McCaughan G, Buti M, et al. Ledipasvir and sofosbuvir plus ribavirin in patients with genotype 1 or 4 hepatitis C virus infection and advanced liver disease: a multicentre, open-label, randomised, phase 2 trial. Lancet Infect Dis. 2016;16(6):685–97.
108. Pan CQ, Duan Z, Dai E, Zhang S, Han G, Wang Y, et al. Tenofovir to prevent hepatitis B transmission in mothers with high viral load. N Engl J Med. 2016;374(24):2324–34.
109. The Korean Association for the Study of the Liver (KASL). KASL clinical practice guidelines for management of chronic hepatitis B. Clin Mol Hepatol. 2019;25(2):93–159.
110. Chauhan R, Lingala S, Gadiparthi C, Lahiri N, Mohanty SR, Wu J, et al. Reactivation of hepatitis B after liver transplantation: current knowledge, molecular mechanisms and implications in management. World J Hepatol. 2018;10(3):352–70.
111. Ceci O, Margiotta M, Marello F, Francavilla R, Loizzi P, Francavilla A, et al. Vertical transmission of hepatitis C virus in a cohort of 2,447 HIV-seronegative pregnant women: a 24-month prospective study. J Pediatr Gastroenterol Nutr. 2001;33(5):570–5.
112. England K, Thorne C, Newell ML. Vertically acquired paediatric coinfection with HIV and hepatitis C virus. Lancet Infect Dis. 2006;6(2):83–90.
113. El-Shabrawi MHF, Kamal NM, Mogahed EA, Elhusseini MA, Aljabri MF. Perinatal transmission of hepatitis C virus: an update. Arch Med Sci: AMS. 2020;16(6):1360–9.
114. Arshad M, El-Kamary SS, Jhaveri R. Hepatitis C virus infection during pregnancy and the newborn period--are they opportunities for treatment? J Viral Hepat. 2011;18(4):229–36.
115. Hughes BL, Page CM, Kuller JA. Hepatitis C in pregnancy: screening, treatment, and management. Am J Obstet Gynecol. 2017;217(5):B2–b12.
116. Lim SG, Baumert TF, Boni C, Gane E, Levrero M, Lok AS, et al. The scientific basis of combination therapy for chronic hepatitis B functional cure. Nat Rev Gastroenterol Hepatol. 2023;20(4):238–53.

Chapter 11
Liver Transplantation for Hepatocellular Carcinoma

Dhiraj Agrawal, Jyoti Wadhwa, Akshay Kulkarni, and Sanjiv Saigal

Abstract Hepatocellular carcinoma (HCC) remains a common indication for liver transplantation (LT) in terms of waitlist registrants and recipients, regardless of underlying etiology. LT is one of the most effective treatments for carefully selected patients with HCC within the Milan criteria (MC) and without evidence of vascular or extrahepatic involvement. The advent of more effective systemic and loco-regional therapies has enabled patients to undergo LT who would otherwise have been considered untransplantable. This review covers the selection criteria, bridging and down-staging strategies, and recent advancements in targeted therapy, as well as how these could be integrated into managing HCC patients undergoing liver transplants.

Keywords Deceased donor liver transplantation · Living donor liver transplantation · Hepatocellular carcinoma · Selection criteria · Down-staging therapy · Bridging therapy

---

D. Agrawal
Department of Gastroenterology and Hepatology, Continental Hospitals, Financial District, Hyderabad, India

J. Wadhwa
Department of Medical and Precision Oncology, Apollo Cancer Centres, Delhi, India

A. Kulkarni
Department of Gastroenterology, Midas Multi-speciality Hospital, Nagpur, Maharashtra, India

S. Saigal (✉)
Hepatology and Liver Transplant Medicine, Max Institute of Liver and Gastrointestinal Sciences, Max Super Speciality Hospital, Saket, New Delhi, India
e-mail: sanjivsaigal@hotmail.com

S. Saigal, D. Jothimani (eds.), *Fundamentals of Transplant Hepatology*,
https://doi.org/10.1007/978-981-95-2624-6_11

Abbreviations

AFP	Alpha-fetoprotein
BCLC	Barcelona Clinic Liver Cancer
CTC	Circulating tumor cells
ctDNA	Circulating tumor DNA
DDLT	Deceased donor LT
DCP	Des-gamma-carboxyprothrombin
DFS	Disease free survival
EBRT	External beam radiation therapy
HCC	Hepatocellular carcinoma
ICI	Immune Checkpoint Inhibitors
LRT	Loco-regional therapy
LT	Liver transplantation
LDLT	Living donor LT
MC	Milan criteria
MORAL	Model of Recurrence after Liver Transplantation
mTOR	Mammalian target of rapamycin inhibitors
MWA	Microwave ablation
MELD	Model for End-Stage Liver Disease
mRECIST	Modified Response Evaluation Criteria in Solid Tumors
NLR	Neutrophil/lymphocyte ratio
NYCA	Newyork/California
OPTN	Organ Procurement and Transplantation Network
PIVKA	Prothrombin-induced by vitamin K absence-II
PVTT	Portal venous tumor thrombus
PET	Positron emission tomography
RFS	Recurrence-free survival
RETREAT	Risk Estimation of Tumor Recurrence After Transplant
RFA	Radiofrequency ablation
SLT	Salvage LT
SBRT	Stereotactic body radiotherapy
TARE	Trans-arterial radioembolization
TACE	Trans-arterial chemoembolization
TRAIN	Time-Radiological-response-Alpha-fetoprotein-INflammation
UNOS	United Network for Organ Sharing
UCSF	University of California—San Francisco
UNOS-DS	UCSF's down-staging

Key Highlights

- Liver cancer is a global health problem, with its incidence rising worldwide.
- For select patients unsuitable for resection or ablation, liver transplantation (LT) is the optimal treatment for hepatocellular carcinoma (HCC).
- Liver transplantation is an effective therapy in HCC patients within the Milan criteria or in those who can be down-staged to within the Milan criteria.

- Expansion of eligibility criteria is being explored to identify the upper limits of tumor burden that can be effectively managed with LT and achieve similar recurrence-free survival.
- Combining new systemic treatments with LT offers a potentially curative therapy to selected patients who previously received palliative care.
- Despite all the efforts to design optimal selection criteria, 8–20% of patients will develop recurrence.
- The unmet needs in the field are refining selection criteria, expanding the donor pool, and defining biomarkers to guide tailored treatment.

11.1 Introduction

Liver transplantation (LT), initially described by Starzl as a treatment for primary liver malignancies, has made significant strides in treating hepatocellular carcinoma (HCC). In the early phase, LT for HCC faced high recurrence rates, leading to a shift in indications to non-oncologic liver diseases. However, patients undergoing LT for other indications and incidentally found to have tumors showed promising survival rates, indicating the need for improved selection criteria. In 1996, Mazzaferro et al. demonstrated 5- and 10-year survival rates of approximately 70% and 55%, respectively, marking a significant milestone [1]. The Milan criteria, established as the gold standard selection criteria, were incorporated into regional and national allocation policies like the United Network for Organ Sharing (UNOS) in 2002. In the subsequent efforts to widen the selection criteria while maintaining acceptable outcomes, most notably, the University of California—San Francisco (UCSF) criteria were published in 2001 [2]. This was followed by the national down-staging policy in December 2017 to address patients initially presenting with HCC beyond the Milan criteria but successfully downsized to within the Milan criteria [3]. The current listing criteria for LT in patients with HCC are undergoing constant refinements to expand the indications for LT while preserving the survival rates comparable to the Milan criteria. Today, the HCC allocation policy worldwide typically relies on the assessment of tumor biology by using tumor size, number of nodules, biomarkers, and responses to therapy.

LT remains the best oncologic treatment strategy for patients with early-stage HCC, and the outcomes following LT are continuously improving, thanks to the evolving patient-centered oncological treatment strategies and new technologies to expand the donor pool, including the option of living donor LT (LDLT) for adults in 1998. Advances in liver-directed therapies used as bridging or down-staging therapy and the approval of modestly effective systemic therapies for advanced HCC aim to improve patient outcomes. In the past, an arbitrary 5-year overall survival (OS) rate of more than 50% has been postulated to be an acceptable outcome following LT. More recently, a 5-year OS rate of 60% has been suggested as a sensible outcome in the setting of LT for HCC.

Especially in Asian countries with organ shortages, the focus has shifted from deceased donor LT deceased donor liver transplantation (DDLT) to LDLT. LDLT emphasizes performing LT in HCC patients most likely to derive significant transplant survival benefits, combining the principles of both urgency and utility. Theoretically, policies that select certain patients to increase post-transplantation survival reduce the likelihood of survival in counter-selected patients. Higher tumor burdens might correlate with a more significant transplantation-associated survival benefit despite worse waitlist and post-transplantation survival. This counterintuitive result is because the adverse effects of higher tumor burdens are more pronounced in patients on the waitlist than in patients who eventually undergo LT. Thus, prioritizing patients with a more significant transplantation-associated survival benefit would increase the total survival of all HCC patients listed for LT to achieve the maximum intention-to-treat survival.

11.2 HCC Staging Systems

Various staging systems have been developed to assess the extent of hepatocellular carcinoma (HCC), though no single globally accepted scoring system exists. The tumor-node-metastasis (TNM) classification is commonly used in patients undergoing surgical resection for HCC, as it is entirely based on pathological data. The Okuda system has limited clinical utility due to its failure to account for multifocal tumors or vascular invasion. The Japanese Integrated Staging system combines TNM staging with Child-Pugh scoring, offering a more comprehensive overview.

The Cancer of the Liver Italian Program (CLIP) score includes tumor morphology features such as unifocal vs. multifocal disease and tumor involvement of <50% vs. >50% of liver volume; however, this system is often too broad for assessing early-stage HCC. In East Asia, the Hong Kong Liver Cancer (HKLC) classification is widely used to guide treatment strategies for HCC.

The Barcelona Clinic Liver Cancer (BCLC) staging system is the most commonly endorsed tool worldwide for stratifying and guiding treatment in patients with HCC, both with and without cirrhosis [4]. It bases treatment recommendations on tumor characteristics, liver function, and performance status. Curative treatments—such as resection, ablation, and liver transplantation (LT)—are primarily reserved for early-stage disease (BCLC stages 0 and A). The updated 2022 BCLC model introduces several advancements, including stratification within the heterogeneous BCLC-B group, integration of immunotherapy as a first-line option for BCLC-C, consideration of transplant for patients meeting locally expanded criteria or after successful down-staging, and the incorporation of a "treatment-stage migration" concept [4].

11.3 Prediction of HCC Recurrence After LT

11.3.1 Radiographic Tumor Burden

Tumor size and number of nodules, as seen on imaging, remain central to determining transplant eligibility. Among these, the largest lesion diameter has the strongest prognostic relevance. The Milan criteria, adopted into UNOS policy (T2 criteria) in 2002, remain the benchmark. Expanded criteria such as the UCSF and "up-to-seven" models have shown comparable post-transplant survival outcomes [5].

11.3.2 Biomarkers

Alpha-fetoprotein (AFP) remains the most widely used serum biomarker for HCC, reflecting tumor differentiation and vascular invasion. However, there is no agreed-upon universal cutoff or standard for assessing dynamic AFP trends. Pre-transplant AFP levels above 1000 ng/mL correlate with poor post-LT survival, independent of tumor size or number. The latest UNOS guidelines require that patients with AFP >1000 ng/mL demonstrate a reduction to <500 ng/mL following loco-regional therapy (LRT) prior to LT [6].

The New York/California (NYCA) score goes a step further by integrating both static AFP levels and their change over time, thus providing a dynamic picture of tumor biology [7]. However, AFP has limitations, including the fact that not all aggressive tumors secrete AFP, and its expression frequency increases with disease stage.

11.3.3 Other Biomarkers

Additional markers associated with HCC recurrence risk include des-gamma-carboxy prothrombin (DCP >7.5 ng/mL), AFP-L3 > 35%, and absolute AFP-L3 levels. Inflammatory markers, such as the neutrophil-to-lymphocyte ratio (NLR) >5 and the platelet-to-lymphocyte ratio, also offer prognostic value. Prothrombin-induced by vitamin K absence-II (PIVKA-II) is emerging as a useful indicator of poorly differentiated or advanced-stage HCC with microvascular invasion.

11.4 Explant Pathology and Imaging Predictors

11.4.1 Microvascular Invasion (MVI)

MVI observed in explant pathology is one of the strongest predictors of post-transplant HCC recurrence and poorer survival outcomes. Risk factors for MVI include tumors >5 cm, multiple lesions, AFP >1000 ng/mL, and increased uptake on Positron emission tomography (PET) imaging.

11.4.2 Tumor Differentiation Grade

Poor tumor differentiation has consistently been identified as a key predictor of HCC recurrence post-LT. Several models, such as those from Padova, Toronto, and Hangzhou, exclude patients with poorly differentiated tumors. However, due to sampling variability and limitations, routine pre-LT liver biopsy is not recommended for eligibility decisions. Recent advances in radiogenomics aim to predict MVI non-invasively.

11.4.3 Functional Imaging (PET Scan)

18F-FDG PET/CT has shown a correlation between tumor uptake and aggressive histological features. Studies from Korea and Japan indicate that PET-negative tumors may allow for relaxed size criteria in LDLT candidates.

11.4.4 Molecular Markers and Liquid Biopsy

Emerging liquid biopsy techniques offer real-time molecular insights into HCC without the need for tissue sampling. These methods may allow for dynamic monitoring of tumor clonal evolution while patients are on the transplant waitlist. Liquid biopsies can overcome the issue of intratumoral heterogeneity that limits single-biopsy reliability. Biomarkers like circulating tumor cells (CTCs) and circulating tumor DNA (ctDNA) are gaining attention for predicting post-LT recurrence [8]. Specific interstitial phenotypes have also been linked to higher recurrence risk. Future research in molecular biomarkers could help stratify transplant candidates, guide treatment decisions, and even support organ allocation strategies.

11.4.5 Selection Criteria for HCC in the DDLT Setting

Liver transplantation is considered the optimal treatment for early-stage HCC (BCLC-A) when patients meet the Milan criteria (MC). However, there is a growing shift toward extending transplant eligibility. Several alternative scoring systems have been proposed and validated, identifying patients beyond MC who can still achieve 5-year survival rates ≥70%. Notable expanded criteria include the UCSF, Toronto, and AFP models, as well as revised criteria up to seven [9] (Table 11.1).

Recurrence prediction models are categorized by the timing of their application—pre-transplant vs. post-transplant. An ideal pre-LT model incorporates both traditional morphological data and biological surrogates (e.g., AFP trends, PET findings) to improve long-term outcomes. Post-transplant models help stratify recurrence risk and identify patients requiring closer follow-up or adjuvant therapy.

11.4.6 Prediction Models Based on Radiologic Factors

Milan criteria are the benchmark for selecting patients with HCC for LT. In 1996, Mazzaferro et al., after analyzing the explant pathology of 48 patients over 3 years, found post-LT OS and recurrence-free survival (RFS) of 85.0% and 92.0%, respectively [1]. The same LT center meta-analyzed 25 articles and showed similar 5-year post-LT patient survival rates of at least 70% in patients within MC [10].

The UCSF criteria, published in 2001, included patients with either a single lesion measuring up to 6.5 cm or up to three lesions, none larger than 4.5 cm, and a total tumor burden of less than 8 cm; these criteria demonstrated a favorable 5-year patient survival rate of 75.2%, based on the explant pathology of 70 patients [2].

11.4.7 Prediction Models Based on Radiological and Serological Factors

AFP model: In 2012, Duvoux et al. proposed AFP scores (Table 11.1), where a score > 2 predicted a 5-year recurrence risk of 50.6% vs. 8.8% ($P < 0.001$) and decreased 5-year survival (47.5% vs. 67.8%; $P < 0.002$) [11]. This model was additionally validated in Asians and LDLT populations. The AFP model discriminates between the low and high risk of recurrence in both patients with HCC within or outside the MC for low overall and disease-free survival.

Updated Up-to-Seven/Metro ticket 2.0 criteria: Mazzaferro et al. presented simple up-to-seven criteria in 2009, where 1156 patients from Europe, the USA, and Brazil met this criterion, showing a 5-year patient survival of 71.2% [5]. The Metro Ticket Investigator Study Group in Milan added AFP value to the "Up to 7 criteria" to form the revised up-to-seven criteria/Metro Ticket 2.0 system. For patients with

Table 11.1 Selection criteria for DDLT for HCC

Author/Year	Criteria name	Criteria	No. of patients	Outcome
Mazzaferro et al. [1]	Milan criteria	Single nodule <5 cm or up to 3 lesions, none larger than 3 cm, no macrovascularinvasion	48	4-year OS: 75.0%
Yao et al. [12]	UCSF criteria	Single lesion ≤6.5 cm OR 2–3 lesions ≤4.5 cm each, or Total tumor diameter ≤ 8 cm	70	5-year OS: 75.2%
Mazzaferro et al. [5]	Up to seven/ Metroticket criteria	Largest tumor diameter (cm) + number of tumors <–7no vascular invasion	1556	5-year OS: 71.2%
DuBay et al. [14]	Toronto criteria	Any size or number of tumors if: No systemic cancer-related symptoms, no extrahepatic disease, no vascular invasion, no poorly differentiated tumors	294	5-year OS 70%, 5-year RFS 66%
Duvoux et al. [11]	AFP model	Low risk: <–2 pointshigh risk: >2 pointslargest diameter (points): <–3 cm (0), 3–6 cm (1), >6 cm (4)number of nodules (points): 1–3 (0), >4 (2)AFP level (points): <100 ng/ml (0), 100–1000 ng/ml (2), >1000 (3)	TC 537; VC: 435	5-year OSlow risk: 67.8%high risk: 47.5%
Yao et al. [15]	UCSF down-staging	Milan or down-staged to Milan; AFP >1000 ng/mLreduced to <500	DS: 118 (34.7%) vs. LT only: 488	5-year OS: 80%
Halazun et al. [17]	Pre-MORAL	Largest tumor size (lowestrisk: ≤3 cm); AFP (lowest risk: < 200 ng/mL); NLR (lower risk <5)	NA	5-yr RFS: 99% low risk70% medium-risk56% high-risk
Mazzaferro et al. [13]	Metro ticket 2.0 criteria	AFP <200 ng/mL AND the sum ofnumber and size of tumors(in cm) <7AFP 200–400 ng/mL AND sum of the number and size oftumors ≤5AFP 400–1000 ng/mL ANDthe sum of the number and sizeof tumors should be ≤4	TC: 1018 VC: 341	TC: 5-year OS 79.7%5-year RFS 89.6%VC 5-year OS 80.8% RFS 86.4%

an AFP < 200 ng/mL, the sum of the number of tumors and size in cm should be less than 7, while for AFP 200 to 400 ng/mL, the sum of tumor number plus size should be less than 5; and if the level of AFP is 400 to 1000 ng/mL, the sum of the number and size of tumors should be not more than 4. This model was developed with multi-institution data from Italy and validated in a population from China. Patients meeting these criteria showed excellent 5-year OS and RFS in training (79.7% and

89.6%, respectively) and validation cohorts (80.8% and 86.4%, respectively) [13]. A Metro Ticket V2.0 calculator is available online. It has been validated in an Asian cohort. The demonstration that the AFP model and Metro Ticket V2.0 outperform the MC benchmark strengthens the position that combining a biomarker with tumor morphology can better predict the risk of recurrence and overall survival after transplantation for HCC (Table 11.1).

11.4.8 Prediction Models Based on Pathological Factors

Pathological factors such as microvascular invasion and tumor differentiation can predict HCC recurrence after LT. Per the expanded Toronto criteria, a pre-LT biopsy is required to exclude poorly differentiated tumors in patients beyond the MC [14]. Additionally, needle biopsy has a relatively lower accuracy for tumor differentiation than explant pathology and also risks cancer seeding.

RETREAT score: The Risk Estimation of Tumor Recurrence After Transplant (RETREAT) score was developed in 2017 based on explant tumor burden (diameter of the largest viable tumor + number of tumors on explant pathology), presence of microvascular invasion, and AFP level at transplantation to predict HCC recurrence accurately. A RETREAT score between 0 and 3 indicates a 1- and 5-year recurrence risk between 10% and 20%, while a score > 5 carries a recurrence risk close to 40% and 75%, respectively [16]. At UCSF, post-operative surveillance intervals are guided by the recipient's RETREAT score.

Model of Recurrence after Liver Transplantation (MORAL): Halazun et al., in 2017, developed the MORAL USA score, including preoperative AFP levels >200 ng/mL, NLR $\geq$ 5, and largest tumor size >3 cm (pre-MORAL score), while on explant pathology, grade 4 tumor, MVI, and size and number > 3 (post-MORAL score) aids tumor recurrence prediction. The low-risk group (score 0–2) had a 5-year RFS of 98.5%, while the very-high-risk group (score > 10) had a 1-year RFS of only 17.9%. The resulting combined combo-MORAL score was found to have a c-statistic of 0.91, with better performance than the MC (0.63) and UCSF criteria (0.57) [17].

11.5 Bridging vs. Down-Staging in HCC Before Liver Transplantation

11.5.1 Bridging Therapy

In patients with hepatocellular carcinoma (HCC) who already meet liver transplant criteria but are awaiting transplantation, "bridging therapy" is used to control tumor progression and minimize the risk of waitlist dropout. In the U.S., approximately 25% of listed patients are removed from the waitlist due to tumor progression.

While there are no standardized recommendations for who should receive bridging therapy, it is generally advised for patients with UNOS T2 HCC who are expected to wait more than 6 months [18].

No single loco-regional therapy (LRT) is preferred, as effectiveness varies. The goal is to achieve a complete response, defined as no viable tumor on imaging and AFP levels below 100 ng/mL. Patients achieving a complete response after their initial LRT, as determined by mRECIST criteria, have lower dropout rates, a greater likelihood of transplantation, and improved outcomes. Monitoring tumor behavior over time post-LRT can aid in refining transplant candidate selection. Additionally, treating underlying liver disease during this period may reduce the risk of hepatic decompensation and enhance tolerance to LRT.

11.5.2 Down-Staging Therapy

Down-staging involves reducing tumor size or AFP levels in patients initially outside transplant criteria to bring them within acceptable thresholds for deceased donor liver transplantation (DDLT). Most studies use the Milan/UNOS T2 criteria as the goal for successful down-staging, although entry criteria vary; outcomes of down-staging correlate strongly with baseline tumor burden, highlighting the importance of selecting appropriate candidates upfront.

To standardize down-staging protocols, UNOS adopted UCSF's inclusion criteria in 2017, allowing patients who do not meet Milan criteria initially but fall within UNOS-DS limits to be eligible for model for end-stage liver disease (MELD) exception once down-staging is successful. Patients with AFP >1000 ng/mL are only considered for exception if their AFP drops below 500 ng/mL. A stable response to LRT for a minimum of 3 months is also seen as a favorable prognostic indicator, reflecting less aggressive tumor biology.

Some propose offering down-staging to all patients without extrahepatic spread or major vascular invasion. However, patients with tumors beyond UNOS-DS criteria ("all-comers") have worse 3-year post-transplant survival [19]. A meta-analysis of 25 studies with nearly 4000 patients confirms that outcomes deteriorate significantly beyond a certain tumor burden threshold. An AFP >100 ng/mL at diagnosis is also linked to reduced down-staging success and poorer post-transplant survival. Collectively, these findings emphasize AFP's role as a surrogate for tumor aggressiveness and prognosis. Patients with T1/T2 HCC who progress or T3 patients who fail down-staging show markedly lower recurrence-free and overall survival.

11.5.3 Down-Staging Procedures and LRT Options

Because sorafenib has historically shown limited efficacy, down-staging has primarily been achieved through liver-directed therapies aimed at reducing tumor size, number, or AFP levels. Candidates for down-staging must maintain adequate liver function and good performance status. Macrovascular invasion on imaging typically excludes patients from down-staging protocols.

11.5.4 Locoregional Therapy

Common LRT techniques include:

- Trans-arterial therapies: Trans-arterial chemoembolization (TACE), DEB-TACE, Trans-arterial radioembolization (TARE) (Y-90), TAE, and hepatic artery infusion (HAI) therapy. Candidates should generally have Child-Pugh class A or B status and total bilirubin ≤3 mg/dL. Although TARE shows longer time to progression and less toxicity compared to TACE, it may cause radiation-induced injury in patients with bilirubin >2 mg/dL.
- Ablation techniques: Radiofrequency ablation (RFA) and microwave ablation (MWA) are standard in select patients.
- Radiation therapy: Advanced external beam radiation methods like stereotactic body radiotherapy (SBRT) and proton-beam therapy are increasingly viable due to their precision. External beam radiation therapy (EBRT) may be preferred over thermal ablation when tumors are in challenging locations or of large size. Radiation can also be used in neoadjuvant or palliative settings, particularly for HCC with macrovascular invasion.

11.5.5 Tumor Response to LRT

The European Hepatocellular Cancer Liver Transplant Study Group identified two key predictors of post-transplant recurrence: AFP slope > 15 ng/mL/month and tumor progression post-LRT [20]. Even meeting Milan criteria offers limited benefit if these high-risk markers are present. Thus, both depth and durability of response are critical. According to mRECIST, complete or partial response signals favorable outcomes, while progressive disease indicates poor prognosis. Active tumors—those with arterial enhancement and venous washout—are considered viable regardless of partial necrosis.

The Time-Radiological-response-Alpha-fetoprotein-INflammation (TRAIN) score, proposed by Lai et al. in 2016, integrates tumor response, AFP dynamics, neutrophil-to-lymphocyte ratio (NLR), and wait time (WT) to predict outcomes [21].

11.6 Systemic Therapy for Bridging or Down-Staging (Table 11.2)

11.6.1 Tyrosine Kinase Inhibitors (TKIs)

Sorafenib was the first systemic therapy for advanced HCC, offering modest survival benefits. Lenvatinib has shown non-inferiority in first-line settings, while regorafenib, cabozantinib, and ramucirumab are available as second-line agents.

11.6.2 Immune Checkpoint Inhibitors (ICIs)

Immune checkpoint blockade has emerged as a promising treatment for advanced HCC. Agents targeting CTLA-4 and PD-1/PD-L1 restore anti-tumor immunity. New combinations like atezolizumab-bevacizumab, tremelimumab-durvalumab, nivolumab, and ipilimumab have been approved and have shown encouraging efficacy.

11.6.3 ICI Use Prior to Transplantation

Initial reports caution against the use of ICIs before transplantation due to the risk of fatal graft rejection. Nordness et al. and Chen et al. described patients who died from acute hepatic necrosis after receiving nivolumab and toripalimab, respectively, prior to LT [22, 23].

However, Tabrizian et al. presented a series of nine patients treated with nivolumab before LT, showing only one mild rejection episode and no graft losses [24]. A broader analysis of 43 patients found a 19% incidence of severe rejection, with 9% mortality [25].

There are also emerging case reports of successful down-staging with atezolizumab-bevacizumab, followed by LT, such as the case reported by Schmiderer et al. [26] In that case, the explant showed an excellent histologic response, reflected

Table 11.2 Approved systemic therapies for hepatocellular carcinoma

First line	Second line
Atezolizumab plus bevacizumab	Regorafenib
Sorafenib	Cabozantinib
Lenvatinib	Ramucirumab
Durvalumab + Tremilimumab	Nivolumab plus ipilimumab
	Dostarlimab-gxly
Nivolumab + Ipilimumab	

in a low RETREAT score indicating low recurrence risk. An ongoing clinical trial (NCT05185505) is evaluating this treatment's safety and feasibility.

Because immunotherapy poses rejection risks, its use in transplant candidates requires caution. Some researchers recommend a washout period—up to 3 months—between the final ICI dose and LT, based on ICI half-lives (e.g., Nivolumab and Atezolizumab: \ ~ 27 days). LDLT offers better coordination opportunities for such regimens due to its elective nature. Graft PD-L1 expression is being explored as a potential predictor of rejection risk.

Living donor liver transplantation offers a unique advantage in timing and coordination, especially for bridging or down-staging strategies. However, emerging therapies, particularly ICIs, must be applied cautiously in transplant candidates due to the potential for severe immune-mediated complications. More research is needed to determine the safest and most effective use of these treatments in the context of liver transplantation, including the identification of predictive biomarkers for rejection and long-term oncologic outcomes.

11.7 LDLT for HCC

LDLT is an effective strategy to address the liver shortage issue, particularly in Asian countries where donation-after-brain-death systems are lacking. LDLT provides planned, timely access to LT in patients with HCC and benefits patients wait-listed for DDLT. In DDLT, liver allocation principles select patients based on urgency and utility schemes. However, in LDLT, there is a "no competition" situation, tending to have pretty liberal tumor burden criteria expanding beyond MC. The "transplant benefit," or the life-years gained with LT compared to the best available alternative therapy, is crucial for LDLT. For HCC beyond Milan criteria, the better OS could be attributed to the shorter waiting time and the low dropout, primarily because of tumor progression. However, controversially, HCC recurrence is more frequent in LDLT, probably due to the fast-tracking of LDLT not allowing sufficient time to evaluate the tumor biology. Secondly, such patients more often have a higher tumor burden outside of acceptable transplant listing criteria.

11.8 Selection Criteria

The selection criteria for patients with HCC may differ in LDLT from those in DDLT. However, this should not adversely affect the double equipoise in LDLT, ensuring both acceptable recipient outcomes and donor safety. Using a Markov model, a minimum 5-year post-LDLT survival of 60% is an adequate benchmark. Also, the hepatitis B virus is associated with more HCC developing in non-cirrhotic livers, and selection criteria are also different in the absence of underlying cirrhosis. Expanded criteria for LDLT (Table 11.3) include: The Japanese 5-5-500 criteria (tumor diameter ≤ 5 cm, tumor number ≤ 5, and AFP ≤ 500 ng/mL) were approved as the national selection criteria for liver transplant candidates with HCC in 2007 [27]. The National Cancer Center of Korea (Asan Medical Center criteria) combined morphological and positron emission tomography (PET) parameters to show excellent in-criteria patient survival in 2008 [28]. The Kyoto criteria include a restriction on the total number of tumors (< 10) as well as the size of the largest tumor (< 5 cm) and PIVKA level < 400 mAU/mL, and for those within these criteria, a meager recurrence rate of just 4% at 5 years [29]. According to the Kyushu criteria, LT is feasible if the tumor diameter is ≤5 cm or PIVKA-II levels ≤300 mAU/mL are satisfied, presenting broad criteria for LT indication [30]. The South Korean MORAL score solely utilizes AFP and DCP serum levels without morphological tumor burden cutoffs to predict tumor recurrence after LDLT (MORAL, Korea). Many Korean centers have developed their selection criteria, with unique experiences handling "far advanced" HCC patients and those with macrovascular invasion. Their studies emphasize the importance of selecting suitable tumor markers and conducting functional studies instead of focusing on tumor size and number. Learnings from Korean centers are vital for broadening liver transplant criteria, especially with the progress in HCC systemic treatment.

Role of Tumor Down-staging in LDLT: Most down-staging studies have been primarily in the DDLT setting, and currently, no consensus exists on down-staging strategies for patients awaiting LDLT. Patients with HCC beyond their "local" criteria should be down-staged to within UCSF criteria with AFP <500 ng/mL and observed for at least 3 months after successful down-staging before LDLT. To summarize, LDLT expanded the use of LT as a treatment for advanced HCC patients who typically lack surgical alternatives. LDLT is a rational and possibly favored choice for HCC patients awaiting LT if the center can provide DDLT and LDLT, and the patient has a prospective liver donor (Fig. 11.1).

Approach to HCC with portal vein tumor thrombosis (PVTT): PVTT is found in 10–40% of patients with HCC at diagnosis and is associated with a median OS of 5–19 months. The BCLC prognosis and treatment strategy algorithm recommends against LT and indicates only palliative treatment. However, a definite benefit of down-staging + LDLT over medical therapies, such as lenvatinib or immunotherapy alone or in combination with TARE/SBRT, has been seen in eligible patients. Down-staging can be done with SBRT with or without TARE or TACE. LT can be offered if patients can be down-staged to meet the acceptable criteria for a transplant, their tumor biology shows a good response, and there is no progression of the disease after treatment during a reasonable waiting period. The Medanta group has transplanted 36 patients, including 20 with segmental (Vp1 and Vp2 PVTT) and 16 with lobar (Vp3 and Vp4) PVTT. The mean time from down-staging to LDLT was 12 weeks (8–23 weeks). At 34 months post-down-staging and 28 months post-LDLT, the 1-year and 5-year OS and RFS rates were 88%, 57%, 79%, and 61%, respectively [31]. Serenari et al. reported outcomes in HCC patients with PVTT who received down-staging with yttrium-90 TARE and underwent DDLT in case of complete and sustained (6 months) radiological response. The 5-year OS rate for DDLT patients post-successful down-staging was 60%, as opposed to 0% in the non-transplant group [32].

Table 11.3 Selection criteria for LDLT for HCC

Author/Year	Criteria name	Criteria	No. of patients	Outcome
Sugawara et al. [38]	Tokyo criteria, Japan	Up to 5 nodules maximum diameter < 5 cm	78	5-year RFS: 90%5-year OS 75.0%
Lee et al. [28]	Asan criteria, Seoul, Korea	Largest tumor diameter < 5 cm number of HCC lesions <6 no gross vascular invasion	221	5-year OS: 76.3%
Taketomi et al. [30]	Kyushu criteria, Japan	Tumor diameter ≤ 5 cm, or PIVKA-II ≤300 mAI/mL	90	5-year OS 82.7%
Takada and Uemoto. [29]	Kyoto criteria, Japan	Number of lesions <10 diameter < 5 cm PIVAK-II < 400 mAU/ml	136	5-year OS: 86.7%, 5-year RR 4.9%
Kim et al. [9]	SMC, Korea	Largest tumor size ≤ 6 cm, number ≤ 7 and AFP ≤1000 ng/mL	180	5-year OS, 90.0%
Lee et al. (2016)	MORAL, Korea	MORAL score ≤ 314.8 score calculation = $11 \times \sqrt{\text{PIVKA-II}} + 2 \times \sqrt{\text{AFP}}$MoRAL score ≤ 314.8score calculation = $11 \times \sqrt{\text{PIVKA-II}} + 2\times \sqrt{\text{AFP}}$	566	66.3% at 5 years 82.6% at 5 years
Shimamura et al. [27]	5–5-500 rule, Japan	Tumor size < 5 cm in diameter tumor number < 5 AFP value <500 ng/ml	965	5-year OS: 75.8%, 5-year RR 7.3%

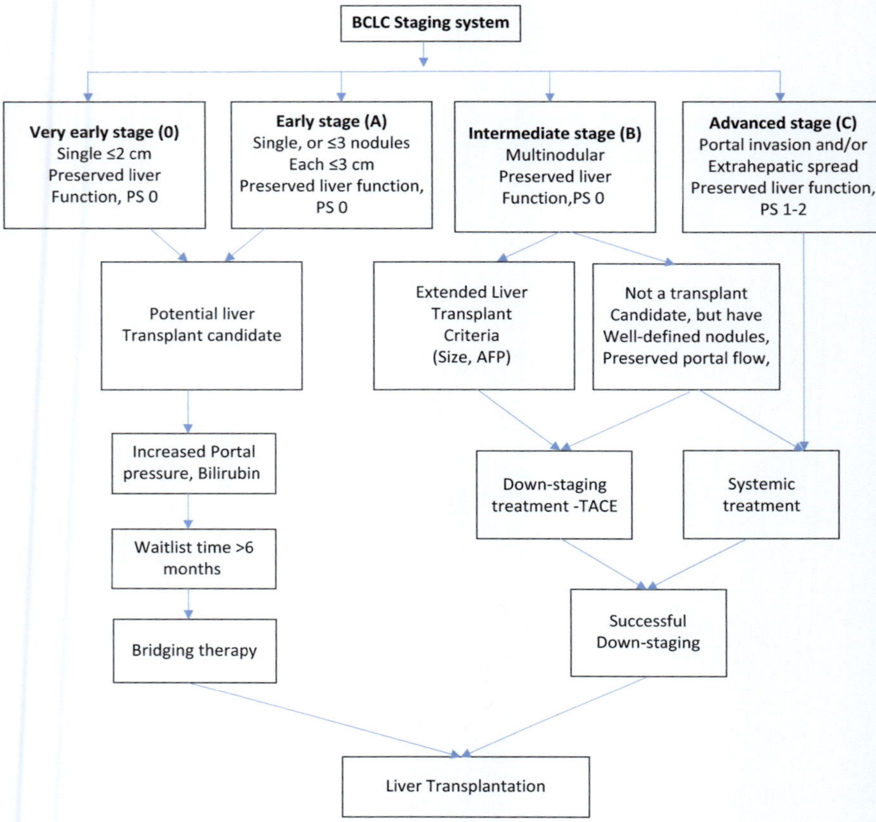

Fig. 11.1 Liver transplantation for HCC-Algorithmic approach

In summary, HCC and PVTT without extrahepatic disease should be considered locally advanced diseases; targeted radiotherapy can result in tumor thrombus resolution and thus help in successful down-staging within transplant criteria. LT 3–4 months later results in acceptable long-term outcomes, although the optimal period between successful down-staging and LT is still unclear. Thus, in selective cases of segmental PVTT with low biological aggressiveness (e.g., low AFP level), LT offers better disease free survival (DFS) and OS than palliative approaches, though still well below the 70% benchmarks achieved for non-malignant LT indications or patients with HCC within the extended criteria. So, whether to accept a graft for a patient with PVTT must be a center-specific decision in the context of organ shortages in DDLT or double equipoise for LDLT [33].

11.9 Management of Recurrent HCC After Liver Transplant

HCC recurrence patterns after LT: Post-transplant HCC recurrence is a significant negative predictor of survival. HCC recurs in about 6–18% of LT recipients. HCC recurrence usually occurs as early as 13 months after LT. Early HCC recurrence could be due to non-detected extrahepatic metastases or circulating HCC clones engrafting and growing in a target organ after LT. Although rare, late recurrence more than 2 years after LT could be due to a second unknown hit during the post-LT period. The pattern of HCC recurrence extends from hepatic to extrahepatic and from single-site to multiple-site. The most common extrahepatic sites are the lungs and bones, followed by the adrenal glands, biopsy tracks, peritoneum, and brain.

Post-LT surveillance for recurrent HCC: There are no standard guidelines for post-LT HCC surveillance. In general, cross-sectional imaging with either multiphase CT or MRI should be performed at least every 6 months for at least 2–3 years post-transplant. Many programs continue surveillance for 5 years based on the likelihood of recurrence. AFP level should be checked every 6 months for 5 years. Imaging for lung metastases with non-contrast CT chest should also be performed every 6 months. Bone metastases may also be a site of recurrence, but given the low sensitivity of bone scans, routine imaging with them is not recommended. Screening based on the RETREAT score could be considered for clinical use.

Immunosuppression management: Preclinical studies indicate mammalian targets of rapamycin inhibitors (mTORi) could control HCC recurrence due to their anti-proliferative and antiangiogenic effects. Reducing calcineurin inhibitors (initial target trough levels <10 ng/ml) and adding an mTOR inhibitor (sirolimus) may reduce HCC recurrence. Data from retrospective studies and two meta-analyses suggest that HCC recurrence was significantly lower in patients treated with mTOR (8%) compared to those using calcineurin inhibitors (CNIs; 3.8%) [34]. Everolimus lacks robust evidence supporting its efficacy in reducing HCC recurrence. Its usage is often weighed against potential risks like hepatic artery thrombosis and impaired wound healing.

Adjuvant systemic therapy: There is no evidence to support the use of adjuvant systemic chemotherapy to prevent post-LT HCC recurrence. Pre-emptive adjuvant therapy with sorafenib likely has minimal added benefit. Immune checkpoint inhibitors in this setting remain an active area of research [35].

Treatment of recurrent HCC after liver transplantation: Recurrent HCC after LT has poor overall survival. Early and multifocal recurrence after LT ($\leq$ 6 months) is associated with worsened survival. After recurrence, the recommendations for patient management do not differ from those applied before transplant. In carefully selected patients, resection of isolated extrahepatic recurrent disease has been shown to have favorable survival outcomes. More recently, liver-directed therapy ablation, trans-arterial chemoembolization, and stereotactic body radiation have been explored in patients with recurrence. Treatment with sorafenib has been studied in combination with an mTOR. However, the role of other kinase inhibitors like lenvatinib, regorafenib, or cabozantinib in the post-LT setting has to be determined.

In the Mayo Clinic experience of PD-1 inhibitor therapy in seven liver transplant recipients, rejection was observed in 2, with a median time to rejection of 24 days after initiation of therapy [36]. Several reports have detailed successful treatment of graft rejection with steroids, mycophenolate mofetil, and anti-thymocyte globulin. Overall, post-LT use of ICIs seems riskier than pre-LT use, and the response rates are lower than those seen in non-transplant patients.

Salvage liver transplantation: Hepatectomy for early-stage HCC in patients without significant fibrosis offers 5-year survival rates of 60%. However, in patients with compensated cirrhosis, the recommendations for resection versus LT are mixed, leading to the ongoing debate. For patients undergoing resection, the strategy of salvage LT (SLT) is recommended only as a second-line treatment for tumor recurrence or post-resection or ablation liver failure [37].

11.10 Conclusions

Liver transplantation for HCC has significantly advanced over the last 30 years, and the future is a rapidly evolving field with many opportunities for innovation and improvement. Selection criteria of HCC patients for LT is expanding with the availability of effective down staging modalities using loco regional therapy and immunotherapy. As we continue to explore these possibilities, it is essential to maintain a patient-centered and multidisciplinary approach.

Conflict of Interest Nothing to report.

Financial Support and Sponsorship None.

Author's Contributions DA, Data acquisition, initial draft, revision, and editing.

SS, Conception, manuscript design, final approval.
AK, editing & proofreading, revisions.
JW, revision, and editing.

References

1. Mazzaferro V, Regalia E, Doci R, et al. Liver transplantation for the treatment of small hepatocellular carcinomas in patients with cirrhosis. N Engl J Med. 1996;334(11):693–9. https://doi.org/10.1056/NEJM199603143341104.
2. Yao FY, Bass NM, Nikolai B, et al. Liver transplantation for hepatocellular carcinoma: analysis of survival according to the intention-to-treat principle and dropout from the waiting list. Liver Transpl. 2002;8(10):873–83. https://doi.org/10.1053/jlts.2002.34923.
3. Mehta N, Dodge JL, Grab JD, Yao FY. National experience on down-staging hepatocellular carcinoma before liver transplant: influence of tumor burden, alpha-fetoprotein, and wait time. Hepatol Baltim Md. 2020;71(3):943–54. https://doi.org/10.1002/hep.30879.

4. Reig M, Forner A, Rimola J, et al. BCLC strategy for prognosis prediction and treatment recommendation: the 2022 update. J Hepatol. 2022;76(3):681–93. https://doi.org/10.1016/j.jhep.2021.11.018.
5. Mazzaferro V, Llovet JM, Miceli R, et al. Predicting survival after liver transplantation in patients with hepatocellular carcinoma beyond the Milan criteria: a retrospective, exploratory analysis. Lancet Oncol. 2009;10(1):35–43. https://doi.org/10.1016/S1470-2045(08)70284-5.
6. Tan DJH, Lim WH, Yong JN, et al. UNOS Down-staging criteria for liver transplantation of hepatocellular carcinoma: systematic review and meta-analysis of 25 studies. Clin Gastroenterol Hepatol. 2023;21(6):1475–84. https://doi.org/10.1016/j.cgh.2022.02.018.
7. Halazun KJ, Rosenblatt RE, Mehta N, et al. Dynamic α-fetoprotein response and outcomes after liver transplant for hepatocellular carcinoma. JAMA Surg. 2021;156(6):559–67. https://doi.org/10.1001/jamasurg.2021.0954.
8. Ye Q, Ling S, Zheng S, Xu X. Liquid biopsy in hepatocellular carcinoma: circulating tumor cells and circulating tumor DNA. Mol Cancer. 2019;18(1):114. https://doi.org/10.1186/s12943-019-1043-x.
9. Kim SJ, Kim JM. Prediction models of hepatocellular carcinoma recurrence after liver transplantation: a comprehensive review. Clin Mol Hepatol. 2022;28(4):739–53. https://doi.org/10.3350/cmh.2022.0060.
10. Mazzaferro V, Bhoori S, Sposito C, et al. Milan criteria in liver transplantation for hepatocellular carcinoma: an evidence-based analysis of 15 years of experience. Liver Transpl. 2011;17(Suppl 2):S44–57. https://doi.org/10.1002/lt.22365.
11. Duvoux C, Roudot-Thoraval F, Decaens T, et al. Liver transplantation for hepatocellular carcinoma: a model including α-fetoprotein improves the performance of Milan criteria. Gastroenterology. 2012;143(4):986–994.e3.; quiz e14–15. https://doi.org/10.1053/j.gastro.2012.05.052.
12. Yao FY, Ferrell L, Bass NM, et al. Liver transplantation for hepatocellular carcinoma: expansion of the tumor size limits does not adversely impact survival. Hepatology. 2001;33(6):1394–1403. https://doi.org/10.1053/jhep.2001.24563.
13. Mazzaferro V, Sposito C, Zhou J, et al. Metroticket 2.0 model for analysis of competing risks of death after liver transplantation for hepatocellular carcinoma. Gastroenterology. 2018;154(1):128–39. https://doi.org/10.1053/j.gastro.2017.09.025.
14. DuBay D, Sandroussi C, Sandhu L, et al. Liver transplantation for advanced hepatocellular carcinoma using poor tumor differentiation on biopsy as an exclusion criterion. Ann Surg. 2011;253(1):166–72. https://doi.org/10.1097/sla.0b013e31820508f1.
15. Yao FY, Mehta N, Flemming J, et al. Downstaging of hepatocellular cancer before liver transplant: long-term outcome compared to tumors within Milan criteria. Hepatology. 2015;61(6):1968–77. https://doi.org/10.1002/hep.27752.
16. Mehta N, Heimbach J, Harnois DM, et al. Validation of a risk estimation of tumor recurrence after transplant (RETREAT) score for hepatocellular carcinoma recurrence after liver transplant. JAMA Oncol. 2017;3(4):493–500. https://doi.org/10.1001/jamaoncol.2016.5116.
17. Halazun KJ, Najjar M, Abdelmessih RM, et al. Recurrence after liver transplantation for hepatocellular carcinoma: a new MORAL to the story. Ann Surg. 2017;265(3):557–64. https://doi.org/10.1097/SLA.0000000000001966.
18. Arvind A, Seif El Dahan K, Malhotra R, et al. Association between bridging therapy and posttransplant outcomes in patients with HCC within Milan criteria: a systematic review and meta-analysis. Liver Transpl. 2024;5 https://doi.org/10.1097/LVT.0000000000000357.
19. Sinha J, Mehta N, Dodge JL, Poltavskiy E, Roberts J, Yao F. Are there upper limits in tumor burden for down-staging of hepatocellular carcinoma to liver transplant? Analysis of the all-comers protocol. Hepatol Baltim Md. 2019;70(4):1185–96. https://doi.org/10.1002/hep.30570.
20. Lai Q, Avolio AW, Graziadei I, et al. Alpha-fetoprotein and modified response evaluation criteria in solid tumors progression after locoregional therapy as predictors of hepatocellular cancer recurrence and death after transplantation. Liver Transpl. 2013;19(10):1108–18. https://doi.org/10.1002/lt.23706.

21. Lai Q, Nicolini D, Inostroza Nunez M, et al. A novel prognostic index in patients with hepatocellular cancer waiting for liver transplantation: time-radiological-response-alpha-fetoprotein--INflammation (TRAIN) score. Ann Surg. 2016;264(5):787–96. https://doi.org/10.1097/SLA.0000000000001881.
22. Nordness MF, Hamel S, Godfrey CM, et al. Fatal hepatic necrosis after nivolumab as a bridge to liver transplant for HCC: are checkpoint inhibitors safe for the pretransplant patient? Am J Transpl. 2020;20(3):879–83. https://doi.org/10.1111/ajt.15617.
23. Chen GH, Wang GB, Huang F, et al. Pretransplant use of toripalimab for hepatocellular carcinoma resulting in fatal acute hepatic necrosis in the immediate postoperative period. Transpl Immunol. 2021;66:101386. https://doi.org/10.1016/j.trim.2021.101386.
24. Tabrizian P, Florman SS, Schwartz ME. PD-1 inhibitor as bridge therapy to liver transplantation? Am J Transpl. 2021;21(5):1979–80. https://doi.org/10.1111/ajt.16448.
25. Liu H, Sethi V, Li X, Xiao Y, Humar A. Liver transplantation for hepatocellular carcinoma: a narrative review and a glimpse into the future. Semin Liver Dis. 2024;44(1):79–98. https://doi.org/10.1055/a-2242-7543.
26. Schmiderer A, Zoller H, Niederreiter M, et al. Liver transplantation after successful downstaging of a locally advanced hepatocellular carcinoma with systemic therapy. Dig Dis Basel Switz. 2023;41(4):641–4. https://doi.org/10.1159/000529023.
27. Shimamura T, Akamatsu N, Fujiyoshi M, et al. Expanded living-donor liver transplantation criteria for patients with hepatocellular carcinoma based on the Japanese nationwide survey: the 5-5-500 rule—a retrospective study. Transpl Int. 2019;32(4):356–68. https://doi.org/10.1111/tri.13391.
28. Lee SG, Hwang S, Moon DB, et al. Expanded indication criteria of living donor liver transplantation for hepatocellular carcinoma at one large-volume center. Liver Transpl. 2008;14(7):935–45. https://doi.org/10.1002/lt.21445.
29. Ito T, Takada Y, Ueda M, et al. Expansion of selection criteria for patients with hepatocellular carcinoma in living donor liver transplantation. Liver Transpl. 2007;13(12):1637–44. https://doi.org/10.1002/lt.21281.
30. Taketomi A, Sanefuji K, Soejima Y, et al. Impact of des-gamma-carboxy prothrombin and tumor size on the recurrence of hepatocellular carcinoma after living donor liver transplantation. Transplantation. 2009;87(4):531–7. https://doi.org/10.1097/TP.0b013e3181943bee.
31. Soin AS, Bhangui P, Kataria T, et al. Experience with LDLT in patients with hepatocellular carcinoma and portal vein tumor thrombosis Postdownstaging. Transplantation. 2020;104(11):2334–45. https://doi.org/10.1097/TP.0000000000003162.
32. Serenari M, Cappelli A, Cucchetti A, et al. Deceased donor liver transplantation after radioembolization for hepatocellular carcinoma and portal vein tumoral thrombosis: a pilot study. Liver Transpl. 2021;27(12):1758–66. https://doi.org/10.1002/lt.26257.
33. Soin A, Lesurtel M, Bhangui P, Cocchi L, Bouattour M, Clavien PA. Are patients with hepatocellular carcinoma and portal vein tumour thrombosis candidates for liver transplantation? J Hepatol. 2023;78(6):1124–9. https://doi.org/10.1016/j.jhep.2023.03.032.
34. Geissler EK, Schnitzbauer AA, Zülke C, et al. Sirolimus use in liver transplant recipients with hepatocellular carcinoma: a randomized, multicenter, open-label phase 3 trial. Transplantation. 2016;100(1):116–25. https://doi.org/10.1097/TP.0000000000000965.
35. Li PJ, Shah S. Mehta N. Recent Advances in Liver Transplantation for Hepatocellular Carcinoma. Curr. Treat. Options in Oncol. 2024;25:1153–62. https://doi.org/10.1007/s11864-024-01247-8.
36. DeLeon TT, Salomao MA, Aqel BA, et al. Pilot evaluation of PD-1 inhibition in metastatic cancer patients with a history of liver transplantation: the Mayo Clinic experience. J Gastrointest Oncol. 2018;9(6):1054–62. https://doi.org/10.21037/jgo.2018.07.05.
37. Guerrini GP, Esposito G, Olivieri T, et al. Salvage versus primary liver transplantation for hepatocellular carcinoma: a twenty-year experience meta-analysis. Cancer. 2022;14(14):3465. https://doi.org/10.3390/cancers14143465.
38. Sugawara Y, Tamura S, Makuuchi M. Living donor liver transplantation for hepatocellular carcinoma: Tokyo University series. Dig Dis. 2007;25(4):310–2. https://doi.org/10.1159/000106910. PMID: 17960065.

Chapter 12
Alcohol-Related Liver Disease

Ameet Mandot and Samir R. Shah

Abstract Alcohol is one of the most common causes of chronic liver disease and cirrhosis of the liver throughout the world. This chapter highlights the major points about epidemiology, natural history, risk factors, clinical features, diagnosis, and treatment of alcohol-related liver disease (ALD) with an emphasis on liver transplantation (LT). The spectrum of disease of ALD is varied. Patients can present with an asymptomatic rise in transaminases, compensated cirrhosis, decompensated cirrhosis, hepatocellular carcinoma, alcoholic hepatitis (AH), or acute-on-chronic liver failure (ACLF); the latter two conditions have a short and severe clinical course with high short-term mortality. This chapter also focuses on the management of ALD, with special focus on living donor liver transplantation (LDLT) and deceased donor liver transplantation (DDLT) in patients with severe alcoholic hepatitis, alcohol-related acute on chronic liver failure and decompensated ALD and their outcomes with regard to survival and post-transplant recidivism.

Keywords Alcoholic hepatitis · Acute-on-chronic liver failure · Liver transplantation in alcoholic hepatitis · Living donor liver transplantation in alcohol-related liver disease · Recidivism post-transplant

Key Highlights

- Alcohol use disorder (AUD) is the most common substance use disorder in the world and the commonest cause of cirrhosis in India, with a 98% male preponderance.

A. Mandot (✉)
Department of Hepatology and LICU, Gleneagles Hospital, Mumbai, India
e-mail: ameetmandot@yahoo.co.in

S. R. Shah
Institute of Liver, Intestine and Pancreas Sciences, Liver Disease Unit,
Nanavati Max Super Speciality Hospital, Mumbai, India

S. Saigal, D. Jothimani (eds.), *Fundamentals of Transplant Hepatology*,
https://doi.org/10.1007/978-981-95-2624-6_12

- Alcohol-related liver disease (ALD) comprises a wide spectrum of conditions that range from the early disease with steatosis or alcoholic steatohepatitis to more advanced stages, which include fibrosis, cirrhosis, and even hepatocellular carcinoma.
- Patients with severe alcoholic hepatitis (AH) have a short-term mortality of up to 30% at 28 days, while the fibrosis stage is the main predictor of long-term mortality in patients with ALD.
- Diagnosing ALD relies on a relevant alcohol drinking history, compatible clinical signs, abnormal laboratory tests, and the exclusion of other alternative causes of liver damage.
- Current guidelines for the management of patients with any form of ALD, including those with non-severe forms of AH, mainly advocate interventions directed at abstinence, nutritional support, and screening of infections.
- Severe alcoholic hepatitis may be treated with medical therapy, including steroids or an early liver transplantation (LT), while liver transplantation is the mainstay of treatment for decompensated cirrhosis of the liver with adequate abstinence.

12.1 Epidemiology

Alcohol use disorder (AUD) is the most prevalent substance use disorder globally, with over one million cases and an estimated 99 million disability-adjusted life years (DALYs) attributed to alcohol consumption in 2016 alone [1]. According to the World Health Organization (WHO), alcohol was responsible for approximately 5.3% of all global deaths—around three million deaths annually [2].

Alcohol is one of the leading causes of end-stage liver disease, with nearly half of cirrhosis-related mortality either directly or indirectly attributed to alcohol consumption [3]. In India, alcohol is the primary cause of cirrhosis, accounting for around 35% of cases, most commonly diagnosed in men between 36 and 56 years of age (98.4% being male) [4].

Approximately 35,000 deaths per year in India are due to alcohol-associated cirrhosis, making alcohol-related liver disease (ALD) one of the top two indications for liver transplantation (LT) [5].

A recent meta-analysis estimated the annual progression rate from alcoholic steatosis to cirrhosis at 3%, with a 6% mortality rate, and found that ALD is more prevalent in men than women [6]. According to a systematic review involving 7528 participants, alcoholic hepatitis (AH) progresses to cirrhosis at a rate of 10% per year, and those with fibrotic liver disease progress at a rate of 8% annually.

Mortality in alcoholic hepatitis ranges from 5% to 15% per year, with the highest rates observed in severe cases [7]. A Global Burden of Disease (2017) analysis estimated the global prevalence of ALD at 23.6 million, with 2.46 million cases of cirrhosis (both compensated and decompensated) [8].

Population studies suggest that the risk of liver disease significantly increases when men consume 40–80 g/day and women 20–40 g/day of alcohol over 10–12 years [9].

12.2 Natural History of Alcohol-Related Liver Disease

ALD encompasses a spectrum of liver conditions that range from early-stage disease, such as steatosis and alcoholic steatohepatitis (ASH), to more advanced stages, including fibrosis, cirrhosis, and hepatocellular carcinoma (HCC).

Patients with ongoing alcohol consumption may experience alcohol-associated hepatitis (AH)—an acute-on-chronic liver injury with a poor prognosis [10]. Roughly 90% of chronic heavy drinkers develop hepatic steatosis, which may reverse with abstinence. However, 20–40% of these individuals progress to inflammatory liver disease and fibrosis, and 10–20% of those with steatohepatitis go on to develop alcoholic cirrhosis, a condition associated with significant morbidity and mortality [10–12].

AH, the most severe manifestation of ALD, is marked by the rapid onset of jaundice and liver decompensation, with histological findings including neutrophilic infiltration and hepatocellular ballooning [13].

- Severe AH carries a 28-day mortality of up to 30% and over 50% mortality at one year [14].
- Even moderate AH presents a significant risk, with short- to mid-term mortality of 3–7% and one-year mortality of 13–20% [15].

  Hepatocellular carcinoma in alcoholic cirrhosis occurs less frequently than in cirrhosis from viral hepatitis or non-alcoholic fatty liver disease (NAFLD), but when it does occur, it is often diagnosed at a later stage, resulting in poorer survival outcomes [16, 17]. The annual incidence of HCC in ALD is estimated at 2.9% [18].

  Among all stages of ALD, fibrosis severity is the strongest predictor of long-term mortality. One study showed 45% mortality in patients with advanced fibrosis (F3–F4) versus 0% in those with minimal fibrosis (F0–F2) (*P* < 0.001) [19].

Alcohol withdrawal has also emerged as a significant prognostic factor and is associated with worse outcomes across all stages of ALD [20, 21]. Within 5 years, up to 30% of individuals with advanced fibrosis develop liver-related complications [22] (Figs. 12.1 and 12.2).

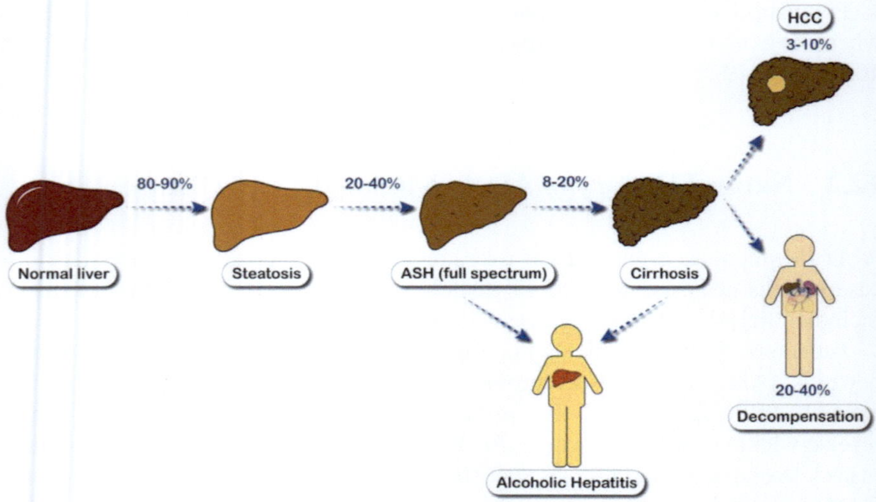

Fig. 12.1 Natural history of alcoholic-related liver disease. Abbreviations: *ASH* alcoholic steatohepatitis, *HCC* hepatocellular carcinoma

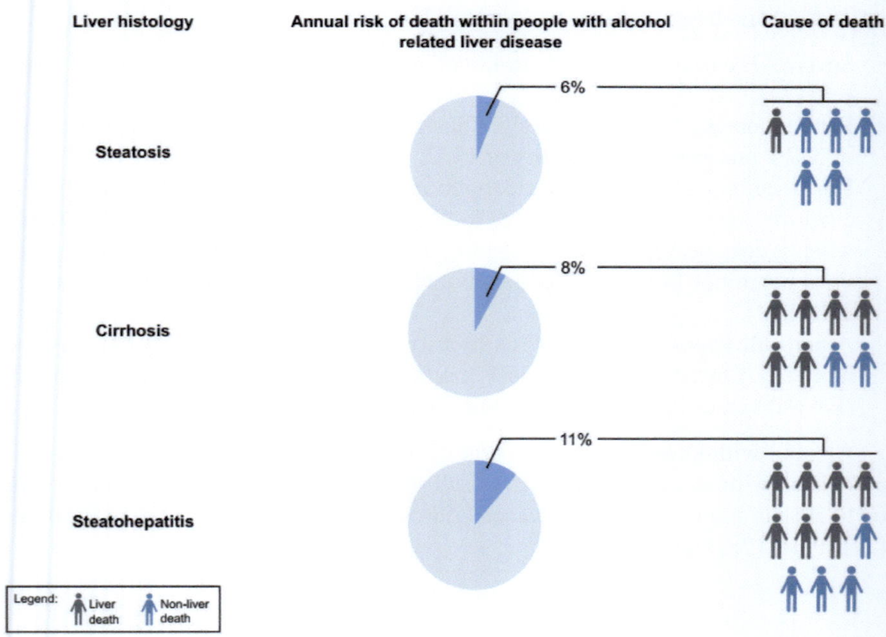

Fig. 12.2 Mortality correlation with stages of ALD

12.3 The Spectrum of Alcohol-Related Liver Diseases

The spectrum of liver diseases associated with AUD ranges from simple steatosis to steatohepatitis, fibrosis, cirrhosis, and cancer [23]. The International Classification of Diseases (ICD-10) recognizes multiple stages of progressive liver damage, including steatosis, steatohepatitis, and early fibrosis, as being considered reversible, while late stages, constituting cirrhosis and liver failure, and cancer, are considered severe and irreversible [24]. Patients with compensated or decompensated cirrhosis of the liver due to alcohol may present with acute-on-chronic liver failure (ACLF), characterized by accelerated worsening of clinical condition associated with high short-term mortality. Lastly, patients with ALD may present with hepatocellular carcinoma, as evidenced by worsening of existing cirrhosis features and imaging studies.

12.4 Risk Factors for ALD

Alcohol consumption has been identified as the most significant risk factor for the development of ALD [25]. However, the individual variability plays a crucial role in the development of cirrhosis, as it happens only in 10–20% of chronic drinkers.

Factors that increase the risk and severity of alcoholic liver disease:

1. Amount of daily alcohol intake
2. Duration of heavy alcohol consumption
3. Female gender
4. Chronic hepatitis C infection
5. Genetic hemochromatosis
6. Genetic factors

- PNPLA3 I148M variant
- TM6SF2 E167K variant
- MBOAT7 rs641738
- C2 allele of cytochrome P4502E1
- Manganese superoxide dismutase valine to alanine variant
- 159 C > T of the promoter for CD14 endotoxin binding receptor
- 167 C > A of cytokine IL10
- 238 G > A in the promoter for TNF-α

12.5 Clinical Features of Alcohol-Related Liver Disease

Early-stage ALD is often identified through laboratory testing or imaging, though physical examination can also offer important clues. In the early stages, patients may present with signs of chronic alcohol use, such as:

- Bilateral parotid or lacrimal gland enlargement
- Muscle wasting
- Malnutrition
- Dupuytren's contracture
- Peripheral neuropathy [26, 27]

As ALD advances to cirrhosis, additional physical signs may appear. Although these findings are not specific to ALD, they include:

- Ascites
- Peripheral edema
- Cognitive dysfunction linked to hepatic encephalopathy
- Visible abdominal collateral veins

Features like gynecomastia and pronounced spider angiomas are more frequently seen in alcohol-related cirrhosis.

In some patients with ongoing heavy drinking, alcoholic hepatitis (AH) may occur. This condition presents acutely with:

- Rapid-onset jaundice
- Fatigue
- Anorexia and weight loss
- Fever
- Right upper quadrant pain from tender hepatomegaly

Most patients with AH already have underlying cirrhosis [28] and may show signs of hepatic decompensation such as:

- Ascites
- Hepatic encephalopathy
- Portal hypertensive bleeding
- Infections

Kidney dysfunction is common in AH and is associated with a worse prognosis [29–32].

12.6 Diagnosis of ALD

Diagnosing ALD involves evaluating a history of alcohol consumption, clinical features, abnormal blood tests, and ruling out other causes of liver injury [33].

12.6.1 Blood-Based Tests

- Gamma-glutamyl transferase (GGT) may be mildly elevated and can indicate hepatic steatosis, often seen after 3–7 days of heavy drinking.
- AST levels are typically elevated 2–6 times the normal range but usually remain under 300–400 IU/L.
- A hallmark of ALD is an AST:ALT ratio > 1 [34].
- Indicators of advanced disease include increased international normalised ratio (INR), high bilirubin, low albumin, and thrombocytopenia.

12.6.2 Fibrosis Biomarkers

Several commercially available blood tests—originally designed for chronic hepatitis C—are also useful in ALD, such as:

- FibroTest
- Fibrometer
- HepaScore

These tests generally offer better diagnostic accuracy than simpler scores like:

- APRI (AST-to-platelet ratio index)
- Forns Index
- FIB-4 [13]

12.6.3 Liver Stiffness Assessment

Transient elastography (TE) is now the most widely used non-invasive tool for assessing liver stiffness and fibrosis. Modern portable devices make point-of-care screening feasible in most clinical settings.

- TE is cost-effective and particularly valuable in primary care for evaluating alcoholic and non-alcoholic liver disease [35].
- Liver stiffness measurements (LSM) strongly correlate with the fibrosis stage.

- Values ≥12–15 kPa suggest advanced fibrosis, provided false positives are ruled out.

  Factors that can falsely elevate TE results include:

- Recent alcohol intake
- Elevated AST (>2x normal)
- Inadequate fasting
- Presence of cholestasis [36–38]

12.6.4 Imaging Techniques

Common imaging modalities include:

- Ultrasound
- Contrast-enhanced CT
- MRI

  These are used to:

- Confirm signs of cirrhosis
- Detect portal hypertension and HCC
- Exclude other causes like biliary obstruction or vascular thrombosis

12.6.4.1 Histology

ALD's histological features vary, largely dependent on the extent and stage of liver injury. Even if they are characteristic, they are not pathognomonic of ALD (Table 12.1 and Fig. 12.3).

Table 12.1 Histological stages of ALD

Stage of ALD	Histological finding
Alcoholic steatosis	Macrovesicular and centrilobular steatosis
Alcoholic Steatohepatitis	Steatosis, hepatocellular damage (characterized by ballooned hepatocytes containing cytoplasmic hyaline inclusions called Mallory-Denk bodies), neutrophilic inflammatory infiltrates, and variable degrees of fibrosis
Alcoholic hepatitis	Above-mentioned changes with superimposed intraparenchymal cholestasis, foamy degeneration in hepatocytes, the presence of megamitochondria, and acute sclerosing hyaline necrosis [39]
Alcoholic cirrhosis	Grading as per salve system for histopathology (SALVE) fibrosis score [40]

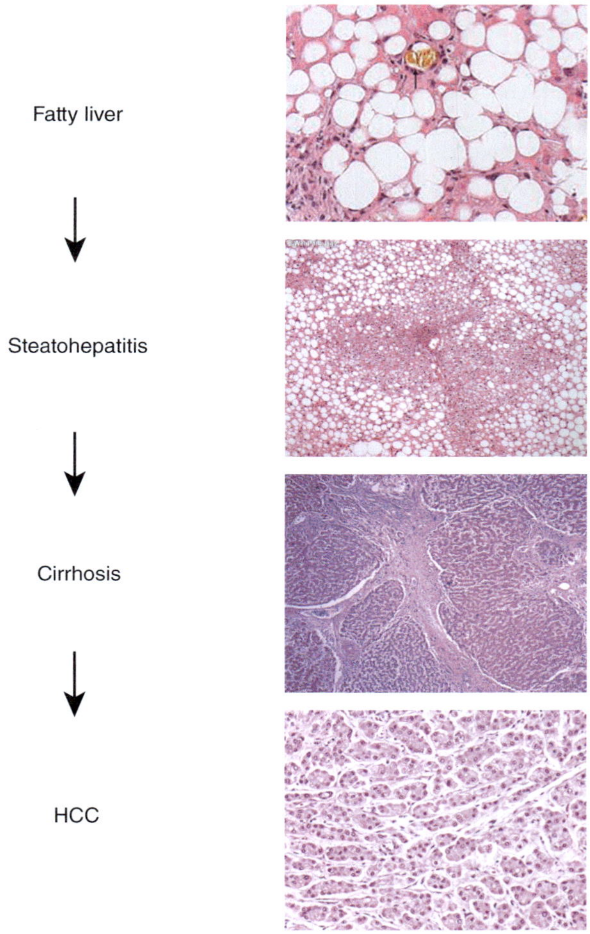

Fig. 12.3 Histologic spectrum of alcohol-associated liver disease

12.7 Treatment of Alcohol-Related Liver Disease

Current clinical guidelines recommend that treatment for all stages of ALD—including mild forms of alcoholic hepatitis (AH)—should prioritize alcohol abstinence, nutritional support, and early specialist referral when indicated [41]. It is critical to manage both components of the illness: the alcohol use disorder (AUD), defined as "a problematic pattern of alcohol use leading to clinically significant impairment or distress" [42], and the liver disease itself [43].

12.7.1 Alcohol Abstinence

Achieving complete abstinence is the cornerstone of ALD management. All patients should be screened for AUD, and if present, considered for behavioral interventions and/or pharmacologic therapy.

12.8 Nutritional Management in ALD

Malnutrition, sarcopenia, and frailty are highly prevalent in ALD, particularly in advanced cirrhosis, affecting 25–56% of cirrhotic patients and up to 90% in end-stage liver disease [44–46]. Sarcopenia (loss of muscle mass or strength) is associated with higher risks of sepsis, hepatic encephalopathy, hyperammonemia, and worse post-LT outcomes [47, 48].

Malnutrition stems from poor intake of macronutrients, influenced by:

- Anorexia, nausea, vomiting, early satiety
- Diet unpalatability (due to sodium/potassium restrictions)
- Mental status changes, hospital fasting, and catabolic stress [49–51]

12.8.1 Assessment of Sarcopenia

- CT-based analysis at the L3/L4 level (e.g., Psoas Muscle Index [PMI]) offers a reliable measure of muscle mass [47].
- Alternatively, Skeletal Muscle Index (SMI) is calculated as muscle area at L3 normalized by height, using Hounsfield unit ranges [52–54].

12.8.2 Nutritional Recommendations

1. Caloric intake: ≥35 kcal/kg/day (for non-obese individuals) [55]
2. Protein intake: 1.2–1.5 g/kg/day; use branched chain amino acids (BCAA) supplements if protein intolerance exists [56]
3. Vitamin & trace element supplementation, especially B-complex vitamins [57–60]
4. Minimize fasting: Frequent small meals, late evening snacks
5. Relax the sodium restriction if it improves intake
6. For obese patients, target 5–10% weight loss with individualized support [61, 62]
7. Diverse protein sources, including dairy and plant-based proteins
8. Aerobic and resistance exercises tailored to the patient's condition

9. Consider testosterone therapy in ALD patients with low levels and no HCC/malignancy/thrombosis—shown to increase muscle mass and improve metabolic parameters [63]
10. Thiamine for Wernicke's encephalopathy:
    - IV 200–500 mg three times a day (TID) for 2–7 days, then 250 mg daily for 3–5 days, taper to 100 mg/day
    - Prophylactic dose: 100–200 mg daily for 3–5 days via IV, IM, or oral [64]

12.8.3 Cirrhosis and Fibrosis Management

- ALD-related cirrhosis is treated similarly to cirrhosis of other etiologies
- Evaluate for compensated vs. decompensated disease
- Test for hepatitis b virus (HBV), hepatitis c virus (HCV), and HIV and consider HBV vaccination if appropriate [65]

Standard practices include:

- Ascites: Paracentesis, sodium restriction, diuretics, SBP screening
- Varices: Endoscopy for prophylactic banding or beta-blockers
- Encephalopathy: Lactulose ± rifaximin
- HCC surveillance: Ultrasound or MRI every 6 months
- Standard prophylaxis for other cirrhosis complications (e.g., SBP, variceal bleeding, HRS) [65]

12.9 Management of Alcoholic Hepatitis (AH)

12.9.1 Diagnostic Criteria National Institute on Alcohol Abuse and Alcoholism (NIAAA) [66]

1. Active alcohol use: >2 drinks/day (women), >3 (men) for >6 months
2. Last drink within 60 days of jaundice onset
3. AST/ALT >50 IU/L but <400 IU/L, with AST:ALT >1.5
4. Sudden onset of jaundice (bilirubin >3 mg/dL)
5. Exclusion of other liver diseases

12.9.2 Assessment of Severity

Maddrey's Discriminant Function (MDF):

- Formula: DF = (4.6 × PT prolongation in seconds) + bilirubin
- Score > 32 = high risk for short term mortality (35% 1-month mortality)

- Model for end stage liver disease (MELD) score: Superior to MDF in prognosis
- AH is severe when MELD ≥20 or associated with encephalopathy
- Mild AH (MELD <20): Managed with abstinence, nutrition, thiamine, and infection monitoring

12.10 Corticosteroid Therapy in AH

- Indicated in AH with MELD ≥20 or MDF ≥32 [67]
- MELD increase ≥2 within 1 week signals poor prognosis and possible ACLF [68, 69]

Evidence from the steroids or pentoxifylline for alcoholic hepatitis (STOPAH) Trial [70, 71]:

- 1103 patients: Prednisolone reduced 28-day mortality (14%) vs. placebo (17%)
- Odds Ratio (OR): 0.72 (CI: 0.52–1.01; $P = 0.06$)
- No mortality difference at 90 days or 1 year
- Infections: 13% on steroids vs 7% on placebo

Treatment Protocol [72, 73]:

- Prednisolone 40 mg/day orally for 28 days
- IV methylprednisolone 32 mg/day if the oral route is not feasible
- Lille Model at Day 7:
  - ≥0.45: Poor response, 6-month survival ~25%
  - <0.45: Good response, 6-month survival ~85% [74]
  - Taper over 16 days if continuing beyond 28 days

Contraindications to Steroids [75–77]:

- Active uncontrolled infections
- Ongoing GI bleeding
- Concurrent HCV infection

12.11 Infection Prevention in AH

Factors contributing to infection risk post-steroid include:

- Older age, impaired liver/kidney function, SIRS, lack of bilirubin improvement [29, 78]
- Bacterial translocation due to gut permeability and endotoxemia from lipopolysaccharide (LPS) is proinflammatory [79, 80]

Management tips:

- Investigate fever, altered mental status, or hemodynamic instability with blood/urine cultures
- Procalcitonin ≥0.45 ng/mL is a useful marker [81]
- Avoid prolonged catheter use
- Consider prophylactic antibiotics in high-risk cases [82–84]

12.12 Pentoxifylline (PTX)

PTX, a TNF-α inhibitor, has been studied in AH, but current data do not support its routine use. Its efficacy in reducing mortality remains unclear, so it is a weakly recommended option [85].

12.12.1 When to Biopsy

Clinical criteria proposed by the NIAAA are useful for the diagnosis; however, they may be inaccurate in up to 46% of cases [86]. The main confounders in patients with diagnostic uncertainty of AH are the presence of factors such as ischemic hepatitis, possible drug-induced liver injury, positive serology for another liver disease etiology, or uncertain alcohol use. Liver biopsy may be required when the diagnosis is uncertain, especially if confounding factors are in place [87]. The transjugular approach enables the measurement of portal pressure, which may also be helpful in estimating short-term prognosis, as the degree of portal hypertension and hyperdynamic circulation relates to AH severity. Liver biopsy may also predict the disease severity and prognosis based on bilirubinostasis, fibrosis, neutrophilic infiltration, and the presence of megamitochondria [88] (Fig. 12.4).

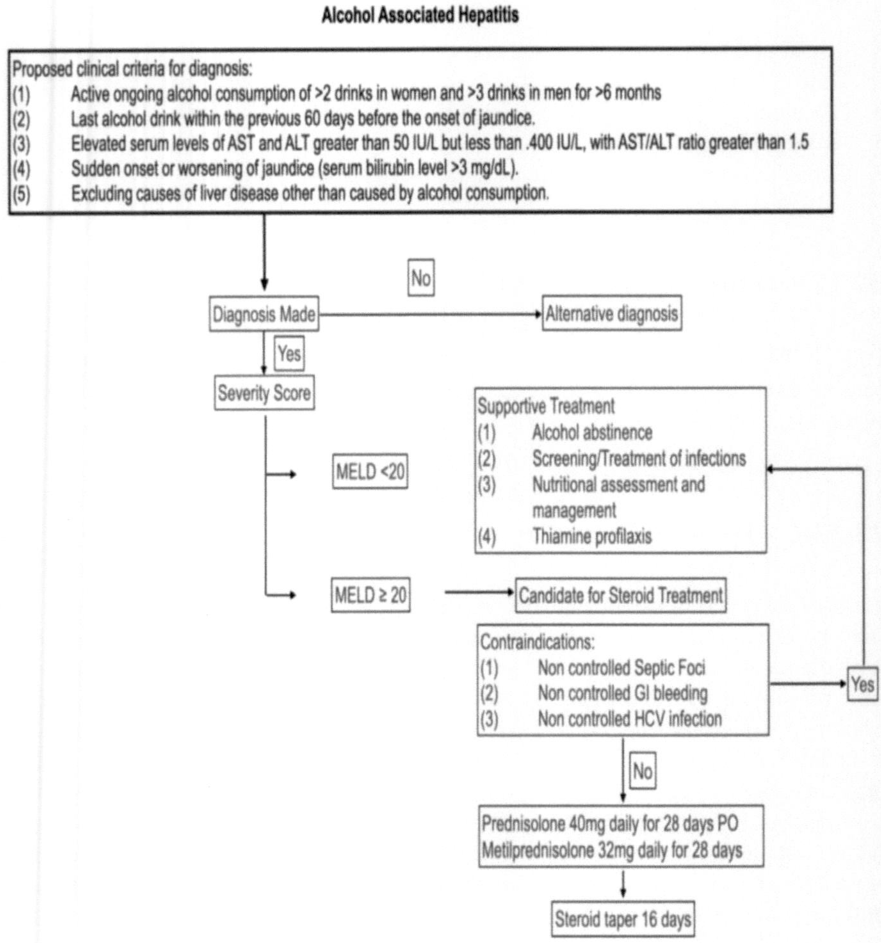

Fig. 12.4 Treatment of alcoholic hepatitis

12.13 Severe Alcoholic Hepatitis and Liver Transplant

Early liver transplant is the definitive and only treatment option that increases survival and improves short- and long-term mortality in patients with severe alcoholic hepatitis, defined as MELD score of ≥20, MDF score of ≥32 on admission, and a non-response to steroid therapy (Lille score of ≥0.45 on day 7).

Early LT was first evaluated in a French–Belgian case–control study by Mathurin et al. [89]. In this study, certain patients were selected based on the following criteria: an absence of comorbidities or psychiatric disorders, no history of underlying cirrhosis, strong family support, and the patient's commitment to lifelong total abstinence from alcohol. Survival at 6 months was significantly higher in early transplanted patients (77 ± 8%) than in patients who did not receive a liver transplant (23 ± 8%). This benefit to survival persisted for 2 years after LT: 71 ± 9% and 23 ± 8% in transplanted and non-transplanted patients, respectively. Two years after LT, 12% of early transplanted patients had alcohol relapse, which was considered to be acceptable when compared with the rate observed after LT in ALD patients who had achieved at least 6 months of sobriety [90, 91]. In a replicative study performed by Im et al. in 2016, higher survival of early transplanted patients compared to non-transplanted matched controls (89% vs. 11%) with an acceptable risk of relapse (25%) was demonstrated [92]. Several other prospective and retrospective studies, including those by Lee et al., Weeks et al., Louvet et al., and Germani et al., have demonstrated similar survival rates in these patients with acceptable relapse rates [93–96].

In the years since these studies, many transplant centers across the world, including united network for organ sharing (UNOS), the UK, France, and Latin America, have relaxed the criteria of 6-month abstinence in patients with severe alcoholic hepatitis with a caveat that patient screening should be stringent and screening for post-transplant relapse should be vigilant.

In the last decade, early transplantation, using a restrictive selection process, has found its place in the therapeutic arsenal for patients with severe alcoholic hepatitis. Early transplantation has gained the support of a growing number of experts from various countries, as evidenced by the recommendations from the European, American, and Latin American regions [97]. A selection approach based on the use of a dedicated score incorporating social and addiction parameters could be interesting and is currently under investigation in a prospective controlled trial (NCT01756794), which is being conducted by the Lille Team (Fig. 12.5).

12.13.1 *Management of Acute-on-Chronic Liver Failure (ACLF) in ALD*

Management of ACLF centers around identifying and treating the precipitating event and providing supportive care for failing organs. Since infections are among the most frequent triggers, broad-spectrum antibiotics should be initiated promptly. Empirical antifungal therapy is reserved for patients—excluding those with pneumonia—who present with septic shock and have known risk factors for invasive fungal infections. Treatment should be tailored to culture results as soon as available [98].

Supportive interventions include:

- Endoscopic variceal ligation and vasopressors for variceal bleeding
- Volume resuscitation (with crystalloids and albumin) and vasoconstrictors like terlipressin or norepinephrine for hypotension

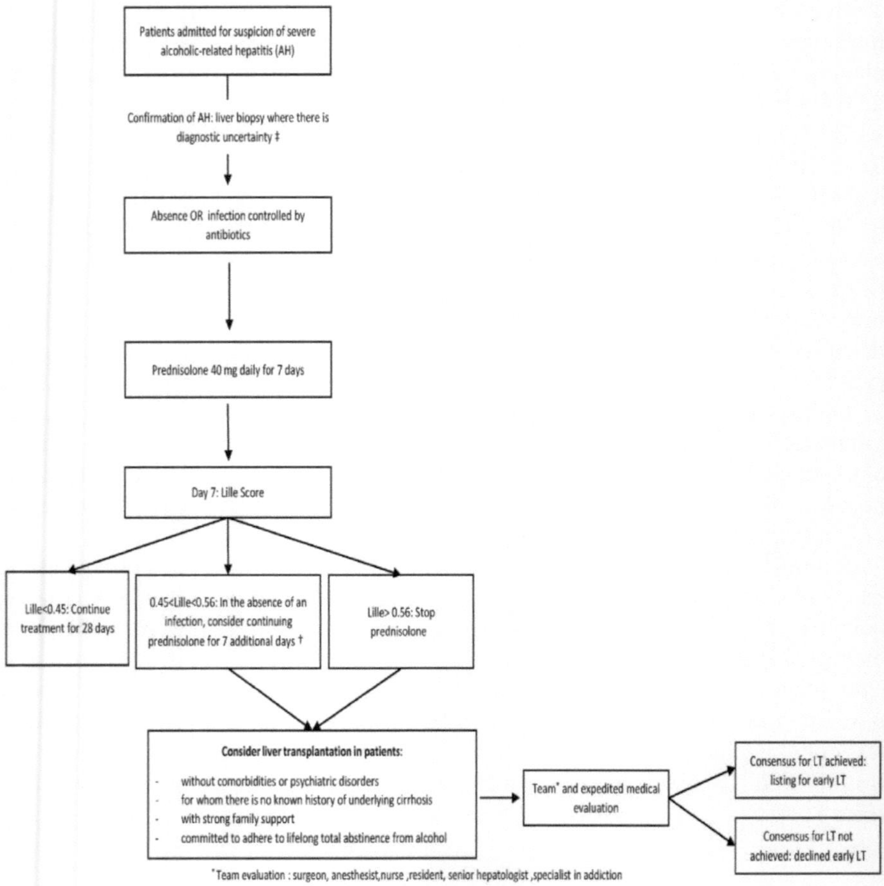

Fig. 12.5 LT in severe alcoholic hepatitis

- Oxygen therapy or mechanical ventilation for respiratory failure
- Renal replacement therapy (RRT) for acute kidney injury

Emerging therapies such as albumin dialysis (MARS), granulocyte colony-stimulating factor (G-CSF), and fecal microbiota transplantation are promising but not yet established as standard care.

Due to poor short-term survival, liver transplantation (LT) is frequently considered for ACLF but remains controversial. While severely ill patients may benefit significantly, LT in these cases may also impact organ allocation equity and result in suboptimal long-term outcomes in deceased donor LT (DDLT) settings [99]. Select studies have shown acceptable 1-year post-LT survival rates (75–84%) in ACLF, including ACLF grade 3 [100, 101].

However, timely psychosocial assessment (e.g., alcohol use patterns, social and family support) is often challenging due to limited timeframes and unstable patient conditions. There is a need for validated fast-track, multidisciplinary assessment models to minimize post-LT relapse.

12.13.2 Living Donor Liver Transplantation (LDLT) in AH and ACLF

LDLT offers a timely solution for critically ill patients with severe alcoholic hepatitis (AH) or ACLF, avoiding delays and waitlist mortality. Although controversial due to concerns about alcohol relapse and the absence of an abstinence period, studies show encouraging outcomes.

For instance, Choudhary et al. reported a relapse rate of only 12.8% among 39 patients with severe AH who received LDLT, likely attributed to strong family support and co-residing donors [102].

Similarly, LDLT in ACLF not responding to medical treatment after 5–10 days can be life-saving. A retrospective study by Yadav et al. showed comparable 1-year survival across ACLF grades (ACLF-1: 92.9%, ACLF-2: 85.4%, ACLF-3: 75.6%; *P* = 0.15), while 90-day survival without transplant in ACLF-3 was only 5.9% vs. 78% post-transplant (*P* < 0.001) [103].

Although consensus on the ideal timing of LT in ACLF is lacking, early intervention—before the onset of sepsis or multiorgan failure—is key [99]. LDLT, being elective, provides an opportunity to stabilize extrahepatic complications, crucial for successful outcomes [103].

12.13.3 Liver Transplantation in Decompensated Cirrhosis (Alcohol-Related)

Given the poor prognosis of decompensated cirrhosis, LT is recommended for patients with a MELD score > 17, particularly if they are abstinent [104]. Survival benefit is more pronounced at higher MELD scores.

While some patients show clinical improvement within 3–6 months after stopping alcohol—resulting in a MELD score reduction—this approach suits less critically ill patients [105, 106]. For others with advanced disease, prolonged observation is neither ethically nor clinically appropriate. Hence, the decision to list for LT should be based not only on the cause of decompensation but also on the anticipated survival benefit.

12.13.4 Addiction Assessment Before Liver Transplant in ALD

Traditionally, a 6-month sobriety period ("6-month rule") was required before considering LT, aimed at identifying those most likely to maintain abstinence [107, 108]. However, newer evidence questions the necessity of this rule.

In a cohort of 163 patients, early LT showed comparable outcomes to those with >6 months of abstinence:

- 1-year survival: 94.1% vs. 95.9%
- Relapse-free survival: 80.4% vs. 83.5%
- Graft survival: 92.7% vs. 90.5% (**P** > 0.4 for all) [109]

Accordingly, US and European guidelines no longer mandate a 6-month abstinence period [110]. Instead, risk factors for relapse—such as psychiatric illness, other substance use, and lack of family support—should be assessed carefully before listing a patient.

12.13.5 Somatic Evaluation Prior to LT in ALD

Given the multisystem effects of chronic alcohol use—ranging from neurological disorders and osteoporosis to malignancies and cardiovascular disease—a comprehensive medical evaluation is essential. Up to 50% of ALD patients are also active smokers, further increasing the risk for aerodigestive and lung cancers [111].

While no standard protocol exists, suggested investigations include:

- Head and neck cancer screening: Clinical exam, neck CT
- Upper GI endoscopy: To detect esophageal cancers
- Chest CT scan
- Cardiac and vascular imaging
- Brain CT/MRI: Especially in patients with hepatic encephalopathy, to exclude other causes [112]

Evaluation must be tailored to disease severity, as delaying LT for extensive work-up in unstable patients may increase mortality risk (Fig. 12.6).

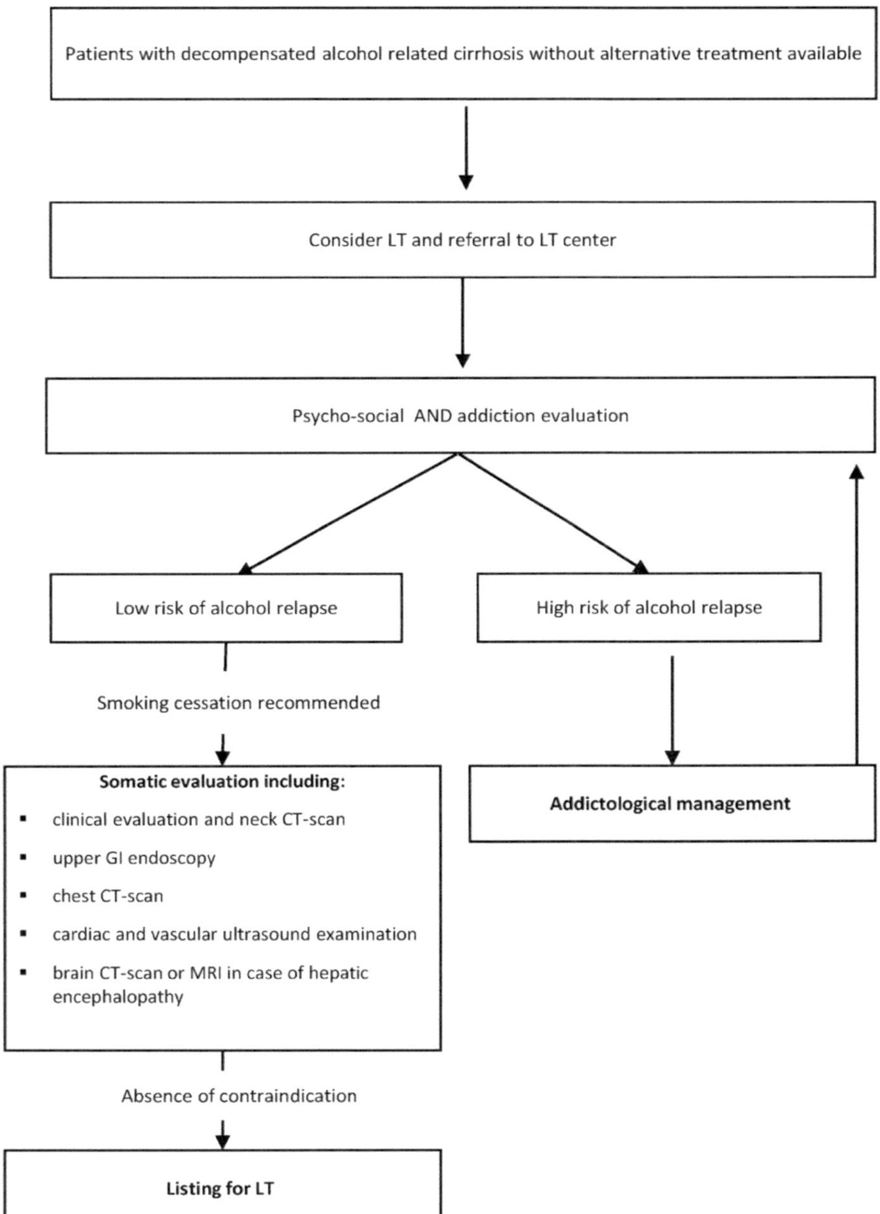

Fig. 12.6 LT in decompensated ALD

12.14 Outcomes of Liver Transplantation for ALD: From the Waiting List to the Period Following Liver Transplantation

Numerous studies have demonstrated that there is a higher probability of delisting from the transplant list of ALD patients due to improvement rather than death following abstinence. These rates are similar to those of patients with cirrhosis of the liver due to HCV, in whom significant improvement is seen following virus eradication due to directly acting antivirals (DAAs). Factors independently associated with delisting following an improvement were a lower MELD score, a higher platelet count, and being a woman. However, the length of abstinence was not statistically different on multivariate analysis ($P = 0.055$), confirming the need to discontinue the 6-month rule [106]. When patients with ALD have access to LT, post-transplant survival is good and has steadily improved in recent years. In fact, they are now at least as good or even better than those of other indications of LT (i.e., hepatocellular carcinoma [HCC] or decompensated HCV-related cirrhosis). The 1-, 5-, and 10-year survival rates are 85%, 74%, and 59%, respectively [110]. Despite these results, with the persistent organ shortage, the main barrier to access to LT for patients with ALD remains the risk of relapse after LT in many centers.

12.15 Alcohol Relapse After Liver Transplantation

In a recent review, Arab et al. propose a three-tier definition of relapse: occasional relapse (less than once per month), mild relapse (continuous drinking at daily and weekly doses within recommended standards of NIAAA, i.e., ≤4 drinks per day for men, ≤3 drinks per day for women, and ≤14 drinks per week for men and ≤7 drinks per week for women), and severe relapse (regular use above recommended standards of the NIAAA or with associated morbidity or mortality, which includes alcohol-related pancreatitis, acute AH, graft loss, or other medical problems directly associated with return to drinking) [113]. Various tools, such as the alcohol use disorders identification test (AUDIT) and AUDIT-C questionnaires, as well as the detection of ethyl glucuronide or phosphatidyl ethanol in blood and urine, can be used for the early detection of relapse [114]. The rate of relapse after LT ranges from 6% to 50% and can lead to graft failure, cirrhosis of the grafted liver, and an overall increase in morbidity and mortality. Therefore, early detection of relapse, psychiatric analysis, and help, along with robust social support, can be useful in the long-term survival of the liver graft and the patient.

12.16 Palliative Care

Unfortunately, some patients with decompensated cirrhosis who may be nonresponsive to therapy may benefit from palliative care (PC) and hospice interventions. PC should be considered for patients who are not candidates for LT; who have ACLF that is unresponsive to treatment, chronic multiorgan failure, or complications of cirrhosis (i.e., HRS, HE, variceal bleeding, or HCC) that are advanced; and who have not responded to or are unlikely to respond to treatment [115]. Therefore, it must be considered in cases where treatment is considered futile (i.e., when clinical reasoning or experience suggests that a life-sustaining treatment is highly unlikely to achieve its purpose) [116]. PC must focus on improving the quality of life for patients and their families through the prevention and relief of suffering. The goal is to neither hasten nor postpone death [116].

12.17 Conclusion

Alcohol use disorder is a major health care burden and is the most common cause of liver cirrhosis in India. Clinical spectrum of alcohol related liver disease can be heterogenous varying from simple steatosis to severe alcohol related hepatitis, ACLF and can lead to cirrhosis and HCC. Holistic approach such as nutritional therapy, abstinence, psychosocial support are integral part of clinical management of these patients. ALD is a major indication for liver transplantation, where appropriate patient selection is strongly recommended.

References

1. GBD 2016 Alcohol Collaborators. Alcohol use and burden for 195 countries and territories, 1990–2016: a systematic analysis for the Global Burden of Disease Study 2016. Lancet. 2018;392:1015–35.
2. Park SH, Kim DJ. Global and regional impacts of alcohol use on public health: emphasis on alcohol policies. Clin Mol Hepatol. 2020;26:652–61.
3. Asrani SK, Devarbhavi H, Eaton J, et al. Burden of liver diseases in the world. J Hepatol. 2019;70:151–71.
4. Mukherjee PS, Vishnubhatla S, Amarapurkar DN, Das K, Sood A, Chawla YK, et al. Etiology and mode of presentation of chronic liver diseases in India: a multi centric study. PLoS One. 2017;12(10):e0187033. https://doi.org/10.1371/journal.pone.0187033.
5. Han S, Yang Z, Zhang T, Ma J, Chandler K, Liangpunsakul S. Epidemiology of alcohol-associated liver disease. Clin Liver Dis. 2021;25:483–92.
6. SAMHSA (2016) National survey on drug use and health. Available from: https://www.samhsa.gov/data/sites/default/files/NSDUHFFR1-2016/NSDUH-FFR1-2016.pdf
7. Jinjuvadia R, Liangpunsakul S. Translational research and evolving alcoholic hepatitis treatment consortium. Trends in alcoholic hepatitis related hospitalizations, financial burden, and mortality in the United States. J Clin Gastroenterol. 2015;49:506–11.

8. Sepanlou SG, Safiri S, Bisignano C, et al. The global, regional, and national burden of cirrhosis by cause in 195 countries and territories, 1990 2017: systematic analysis for the Global Burden of Disease Study 2017. Lancet Gastroenterol Hepatol. 2020;5:245–66.
9. Becker U, Deis A, Sorensen T, et al. Prediction of risk of liver disease by alcohol intake, sex, and age: a prospective population study. Hepatology. 1996;23:1025–9.
10. Altamirano J, Bataller R. Alcoholic liver disease: pathogenesis and new targets for therapy. Nat Rev Gastroenterol Hepatol. 2011;8:491–501.
11. Adachi M, Brenner DA. Clinical syndromes of alcoholic liver disease. Dig Dis. 2005;23:255–63.
12. Hagstrom H, Thiele M, Roelstraete B, Soderling J, Ludvigsson JF. Mortality in biopsy-proven alcohol-related liver disease: a population-based nationwide cohort study of 3453 patients. Gut. 2021;70:170–9.
13. Altamirano J, Miquel R, Katoonizadeh A, et al. A histologic scoring system for prognosis of patients with alcoholic hepatitis. Gastroenterology 2014; 146:1231–1239.e16.
14. Seitz HK, Bataller R, Cortez-Pinto H, et al. Alcoholic liver disease. Nat Rev Dis Primers. 2018;4:16.
15. Clemente-Sanchez A, Oliveira-Mello A, Bataller R. Moderate alcoholic hepatitis. Clin Liver Dis. 2021;25:537–55.
16. Golabi P, Fazel S, Otgonsuren M, Sayiner M, Locklear CT, Younossi ZM. Mortality assessment of patients with hepatocellular carcinoma according to underlying disease and treatment modalities. Medicine. 2017:96e5904.
17. Bucci L, Garuti F, Camelli V, et al. Comparison between alcohol and hepatitis C virus-related hepatocellular carcinoma: clinical presentation, treatment and outcome. Aliment Pharmacol Ther. 2016;43:385–99.
18. Ganne-Carrie N, Chaffaut C, Bourcier V, et al. Estimate of hepato-cellular carcinoma incidence in patients with alcoholic cirrhosis. J Hepatol. 2018;69:1274–83.
19. Lackner C, Spindelboeck W, Haybaeck J, et al. Histological parameters and alcohol abstinence determine long-term prognosis in patients with alcoholic liver disease. J Hepatol. 2017;66:610–8.
20. Muntaner L, Altamirano JT, Augustin S, et al. High doses of betablockers and alcohol abstinence improve long-term rebleeding and mortality in cirrhotic patients after an acute variceal bleeding. Liver Int. 2010;30:1123–30.
21. EASL Clinical Practice Guidelines. Management of alcohol-related liver disease. J Hepatol. 2018;69:154–81.
22. Delacote C, Bauvin P, Louvet A, et al. A model to identify heavy drinkers at high risk for liver disease progression. Clin Gastroenterol Hepatol. 2020;18:2315–2323.e6.
23. Frazier TH, Stocker AM, Kershner NA, Marsano LS, McClain CJ. Treatment of alcoholic liver disease. Ther Adv Gastroenterol. 2011;4:63–81.
24. O'Shea RS, Dasarathy S, McCullough AJ. Practice guideline committee of the American association for the study of liver diseases, practice parameters committee of the American college of gastroenterology. Alcoholic liver disease. Hepatol Baltim Md. 2010;51:307–28.
25. Savolainen VT, Liesto K, Mannikko A, Penttila A, Karhunen PJ. Alcohol consumption and alcoholic liver disease: evidence of a threshold level of effects of ethanol. Alcohol Clin Exp Res. 1993;17:1112–7.
26. Bush K, Kivlahan DR, McDonell MB, Fihn SD, Bradley KA. The AUDIT alcohol consumption questions (AUDIT-C): an effective brief screening test for problem drinking. Ambulatory Care Quality Improvement Project (ACQUIP). Alcohol use disorders identification test. Arch Intern Med. 1998;158:1789–95.
27. Arab JP, Atkinson SR, Bataller R. Alcohol-related liver disease. In: Yamada's Textbook of Gastroenterology. 7th ed. Wiley; 2022. p. 1966–78. Print ISBN: 9781119600169 | Online ISBN: 9781119600206.

28. Degre D, Stauber RE, Englebert G, et al. Long-term outcomes in patients with decompensated alcohol-related liver disease, steatohepatitis and Maddrey's discriminant function <32. J Hepatol. 2020;72:636–42.
29. Michelena J, Altamirano J, Abraldes JG, et al. Systemic inflammatory response and serum lipopolysaccharide levels predict multiple organ failure and death in alcoholic hepatitis. Hepatology. 2015;62:762–72.
30. Vergis N, Atkinson SR, Knapp S, et al. In patients with severe alcoholic hepatitis, prednisolone increases susceptibility to infection and infection-related mortality, and is associated with high circulating levels of bacterial DNA. Gastroenterology. 2017;152:1068–1077.e4.
31. Altamirano J, Fagundes C, Dominguez M, et al. Acute kidney injury is an early predictor of mortality for patients with alcoholic hepatitis. Cli Gastroenterol Hepatol. 2012;10:65–71.e3.
32. Sujan R, Cruz-Lemini M, Altamirano J, et al. A validated score predicts acute kidney injury and survival in patients with alcoholic hepatitis. Liver Transpl. 2018;24:1655–64.
33. Arab JP, Roblero JP, Altamirano J, et al. Alcohol-related liver disease: clinical practice guidelines by the Latin American association for the study of the liver (ALEH). Ann Hepatol. 2019;18:518–35.
34. Alatalo P, Koivisto H, Puukka K, et al. Biomarkers of liver status in heavy drinkers, moderate drinkers and abstainers. Alcohol Alcohol. 2009;44:199–203.
35. Serra-Burriel M, Graupera I, Toran P, et al. Transient elastography for screening of liver fibrosis: cost-effectiveness analysis from six prospective cohorts in Europe and Asia. J Hepatol. 2019;71:1141–51.
36. Thiele M, Detlefsen S, Sevelsted Mùller L, et al. Transient and 2- dimensional shear-wave elastography provide comparable assessment of alcoholic liver fibrosis and cirrhosis. Gastroenterology. 2016;150(123):133.
37. Thiele M, Madsen BS, Hansen JF, Detlefsen S, Antonsen S, Krag A. Accuracy of the enhanced liver fibrosis test vs FibroTest, elastography, and indirect markers in detection of advanced fibrosis in patients with alcoholic liver disease. Gastroenterology. 2018;154:1369–79.
38. Pavlov CS, Casazza G, Nikolova D, et al. Transient elastography for diagnosis of stages of hepatic fibrosis and cirrhosis in people with alcoholic liver disease. Cochrane Database Syst Rev. 2015;1:Cd010542.
39. Lucey MR, Mathurin P, Morgan TR. Alcoholic hepatitis. N Engl J Med. 2009;360:2758–69.
40. Lackner C, Stauber RE, Davies S, et al. Development and prognostic relevance of a histologic grading and staging system for alcohol-related liver disease. J Hepatol. 2021;75:810–9.
41. Simonetto DA, Shah VH, Kamath PS. Outpatient management of alcohol-related liver disease. Lancet Gastroenterol Hepatol. 2020;5:485–93.
42. American Psychiatric Association. Diagnostic and Statistical Manual of Mental Disorders (DSM-5). American Psychiatric Pub; 2013.
43. Singal AK, Bataller R, Ahn J, Kamath PS, Shah VH. ACG clinical guideline: alcoholic liver disease. Am J Gastroenterol. 2018;113:175–94.
44. Huynh DK, Selvanderan SP, Harley HAJ, Holloway RH, Nguyen NQ. Nutritional care in hospitalized patients with chronic liver disease. World J Gastroenterol. 2015;21:12835–42.
45. Yao CK, Fung J, Chu NHS, Tan VPY. Dietary interventions in liver cirrhosis. J Clin Gastroenterol. 2018;52:663–73.
46. Henkel AS, Buchman AL. Nutritional support in patients with chronic liver disease. Nat Clin Pract Gastroenterol Hepatol. 2006;3:202–9.
47. Anand AC. Nutrition and muscle in cirrhosis. J Clin Exp Hepatol. 2017;7:340–57.
48. Singal AK, Charlton MR. Nutrition in alcoholic liver disease. Clin Liver Dis. 2012;16:805–26.
49. Bunchorntavakul C, Reddy KR. Review article: malnutrition/sarcopenia and frailty in patients with cirrhosis. Aliment Pharmacol Ther. 2020;51:64–77.
50. Tandon P, Montano-Loza AJ, Lai JC, Dasarathy S, Merli M. Sarcopenia and frailty in decompensated cirrhosis. J Hepatol. 2021;75(Suppl 1):S147–62.

51. Cruz-Jentoft AJ, Bahat G, Bauer J, et al. Sarcopenia: revised European consensus on definition and diagnosis. Age Ageing. 2019;48:16–31.
52. Paris MT, Tandon P, Heyland DK, et al. Automated body composition analysis of clinically acquired computed tomography scans using neural networks. Clin Nutr. 2020;39:3049–55.
53. Carey EJ, Lai JC, Wang CW, et al. A multicenter study to define sarcopenia in patients with end-stage liver disease. Liver Transplant. 2017;23:625–33.
54. Mitsiopoulos N, Baumgartner RN, Heymsfield SB, Lyons W, Gallagher D, Ross R. Cadaver validation of skeletal muscle measurement by magnetic resonance imaging and computerized tomography. J Appl Physiol. 1998;85:115–22. https://doi.org/. https://doi.org/10.1152/jappl.1998.85.1.115.
55. Bemeur C, Butterworth RF. Reprint of: nutrition in the management of cirrhosis and its neurological complications. J Clin Exp Hepatol. 2015;5(Suppl 1):S131–40.
56. Matsuoka S, Tamura A, Nakagawara H, Moriyama M. Improvement in the nutritional status and clinical conditions of patients with liver failure using a liver diet combined with a branched chain amino acids-enriched elemental diet. Hepato-Gastroenterology. 2014;61:1308–12.
57. Mills PR, Shenkin A, Anthony RS, et al. Assessment of nutritional status and in vivo immune responses in alcoholic liver disease. Am J Clin Nutr. 1983;38:849–59.
58. Schenker S, Halff GA. Nutritional therapy in alcoholic liver disease. Semin Liver Dis. 1993;13:196–209.
59. Lieber CS. Alcohol, liver, and nutrition. J Am Coll Nutr. 1991;10:602–32.
60. Lindor KD. Management of osteopenia of liver disease with special emphasis on primary biliary cirrhosis. Semin Liver Dis. 1993;13:367–73.
61. Puri P, Dhiman RK, Taneja S, et al. Nutrition in chronic liver disease: consensus statement of the Indian national association for study of the liver. J Clin Exp Hepatol. 2021;11:97–143.
62. Wharton S, Lau DCW, Vallis M, et al. Obesity in adults: a clinical practice guideline. CMAJ. 2020;192:E875–91.
63. Sinclair M, Grossmann M, Hoermann R, Angus PW, Gow PJ. Testosterone therapy increases muscle mass in men with cirrhosis and low testosterone: a randomised controlled trial. J Hepatol. 2016;65:906–13.
64. Ganatra RB, Breu AC, Ronan MV. Clinical guideline highlights for the hospitalist: 2020 American society of addiction medicine clinical practice guideline on alcohol withdrawal management. J Hosp Med. 2021;17:47.
65. European Association for the Study of the Liver. Electronic address: easloffice@easloffice.eu, European association for the study of the liver. EASL clinical practice guidelines: management of alcohol-related liver disease. J Hepatol. 2018;69:154.
66. EASL clinical practical guidelines. Management of alcoholic liver disease. J Hepatol. 2012;57:399–420.
67. Pavlov CS, Varganova DL, Casazza G, Tsochatzis E, Nikolova D, Gluud C. Glucocorticosteroids for people with alcoholic hepatitis. Cochrane Database Syst Rev. 2017;11:CD001511.
68. Srikureja W, Kyulo NL, Runyon BA, Hu KQ. MELD score is a better prognostic model than child-Turcotte-Pugh score or discriminant function score in patients with alcoholic hepatitis. J Hepatol. 2005;42:700–6.
69. Singal AK, Mathurin P. Diagnosis and treatment of alcohol associated liver disease: a review. JAMA. 2021;326:165–76.
70. Singal AK, Shah VH. Therapeutic strategies for the treatment of alcoholic hepatitis. Semin Liver Dis. 2016;36:56–68.
71. Thursz MR, Richardson P, Allison M, et al. Prednisolone or pentoxifylline for alcoholic hepatitis. N Engl J Med. 2015;372:1619–28.
72. Singal AK, Kamath PS, Gores GJ, Shah VH. Alcoholic hepatitis: current challenges and future directions. Clin Gastroenterol Hepatol. 2014;12:555–64. quiz e31 e32
73. Singal AK, Shah VH. Alcoholic hepatitis: prognostic models and treatment. Gastroenterol Clin N Am. 2011;40:611–39.

74. Louvet A, Naveau S, Abdelnour M, et al. The Lille model: a new tool for therapeutic strategy in patients with severe alcoholic hepatitis treated with steroids. Hepatology. 2007;45:1348–54. https://doi.org/10.1002/hep.21607.
75. Singal AK, Kuo YF, Anand BS. Hepatitis C virus infection in alcoholic hepatitis: prevalence patterns and impact on in-hospital mortality. Eur J Gastroenterol Hepatol. 2012;24:1178–84.
76. Segev DL, Sozio SM, Shin EJ, et al. Steroid avoidance in liver transplantation: meta-analysis and meta-regression of randomized trials. Liver Transplant. 2008;14:512–25.
77. Shoreibah M, Anand BS, Singal AK. Alcoholic hepatitis and concomitant hepatitis C virus infection. World J Gastroenterol. 2014;20:11929–34.
78. Louvet A, Wartel F, Castel H, et al. Infection in patients with severe alcoholic hepatitis treated with steroids: early response to therapy is the key factor. Gastroenterology. 2009;137:541–8.
79. Kwong EK, Puri P. Gut microbiome changes in nonalcoholic fatty liver disease & alcoholic liver disease. Transl Gastroenterol Hepatol. 2021;6:3.
80. Tornai D, Szabo G. Emerging medical therapies for severe alcoholic hepatitis. Clin Mol Hepatol. 2020;26:686–96.
81. Karakike E, Moreno C, Gustot T. Infections in severe alcoholic hepatitis. Ann Gastroenterol Hepatol. 2017;30:152–60.
82. Templeton A, Schlegel M, Fleisch F, et al. Multilumen central venous catheters increase risk for catheter-related bloodstream infection: prospective surveillance study. Infection. 2008;36:322–7.
83. Kulkarni AV, Tirumalle S, Premkumar M, et al. Primary norfloxacin prophylaxis for APASL-defined acute-on-chronic liver failure: a placebo-controlled double-blind randomized trial. Am J Gastroenterol. 2022. Published online January 17;117:607.
84. Website. https://easl.eu/wp-content/uploads/2021/06/EASL_2021_Version-5-new.pdf
85. Subramaniyan V, Chakravarthi S, Jegasothy R, et al. Alcohol-associated liver disease: a review on its pathophysiology, diagnosis and drug therapy. Toxicol Rep. 2021;8:376–85.
86. Hamid R, Forrest EH. Is histology required for the diagnosis of alcoholic hepatitis? A review of published randomised controlled trials. Gut. 2011;60(Suppl 1):A233. https://doi.org/10.1136/gut.2011.239301.492.A233.
87. Forrest E, Goldin R. Letter: the diagnostic and prognostic significance of liver histology in alcoholic hepatitis—authors' reply. Aliment Pharmacol Ther. 2021;54:864. https://doi.org/10.1111/apt.16559864.
88. Arab JP, Arrese M, Singal AK. Diagnosis of alcohol-associated hepatitis: when is liver biopsy required? Clin Liver Dis. 2021;25:571–84.
89. Mathurin P, Moreno C, Samuel D, et al. Early liver transplantation for severe alcoholic hepatitis. N Engl J Med. 2011;365:1790–800.
90. DiMartini A, Dew MA, Day N, et al. Trajectories of alcohol consumption following liver transplantation. Am J Transplant. 2010;10:2305–12.
91. Rogal S, Shenai N, Kruckenberg K, Rosenberger E, Dew MA, DiMartini A. Post-transplant outcomes of persons receiving a liver graft for alcoholic liver disease. Alcohol Alcohol. 2018;53:157–65.
92. Im GY, Kim-Schluger L, Shenoy A, et al. Early liver transplantation for severe alcoholic hepatitis in the United States—a single-center experience. Am J Transplant. 2016;16:841–9.
93. Louvet A, Labreuche J, Moreno C, et al. Early liver transplantation for severe alcohol-related hepatitis not responding to medical treatment: a prospective controlled study. Lancet Gastroenterol Hepatol. 2022;7:416–25.
94. Lee BP, Chen PH, Haugen C, et al. Three-year results of a pilot program in early liver transplantation for severe alcoholic hepatitis. Ann Surg. 2017;265:20–9.
95. Weeks SR, Sun Z, McCaul ME, et al. Liver transplantation for severe alcoholic hepatitis, updated lessons from the world's largest series. J Am Coll Surg. 2018;226:549–57.
96. Germani G, Angrisani D, Addolorato G, et al. Liver transplantation for severe alcoholic hepatitis: a multicenter Italian study. Am J Transplant. 2022;22:1191–200.

97. Philippe Mathurin. Early liver transplantation for acute alcoholic hepatitis: we can't say no. J Hepatol. 2021;75(3):718.
98. Arroyo V, Moreau R, Jalan R. Acute-on-chronic liver failure. N Engl J Med. 2020;382:2137–45. https://doi.org/10.1056/NEJMra1914900.
99. Putignano A, Gustot T. New concepts in acute-on-chronic liver failure: implications for liver transplantation. Liver Transpl. 2017;23:234–43. https://doi.org/10.1002/lt.24654.
100. Artru F, Louvet A, Ruiz I, Levesque E, Labreuche J, Ursic-Bedoya J, et al. Liver transplantation in the most severely ill cirrhotic patients: a multicenter study in acute-on-chronic liver failure grade 3. J Hepatol. 2017;67:708–15. https://doi.org/10.1016/j.jhep.2017.06.009.
101. Thuluvath PJ, Thuluvath AJ, Hanish S, Savva Y. Liver transplantation in patients with multiple organ failures: feasibility and outcomes. J Hepatol. 2018;69:1047–56. https://doi.org/10.1016/j.jhep.2018.07.007.
102. Choudhary NS, Saigal S, Gautam D, Saraf N, Rastogi A, Goja S, Bhangui P, Thiagrajan S, Yadav SK, Mehrotra S, Rastogi V, Soin AS. Good outcome of living donor liver transplantation for severe alcoholic hepatitis not responding to medical management: a single center experience of 39 patients. Alcohol. 2018; https://doi.org/10.1016/j.alcohol.2018.07.009.
103. Yadav SK, et al. Living donor liver transplantation for acute-on-chronic liver failure. Liver Transpl. 2019;25(3):459–68.
104. Wiesner R, Edwards E, Freeman R, et al. Model for end-stage liver disease (MELD) and allocation of donor livers. Gastroenterology. 2003;124:91–6.
105. Veldt BJ, Laine F, Guillygomarc'h A, et al. Indication of liver transplantation in severe alcoholic liver cirrhosis: quantitative evaluation and optimal timing. J Hepatol. 2002;36:93–8.
106. Giard JM, Dodge JL, Terrault NA. Superior wait-list outcomes in patients with alcohol-associated liver disease compared with other indications for liver transplantation. Liver Transplant. 2019;25:1310–20.
107. Antonini TM, Guillaud O, Dumortier J, et al. Impact of a first study of early transplantation in acute alcoholic hepatitis: results of a nationwide survey in French liver transplantation programs. Liver Transplant. 2018;24:841–4.
108. Tandon P, Goodman KJ, Ma MM, et al. A shorter duration of pretransplant abstinence predicts problem drinking after liver transplantation. Am J Gastroenterol. 2009;104:1700–6.
109. Herrick-Reynolds KM, Punchhi G, Greenberg RS, et al. Evaluation of early vs standard liver transplant for alcohol-associated liver disease. JAMA Surg. 2021;156:1026–34.
110. European Association for the Study of the Liver, Electronic Address, European Association for the Study of the L. EASL Clinical Practice Guidelines: management of alcohol-related liver disease. J Hepatol. 2018;69:154–81.
111. Martin P, DiMartini A, Feng S, Brown R Jr, Fallon M. Evaluation for liver transplantation in adults: 2013 practice guideline by the American Association for the Study of Liver Diseases and the American Society of Transplantation. Hepatology. 2014;59:1144–65.
112. Pelletier S, Alarcon R, Ewert V, Forest M, Nalpas B, Perney P. Comparison of the MoCA and BEARNI tests for detection of cognitive impairment in in-patients with alcohol use disorders. Drug Alcohol Depend. 2018;187:249–53.
113. Arab JP, Izzy M, Leggio L, Bataller R, Shah VH. Management of alcohol use disorder in patients with cirrhosis in the setting of liver transplantation. Nat Rev Gastroenterol Hepatol. 2022;19:45–59.
114. Bradley KA, DeBenedetti AF, Volk RJ, Williams EC, Frank D, Kivlahan DR. AUDIT-C as a brief screen for alcohol misuse in primary care. Alcohol Clin Exp Res. 2007;31:1208–17.
115. Lucey MR. Alcohol-associated cirrhosis. Clin Liver Dis. 2019;23:115–26.
116. Kim DJ, Choi MS. Life-sustaining treatment and palliative care in patients with liver cirrhosis—legal, ethical, and practical issues. Clin Mol Hepatol. 2017;23:115–22.

Chapter 13
Metabolic Dysfunction-Associated Steatotic Liver Disease

Arka De and Ajay Duseja

Abstract Non-alcoholic fatty liver disease (NAFLD), recently renamed as metabolic dysfunction-associated steatotic liver disease (MASLD), is a major cause of end-stage liver disease and hepatocellular carcinoma (HCC), necessitating liver transplantation (LT). Despite initial concerns, recent data suggest that patients with MASLD do not face higher risks of waitlist drop-out or mortality compared to other etiologies. While peri-transplant complications, particularly infections, may be more frequent in patients transplanted for MASLD, overall graft and patient survival rates are comparable to other etiologies. However, other long-term complications such as diabetes, hypertension, dyslipidemia, and cardiovascular events are more common. Comprehensive pre-transplant assessments focusing on cardiovascular risk, metabolic comorbidities, and renal dysfunction are essential to optimize overall outcomes. In this chapter, we have clarified the change in nomenclature from NAFLD to MASLD and highlighted the challenges in diagnosing MASLD as the etiology of cirrhosis or hepatocellular carcinoma. We also discuss the epidemiology of MASLD with reference to LT, the strategies for pre-LT assessment, medical optimization of metabolic comorbidities, and post-LT immunosuppression.

Keywords Non-alcoholic fatty liver disease · Metabolic-dysfunction-associated fatty liver disease · NAFLD · MASLD · Non-alcoholic steatohepatitis

Key Highlights

- Metabolic dysfunction-associated steatotic liver disease (MASLD) is a leading cause of end-stage liver disease and hepatocellular carcinoma requiring liver transplant (LT).

A. De · A. Duseja (✉)
Department of Hepatology, Postgraduate Institute of Medical Education and Research, Chandigarh, India
e-mail: ajayduseja@yahoo.co.in

S. Saigal, D. Jothimani (eds.), *Fundamentals of Transplant Hepatology*,
https://doi.org/10.1007/978-981-95-2624-6_13

- Unlike NAFLD, MASLD is not a diagnosis of exclusion. Diagnosis of MASLD requires the presence of hepatic steatosis along with at least one cardiometabolic risk factor in the absence of significant alcohol intake.
- Diagnosis of MASLD as the etiology of cirrhosis or HCC may be challenging due to the impact of cirrhosis per se on metabolic parameters. Past history of metabolic risk factors, particularly obesity or diabetes, may often be the only clue.
- Post-transplant graft and patient survival in MASLD is similar to that of other etiologies. However, long-term medical complications like diabetes mellitus, hypertension, dyslipidemia, weight gain, recurrent Metabolic dysfunction-assocciated steatphepatitis (MASH), cardiovascular events, and malignancies are more common in patients transplanted for MASLD.
- Pre-transplant evaluation should ffocus particularly on assessing cardiovascular risk, metabolic comorbidities, and renal dysfunction.
- Holistic management of cardiometabolic risk factors, including obesity, diabetes mellitus, hypertension, and dyslipidemia both pre- and post-transplant is crucial.
- Caution about long-term metabolic adverse effects of commonly used immunosuppressants in the post-transplant setting.

13.1 Introduction and Clarification of Terminology

The global prevalence of non-alcoholic fatty liver disease (NAFLD) among the general adult population is estimated to be 30% [1]. It is thus unsurprising that NAFLD is emerging as a major cause of end-stage liver disease and hepatocellular carcinoma (HCC) requiring liver transplant (LT). Histologically, NAFLD includes a spectrum ranging from simple steatosis, non-alcoholic steatohepatitis (NASH) with or without fibrosis, cirrhosis, and HCC [2]. Traditionally, NAFLD has been a diagnosis of exclusion requiring the absence of significant alcohol intake and other etiologies of hepatic steatosis. Recently, an international Delphi consensus has recommended a change in the nomenclature of NAFLD and NASH to metabolic-dysfunction-associated steatotic liver disease (MASLD) and metabolic-dysfunction-associated steatohepatitis (MASH), respectively. In a nutshell, MASLD can now be diagnosed as a cause of hepatic steatosis in the presence of any one of the five metabolic risk factors shown in Table 13.1 in the absence of significant alcohol

Table 13.1 Metabolic risk factors for defining MASLD

1. Overweight/obese (as per BMI[1]) *OR* central obesity (as per waist circumference[2])
2. Fasting serum glucose $\geq$ 100 mg/dL *OR* 2-hour post-load serum glucose $\geq$ 140 mg/dL *OR* HbA1c $\geq$ 5.6% *OR* type 2 diabetes mellitus *OR* antidiabetic treatment
3. Blood pressure $\geq$ 130/85 mm of Hg or antihypertensive medication
4. Triglycerides $\geq$ 150 mg/dl or lipid-lowering treatment
5. HDL $\leq$ 50 in females or $\leq$ 40 in males or lipid-lowering treatment

[1]BMI cut-off for overweight and obesity in Indians: $\geq$ 23 kg/m^2 and $\geq$ 25 kg/m^2, respectively
[2]Waist circumference cut-offs for central obesity in Indians: > 90 cm in males and > 80 cm in females

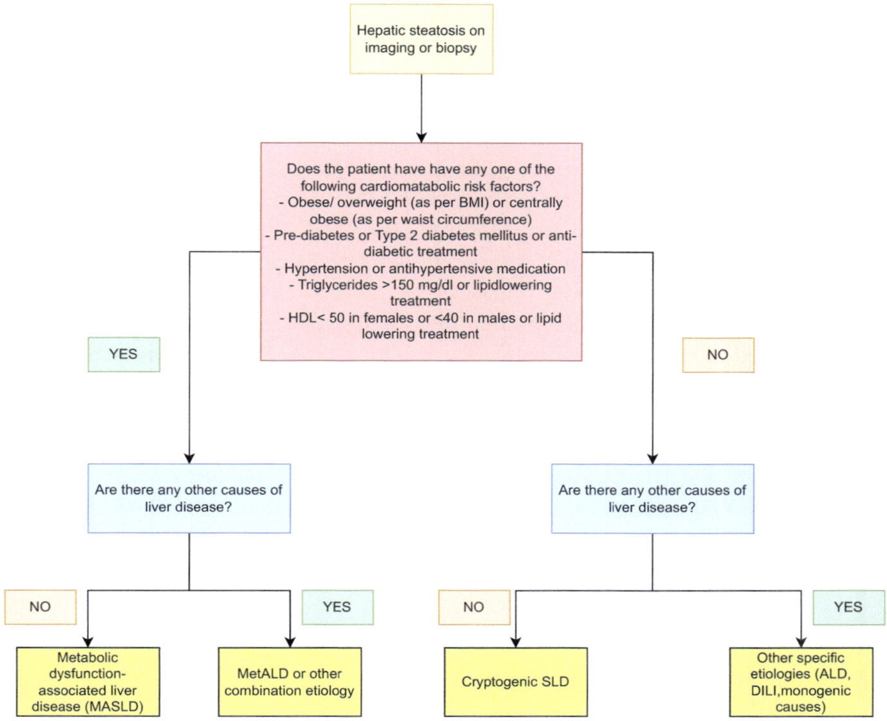

Fig. 13.1 Framework for classifying steatotic liver disease (SLD)

intake (<20 g/day in females and <30 g/day in males). MASLD is thus no longer a diagnosis of exclusion and can coexist with other etiologies (Fig. 13.1) [3]. It has been shown that most patients with NAFLD fulfill the MASLD criteria; hence, it has been suggested that data on NAFLD patients may be extrapolated for MASLD. To avoid confusion, we will use both terms throughout the chapter. In this chapter, we will discuss the epidemiology of MASLD with reference to LT, strategies for pre-LT assessment and medical optimization, and post-LT immunosuppression. We will not be discussing long-term post-LT complications, including new-onset or worsening metabolic risk factors, recurrent MASLD, etc., which have been covered in other chapters.

13.2 Liver Transplant in MASLD: Epidemiology

MASLD is the second leading cause of LT in the United States, accounting for 21.5% of all LTs in 2018 [4]. Data from both the European Liver Transplant Registry (ELTR) and the United Network for Organ Sharing (UNOS) databases confirm that

MASLD has been the most rapidly growing indication for LT over the past two decades [4, 5]. Data from India on this aspect is limited. A single center review from North India reported MASLD to be the etiology in 26.5% of 2137 adult LTs at their center [6].

MASLD has also emerged as a major cause of HCC, which can sometimes occur even in the absence of cirrhosis. A modeling study has estimated that the incidence of MASLD-related HCC will increase by over 135% from 2015 to 2030 [7]. A similar trend of increasing incidence of MASLD-related HCC over the past two decades has also been noted in India [8]. A large multicentric review of records from 5798 HCC patients in 11 participating Indian tertiary centers from 2017 to 2022 reported that MASLD was the commonest etiology, being seen in 35.5% of patients [9]. Among patients on the LT waitlist in the United States, MASLD has been recognized as the most rapidly increasing cause of HCC, with an almost eight-fold rise from 2002 to 2016 [10].

There has been some controversy about increased drop-out and mortality among patients with MASLD cirrhosis or HCC on the LT waitlist. However, a recent analysis of the UNOS database has disproved this fear, and patients with MASLD do not appear to be at a higher risk of waitlist drop-out, and transplantation rates are comparable with those of other etiologies [11].

13.3 Outcomes of LT in MASLD

Peri-transplant complications, particularly infections, may be more common in patients with MASLD [12]. However, major complications are comparable to those of other etiologies with similar graft and patient survival rates at 1 year (85–90%) and 5 years (70–80%) [13]. In patients transplanted for HCC, patient and graft survival, as well as tumor recurrence, are comparable between MASLD and other etiologies [14, 15]. However, long-term medical complications like DM, hypertension, dyslipidemia, weight gain, recurrent MASH, cardiovascular events, and malignancies are more common in patients transplanted for MASLD-related cirrhosis or HCC. These long-term complications have been dealt with in detail in other chapters.

13.4 Pre-Transplant Considerations

The pre-transplant assessment of patients with MASLD requires a thorough holistic evaluation with particular focus on cardiovascular risk, metabolic comorbidities, and renal dysfunction (Table 13.2).

Table 13.2 Pre-transplant evaluation and optimization of patients with MASLD-related cirrhosis

Diabetes mellitus	The Oral Glucose Tolerance Test (OGTT) is the most reliable method to diagnose DM HbA1c is helpful for monitoring glycemic control, but may be falsely low Proper control of blood sugar levels is essential before undergoing LT Only insulin is recommended in CTP-C cirrhosis Oral antidiabetic agents like metformin may be used in CTP-A and B cirrhosis Insulin secretagogues should be avoided
Obesity	The first-line intervention for obese individuals is lifestyle change Plan a nutritional and lifestyle program to achieve progressive weight loss (>5–10%) in obese cirrhotic patients An individualized, moderately hypocaloric (~500–800 kcal/d) diet should be supplemented with adequate protein intake (>1.5 g /kg/day) to attain gradual weight loss without compromising protein stores Exercise as per patient's ability; the minimum goal of physical activity should be to maintain residual mobility Resistance exercise can supplement aerobic exercises Pre-LT bariatric surgery is contraindicated in cirrhosis with clinically significant portal hypertension; however, it may be considered at the time of LT or after it
Cardiovascular disease	Pre-LT cardiovascular risk stratification is mandatory Specific algorithm of cardiac workup should be followed The latest scientific statement from the American Heart Association suggests considering NASH as an independent high-risk factor for cardiovascular events. Stress tests alone are not sufficient, and all patients should undergo coronary angiography (initial CT coronary angiography)
Kidney dysfunction	Ensure proper monitoring of kidney function prior to LT Treatment of comorbidities like DM and hypertension Avoiding nephrotoxic drugs Properly select individuals for combined liver and kidney transplantation as per established criteria Minimize calcineurin inhibitors post-LT
Arterial Hypertension	Diuretics, particularly in patients with ascites Non-selective beta-blockers (carvedilol>propranolol) Angiotensin-converting enzyme (ACE) inhibitors, if no impaired renal function or refractory ascites Calcium Channel Blockers
Dyslipidemia	Omega-3 fatty acids are helpful for hypertriglyceridemia; fFish oil and nuts are good natural sources of omega-3 fatty acids When indicated, statins are safe in CTP-A and CTP-B cirrhosis. However, it should be avoided in CTP-C cirrhosis
NASH-specific pharmacotherapy	NASH-specific pharmacotherapy is currently not recommended in patients with cirrhosis

DM Diabetes mellitus, *LT* Liver transplant, *CTP* Child-Turcotte-Pugh

13.4.1 Diagnosing MASLD in Patients with Cirrhosis or HCC

Establishing MASLD as the etiology in patients with cirrhosis or HCC may sometimes be tricky, and many of these patients had been labeled as cryptogenic cirrhosis in the past. This is because there is a tendency for hepatic steatosis to decrease as fibrosis progresses. Thus, steatosis may not be detectable in patients with established cirrhosis. Another point to consider is that the onset of cirrhosis per se has a variable influence on metabolic comorbidities. For instance, weight loss is common in cirrhosis, and systemic vasodilatation in end-stage liver disease may mask years of hypertension. Cirrhosis itself may lead to the onset of hepatogenous diabetes, and it also impacts lipid profile with a decrease in high-density lipoprotein (HDL). Thus, the past history and duration of metabolic comorbidities should also be considered and not just the current status [3, 16]. As such, the diagnosis of MASLD should be considered in patients with the presence or history of metabolic comorbidities without significant alcohol intake, even in the absence of demonstrable steatosis. The current Indian National Association for Study of the Liver (INASL) guidelines require the presence or history of obesity (including central obesity) and another metabolic risk factor in the absence of other etiologies for the diagnosis of NASH-cirrhosis or NASH-HCC [16].

13.4.2 Cardiopulmonary Risk Assessment

Compared to other etiologies, MASLD has been associated with an increased risk of major adverse cardiovascular events, critical coronary stenosis, and worse outcomes after cardiac events independent of the presence of other metabolic comorbidities like DM [17]. It has also been shown to be an independent risk factor for obstructive coronary artery disease (CAD) and adverse cardiac outcomes after LT [18, 19]. Apart from coronary artery disease (CAD), many of these patients also have asymptomatic cirrhotic cardiomyopathy with prolonged QTc, which may predispose them to ventricular arrhythmias. Obstructive sleep apnea is also independently associated with MASLD and may pose anesthetic challenges. A detailed cardiopulmonary evaluation is thus mandatory in MASLD patients listed for LT as is indeed true for other etiologies as well.

At the very least, all patients being evaluated for LT should undergo a thorough clinical evaluation, ECG, transthoracic echocardiography with bubble-contrast study, chest X-ray, and pulmonary function tests. Furthermore, cardiovascular evaluation depends on the patient's estimated cardiovascular risk. There is substantial variation in the investigation protocols for cardiovascular risk assessment that are followed in various institutes, which is partially attributable to differences in cardiovascular risk stratification. The Framingham risk score has been shown to correlate with cardiovascular risk after LT and may be used for tailoring further diagnostic or therapeutic decisions. Scores have also been developed specifically for predicting cardiovascular risk in patients listed for LT, including the cardiovascular risk in orthotopic liver transplantation (CAR-OLT), cardiac arrest risk index (CARI), and CAD in LTx (CAD-LT) scores [17]. However, they need further validation, particularly in Indian patients.

The details of cardiovascular risk stratification and assessment prior to LT have been covered elsewhere in the book. From the point of view of MASLD patients listed for LT, it is relevant to note that the recent scientific statement of the American

Heart Association recognizes NASH as an independent high-risk factor for CAD risk stratification [17]. It suggests that patients with NASH or DM or ≥ 2 CAD risk factors (dyslipidemia, hypertension, chronic kidney disease (CKD), left ventricular hypertrophy, family history of CAD, tobacco use) are at high risk for significant CAD and should undergo coronary angiography (non-invasive CT coronary angiography preferred for initial evaluation). Stress testing alone is not recommended in these high-risk patients as per this guidance document, although real-life practice varies from center to center. Indeed, most centers in India follow a similar protocol for cardiovascular risk assessment in patients with MASLD cirrhosis being evaluated for LT as for other etiologies of liver disease. Cardiovascular risk assessment, at least an ECG and a transthoracic echocardiogram, should be repeated annually.

13.4.3 Obesity

Overweight, obesity, and central obesity are the most common metabolic comorbidities in patients with MASLD. More than 80–90% of obese patients have underlying MASLD. Obesity is an independent risk factor for decompensation and infections in cirrhosis [20, 21]. It is important to remember that in decompensated cirrhotics, the measured body weight should be corrected for the presence of ascites or pedal edema, i.e., 5–15% for grade 1 to grade 3 ascites with an additional correction of 5% for pedal edema [22]. From a surgical perspective, high body mass index (BMI) may make the transplant technically challenging with a possible increased rate of peri-transplant complications, including infections and longer ICU admission [23]. However, the long-term outcomes of LT are similar in obese and non-obese patients. As such, very high BMI is not an absolute contraindication for LT, provided the patient has acceptable cardiorespiratory fitness to tolerate the procedure. However, in real-world settings, many centers use their own BMI thresholds for making the decision to proceed with LT.

Weight loss through lifestyle interventions, including dietary modifications and exercise, constitutes the central pillar in the management of MASLD [16]. However, there is an important caveat to weight loss in patients with cirrhosis. Despite being overweight or obese, underlying myosteatosis and sarcopenia are also prevalent in patients with MASLD cirrhosis and can lead to poor outcomes post-LT [24, 25]. Thus, calorie restriction should be supplemented with adequate protein intake of 1.5 g/kg/day to avoid exacerbating muscle loss [26, 27]. Protein restriction is not necessary even in patients with a history of hepatic encephalopathy, although plant, dairy, or fish proteins may be preferred. Red meat should be best avoided. Current evidence suggests that previous concerns about worsening portal hypertension with exercise are unfounded. In the SportDiet study, dietary intervention and exercise were well tolerated, with a decrease in body weight of >5% and hepatic venous pressure gradient (HVPG) of >10% being noted in 52% and 42% of patients with cirrhosis, respectively [28]. Intensity and duration of exercise in decompensated cirrhosis should be tailored according to the individual's levels of tolerance.

Resistance exercise may be particularly helpful for cirrhotics, who often have poor cardiorespiratory reserve and may be unable to carry out aerobic exercises due to obesity and related complications. Guidelines from INASL and other international expert societies suggest a target weight loss of 5–10% in obese patients with cirrhosis [16, 26, 27].

In general, pharmacotherapy for weight loss is not recommended in patients with cirrhosis. There is much excitement about the use of drugs targeting the incretin axis for the management of obesity in general. Semaglutide, a glucagon-like peptide-1 (GLP-1) agonist, has been shown to be safe in compensated cirrhosis. In a recent randomised controlled trial (RCT), weekly injectable semaglutide (2.4 mg) led to a mean weight loss of 9% over 48 weeks in patients with NASH-cirrhosis without any substantial safety or tolerability issues [29]. However, there was no difference in histological improvement in NASH or fibrosis as compared to placebo. Further, body composition was not assessed in the study, and there is no information on sarcopenia or myosteatosis. Finally, it should be noted that patients with decompensated cirrhosis or HCC were excluded from this RCT on semaglutide in MASH-cirrhosis.

Bariatric surgery is relatively contraindicated in compensated cirrhosis and absolutely contraindicated in decompensated cirrhosis with an adjusted odds ratio for mortality of 2.17 and 21.2, respectively, compared to non-cirrhotic patients [30, 31]. However, bariatric surgery may be performed at the time of LT in settings where the expertise is available or after LT [32]. Sleeve gastrectomy is preferred over Roux-en-Y gastric bypass, as it preserves endoscopic access to the papilla for management of biliary complications and avoids the risk of malabsorption of immunosuppressive drugs [32]. A long-term follow-up (≥3 years) of 13 patients who underwent simultaneous sleeve gastrectomy and LT at Mayo Clinic had a significantly higher weight loss with lower prevalence of hepatic steatosis, insulin resistance, and metabolic complications like hypertension compared to 36 control patients who underwent LT alone with lifestyle interventions [33]. The feasibility of bariatric surgery performed after LT has been reported in small case series, although there are concerns regarding the anticipated difficult surgery due to peritoneal adhesions.

Endoscopic bariatric and metabolic therapies are an evolving field. While data is emerging in patients with compensated cirrhosis, there is negligible data in patients with decompensated cirrhosis or on the transplant waitlist [34, 35]. Some procedures, like duodenal mucosal resurfacing, may potentially interfere with the absorption of immunosuppressive drugs. As a temporizing measure, intragastric balloons have been used in small case series to induce weight loss and stabilize the patient prior to LT [36]. However, more data needs to be generated before such procedures can be employed as a routine practice in transplant waitlist patients due to fears that rapid weight loss may paradoxically worsen sarcopenia and post-LT outcomes.

13.4.4 Diabetes Mellitus

Type 2 DM is estimated to be present in 33–66% of patients with MASLD. Pre-LT DM has been associated with poorer outcomes after LT, including a higher risk of infections and cardiovascular complications, longer hospital stays, and decreased graft and overall survival. In the setting of cirrhosis, type 2 DM needs to be differentiated from hepatogenous diabetes [37]. Type 2 DM occurs due to insulin resistance, is present for a long duration, and is considered a risk factor for developing MASLD cirrhosis. On the other hand, hepatogenous diabetes is of recent onset and occurs only in the presence of cirrhosis. The pathophysiology is speculative and involves pancreatic beta-cell atrophy and insulin resistance. Hepatogenous diabetes should not be considered as a risk factor while considering the diagnosis of MASLD as the etiology in a patient with cirrhosis. It should be noted that glycosylated hemoglobin (HbA1c) may be falsely low in cirrhotic patients due to concurrent splenomegaly and anemia. Although HbA1c is commonly used for both diagnosis and monitoring in clinical practice, the ideal (gold standard) diagnostic test in patients with cirrhosis is the oral glucose tolerance test (OGTT).

Patients with cirrhosis have been excluded from trials of antidiabetic drugs. The various factors that should be kept in mind while choosing an antidiabetic agent in a patient with cirrhosis include the severity of liver disease (Child-Turcotte-Pugh (CTP) class), risk of hypoglycemia, and kidney injury. Only insulin is safe for patients in CTP class C. Oral antidiabetic agents may be used with caution in CTP classes A and B with close monitoring. Metformin is likely the safest and may have additional benefits by decreasing insulin resistance. Although data are scant, GLP-1 receptor agonists, dipeptidyl peptidase-4 (DPP-4) inhibitors, or sodium-glucose cotransporter-2 (SGLT2) inhibitors may also be used in patients with compensated cirrhosis. The recent RCT on the use of weekly injectable semaglutide in patients with NASH-related compensated cirrhosis has already been alluded to in the previous section [29]. Insulin secretagogues like sulphonylureas, which can lead to hypoglycemia, should be preferably avoided in cirrhosis, particularly the long-acting formulations.

13.4.5 Other Metabolic Comorbidities

Apart from the diuretic action of mineralocorticoid receptor antagonists, non-selective beta-blockers like propranolol and carvedilol are also suitable for managing hypertension in patients with cirrhosis due to their additional effect on the reduction of portal pressure. A higher decrease in mean arterial pressure is attained with carvedilol compared to propranolol. ACE inhibitors and angiotensin receptor blockers are first-line antihypertensive agents in the general population and have renoprotective and cardioprotective effects. In cirrhotic patients with refractory or recurrent ascites, they should best be avoided due to the fear that blocking the renin-angiotensin-aldosterone system (RAAS) pathway may further decrease the already perturbed renal perfusion, thereby precipitating acute kidney injury or hypotension. However, ACE inhibitors and angiotensin receptor blockers may be used with caution in patients with grade 1–2 ascites, particularly in patients who have already been on these agents for management of hypertension [22].

Omega-3 fatty acid supplementation, including its natural sources like fish oil and walnuts, may be helpful for hypertriglyceridemia. Statins, when indicated, are safe in patients with CTP-A and -B cirrhosis. However, they should be avoided in decompensated cirrhosis due to an increased risk of rhabdomyolysis, as has been reported with simvastatin [38, 39].

13.4.6 Renal Dysfunction

Among the various extrahepatic associations of MASLD, chronic kidney disease (CKD) is particularly relevant in the transplant setting. Pre-LT CKD is an independent predictor of post-transplant mortality with a hazard ratio of 1.14 [40]. Further, MASLD has also been shown to be an independent predictor of post-LT CKD [41]. Simultaneous liver-kidney transplants should be considered in patients fulfilling established criteria, like CKD with eGFR <30 ml/min for more than 3 months [42]. Particular attention should be paid to immunosuppressive strategies in patients with deranged renal function prior to LT, with the minimization of calcineurin inhibitors (CNIs) and the avoidance of other nephrotoxic drugs. The medical management of other risk factors for CKD, including DM and hypertension, should also be optimized.

13.4.7 MASLD-Specific Pharmacotherapy

In general, no disease-specific pharmacotherapy is recommended in patients with MASLD cirrhosis. Some retrospective data suggest that vitamin E and metformin may reduce the risk of decompensation in MASLD patients with decompensated cirrhosis [43, 44]. Belapectin (galectin-3 inhibitor) and emricasan (pan-caspase inhibitor) have been evaluated in multicentric phase 2 trials in patients with cirrhosis and portal hypertension, although no significant improvement in hepatic venous pressure gradient was observed with either drug [45, 46]. Weekly injectable semaglutide has been recently evaluated in compensated cirrhosis. Despite significant weight reduction, no histological improvement was observed in MASLD or fibrosis at 48 weeks in comparison to placebo [29]. Only emricasan has been evaluated in patients with decompensated cirrhosis. Although safe, it did not prevent further decompensations, and there was no change in disease severity scores as compared to placebo [47].

13.5 Immunosuppression Strategy in LT for MASLD

Immunosuppression strategies in patients transplanted for MASLD cirrhosis or HCC should take into account the increased risk of these patients developing new-onset or worsening metabolic comorbidities, renal dysfunction, and recurrent MASLD. Steroids should be tapered and withdrawn early, at the latest by 3 months. Barring steroids, adverse metabolic effects are most common with calcineurin inhibitors (CNIs), which also have nephrotoxic effects. DM is more common with tacrolimus, while hypertension and dyslipidemia are more common with cyclosporine. Mammalian target of rapamycin (mTOR) inhibitors can cause hypertriglyceridemia and proteinuria. Among the various classes of immunosuppressive agents, antimetabolites like mycophenolate appear to be the safest from a metabolic and renal point of view. Thus, many centers currently practice a maintenance immunosuppression protocol that uses antimetabolites with or without mTOR inhibitors, along with dose minimization or complete withdrawal of tacrolimus, in patients transplanted for MASLD-related cirrhosis or HCC [16, 48].

13.6 Conclusion

MASLD-related cirrhosis and HCC are the fastest-growing indications for LT globally. Identification and adequate management of metabolic comorbidities like obesity and diabetes are paramount for optimizing outcomes in this group of patients. Patients with MASLD are also at high risk of cardiovascular adverse events and chronic kidney disease. A meticulous cardiovascular assessment is an essential component of the pre-LT workup in these patients.

Declaration of Interest All authors declare that they have no conflict of interest and have no financial disclosures.

FundingNone

References

1. Younossi ZM, Golabi P, Paik JM, Henry A, Van Dongen C, Henry L. The global epidemiology of nonalcoholic fatty liver disease (NAFLD) and nonalcoholic steatohepatitis (NASH): a systematic review. Hepatology. 2023;77(4):1335–47.
2. De A, Duseja A. Natural history of simple steatosis or nonalcoholic fatty liver. J Clin Exp Hepatol. 2020;10(3):255–62.
3. Rinella ME, Lazarus JV, Ratziu V, et al. A multi-society Delphi consensus statement on new fatty liver disease nomenclature [published online ahead of print, 2023 Jun 20]. J Hepatol. 2023;S0168-8278(23):00418-X. https://doi.org/10.1016/j.jhep.2023.06.003.
4. Cotter TG, Charlton M. Nonalcoholic steatohepatitis after liver transplantation. Liver Transpl. 2020;26(1):141–59.

5. Adam R, Karam V, Cailliez V, Grady JGO, Mirza D, Cherqui D. 2018 Annual report of the European Liver Transplant Registry (ELTR) - 50-year evolution of liver transplantation. Transpl Int. 2018;31(12):1293–317.
6. Choudhary NS, Bhangui P, Soin AS. Liver transplant outcomes in India. Clin Liver Dis (Hoboken). 2022;19(1):32–5.
7. Estes C, Razavi H, Loomba R, Younossi Z, Sanyal AJ. Modeling the epidemic of nonalcoholic fatty liver disease demonstrates an exponential increase in burden of disease. Hepatology. 2018;67(1):123–33.
8. Tohra S, Duseja A, Taneja S, et al. Experience with changing etiology and nontransplant curative treatment modalities for hepatocellular carcinoma in a real-life setting-a retrospective descriptive analysis. J Clin Exp Hepatol. 2021;11(6):682–90.
9. Prabhakar T, Kaushal K, Prasad M, et al. Etiologic fractions in patients of hepatocellular carcinoma in India with and without a background of cirrhosis: a multi-centric study. Hepatol Int. 2023;17(3):745–52.
10. Younossi Z, Stepanova M, Ong JP, Jacobson IM, Bugianesi E, Duseja A. Nonalcoholic steatohepatitis is the fastest growing cause of hepatocellular carcinoma in liver transplant candidates. Clin Gastroenterol Hepatol. 2019;17(4):748–755 e3.
11. Thuluvath PJ, Hanish S, Savva Y. Waiting list mortality and transplant rates for NASH cirrhosis when compared with cryptogenic, alcoholic, or AIH cirrhosis. Transplantation. 2019;103(1):113–21.
12. van den Berg EH, Douwes RM, de Meijer VE, Schreuder T, Blokzijl H. Liver transplantation for NASH cirrhosis is not performed at the expense of major post-operative morbidity. Dig Liver Dis. 2018;50(1):68–75.
13. Burra P, Becchetti C, Germani G. NAFLD and liver transplantation: disease burden, current management and future challenges. JHEP Rep. 2020;2(6):100192.
14. Haldar D, Kern B, Hodson J, Armstrong MJ, Adam R, Berlakovich G. Outcomes of liver transplantation for non-alcoholic steatohepatitis: a European Liver Transplant Registry study. J Hepatol. 2019;71(2):313–22.
15. Sadler EM, Mehta N, Bhat M, Ghanekar A, Greig PD, Grant DR. Liver transplantation for NASH-related hepatocellular carcinoma versus non-NASH etiologies of hepatocellular carcinoma. Transplantation. 2018;102(4):640–7.
16. Duseja A, Singh SP, De A, et al. Indian National Association for Study of the Liver (INASL) guidance paper on Nomenclature, Diagnosis and Treatment of Nonalcoholic Fatty Liver Disease (NAFLD). J Clin Exp Hepatol. 2023;13(2):273–302.
17. Cheng XS, VanWagner LB, Costa SP, et al. Emerging evidence on coronary heart disease screening in kidney and liver transplantation candidates: a scientific statement from the American Heart Association: endorsed by the American Society of Transplantation. Circulation. 2022;146(21):e299–324.
18. VanWagner LB, Serper M, Kang R, et al. Factors associated with major adverse cardiovascular events after liver transplantation among a national sample. Am J Transplant. 2016;16:2684–94.
19. Patel SS, Nabi E, Guzman L, et al. Coronary artery disease in decompensated patients undergoing liver transplantation evaluation. Liver Transpl. 2018;24:333–42.
20. Berzigotti A, Garcia-Tsao G, Bosch J, Grace ND, Burroughs AK, Morillas R. Obesity is an independent risk factor for clinical decompensation in patients with cirrhosis. Hepatology. 2011;54(2):555–61.
21. Sundaram V, Kaung A, Rajaram A, Lu SC, Tran TT, Nissen NN. Obesity is independently associated with infection in hospitalised patients with end-stage liver disease. Aliment Pharmacol Ther. 2015;42(11–12):1271–80.
22. Singh V, De A, Mehtani R, et al. Asia-Pacific association for study of liver guidelines on management of ascites in liver disease. Hepatol Int. 2023;17(4):792–826.
23. LaMattina JC, Foley DP, Fernandez LA, Pirsch JD, Musat AI, D'Alessandro AM. Complications associated with liver transplantation in the obese recipient. Clin Transpl. 2012;26(6):910–8.

24. Hegyi PJ, Soós A, Hegyi P, et al. Pre-transplant sarcopenic obesity worsens the survival after liver transplantation: a meta-analysis and a systematic review. Front Med (Lausanne). 2020;7:599434.
25. Carias S, Castellanos AL, Vilchez V, et al. Nonalcoholic steatohepatitis is strongly associated with sarcopenic obesity in patients with cirrhosis undergoing liver transplant evaluation. J Gastroenterol Hepatol. 2016;31(3):628–33.
26. European Association for the Study of the Liver. EASL Clinical Practice Guidelines on nutrition in chronic liver disease. J Hepatol. 2019;70(1):172–93.
27. Puri P, Dhiman RK, Taneja S, et al. Nutrition in chronic liver disease: consensus statement of the Indian National Association for Study of the Liver. J Clin Exp Hepatol. 2021;11(1):97–143.
28. Berzigotti A, Albillos A, Villanueva C, et al. Effects of an intensive lifestyle intervention program on portal hypertension in patients with cirrhosis and obesity: the SportDiet study. Hepatology. 2017;65(4):1293–305.
29. Loomba R, Abdelmalek MF, Armstrong MJ, et al. Semaglutide 2·4 mg once weekly in patients with non-alcoholic steatohepatitis-related cirrhosis: a randomised, placebo-controlled phase 2 trial. Lancet Gastroenterol Hepatol. 2023;8(6):511–22.
30. Mosko JD, Nguyen GC. Increased perioperative mortality following bariatric surgery among patients with cirrhosis. Clin Gastroenterol Hepatol. 2011;9(10):897–901.
31. Patton H, Heimbach J, McCullough A. AGA clinical practice update on bariatric surgery in cirrhosis: expert review. Clin Gastroenterol Hepatol. 2021;19(3):436–45.
32. Diwan TS, Rice TC, Heimbach JK, Schauer DP. Liver transplantation and bariatric surgery: timing and outcomes. Liver Transpl. 2018;24(9):1280–7.
33. Zamora-Valdes D, Watt KD, Kellogg TA, Poterucha JJ, Di Cecco SR, Francisco-Ziller NM. Long-term outcomes of patients undergoing simultaneous liver transplantation and sleeve gastrectomy. Hepatology. 2018;68(2):485–95.
34. Ren M, Zhou X, Zhang Y, et al. Effects of bariatric endoscopy on non-alcoholic fatty liver disease: a comprehensive systematic review and meta-analysis. Front Endocrinol (Lausanne). 2022;13:931519.
35. Vijayaraghavan R, Sarin SK, Bharadwaj A, et al. Intragastric balloon in obese compensated nonalcoholic steatohepatitis cirrhosis patients is safe and achieves significant weight reduction at 6-months. Dig Dis Sci. 2023;68(3):1035–41.
36. Choudhary NS, Puri R, Saraf N, et al. Intragastric balloon as a novel modality for weight loss in patients with cirrhosis and morbid obesity awaiting liver transplantation. Indian J Gastroenterol. 2016;35(2):113–6.
37. Kumar R, García-Compeán D, Maji T. Hepatogenous diabetes: knowledge, evidence, and skepticism. World J Hepatol. 2022;14(7):1291–306.
38. Muñoz AE, Pollarsky FD, Marino M, Cartier M, Vázquez H, Salgado P, Romero G. Addition of statins to the standard treatment in patients with cirrhosis: safety and efficacy. World J Gastroenterol. 2021;27:4639–52.
39. Pose E, Napoleone L, Amin A, et al. Safety of two different doses of simvastatin plus rifaximin in decompensated cirrhosis (LIVERHOPE-SAFETY): a randomised, double-blind, placebo-controlled, phase 2 trial. Lancet Gastroenterol Hepatol. 2020;5:31–41.
40. Musso G, Gambino R, Tabibian JH, Ekstedt M, Kechagias S, Hamaguchi M. Association of non-alcoholic fatty liver disease with chronic kidney disease: a systematic review and meta-analysis. PLoS Med. 2014;11(7):e1001680.
41. Fussner LA, Charlton MR, Heimbach JK, Fan C, Dierkhising R, Coss E. The impact of gender and NASH on chronic kidney disease before and after liver transplantation. Liver Int. 2014;34(8):1259–66.
42. Arora A, Kumar A, Prasad N, et al. INASL-ISN joint position statements on management of patients with simultaneous liver and kidney disease. J Clin Exp Hepatol. 2021;11(3):354–86.
43. Vilar-Gomez E, Vuppalanchi R, Gawrieh S, et al. Vitamin E improves transplant-free survival and hepatic decompensation among patients with nonalcoholic steatohepatitis and advanced fibrosis. Hepatology. 2020;71:495–509.

44. Vilar-Gomez E, Vuppalanchi R, Desai AP, et al. Long-term metformin use may improve clinical outcomes in diabetic patients with non-alcoholic steatohepatitis and bridging fibrosis or compensated cirrhosis. Aliment Pharmacol Ther. 2019;50:317–28.
45. Chalasani N, Abdelmalek MF, Garcia-Tsao G, et al. Effects of Belapectin, an inhibitor of Galectin-3, in patients with nonalcoholic steatohepatitis with cirrhosis and portal hypertension. Gastroenterology. 2020;158(5):1334–1345.e5.
46. Garcia-Tsao G, Bosch J, Kayali Z, et al. Randomized placebo-controlled trial of emricasan for non-alcoholic steatohepatitis-related cirrhosis with severe portal hypertension. J Hepatol. 2020;72(5):885–95.
47. Frenette C, Kayali Z, Mena E, et al. Emricasan to prevent new decompensation in patients with NASH-related decompensated cirrhosis. J Hepatol. 2021;74(2):274–82.
48. De Simone P, Fagiuoli S, Cescon M, De Carlis L, Tisone G, Volpes R. Use of everolimus in liver transplantation: recommendations from a working group. Transplantation. 2017;101(2):239–51.

Chapter 14
Management of Variceal Bleed in Waitlisted Patients

Pankaj Singh and Kaushal Madan

Abstract Management of variceal bleeding in patients on a liver transplantation (LT) waitlist is highly challenging. Treatment approach varies depending on the listing for the type of LT protocol (living donor liver transplant [LDLT]/diseased donor liver transplant [DDLT]). The initial steps of treatment in both protocols are the same. After an episode of controlled index bleed, LDLT candidates should be considered for an early transplant. Delay in transplant due to any reason necessitates initiation of standard treatment in these patients, since recurrent bleeding may lead to further decompensation and other life-threatening complications. DDLT candidates also need to be prioritized in the waitlist, though the timing of transplant still depends on the availability of deceased donors. Hence, these patients should be treated with the standard treatment of care for variceal bleeding. Those with refractory variceal bleed should undergo immediate LT; if immediate LT not possible, rescue therapies like balloon tamponade, self-expanding metal stents (SEMS), or transjugular intrahepatic portosystemic shunt (TIPS) can be used to achieve hemostasis and as a bridge to LT. Preemptive TIPS should be considered early in high-risk patients for recurrent or refractory bleed. For refractory gastric variceal bleed, balloon-occluded retrograde transvenous obliteration (BRTO) and endoscopic ultrasound (EUS)-guided coiling are highly effective in controlling bleeding till liver transplant can be carried out. Appropriate prevention, early recognition, and timely intervention for variceal bleeding in the patient awaiting LT are the keys to a positive outcome in the peri-transplantation period.

Keywords Portal hypertension · Esophageal varices · Fundal varices · Variceal Bleeding · Beta-blocker · Upper gastrointestinal endoscopy · Transjugular Intrahepatic Portosystemic Shunts

---

P. Singh · K. Madan (✉)
Centre for Gastroenterology, Hepatology & Endoscopy, Max Super Specialty Hospital, Saket, New Delhi, India
e-mail: k_madan_2000@yahoo.com

S. Saigal, D. Jothimani (eds.), *Fundamentals of Transplant Hepatology*,
https://doi.org/10.1007/978-981-95-2624-6_14

Key Highlights

- Gastroesophageal varices occur in up to 85% of patients awaiting liver transplantation.
- Acute variceal bleed is a medical emergency where initial fluid resuscitation is mandatory with a target hemoglobin between 7 and 8 g/dL.
- A combination of endoscopic variceal ligation (EVL) and vasoactive drugs (terlipressin) achieves effective hemostasis in 85–90% of the cases.
- SEMS or early TIPS should be considered in patients with refractory variceal bleeding. Decision-making may be challenging in a sick liver patient with multi-organ failure.
- BRTO and EUS-guided coiling are recent modalities in the treatment of refractory gastric variceal bleeding.
- Early liver transplantation should be considered in patients with worsening liver failure following a variceal bleed.

14.1 Introduction

Over the last two decades, liver transplantation (LT) has emerged as the only curative treatment for decompensated liver cirrhosis, acute liver failure, acute-on-chronic liver failure (ACLF), and hepatocellular carcinoma. Worldwide the two LT protocols followed include living donor liver transplant (LDLT) and deceased donor liver transplant (DDLT). European countries and the United States, where the most liver transplants are DDLT, follow a centralized standard criterion for organ allocation and listing patients for liver transplantation depending on the clinical situations and priority for transplant [1]. In India, around 80% of transplantations are LDLT, and there is still a gross inequity in access to liver transplantation. Those registered for DDLT may have to wait for months to years till the cadaveric donors are available [2]. Even in the LDLT settings, the wait time between the decision to transplant and the performance of a transplant may vary from a few days to a few months. Comprehensive management of the waitlisted patients is essential to prevent death or dropout due to worsening in their conditions. It is also imperative to keep them in the best physical and mental state prior to transplant to have better outcomes in the post-transplant period.

Gastroesophageal varices are present in 40–85% of patients with decompensated cirrhosis who are on the waiting list for liver transplant [3]. Despite the best of preventive therapy, acute variceal bleeding tends to occur in approximately 50% of them before transplant and is the leading cause of death in the pre-transplant period, with mortality extending up to 15–20% after the index bleed [4, 5]. The estimated risk of bleeding for the small and large varices is 5% and 15% per year, respectively [6]. The varices usually develop when there is clinically significant portal hypertension, defined as portal pressure as measured by the hepatic venous pressure gradient (HVPG) >10 mmHg; those with HVPG >12 mmHg are at a higher risk of variceal bleeding and those with HVPG >16 have the highest risk of mortality. HVPG reduction by ≥20% or to ≤12 mm Hg is associated with significant reduction in the risk of bleeding and mortality [7]. The risk is even higher in ACLF patients who tend to have a higher HVPG triggered by the associated pro-inflammatory state [8]. All waitlisted patients must have an upper gastrointestinal endoscopy done to screen for varices. Due to limited data on variceal bleeding in the patients awaiting liver transplantation, the preliminary management of variceal bleeding stays the same as in patients with cirrhosis who have not been listed for transplant.

14.2 Management

14.2.1 Primary Prophylaxis of Variceal Bleeding

On screening endoscopy, if no varices are found, no specific therapy is required. But if the patients remain on the waitlist, a repeat endoscopy should be performed in 1 year. If only small varices are present and there is no history of variceal bleeding, primary prophylaxis is not required. If small varices with red color signs are present or with Child-Pugh B or Child-Pugh C liver disease status, non-selective beta-blocker (NSBB) prophylaxis should be started with either carvedilol at a starting dose of 6.25 mg/day and titrated up to a maximum of 12.5 mg/day or propranolol at a starting dose of 20–40 mg twice daily and a maximum of 160 mg/day in patients with ascites and 320 mg/day in patients without ascites [9]. Carvedilol maximal dose titration should be done with the target to maintain systolic blood pressure >90 mmHg, and propranolol dose titration should be done till that target resting heart rate of 55–60 beats/min or systolic blood pressure >90 mmHg is achieved. Beta-blockers act by blocking β1 receptors with a reduction in cardiac output and β2 receptors, causing splanchnic vascular constriction. In a waitlisted patient with medium- or large-sized varices, a reasonable approach should be an early liver transplant if feasible. There are recent studies among waitlisted patients for liver transplantation, where use of beta-blockers has been shown to be associated with better survival. In a study among 322 patients listed for liver transplantation and having ascites (117 with refractory ascites), Leithead et al. demonstrated better transplant-free survival at doses of propranolol 80 mg/day or carvedilol 6.25 mg/day (HR: 0.55; CI: 0.32–0.95; $p = 0.032$) [10].

In another study, 316 patients, 39% with refractory ascites, were being assessed for liver transplantation. Mortality was lower in the group on NSBB (HR: 0.55; CI: 0.33–0.94), but the mortality was not different in the subgroup with refractory ascites. [11]

However, caution should be exercised, or lower doses of beta-blockers (up to 80 mg per day of propranolol or up to 12.5 mg/day of carvedilol) should be used among patients with refractory ascites, and especially those with recent AKI or SBP or sepsis. In such patients, beta-blockers may further reduce the already lower mean arterial pressure and precipitate worsening of the clinical situation. A recent study by Lai et al. concluded that NSBB use is associated with stage 2 AKI and waitlist mortality in patients awaiting liver transplant with Child-Pugh class C cirrhosis [12]. If there is a short delay in transplant, these patients should be started with beta-blockers (if not contraindicated), since endoscopic ligation can be associated with complications like post-ligation ulcer bleeding, which can be life-threatening at times [13]. In those with significant delay in transplant, contraindications to beta-blockers, large varices with high-risk signs (nipple sign/hematocystic spots) or large varices with remote access to endoscopy facility should be offered endoscopic variceal ligation [14, 15]. Repeated variceal ligation should be performed every 3–4 weeks until obliteration of the varices, which may be achieved after two to four sessions.

14.2.2 Acute Variceal Bleeding

Acute variceal bleeding in a waitlisted patient is a medical emergency and should be managed as per the standard guidelines. The patient should be admitted in an intensive care setting, preferably in a liver intensive care unit if available. The management should ideally be aimed at first resuscitating the patient, controlling the bleeding, preventing infection, preventing rebleeding, preventing hepato-renal decompensation, and preventing ACLF.

14.2.3 Resuscitation

Airway protection by means of intubation should be considered in those who are actively bleeding, especially with associated hepatic encephalopathy. A restrictive blood transfusion strategy with a target hemoglobin of 7–9 g/dL is preferred over aggressive transfusion [16]. In patients with decompensated liver cirrhosis, prothrombin time (PT), and international normalized ratio (INR) do not reflect the bleeding tendency; hence, correction of INR in all variceal bleeding with fresh frozen plasma is not recommended. Thromboelastography (TEG)-guided transfusion of blood products is the preferred approach to correct coagulopathy in these patients without compromising hemostasis. A recent randomized trial of 60 patients by Rout et al. has shown a reduced requirement of blood product transfusion in the TEG-guided approach compared to conventional parameters (13% vs. 100%, respectively) [17]. Even among patients of cirrhosis with non-variceal gastrointestinal bleeding, TEG-based correction of coagulopathy (versus standard of care), in an RCT, resulted in lower use of blood products (26.5% vs. 87.2%) without compromising the hemostasis or survival. [18]

Correction of coagulopathy with recombinant activated factor VII (rFVIIa) has not shown any beneficial effect compared to standard therapy in two recent RCTs; hence, it is not recommended [19, 20]. There is no recommendation for management of thrombocytopenia in variceal bleeding. The principle is to control the bleeding source rather than the bleeding tendency.

14.2.4 Pharmacological Management

14.2.4.1 Vasoactive Drugs

Pharmacotherapy with vasoactive agents is meant to decrease portal pressure and should be initiated as soon as possible and prior to endoscopy. Three recommended drugs for this purpose include terlipressin, somatostatin, and octreotide [21]. Early initiation of vascocontrictors is associated with a reduced rate of failure to control bleeding, lower transfusion requirement, and a lower 7-day all-cause mortality. Of all three, terlipressin (2 mg every 4 hours for the first 48 h, followed by 1 mg every 4 h for 5 days) should be the first choice, as it is the only vasoconstrictor with a mortality benefit over placebo [22]. Continuous infusion of terlipressin has shown to be superior to intermittent boluses, not only in terms of achieving early HVPG reduction (71.5% vs. 49.1%) and initial control of bleeding (85.4% vs. 58.2%) but also in terms of fewer adverse events (36.3% vs. 56.4%). [23]

An alternate option if terlipressin is not available or contraindicated is somatostatin (250 mg IV bolus, followed by an infusion of 250 mg/h for 5 days) or octreotide (50–100 mg IV bolus followed by 50 mg/h for 5 days) [24]. The feasibility of a shorter course of vasoconstrictor (1–2 days vs. 3–5 days) [25] was evaluated in a recent meta-analysis in 2018; 42-day mortality was not significantly different. Another RCT in 2015, comparing octreotide therapy for 2 days versus 5 days, showed better cost-effectiveness in the 2-day group but without any statistically significant difference in rebleeding or survival rates [26]. Terlipressin is found to control variceal bleeding in 75–80% of cases in 2 days and around 70% at 5 days [27]. Hence, till further studies are available, the current guidelines recommend IV vasoconstrictors to be continued for 2–5 days. However, the use of terlipressin is not without associated adverse events, and this is an important consideration among patients who are waiting for a liver transplantation. Ischemic complications, such as limb ischemia, mesenteric ischemia, and acute coronary syndrome, have classically been described due to its avid vasoconstrictor properties. A recent RCT highlighted the significant risk of pulmonary complications such as acute respiratory distress syndrome (ARDS) with the use of terlipressin. Of a total of 300 patients with type 1 hepatorenal syndrome (HRS) (199 in the terlipressin group and 101 in the placebo group), respiratory disorders were responsible for death in 22 (11%) patients receiving terlipressin [28].

Therefore, these adverse events should be kept in mind to decide on the duration of therapy, especially among patients who are awaiting liver transplant. In our practice we usually do not continue terlipressin beyond 2–3 days after the initial hemostasis.

14.2.4.2 Antibiotics

Bacterial infection is seen in up to 50% of patients with cirrhosis who present with GI bleeding and is associated with poor outcome [29, 30]. A Cochrane meta-analysis of 12 placebo-controlled trials has shown that antibiotics with gram-negative coverage positively influence survival in variceal bleeding and reduce bacterial infections and early rebleeding [31]. Hence, a short course of prophylactic antibiotics is recommended in all of these patients after admission irrespective of confirmed infection [32]. The best choice of antibiotics in waitlisted patient is intravenous third-generation cephalosporins. Ceftriaxone 1 g/day for a maximum of 7 days is better than oral antibiotics [33]. However, local microbial resistance patterns should be considered in deciding the effective choice of antibiotic in different centers.

14.2.4.3 Proton Pump Inhibitors

In cases of confirmed bleeding due to portal hypertension, PPIs should not be used, since PPIs are found to be associated with increased risk of hepatic encephalopathy and spontaneous bacterial peritonitis [34, 35]. This aspect is particularly important among the patients who are awaiting liver transplantation. Limited evidence suggests that a short course of proton pump inhibitors after endoscopic variceal ligation (EVL) might reduce post-EVL ulcer size without having s significant effect on bleeding or survival [36].

14.2.5 Endoscopic Management

Endoscopic therapy is the cornerstone of the management of variceal bleeding; it should be done as early as possible once hemodynamic stability is achieved and preferably within 12 h of the index bleed [15]. Combination therapy with endoscopic variceal ligation (EVL) and vasoactive drugs is the standard of care and is effective in achieving hemostasis in 85–90% of the cases, reduced 7-day mortality, transfusion requirement, and duration of hospital stay [9]. Endoscopic sclerotherapy is associated with a higher risk for complications; hence, has fallen out of favor over EVL, except when EVL is not technically feasible. On endoscopy, the site of an actively bleeding varix or high-risk stigmata such as a fibrin plug (nipple sign) or red wale sign should be targeted first. Subsequent EVL should be done in spiral fashion proximally from the gastroesophageal junction [37]. Other modalities of endotherapy like endoscopic clipping, argon plasma coagulation, and cyanoacrylate glue have no established role in the management of esophageal variceal bleeding. A 2020 metanalysis including five retrospective studies found that there was no effect of the timing of endoscopy on mortality or rebleeding rates, suggesting that initial resuscitation is critical before performing an endoscopic procedure [38]. Another study showed that urgent endoscopy could be harmful to the patients, possible due to suboptimal resuscitation [39]. Hence suggesting that timing may be individualized according to the patient's clinical condition.

14.3 Refractory Variceal Bleeding

Approximately 20% of the variceal bleeding will be refractory to the conventional endoscopic therapy. Refractory variceal bleeding is defined as either failure to control the bleed or failure of secondary prophylaxis [40].

14.3.1 Rescue Therapy in Refractory Variceal Bleeding

In waitlisted patients with refractory bleeding, the best treatment approach should be consideration for an early liver transplant. Rescue therapies are meant for those who are going to have a delay in transplant due to any reason and cannot be stabilized before transplant because of the ongoing or recurrent bleeds. If the patient is hemodynamically stable and if the initial endoscopy attempt was not done under ideal circumstances, a second endoscopic therapy should always be attempted. If it fails or if the bleeding is severe and the patient is hemodynamically unstable, rescue therapy should be considered. The rescue therapies include balloon tamponade, self-expanding metal stent (SEMS) placement, and shunt procedures (transjugular intrahepatic portosystemic shunt [TIPS]/surgical shunts). Hemostatic powder has also been found to be an effective short-duration (~24 h) rescue therapy or a bridge to a more definitive therapy [41].

14.3.2 Balloon Tamponade and Self-Expanding Metal Stents (SEMS)

Both the balloon tamponade and fully covered SEMS work by the similar principle of the tamponade effect by compressing the bleeding varices in the lower esophagus and aim to achieve temporary hemostasis. Three types of balloons are available: (a) the Sengstaken-Blakemore (SB) tube, most commonly used; (b) the Minnesota tube; and (c) the Linton-Nachlas tube. Balloon tamponade has a high initial success in stopping bleeding (90% hemostasis rate), but recurrent bleeding is seen in approximately half of them within 24 h after deflating the balloon. Esophageal balloon tamponade carries a high risk of complication (20–60%), which increases with duration of placement; hence, its placement should be limited to less than 24 h. The common complications associated with balloon tamponade are esophageal rupture (6–20%), aspiration pneumonitis, asphyxia, and ala-nasi necrosis (since the traction is applied by holding it against the external nares [42]. The recently available SEMS is found to be associated with greater control of bleeding (66% vs. 25% with balloon), fewer complications, reduced requirement for transfusion, and TIPS utilization when compared with balloon tamponade [43]. The pooled clinical and technical success rate of SEMS in controlling the variceal bleed was 96% and 97%, respectively [44]. SX-Ella Danis stent is the most popular SEMS used for uncontrolled esophageal variceal bleeding, it can be easily deployed and removed at endoscopy. As an emergency procedure, the stent can even be placed at the bedside without any fluoroscopic or endoscopic guidance. A meta-analysis including 12 studies of fully covered SEMS for refractory variceal bleeding showed a success rate of 96%, adverse events of 36%, and 30-days survival of 68% [44]. The only disadvantage of SEMS in comparison to Sengstaken-Blakemore tubes is higher cost and inability to use in bleeding from gastric varices. SEMS placement does have associated risks of ulceration, migration (28%), and rebleeding after removal (16%). These stents can be kept in place for up to 7 days, and hence allow more time to plan for a definitive therapy [45]. Therefore, SEMS should be preferred over balloon tamponade when available. Both the balloon tamponade and self-expanding metal stents aim to achieve temporary hemostasis; hence, once the patient is hemodynamically stabilized, a more definitive therapy such as transjugular intrahepatic portosystemic shunt (TIPS) or liver transplant should be planned.

14.3.3 Transjugular Intrahepatic Portosystemic Shunt (TIPS)

Utilization of TIPS after balloon tamponade is effective in controlling bleeding in 90–95% of these patients. The TIPS procedure involves the formation of a radiological shunt by the placement of a stent or graft between a portal vein branch and a hepatic vein, directing the portal blood flow directly into hepatic veins, bypassing the liver. This shunt procedure is highly effective in reducing the portal hypertension and is now considered as the gold standard for refractory variceal bleeding. The complications of TIPS can be stent-related complications like shunt occlusion, stent migration, and hepatic encephalopathy and procedure-related complications are fever, deranged liver function, haemobilia, hepatic capsular laceration, carotid artery puncture, right atrial perforation, and mal-deployment of stent. The use of polytetrafluoroethylene (PTFE)-covered metal stents is preferred over uncovered stents, as it has improved patency and survival and reduced chances of hepatic encephalopathy [46].

14.3.3.1 Rescue/Salvage TIPS

Rescue TIPS is the first-line therapy in patients who fail standard conventional therapy for variceal bleeding and present with persistent severe bleeding or early variceal rebleeding resulting in high mortality. Although in this setting TIPS may be the only means of arresting bleeding, which can be achieved in 90–100% of patients, it may be associated with higher mortality rates. [47] A study by Maimone et al. has shown the 6 and 12 weeks mortality rates of 36% and 42% in patients undergoing salvage TIPS [48]. Hence, proper patient selection is the key to success with this intervention. Rescue/salvage TIPS may be a futile exercise in patients with a Child-Pugh score of more than 13 and should be rather avoided [49]. A recent multicentre study by Walter et al. proposed the combination of MELD score and lactate to predict the 6-week mortality in patients undergoing salvage TIPS and has shown more than 90%, 6-week mortality in patients with a MELD score of ≥30 and serum lactate of ≥12 mmol/L. [50]

14.3.3.2 Preemptive TIPS

The role of TIPS has now evolved from rescue therapy to preemptive TIPS for patients at high risk for treatment failure. Early/preemptive TIPS, within 72 h of variceal bleed in patients with high risk for rebleeding like Child-Pugh C status, Child-Pugh B status with active bleed at endoscopy, HVPG ≥20 after initial control, or MELD score ≥19 has been shown to improve 1-year survival, reduce treatment failure, and improve transplant-free survival [51]. Early PTFE-covered TIPS, in addition to standard therapy (vasoactive drugs plus endoscopic band ligation), followed later by beta-blocker/isosorbide-mononitrate plus endoscopic band ligation (EBL), resulted in a significant reduction in failure to control bleeding, rebleeding, and mortality than those treated with drugs plus EBL. Six-week mortality was reduced from 33% in the drug plus EBL group to 4% in the early TIPS group. Delaying the TIPS and using it as salvage resulted in the loss of 64% of patients in the EBL group [52]. Monescillo et al., demonstrated that early TIPS in patients with HVPG >20 mm Hg have reduced the risk of treatment failure with better survival rates [53]. However, the favorable effect on survival of early TIPS was subsequently found to apply only to patients in the Child-Pugh C status but not to those in the Child-Pugh B status with active bleeding at endoscopy [54, 55]. Another recent prospective study showed lower rebleeding rates for early TIPS when compared with standard therapy; however, the trial failed to show a survival benefit [56]. Another RCT among 117 patients with advanced cirrhosis, demonstrated higher transplant-free survival at 6 weeks and 1 year in the early TIPS group as compared to the standard of care[57].

A 2020 systemic review and meta-analysis (5 studies with 1754 patients), evaluating the role of early TIPS in high-risk patients, found a significant reduction in treatment failure rates in the early TIPS group of 2% compared to 17% in the standard treatment group [58]. The fear that placement of TIPS may make the transplant surgery difficult or post-LT outcomes inferior has not been debunked. A meta-analysis, which analyzed 13 studies, showed that operative times, PRBS transfusions, ICU stays, vascular complications and reinterventions were similar in the groups with or without preoperative TIPS [59].

14.3.4 Secondary Prophylaxis

After an episode of index variceal bleeding, the rebleeding rate at 1 year is around 60%, and mortality from each such episode is 20%. So, Unless the LT is going to be performed early (within a month), the patients on the waitlist, after a bleed, should definitely be put on secondary prophylaxis.

Current guidelines recommend combined therapy with endoscopic variceal ligation plus non-selective beta-blockers (NSBB) as the first-line therapy in the prevention of rebleeding [21]. A large meta-analysis of 23 trials in 1860 patients evaluated the role of combination therapy (EVL plus NSBB) versus either therapy alone, and revealed that the combination therapy group had a higher reduction in overall rebleeding rate than either therapy alone without any difference in survival [60]. In patients with refractory ascites, NSBB should be used with caution and should be discontinued in those with circulatory dysfunction defined by systolic blood pressure <90 mm Hg, serum sodium <130 meq/L, or acute kidney injury [61]. Those patients who rebleed despite being on secondary prophylaxis with NSBB plus EVL should be offered TIPS [62]. Post-TIPS patients do not need further endoscopic or medical therapy for secondary prophylaxis but should be referred for liver transplant in case they have other complications. Patients who have variceal bleeding despite primary prophylaxis with beta-blockers have a higher risk of rebleeding and mortality compared to those who bleed while not on beta-blockers. Though the best approach in these patients is still unknown, preemptive TIPS should be considered instead of NSBB/EVL. In patients with cirrhosis with portal vein thrombosis (PVT), TIPS has been shown to be more effective than EVL plus NSBB in the prevention of rebleeding with a higher likelihood of thrombus resolution, particularly in those awaiting liver transplantation, in whom the presence of PVT has been associated with a high risk of post-transplant mortality [63, 64].

14.4 Gastric Varices

Gastric varices occur in nearly 20% of patients with cirrhosis. First-line treatment for bleeding gastric varices is injection of *N*-butyl-2-cyanoacrylate glue, and this is effective in over 90–95% of patients. Refractory gastric varices bleeding is often severe and difficult to control; hence, should be referred for TIPS. Recent studies of salvage TIPS in refractory gastric variceal bleeding have shown good initial control (96.4% and 90%), but the rebleeding rates were slightly higher as compared with TIPS done for esophageal varices: 29% at 7 months and 31% at 1 year. [65, 66] Hence, ideal approach is to combine TIPS with percutaneous transhepatic variceal embolization (PTVE) or balloon-occluded retrograde transvenous obliteration (BRTO). A prospective comparative study of BRTO versus TIPS with a follow-up of 1 year has shown a much lower rebleeding rate in the BRTO group (8.6%) as compared to the TIPS group (19.8%), with similar rates of mortality [67]. Among

55 patients with failure of endotherapy for gastric variceal bleed, BRTO was able to provide a transplant-free survival rate of 90.4% [68].

In a retrospective review by Saad et al. BRTO in the presence of TIPS (i.e., BTRO+TIPS) reduces the risk of ascites and recurrent post-BRTO bleed as compared to patients who underwent BRTO alone. However, there was no survival benefit between the two groups [69]. Due to the lower risk of ascites, combining BRTO with TIPSS may be a better option among patients awaiting liver transplantation.

Recent evidences suggest endoscopic ultrasound (EUS)-guided endotherapy to be more safer and effective treatment option than direct endoscopic glue injection [70]. The combination of coil embolization and glue injection is associated with lower recurrence rate, requirement of a smaller number of coils, and lesser volume of glue when compared to EUS-guided monotherapy; hence, it is now the preferred modality of treatment for gastric varices [71]. For secondary prophylaxis in patients with isolated gastric varices type 1 (IGV1) and gastroesophageal varices type 2 (GOV2), balloon occluded retrograde transvenous obliteration (BRTO) can be done if gastro/lieno-renal shunts are present [72].

14.4.1 Surgery

14.4.1.1 TIPS Versus Surgical Shunts

TIPS is preferred over shunt surgery because it is associated with less operative morbidity and mortality. Moreover, in patients awaiting liver transplantation, TIPS appears to be a better option than surgery. Rosemurgy et al. compared TIPS with surgical H-graft shunt in a total of 132 patients as a rescue therapy for variceal bleeding. The rebleeding rate was 16% in the TIPS group versus 3% in the surgery group. Thirty-day and total mortality were 15% versus 20% and 43% versus 30% in the TIPS and surgery groups, respectively. This study finally recommended surgery as the best rescue treatment option for refractory variceal bleeding. Limitations of this study were the lack of randomization and the use of uncovered stents for TIPS [73–75]. Several recent studies (especially those using the PTFE-covered stents) with TIPS have reported high success in controlling bleeding in patients with acute treatment failure (90–100%) [76–79]. In the current clinical practice, there is no role for surgical shunts, and the only surgery that should be done in such patients is liver transplantation. Further bridging to transplant can be done with TIPS or BRTO, rather than a surgical shunt.

14.5 Liver Transplantation

Controlled trials comparing EVL or TIPS placement with urgent liver transplant in patients who bleed while on the waiting list are lacking; till then, early or urgent liver transplant, when feasible, is probably the most appropriate approach. Needless to say, that option for urgent liver transplant is valid only for those planned for LDLT and with complete or near-complete donor workup. Those on the waitlist for DDLT still may have to be managed with the best available modality, EVL or TIPS. For high-risk patients (where standard therapy for variceal bleed is likely to fail), preemptive TIPS has the highest success in controlling bleeding with improved 1-year and transplant-free survival. Several prognostic factors in patients with liver cirrhosis with variceal bleed awaiting transplant, such as high Child-Pugh/MELD score, elevated aspartate aminotransferase (AST) levels, shock at admission, portal vein thrombosis, hepatocellular carcinoma, active bleeding at endoscopy on admission, and hepatic venous pressure gradient (HVPG) of 20 mm Hg help in identifying the high-risk patients who should undergo TIPS [80]. Ideal timing of transplantation after an episode of bleeding is still unknown; however, most centers prefer to wait for at least 2 weeks for elective transplantation [81].

14.6 Conclusion

Variceal bleeding in the waitlisted patients is the leading cause of mortality and dropout in the pre-transplant period and is an important predictor of poor outcomes in the post-transplant period. Among those listed for LDLT, the best treatment option is to consider early liver transplant. The increasing need for cadaveric donors continues to put those listed for DDLT to spend a long time on the waiting list, increasing the risk for further decompensation and death. Effective treatment for acute variceal bleeding in waitlisted patients should include optimal resuscitation, early initiation of vasoactive drugs, and timely endoscopic interventions. For secondary prophylaxis, EVL should be combined with a non-selective beta-blocker along with continued treatment of the underlying cause like hepatitis B or C, and alcohol cessation. In the setting of refractory variceal bleeding with significant delay in liver transplant, rescue therapy with temporary placement of balloon tamponade or SEMS is recommended as a bridge to definitive treatment, TIPS, or liver transplant (Fig. 14.1). High-risk individuals should be identified and subjected to preemptive TIPS. Patients who do not undergo TIPS should undergo periodic endoscopic surveillance and EVL to ensure complete eradication of the varices.

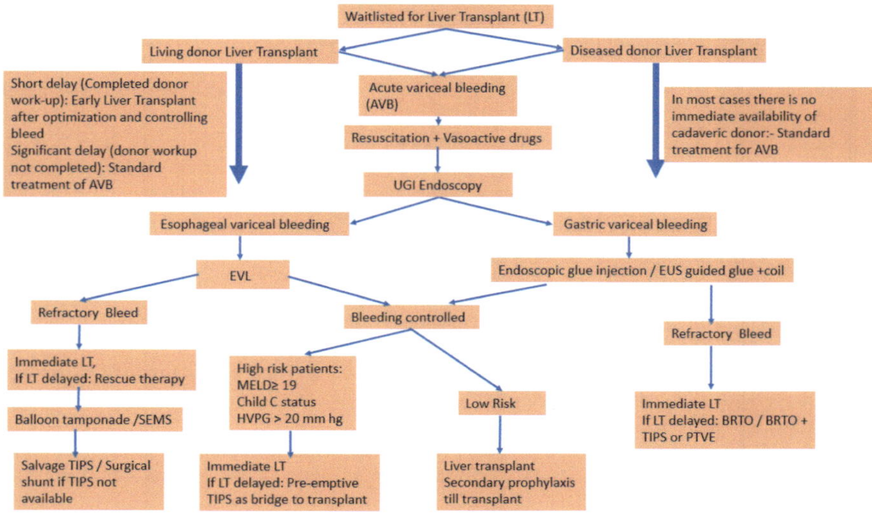

Fig. 14.1 Schematic flowchart for management of variceal bleeding in waitlisted patients

References

1. Kalra A, Biggins SW. New paradigms for organ allocation and distribution in liver transplantation. Curr Opin Gastroenterol. 2018;34:123–31.
2. Narasimhan G, Kota V, Rela M. Liver transplantation in India. Liver Transpl. 2016;22:1019–24.
3. Kovalak M, Lake J, Mattek N, Eisen G, Lieberman D, Zaman A. Endoscopic screening for varices in cirrhotic patients: data from a national endoscopic database. Gastrointest Endosc. 2007;65:82–8.
4. Carbonell N, Pauwels A, Serfaty L, et al. Improved survival after variceal bleeding in patients with cirrhosis over the past two decades. Hepatology. 2004;40:652–9.
5. Reverter E, Tandon P, Augustin S, et al. A MELD-based model to determine risk of mortality among patients with acute variceal bleeding. Gastroenterology. 2014;146:412–9.
6. Garcia-Tsao G, Abraldes JG, Berzigotti A, Bosch J. Portal hypertensive bleeding in cirrhosis: risk stratification, diagnosis, and management: 2016 practice guidance by the American Association for the study of liver diseases. Hepatology. 2017;65:310–35.
7. D'Amico G, Garcia-Pagan JC, Luca A, Bosch J. Hepatic vein pressure gradient reduction and prevention of variceal bleeding in cirrhosis: a systematic review. Gastroenterol. 2006;131:1611–24.
8. Garg H, Kumar A, Garg V, et al. Hepatic and systemic hemodynamic derangements predict early mortality and recovery in patients with acute-on-chronic liver failure. J Gastroenterol Hepatol. 2013;28:1361–7.
9. Garcia-Tsao G, Bosch J. Management of varices and variceal hemorrhage in cirrhosis. N Engl J Med. 2010;362:823–32.
10. Leithead JA, Rajoriya N, Tehami N, Hodson J, et al. Non-selective β-blockers are associated with improved survival in patients with ascites listed for liver transplantation. Gut. 2015;64:1111–9.
11. Onali S, Kalafateli M, Majumdar A, Westbrook R, et al. Non-selective beta-blockers are not associated with increased mortality in cirrhotic patients with ascites. Liver Int. 2017;37:1334–44.

12. Lai M, Fenton C, Ge J, Rubin J, Lai JC, Cullaro G. Nonselective beta-blockers may lead to stage 2 acute kidney injury and wailist mortality in child C cirrhosis. Hepatol Commun. 2023;7:e 0255. https://doi.org/10.1097/HC9.0000000000000255.
13. Albillos A, Penas B, Zamora J. Role of endoscopy in primary prophylaxis for esophageal variceal bleeding. Clin Liver Dis. 2010;14:231–50.
14. Garcia-Tsao G, Sanyal AJ, Grace ND, et al. Practice Guidelines Committee of the American Association for the Study of Liver Diseases; Practice Parameters Committee of the American College of Gastroenterology. Prevention and management of gastroesophageal varices and variceal hemorrhage in cirrhosis. Hepatology. 2007;46:922–38.
15. de Franchis R. Evolving consensus in portal hypertension: report of the Baveno IV consensus workshop on methodology of diagnosis and therapy in portal hypertension. J Hepatol. 2005;43:167–76.
16. Villanueva C, Colomo A, Bosch A, et al. Transfusion strategies for acute upper gastrointestinal bleeding. N Engl J Med. 2013;368:11–21.
17. Rout G, Shalimar GD, et al. Thromboelastography-guided blood product transfusion in cirrhosis patients with variceal bleeding: a randomized controlled trial. J Clin Gastroenterol. 2020;54:255–62.
18. Kumar M, Ahmad J, Maiwall R, Choudhury A, et al. Thromboelastography-guided blood component use in patients with cirrhosis with nonvariceal bleeding: a randomized controlled trial. Hepatology. 2020;71:235–46.
19. Bosch J, Thabut D, Albillos A, et al. Recombinant factor VIIa for variceal bleeding in patients with advanced cirrhosis: a randomized, controlled trial. Hepatology. 2008;47:1604–14.
20. Bosch J, Thabut D, Bendtsen F, et al. Recombinant factor VIIa for upper gastrointestinal bleeding in patients with cirrhosis: a randomized, double-blind trial. Gastroenterology. 2004;127:1123–30.
21. European Association for the Study of the Liver. EASL Clinical Practice Guidelines for the management of patients with decompensated cirrhosis. J Hepatol. 2018;69:406–60.
22. Levacher S, Letoumelin P, Pateron D, et al. Early administration of terlipressin plus glyceryl trinitrate to control active upper gastrointestinal bleeding in cirrhotic patients. Lancet. 1995;346:865–8.
23. Arora V, Choudhary SP, Maiwall R, Vijayaraghavan R, et al. Low-dose continuous terlipressin infusion is effective and safer than intravenous bolus injections in reducing portal pressure and control of acute variceal bleeding. Hepatol Int. 2023;17:131–8.
24. Corley DA, Cello JP, Adkisson W, et al. Octreotide for acute esophageal variceal bleeding: a meta-analysis. Gastroenterology. 2001;120:946–54.
25. Yan P, Tian X, Li J. Is additional 5-day vasoactive drug therapy necessary for acute variceal bleeding after successful endoscopic hemostasis? A systematic review and meta-analysis. Medicine (Baltimore). 2018;97:e12826.
26. Rengasamy S, Ali SM, Sistla SC, Lakshmi CP, Harichandra Kumar KT. Comparison of 2 days versus 5 days of octreotide infusion along with endoscopic therapy in preventing early rebleed from esophageal varices: a randomized clinical study. Eur J Gastroenterol Hepatol. 2015;27:386–92.
27. Ioannou G, Doust J, Rockey DC. Terlipressin for acute variceal hemorrhage. Cochrane Database Syst Rev. 2003:CD002147.
28. Wong F, Pappas SC, Curry MP, Reddy KR, et al. CONFIRM study investigators. Terlipressin plus albumin for the treatment of type 1 Hepatorenal syndrome. N Engl J Med. 2021;384:818-828.
29. Hou MC, Lin HC, Liu TT, et al. Antibiotic prophylaxis after endoscopic therapy prevents rebleeding in acute variceal hemorrhage: a randomized trial. Hepatology. 2004;39:746–53.
30. Pauwels A, Mostefa-Kara N, Debenes B, et al. Systemic antibiotic prophylaxis after gastrointestinal hemorrhage in cirrhotic patients with a high risk of infection. Hepatology. 1996;24:802–6.

31. Chavez-Tapia NC, Barrientos-Gutierrez T, Tellez-Avila F, et al. Meta-analysis: antibiotic prophylaxis for cirrhotic patients with upper gastrointestinal bleeding—an updated Cochrane review. Aliment Pharmacol Ther. 2011;34:509–18.
32. Bernard B, Grange JD, Nguyen K, et al. Antibiotics prophylaxis in cirrhotic patients with gastrointestinal bleeding: a meta-analysis. Hepatology. 1999;29:1655–61.
33. Ferna'ndez J, Ruiz del Arbol L, Gomez C, et al. Norfloxacin versus ceftriaxone in the prophylaxis of infections in patients with advanced cirrhosis and hemorrhage. Gastroenterology. 2006;131:1049–56.
34. Dam G, Vilstrup H, Watson H, et al. Proton pump inhibitors as a risk factor for hepatic encephalopathy and spontaneous bacterial peritonitis in patients with cirrhosis with ascites. Hepatology. 2016;64:1265–72.
35. Janka T, Tornai T, Borbely B, et al. Deleterious effect of proton pump inhibitors on the disease course of cirrhosis. Eur J Gastroenterol Hepatol. 2020;32:257–64.
36. Shaheen NJ, Stuart E, Schmitz SM, et al. Pantoprazole reduces the size of post banding ulcers after variceal band ligation: a randomized, controlled trial. Hepatology. 2005;41:588–94.
37. Poza Cordon J, Froilan Torres C, Burgos Garcia A, et al. Endoscopic management of esophageal varices. World J Gastrointest Endosc. 2012;4:312–22.
38. Jung DH, Huh CW, Kim NJ, Kim BW. Optimal endoscopy timing in patients with acute variceal bleeding: a systematic review and meta-analysis. Sci Rep. 2020;10(1):4046.
39. Huh CW, Kim JS, Jung DH, et al. Optimal endoscopy timing according to the severity of underlying liver disease in patients with acute variceal bleeding. Dig Liver Dis. 2019;51(7):993–8.
40. de Franchis R. Revising consensus in portal hypertension: report of the Baveno V consensus workshop on methodology of diagnosis and therapy in portal hypertension. J Hepatol. 2010;53:762–8.
41. Ibrahim M, El-Mikkawy A, Mostafa I, Devière J. Endoscopic treatment of acute variceal hemorrhage by using hemostatic powder TC-325: a prospective pilot study. Gastrointest Endosc. 2013;78:769–73.
42. D'Amico G, Pagliaro L, Bosch J. The treatment of portal hypertension: a meta-analytic review. Hepatology. 1995;22:332–54.
43. Escorsell À, Pavel O, Cárdenas A, et al. Esophageal balloon tamponade versus esophageal stent in controlling acute refractory variceal bleeding: a multicenter randomized, controlled trial. Hepatology. 2016;63:1957–67.
44. McCarty TR, Njei B. Self-expanding metal stents for acute refractory esophageal variceal bleeding: a systematic review and meta-analysis. Dig Endosc. 2016;28:539–47.
45. Marot A, Trepo E, Doerig C, et al. Self-expanding metal stent should be considered in patients with cirrhosis and uncontrolled variceal bleeding. Hepatology. 2016;64:2273.
46. Bureau C, Garcia Pagan JC, Layrargues GP, et al. Patency of stents covered with polytetrafluoroethylene in patients treated by transjugular intrahepatic portosystemic shunts: long-term results of a randomized multicentre study. Liver Int. 2007;27:742–7.
47. Vangeli M, Patch D, Burroughs AK. Salvage tips for uncontrolled variceal bleeding. J Hepatol. 2002;37:703–4.
48. Maimone S, Saffioti F, Filomia R, et al. Predictors of re-bleeding and mortality among patients with refractory variceal bleeding undergoing salvage transjugular intrahepatic portosystemic shunt (TIPS). Dig Dis Sci. 2019;64:1335–45.
49. Tandon P, Abraldes JG, Keough A, et al. Risk of bacterial infection in patients with cirrhosis and acute variceal hemorrhage, based on child-Pugh class, and effects of antibiotics. Clin Gastroenterol Hepatol. 2015;13:1189–96.
50. Walter A, Rudler M, Olivas P, et al. Combination of model for end stage liver disease and lactate predicts death in patients treated with salvage transjugular intrahepatic portosystemic shunt for refractory variceal bleeding. Hepatology. 2021;74:2085–101.
51. Tripathi D, Stanley AJ, Hayes PC, et al. Transjugular intrahepatic portosystemic stent-shunt in the management of portal hypertension. Gut. 2020;69:1173–92.

52. Garcia-Pagan JC, Caca K, Bureau C, et al. An early decision for PTFE-TIPS improves survival in high-risk cirrhotic patient admitted with an acute variceal bleeding. A multicenter RCT. Hepatology. 2008;48:373A.
53. Monescillo A, Martnez-Lagares F, Ruiz-del-Arbol L, et al. Influence of portal hypertension and its early decompression by TIPS placement on the outcome of variceal bleeding. Hepatology. 2004;40:793–801.
54. Hernández-Gea V, Procopet B, Giráldez Á, et al. Preemptive-TIPS improves outcome in high-risk variceal bleeding: an observational study. Hepatology. 2019;69:282–93.
55. Thabut D, Pauwels A, Carbonell N, et al. Cirrhotic patients with portal hypertension-related bleeding and an indication for early-TIPS: a large multicentre audit with real-life results. J Hepatol. 2017;68:73–81.
56. Dunne PDJ, Sinha R, Stanley AJ, et al. Randomised clinical trial: standard of care versus early-transjugular intrahepatic Porto-systemic shunt (TIPSS) in patients with cirrhosis and oesophageal variceal bleeding. Aliment Pharmacol Ther. 2020;52:98–106.
57. Lv Y, Yang Z, Liu L, Li K, et al. AVB-TIPS Study Group. Early TIPS with covered stents versus standard treatment for acute variceal bleeding in patients with advanced cirrhosis: a randomised controlled trial. Lancet Gastroenterol Hepatol. 2019;4:587–98.
58. Li S, Zhang C, Lin LL, et al. Early-TIPS versus current standard therapy for acute variceal bleeding in cirrhosis patients: a systemic review with meta-analysis. Front Pharmacol. 2020;11:603.
59. Hinojosa-Gonzalez DE, Tellez-Garcia E, Salgado-Garza G, Roblesgil-Medrano A, et al. Intraoperative and postoperative impact of pre-transplantation transjugular intrahepatic portosystemic shunts in orthotopic liver transplantations: a systematic review and meta-analysis. Turk J Surg. 2022;38:121–33.
60. Gonzalez R, Zamora J, Gomez-Camarero J, et al. Meta-analysis: combination endoscopic and drug therapy to prevent variceal rebleeding in cirrhosis. Ann Intern Med. 2008;149:109–22.
61. de Franchis R, Baveno VIF. Expanding consensus in portal hypertension: report of the Baveno VI Consensus Workshop: stratifying risk and individualizing care for portal hypertension. J Hepatol. 2015;63:743–52.
62. Garcia-Tsao G, Abraldes JG, Berzigotti A, et al. Portal hypertensive bleeding in cirrhosis: risk stratification, diagnosis, and management: 2016 practice guidance by the American Association for the study of liver diseases. Hepatology. 2017;65:310–35.
63. Lv Y, Qi X, He C, et al. Covered TIPS versus endoscopic band ligation plus propranolol for the prevention of variceal rebleeding in cirrhotic patients with portal vein thrombosis: a randomised controlled trial. Gut. 2018;67:2156–68.
64. Zanetto A, Rodriguez-Kastro KI, Germani G, et al. Mortality in liver transplant recipients with portal vein thrombosis—an updated meta-analysis. Transpl Int. 2018;31:1318–2.
65. Chau TN, Patch D, Chan YW, Nagral A, Dick R, Burroughs AK. "Salvage" transjugular intrahepatic portosystemic shunts: gastric fundal compared with esophageal variceal bleeding. Gastroenterology. 1998;114:981–7.
66. Barange K, Péron JM, Imani K, Otal P, et al. Transjugular intrahepatic portosystemic shunt in the treatment of refractory bleeding from ruptured gastric varices. Hepatology. 1999;30:1139–43.
67. Lee SJ, Kim SU, Kim MD, et al. Comparison of treatment outcomes between balloon-occluded retrograde transvenous obliteration and transjugular intrahepatic portosystemic shunt for gastric variceal bleeding hemostasis. J Gastroenterol Hepatol. 2017;32:1487–94.
68. Mukund A, Rangarh P, Shasthry SM, Patidar Y, Sarin SK. Salvage balloon occluded retrograde transvenous obliteration for gastric variceal bleed in cirrhotic patients with endoscopic failure to control bleed/very early rebleed: long-term outcomes. J Clin Exp Hepatol. 2020;10:421–8.
69. Saad WE, Wagner CC, Lippert A, et al. Protective value of TIPS against the development of hydrothorax/ascites and upper gastrointestinal bleeding after balloon-occluded retrograde transvenous obliteration (BRTO). Am J Gastroenterol. 2013;108:1612–9.

70. Bick BL, Al-Haddad M, Liangpunsakul S, Ghabril MS, DeWitt JM. EUS-guided fine needle injection is superior to direct endoscopic injection of 2-octyl cyanoacrylate for the treatment of gastric variceal bleeding. Surg Endosc. 2019;33:1837–45.
71. Bhat YM, Weilert F, Fredrick RT, et al. EUS-guided treatment of gastric fundal varices with combined injection of coils and cyanoacrylate glue: a large U.S. experience over 6 years (with video). Gastrointest Endosc. 2016;83:1164–72.
72. Fukuda T, Hirota S, Sugimura K. Long-term results of balloon-occluded retrograde transvenous obliteration for the treatment of gastric varices and hepatic encephalopathy. J Vasc Interv Radiol. 2001;12:327–36.
73. Rosemurgy AS, Goode SE, Zwiebel BR, et al. A prospective trial of transjugular intrahepatic portasystemic stent shunts versus small-diameter prosthetic H-graft portacaval shunts in the treatment of bleeding varices. Ann Surg. 1996;224:378–84.
74. Rosemurgy AS, Serafini FM, Zweibel BR, et al. Transjugular intrahepatic portosystemic shunt vs. small-diameter prosthetic H-graft portacaval shunt: extended follow-up of an expanded randomized prospective trial. J Gastrointest Surg. 2000;4:589–97.
75. Bureau C, Garcia-Pagan JC, Pomier-layrargues G, et al. Improved clinical outcome using polytetrafluoroethylene-coated stents for TIPS: results of a randomized study. Gastroenterology. 2004;126:469–75.
76. Gerbes AL, Gulberg V, Waggershauser T, et al. Transjugular intrahepatic portosystemic shunt (TIPS) for variceal bleeding in portal hypertension: comparison of emergency and elective interventions. Dig Dis Sci. 1998;43:2463–9.
77. Chau TN, Patch D, Chan YW, et al. "Salvage" transjugular intrahepatic portosystemic shunts: gastric fundal compared with esophageal variceal bleeding. Gastroenterology. 1998;114:981–7.
78. LaBerge JM, Somberg KA, Lake JR, et al. Two-year outcome following transjugular intrahepatic portosystemic shunt for variceal bleeding: results in 90 patients. Gastroenterology. 1995;108:1143–51.
79. Sanyal AJ, Freedman AM, Luketic VA, et al. Transjugular intrahepatic portosystemic shunts for patients with active variceal hemorrhage unresponsive to sclerotherapy. Gastroenterology. 1996;111:138–46.
80. Bambha Kiran, Ray Kim W, Pedersen Rachel A, et al. Predictors of rebleeding and mortality following acute variceal hemorrhage in patients with cirrhosis. Gut. 2008;57:814–20.
81. Sharma M, Alla M, Kulkarni A, Nagaraja Rao P, Nageshwar Reddy D. Managing a prospective liver transplant recipient on the waiting list. J Clin Exp Hepatol. https://doi.org/10.1016/j.jceh.2023.06.003.

Chapter 15
Renal Dysfunction in Liver Disease

Satender Pal Singh and Rakhi Maiwall

Abstract Reduced renal blood flow and glomerular filtration rate are the hallmarks of hepatorenal syndrome (HRS), the manifestation of renal dysfunction in cirrhotic patients. When kidney function tests are deranged, yet there is no sign of intrinsic kidney disease, such as proteinuria, hematuria, or abnormal kidney ultrasonography, the condition is known as hepatorenal syndrome. Hepatorenal syndrome, which results from functional alterations in the renal circulation and is treatable with vasoconstrictor medications, is different from other causes of acute kidney injury (AKI). Depending on how severe and rapidly the kidney injury is progressing, there are two distinct types of hepatorenal syndrome. The first, HRS-AKI, is an acute kidney dysfunction, whereas the second, HRS-chronic kidney disease (CKD), is a more persistent kidney dysfunction. In this review, we discuss the definition, pathophysiology, assessment, management, and future perspective of renal dysfunction in cirrhosis.

Keywords Renal dysfunction · Hepatorenal syndrome · Cirrhosis · Albumin · Terlipressin · Noradrenaline

Abbreviations

ACLF	Acute on chronic liver failure
AKD	Acute kidney disease
AKI	Acute kidney injury
AKIN	Acute kidney injury network
ATN	Acute tubular necrosis

S. P. Singh
Department of Transplant Hepatology, Institute of Liver and Biliary Sciences, New Delhi, India

R. Maiwall (✉)
Department of Hepatology, Institute of Liver and Biliary Sciences, New Delhi, India
e-mail: rakhi_2011@yahoo.co.in

S. Saigal, D. Jothimani (eds.), *Fundamentals of Transplant Hepatology*,
https://doi.org/10.1007/978-981-95-2624-6_15

BUN	Blood urea nitrogen
CKD	Chronic kidney disease
CTP	Child-Turcotte-Pugh
DAMP	Damage-associated molecular pattern
GFR	Glomerular filtration rate
HRS	Hepatorenal syndrome
ICA	International club of ascites
KDIGO	Kidney disease improving global outcomes
KIM	Kidney injury molecule
LT	Liver transplantation
MAP	Mean arterial pressure
MDRD	Modification of diet in renal disease
MELD	Model for end stage liver disease
NGAL	Neutrophil Gelatinase-associated lipocalin
OPN	Osteopontin
PAMP	Pathogen-associated molecular patterns
PRA	Plasma renin activity
RIFLE	Risk, Injury, Failure, Loss, End-stage renal failure
SMT	Standard medical therapy
sCr	Serum creatinine
TERLI	Terlipressin
TIMP	Tissue inhibitors of metalloproteinases

Key Highlights
- Hepatorenal syndrome (HRS-AKI) is a specific form of renal dysfunction in patients with cirrhosis.
- There has been a paradigm change in the definition and management of HRS-AKI.
- Patients with HRS-AKI may develop repeated episodes and chronic kidney disease.
- Liver transplantation is recommended for patients with HRS-AKI.
- Biomarkers of tubular injury could guide the diagnosis of HRS-AKI and differentiation from acute tubular necrosis.

15.1 Introduction

Renal dysfunction is a common, life-threatening complication in patients with liver disease. Types of renal dysfunction include HRS-AKI and HRS-NAKI. NAKI-HRS is further subdivided into AKD and CKD. Hepatorenal syndrome (HRS) has been defined as a purely "functional" type of renal dysfunction that often occurs in patients with cirrhosis in the setting of marked abnormalities in arterial circulation, as well as overactivity of the endogenous vasoactive systems [1]. Around 20% of the patients who are hospitalized with liver cirrhosis and ascites gradually progress to develop acute kidney injury (AKI), and 20% among these develop hepatorenal syndrome (HRS) [2]. AKI is defined as an increase in serum creatinine ≥0.3 mg/dl within 48 h or >50% from baseline value in the last 7 days, according to the ICA consensus document and/or urinary output <0.5 ml/kg B.W. >6 h. Acute kidney disease (AKD) is defined as structural and/or functional abnormalities characterised by GFR <60 mL/min/ 1.73 m^2 for less than 3 months or an increase in serum creatinine level by >50% for less than 3 months. AKI is a subset of AKD; therefore, any patient with AKI, by definition, has AKD. Chronic kidney disease (CKD) is defined as abnormalities in kidney structure or function (GFR <60 ml/min/1.72 m^2) that persist for >90 days. Apart from known factors, older age, presence of diabetes, obesity, hypertension, and recurrent AKI predispose cirrhosis patients to the risk of CKD [3].

15.2 Evolving Definitions of AKI

In May 2004, the RIFLE criteria were introduced, incorporating the terms risk, injury, failure, loss, and end-stage renal disease (ESRD) to assess kidney function [4]. These classifications were based on changes in serum creatinine (sCr) levels and/or urine output. However, limitations included the equal weighting of sCr and urine output in evaluating kidney function and the instability of glomerular filtration rate (GFR) measurements. To address these issues, the Acute Kidney Injury Network (AKIN) revised the RIFLE criteria in 2007, aiming to improve the recognition and understanding of AKI. The AKIN system also categorizes AKI into three stages—risk, injury, and failure—but omits GFR as a diagnostic parameter [5].

In 2012, the Kidney Disease: Improving Global Outcomes (KDIGO) guidelines were introduced, drawing upon both the AKIN and RIFLE criteria. KDIGO combines elements from both systems, aiming to enhance diagnostic utility, though its reliability and sensitivity still require further validation in clinical settings. The International Ascites Club (IAC) also proposed a definition for AKI, excluding urine output due to challenges in measurement accuracy, diuretic influence, and collection difficulties. A study by Amathieu et al. highlighted the importance of oliguria in critically ill patients with chronic liver disease, showing that including urine output in diagnostic criteria increased AKI detection rates and that stage 2–3 AKI identified through urine output (AKI-UO) was significantly associated with higher hospital mortality [6]. As a result, experts have emphasized the importance of retaining urine output criteria for patients with cirrhosis. (See Table 15.1 for a summary of criteria.)

Table 15.1 Evolving diagnostic criteria in AKI

Rifle criteria	AKIN criteria	KDIGO criteria
Diagnostic criteria		
Increase in sCr to ≥1.5 times baseline within 7 days; GFR decrease >25%; or urine volume	Increase in sCr by ≥0.3 mg/dl (26.5 μmol/L) within 48 h; increase in sCr ≥ 1.5 times baseline within 48 h; or urine volume < 0.5 ml/kg/h for 6 h	Increase in sCr by 0.3 mg/dl (26.5 μmol/L) within 48 h; increase in sCr to ≥1.5 times baseline that is known or presumed to have occurred within the previous 7 days; or urine volume < 0.5 ml/kg/h for 6 h
Staging criteria		
Risk: sCr increase of 1.5–1.9 times baseline; GFR decrease of 25–50%; or urine output <0.5 ml/kg/h for 6 h Injury: sCr increase of 2.0–2.9 times baseline; GFR decrease of 50–75%; or urine output <0.5 ml/kg/h for 12 h Failure: Scr increase ≥3.0 times baseline; GFR decrease of 50–75%; Scr increase ≥4.0 mg/dl (353.6 μmol/L) with an acute increase of at least 0.5 mg/dl (44 μmol/L); urine output <0.3 ml/kg/h for ≥24 h; or anuria for ≥12 h	Stage 1: sCr increase of 1.5–1.9 times baseline; sCr increase ≥0.3 mg/dl (26.5 μmol/L); or urine output <0.3 ml/kg/h for ≥24 h; or anuria for ≥12 h Stage 2: sCr increase of 2.0–2.9 times baseline or urine output <0.3 ml/kg/h for ≥24 h; or anuria for ≥12 h Stage 3: sCr increase of 3.0 times baseline; sCr increase ≥4.0 mg/dl (353.6 μmol/L) with an acute increase of at least 0.5 mg/dl (44 μmol/L); urine output <0.3 ml/kg/h for ≥24 h; or anuria for ≥12 h	Stage 1: sCr increase of 1.5–1.9 times baseline; sCr increase ≥0.3 mg/dl (26.5 μmol/L); or urine output <0.5 ml/kg/h for 6–12 h Stage 2: sCr increase of 2.0–2.9 times baseline or urine output <0.5 ml/kg/h for ≥12 h Stage 3: sCr increase of 3.0 times baseline; sCr increase to ≥4.0 mg/dl (353.6 μmol/L); initiation of renal replacement therapy; urine output <0.3 ml/kg/h for ≥24 h; or anuria for ≥12 h

AKD acute kidney disease, *AKI* acute kidney injury, *CKD* chronic kidney disease, *eGFR* estimated GFR, *HRS* hepatorenal syndrome, *sCr* serum creatinine

15.3 Spectrum of Renal Dysfunction in Liver Cirrhosis

HRS is often precipitated by hepatic (alcohol abuse, drugs, or flare of hepatitis) and/or extrahepatic (bacterial infections and/or bacterial translocation) factors. The definition of subtypes of HRS is based on whether renal dysfunction is acute (AKI), sub-acute (AKD), or chronic (CKD).

15.3.1 Acute Kidney Injury

Acute kidney injury (AKI) is caused by a number of etiologies that either cause direct injury to the kidney (structural injury) or temporarily limit its function (functional injury). AKI can have prerenal, intrarenal, intrinsic (acute tubular necrosis, acute interstitial nephritis, acute glomerular and vasculitis renal disorders), and/or post-renal (acute obstructive nephropathy) causes in individuals with cirrhosis in the same way it can in patients without cirrhosis [7]. The next step in the assessment of AKI in cirrhosis is to diagnose AKI phenotypes, namely, acute tubular necrosis AKI (ATN-AKI), prerenal AKI, HRS-AKI, and post-renal AKI. The majority of prerenal AKI cases may be treated with plasma volume expansion, and post-renal AKI is uncommon; therefore, the clinical problem is in separating HRS-AKI from HRS-NAKI. As a marker of renal injury, sCr has a diagnostic disadvantage in that it cannot differentiate between functional and structural etiologies of AKI. Tubular injury biomarkers reflect structural injury and, thus, when appearing in conjunction with a decrease in GFR, should indicate that the change is attributable to structural damage [8].

15.3.2 *Acute and Chronic Kidney Disease*

KDIGO guidelines define CKD as abnormalities in kidney structure or function (GFR <60 ml/min/1.72 m^2) that persist for >90 days, and AKD as AKI or as abnormalities in kidney structure or function (GFR <60 ml/min/1.72 m^2) that persist for <90 days [9]. It is challenging to arrive at a new, more precise definition of HRS-2 because it wasn't defined clearly and was simply assumed to be higher chronic abnormalities in sCr without a clear timeline [10]. Recently, the acute disease quality initiative (ADQI) proposed considering AKI and AKD as a continuum, where AKI is considered to have evolved to AKD when it persists for ≥7 days after the precipitating event [11].

Importantly, the new definition helps clinicians to define the presence of HRS-AKI superimposed on CKD in a patient with structural damage of the kidney, as evidenced by an abnormal biopsy, renal ultrasonography, or significant proteinuria (i.e., diabetic nephropathy) [12]. The rising prevalence of cirrhosis caused by Non-alcoholic steatohepatitis/Metabolic dysfunction-assocated steatohepatitis is associated with comorbidities such as diabetes mellitus and arterial hypertension, which can lead to structural CKD. Classification is summarized in Table 15.2.

Table 15.2 Classification of HRS-AKI and HRS-NAKI

Old classification	New classification		Criteria
HRS 1	HRS-AKI		a. Absolute increase in sCr ≥0.3 mg/dl within 48 h and/or b. Urinary output ≤0.5 ml/kg B.W. ≥6 h c. Percent increase in sCr 50% using the last available value of outpatient sCr within 3 months as the baseline
HRS 2	HRS-NAKI	HRS-AKD	a. eGFR <60 ml/min per 1.73 m^2 for <3 months in the absence of other (structural) causes b. Percent increase in sCr <50% using the last available value of outpatient sCr within 3 months as the baseline
		HRS-CKD	eGFR <60 ml/min per 1.73 m^2 for ≥3 months in the absence of other (structural) causes

AKD acute kidney disease, *AKI* acute kidney injury, *CKD* chronic kidney disease, *eGFR* estimated GFR, *HRS* hepatorenal syndrome, *sCr* serum creatinine

15.4 Pathophysiology of Hepatorenal Syndrome

The primary contributor to renal dysfunction in cirrhosis is a hyperdynamic circulatory state. Portal hypertension triggers the increased synthesis and release of endogenous vasodilators—such as nitric oxide, carbon monoxide, and cannabinoids—primarily into the splanchnic arterial system. This results in an expanded plasma volume and enhanced splanchnic blood flow, ultimately causing a decline in effective arterial blood volume and a reduction in mean arterial pressure (MAP) [13].

Understanding the pathogenesis and management of HRS also involves recognizing the roles of cirrhotic cardiomyopathy and relative adrenal insufficiency, both of which are associated with worsening renal function and increased mortality [14]. Cirrhotic patients often exhibit subclinical signs of cardiac abnormalities, including diastolic dysfunction, and a blunted response to both inotropic and chronotropic stimulation.

Initially, compensatory mechanisms activate to preserve perfusion to vital organs—these include an increase in cardiac output (CO) and stimulation of vasoconstrictive systems such as the renin-angiotensin-aldosterone system, the sympathetic nervous system, and secretion of arginine vasopressin. In advanced cases, the heart fails to sustain an adequate CO, leading to compromised MAP and systemic circulation. As a result, renal hypoperfusion and dysfunction arise due to both decreased MAP and intensified renal vasoconstriction [15].

Infections, particularly spontaneous bacterial peritonitis, and the systemic circulatory disturbances characteristic of HRS are largely driven by bacterial translocation [16]. This process activates monocytes via pathogen-associated molecular patterns (PAMPs), including bacterial endotoxins and DNA. Activated monocytes release proinflammatory cytokines such as tumor necrosis factor-alpha (TNF-α), interleukin-6 (IL-6), and interleukin-1 beta (IL-1β). This inflammatory cascade, coupled with microvascular dysfunction, intensifies the impact of both PAMPs and damage-associated molecular patterns (DAMPs) on proximal tubule epithelial cells, further contributing to renal injury [17] as shown in Fig. 15.1.

15.5 Assessment of Renal Dysfunction in Cirrhosis

Urinalysis: A clean-catch specimen is used for analysis. Glomerular diseases often manifest as proteinuria and microscopic hematuria and are commonly accompanied by hypertension and edema. Findings may include red and white blood cells, cellular casts, proteinuria, and—if infection is present—bacteria, positive nitrites, and leukocyte esterase.

Complete Blood Count (CBC): Anemia may indicate chronic kidney disease, bleeding, or acute inflammation. Elevated white blood cell counts suggest possible

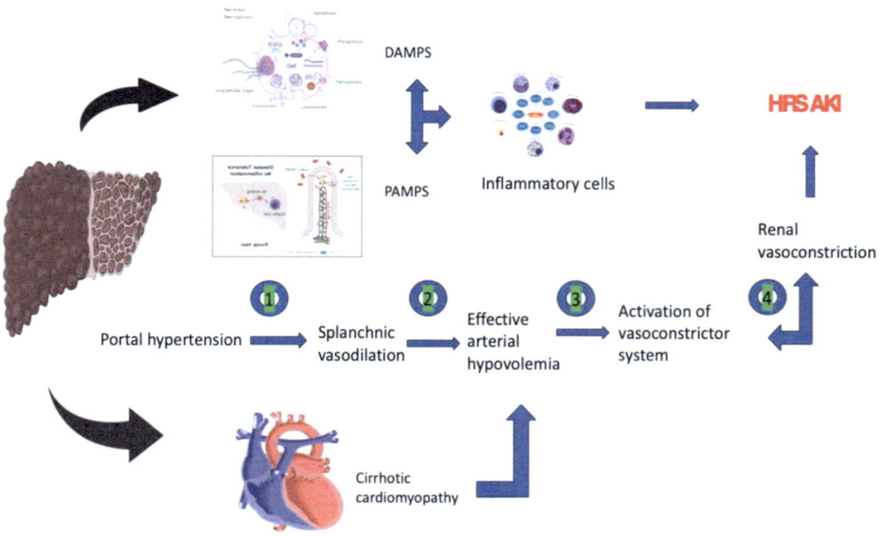

Fig. 15.1 Pathogenesis of HRS and AKI in cirrhosis (1). Patients with cirrhosis present with a marked splanchnic arterial vasodilation due to portal hypertension; (2) Splanchnic vasodilation causes a decrease in systemic vascular resistance leading to effective arterial hypovolemia; (3) There is activation of endogenous vasoconstrictors such as the renin-angiotensin-aldosterone system, sympathetic nervous system, and arginine vasopressin; and (4) The activation of these systems leads to renal vasoconstriction, inducing a decrease in GFR and development of HRS. A decrease in CO may contribute to a decrease in effective arterial blood volume. PAMPs and DAMPs, derived from bacterial translocation and from injured liver, may activate circulating innate immune cells, leading to an inflammatory response. The inflammatory mediators may lead to impairment of circulatory dysfunction and, consequently, kidney tissue damage

infection. Thrombocytopenia can occur in rare conditions such as cryoglobulinemia, hemolytic uremic syndrome, or thrombotic microangiopathy.

Fractional Excretion of Sodium (FENa): Useful in differentiating types of renal dysfunction. A low FENa (<1%) supports a diagnosis of prerenal azotemia and is typically <0.2% in hepatorenal syndrome, provided tubular function is intact. Elevated FENa can also result from diuretic use [18]. The formula is:

$$\text{FENa} = \left(\text{Urine Na} \times \text{Serum Creatinine}\right) / \left(\text{Serum Na} \times \text{Urine Creatinine}\right) \times 100\%$$

Urine Osmolality: Assesses tubular response to antidiuretic hormone and overall tubular function during hypovolemia. It is elevated in prerenal azotemia (though the influence of substances like dyes and mannitol should be excluded) and approximates serum osmolality in acute tubular necrosis.

Urine Sodium and Protein-to-Creatinine Ratio (PCR) [19]:

- Urine Na >20 mEq/L: Suggests acute tubular necrosis, though not diagnostic by itself.
- Urine Na <20 mEq/L: Indicates sodium retention, often seen in prerenal azotemia due to renal hypoperfusion.
- Urine PCR values:
  - <0.3: Suggestive of acute kidney injury (AKI)
  - 0.3–3.0: Indicates mixed etiology
  - >3.0: Suggests structural kidney damage

GFR Estimation Equations: Formulas such as Cockcroft-Gault, MDRD, and CKD-EPI are commonly used to estimate glomerular filtration rate (GFR). However, these often overestimate GFR in cirrhotic patients. The Cockcroft-Gault equation is particularly unreliable due to its dependence on body weight, which can be distorted by ascites and edema in cirrhosis. Alternative methods, including CKD-EPI equations using cystatin C, have demonstrated improved accuracy in assessing renal function in this population [20].

Renal Biopsy: Typically performed when serologic tests suggest glomerulonephritis or when the cause of kidney injury remains unclear. Biopsy can help confirm diagnoses like acute tubular necrosis, glomerulonephritis, vasculitis, or other intrinsic renal diseases, although it is not routinely used for diagnosing acute tubular necrosis alone.

15.5.1 Biomarkers

Timely identification of acute kidney injury (AKI) and accurate assessment of renal function are essential in the management of patients with cirrhosis. However, AKI is often underdiagnosed in this population due to underlying abnormalities. Urine output is not a reliable indicator of renal function or glomerular filtration rate (GFR) in cirrhotic patients. Factors like third-spacing can lead to reduced urine output, giving a false impression of impaired renal function, while diuretic use may mask dysfunction by falsely elevating urine output.

Serum creatinine (sCr) remains the most commonly used marker for estimating GFR due to its availability, affordability, and general reliability. Nevertheless, its accuracy is affected by variables such as age, race, gender, and muscle mass. Cirrhotic patients often suffer from malnutrition, muscle wasting, and sarcopenia, resulting in low creatinine levels that may overestimate true GFR and kidney function [21].

This issue has raised concerns over the inclusion of sCr in MELD-based scoring systems (MELD, MELD-Na, and MELD 3.0), as it may lead to misrepresentation of renal function and inappropriate prioritization for liver transplantation [22]. Additionally, elevated bilirubin levels in cirrhotic patients can interfere with Jaffe's kinetic assay, producing falsely low sCr readings and further distorting the assessment of renal function.

Research by Solé et al. demonstrated the potential of kidney injury biomarkers to detect tubular damage. These biomarkers could be instrumental in guiding clinical decisions regarding whether to proceed with combined liver-kidney transplantation or liver transplantation alone in cirrhotic patients with AKI being evaluated for transplant [23].

Cystatin C is a low-molecular-weight protein that is produced by all nucleated cells. It is filtered by the glomerulus and mainly reabsorbed by the proximal tubule. Despite the limitations, cystatin C is not affected by age, muscle mass, malignancy, or inflammation. The assay, unlike sCr, is not affected by high levels of serum bilirubin. Maiwall et al. studied 531 patients with cirrhosis and showed cystatin C but not sCr as an independent predictor of new AKI on multivariate analysis. Incorporation of cystatin C into components of MELD, that is, the "MELD-Cystatin" score, predicted the development of AKI and mortality and performed significantly better than the MELD and CTP scores [24]. In a recent meta-analysis of 25 studies, estimating GFR in cirrhosis using creatinine-based and cystatin C-based equations showed that creatinine-based equations overestimated GFR as compared to cystatin C-based equations. Also, equations based on both creatinine and cystatin C were the least biased. All equations significantly overestimated GFR (+21.7 mL/minute/1.73 m^2; 95% CI, 17.7–25.7) at GFR <60 mL/minute/1.73 m^2; of these, chronic kidney disease-Epi-cystatin C and GFR Assessment in Liver Disease were the least biased, followed by Royal Free Hospital and Modification of Diet in Renal Disease 6 [25].

NGAL is a small protein made by the kidney, lung, stomach, and colon. Previous studies have shown that NGAL was upregulated in prerenal AKI and ATN settings and that increased urinary NGAL could be detected within 2 h of initial renal injury. Multiple studies have evaluated the efficacy and utility of urinary NGAL in cirrhotic patients with AKI. Studies have found that urinary NGAL is superior to cystatin C in the utility for the diagnosis of AKI or ATN. Barreto et al. showed patients with AKI ($n = 65$) had significantly higher levels of uNGAL compared to patients without AKI (203 ± 390 vs. 79 ± 126 μg/g creatinine, $p < 0.001$). Moreover, uNGAL levels were significantly higher in patients who developed persistent AKI ($n = 40$), compared to those with transient AKI ($n = 25$) (281 ± 477 vs. 85 ± 79 μg/g creatinine, $p < 0.001$). Among patients with persistent AKI, uNGAL was able to discriminate type-1 HRS from other causes of AKI (59 ± 46 vs. 429 ± 572 μg/g creatinine, respectively; $p < 0.001$) [26]. Kim et al studied urinary NGAL and cystatin C in 328 decompensated cirrhosis patients (41 patients with AKI). The authors found that urinary NGAL is a predictor of AKI and outcomes (including mortality) [27]. Recently, Huelin et al studied urinary NGAL and IL-18 in 320 cirrhosis patients with AKI. Urinary NGAL was elevated in AKI progression during hospitalization and was predictive of AKI progression in conjunction with the MELD score [28]. Yewale et al. studied urine NGAL in 147 patients for complications of decompensated cirrhosis, showing that urine NGAL was highest in acute tubular necrosis (ATN), lowest in prerenal azotemia, and intermediate in hepatorenal syndrome (HRS-AKI). A cut-off of 203.9 ng/mL discriminated between HRS and PRA with 77.8% sensitivity and 68.7% specificity. Urine NGAL correlated with MELD-Na score, need for ICU stay, in-hospital mortality, and mortality at 3 and 6 months [29]. Allegreti et al. also studied urinary NGAL in a prospective cohort of 213 US hospitalized patients with decompensated cirrhosis (161 with AKI and 52 reference patients without AKI). At an optimal cut point of 244 μg/g creatinine, NGAL distinguished ATN (344 [132–1429] μg/g creatinine) from prerenal AKI (45 [0–154] μg/g) or HRS (110 [50–393] μg/g; $P < 0.001$), with a C statistic of 0.762 [30].

Interleukin-18 (IL-18) is a proinflammatory cytokine produced in the proximal tubules and is released into the urine when these cells are damaged during acute kidney injury (AKI). Urinary IL-18 levels are notably elevated in AKI caused by ischemic injury, but they typically remain normal in cases involving urinary tract infections, nephrotoxic damage, or chronic kidney disease (CKD). A study by Tsai et al. in 2013 assessed 168 cirrhotic patients with AKI and severe sepsis. The researchers observed that urinary IL-18 levels were significantly higher in those with acute tubular necrosis (ATN) compared to patients with functional AKI. They proposed a diagnostic threshold of 708.5 pg/mg creatinine to distinguish between these two conditions. Urinary IL-18 proved to be a more reliable marker for ATN than serum IL-18, and higher urinary IL-18 concentrations were also linked to increased hospital mortality [31].

KIM-1 is elevated in AKI from ischemic injury to the proximal tubule. Belcher et al evaluated KIM-1 in patients with AKI with other etiologies (PRA, ATN, and HRS) and found that ATN was the most elevated, with overlap with HRS [32]. Other studies found that in patients with cirrhosis, elevations in urinary KIM-1 levels were increased mainly in ATN compared to other AKI presentations and could serve as a prognostic indicator. Lei et al. showed that urinary KIM-1, urinary NGAL, serum Cys C, and the combined detection factor can help in the early diagnosis of AKI secondary to decompensated cirrhosis [33].

L-FABP is a small protein found in the proximal tubular epithelium and binds to free fatty acids when reabsorbed in the proximal tubule. L-FABP may be elevated in sepsis and specific etiologies of CKD (diabetic nephropathy or glomerulonephritis). Eguchi et al studied L-FABP in 242 chronic liver disease patients (chronic hepatitis, liver cirrhosis, and hepatocellular carcinoma). The authors found that serum L-FABP increased in liver cirrhosis compared to chronic hepatitis and is higher in the presence of hepatocellular carcinoma [34]. Kulkarni et al. studied 25 patients with alcohol-ACLF and showed adipocyte-FABP is highly sensitive at predicting mortality and outcome. L-FABP correlates with kidney function markers, especially BUN, creatinine, and GFR. This study demonstrates the potential of L-FABP for predicting outcomes in chronic liver disease and other complications, including AKI [35].

15.5.2 Recovery and Non-recovery Markers

Levitsky J in 2014 used a combined model including elevated OPN and TIMP-1 levels, age <57, and absence of diabetes and showed that plasma protein profiles might improve the prediction of pre-LT kidney injury recovery after LT [36]. Later in 2019, Levitsky J used a cohort of patients undergoing LT to independently validate a published pre-LT model predictive of post-transplant renal recovery [Renal Recovery Assessment at Liver Transplant (REVERSE)]. A study showed that patients with elevated pre-LT serum levels of OPN and TIMP-1 had recovery of renal function correlated with decreases in the levels of both proteins. At 4 weeks post-LT (n = 77 subset), the largest decline in OPN and TIMP-1 was seen in the recovered AKI group [37]. Maiwall et al. also studied that non-resolution of acute kidney injury in the first week predicts the development of chronic kidney disease in critically ill patients with cirrhosis. A study showed that higher NGAL, renal tubular epithelial cells, or granular casts were independent predictors of AKI-NR and CKD development [38].

15.5.3 Other Markers

Two new biomarkers being studied for potential benefits are insulin-like growth factor binding protein-7 and tissue matrix metalloproteinase inhibitor-2 by Zhang et al. They showed that TIMP-2.IGFBP7 is not suitable for the diagnosis of HRS or prediction of therapy responses. Still, it can play a prognostic role in predicting mortality in liver cirrhosis patients [39]. Kerbert et al. studied extracellular matrix biomarkers in cirrhosis with acute decompensation, stable cirrhosis, and healthy controls and showed disrupted turnover of collagen types III and VI in decompensated cirrhosis with or without ACLF. Plasma biomarkers of these collagens (PRO-C3 and PRO-C6) were associated with the severity of liver dysfunction and inflammation. PRO-C6, also known as the hormone endotrophin, was also found to be associated with multi-organ failure and prognosis in acute decompensation and ACLF [40].

15.6 Treatment

15.6.1 Albumin

Albumin has pleiotropic effects, the most important being oncotic action and anti-inflammatory properties. Also, albumin is capable of maintaining or increasing the CO even in the most advanced phases of liver disease [41]. To date, the correct dose of albumin to be given to a patient of decompensated cirrhosis, HRS-AKI, is a mystery because of the non-tolerability of albumin injection as given in previous guidelines. So, the limitations of using albumin alone, first, are that the dose needed to obtain and to maintain an effective improvement of the cardio-circulatory function as well as an anti-inflammatory effect is quite high (1.5 g/kg of bodyweight/week). The second is that while exerting its non-oncotic actions, the albumin molecule undergoes post-translational changes that reduce its biological potential; as a result, either the pre-treatment concentration of endogenous effective albumin or the dose of exogenous effective albumin administered is the need of the hour in HRS [42]. Table 15.3 provides a summary of the albumin studies conducted in cirrhosis.

15.6.2 Vasoconstrictors

15.6.2.1 Terlipressin

Randomized controlled trials have demonstrated that the combination of terlipressin plus albumin is more effective than albumin alone in the treatment of HRS. Terlipressin can be administered both as intravenous boluses (starting from 0.5–1 mg every 4–6 h to a maximum dose of 2 mg every 4 h) and as continuous intravenous infusions (starting from 2 mg/day to a maximum dose of 12 mg/day). The latter administration has been associated with a significantly lower incidence of severe side effects, which include persistent diarrhea, abdominal ischemia, peripheral ischemia, angina pectoris, and circulatory overload. These findings are probably consistent with the short-term effect (3–4 h) of terlipressin on portal pressure. The dose of terlipressin should be increased in a stepwise manner if sCr does not decrease by at least 25% after 3 days of treatment. In patients with no response or partial response, the treatment should be discontinued within 14 days. Despite higher rates of response to terlipressin and albumin in patients with type 2 HRS, recurrence of HRS is quite common. HRS-2, now termed HRS-NAKI, cannot be considered an indication for the use of terlipressin plus albumin even in patients who are on the waiting list for LT [41].

15.6.2.2 Noradrenaline

Noradrenaline has demonstrated a favorable safety profile, is widely accessible, and is more cost-effective compared to other options, making it a potentially advantageous treatment for hepatorenal syndrome (HRS). As a catecholamine, it primarily acts on alpha-adrenergic receptors. Adverse effects are generally mild and self-limiting, with some patients reporting atypical chest pain despite a normal electrocardiogram and cardiac enzyme findings.

In a study by Alessandria et al., HRS reversal was achieved in 70% (7 out of 10) of patients treated with noradrenaline, compared to 83% (10 out of 12) with

Table 15.3 Studies of albumin in Cirrhosis

Study	Methodology	Renal dysfunction	Conclusion
Caraceni et al. [43] ANSWER study	Patients were randomized to SMT or SMT plus HA (40 g twice weekly for 2 weeks and then 40 g weekly) for up to 18 months	The incidence rate ratio of HRS type 1 with its 95% CI was <0.5, indicating a significant reduction in the SMT plus HA group	Long-term HA administration prolongs overall survival and acts as a disease-modifying treatment in patients with decompensated cirrhosis
Sanyal et al. [44] REVERSE trial	Patients received intravenous terlipressin 1–2 mg every 6 h plus albumin or placebo plus albumin for up to 14 days	HRS reversal was significantly more frequent with terlipressin vs. placebo (27% vs. 14%; $P = 0.004$)	Terlipressin plus albumin resulted in a significantly higher rate of HRS reversal vs. albumin alone in patients with HRS-1
Cavallin et al. [45] Italian study group	To compare the effectiveness of terlipressin plus albumin versus midodrine and octreotide plus albumin in the treatment of HRS	There was a higher rate of recovery of renal function in the TERLI group (19/27, 70.4%) compared to the MID/OCT group (6/21, 28.6%)	Terlipressin plus albumin is more effective than midodrine and octreotide plus albumin in improving renal function in patients with HRS
Wong et al. [46] CONFIRM investigators	Patients were randomly assigned in a 2:1 ratio to receive terlipressin plus albumin or placebo plus albumin.	Reversal of HRS was reported in 63 patients (32%) in the terlipressin group and 17 patients (17%) in the placebo group ($P = 0.006$).	Terlipressin and albumin infusion were more effective than placebo in improving renal function.
China et al. [47] ATTIRE investigators	Patients were randomly assigned to the targeted 20% albumin solution arm till 14 days or discharge and to standard-care arm	Kidney dysfunction occurred in (10.5%) the albumin group and (14.4%) of the standard-care group	Albumin infusions to a target of 30 g per liter or more were not more beneficial than the current standard care
Sola et al. [48] MACHT investigators	Patients were randomly assigned to receive midodrine (15–30 mg/day) and albumin (40 g/15 days) or matching placebos for one year	Treatment with midodrine and albumin was associated with HRS reversal and a decrease in plasma renin activity and aldosterone compared to placebo	Treatment with midodrine and albumin slightly suppressed the activity of vasoconstrictor systems

Studies of albumin in cirrhosis. *SMT* Standard medical therapy, *HA* Human albumin, *HRS* Hepatorenal syndrome, *Terli* Terlipressin, Mid: Midodrine, *OCT* Octreotide

terlipressin [49]. Similarly, Duvoux et al. reported HRS reversal in 83% of patients (10 out of 12; 95% CI: 52%–98%) after a median treatment duration of 7 days (range: 5–10 days) [50].

Sharma et al. found noradrenaline to be an effective and safe alternative to terlipressin for improving renal function. Their multivariate analysis identified baseline creatinine clearance, mean arterial pressure (MAP), and plasma renin activity as independent predictors of treatment response [51]. Additionally, a randomized controlled trial by Singh et al. concluded that noradrenaline was as effective and safe as terlipressin in treating HRS, with the added benefit of lower cost. The study also found that the baseline Child-Turcotte-Pugh (CTP) score could predict treatment response [52].

15.6.3 Midodrine

Midodrine (an a1-agonist drug) combined with octreotide (a somatostatin analogue), together with albumin infusion, has been shown to be effective in treating HRS-1. However, in a small, single center, randomized controlled trial, the combination of terlipressin plus albumin was shown to be significantly more effective than the combination of midodrine plus octreotide and albumin in the treatment of HRS (improvement of renal function in 70 vs. 29%, respectively; $p = 0.01$) [45]. Esrailian compared the survival of HRS patients who received octreotide and midodrine treatment at Rancho Los Amigos Medical Center with a concurrent untreated control group of HRS patients who did not receive this treatment. Of the 81 patients, 60 were treated with octreotide/midodrine and 21 were controls. Mortality was significantly lower in the treatment group (43%) than in the controls (71%; $P < 0.05$). Furthermore, 24 study patients (40%) had a sustained reduction of serum creatinine compared with only 2 controls (10%; $P < 0.05$). The study suggested that octreotide/midodrine treatment appears to improve 30-day survival [53]. Transjugular intrahepatic portosystemic shunt (TIPS) has been shown to improve kidney function and clinical outcomes in patients with functional kidney disease and refractory ascites. Kidney function improves after TIPS in patients with HRS-NAKI, while combining midodrine, octreotide, and albumin with TIPS might improve kidney function in selected patients with HRS-AKI.

15.6.4 Transplantation

The use of creatinine in the MELD score has demonstrated the increased importance for patients with renal dysfunction (HRS-AKI or HRS-CKD) to undergo LT. In the setting of HRS, Boyer et al. reported a survival advantage of 100% vs. 34% in patients with HRS treated with terlipressin and LT compared to patients treated with terlipressin alone [41]. Although LT remains the only definitive treatment of HRS-AKI, the role of the liver and even simultaneous liver-kidney transplant (SLK) remains unclear in the setting of non-HRS-AKI. In a large retrospective study comparing survival in HRS-AKI patients after undergoing SLK vs cirrhotic patients with non-HRS-AKI undergoing the same, HRS-AKI patients' survival post-transplant was significantly superior to that in the non-HRS-AKI group [54]. For patients with cirrhosis and CKD, SLK was recommended for patients with epidermal GFR (eGFR) less than 60 mL/min for at least 90 d before listing or eGFR less than 35 mL/min during the time of listing or inherited metabolic disease. In patients with cirrhosis and AKI, there must be a combination of dialysis and eGFR <25 mL/min for 6 weeks [55].

15.7 Renal Replacement Therapy

The start of renal replacement therapy (RRT) in cirrhosis should be tailored to the individual, guided by the evolving status of both kidney and liver function, and ideally instituted before clear-cut complications emerge. Early RRT is reasonable when there is clinical or investigational evidence of intravascular fluid overload unresponsive to diuretics—even without overt AKI [56]. Because cirrhotic patients are predisposed to hepatic encephalopathy, and uremic features can mimic uraemia, consider an earlier threshold for RRT when encephalopathy persists despite appropriate therapy. Selection of modality should reflect local expertise and infrastructure, balanced against procedure-specific risks. In those listed for, or being assessed for, liver transplantation, RRT should be used proactively to stabilise physiology and serve as a bridge to transplant. For patients ineligible for transplantation, engage the patient and caregivers in frank goals-of-care discussions, emphasising the guarded prognosis and the very low transplant-free survival, particularly at high MELD scores [57]. DIALIVE, a novel extracorporeal liver support system, demonstrated modest improvements in kidney function in patients with liver disease. By exchanging dysfunctional albumin and removing inflammatory mediators, DIALIVE directly targets key pathophysiological mechanisms but needs further validation. In contrast, albumin dialysis using the molecular adsorbent recirculating system and Prometheus in cirrhosis showed no significant survival benefit [58].

15.8 Future Perspective

Metabolomic profiling may be a new tool for identifying biomarkers of renal dysfunction in patients with cirrhosis, allowing for the early diagnosis of HRS, predicting response to HRS treatment, and native kidney recovery after liver transplantation, all of which are important in decision-making regarding the need for SLKT. The future should also see further developments in the prediction models of morbidity and mortality in patients with cirrhosis and HRS-AKI so as to improve our management of these patients.

15.9 Conclusion

HRS-AKI is a form of AKI in cirrhosis. It is a diagnosis of exclusion. Recent changes in diagnostic criteria now allow HRS-AKI to be diagnosed at a lower level of sCr, facilitating the earlier institution of treatment. Vasoconstrictors are the mainstay of treatment, with terlipressin being the most commonly used worldwide. Vasoconstrictors are usually given in conjunction with albumin, but care needs to be taken not to overdose patients with albumin. Timely assessment for liver transplant is necessary, as these patients still have a high mortality rate despite responding to pharmacotherapy because of their advanced liver dysfunction. Combined liver-kidney transplant should be considered for patients with underlying CKD or with prolonged pre-transplant RRT.

Conflict of Interest None of the authors has any relevant conflict of interest as it relates to this work.

Financial Support Statement None.

References

1. Bucsics T, Krones E. Renal dysfunction in cirrhosis: acute kidney injury and the hepatorenal syndrome. Gastroenterol Rep (Oxf). 2017;5(2):127–37. https://doi.org/10.1093/gastro/gox009. Epub 2017 Apr 24. PMID: 28533910
2. Ripoll C, Platzer S, Franken P, et al. Liver-HERO Study Group. Liver-HERO: hepatorenal syndrome-acute kidney injury (HRS-AKI) treatment with transjugular intrahepatic portosystemic shunt in patients with cirrhosis-a randomized controlled trial. Trials. 2023;24(1):258. https://doi.org/10.1186/s13063-023-07261-9. PMID: 37020315; PMCID: PMC10077612
3. Angeli P, Garcia-Tsao G, Nadim MK, Parikh CR. News in pathophysiology, definition and classification of hepatorenal syndrome: a step beyond the International Club of Ascites (ICA) consensus document. J Hepatol. 2019;71(4):811–22. https://doi.org/10.1016/j.jhep.2019.07.002. Epub 2019 Jul 11. PMID: 31302175
4. Lopes JA, Jorge S. The RIFLE and AKIN classifications for acute kidney injury: a critical and comprehensive review. Clin Kidney J. 2013;6(1):8–14. https://doi.org/10.1093/ckj/sfs160. Epub 2012 Jan 1. PMID: 27818745; PMCID: PMC5094385
5. Kim JH, Kim YS, Choi MS, et al. Prediction of clinical outcomes after kidney transplantation from deceased donors with acute kidney injury: a comparison of the KDIGO and AKIN criteria. BMC Nephrol. 2017;18(1):39. https://doi.org/10.1186/s12882-017-0461-5. Published 2017 Jan 27
6. Amathieu R, Al-Khafaji A, Sileanu FE, et al. Significance of oliguria in critically ill patients with chronic liver disease. Hepatology. 2017;66(5):1592–600. https://doi.org/10.1002/hep.29303. Epub 2017 Sep 26. PMID: 28586126
7. Rosi S, Piano S, Frigo AC, et al. New ICA criteria for the diagnosis of acute kidney injury in cirrhotic patients: can we use an imputed value of serum creatinine? Liver Int. 2015;35(9):2108–14. https://doi.org/10.1111/liv.12852. Epub 2015 May 7. PMID: 25900355
8. Francoz C, Nadim MK, Durand F. Kidney biomarkers in cirrhosis. J Hepatol. 2016;65(4):809–24. https://doi.org/10.1016/j.jhep.2016.05.025. Epub 2016 May 26. PMID: 27238754

9. Khwaja A. KDIGO clinical practice guidelines for acute kidney injury. Nephron Clin Pract. 2012;120(4):c179–84. https://doi.org/10.1159/000339789. Epub 2012 Aug 7. PMID: 22890468
10. Wong F, Nadim MK, Kellum JA, et al. Working party proposal for a revised classification system of renal dysfunction in patients with cirrhosis. Gut. 2011;60(5):702–9. https://doi.org/10.1136/gut.2010.236133. Epub 2011 Feb 15. PMID: 21325171
11. Chawla LS, Bellomo R, Bihorac A, et al. Acute disease quality initiative workgroup 16. Acute kidney disease and renal recovery: consensus report of the acute disease quality initiative (ADQI) 16 workgroup. Nat Rev Nephrol. 2017;13(4):241–57. https://doi.org/10.1038/nrneph.2017.2. Epub 2017 Feb 27. PMID: 28239173
12. Subedi A, Suresh Kumar VC, Sharma Subedi A, et al. A review of hepatorenal syndrome. Cureus. 2021;13(7):e16084. https://doi.org/10.7759/cureus.16084. PMID: 34367745; PMCID: PMC8330394
13. Yeung E, Yong E, Wong F. Renal dysfunction in cirrhosis: diagnosis, treatment and prevention. MedGenMed. 2004;6(4):9. PMID: 15775836; PMCID: PMC1480573
14. Singh SP, Mondia N. Adrenal insufficiency associated with low high-density lipoprotein (HDL) in patients of chronic liver disease. Ind J Clin Med. 2023;13(1):6–10. https://doi.org/10.1177/26339447221142358.
15. Gassanov N, Caglayan E, Semmo N, et al. Cirrhotic cardiomyopathy: a cardiologist's perspective. World J Gastroenterol. 2014;20(42):15492–8. https://doi.org/10.3748/wjg.v20.i42.15492. PMID: 25400434; PMCID: PMC4229515
16. Hartleb M, Gutkowski K. Kidneys in chronic liver diseases. World J Gastroenterol. 2012;18(24):3035–49. https://doi.org/10.3748/wjg.v18.i24.3035. PMID: 22791939; PMCID: PMC3386317
17. Kany S, Vollrath JT, Relja B. Cytokines in inflammatory disease. Int J Mol Sci. 2019;20(23):6008. https://doi.org/10.3390/ijms20236008. PMID: 31795299; PMCID: PMC6929211
18. Urrunaga NH, Mindikoglu AL, Rockey DC. Renal dysfunction in cirrhosis. Curr Opin Gastroenterol. 2015;31(3):215–23. https://doi.org/10.1097/MOG.0000000000000168. PMID: 25763790; PMCID: PMC4416403
19. Rognant N, Lemoine S. Evaluation of renal function in patients with cirrhosis: where are we now? World J Gastroenterol. 2014;20(10):2533–41. https://doi.org/10.3748/wjg.v20.i10.2533. PMID: 24627589; PMCID: PMC3949262
20. El-Makarem, M.A.ER.A, Mousa, et al. Comparative study of various glomerular filtration rate estimating equations in Egyptian patients with hepatitis C virus-related liver cirrhosis: a single-center observational study. Egypt Liver J. 2021;11:23. https://doi.org/10.1186/s43066-021-00093-9.
21. Gupta K, Bhurwal A, Law C, et al. Acute kidney injury and hepatorenal syndrome in cirrhosis. World J Gastroenterol. 2021;27(26):3984–4003. https://doi.org/10.3748/wjg.v27.i26.3984. PMID: 34326609; PMCID: PMC8311533
22. Singh SP, Maiwall R. MELD 3.0: a better score for liver allocation? Liver Transpl. 2023;23 https://doi.org/10.1097/LVT.0000000000000180. Epub ahead of print. PMID: 37212479
23. Solé C, Ma AT, Solà E, et al. Sequential changes in urinary biomarker levels in patients with cirrhosis and severe hepatorenal syndrome. Liver Int. 2021;41(11):2729–32. https://doi.org/10.1111/liv.15069. Epub 2021 Oct 5. PMID: 34569697
24. Maiwall R, Kumar A, Bhardwaj A, et al. Cystatin C predicts acute kidney injury and mortality in cirrhotics: a prospective cohort study. Liver Int. 2018;38(4):654–64. https://doi.org/10.1111/liv.13600. Epub 2017 Oct 19. PMID: 28941301
25. Singapura P, Ma TW, Sarmast N, et al. Estimating glomerular filtration rate in cirrhosis using creatinine-based and cystatin C-based equations: systematic review and meta-analysis. Liver Transpl. 2021;27(11):1538–52. https://doi.org/10.1002/lt.26216. Epub 2021 Aug 1. PMID: 34143570

26. Barreto R, Elia C, Solà E, et al. Urinary neutrophil gelatinase-associated lipocalin predicts kidney outcome and death in patients with cirrhosis and bacterial infections. J Hepatol. 2014;61(1):35–42. https://doi.org/10.1016/j.jhep.2014.02.023. Epub 2014 Mar 5. PMID: 24613364
27. Kim TH, Seo YS, Kang SH, et al. Korean Study Group of Portal Hypertension. Prognosis predictability of serum and urine renal markers in patients with decompensated cirrhosis: a multicentre prospective study. Liver Int. 2020;40(12):3083–92. https://doi.org/10.1111/liv.14631. PMID: 32750739
28. Huelin P, Solà E, Elia C, et al. Neutrophil gelatinase-associated Lipocalin for assessment of acute kidney injury in cirrhosis: a prospective study. Hepatology. 2019;70(1):319–33. https://doi.org/10.1002/hep.30592. Epub 2019 Apr 25. PMID: 30810244
29. Yewale RV, Ramakrishna BS, Venugopal G, et al. Urine neutrophil gelatinase-associated lipocalin as a biomarker of acute kidney injury and prognosis in decompensated chronic liver disease: a prospective study. Indian J Gastroenterol. 2023;42(1):106–17. https://doi.org/10.1007/s12664-022-01312-w. Epub 2023 Feb 10. PMID: 36763249; PMCID: PMC9913035
30. Allegretti AS, Parada XV, Endres P, et al. HRS-HARMONY study investigators. Urinary NGAL as a diagnostic and prognostic marker for acute kidney injury in cirrhosis: a prospective study. Clin Transl Gastroenterol. 2021;12(5):e00359. https://doi.org/10.14309/ctg.0000000000000359. PMID: 33979307; PMCID: PMC8116001
31. Tsai MH, Chen YC, Yang CW, et al. Acute renal failure in cirrhotic patients with severe sepsis: value of urinary interleukin-18. J Gastroenterol Hepatol. 2013;28(1):135–41. https://doi.org/10.1111/j.1440-1746.2012.07288.x. PMID: 23034155
32. Belcher JM, Sanyal AJ, Peixoto AJ, et al. TRIBE-AKI Consortium. Kidney biomarkers and differential diagnosis of patients with cirrhosis and acute kidney injury. Hepatology. 2014;60(2):622–32. https://doi.org/10.1002/hep.26980. Epub 2014 Jun 26. PMID: 24375576; PMCID: PMC4065642
33. Lei L, Li LP, Zeng Z, et al. Value of urinary KIM-1 and NGAL combined with serum Cys C for predicting acute kidney injury secondary to decompensated cirrhosis. Sci Rep. 2018;8(1):7962. https://doi.org/10.1038/s41598-018-26226-6. PMID: 29784944; PMCID: PMC5962573
34. Eguchi A, Hasegawa H, Iwasa M, et al. Serum liver-type fatty acid-binding protein is a possible prognostic factor in human chronic liver diseases from chronic hepatitis to liver cirrhosis and hepatocellular carcinoma. Hepatol Commun. 2019;3(6):825–37. https://doi.org/10.1002/hep4.1350. PMID: 31168516; PMCID: PMC6545868
35. Kulkarni AV, Sharma M, Kumar P, et al. Adipocyte fatty acid-binding protein as a predictor of outcome in alcohol-induced acute-on-chronic liver failure. J Clin Exp Hepatol. 2021;11(2):201–8. https://doi.org/10.1016/j.jceh.2020.07.010. Epub 2020 Jul 28. PMID: 33746445; PMCID: PMC7953014
36. Levitsky J, Baker TB, Jie C, et al. Plasma protein biomarkers enhance the clinical prediction of kidney injury recovery in patients undergoing liver transplantation. Hepatology. 2014;60(6):2017–26. https://doi.org/10.1002/hep.27346. Epub 2014 Oct 29. PMID: 25078558
37. Levitsky J, Asrani SK, Abecassis M, et al. External validation of a Pretransplant biomarker model (REVERSE) predictive of renal recovery after liver transplantation. Hepatology. 2019;70(4):1349–59. https://doi.org/10.1002/hep.30667. Epub 2019 May 28. PMID: 31002431
38. Maiwall R, Pasupuleti SSR, Hidam AK, et al. Non-resolution of acute kidney injury in the first week portends the development of chronic kidney disease in critically ill patients with cirrhosis. Aliment Pharmacol Ther. 2023; https://doi.org/10.1111/apt.17639. Epub ahead of print. PMID: 37455381
39. Zhang CC, Hoffelt DAA, Merle U. Urinary cell cycle arrest biomarker [TIMP-2]·[IGFBP7] in patients with hepatorenal syndrome. Biomarkers. 2019;24(7):692–9. https://doi.org/10.1080/1354750X.2019.1652347. Epub 2019 Aug 22. PMID: 31389249
40. Kerbert AJC, Gupta S, Alabsawy E, et al. Biomarkers of extracellular matrix formation are associated with acute-on-chronic liver failure. JHEP Rep. 2021;3(6):100355. https://doi.org/10.1016/j.jhepr.2021.100355. PMID: 34805815; PMCID: PMC8581571

41. Boyer TD, Sanyal AJ, Wong F, et al. REVERSE study investigators. Terlipressin plus albumin is more effective than albumin alone in improving renal function in patients with cirrhosis and Hepatorenal syndrome type 1. Gastroenterology. 2016;150(7):1579–1589.e2. https://doi.org/10.1053/j.gastro.2016.02.026. Epub 2016 Feb 16. PMID: 26896734
42. Bernardi M, Maggioli C, Zaccherini G. Human albumin in the management of complications of liver cirrhosis. Crit Care. 2012;16(2):211. https://doi.org/10.1186/cc11218. PMID: 22429536; PMCID: PMC3681351
43. Caraceni P, Riggio O, Angeli P, et al. ANSWER Study Investigators. Long-term albumin administration in decompensated cirrhosis (ANSWER): an open-label randomised trial. Lancet. 2018;391(10138):2417–29. https://doi.org/10.1016/S0140-6736(18)30840-7. Epub 2018 Jun 1. Erratum in: Lancet. 2018 Aug 4;392(10145):386. PMID: 29861076
44. Sanyal AJ, Boyer T, Garcia-Tsao G, et al. Terlipressin Study Group. A randomized, prospective, double-blind, placebo-controlled trial of terlipressin for type 1 hepatorenal syndrome. Gastroenterology. 2008;134(5):1360–8. https://doi.org/10.1053/j.gastro.2008.02.014. Epub 2008 Feb 13. PMID: 18471513; PMCID: PMC3730280
45. Cavallin M, Kamath PS, Merli M, et al. Italian Association for the Study of the liver study group on hepatorenal syndrome. Terlipressin plus albumin versus midodrine and octreotide plus albumin in the treatment of hepatorenal syndrome: a randomized trial. Hepatology. 2015;62(2):567–74. https://doi.org/10.1002/hep.27709. Epub 2015 Feb 13. PMID: 25644760
46. Wong F, Pappas SC, Curry MP, et al. CONFIRM Study Investigators. Terlipressin plus albumin for the treatment of type 1 hepatorenal syndrome. N Engl J Med. 2021;384(9):818–28. https://doi.org/10.1056/NEJMoa2008290. PMID: 33657294
47. China L, Freemantle N, Forrest E, et al. ATTIRE trial investigators. A randomized trial of albumin infusions in hospitalized patients with cirrhosis. N Engl J Med. 2021;384(9):808–17. https://doi.org/10.1056/NEJMoa2022166. PMID: 33657293
48. Solà E, Solé C, Simón-Talero M, et al. Midodrine and albumin for prevention of complications in patients with cirrhosis awaiting liver transplantation. A randomized placebo-controlled trial. J Hepatol. 2018;69(6):1250–9. https://doi.org/10.1016/j.jhep.2018.08.006. Epub 2018 Aug 21. PMID: 30138685
49. Alessandria C, Ottobrelli A, Debernardi-Venon W, et al. Noradrenalin vs terlipressin in patients with hepatorenal syndrome: a prospective, randomized, unblinded, pilot study. J Hepatol. 2007;47(4):499–505. https://doi.org/10.1016/j.jhep.2007.04.010. Epub 2007 May 24. PMID: 17560680
50. Duvoux C, Zanditenas D, Hézode C, et al. Effects of noradrenalin and albumin in patients with type I hepatorenal syndrome: a pilot study. Hepatology. 2002;36(2):374–80. https://doi.org/10.1053/jhep.2002.34343. PMID: 12143045
51. Sharma P, Kumar A, Shrama BC, Sarin SK. An open label, pilot, randomized controlled trial of noradrenaline versus terlipressin in the treatment of type 1 hepatorenal syndrome and predictors of response. Am J Gastroenterol. 2008;103(7):1689–97. https://doi.org/10.1111/j.1572-0241.2008.01828.x. Epub 2008 Jun 28. PMID: 18557715
52. Singh V, Ghosh S, Singh B, et al. Noradrenaline vs. terlipressin in the treatment of hepatorenal syndrome: a randomized study. J Hepatol. 2012;56(6):1293–8. https://doi.org/10.1016/j.jhep.2012.01.012. Epub 2012 Feb 6. PMID: 22322237
53. Esrailian E, Pantangco ER, Kyulo NL, et al. Octreotide/Midodrine therapy significantly improves renal function and 30-day survival in patients with type 1 hepatorenal syndrome. Dig Dis Sci. 2007;52(3):742–8. https://doi.org/10.1007/s10620-006-9312-0. PMID: 17235705
54. Modi RM, Patel N, Metwally SN, Mumtaz K. Outcomes of liver transplantation in patients with hepatorenal syndrome. World J Hepatol. 2016;8(24):999–1011. https://doi.org/10.4254/wjh.v8.i24.999. PMID: 27648152; PMCID: PMC5002501
55. Enestvedt CK. PRO: simultaneous liver-kidney transplantation in the current era: still the best option. Clin Liver Dis (Hoboken). 2021;16(6):266–71. https://doi.org/10.1002/cld.980. PMID: 33489100; PMCID: PMC7805296

56. Maiwall R, Singh SP, Angeli P, et al. APASL clinical practice guidelines on the management of acute kidney injury in acuteon-chronic liver failure. Hepatol Int. 2024;18(3):833–869. https://doi.org/10.1007/s12072-024-10650-0.
57. Nadim MK, Kellum JA, Forni L, et al. Acute kidney injury in patients with cirrhosis: Acute Disease Quality Initiative (ADQI) and International Club of Ascites (ICA) joint multidisciplinary consensus meeting. J Hepatol. 2024;81(1):163–183. https://doi.org/10.1016/j.jhep.2024.03.031.
58. Agarwal B, Cañizares RB, Saliba F, Ballester MP, Tomescu R, Martin D, et al. Randomised, controlled clinical trial of the DIALIVE liver dialysis device versus standard of care in patients with acute-on-chronic liver failure. J Hepatol 2023;79:79–92.

Chapter 16
Sepsis in Cirrhosis: Challenges, Timely Diagnosis, and Optimal Antibiotic Strategies

Satender Pal Singh, Omkar Rudra, and Dinesh Jothimani

Abstract Sepsis is a major complication in patients with liver cirrhosis, leading to worsening of hepatic decompensation and acute on-chronic liver failure, with an associated mortality ranging between 38% and 70%. The underlying pathogenesis involves cirrhosis-associated immune dysfunction (CAID), altered gut microbiota, and intestinal permeability, leading to systemic inflammation. Assessment and management strategies for sepsis in cirrhotic patients are complex, necessitating early identification and aggressive treatment. Fluid resuscitation, vasopressor therapy, and antibiotic administration are critical components of care, but response to treatment may not be achievable in sick liver patients. Early initiation of broad-spectrum antibiotics followed by appropriate antibiotics is important to reduce bacterial resistance. Future directions include the potential of metagenomics for rapid pathogen identification and innovative therapies to address antibiotic resistance. This comprehensive review highlights the intricate relationship between liver cirrhosis and sepsis, emphasizing the need for tailored management approaches to improve patient outcomes.

Keywords Cirrhosis · Sepsis · Infection

S. P. Singh · O. Rudra
Department of Transplant Hepatology, Institute of Liver and Biliary Sciences, New Delhi, India

D. Jothimani (✉)
Institute of Liver Disease and Transplantation, Dr Rela Institute and Medical Centre, Chennai, Tamil Nadu, India
e-mail: dinesh.jothimani@relainstitute.com

S. Saigal, D. Jothimani (eds.), *Fundamentals of Transplant Hepatology*,
https://doi.org/10.1007/978-981-95-2624-6_16

Abbreviations

ACLF	Acute-on-chronic liver failure
AKI	Acute kidney injury
CAID	Cirrhosis-associated immune dysfunction
EGDT	Early goal-directed therapy
FMT	Fecal microbiota transplantation
MAP	Mean arterial pressure
MDR	Multidrug resistant
PIRO	Predisposition infection response organ dysfunction
SBP	Spontaneous bacterial peritonitis
SIRS	Systemic inflammatory response syndrome
SOFA	Sequential organ failure assessment
SSC	Surviving sepsis campaign
XDR	Extensive drug resistance

Key Highlights

- Sepsis precipitates acute decompensation and acute-on-chronic liver failure in patients with background cirrhosis.
- Gut dysbiosis and immune dysfunction augment inflammation and liver injury, reducing autochthonous, or "beneficial," taxa and increasing pathobionts, or pathogenic organisms.
- Assessment of sepsis should be done simultaneously while managing the patient.
- PCR-based diagnostic kits can aid in the identification of multiple microbial pathogens.
- Fluid resuscitation should be according to early goal-directed therapy with hemodynamic monitoring.
- Antibiotics should be started with a broad-spectrum and later should be culture-based.
- Antifungals should be added to antibiotics in case of non-response.
- Microbe-targeted therapy is a future approach to deal with patients with cirrhosis and sepsis.

16.1 Introduction

Sepsis is the leading cause of hospitalization among patients with liver cirrhosis. It often triggers hepatic decompensation and can lead to acute-on-chronic liver failure (ACLF), involving failure of multiple organs in more than two-thirds of affected individuals. The prolonged hospital stays that follow significantly escalate healthcare costs, nearly tripling them compared to patients without cirrhosis [1].

Research indicates that liver cirrhosis itself is an independent risk factor for bacterial infections, with associated mortality rates ranging from 38% to 70%, much higher than in the general population [2, 3]. Despite progress in medical care, bacterial infections still affect approximately 32% of cirrhotic patients, and sepsis-related mortality has risen in recent years (incidence risk ratio: 4.70; 95% CI: 4.61–4.79) [4]. One contributing factor is the shifting epidemiology of bacterial infections, most notably the growing incidence of multidrug resistant (MDR) and extensively drug-resistant (XDR) organisms in patients with cirrhosis and ACLF [5].

The likelihood of developing sepsis increases with the severity of liver disease and the extent of organ dysfunction. Common sources of infection in patients with cirrhosis and ACLF include spontaneous bacterial peritonitis (SBP), urinary tract infections, bloodstream infections, pneumonia, and cellulitis [5, 6].

16.2 Pathogenesis

Cirrhosis is linked to several factors that increase vulnerability to infections. Recent research has highlighted the role of *cirrhosis-associated immune dysfunction (CAID)*, alterations in gut microbiota, increased intestinal permeability, and changes in bile acid composition as key contributors to the development of sepsis [7].

CAID is a distinct immune disorder observed in cirrhotic patients, marked by the paradoxical coexistence of heightened systemic inflammation and weakened immune defenses. It impacts both innate and adaptive immune cells (see Fig. 16.1). This immune dysregulation promotes microbial imbalances (dysbiosis) across various body sites—including stool, mucosal surfaces of the gastrointestinal tract, blood, skin, and saliva.

In the gut, dysbiosis involves a decline in beneficial, autochthonous bacteria and an overgrowth of harmful pathobionts such as gram-negative Enterobacteriaceae (e.g., *Escherichia*, *Klebsiella*) and gram-positive organisms like *Streptococci* and *Enterococci*. These microbial changes, along with impaired intestinal barrier function, result in endotoxemia and systemic inflammation, paving the way for sepsis [8].

Emerging evidence suggests that gut dysbiosis not only contributes to sepsis but also accelerates the progression of various chronic liver conditions—such as nonalcoholic fatty liver disease, alcoholic liver disease, viral hepatitis, and autoimmune liver disease—toward end-stage liver failure.

Bile acids also play a critical role in maintaining intestinal health by supporting digestion and regulating the gut microbiome. In cirrhosis, there is disruption in bile acid metabolism, including decreased production and reduced conversion to secondary bile acids. This limits the production of antimicrobial peptides and promotes the downward migration of oral bacteria into the lower gut, encouraging small intestinal bacterial overgrowth [9].

Additionally, external factors such as continued alcohol use, excessive proton pump inhibitor (PPI) consumption, physical frailty, repeated antibiotic exposure,

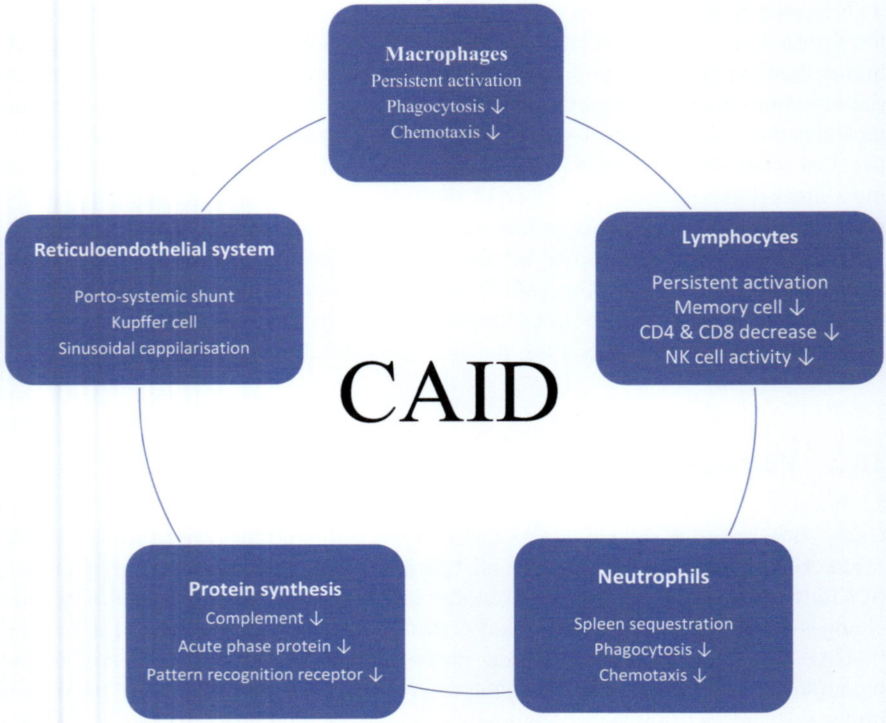

Fig. 16.1 Cirrhosis-associated immune dysfunction (CAID). It involves the activation of macrophages, lymphocytes, neutrophils, and the reticuloendothelial system, thereby dysregulating protein synthesis

frequent hospitalizations, and invasive medical procedures further increase susceptibility to bacterial—and increasingly, fungal—infections in cirrhotic patients [10, 11].

16.2.1 Assessment of Sepsis

Assessment starts simultaneously while managing the patient with sepsis, including securing the airway, correcting hypoxemia, and establishing venous access.

An initial brief history and examination, laboratory tests (including blood cultures), and imaging studies are obtained. This brief assessment yields clues to the suspected source and complications of sepsis and, therefore, helps guide empiric therapy and additional testing. Investigations include complete blood counts with differential counts, liver and renal function tests, and coagulation studies, including D-dimer level. Evaluation of arterial blood gas (ABG) aids in determining the acid-base status, oxygenation, and lactate. An elevated lactate (e.g., >2 mmol/L or greater than the laboratory upper limit of normal) may indicate the severity of sepsis and is used to follow the therapeutic response [12]. Peripheral blood cultures (aerobic and anaerobic cultures from at least two different sites), urinalysis, and microbiologic cultures from suspected sources (e.g., sputum, urine, intravascular catheter, wound or surgical site, body fluids) aid in the identification of the organism. Imaging targeted at the suspected site of infection is warranted (e.g., chest radiography, computed tomography of chest and/or abdomen). While the diagnostic value of procalcitonin in patients with sepsis is doubtful, its value in de-escalating antibiotic therapy is well established [12].

16.3 Evolving Definitions and Scoring Systems

While infections initiate sepsis, the body's response to sepsis is highly variable, leading to evolving definitions over time. Initially, sepsis was described as an exaggerated inflammatory response to microbial infection, characterized by a cytokine storm. Based on this understanding, the Sepsis-1 definition described sepsis as a "systemic inflammatory response syndrome (SIRS) to infection." [13] Although SIRS criteria were easy to apply, they lacked specificity and were overly sensitive.

To address these limitations, the Sepsis-2 definition introduced the PIRO model—an acronym for Predisposition, Insult (infection), Response, and Organ dysfunction [14]. This framework helped clinicians distinguish between primary organ dysfunction related to liver disease and secondary dysfunction involving extrahepatic organs. The PIRO model enabled better risk stratification in cirrhotic patients, identifying those at higher risk for sepsis, subsequent organ failure, and recurrent infections. It also defined key therapeutic windows to intervene and potentially prevent further clinical deterioration.

The Sepsis-3 definition further refined the concept by shifting focus to "life-threatening organ dysfunction caused by a dysregulated host response to infection," replacing the terms SIRS and severe sepsis [15]. In this updated framework, organ dysfunction is quantified as a rise in the Sequential Organ Failure Assessment (SOFA) score by ≥2 points (see Table 16.1). Septic shock is now defined by the need for vasopressor support to maintain a mean arterial pressure (MAP) of ≥65 mm Hg, along with a serum lactate level exceeding 2 mmol/L [16].

16.3.1 *Other Modalities of Sepsis Assessment*

Additional investigations targeted at the suspected source(s) should be considered in patients with sepsis as promptly as is feasible. Multiplex PCR panels can help in the identification of the causative organism and assist in targeted therapy while awaiting culture reports. Both bacterial and viral panels are currently available. In patients not responding to targeted antibiotic therapy, evaluation for underlying

Table 16.1 Sequential Organ Failure Assessment (SOFA) score

Parameters/score	1	2	3	4
Respiratory (PaO2 /FiO2)	<400	<300	<200	<100
Coagulation (platelets ×103 /μ/L)	<150	<100	<50	<20
Liver bilirubin (mg/dL)	1.2–1.9	2.0–5.9	6.0–11.9	>12.0
Cardiovascular hypotension or vasoactive agents (μg/kg/min)	MAP <70 mm Hg	Dopamine ≤5 or dobutamine (any dose)	Dopamine >5, epinephrine ≤0.1 or norepinephrine ≤0.1†	Dopamine >15, epinephrine >0.1, or norepinephrine >0.1
Central nervous system Glasgow Coma Scale	13–14	10–12	6–9	<6
Renal creatinine (mg/dL) or urine output (mL/day)	1.2–1.9	2.0–3.4	3.5–4.9 or <500	>5.0 or <200

The Sequential Organ Failure Assessment (SOFA) score is a tool used to assess organ dysfunction in critically ill patients, including those with sepsis. The SOFA score evaluates six organ systems: respiratory, coagulation, liver, cardiovascular, central nervous system, and renal. Each system is scored from 0 to 4 based on specific criteria, and the total SOFA score ranges from 0 to 24, with higher scores indicating more severe organ dysfunction

fungal infections should be undertaken. The use of serological assays like 1,3 beta-D-glucan, galactomannan, and anti-mannan antibodies, if available, is warranted and would provide insight into the presence of invasive *Candida* or *Aspergillus* infections.

16.3.2 Management of Patients with Cirrhosis and Sepsis

Hemodynamics in cirrhosis are characterized by profound splanchnic arteriolar vasodilatation and peripheral vasoconstriction, which complicates sepsis management. Like patients without cirrhosis, early administration of antibiotics, fluid management, vasopressors, and infectious source control are the foundation of sepsis management.

16.4 Hemodynamic Monitoring

The primary objective of fluid resuscitation in sepsis is to promptly restore tissue perfusion and prevent or limit end-organ damage. The current standard approach combines Early Goal-Directed Therapy (EGDT) with physiological indicators—such as urine output, lactate clearance, and timely antibiotic administration within the first hour of presentation [17].

In cirrhotic patients, physiological abnormalities such as vascular hyporesponsiveness, a hyperdynamic circulatory state, low systemic vascular resistance, elevated cardiac output, reduced mean arterial pressure (MAP), and high central venous oxygen saturation complicate fluid status evaluation [18, 19]. Central venous pressure (CVP), often used to assess intravascular volume, may instead reflect elevated intra-abdominal pressure in these patients, making static measurements potentially misleading [20].

For cirrhotic patients without ascites, respiratory variation in the inferior vena cava (IVC) diameter is considered one of the most reliable noninvasive indicators of fluid responsiveness. Cardiac ultrasound is now recommended to guide fluid resuscitation in sepsis; however, its utility in cirrhosis is not clearly established [21, 22].

Serum lactate is routinely used as a surrogate marker of tissue hypoxia in sepsis and is integrated into the current definition of septic shock. In cirrhosis, however, impaired hepatic clearance leads to higher baseline lactate levels, making interpretation more complex [23]. Serial lactate monitoring may offer better clinical insights, as trends in lactate correlate more closely with outcomes [24]. Nevertheless, a lactate level exceeding 2 mmol/L in a hemodynamically unstable cirrhotic patient should be presumed to reflect septic shock unless another cause is identified [24].

Other potential markers of tissue hypoperfusion—such as a skin mottling score ≥ 2 and tissue oxygen saturation $< 60\%$ assessed via laser Doppler—have recently been proposed in cirrhotic patients with septic shock. These markers are associated with poor prognosis, although their exact role in clinical management remains to be defined [25].

Implementation of the Surviving Sepsis Campaign (SSC) protocol, despite being evidence-based, has not demonstrated improved survival in cirrhotic patients with septic shock [26]. International consensus guidelines for managing critically ill cirrhotic patients recommend targeting a lower MAP (around 60 mmHg) [20]. In such patients, placement of an arterial line and central venous catheter is advised, along with monitoring via pulmonary artery catheter (PAC) or echocardiography during resuscitation. PAC use may be specifically helpful in patients with right ventricular dysfunction or pulmonary hypertension, although no definitive targets for ventricular filling pressure, intravascular volume, lactate, or central venous oxygen saturation ($ScvO_2$) were proposed [20].

Each modality has limitations in cirrhotic patients. Echocardiography is highly operator-dependent, lacks continuous monitoring capability, and may be inaccurate in assessing cardiac function under hyperdynamic conditions. Meanwhile, PAC, although informative, carries significant risks due to its invasive nature and is less favored due to the bleeding and infection risks common in this population [27].

Urine output remains a key early indicator of fluid status. However, in cirrhosis, it is crucial to recognize that oliguria may be the only sign of renal dysfunction. Serum creatinine often underestimates renal impairment due to the high prevalence of sarcopenia and malnutrition in these patients [20].

16.5 Fluid Resuscitation

Fluid administration is a cornerstone in the management of sepsis, aiming to restore tissue perfusion and prevent organ failure. The optimal type of intravenous fluid for resuscitation in ICU settings remains a subject of debate. Multiple studies have compared normal saline (0.9% sodium chloride), balanced crystalloids (e.g., Ringer's lactate), and colloids such as human albumin [28].

While individual trials have not consistently shown albumin to be superior to saline, meta-analyses have reported reduced mortality with albumin compared to crystalloids or starches in adult septic patients [29]. Furthermore, albumin has been associated with a significant reduction in 90-day mortality in patients with septic shock when compared with crystalloids. Albumin infusion has also demonstrated mortality benefits in patients with spontaneous bacterial peritonitis [30] and hepatorenal syndrome [31], and it has improved outcomes after large-volume paracentesis [32].

Although current evidence does not firmly support albumin as the first-line fluid for initial resuscitation in cirrhotic patients, it is increasingly recommended for those with suspected infection. A suggested dosing range is 50–100 grams per day [20]. Despite its benefits, cost may limit its widespread use. Regardless of the fluid type, prompt and adequate volume resuscitation remains critical in the treatment of septic shock.

16.6 Vasopressors

The effectiveness of various vasopressors in cirrhotic patients with septic shock has not been thoroughly investigated. Norepinephrine is considered the first-line agent in sepsis management due to its favorable safety profile when compared with dopamine, which is no longer recommended [33]. Norepinephrine works by inducing vasoconstriction, which increases venous return and cardiac preload. It also enhances cardiac contractility via beta-adrenergic stimulation [34]. However, prolonged use can result in side effects such as reflex bradycardia, arrhythmias, and tissue ischemia [34].

Epinephrine, while similar in action, carries a higher risk of adverse effects like arrhythmias, myocardial ischemia, pulmonary hypertension, lactic acidosis, and hyperglycemia [35]. These complications are particularly concerning in cirrhotic patients who already have impaired lactate clearance [36, 37].

Inotropes like dobutamine are used in sepsis with myocardial dysfunction, but cirrhotic patients—who typically have high cardiac output—may derive limited benefit from them. The hyperdynamic state seen in both cirrhosis and septic shock is also associated with a deficiency of endogenous vasopressin [38]. While the Surviving Sepsis Campaign (SSC) does not endorse vasopressin as first-line or monotherapy for septic shock [20], it may offer added benefit in cirrhotic patients by promoting splanchnic vasoconstriction and improving circulatory dynamics.

Nonetheless, vasopressin use is not without risk. At higher doses (above 0.4 U/min), it can cause arrhythmias, reduced cardiac output, and tissue ischemia [35]. These risks must be carefully weighed in a population already prone to hemodynamic instability and complications.

16.6.1 Steroids

Adrenal insufficiency is common in patients with cirrhosis presenting with sepsis and septic shock, although it can also be present in patients with stable or decompensated cirrhosis [39, 40]. In critical illness, adrenal insufficiency is associated with hemodynamic instability, reduced response to vasoactive drugs, and increased mortality. Corticosteroids are commonly used in patients with septic shock, particularly those with an unsatisfactory response to vasopressors [40]. Addition of corticosteroids results in faster shock resolution and lower vasopressor requirements, whereas their effect on survival remains unsettled. A recent large, multicenter trial showed that hydrocortisone alone does not reduce mortality compared to placebo [41], whereas another recent study demonstrated that a combination of hydrocortisone plus fludrocortisone may improve 90-day survival in patients with septic shock [42]. Steroids are indicated in patients with sepsis and absolute or relative adrenal insufficiency.

16.6.2 Antibiotics

Diagnosing sepsis in cirrhosis can be challenging and requires a high index of suspicion. This often leads to delays in the initiation of empiric antibiotics, which, in turn, are associated with worse outcomes. Therefore, both the choice of antibiotics and the timing of administration are crucial. Each hour of delay in antimicrobial therapy increases mortality by 1.86 times [43]. Factors such as the source of infection (community or hospital acquired), recent antibiotic use, and history of colonization or infection by multidrug resistant organisms determine the choice of antibiotics [44].

When prescribing antibiotics for patients with cirrhosis, several factors must be considered due to the increased risk of complications, such as hepatic encephalopathy, renal impairment, and heightened susceptibility to infections [45]. Here are some general principles and antibiotic recommendations for patients with cirrhosis:

- *Consideration of Liver Function*: Since patients with cirrhosis often have impaired liver function, it is essential to choose antibiotics with minimal hepatotoxicity and those primarily eliminated by the kidneys. Avoid hepatotoxic antibiotics, such as certain cephalosporins (e.g., ceftriaxone) and fluoroquinolones (e.g., ciprofloxacin), unless no suitable alternatives exist.
- *Use of Narrow-Spectrum Antibiotics*: Whenever possible, opt for narrow-spectrum antibiotics to minimize the disruption of normal flora and reduce the risk of antibiotic-associated complications, such as *Clostridium difficile* infection.
- *Assessment of Renal Function*: Renal impairment is common in cirrhosis, so renal function should be assessed before prescribing antibiotics. Dosages of antibiotics should be adjusted based on renal function, and antibiotics with minimal renal excretion should be considered for patients with renal impairment.
- *Guided Therapy*: Whenever feasible, follow antibiotic stewardship principles by obtaining cultures before initiating antibiotic therapy. This helps guide antibiotic selection and allows treatment to be tailored to the identified pathogen's susceptibility profile.
- *Avoidance of Nephrotoxic Agents*: Nephrotoxic antibiotics should be avoided, particularly in patients with cirrhosis who may already have compromised renal function. Examples include aminoglycosides and vancomycin, although vancomycin may be necessary in certain situations.
- *Consideration of the Infection Site*: The choice of antibiotic should be guided by the suspected site of infection and the likely pathogens involved. For example, in spontaneous bacterial peritonitis (SBP), the first-line treatment is typically a third generation cephalosporin (e.g., cefotaxime) or a fluoroquinolone (e.g., levofloxacin) if the patient is not allergic.
- *Consultation with an Infectious Disease Specialist*: In cases of severe infections or uncertainty regarding antibiotic selection, consultation with an infectious disease specialist may be prudent.
- *Avoidance of Drug Interactions*: Be cautious of potential drug interactions, especially with medications used to manage cirrhosis-related complications, such as diuretics, beta-blockers, and medications for hepatic encephalopathy.
- *Monitoring for Adverse Effects*: Patients should be closely monitored for signs of adverse effects related to antibiotic therapy, including renal impairment, hepatic decompensation, and allergic reactions.

For hospital acquired and nosocomial infections, it is essential to consider local patterns of antibiotic resistance. In high-risk patients, broad-spectrum antibiotics with activity against vancomycin-susceptible enterococci (VSE), vancomycin-resistant enterococci (VRE), and methicillin-resistant *Staphylococcus aureus* (MRSA)—such as daptomycin and linezolid—should be used [46]. Once the infectious source and causative organism are confirmed, treatment should be de-escalated to a targeted, pathogen-specific antibiotic. Recommended antibiotic options are outlined in Table 16.2.

Table 16.2 Antibiotic recommendations in patients with cirrhosis

Infection	AASLD	EASL
Peritonitis, Bacteremia	Community acquired: Third-generation cephalosporins	Community acquired: Third-generation cephalosporins or Piperacillin/tazobactam
	Nosocomial: Piperacillin/tazobactam and daptomycin (VRE in the past or evidence of GI colonization) Meropenem (if MDR gram-negative infection)	Nosocomial: Carbapenems alone Carbapenems and daptomycin, vancomycin, or linezolid (high prevalence of MDR gram-positive bacteria or sepsis)
Pyelonephritis/ urinary tract infection	Uncomplicated pyelonephritis: Fluoroquinolones (ciprofloxacin or levofloxacin). Severe pyelonephritis: Third-generation cephalosporins (e.g., ceftriaxone). H/o recent antibiotic exposure: Piperacillin/tazobactam or carbapenem	Community acquired: Uncomplicated: Ciprofloxacin or cotrimoxazole. Sepsis: Third-generation cephalosporins or piperacillin/ tazobactam
		Nosocomial: Uncomplicated: Fosfomycin or nitrofurantoin. Sepsis: Meropenem and teicoplanin or vancomycin
Pneumonia	Community acquired: Non-severe: B-lactam and macrolide or respiratory fluoroquinolones Severe: B-lactam and macrolide or B-lactam and fluoroquinolones. Vancomycin—added if prior respiratory isolation of MRSA	Community acquired: Piperacillin/tazobactam or ceftriaxone and macrolide or levofloxacin or moxifloxacin
	Hospital-acquired (not ventilator associated): Non-severe (no sepsis, no intubation): One of the following: Piperacillin/tazobactam or cefepime or levofloxacin Severe (septic or needing to be intubated). One of the following: Piperacilin tazobactam or cefepime or meropenem and levofloxacin Vancomycin—added if MRSA isolated in last 90 d or if antibiotics were used in the last 90 d Pseudomonas coverage: prior respiratory isolation of pseudomonas or recent use of parenteral antibiotics or hospitalization	Nosocomial: Ceftazidime or meropenem and levofloxacin ± glycopeptides or linezolid

(continued)

Table 16.2 (continued)

Infection	AASLD	EASL
Cellulitis	Moderate (systemic signs of infection): Penicillin or ceftriaxone or cefazolin or clindamycin. Severe (failed antibiotics, presence of sepsis): Vancomycin and piperacillin / tazobactam	Community acquired: Piperacillin/tazobactam or third-generation cephalosporins and oxacillin
		Nosocomial: Third-generation cephalosporin or meropenem and oxacillin or glycopeptides or daptomycin or linezolid

Antibiotic recommendations in patients with cirrhosis: Antibiotic selection in patients with cirrhosis should be individualized based on factors such as the type and severity of infection, the patient's liver and renal function, drug allergies, and local antimicrobial resistance patterns. Close monitoring and interdisciplinary collaboration are essential for optimizing antibiotic therapy while minimizing the risk of complications in this patient population [54–56]

If patients show no clinical improvement within 48 to 72 hours of broad-spectrum antibiotic therapy, empiric antifungal treatment should be considered [20].

There are four major classes of antifungal agents:

- The polyenes (amphotericin B),
- The triazoles (fluconazole, itraconazole, voriconazole, and posaconazole),
- The echinocandins (caspofungin, anidulafungin, and micafungin),
- Flucytosine.

The commonly prescribed antifungal medications are the triazole class of drugs. Recent studies, however, have reported an increasing prevalence of resistance to azoles among non-albicans spp.

In critically ill patients, echinocandins have been recommended as the first-line treatment. Echinocandins are noted to have minimal hepatotoxicity and nephrotoxicity compared to azoles. Their adverse effects are also noted to be minimal. These added advantages have made Echinocandins to be used as the first-line treatments for patients with cirrhosis and nosocomial SFP or critically ill patients with liver cirrhosis and community-acquired SFP. Caspofungin and micafungin undergo minimal hepatic metabolism. Dose adjustments are not required in moderate and severe liver disease except for Caspofungin [47–52].

Procalcitonin levels have been studied as a bacterial infection biomarker and as a tool to guide antibiotic therapy. It has been proposed that in stable critically ill patients, procalcitonin levels of <0.5 μg/L or a decrease of $\geq 80\%$ from peak can be used as supportive data in the discontinuation of antibiotic treatment. Although procalcitonin is an established inflammatory biomarker of bacterial infection, its role in cirrhosis needs clarity [53].

Since the majority of the drugs are metabolized in the liver, most require dose modifications in the presence of liver dysfunction. The degree of dysfunction and the need for modification are based on the CTP score. Dosage modifications routinely undertaken are mentioned in Table 16.3.

Table 16.3 Dose adjustment of antibiotics in cirrhosis

Antibiotic	Interaction	Recommendation
Cefotaxime	Liver metabolizes about 40–50% of the drug to an active deacetylated metabolite. Very high therapeutic index of the antibiotic.	Dose adjustment is not necessary for patients with hepatic impairment
Amoxicillin-clavulanate	Eliminated via renal tubular secretion	Does not require dose adjustment
Ampicillin	Unchanged pharmacokinetic parameters in cirrhotic	Dose reduction is recommended in renal impairment
Ciprofloxacin and Norfloxacin	Eliminated via renal and hepatic routes. Hepatic biotransformation—metabolites with partial antibacterial action.	Ciprofloxacin and norfloxacin doses need not be adjusted. In patients with TIPS, prolongation of QTc intervals may be caused by fluoroquinolones—needs appropriate care and monitoring.
Ofloxacin	Renal dysfunction in patients with ascites alters the metabolism of the drug, and lower renal elimination is noted in cirrhotics.	Dose adjustment needed in renal dysfunction.
Glycopeptides (e.g., vancomycin, teicoplanin)	Nephrotoxic. Increased risk of AKI in patients with ALF	Needs to be used with caution.
Tigecycline	No change in pharmacokinetic properties was noted in C-P class A or B C-P class C: drug clearance is reduced by half	Mild to moderate liver cirrhosis—no dose adjustment severe disease—maintenance dose reduced by 50%
Aminoglycosides (neomycin and paromomycin)	Ototoxicity and nephrotoxicity are major concern.	Use is reserved for severe bacterial infections not responsive to other antibiotics.
Metronidazole	Prolonged rate of elimination in patients with HE Increased risk for irreversible peripheral neurotoxicity Limited studies on efficacy Disulfiram-like reactions in patients consuming ethanol or ethanol-containing medications	Not recommended for the management of DCLD with HE

Antibiotics in Hepatic Dysfunction: Antibiotic dose modification is crucial in patients with hepatic dysfunction (such as cirrhosis) to prevent drug toxicity and ensure therapeutic efficacy. Hepatic dysfunction can alter the metabolism and elimination of drugs, leading to increased drug levels and potential adverse effects [57–73]

16.7 Liver Transplantation

Liver transplantation (LT) offers a survival benefit for patients with decompensated cirrhosis and acute-on-chronic liver failure (ACLF). However, active sepsis remains a strict contraindication to transplantation. These patients should be evaluated for early transplant candidacy once the infection has been effectively treated. Currently, there are no standardized criteria for delisting critically ill patients, and decisions are often made subjectively, varying between transplant centers.

In this population, the timing for considering LT is critical and often limited. Patients who have controlled infections and two or fewer organ failures may be suitable candidates for transplantation. In addition to organ support requirements, both the severity and duration of organ dysfunction should be factored into the decision-making process, as they can significantly impact post-transplant outcomes.

16.8 Prevention

Low albumin levels in ascitic fluid are a recognized risk factor for spontaneous bacterial peritonitis (SBP); therefore, such patients benefit from primary prophylaxis. Episodes of variceal bleeding can trigger bacterial translocation and bloodstream infections, so prophylactic antibiotics are recommended in these cases to reduce the risk of sepsis. Notably, patients who develop sepsis after a variceal bleed have higher rates of rebleeding.

At present, prophylactic probiotics do not have an established role in sepsis prevention among cirrhotic patients. However, recent studies suggest that rifaximin—a non-absorbable antibiotic that modulates gut microbiota—may offer benefit in this population.

16.9 Future Directions

16.9.1 Culture-Independent Pathogen Detection

New diagnostic approaches, such as multiplex polymerase chain reaction (PCR) syndromic panels, allow for rapid, simultaneous detection of multiple pathogens commonly associated with bloodstream, respiratory, gastrointestinal, or central nervous system infections [74]. These tools may prove valuable in cirrhotic patients, where early and accurate diagnosis is crucial.

Another emerging approach is metagenomics, which involves sequencing the collective genetic material from mixed microbial communities. This technique may help identify infections, especially when traditional cultures are negative. Notably, studies have shown that the microbiome profile at hospital admission differs between infected and uninfected cirrhotic patients [75].

Challenges with metagenomics include high costs, longer turnaround times, contamination with host DNA, difficulty distinguishing live from dead organisms, and the need for advanced bioinformatics support. Despite these limitations, ongoing advancements have improved its feasibility. At present, metagenomics can be considered in cases where infection is suspected but standard cultures fail to identify a pathogen.

16.10 Microbe-Targeted Therapies

Microbe-targeted therapies for infections in patients with cirrhosis include probiotics and prebiotics, fecal microbiota transplantation, and phage therapy.

16.10.1 Probiotics and Prebiotics

Multiple studies involving outpatients colonized with MDR organisms have failed to show the benefit of using multistrain or single-strain probiotics [76]. Lactulose, which is a prebiotic used to treat hepatic encephalopathy, is not associated with any appreciable change in infection rates or carriage of MDR organisms [77].

16.10.2 Fecal Microbiota Transplantation (FMT)

FMT involves the safe transfer of filtrated fecal material, in capsular or liquid formulations, from a donor to a recipient [78]. Studies involving patient groups with high rates of infection due to MDR bacteria, such as patients with neutropenia undergoing bone marrow transplantation, have shown that fecal transplantation results in a reduced risk of antibiotic-resistant infection [79]. Fecal transplantation is safe in patients with cirrhosis, resolves antibiotic-associated structural and functional collapse of the microbiome, and reduces the abundance of antibiotic-resistance genes in recipients [80].

16.10.3 Phage Therapy

Bacteriophages have been used therapeutically for antibiotic-resistant infections with varying degrees of success [81]. The advantages are their bactericidal nature and penetration of biofilms, whereas the disadvantages are related to strain specificity and the risk of resistance [82]. Phage therapy can be administered topically, intravenously, or orally. The lack of regulatory approval for phage therapy in patients with cirrhosis and infection, as well as the need to individualize treatment, makes widespread application of phage therapy difficult at present.

16.11 Conclusion

Sepsis remains the most dreadful complication in patients with liver cirrhosis, with associated significant morbidity and mortality. Septic cirrhotic patients develop progression of liver disease and may require intensive care therapy and organ support. Prompt and early identification of septic complications would prevent progression of liver disease and may improve clinical outcomes. These patients should often be managed by a multidisciplinary team consisting of a hepatologist, intensivist, and infectious disease specialist. Patients with progressive hepatic decompensation and acute-on-chronic liver failure benefit from early liver transplantation following the resolution of sepsis. An algorithmic approach to sepsis in cirrhosis is proposed in Fig. 16.2.

16.12 Approach

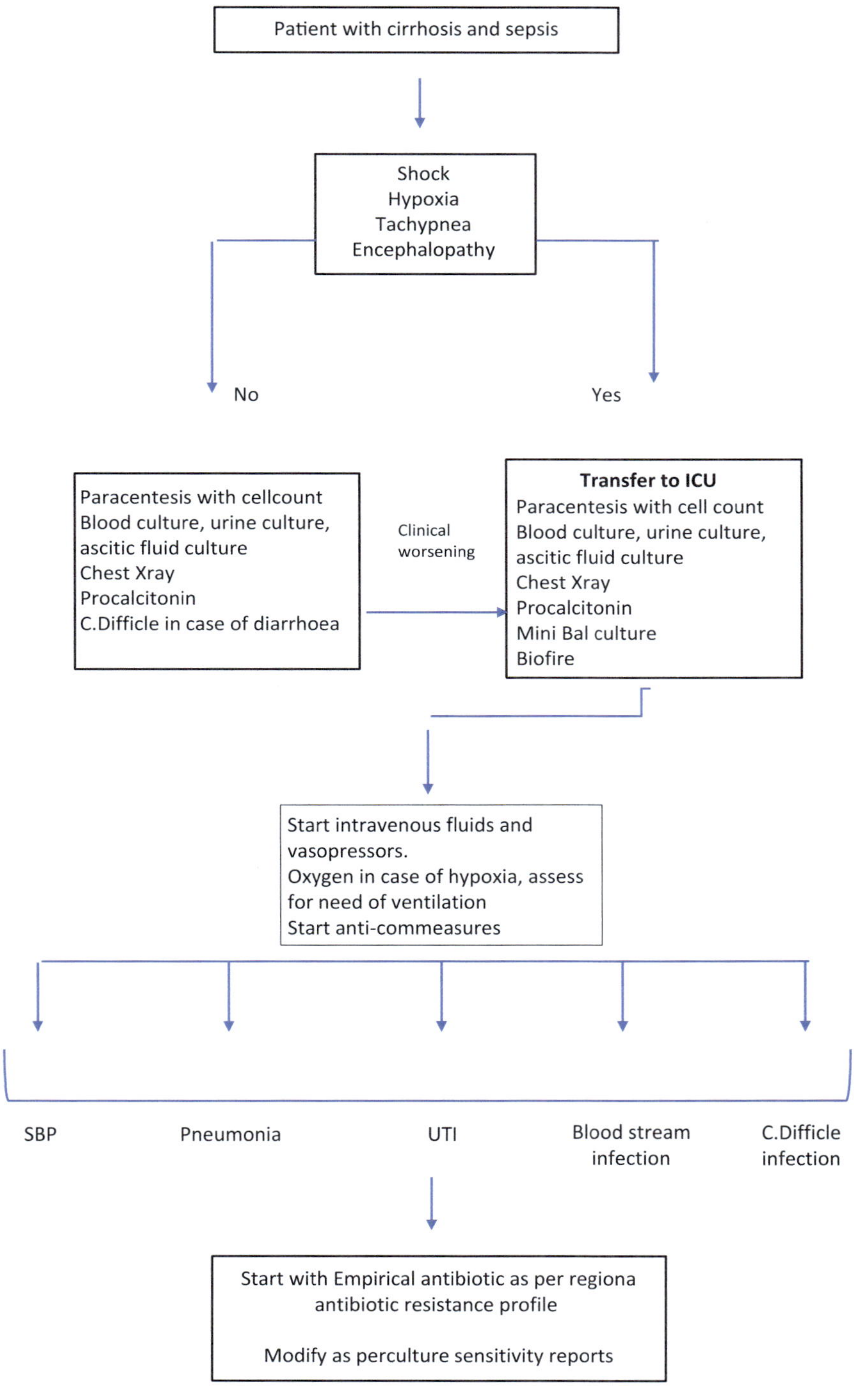

Fig. 16.2 Algorithmic approach to sepsis in cirrhosis

Conflict of Interest None.

Financial Disclosure None to disclose.

References

1. Allen AM, Kim WR, Moriarty JP, Shah ND, Larson JJ, Kamath PS. Time trends in the health care burden and mortality of acute on chronic liver failure in the United States. Hepatology. 2016;64:2165–72.
2. Gustot T, Felleiter P, Pickkers P, Sakr Y, Rello J, Velissaris D. Impact of infection on the prognosis of critically ill cirrhotic patients: results from a large worldwide study. Liver Int. 2014;34:1496–503.
3. Singer M, Deutschman CS, Seymour CW, et al. The third international consensus definitions for sepsis and septic shock (sepsis-3). JAMA. 2016;315:801–10.
4. Schmidt ML, Barritt AS, Orman ES, Hayashi PH. Decreasing mortality among patients hospitalized with cirrhosis in the United States from 2002 through 2010. Gastroenterology. 2015;148:967–77.
5. Piano S, Singh V, Caraceni P, et al. International Club of Ascites Global Study Group. Epidemiology and effects of bacterial infections in patients with Cirrhosis worldwide. Gastroenterology. 2019;156(5):1368–80.e10.
6. Singh SP, Bhatia V, Kale P, Kumar G, Khillan V, Vijayaraghavan R. Bowel colonization with carbapenem-resistant bacteria is associated with short-term outcomes in patients with acute-on-chronic liver failure. J Gastroenterol Hepatol. 2025;40(2):528–36. https://doi.org/10.1111/jgh.16830.
7. Bonnel AR, Bunchorntavakul C, Reddy KR. Immune dysfunction and infections in patients with cirrhosis. Clin Gastroenterol Hepatol. 2011;9:727–38.
8. Albillos A, Lario M, Álvarez-Mon M. Cirrhosis-associated immune dysfunction: distinctive features and clinical relevance. J Hepatol. 2014;61:1385–96.
9. Bajaj JS, Heuman DM, Hylemon PB, et al. Altered profile of human gut microbiome is associated with cirrhosis and its complications. J Hepatol. 2014;60:940–7.
10. O'Leary JG, Reddy KR, Wong F, et al. Long-term use of antibiotics and proton pump inhibitors predict development of infections in patients with cirrhosis. Clin Gastroenterol Hepatol. 2015;13(4):753.e1–9.e1.
11. FernÁndez J, Acevedo J, Wiest R, et al. Bacterial and fungal infections in acute- on-chronic liver failure: prevalence, characteristics and impact on prognosis. Gut. 2018;67:1870–80.
12. Thompson K, Venkatesh B, Finfer S. Sepsis and septic shock: current approaches to management. Intern Med J. 2019;49(2):160–70. https://doi.org/10.1111/imj.14199. PMID: 30754087.
13. Rhodes A, Evans LE, Alhazzani W, et al. Surviving sepsis campaign: international guidelines for management of sepsis and septic shock: 2016. Intensive Care Med. 2017;43(3):304–77. https://doi.org/10.1007/s00134-017-4683-6.
14. Scala R, Schultz M, Bos LDJ, Artigas A. New Surviving Sepsis Campaign guidelines: back to the art of medicine. Eur Respir J. 2018;52(1):1701818. Published 2018 Jul 11. https://doi.org/10.1183/13993003.01818-2017.
15. Medlej K. Calculated decisions: qSOFA (quick SOFA) score for sepsis. Emerg Med Pract. 2018;20(Suppl 10):CD2–4. Published 2018 Oct 1.
16. Marik PE, Taeb AM. SIRS, qSOFA and new sepsis definition. J Thorac Dis. 2017;9(4):943–5. https://doi.org/10.21037/jtd.2017.03.125.
17. Rivers E, Nguyen B, Havstad S, et al. Early goal-directed therapy in the treatment of severe sepsis and septic shock. N Engl J Med. 2001;345:1368–77.

18. Moreau R, Lee SS, Soupison T, Roche-Sicot J, Sicot C. Abnormal tissue oxygenation in patients with cirrhosis and liver failure. J Hepatol. 1988;7:98–105.
19. Moreau R, Hadengue A, Soupison T, et al. Septic shock in patients with cirrhosis: hemodynamic and metabolic characteristics and intensive care unit outcome. Crit Care Med. 1992;20:746–50.
20. Nadim MK, Durand F, Kellum JA, et al. Management of the critically ill patient with cirrhosis: a multidisciplinary perspective. J Hepatol. 2016;64:717–35.
21. Levitov A, Frankel HL, Blaivas M, et al. Guidelines for the appropriate use of bedside general and cardiac ultrasonography in the evaluation of critically ill patients–part II: cardiac ultrasonography. Crit Care Med. 2016;44:1206–27.
22. Via G, Tavazzi G, Price S. Ten situations where inferior vena cava ultrasound may fail to accurately predict fluid responsiveness: a physiologically based point of view. Intens Care Med. 2016;42:1164–7.
23. Sterling SA, Puskarich MA, Jones AE. The effect of liver disease on lactate normalization in severe sepsis and septic shock: a cohort study. Clin Exp Emerg Med. 2015;2:197–202.
24. Funk GC, Doberer D, Kneidinger N, Lindner G, Holzinger U, Schneeweiss B. Acid-base disturbances in critically ill patients with cirrhosis. Liver Int. 2007;27:901–9.
25. Galbois A, Bige N, Pichereau C, et al. Exploration of skin perfusion in cirrhotic patients with septic shock. J Hepatol. 2015;62:549–55.
26. Dellinger RP, Levy MM, Carlet JM, et al. Surviving Sepsis Campaign: international guidelines for management of severe sepsis and septic shock: 2008. Crit Care Med. 2008;36:296–327.
27. Huygh J, Peeters Y, Bernards J, Malbrain ML. Hemodynamic monitoring in the critically ill: an overview of current cardiac output monitoring methods. F1000Res. 2016;5. pii:F1000 Faculty Rev-2855.
28. Finfer S, Bellomo R, Boyce N, French J, Myburgh J, Norton R. A comparison of albumin and saline for fluid resuscitation in the intensive care unit. N Engl J Med. 2004;350:2247–56.
29. Rochwerg B, Alhazzani W, Sindi A, et al. Fluid resuscitation in sepsis: a systematic review and network meta-analysis. Ann Intern Med. 2014;161:347–55.
30. Salerno F, Navickis RJ, Wilkes MM. Albumin infusion improves outcomes of patients with spontaneous bacterial peritonitis: a meta-analysis of randomized trials. Clin Gastroenterol Hepatol. 2013;11:123–130.e1.
31. Ortega R, Gines P, Uriz J, et al. Terlipressin therapy with and without albumin for patients with hepatorenal syndrome: results of a prospective, nonrandomized study. Hepatology. 2002;36(4 Pt 1):941–8.
32. Bernardi M, Caraceni P, Navickis RJ, Wilkes MM. Albumin infusion in patients undergoing large-volume paracentesis: a meta-analysis of randomized trials. Hepatology. 2012;55:1172–81.
33. De Backer D, Aldecoa C, Njimi H, Vincent JL. Dopamine versus norepinephrine in the treatment of septic shock: a metaanalysis. Crit Care Med. 2012;40:725–30.
34. Stratton L, Berlin DA, Arbo JE. Vasopressors and inotropes in sepsis. Emerg Med Clin N Am. 2017;35:75–91.
35. Herget-Rosenthal S, Saner F, Chawla LS. Approach to hemodynamic shock and vasopressors. Clin J Am Soc Nephrol. 2008;3:546–53.
36. Overgaard CB, Dzavik V. Inotropes and vasopressors: review of physiology and clinical use in cardiovascular disease. Circulation. 2008;118:1047–56.
37. Ellender TJ, Skinner JC. The use of vasopressors and inotropes in the emergency medical treatment of shock. Emerg Med Clin N Am. 2008;26(759–786):ix.
38. Wagener G, Bakker J. Vasopressin in cirrhosis and sepsis: physiology and clinical implications. Minerva Anestesiol. 2015;81:1377–83.
39. Singh SP, Mondia N. Adrenal insufficiency associated with low high-density lipoprotein (HDL) in patients of chronic liver disease. Indian J Clin Med. 2023;13(1):6–10. https://doi.org/10.1177/26339447221142358.
40. Fede G, Spadaro L, Tomaselli T, et al. Adrenocortical dysfunction in liver disease: a systematic review. Hepatology. 2012;55:1282–91.

41. Venkatesh B, Finfer S, Cohen J, et al. Adjunctive glucocorticoid therapy in patients with septic shock. N Engl J Med. 2018;378:797–808.
42. Annane D, Renault A, Brun-Buisson C, et al. Hydrocortisone plus fludrocortisone for adults with septic shock. N Engl J Med. 2018;378:809–18.
43. Karvellas CJ, Abraldes JG, Arabi YM, Kumar A. Appropriate and timely antimicrobial therapy in cirrhotic patients with spontaneous bacterial peritonitis-associated septic shock: a retrospective cohort study. Aliment Pharmacol Ther. 2015;41:747–57.
44. Fernandez J, Gustot T. Management of bacterial infections in cirrhosis. J Hepatol. 2012;56(Suppl 1):S1–S12.
45. Bunchorntavakul C, Chavalitdhamrong D. Bacterial infections other than spontaneous bacterial peritonitis in cirrhosis. World J Hepatol. 2012;4:158–68.
46. Fernandez J, Arroyo V. Bacterial infections in cirrhosis: a growing problem with significant implications. Clin Liver Dis. 2013;2:102–5.
47. Cornely OA, Bassetti M, Calandra T, Garbino J, Kullberg BJ, Lortholary O, et al. ESCMID* guideline for the diagnosis and management of Candida diseases 2012: non-neutropenicadultpatients. Clin Microbiol Infect. 2012;18(Suppl 7):19–37.
48. Pappas PG, Kauffman CA, Andes DR, Clancy CJ, Marr KA, Ostrosky-Zeichner L, et al. Clinical practice guideline for the management of candidiasis: 2016 update by the Infectious Dis-eases Society of America. Clin Infect Dis. 2016;62(4):e1–50.
49. Mistry GC, Migoya E, Deutsch PJ, Winchell G, Hesney M, et al. Single- and multiple-dose administration of caspo-fungin in patients with hepatic insufficiency: implicationsfor safety and dosing recommendations. J Clin Pharmacol 2007;47:951—961.
50. Yeoh SF, Lee TJ, Chew KL, Lin S, Yeo D, Setia S. Echinocan-dins for management of invasive candidiasis in patients withliver disease and liver transplantation. Infect Drug Resist. 2018;11:805–19.
51. Tacconelli E, Buhl M, Humphreyx H, Malek V, Presterl E, Rodriguez-Bano J, et al. Analysis of the challange in implemnting guidelines to prevent the spread of multidrug-resistant gram negatives in Europe. BMJ Open. 2019;9(5):e027683.
52. Allaire M, et al. Management of infections in patients with cirrhosis in the context of increasing therapeutic resistance: a systematic review, vol. 44. Clin Res Hepatol Gastroenterol; 2019. p. 264–74.
53. Piano S, Morando F, Carretta G, et al. Predictors of early readmission in patients with cirrhosis after the resolution of bacterial infections. Am J Gastroenterol. 2017;112:1575–83.
54. Biggins SW, Angeli P, Garcia-Tsao G, Ginès P, Ling SC, Nadim MK, Wong F, Kim WR. Diagnosis, evaluation, and Management of Ascites, spontaneous bacterial peritonitis and Hepatorenal syndrome: 2021 Practice Guidance by the American Association for the Study of Liver Diseases. Hepatology. 2021;74:1014–48.
55. European Association for the Study of the Liver. EASL Clinical Practice Guidelines for the management of patients with decompensated cirrhosis. J Hepatol. 2018;69:406–60.
56. Dirchwolf M, Gomez Perdiguero G, Grech IM, Marciano S. Challenges and recommendations when selecting empirical antibiotics in patients with cirrhosis. World J Hepatol. 2023;15(3):377–85.
57. Lefrock JL, Prince RA, Left RD. Mechanism of action, antimicrobial activity, pharmacology, adverse effects, and clinical efficacy of cefotaxime. Pharmacother J Hum Pharmacol Drug Ther. 1982;2:174–84.
58. Ko RJ, Sattler FR, Nichols S, Akriviadis E, Runyon B, Appleman M, Cohen JL, Koda RT. Pharmacokinetics of cefotaxime and desacetylcefotaxime in patients with liver disease. Antimicrob Agents Chemother. 1991;35:1376–80.
59. Graninger W, Uihlein M, Ferenci P, Moser C, Georgopoulos A. Cefotaxime and desacetylcefotaxime blood levels in hepatic dysfunction. J Antimicrob Chemother. 1984;14:143–6.
60. Hary L, Andrejak M, Leleu S, Orfila J, Capron JP. The pharmacokinetics of ceftriaxone and cefotaxime in cirrhotic patients with ascites. Eur J Clin Pharmacol. 1989;36:613–6.

61. Verbeeck RK. Pharmacokinetics and dosage adjustment in patients with hepatic dysfunction. Eur J Clin Pharmacol. 2008;64:1147–61.
62. Elbekai R, Korashy H, El-Kadi A. The effect of liver cirrhosis on the regulation and expression of drug metabolizing enzymes. Curr Drug Metab. 2004;5:157–67.
63. Westphal J-F, Brogard J-M. Drug administration in chronic liver disease. Drug Saf. 1997;17:47–73.
64. Shirali A, Pazhayattil GS. Drug-induced impairment of renal function. Int J Nephrol Renov Dis. 2014;7:457–68.
65. Lewis GP, Jusko WJ. Pharmacokinetics of ampicillin in cirrhosis. Clin Pharmacol Ther. 1975;18:475–84.
66. Acevedo J, Prado V, Fernández J. Changing options for prevention and treatment of infections in cirrhosis. Curr Treat Options Gastroenterol. 2014;12:256–67.
67. Korth-Bradley JM, Baird-Bellaire SJ, Patat AA, Troy SM, Böhmer GM, Gleiter CH, Buecheler R, Morgan MY. Pharmacokinetics and safety of a single intravenous dose of the antibiotic tigecycline in patients with cirrhosis. J Clin Pharmacol. 2011;51:93–101.
68. Delcò F, Tchambaz L, Schlienger R, Drewe J, Krähenbühl S. Dose adjustment in patients with liver disease. Drug Saf. 2005;28:529–45.
69. Montay G, Gaillot J. Pharmacokinetics of fluoroquinolones in hepatic failure. J Antimicrob Chemother. 1990;26:61–7.
70. Sambatakou H, Giamarellos-Bourboulis EJ, Galanakis N, Giamarellou H. Pharmacokinetics of fluoroquinolones in uncompensated cirrhosis: the significance of penetration in the ascitic fluid. Int J Antimicrob Agents. 2001;18:441–4.
71. Patidar KR, Bajaj JS. Antibiotics for the treatment of hepatic encephalopathy. Metab Brain Dis. 2013;28:307–12.
72. Loft S, Sonne J, Døssing M, Andreasen PB. Metronidazole pharmacokinetics in patients with hepatic encephalopathy. Scand J Gastroenterol. 1987;22:117–23.
73. Zoratti C, Moretti R, Rebuzzi L, Albergati IV, Di Somma A, Decorti G, Di Bella S, Crocè LS, Giuffrè M. Antibiotics and liver cirrhosis: what the physicians need to know. Antibiotics. 2022;11(1):31.
74. Cao MD, Ganesamoorthy D, Elliott AG, Zhang H, Cooper MA, Coin LJM. Streaming algorithms for identification of pathogens and antibiotic resistance potential from real-time MinION sequencing. Gigascience. 2016;5:32.
75. Bajaj JS, Vargas HE, Reddy KR, et al. Association between intestinal microbiota collected at hospital admission and outcomes of patients with cirrhosis. Clin Gastroenterol Hepatol. 2019;17(4):756.e3–65.e3.
76. Libertucci J, Young VB. The role of the microbiota in infectious diseases. Nat Microbiol. 2019;4:35–45.
77. Vilstrup H, Amodio P, Bajaj J, et al. Hepatic encephalopathy in chronic liver disease: 2014 practice guideline by the American Association for the Study of Liver Diseases and the European Association for the Study of the Liver. Hepatology. 2014;60:715–35.
78. Allegretti JR, Mullish BH, Kelly C, Fischer M. The evolution of the use of faecal microbiota transplantation and emerging therapeutic indications. Lancet. 2019;394:420–31.
79. Manges AR, Steiner TS, Wright AJ. Fecal microbiota transplantation for the intestinal decolonization of extensively antimicrobial-resistant opportunistic pathogens: a review. Infect Dis (Lond). 2016;48:587–92.
80. Bajaj JS, Kassam Z, Fagan A, et al. Fecal microbiota transplant from a rational stool donor improves hepatic encephalopathy: a randomized clinical trial. Hepatology. 2017;66:1727–38.
81. Crofts TS, Gasparrini AJ, Dantas G. Next-generation approaches to understand and combat the antibiotic resistome. Nat Rev Microbiol. 2017;15:422–34.
82. Kutter E, De Vos D, Gvasalia G, et al. Phage therapy in clinical practice: treatment of human infections. Curr Pharm Biotechnol. 2010;11:69–86.

Chapter 17
Critical Care Management of Patients Awaiting Liver Transplantation

Akila Rajakumar and Susan Paulin

Abstract Patients on the waitlist for liver transplantation (LT) can develop acute decompensation or acute-on-chronic liver failure (ACLF) necessitating management in the critical care unit. It has also been shown that downstaging ACLF grade before transplantation improves outcomes, thus emphasizing the importance of *appropriate management of* these patients during admissions to critical care units. This cohort of patients has a very delicate reserve and fine balance with other organ functions. Any form of decompensation can rapidly result in other organ failures. Prompt and aggressive management of the precipitating cause and supporting existing organ failures is essential to avoid cascading organ failures in this group of patients. To address the common causes for admission to liver intensive care, we present an outline on critical care management of patients presenting with hypovolemic shock due to gastrointestinal bleeding, altered sensorium, acute kidney Injury, and septic shock.

Keywords Hepatic encephalopathy · Upper GI bleed · AKI in cirrhosis · Sepsis in cirrhosis

Key Highlights
- Appropriate and timely identification and management of patients with end-stage liver disease presenting to the critical care unit is imperative to prevent further deterioration and organ failures.
- Treatment strategies based on current recommendations and guidelines can aid in improving patient outcomes.
- A protocol-based approach can help in prompt, early intervention and safely lead to transplantation.

A. Rajakumar (✉) · S. Paulin
Liver anesthesia and Intensive Care, Institute of Liver Disease and Transplantation, Dr. Rela Institute and Medical Centre, Chennai, India
e-mail: akila.rajakumar@relainstitute.com

S. Saigal, D. Jothimani (eds.), *Fundamentals of Transplant Hepatology*, https://doi.org/10.1007/978-981-95-2624-6_17

Liver transplantation (LT) is now recognized as the standard of care for patients with decompensated cirrhosis. With progressively improving success rates, the number of patients referred for LT is also increasing. Patients on the waitlist for LT can develop acute decompensation (AD) or acute-on-chronic liver failure (ACLF), necessitating management in critical care unit. AD refers to the development of one or more of the following complications: tense ascites, hepatic encephalopathy, and gastrointestinal bleeding [1, 2]. The European Association for the Study of Chronic Liver Failure (EASL-CLIF) Consortium defines ACLF as an acute decompensation of cirrhosis associated with organ failures and high short-term mortality (28-day mortality ≥15%) [1]. The common precipitating triggers for ACLF are bacterial infections, active alcoholism, exacerbation of hepatitis B and other viral hepatitis, GI hemorrhage, transjugular intrahepatic portosystemic shunt (TIPSS), other surgeries, non-liver surgeries, and large volume paracentesis without albumin cover. About 20–40% patients develop ACLF without an obvious trigger. [1, 3] The CLIF-C ACLF score developed by the EASL-CLIF Consortium from the CANONIC study has superior performance in the prediction of mortality in patients with ACLF when compared to well-validated scores in cirrhotic patients like Child–Turcotte–Pugh score(CTP), Model for End-Stage Liver Disease (MELD), and MELD-Sodium (MELD-Na) scores in predicting 28-day mortality [4]. Although ACLF, by definition, is associated with high short-term mortality, which increases with increasing number of organ failure scores, good outcomes have been demonstrated following transplantation with ACLF 3 [5]. It has also been shown that downstaging ACLF grade before transplantation improves outcomes [6], thus emphasizing the importance of appropriate management of these patients during admissions to critical care units.

This cohort of patients has a very delicate reserve and fine balance with other organ functions. Any form of decompensation can rapidly result in other organ failures. Prompt and aggressive management of the precipitating cause and supporting existing organ failures is essential to avoid cascading organ failures in this group of patients. To address the common causes for admission to liver intensive care, we present an outline on critical care management of patients presenting with (1) hypovolemic shock due to gastrointestinal bleeding, (2) altered sensorium, (3) septic shock, and (4) acute kidney injury.

17.1 Hypovolemic Shock Due to Gastrointestinal Bleed

One of the frequent inciting events for the onset of ACLF is upper gastrointestinal (UGI) bleed [7]. Rapid recognition and aggressive management is essential to avoid failure of other organs and successful bridging to LT.

Life-threatening hemorrhage occurs following rupture of the varix in the background of portal hypertension. Gastroesophageal varices are found in almost 72% of Child B/C cirrhosis [8]. Despite the availability of advanced therapeutic modalities, an overall mortality of 15–25% is observed at 6 weeks with each episode of variceal bleed. Mortality risk is especially greater in the presence of acute kidney injury (AKI) and infections [9]. Isolated gastric varices located in the fundus, which are referred to as the cardio fundal varices, are shown to be associated with a higher risk of bleeding [10].

17.1.1 Initial Management

There must be a high suspicion of acute variceal bleeding in any cirrhotic patient presenting with acute GI bleeding, along with a drop in hemoglobin, and treatment must be initiated regardless of confirmation by endoscopy. The goals of therapy in the event of acute variceal bleed include control of acute bleeding with prevention of early recurrence (within 5 days) and 6-week mortality.

Initial therapy should be aimed at restoring euvolemia and thereby hemodynamic stability, to ensure adequate tissue perfusion and oxygenation.

For resuscitation, two wide-bore cannulas must be secured for rapid volume expansion. Balanced salt solutions are recommended as initial fluids of choice, and resuscitation with colloids has not been found to be superior to crystalloids. In the presence of severe anemia, packed red blood cells can be used. A restrictive transfusion strategy with a hemoglobin threshold of 7 g/dL and target range after transfusion of 7–9 g/dL has been found to have mortality benefits with lesser chances of rebleeding, need for rescue therapy, and reduced hospital stay. In the event of massive hemorrhage and in the presence of cardiac comorbidities, transfusions can be performed at the discretion of the attending intensivists to maintain an appropriate physiological status [11]. In two randomized controlled trials, one performed in variceal and another in nonvariceal bleeding cirrhotics, thromboelastogram-guided correction of coagulopathy—in comparison to correction-based conventional tests of coagulation—significantly reduced the volume of blood products transfused without increasing risk of rebleeding, failure to control bleeding, or mortality. The correction of intrenational normalised ratio (INR) with fresh frozen plasma (FFP) and Factor VIIa is not recommended since INR is not a reliable indicator of coagulation status in cirrhosis [10]. The presence of portal vein and/or splenic vein thrombosis is frequently found in association with cardio fundal varices and hence need prompt investigation and intervention [10].

17.1.2 Airway and Breathing

Routine prophylactic intubation is not recommended in all patients with UGI bleed since current evidence on its application show no reduction in the incidence of pneumonia, hospital stay, and mortality risk [12]. The European Non-Variceal UGI Bleed guidelines recommend prophylactic intubation in severe hematemesis, agitation, or inability to protect the airway [13]. The Baveno VII guidance for variceal bleed suggests intubation in the presence of altered sensorium and active hematemesis with a rapid extubation plan following endoscopy [14]. In the event of inability to tolerate endoscopy under conscious sedation, intubation can be provided.

17.1.3 Pharmacological Treatment of UGI Bleeding

The use of vasoactive agents in acute UGI bleed has shown to be associated with a lower 7-day all-cause mortality and lower transfusion requirements. Hence, they should be started as soon as possible upon admission and prior to diagnostic endoscopy [10]. The two classes of drugs widely used in the control of acute variceal bleeding are vasopressin and its analogs and somatostatin and its analogs. Terlipressin, octreotide, and somatostatin are frequently used pharmacological agents in the event of UGI bleed. Though no difference in efficacy has been demonstrated with these agents, terlipressin is the only drug shown to have a survival benefit [15].

Vasopressin is a potent splanchnic vasoconstrictor that reduces blood flow to the splanchnic circulation, thereby decreasing portal and collateral blood flow and eventually reducing the variceal pressure. However, the clinical utility of vasopressin is limited by its multiple adverse effects including arrhythmias, peripheral and bowel ischemia, and hypertension. Nitroglycerin enhances the effect of vasopressin on portal pressures and reduces cardiovascular side effects. The addition of nitroglycerin to vasopressin has shown a significant reduction in failure to control bleeding when compared with Vasopressin alone [15].

Terlipressin is a synthetic analogue of vasopressin, which has an immediate systemic vasoconstrictor effect followed by portal hemodynamic effects due to delayed conversion to vasopressin. The recommended dose of terlipressin is 2 mg IV every 4 hours during the first 48 hours, followed by 1 mg/4 hours thereafter. The optimal dosage is often determined by the onset of peripheral ischemia which needs careful monitoring. It has been observed that continuous infusions of terlipressin are associated with lower cumulative doses and fewer adverse effects compared to intermittent boluses [16]. The Baveno V guidelines advocate 5 days of terlipressin treatment to avoid early rebleeding; however, few trials have shown efficacy with even 24 hours of therapy after satisfactory hemostasis with endoscopy, following esophageal variceal bleeding [15]. Terlipressin, when given as a continuous infusion, was better tolerated than intermittent boluses and also resulted in lower effective doses [16].

Somatostatin is given as a continuous infusion of 250-500microgram/hour with an initial bolus of 250 microgram. The recommended dose of octreotide is a continuous infusion of 50 microgram/hour following an initial bolus of 50 microgram.

In order to improve endoscopic visualization, prokinetics may be of use. They help in better visualization by inducing gastric emptying. The European Society of Gastrointestinal Endoscopy recommends pre-endoscopy administration of intravenous erythromycin in selected patients with clinically severe or ongoing active UGIH. A single IV dose of 250 mg of erythromycin infused over 30–120 minutes appears to be safe and well tolerated with no adverse events. [11] The presence of QT prolongation is a relative contraindication. However, recommendations with regard to other prokinetic agents, such as metoclopramide, have not been made due to insufficient clinical data.

17.1.4 Antibiotics

Infections are frequently observed in patients admitted with UGI bleed, and in many instances, they act as the precipitating event for decompensation. The presence of bacterial Infection has been identified as an independent predictor of mortality following UGI bleed [9]. Hence, these patients must be initiated on antibiotic prophylaxis as soon as they are admitted with an acute UGI bleed. Antibiotic prophylaxis is best administered as per local antibiogram and must be restricted to a maximum of 7 days [10].

17.1.5 Proton Pump Inhibitor Therapy

Pre-endoscopy PPI therapy can be considered in the event of acute UGI bleed to downstage endoscopic stigmata, especially in settings where endoscopy is not readily available. A short course of PPI after endoscopic variceal ligation (EVL) has been found to reduce the size of post-EVL ulcers. An intravenous bolus of 80 mg of pantoprazole followed by a continuous infusion at 8 mg/hour over 72 hours can be administered in this setting. High-dose IV bolus as twice daily dosing can be considered alternatively [13]. Since long-term use of PPI has been found to be associated with an increased risk of hepatic encephalopathy, *Clostridium difficile* infection and spontaneous bacterial peritonitis (SBP), it must be used with caution [17].

17.1.6 Miscellaneous Care

Acute UGI bleed has been recognized as a precipitant for hepatic encephalopathy (HE). Hence, these patients should be closely monitored for the onset of overt HE, started on oral nonabsorbable dissaccharides for prophylaxis, and treated with lactulose or lactitol when encephalopathy sets in [9].

For patients on low-dose aspirin as monotherapy for primary cardiovascular prophylaxis, temporary interruption is advocated, and the medication can be restarted when clinically appropriate. However, in cases of secondary cardiovascular prophylaxis, aspirin should not be interrupted or should be restarted as soon as possible, preferably within 3–5 days.

17.1.7 Endoscopy

Upper GI endoscopy should be performed as early as possible, within the first 12 hours after admission, in the event of acute UGI bleed. Once the source of bleeding is confirmed, EVL should be performed within the same setting. EVL has been found to have high efficacy with low complication rates and is preferred as the standard of care, along with vasoconstrictors for variceal bleed [18, 19]. Sclerotherapy is preferred when banding is not feasible and in cases of isolated gastric varices and those gastroesophageal varices that extend beyond the cardia [18]. To prevent rebleeding from gastric varices, additional glue injections must be considered after 2–4 weeks, along with the addition of beta-blocker therapy [18]. Other rapidly emerging endoscopic tools with a greater safety profile and efficacy are endoscopic ultrasound–guided insertion of coils and cyanoacrylate injections. These modalities are currently under review.

Up to 10–15% of patients with acute UGI bleed are found to have persistent bleeding or early rebleeding and are associated with a high risk of mortality [20]. In the case of esophageal varices, if the patient is stable, a second therapeutic endoscopy can be performed. In refractory cases, transjugular intrahepatic portosystemic shunt (TIPS) can be considered as a rescue therapy of choice [18]. Rescue TIPS has to be offered in select patients only and has been found to be futile in patients with advanced liver disease with child-turcotte-pugh (CTP) score of 14 to 15 [21].

In patients refractory to standard therapy, a bridge therapy such as balloon tamponade with the Linton Nachlas tube can be used to acutely control hemorrhage, especially from gastric varices until a more definite therapy such as TIPS can be done. In the case of the use of Sengstaken-Blakemore or Minnesota tube,

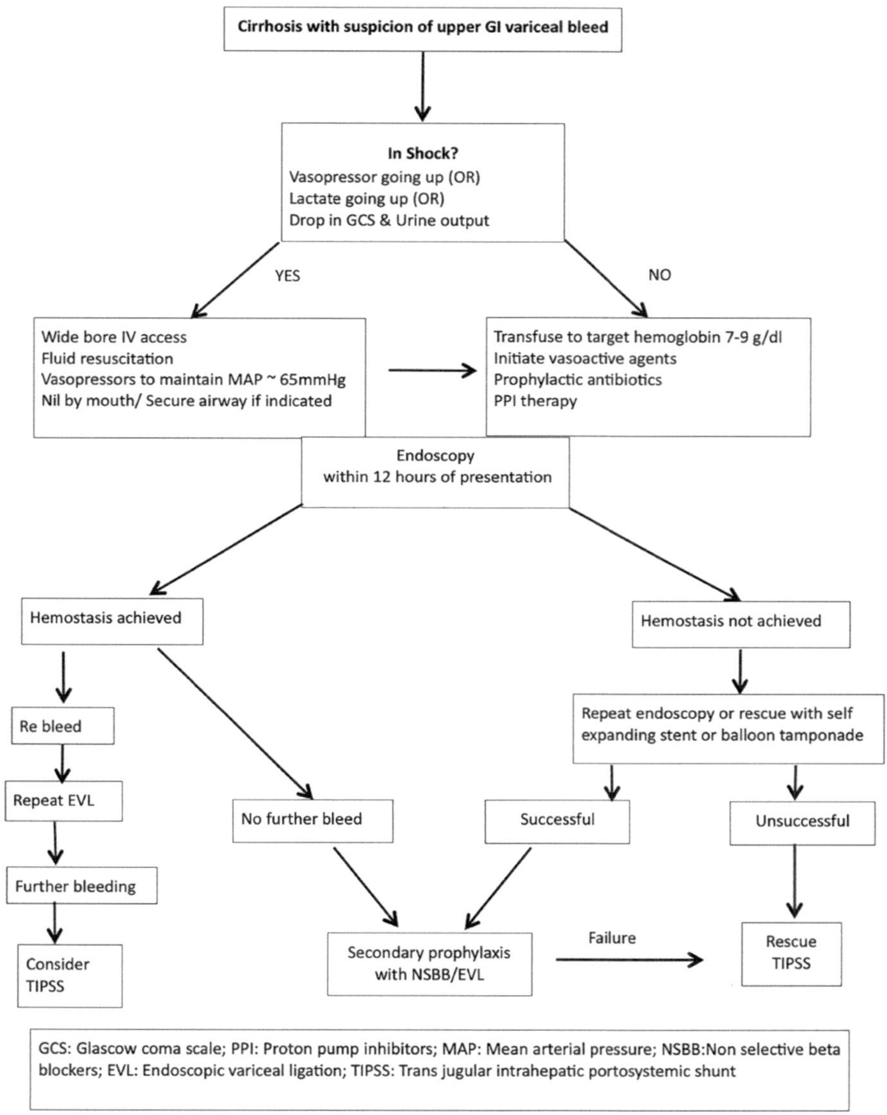

Fig. 17.1 Algorithm 1. Management of Upper Gastrointestinal bleed

inflation of just the gastric balloon and anchoring it against the gastroesophageal junction could provide adequate tamponade for hemostasis. Since balloon tamponade is associated with high rates of severe adverse events, its use should not exceed 24 hours. A new therapeutic option under evaluation is the endoscopic placement of self-expandable metallic stents which can be left in situ for 7 days. A multicenter RCT has shown better control of bleeding with lesser side effects with these stents in comparison to balloon tamponade; however, no survival benefit was noted. [22]

17.1.8 Follow-Up

Patients with cirrhosis who recover from an episode of active variceal hemorrhage should receive secondary prophylaxis in the form of combination of nonselective β-blockers plus EVL to prevent recurrence of variceal hemorrhage. Patients who receive TIPS need no further preventive measures but require frequent screening for shunt patency. Referral to a transplant center should be considered when indicated [23].

A quick overview of the management of upper GI bleed is elaborated in Fig. 17.1.

17.2 Management of Altered Sensorium

Altered sensorium due to hepatic encephalopathy is a frequent complication among patients with cirrhosis necessitating frequent hospital and ICU admissions.

Hepatic encephalopathy (HE) is brain dysfunction caused by severe liver dysfunction and/or presence of portosystemic shunts (PSS). HE can manifest as a wide spectrum of neurological or psychiatric abnormalities ranging from subclinical alterations to coma and these changes are usually reversible [24]. Concomitant disorders as an additional cause for cerebral dysfunction should to be considered in cirrhosis. Factors such as electrolyte disturbances especially hyponatremia, uremia, and thiamine deficiency; sepsis; use of psychoactive medications such as benzodiazepines and opioids; drug withdrawal especially alcohol; respiratory failure; and rarely intracranial hemorrhage can also contribute to the development of altered sensorium in this group. Therefore, management of HE should follow the four-pronged approach: (1) prompt initiation of supportive care for patients with altered consciousness; (2) evaluation and treatment for alternative causes of altered mental status; (3) identification of precipitating factors and their correction; and (4) commencement of empirical HE treatment [24].

Patients with persistent higher grades of HE will require airway protection in the critical care unit. Management of precipitating factors should happen simultaneously. Lactulose is the first choice for treatment of episodic overt HE. In acute exacerbation 30 g of lactulose orally or through the nasogastric tube, every hour until bowel movement, should be administered and subsequent doses can be modified to target two to three soft bowel movements per day. Lactulose enemas are an alternative option in cases of severe HE where enteral route is not recommended. Rifaximin is an effective add-on therapy to lactulose for prevention of OHE recurrence and the combination with lactulose has been demonstrated to be better compared to lactulose alone. Polyethylene glycol has also shown promising outcomes [25] and can serve as a good alternative to reduce the risk of ileus. Alternative agents, in cases not responding to conventional therapy, include oral branched chain amino acids and intravenous L-ornithine-L-aspartate which require further large scale studies [26]. Brain imaging is to be considered for overt HE, if the onset of the symptoms is abrupt and severe, presence of focal neurological signs or there is limited or no response to empirical treatment of HE and the precipitating factor. Electroencephalography should also be considered in refractory HE to rule out other cases of altered mental status. Although ammonia levels, trends and cut off are not as useful for managing HE in this group of patients as in acute liver failure, a low level in a patient with altered mental status implies causes other than HE [27].

Recent studies have shown that restricting protein intake could actually be detrimental [28] since patients with cirrhosis have increased protein requirements generally to achieve balanced nitrogen metabolism. This stimulates protein breakdown from muscle leading to rise in plasma ammonia levels. On the other hand, hepatic regeneration is assisted by a positive nitrogen balance along

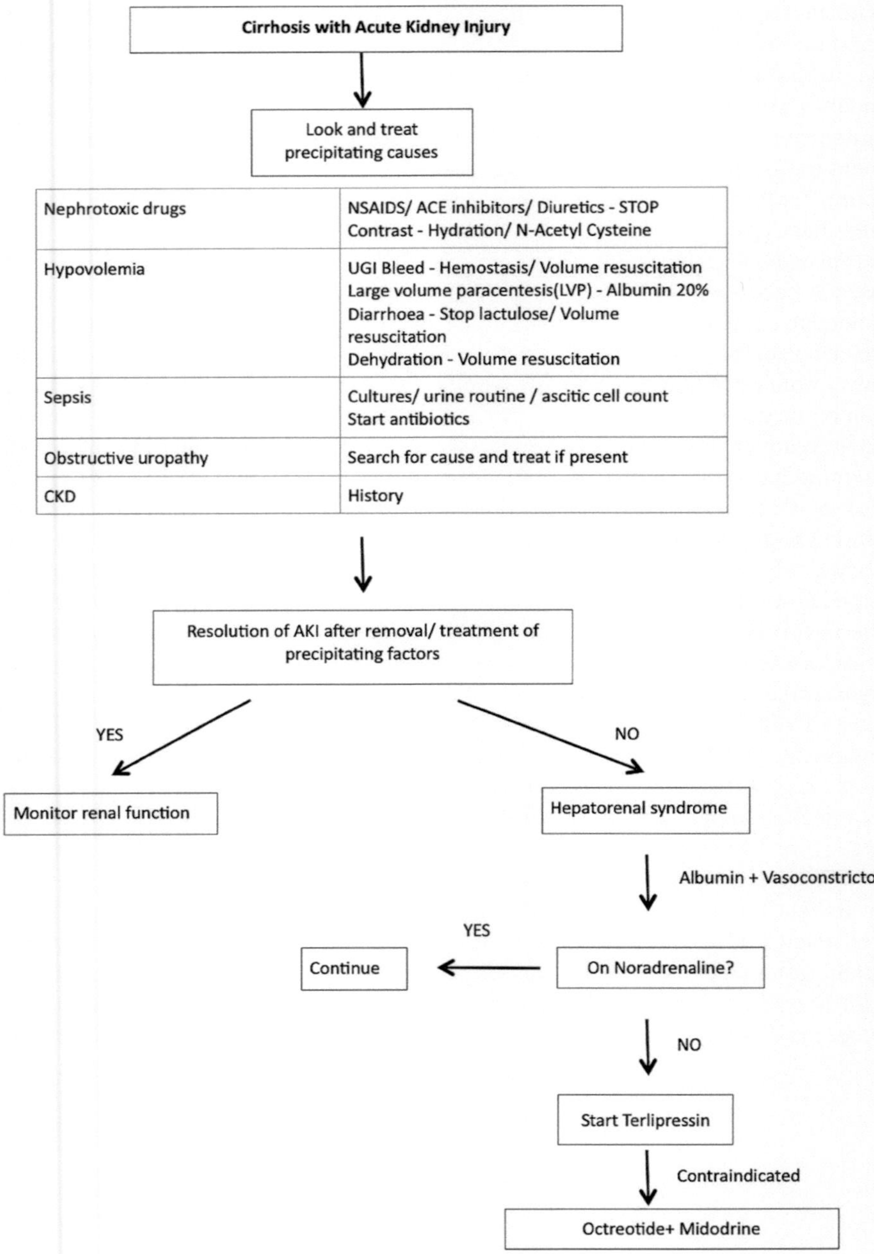

Fig. 17.2 Algorithm 2. Management of altered mental status

with increased muscle capacity to detoxify ammonia. Hence adequate protein intake and not low protein diet should be advocated in patients HE. All patients with HE should undergo a proper assessment of nutritional status and nutritional rehabilitation should be initiated as soon as clinically appropriate [24, 28, 29].

Short-acting agents like propofol or dexmedetomidine are preferred if sedation is required for these patients on ventilator. Low tidal volume lung protective ventilatory strategies should be applied with adequate precautions to prevent ventilator associated pneumonia. An assessment of mental status can be challenging in mechanically ventilated patients under sedation. Prolonged effect of sedatives has been observed in patients with cirrhosis long after their discontinuation. However, daily sedation break should be provided for assessment of sensorium. Benzodiazepine receptor antagonist such as flumazenil has been shown to provide short-term improvement of HE but without any survival or recovery benefit [30]. There is no evidence supporting the role of renal replacement therapy for refractory HE. Liver support devices have a role in reversal of encephalopathy but do not improve survival outcomes.

Liver transplantation is the only curative option for recurrent overt HE especially in refractory cases. It is important to distinguish HE from other causes of mental impairment, such as Alzheimer's disease and small-vessel cerebrovascular disease. Large PSSs may cause neurological disturbances and persistent HE, even after LT. Therefore, shunts should be identified and embolization considered before or during transplantation [31]. Figure 17.2 gives an outline of the management of cirrhotic patients with altered mental status.

17.3 Management of Patients with Sepsis/Septic Shock

The term "cirrhosis-associated immune dysfunction" [32] is used to describe the combined presentation of systemic inflammation and immune deficiency. High-grade systemic inflammatory response seems to be the key driver of ACLF, which cause significant functional immune paresis, making these patients highly susceptible to infections [33]. Dysregulation of the gut–liver axis also leads to a higher risk of bacterial translocation [34]. Sepsis seems to be responsible for precipitating ACLF in up to 30% of cases [1]. Sepsis and progression to septic shock significantly increase the risk of dying in these patients and are reported to be as high as 65% [35]. Physiological changes like tachycardia and hyperdynamic circulation, hypersplenism-induced leucopenia and thrombocytopenia, and blunted temperature regulation interfere with the accuracy of early diagnosis of sepsis and septic shock [36]. Therefore, a high index of suspicion is required to avoid delay in the administration of antibiotic therapy.

17.3.1 Management Principles

Management principles are similar to the general population and include early and appropriate administration of antibiotics after taking samples for cultures, fluid resuscitation and/or vasopressors to maintain tissue perfusion, and oxygenation and source control. Establishing optimal endpoints in resuscitation, like urine output and lactate clearance, will be challenging due to baseline abnormalities in these parameters [37].

17.3.2 Fluid Resuscitation

It has been well demonstrated and understood that a significant increase in central blood volume cannot be achieved by standard volume expansion including albumin administration in advanced cirrhosis. Increased fluid administration can result in deleterious effects like distension of collaterals, causing worsening bleeding, ascites, and peripheral edema [38–40].

Crystalloids, preferentially buffered solutions, are recommended by Surviving Sepsis Guidelines for resuscitation in septic shock [41]. Albumin has also been suggested in patients requiring large volumes of crystalloids, especially in patients with hypoalbuminemia; the same recommendation has also been endorsed by the Expert Consensus Committee in ACLF [42]. In the general critical care population, large-scale randomized controlled trials have failed to demonstrate a survival benefit with the use of albumin for resuscitation. Albumin has been extensively studied in cirrhosis for its beneficial effects on hepatorenal syndrome (HRS), SBP, and post-paracentesis circulatory dysfunction. It might have a beneficial role due to its additional effect on modulating the systemic inflammation. About 20% albumin has been shown to be superior to plasmalyte in earlier achievement of target mean arterial blood pressure (MAP) in a recent RCT although no survival benefit was seen. Of interest to note were the increased pulmonary complications in the albumin group [43]. When choosing crystalloids, balanced salt solutions like plasmalyte should be used. Studies have clearly demonstrated increased mortality with the use of saline for fluid resuscitation in the general population [44]. It can be assumed that the deleterious effects will be more pronounced in cirrhosis due to markedly reduced buffering capacity. Hydroxyethyl starches are not recommended for resuscitation due to the increased risks of nephrotoxicity [45].

Therefore, with the available limited evidence, an initial volume expansion with 5–10 mL/kg of plasmalyte or 5% albumin should be considered for initial resuscitation of sepsis and failure to respond should prompt initiating vasopressors for maintaining the target MAP. Further fluid management should, ideally, be based on hemodynamic monitoring only.

17.3.3 Vasopressors

Norepinephrine has emerged as the first vasopressor of choice in septic shock both in the general population and in patients with advanced cirrhosis [41, 42, 45]. Epinephrine should be avoided because of profound vasoconstriction, which can cause tissue ischemia leading to impaired lactate clearance and dysrhythmias [42, 46]. Endogenous vasopressin deficiency has been demonstrated in cirrhotic patients presenting for liver transplantation [47], emphasizing an important role as a second-line vasopressor in cirrhotic patients with sepsis. The additional effect of vasopressin in the redistribution of blood from the splanchnic pool to the central compartment might be beneficial, although careful monitoring for digital ischemia due to poor peripheral perfusion has to be done, especially, in doses in excess of 0.4 units/minute [46]. Angiotensin II has demonstrated significant benefit in refractory septic shock; however, this is yet to be evaluated in patients with cirrhosis [48]. In patients with impaired cardiac contractility, dobutamine is preferred, although such instances are not very frequent in cirrhotic patients due to the hyperdynamic circulation.

17.3.4 Assessment of Fluid Responsiveness

Altered distribution of the circulatory volume and other associated changes make usual parameters used for bedside assessment of hypovolemia less useful in these patients. Measurement of central venous pressure can also be misleading in the presence of increased intra-abdominal pressure. The point-of-care ultrasound (POCUS) and bedside echocardiography seem to be emerging as very useful noninvasive tools to assess volume status and fluid responsiveness in these patients. Inferior vena cava diameter and collapsibility are good dynamic measures of fluid responsiveness, although their assessment can be difficult in patients with massive ascites. Presence of more than 40% variability in inferior venacava (IVC) diameter in patients on spontaneous breathing and > 12–18% in patients on mechanical ventilator are good indicators of fluid responsiveness [49]. An increase in left ventricular outflow tract velocity time integral >12% during passive leg raising also helps in identifying fluid responders [50]. Pulse pressure variation and stroke volume variation are useful predictors in mechanically ventilated patients with good lung compliance. Invasive measures like pulse contour cardiac output analysis could be considered in critically ill patients who are poorly responding to initial resuscitative measures.

17.3.5 Role of Steroids

Adrenal insufficiency has been reported in patients with cirrhosis, which, in the presence of critical illness, can lead to profound hemodynamic instability, reduced response to vasoactive drugs, and increased mortality [51]. Although results from various studies regarding the benefit of steroids in the management of refractory hypotension are conflicting, expert consensus recommend a trial of hydrocortisone 200–300 mg/day in divided doses until improvement in hemodynamics is observed [45].

Table 17.1 Considerations for management and relisting patients for liver transplantation after common infections [56]

Infection	Characteristics	Recommendations
Urine	Asymptomatic bacteriuria	Not a contraindication Peritransplant antibiotic cover
	Asymptomatic candiduria	Not a contraindication
	UTI with negative blood cultures	Not a contraindication Peritransplant antibiotic cover
SBP	Bacterial SBP	5 days of treatment Reactivate if repeat tap shows a $>$ 25% decrease in PMN count $\geq$48 hours after treatment initiation, and other clinical parameters improve.
	Fungal SBP	Full course of therapy A repeat PMN count $<$250 cells/mm [3] of treatment required. Secondary causes need to be ruled out
Pneumonia	Pneumonia	Can list after $\geq$7 days of therapy when clinical improvement is documented. In patients without clinical improvement, imaging required Empyema requires drainage and a complete course of antibiotics, VATS to be considered
Bacteremia	Central line	Remove the catheter and treat with appropriate antibiotics for 7–14 days Can be listed based on clinical improvement
	Spontaneous	Antibiotics for 7–14 days Likely source: bacterial translocation or skin Can be listed based on clinical improvement with negative repeat blood cultures after 48 hours
	Fungemia	Full course of therapy Secondary causes need to be ruled out Repeat negative blood cultures off therapy is required

(continued)

Table 17.1 (continued)

Infection	Characteristics	Recommendations
Cloatridium Difficile	Diarrhea	At least 7 days of therapy Clinical improvement and normalization of WBC prior to listing is required Sigmoidoscopy can help assess mucosal healing in uncertain cases
Cholecystitis	Operative candidates	Surgical intervention
	Nonoperative candidates	IV antibiotics: First-line therapy. C-tube placement for those without a clinical response Endoscopic gallbladder stenting or aspiration when C-tube placement is absolutely contraindicated and IV antibiotics are failing Transplant reactivation after adequate clinical response

UTI urinary tract infection, *SBP* spontaneous bacterial peritonitis, *PMN* Polymorphonuclear lymphocytes, *WBC* white blood cells, *C- Tube* Cholecystostomy tube, *IV* intravenous

17.3.6 Antibiotic Administration

Patients with advanced cirrhosis are complicated by altered gut microbiota along with increased risk of bacterial translocation. In addition to their immunocompromised states, they are at increased risk of colonization by resistant organisms [36]. Thus, the choice of antibiotics and the timing of administration play a vital role here.

Screening for the source of infection is imperative in the management of sepsis. Spontaneous bacterial peritonitis, urinary tract infection, and pneumonia are more frequently encountered in patients admitted to the ICU with sepsis. Other causes include bacteremias following invasive procedures such as endoscopy and TIPS, cellulitis, catheter-related infections, and fungal sepsis.

Patients with suspicion of sepsis should be initiated on empirical antibiotics at the earliest, since delay by each hour affects the outcomes. Simultaneously, a thorough evaluation should be started [52]. The choice of the antibiotic should be based on the following factors: presumed source, hospital- or community-acquired, history of previous infection or colonization with multidrug-resistant organisms, and the local antibiogram. A robust antimicrobial stewardship is required to monitor use and to recommend de-escalation of broad-spectrum antibiotics if the susceptibility pattern allows. Lack of improvement despite being on appropriate broad-spectrum antibacterial therapy mandates empirical antifungal therapy. Screening for fungal sepsis with Beta-D-glucan and galactomannan assays should be performed whenever possible.

During the workup of patients with suspected infections, inflammatory biomarkers such as C-reactive protein (CRP) or procalcitonin can be utilized to identify infection and assess clinical improvement. In the general population, serum procalcitonin is found to be valuable in monitoring the response to antibiotic therapy and rationalizing antibiotic duration, but its role in cirrhotic patients has not been extensively studied. In a small prospective cohort study, in patients with advanced cirrhosis, it was demonstrated that serum procalcitonin can serve as a noninvasive biomarker in diagnosing SBP with a high degree of accuracy [53]. Therefore, it should only be used as an adjunct to clinical features and other indicators for decision-making in septic patients with cirrhosis [54]. C-reactive protein was also found to be a reliable marker for bacterial infections in a small study of cirrhotic patients at levels higher than 29.5 mg/L [55]. Once patients recover from the septic episode, they should be expedited for liver transplantation at the earliest available opportunity. Table 17.1 gives a summary of management and relisting of cirrhotic patients for liver transplantation following an episode of infection [56].

17.4 Management of Patients with Acute Kidney Injury

It has been observed that the mortality of patients who develop AKI or AKI superimposed on chronic kidney disease is three times greater than those without renal dysfunction, signifying the need for aggressive optimisation [57, 58]. A thorough etiological assessment and evaluation is essential to initiate targeted interventions to avert progression of renal dysfunction and this has been shown to decrease mortality [59, 60] Prerenal causes seem to responsible for more than half of the AKI; acute tubular necrosis due to intrinsic causes account for 30% with less than 1% due to post renal obstruction. Hepatorenal syndrome (HRS) contributes to 15–20% of AKI cases in cirrhosis [61].

Hypovolemia leading to AKI usually results from (1) rapid fluid losses including gastrointestinal (GI) losses from excessive laxatives, excessive diuresis due to drugs, and GI bleeding; (2) drug induced hypotension—overdosage of beta blockers; (3) circulatory dysfunction due to large volume paracentesis; and (4) worsening vasodilatation or direct effect of systemic inflammatory response due to infections. Workup should search for and exclude these and other intrinsic (sepsis, bile cast nephropathy and nephrotoxic medications) and post-renal causes.

Volume expansion is the key to prevent further progression and reversal of hypovolemic AKI. All contributing offending agents are to be discontinued. Volume resuscitation is recommended in hypovolemic patients with crystalloids and euvolemic patients with 20–25% albumin, and further fluid administration has to be

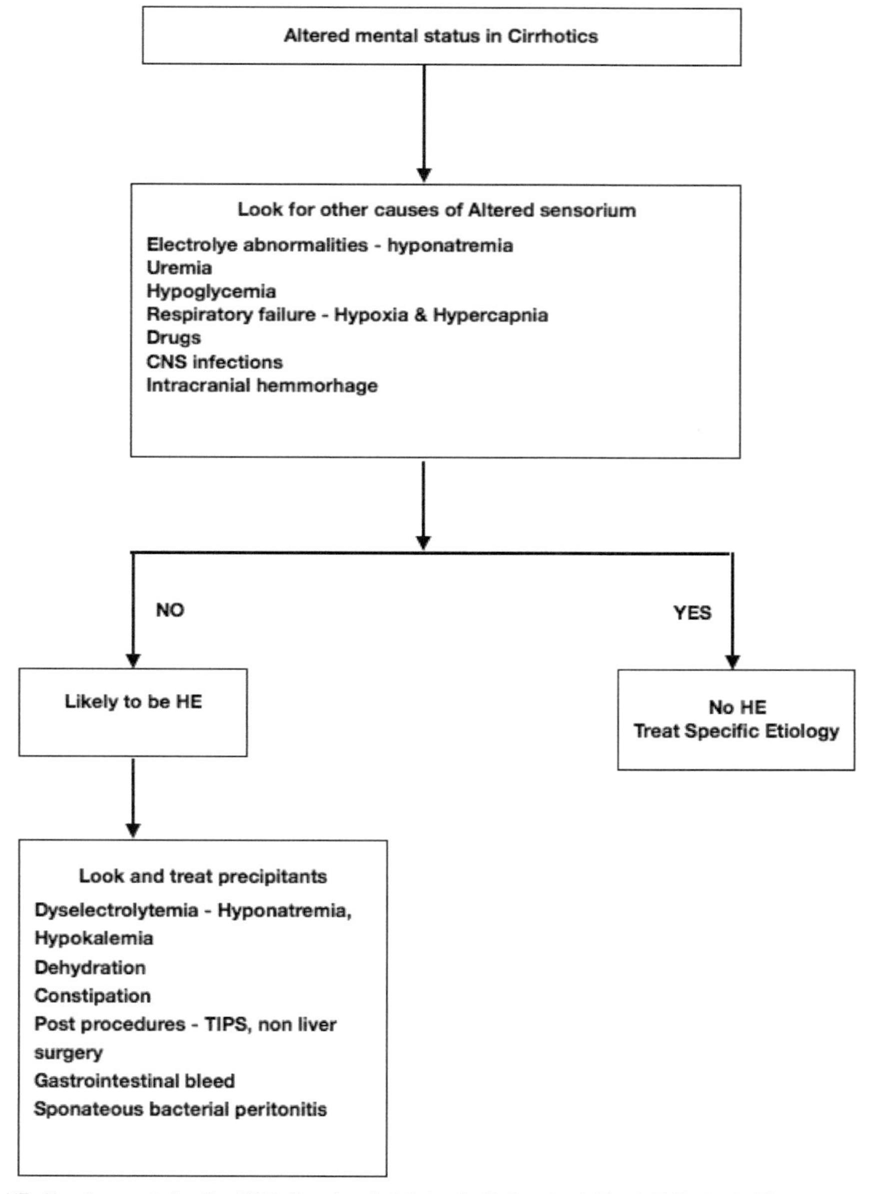

Fig. 17.3 Algorithm 3. Management of Acute kidney Injury

titrated based on volume responsiveness. The role of various cardiac output monitoring devices in the assessment of fluid responsiveness has been described above.

Hemodynamic monitoring tools and volume targets are yet to be validated and clearly defined in patients with cirrhosis; however, echocardiography has been shown to be useful and promising for bedside assessment of fluid status and responsiveness. [37] Caution needs to be exercised to avoid pulmonary edema in these patients with overzealous volume expansion because of their contracted central compartment, and therefore, regular assessment of volume responsiveness is recommended.

Those with sepsis-induced hypotension are seen to be less fluid responsive in cirrhosis and early initiation of vasopressors to restore mean arterial blood pressure (MAP) is recommended with norepinephrine being the first choice [37]. Aggressive treatment of the precipitating cause also should be initiated simultaneously including initiation of broad-spectrum antibiotics.

When the diagnosis of HRS-AKI is made, combination of albumin with vasoconstrictors is the first-line therapy [62, 63]. It was found that terlipressin was superior to midodrine and octreotide in HRS reversal, and it is recommended to initiate norepinephrine for this effect when terlipressin is not available [63]. Terlipressin use has been shown to be associated with an increased incidence of respiratory failure due to pulmonary edema [64], and therefore, the combination of albumin + terlipressin should not be used in patients with clinical evidence of intravascular volume overload. It has been observed that continuous infusions of terlipressin are associated with lower cumulative doses and fewer adverse effects compared to intermittent boluses [16].

17.4.1 Role of Renal Replacement Therapy (RRT)

Initial consensus was to not offer RRT to patients who are not suitable for liver transplantation. However, currently, a short trial of RRT is being recommended in selected patients with HRS-AKI even if they are not transplant candidates. There is no consensus on when to initiate RRT in this cohort of AKI patients. Data on the critically ill patients have not demonstrated significant benefits of early versus late initiation of RRT [65–68]. Nevertheless, RRT should be considered in the usual life-threatening indications refractory to medical therapy like hyperkalemia, worsening metabolic acidosis, volume overload, and complications from uremia [69].

Figure 17.3 provides a brief outline on the management of acute kidney injury in patients with cirrhosis.

17.5 Conclusion

Patients with cirrhosis on the waitlist are prone to develop complications. Hence, careful and aggressive management of such complications in specialized intensive care units with attention to detail is required. Preventive strategies should be used to avoid such complications in future, whenever feasible.

References

1. Moreau R, Jalan R, Gines P, et al. Acute-on-chronic liver failure is a distinct syndrome that develops in patients with acute decompensation of cirrhosis. Gastroenterology. 2013;144(7):1426–37, 1437.e1–9. (In eng). https://doi.org/10.1053/j.gastro.2013.02.042.
2. Sarin SK, Choudhury A, Sharma MK, et al. Acute-on-chronic liver failure: consensus recommendations of the Asian Pacific association for the study of the liver (APASL): an update. Hepatol Int. 2019;13(4):353–90. (In eng). https://doi.org/10.1007/s12072-019-09946-3.
3. Shi Y, Yang Y, Hu Y, et al. Acute-on-chronic liver failure precipitated by hepatic injury is distinct from that precipitated by extrahepatic insults. Hepatology. 2015;62(1):232–42. (In eng). https://doi.org/10.1002/hep.27795.
4. Jalan R, Saliba F, Pavesi M, et al. Development and validation of a prognostic score to predict mortality in patients with acute-on-chronic liver failure. J Hepatol. 2014;61(5):1038–47. (In eng). https://doi.org/10.1016/j.jhep.2014.06.012.
5. Artru F, Louvet A, Ruiz I, et al. Liver transplantation in the most severely ill cirrhotic patients: a multicenter study in acute-on-chronic liver failure grade 3. J Hepatol. 2017;67(4):708–15. (In eng). https://doi.org/10.1016/j.jhep.2017.06.009.
6. Sundaram V, Kogachi S, Wong RJ, et al. Effect of the clinical course of acute-on-chronic liver failure prior to liver transplantation on post-transplant survival. J Hepatol. 2020;72(3):481–8. (In eng). https://doi.org/10.1016/j.jhep.2019.10.013.
7. EASL Clinical Practice Guidelines on acute-on-chronic liver failure. J Hepatol. 2023;79(2):461–91. (In eng). https://doi.org/10.1016/j.jhep.2023.04.021.
8. Merli M, Nicolini G, Angeloni S, et al. Incidence and natural history of small esophageal varices in cirrhotic patients. J Hepatol. 2003;38(3):266–72. (In eng). https://doi.org/10.1016/s0168-8278(02)00420-8.
9. EASL Clinical Practice Guidelines for the management of patients with decompensated cirrhosis. J Hepatol. 2018;69(2):406–60. (In eng). https://doi.org/10.1016/j.jhep.2018.03.024.
10. Garcia-Tsao G, Abraldes JG, Berzigotti A, Bosch J. Portal hypertensive bleeding in cirrhosis: risk stratification, diagnosis, and management: 2016 practice guidance by the American Association for the study of liver diseases. Hepatology. 2017;65(1):310–35. (In eng). https://doi.org/10.1002/hep.28906.
11. Villanueva C, Colomo A, Bosch A, et al. Transfusion strategies for acute upper gastrointestinal bleeding. N Engl J Med. 2013;368(1):11–21. (In eng). https://doi.org/10.1056/NEJMoa1211801.
12. Orpen-Palmer J, Stanley AJ. A review of risk scores within upper gastrointestinal bleeding. J Clin Med. 2023;12(11):3678. https://doi.org/10.3390/jcm12113678.
13. Gralnek IM, Stanley AJ, Morris AJ, et al. Endoscopic diagnosis and management of nonvariceal upper gastrointestinal hemorrhage (NVUGIH): European Society of Gastrointestinal Endoscopy (ESGE) Guideline - Update 2021. Endoscopy. 2021;53(3):300–32. (In eng). https://doi.org/10.1055/a-1369-5274.
14. de Franchis R, Bosch J, Garcia-Tsao G, Reiberger T, Ripoll C. Baveno VII - Renewing consensus in portal hypertension. J Hepatol. 2022;76(4):959–74. (In eng). https://doi.org/10.1016/j.jhep.2021.12.022.

15. Tripathi D, Stanley AJ, Hayes PC, et al. U.K. guidelines on the management of variceal haemorrhage in cirrhotic patients. Gut. 2015;64(11):1680–704. (In eng). https://doi.org/10.1136/gutjnl-2015-309262.
16. Cavallin M, Piano S, Romano A, et al. Terlipressin given by continuous intravenous infusion versus intravenous boluses in the treatment of hepatorenal syndrome: a randomized controlled study. Hepatology. 2016;63(3):983–92. (In eng). https://doi.org/10.1002/hep.28396.
17. Janka T, Tornai T, Borbély B, et al. Deleterious effect of proton pump inhibitors on the disease course of cirrhosis. Eur J Gastroenterol Hepatol. 2020;32(2):257–64. (In eng). https://doi.org/10.1097/meg.0000000000001499.
18. de Franchis R. Expanding consensus in portal hypertension: report of the Baveno VI Consensus Workshop: Stratifying risk and individualizing care for portal hypertension. J Hepatol. 2015;63(3):743–52. (In eng). https://doi.org/10.1016/j.jhep.2015.05.022.
19. Edelson J, Basso JE, Rockey DC. Updated strategies in the management of acute variceal haemorrhage. Curr Opin Gastroenterol. 2021;37(3):167–72. (In eng). https://doi.org/10.1097/mog.0000000000000723.
20. Garcia-Tsao G, Bosch J. Management of varices and variceal hemorrhage in cirrhosis. N Engl J Med. 2010;362(9):823–32. (In eng). https://doi.org/10.1056/NEJMra0901512.
21. Maimone S, Saffioti F, Filomia R, et al. Predictors of re-bleeding and mortality among patients with refractory Variceal bleeding undergoing salvage Transjugular Intrahepatic Portosystemic Shunt (TIPS). Dig Dis Sci. 2019;64(5):1335–45. (In eng). https://doi.org/10.1007/s10620-018-5412-x.
22. Escorsell À, Pavel O, Cárdenas A, et al. Esophageal balloon tamponade versus esophageal stent in controlling acute refractory variceal bleeding: a multicenter randomized, controlled trial. Hepatology. 2016;63(6):1957–67. (In eng). https://doi.org/10.1002/hep.28360.
23. Garcia-Tsao G, Sanyal AJ, Grace ND, Carey W. Prevention and management of gastroesophageal varices and variceal hemorrhage in cirrhosis. Hepatology. 2007;46(3):922–38. (In eng). https://doi.org/10.1002/hep.21907.
24. Vilstrup H, Amodio P, Bajaj J, et al. Hepatic encephalopathy in chronic liver disease: 2014 Practice Guideline by the American Association for the Study of Liver Diseases and the European Association for the Study of the Liver. Hepatology. 2014;60(2):715–35. (In eng). https://doi.org/10.1002/hep.27210.
25. Rahimi RS, Singal AG, Cuthbert JA, Rockey DC. Lactulose vs polyethylene glycol 3350--electrolyte solution for treatment of overt hepatic encephalopathy: the HELP randomized clinical trial. JAMA Intern Med. 2014;174(11):1727–33. (In eng). https://doi.org/10.1001/jamainternmed.2014.4746.
26. Rahimi RS, Safadi R, Thabut D, et al. Efficacy and safety of ornithine Phenylacetate for treating overt hepatic encephalopathy in a randomized trial. Clin Gastroenterol Hepatol. 2021;19(12):2626–2635.e7. (In eng). https://doi.org/10.1016/j.cgh.2020.10.019.
27. Cordoba J, Ventura-Cots M, Simón-Talero M, et al. Characteristics, risk factors, and mortality of cirrhotic patients hospitalized for hepatic encephalopathy with and without acute-on-chronic liver failure (ACLF). J Hepatol. 2014;60(2):275–81. (In eng). https://doi.org/10.1016/j.jhep.2013.10.004.
28. Córdoba J, López-Hellín J, Planas M, et al. Normal protein diet for episodic hepatic encephalopathy: results of a randomized study. J Hepatol. 2004;41(1):38–43. (In eng). https://doi.org/10.1016/j.jhep.2004.03.023.
29. Findlay JY, Fix OK, Paugam-Burtz C, et al. Critical care of the end-stage liver disease patient awaiting liver transplantation. Liver Transpl. 2011;17(5):496–510. (In eng). https://doi.org/10.1002/lt.22269.
30. Als-Nielsen B, Gluud LL, Gluud C. Benzodiazepine receptor antagonists for hepatic encephalopathy. Cochrane Database Syst Rev. 2004(2):Cd002798. (In eng). https://doi.org/10.1002/14651858.CD002798.pub2.
31. Lynn AM, Singh S, Congly SE, et al. Embolization of portosystemic shunts for treatment of medically refractory hepatic encephalopathy. Liver Transpl. 2016;22(6):723–31. (In eng). https://doi.org/10.1002/lt.24440.

32. Albillos A, Martin-Mateos R, Van der Merwe S, Wiest R, Jalan R, Álvarez-Mon M. Cirrhosis-associated immune dysfunction. Nat Rev Gastroenterol Hepatol. 2022;19(2):112–34. (In eng). https://doi.org/10.1038/s41575-021-00520-7.
33. Martin-Mateos R, Alvarez-Mon M, Albillos A. Dysfunctional immune response in acute-on-chronic liver failure: it takes two to tango. Front Immunol. 2019;10:973. (In eng). https://doi.org/10.3389/fimmu.2019.00973.
34. Albillos A, de Gottardi A, Rescigno M. The gut-liver axis in liver disease: pathophysiological basis for therapy. J Hepatol. 2020;72(3):558–77. (In eng). https://doi.org/10.1016/j.jhep.2019.10.003.
35. Galbois A, Aegerter P, Martel-Samb P, et al. Improved prognosis of septic shock in patients with cirrhosis: a multicenter study*. Crit Care Med. 2014;42(7):1666–75. (In eng). https://doi.org/10.1097/ccm.0000000000000321.
36. Simonetto DA, Piccolo Serafim L, Gallo de Moraes A, Gajic O, Kamath PS. Management of Sepsis in patients with cirrhosis: current evidence and practical approach. Hepatology. 2019;70(1):418–28. (In eng). https://doi.org/10.1002/hep.30412.
37. Durand F, Kellum JA, Nadim MK. Fluid resuscitation in patients with cirrhosis and sepsis: a multidisciplinary perspective. J Hepatol. 2023;79(1):240–6. (In eng). https://doi.org/10.1016/j.jhep.2023.02.024.
38. Brinch K, Møller S, Bendtsen F, Becker U, Henriksen JH. Plasma volume expansion by albumin in cirrhosis. Relation to blood volume distribution, arterial compliance and severity of disease. J Hepatol. 2003;39(1):24–31. (In eng). https://doi.org/10.1016/s0168-8278(03)00160-0.
39. Hoste EA, Maitland K, Brudney CS, et al. Four phases of intravenous fluid therapy: a conceptual model. Br J Anaesth. 2014;113(5):740–7. (In eng). https://doi.org/10.1093/bja/aeu300.
40. Møller S, Bendtsen F, Henriksen JH. Effect of volume expansion on systemic hemodynamics and central and arterial blood volume in cirrhosis. Gastroenterology. 1995;109(6):1917–25. (In eng). https://doi.org/10.1016/0016-5085(95)90759-9.
41. Evans L, Rhodes A, Alhazzani W, et al. Surviving sepsis campaign: international guidelines for management of sepsis and septic shock 2021. Intensive Care Med. 2021;47(11):1181–247. (In eng). https://doi.org/10.1007/s00134-021-06506-y.
42. Nanchal R, Subramanian R, Karvellas CJ, et al. Guidelines for the management of adult acute and acute-on-chronic liver failure in the ICU: cardiovascular, endocrine, hematologic, pulmonary, and renal considerations. Crit Care Med. 2020;48(3):e173–91. (In eng). https://doi.org/10.1097/ccm.0000000000004192.
43. Maiwall R, Kumar A, Pasupuleti SSR, et al. A randomized-controlled trial comparing 20% albumin to plasmalyte in patients with cirrhosis and sepsis-induced hypotension [ALPS trial]. J Hepatol. 2022;77(3):670–82. (In eng). https://doi.org/10.1016/j.jhep.2022.03.043.
44. Finfer S, Micallef S, Hammond N, et al. Balanced multielectrolyte solution versus saline in critically ill adults. N Engl J Med. 2022;386(9):815–26. (In eng). https://doi.org/10.1056/NEJMoa2114464.
45. Nadim MK, Durand F, Kellum JA, et al. Management of the critically ill patient with cirrhosis: a multidisciplinary perspective. J Hepatol. 2016;64(3):717–35. (In eng). https://doi.org/10.1016/j.jhep.2015.10.019.
46. Overgaard CB, Dzavík V. Inotropes and vasopressors: review of physiology and clinical use in cardiovascular disease. Circulation. 2008;118(10):1047–56. (In eng). https://doi.org/10.1161/circulationaha.107.728840.
47. Wagener G, Bakker J. Vasopressin in cirrhosis and sepsis: physiology and clinical implications. Minerva Anestesiol. 2015;81(12):1377–83. (In eng).
48. Khanna A, English SW, Wang XS, et al. Angiotensin II for the treatment of Vasodilatory shock. N Engl J Med. 2017;377(5):419–30. (In eng). https://doi.org/10.1056/NEJMoa1704154.
49. De Backer D, Fagnoul D. Intensive care ultrasound: VI. Fluid responsiveness and shock assessment. Ann Am Thorac Soc. 2014;11(1):129–36. (In eng). https://doi.org/10.1513/AnnalsATS.201309-320OT.
50. Levitov A, Frankel HL, Blaivas M, et al. Guidelines for the appropriate use of bedside general and cardiac ultrasonography in the evaluation of critically ill patients-part II: cardiac

ultrasonography. Crit Care Med. 2016;44(6):1206–27. (In eng). https://doi.org/10.1097/ccm.0000000000001847.

51. Fede G, Spadaro L, Tomaselli T, et al. Adrenocortical dysfunction in liver disease: a systematic review. Hepatology. 2012;55(4):1282–91. (In eng). https://doi.org/10.1002/hep.25573.
52. Singer M, Deutschman CS, Seymour CW, et al. The third international consensus definitions for sepsis and septic shock (Sepsis-3). JAMA. 2016;315(8):801–10. (In eng). https://doi.org/10.1001/jama.2016.0287.
53. Verma R, Satapathy SK, Bilal M. Procalcitonin and C-reactive protein in the diagnosis of spontaneous bacterial peritonitis. Transl. Gastroenterol Hepatol. 2022;7:36(In eng). https://doi.org/10.21037/tgh-19-297.
54. Dong R, Wan B, Lin S, et al. Procalcitonin and liver disease: a literature review. J Clin Transl Hepatol. 2019;7(1):51–5. (In eng). https://doi.org/10.14218/jcth.2018.00012.
55. Lazzarotto C, Ronsoni MF, Fayad L, et al. Acute phase proteins for the diagnosis of bacterial infection and prediction of mortality in acute complications of cirrhosis. Ann Hepatol. 2013;12(4):599–607. (In eng).
56. Fagiuoli S, Colli A, Bruno R, et al. Management of infections in cirrhotic patients: report of a consensus conference. Dig Liver Dis. 2014;46(3):204–12. (In eng). https://doi.org/10.1016/j.dld.2013.07.015.
57. Cullaro G, Rubin JB, Fortune BE, et al. Association between kidney dysfunction types and mortality among hospitalized patients with cirrhosis. Dig Dis Sci. 2022;67(7):3426–35. (In eng). https://doi.org/10.1007/s10620-021-07159-z.
58. Cullaro G, Verna EC, Lai JC. Association between renal function pattern and mortality in patients with cirrhosis. Clin Gastroenterol Hepatol. 2019;17(11):2364–70. (In eng). https://doi.org/10.1016/j.cgh.2019.01.043.
59. Fede G, D'Amico G, Arvaniti V, et al. Renal failure and cirrhosis: a systematic review of mortality and prognosis. J Hepatol. 2012;56(4):810–8. (In eng). https://doi.org/10.1016/j.jhep.2011.10.016.
60. Rajakumar A, Appuswamy E, Kaliamoorthy I, Rela M. Renal dysfunction in cirrhosis: critical care management. Indian J Crit Care Med. 2021;25(2):207–14. (In eng). https://doi.org/10.5005/jp-journals-10071-23721.
61. Garcia-Tsao G, Parikh CR, Viola A. Acute kidney injury in cirrhosis. Hepatology. 2008;48(6):2064–77. (In eng). https://doi.org/10.1002/hep.22605.
62. Mohamed MMG, Rauf A, Adam A, Kheiri B, Lacasse A, El-Halawany H. Terlipressin effect on hepatorenal syndrome: updated meta-analysis of randomized controlled trials. JGH Open. 2021;5(8):896–901. (In eng). https://doi.org/10.1002/jgh3.12600.
63. Pitre T, Kiflen M, Helmeczi W, et al. The comparative effectiveness of vasoactive treatments for Hepatorenal syndrome: a systematic review and network meta-analysis. Crit Care Med. 2022;50(10):1419–29. (In eng). https://doi.org/10.1097/ccm.0000000000005595.
64. Wong F, Pappas SC, Curry MP, et al. Terlipressin plus albumin for the treatment of type 1 Hepatorenal syndrome. N Engl J Med. 2021;384(9):818–28. (In eng). https://doi.org/10.1056/NEJMoa2008290.
65. Barbar SD, Clere-Jehl R, Bourredjem A, et al. Timing of renal-replacement therapy in patients with acute kidney injury and sepsis. N Engl J Med. 2018;379(15):1431–42. https://doi.org/10.1056/NEJMoa1803213.
66. Gaudry S, Hajage D, Benichou N, et al. Delayed versus early initiation of renal replacement therapy for severe acute kidney injury: a systematic review and individual patient data meta-analysis of randomised clinical trials. Lancet. 2020;395(10235):1506–15(In eng). https://doi.org/10.1016/s0140-6736(20)30531-6.
67. Gaudry S, Hajage D, Schortgen F, et al. Initiation strategies for renal-replacement therapy in the intensive care unit. N Engl J Med. 2016;375(2):122–33. https://doi.org/10.1056/NEJMoa1603017.
68. Timing of initiation of renal-replacement therapy in acute kidney injury. N Engl J Med. 2020;383(3):240–51. https://doi.org/10.1056/NEJMoa2000741.
69. Gaudry S, Palevsky PM, Dreyfuss D. Extracorporeal kidney-replacement therapy for acute kidney injury. N Engl J Med. 2022;386(10):964–75. (In eng). https://doi.org/10.1056/NEJMra2104090.

Chapter 18
Coagulation Issues in Liver Patients

Naveen Bhagat and Arka De

Abstract Patients with chronic liver disease (CLD) experience complicated hemostatic alterations that impact all facets of coagulation, including the formation and disintegration of clots. Although it is a widely held idea that liver disease raises the risk of bleeding, thrombosis and hypercoagulability are also frequently linked to liver disease. The coagulation system shows signs of "rebalancing" in compensated liver disease, which can be influenced by a number of internal and external variables that lead to thrombosis or bleeding. Events such as bacterial infections and kidney failure can cause significant hemostatic changes that increase the risk of bleeding diathesis. Therefore, patients experiencing decompensation, infections, or acute-on-chronic liver failure (ACLF) are at a heightened risk of bleeding.

Because conventional coagulation tests (CCTs) do not offer information on the interplay between different blood components, the rate of clot formation, the strength of the clot, or thrombolysis, they are unable to accurately reflect the hemostasis derangement in CLD. Global coagulation assays like thrombin generation and viscoelastic point-of-care (POC) devices better reflect the interaction between procoagulants, anticoagulants, platelets, and the fibrinolytic system. This chapter summarizes the changes in hemostasis in CLD, the limitations of conventional laboratory tests that are used to assess bleeding risk, and clinical implications for preventing and managing bleeding.

Keywords Coagulopathy · Cirrhosis · Hemostasis · Bleeding · Hemostasis

---

N. Bhagat · A. De (✉)
Department of Hepatology, Postgraduate Institute of Medical Education and Research, Chandigarh, India
e-mail: arkascore@gmail.com

S. Saigal, D. Jothimani (eds.), *Fundamentals of Transplant Hepatology*,
https://doi.org/10.1007/978-981-95-2624-6_18

Key Highlights

- The notion of "rebalanced hemostasis" in chronic liver disease (CLD) highlights the maintained equilibrium despite changes in procoagulant, anticoagulant, and fibrinolytic factors. This balance can shift toward thrombosis or bleeding due to contextual factors like infections or acute renal failure.
- Thrombocytopenia and impaired platelet function are common in CLD patients. Despite these, increased vWF levels promote platelet adhesion, leading to a procoagulant state.
- Conventional coagulation tests PT/INR do not accurately reflect hemostatic derangement or bleeding risk in liver disease. These conventional tests focus on procoagulant factors but overlook the interplay of anticoagulants and fibrinolytic systems.
- Bleeding in CLD is more commonly a consequence of portal hypertension (e.g., variceal bleed) rather than coagulopathy. On balance, CLD is more often a prothrombotic state.
- In advanced CLD, fibrinolysis may be accelerated due to increased tissue plasminogen activator and impaired antifibrinolytic mechanisms, resulting in hyperfibrinolysis and a risk of bleeding.
- Global coagulation assays and point-of-care (POC) tests, including thrombin generation tests (TGT) and viscoelastic tests (like TEG and ROTEM), provide dynamic insights into clot initiation, clot formation, and fibrinolysis. They hold promise in assessing bleeding risks and guiding transfusion strategies.

18.1 Overview of Changes in the Coagulation System in Liver Disease

Hepatic synthetic dysfunction and portal hypertension (comprising portosystemic shunting and endothelial dysfunction) are the two main causes of alterations in all phases of hemostasis that characterize hepatic disease. In individuals with hepatic disease, compensatory mechanisms "rebalance" the coagulation system by counteracting these abnormalities [1].

There are three stages to the hemostatic process. Primary hemostasis, or active platelets, first seals the vascular breach. Coagulation, the formation of fibrin mesh, and clot fortification by plasma procoagulant proteins occur next. Ultimately, fibrinolysis, or the disintegration of the fibrin mesh by plasma anticoagulant proteins, takes place following the completion of vascular healing (Fig. 18.1) [2].

Reduced synthesis of procoagulant proteins (FII, FV, FVII, FIX, FX, and FXI) is a hallmark of CLD. Although levels vary greatly, clotting factor levels often follow the course of liver disease [3]. Approximately 50–78% of patients with chronic liver illness develop an acquired dysfibrinogenemia. The polymerization of fibrin monomers is hampered by aberrant fibrinogen produced by regenerating hepatocytes, which has more sialic acid residues. In individuals

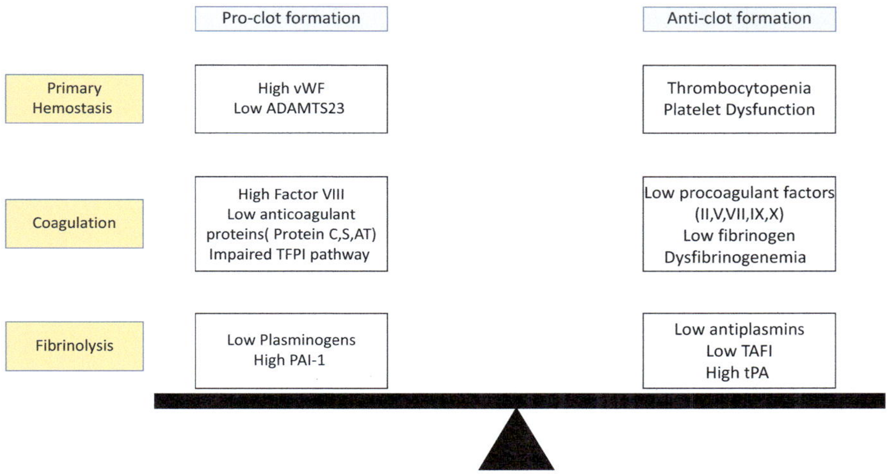

Fig. 18.1 Rebalanced hemostasis in cirrhosis

with stable cirrhosis, FVIII levels are frequently raised multiple times. Increased production in response to cytokine release from necrotic tissue, decreased clearance because of defective hepatic expression of the low-density lipoprotein receptor, and stability due to high VWF levels indicative of hepatic dysfunction can all contribute to elevated FVIII levels [4, 5].

Protein C, protein S, and antithrombin levels are reduced to 10–65% of normal, which is comparable to the values observed in individuals with hereditary deficiencies [3, 6]. Endothelial cells synthesize the tissue factor pathway inhibitor (TFPI). Patients with CLD either have regular or high TFPI levels. Reduced amounts of protein S, a cofactor for TFPI-mediated down-regulation of thrombin production, however, compromise the functional integrity of the TFPI anticoagulant pathway [7].

18.1.1 Primary Hemostasis

Von Willebrand factor (vWF), an adhesive protein that selectively binds and activates platelets, is released by damaged endothelium during primary hemostasis. By connecting neighboring platelets via the long-length serum fibrinogen and vWF strands, the joined platelets create a thrombus.

Liver disease can have a negative impact on platelets' quantity and function. Thrombocytopenia can be observed in as many as 76% of cirrhosis patients and has a complex etiology:

- The redistribution of circulating platelets to the splenic pool characterizes platelet sequestration due to congestive splenomegaly, which is indicative of portal hypertension.

- Treatment with antivirals, alcohol, or low folate inhibits platelet formation.
- One possible cause of thrombocytopenia is decreased hepatic synthesis of thrombopoietin (TPO), the main physiological regulator of platelet formation.
- In CLD, increased platelet turnover might be a factor in thrombocytopenia [1]. "Hypersplenism" refers to the splenic macrophages' enhanced ability to eliminate senescent cells.
- Patients with primary biliary cirrhosis and hepatitis C experience immune-mediated platelet destruction.
- Hypercoagulability associated with cirrhosis may also lead to platelet consumption, which in turn triggers platelet activation.

The reduced serum activity of ADAMTS 13, a metalloprotease enzyme that breaks down vvWF, along with improved platelet adhesion due to increased endothelial synthesis of vWF, helps counteract thrombocytopenia and platelet dysfunction in CLD. Patients with cirrhosis have lower plasma levels of this enzyme, which is only produced in the liver [6]. Despite the deregulated CCTs, there is a procoagulant condition because of increased endothelium production, decreased hepatic clearance of factor VIII and vWF, and decreased synthesis of inhibitors (protein C, protein S, and antithrombin) [7–9].

Primary hemostasis defects result in mucocutaneous hemorrhage. This includes bleeding from the nose and gums, petechiae or tiny ecchymoses, melena, hematuria, and prolonged bleeding following minor lacerations or venipunctures [2, 7].

18.1.2 Secondary Hemostasis

The platelet plug is maintained during secondary hemostasis by the production of fibrin.

During the initial stage, a little thrombin clot quickly forms. In the ensuing amplification phase, this early thrombin quickly produces more thrombin on platelet surfaces in a positive feedback loop known as the thrombin burst. Ultimately, fibrinogen is transformed into a stable, cross-linked fibrin clot by thrombin. Deep tissue bleeding, such as massive subcutaneous hematomas, muscle and joint hematomas, and bleeding into bodily cavities, is typically associated with secondary hemostasis-type coagulopathic bleeding.

18.1.3 Fibrinolysis

Fibrinolysis resorbs the clot after hemostasis has been established. The liver is responsible for the synthesis of all profibrinolytic and antifibrinolytic proteins, with the exception of tissue plasminogen activator (tPA) and PAI-1, which are produced by endothelial cells. In chronic liver illness, levels of plasminogen, antiplasmin, thrombin-activatable fibrinolysis inhibitor (TAFI), and FXIII are typically decreased. On the other hand, decreased hepatic clearance and the production of tPA by activated endothelial cells typically result in elevated tPA plasma. Levels of PAI-1 may be elevated or normal [10].

Between people, fibrinolytic activity varies significantly. Fibrinolytic activity is present in ascitic fluid in CLD. In certain cases, substantial quantities of ascitic fluid reabsorption into the systemic circulation may have an acceleration of fibrinolysis [11]. Accelerated intravascular coagulation (AVIC) is the term for the hyperfibrinolysis condition that characterizes advanced CLD and results in persistent lysed microthrombi. Mild mucocutaneous bleeding accompanied by decreased platelet aggregation due to increased fibrin degradation products is how the condition presents itself.

Chronic consumptive coagulopathy progresses with increasing severity of liver disease due to deteriorating endotoxemia, systemic inflammation, reticuloendothelial dysfunction, and bigger portosystemic shunts. Patients with advanced cardiac failure are at risk for bleeding during procedures because of their severe sickness, concomitant renal dysfunction, and substantial hyperfibrinolysis. Elevated fibrin breakdown products significantly impair platelet function, since they overpower fragile fibrinolytic compensatory mechanisms and compound with renal impairment. Important clinical findings include late bleeding following a surgery and new or worsening mucocutaneous hemorrhage.

18.2 Rebalanced Hemostasis

The notion that "rebalanced hemostasis has replaced the classical interpretation of coagulopathy of liver disease" refers to the new equilibrium that is created between the procoagulant, anticoagulant, and fibrinolytic systems as a result of the hemostatic changes [4]. Depending on the triggering contextual risk factors, a relative shortage in procoagulant and anticoagulant factors may tilt the scales toward bleeding or thrombosis [10].

The severity of liver illness is strongly correlated with vWF levels, which are significantly higher in cirrhotics [11]. Elevated amounts of vWF compensate for the deficiencies in initial hemostasis resulting from thrombocytopenia and platelet dysfunction. Extremely high vWF levels may restore platelet adherence to subendothelium at arterial damage sites, according to in vitro investigations [11]. Hepatic cells produce ADAMTS13, a plasma metalloproteinase that breaks down multimeric vWF into smaller, less sticky multimers. Normal platelet function is promoted by a decrease in ADAMTS13 levels with increasing severity of liver disease [12]. Parallel alterations in the profibrinolytic and antifibrinolytic proteins also cause a rebalancing of fibrinolysis.

18.2.1 Hemostasis in Acute Liver Failure

In addition to increased factor VII, fibrinogen, platelets, and plasminogen activator inhibitor type 1 as acute phase reactants, hemostasis is maintained in ALF via the same mechanisms as in CLD. Using thromboelastography, it has been found that clot formation in ALF is normal despite noticeably extended INRs of 1.5–9.6 [13, 14].

18.3 Bleeding Risk in Chronic Liver Disease and Its Management

Overall, hemostatic function in CLD patients might not be as compromised as has long been thought. The most frequent reason why patients are admitted to the intensive care unit (ICU) is upper gastrointestinal bleeding caused by esophageal and/or stomach varices. In addition, thrombosis is more common in cirrhosis patients, particularly in those with cholestatic liver disease [10, 11].

Stable CLD patients are frequently scheduled as outpatients for non-emergent treatments like liver core biopsy staging. Even though preprocedural correction of coagulation abnormalities is not always necessary, serious procedure-related coagulopathic bleeding is rare and almost exclusively limited to primary hemostasis-type bleeding resulting from severe hyperfibrinolysis and acute platelet dysfunction [15]. The majority of CLD patients experiencing acute decompensation may exhibit clinical signs of acute, severe hyperfibrinolysis.

The conventional tests for coagulation, like the international normalized ratio (INR), are the most problematic because of their entrenched but unfounded position in traditional medical teaching. The test is a mathematical manipulation of the prothrombin time and measures procoagulant factors I, II, V, VII, and X; however, it does not measure the deficit of liver-derived anticoagulant factors, such as protein C. Moreover, the test is “normalized” against warfarin-treated patients based on the activity of an added commercially available thromboplastin reagent. This causes significant variation in the INR in cirrhosis between different hospitals, depending on which thromboplastin is used in the test. Furthermore, the use of fresh frozen plasma to “correct” a prolonged INR in cirrhosis does not actually change thrombin production (factor II) but does exacerbate portal hypertension.

According to the American Association for the Study of Liver Disease (AASLD) Practice Guidelines for liver biopsy, bleeding problems cannot be accurately anticipated at any certain PT/INR cut-off or above [16]. Compared to INR, platelet count is thought to be a more accurate indicator of bleeding risk.

Platelet counts between 60,000 and 75,000 have been linked in multiple studies to a markedly higher incidence of bleeding following surgery [17]. It is unclear, therefore, what platelet count threshold might raise the danger of bleeding. Because the endpoint of CCTs such as PT/INR and PTT is the commencement of fibrin polymerization, which happens at inadequate thrombin production levels, these tests are unable to determine clot strength and stability. Global coagulation assays, on the other hand, show the relationships between procoagulants, natural anticoagulants, and fibrinolytic systems. TGT measure the total thrombin produced during in vitro coagulation in a dynamic manner [18]. TGT assess the equilibrium between procoagulant and anticoagulant variables in liver disease when thrombomodulin (the main physiologic activator of protein C) is present. Despite extended PT/INR and PTT readings, TGT was utilized to show that plasma from patients with stable cirrhosis produces thrombin at an average or even increasing rate [19, 20]. Still, it is mainly a research tool and has not been proven to accurately forecast the risk of bleeding in patients with liver disease.

18.4 Viscoelastic "Point-of-Care" Tests

Viscoelastic POC tests include thromboelastography (TEG, Hemonetics Corporation, Braintree, MA), rotation thrombelastometry (ROTEM, TEM International GmbH, Munich, Germany), and Sonoclot (Sienco Inc., Morrison). Changes in a "resistance to motion" measure (TEG, ROTEM) or ultrasonic density (sonorheometry) are what allow these tests to gauge the thickness of a clot that is forming. Through the use of a tiny cuvette containing whole blood, ROTEM and TEG demonstrate how resistance to stirring can be transduced when soluble components turn into insoluble fibrin, platelet, or red blood cell clots, and how resistance can then be reduced when a clot experiences plasmin-driven breakdown, or fibrin clot lysis. To concentrate on distinct facets of clot formation and dissolution, the reactions can be conducted with a range of clot stimulators and additives. The available aggregometric POC tests (Multiplate®, PFA-100®, TEG® Platelet Mapping TM Assay, VerifyNow®) differ in the agonists that are used to activate the platelets in the test cells, such as collagen, adenosine phosphate, epinephrine, arachidonic acid, and thrombin, and also differ in the shearing forces that are generated in the test cells.

Coagulation monitoring devices that are used at the point-of-care (POC) measure the complete clotting process in a whole blood sample at the patient's bedside. The coagulation factors found in plasma interact with red blood cells and platelets, resulting in the creation of fibrin and subsequent clot retraction and fibrinolysis, which are shown graphically.

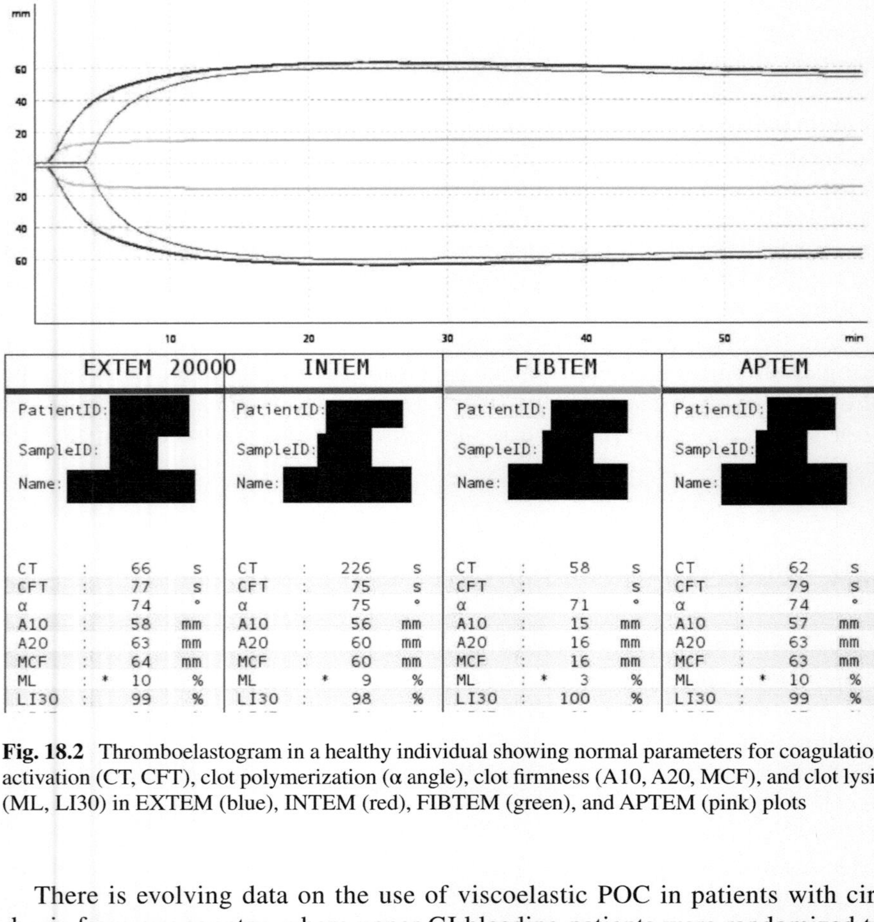

Fig. 18.2 Thromboelastogram in a healthy individual showing normal parameters for coagulation activation (CT, CFT), clot polymerization (α angle), clot firmness (A10, A20, MCF), and clot lysis (ML, LI30) in EXTEM (blue), INTEM (red), FIBTEM (green), and APTEM (pink) plots

There is evolving data on the use of viscoelastic POC in patients with cirrhosis from our country, where upper GI bleeding patients were randomized to CCTs or viscoelastic-based POC tests and have shown that control of bleeding and early rebleeding rates were similar, with improved late rebleeding rates, and also FFP and platelet transfusions were decreased in the viscoelastic POC test groups [21, 22].

Representative thromboelastograms obtained using TEG, ROTEM, and Sonoclot are shown in Figs. 18.2, 18.3, and 18.4 [22]. Table 18.1 denotes the various

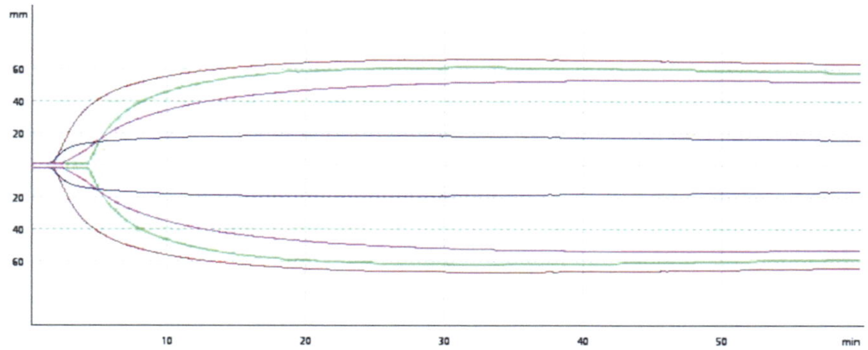

EXTEM 20000	INTEM	FIBTEM	APTEM
PatientID: [redacted]	PatientID: [redacted]	PatientID: [redacted]	PatientID: [redacted]
SampleID:	SampleID:	SampleID:	SampleID:
Name: , [redacted]	Name: , [redacted]	Name: , [redacted]	Name: , [redacted]
CT : 102 s	CT : 252 s	CT : 92 s	CT : 144 s
CFT : 65 s	CFT : 69 s	CFT : s	CFT : 193 s
α : 77 °	α : 77 °	α : 65 °	α : 54 °
A10 : 58 mm	A10 : 55 mm	A10 : 18 mm	A10 : 40 mm
A20 : 65 mm	A20 : 61 mm	A20 : 19 mm	A20 : 49 mm
MCF : 67 mm	MCF : 62 mm	MCF : 19 mm	MCF : 54 mm
ML : * 4 %	ML : * 5 %	ML : * 13 %	ML : * 2 %
LI30 : 100 %	LI30 : 100 %	LI30 : 98 %	LI30 : 100 %

Fig. 18.3 Thromboelastogram in a patient with extrahepatic portal venous obstruction with JAK2V617F mutation on apixaban (factor Xa inhibitor). Prolonged CT on both EXTEM (red) and INTEM (green) plots suggests a delay in coagulation activation due to the involvement of both extrinsic and intrinsic pathways. Clot polymerization, firmness, and lysis parameters are within normal limits in EXTEM, INTEM, FIBTEM (blue), and APTEM (pink) plots

therapeutic agents used for various roles in liver diseases, describing their dose, route, mechanism of action, advantages, and disadvantages. Tables 18.2, 18.3, and 18.4 show comments on the latest American Gastroenterology Association (AGA) recommendations on interventions for hemostasis management are summarized in Tables 18.2, 18.3, and 18.4 [23].

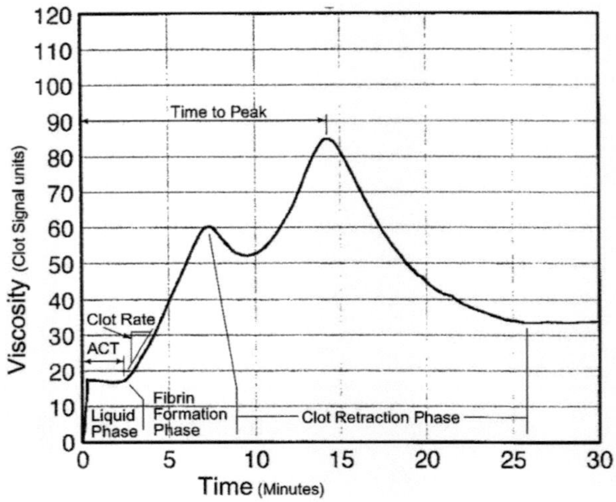

Test	Result	Normal Range
gbACT	ACT	(100.0 – 155.0)
	Clot Rate	(9.0 – 35.0)
	Platelet Function	(>1.5)

Fig. 18.4 Sonoclot signature obtained with glass bead activated clotting time test (gbACT). Depending on the analyzer used, the machine also displays an automatic quantitative result of activated clotting time (ACT), clotting rate (CR), and platelet function (PF), which helps to decide the type of transfusion component required. If transfusion is clinically indicated, a prolonged ACT indicates coagulation factor deficiency, which may be replaced with fresh frozen plasma, shallow CR indicates low/poor fibrinogen with slow fibrin formation, and consideration should be given to fibrinogen or cryoprecipitate, and low PF suggests the need for platelets

Table 18.1 Blood products and drugs used for the correction of various coagulation parameters

Therapeutic agent	Dose and route of administration	Mechanism of action	Advantages	Disadvantages
Agents for hemostasis				
FFP	15–30 mL/kg IV	Partial correction of deficient coagulation factors	Cost-effective and available at all blood banks as a product of fractionating whole blood	Volume overload
Cryoprecipitate	10–20 mL plasma IV	FVIII, FXIII, fibrinogen, fibronectin, and vWF replacement	Same as FFP and provides ample doses of fibrinogen in patients with DIC	Transfusion reactions
Single-donor apheresis platelet unit	Platelets in a dose of 8000–12,000 cells/unit IV	Platelet boost to improve the number and function	Small volume	Transfusion reactions and TRALI
PCCs	A typical dose is 25–30 units of FIX per kg body weight IV	Three-factor (II, IX, X) and four-factor (II, IX, X, with the addition of FVII) products. Also have proteins C and S	Concentrated volume	Expensive Risk for thrombosis
rFVIIa	40–90 μg/kg IV	FVII as a driver of the coagulation cascade	Concentrated volume	Expensive Risk for thrombosis
Thrombopoietin agonists				
Eltrombopag	25–75 mg qd po × 10–20 days	Increases PLT		Expensive Short-lived effect; risk for PVT
Antifibrinolytic agents				
Tranexamic acid	500 mg q6 hours IV or po	Disrupts the plasminogen/plasmin interaction with fibrin, preventing lysis of the clot	Relatively inexpensive, effective topically	Doubtful risk for thrombosis or urinary clots if used in hematuria

(continued)

Table 18.1 (continued)

Therapeutic agent	Dose and route of administration	Mechanism of action	Advantages	Disadvantages
EACA	Initial: 4–5 g IV/po during the first hour maintenance: 1–4 g po/IV q4–8 h	Inhibits fibrinolysis through inhibition of plasminogen binding to fibrin and conversion to plasmin, which causes fibrinolysis	Effective topically	
Anticoagulation in liver disease				
Unfractionated heparin	IV or SQ injection	Inactivates FXa and thrombin	Not well studied in cirrhosis but commonly used	Needs frequent monitoring of aPTT
LMWH (enoxaparin, dalteparin)	SQ injection	Inactivates FXa and thrombin	Monitoring not needed	Extensively used in cirrhosis, but it is expensive, and there is the possibility of heparin-induced thrombocytopenia
VKA	P/O	Inhibits vitamin K-dependent FII, FVII, FIX, and FX	Cost-effective	Dosing requirement varies
DOACs	P/O	Direct thrombin inhibition by drugs such as dabigatran	Oral drugs	Role in PVT
FXa inhibitors	Fondaparinux 7.5 mg qd S/C Rivaroxaban 10 mg qd P/O	Direct inhibition of FXa	po or SQ administration	Role in heparin-induced thrombocytopenia

Table 18.2 Key interventions in procedural bleeding risk mitigation in Cirrhosis

Bleeding prophylaxis	Comment
Platelets _50,000 by infusion or with a TPO agonist if elective	Whether or not to recheck platelets is debated but recommended when bleeding risk is assessed as greater than minimal
Fibrinogen >120 mg/dl	Best achieved with cryoprecipitate. Weight-based dose usually raises fibrinogen level by 50 mg/dL.
Control infection	Active infection may cause release of endothelial derived "heparinoids," which can have an anticoagulant effect
Optimize renal function	Superimposed renal failure is associated with uremic platelet dysfunction, volume issues, and changes in hemostatic cascade
Hematocrit of >25% is suggested	Improves platelet margination

Table 18.3 Key interventions in active bleeding in Cirrhosis

Active bleeding	Comment
Portal hypertension related	Anti-portal hypertension interventions minimize volume expansion and blood product transfusions due to effects on portal pressure.
Wound or mucosal oozing suspicious for AIC or hyperfibrinolysis	Platelets to >50,000, fibrinogen >120 mg/dl. Consider anti-fibrinolytic agent (aminocaproic acid or tranexamic acid). The role of other agents, like prothrombin complex concentrate, is not yet defined.
Control infection	Active infection may cause the release of endothelial derived "heparinoids," which can have an anticoagulant effect
Optimize renal function	Superimposed renal failure is associated with uremic platelet dysfunction, volume issues, and changes in the hemostatic cascade
Hematocrit of >25% is suggested	Improves platelet margination

Table 18.4 Key interventions in thrombotic complications in Cirrhosis

Anticoagulant therapy	Comment
Acute settings such as new (especially if symptomatic) PVT or extension of prior thrombosis	Systemic anticoagulation with IV heparin or LMWH. Note, asymptomatic incidentally discovered PVT does not invariably warrant therapy. Spontaneous resolution may occur, especially if partial.
Chronic PVT, especially in patients listed for transplantation or with history of symptomatic PVT or mesenteric thrombosis	DOACs are reported as safe and effective in Child–Pugh class A and early class B. Vitamin K antagonists (e.g., warfarin) are extensively reported but problematic due to the uncertainty of the target INR.
DVT prophylaxis in hospitalized patients with cirrhosis is indicated	In the absence of bleeding, routine DVT prophylaxis measures are recommended.

18.5 Conclusion

It is widely accepted that CLD patients have rebalanced hemostasis and that additional insults such as infection or renal failure have the potential to tip this delicate balance to either side. PT/INR and platelet counts are examples of CCTs that are frequently used in clinical settings. However, they are not intended to capture the intricate relationships that exist between cells and coagulation proteins, particularly when it comes to controlling or preventing procedural bleeding. Hemostasis global assays and POC viscoelastic tests are becoming generally acknowledged and included in guidelines because they are useful in determining bleeding risk and directing therapy. In addition to hemostasis problems, hemodynamic and mechanical variables also frequently contribute to bleeding in patients with CLD, and these issues also need to be treated.

Disclosures All authors declare no conflict of interest and have no financial disclosures.

References

1. Lisman T, Porte RJ. Rebalanced hemostasis in patients with liver disease: evidence and clinical consequences. Blood. 2010;116(6):878–85.
2. Pradella P, Bonetto S, Turchetto S, et al. Platelet production and destruction in liver cirrhosis. J Hepatol. 2011;54:894–900.
3. Ewe K. Bleeding after liver biopsy does not correlate with indices of peripheral coagulation. Dig Dis Sci. 1981;26(5):388–93.
4. Tripodi A, Salerno F, Chantarangkul V, et al. Evidence of normal thrombin generation in cirrhosis despite abnormal conventional coagulation tests. Hepatology. 2005;41(3):553–8.
5. Zhao Y, Weyand AC, Shavit JA. Novel treatments for hemophilia through rebalancing of the coagulation cascade. Pediatr Blood Cancer. 2021;68(5):e28934.
6. Lisman T, Bongers TN, Adelmeijer J, et al. Elevated levels of von Willebrand factor in cirrhosis support platelet adhesion despite reduced functional capacity. Hepatology. 2006;44:53–61.
7. Northup PG. Hypercoagulation in liver disease. Clin Liver Dis. 2009;13:109–16.
8. Tripodi A, Primignani M, Chantarangkul V, et al. An imbalance of pro- vs anti-coagulation factors in plasma from patients with cirrhosis. Gastroenterology. 2009;137:2105–11.
9. Potze W, Arshad F, Adelmeijer J, Blokzijl H, van den Berg AP, Meijers JCM, et al. Decreased tissue factor pathway inhibitor (TFPI)-dependent anticoagulant capacity in patients with cirrhosis who have decreased protein S but normal TFPI plasma levels. Br J Haematol. 2013;162:819–26.
10. Rijken DC, Kock EL, Guimarães AHC, et al. Evidence for an enhanced fibrinolytic capacity in cirrhosis as measured with two different global fibrinolysis tests. J Thromb Haemost. 2012;10:2116–22.
11. Agarwal S, Joyner KA, Swaim MW. Ascites fluid as a possible origin for hyperfibrinolysis in advanced liver disease. Am J Gastroenterol. 2000;95:3218–24.
12. Asakura H. Classifying types of disseminated intravascular coagulation: clinical and animal models. J Intensive Care. 2014;2:20–7.
13. Agarwal B, Wright G, Gatt A, et al. Evaluation of coagulation abnormalities in acute liver failure. J Hepatol. 2012;57:780–6.
14. Stravitz RT, Lisman T, Luketic VA, et al. Minimal effects of acute liver injury/acute liver failure on hemostasis as assessed by thromboelastography. J Hepatol. 2012;56:129–36.
15. Singh SA, Sharma S, Singh A, Singh AK, Sharma U, Bhadoria AS. The safety of ultrasound guided central venous cannulation in patients with liver disease. Saudi J Anaesth. 2015;9(2):155–60.
16. Rockey DC, Caldwell SH, Goodman ZD, Nelson RC, Smith AD, American Association for the Study of Liver Diseases. Liver biopsy. Hepatology. 2009;49:1017–44.
17. Giannini EG, Greco A, Marenco S, Andorno E, Valente U, Savarino V. Incidence of bleeding following invasive procedures in patients with thrombocytopenia and advanced liver disease. Clin Gastroenterol Hepatol. 2010;8:899–902; quiz e109.
18. Mallett SV, Chowdary P, Burroughs AK. Clinical utility of viscoelastic tests of coagulation in patients with liver disease. Liver Int. 2013;33:961–74.
19. Tripodi A, Primignani M, Lemma L, Chantarangkul V, Mannucci PM. Evidence that low protein C contributes to the procoagulant imbalance in cirrhosis. J Hepatol. 2013;59:265–70.
20. Gatt A, Riddell A, Calvaruso V, Tuddenham EG, Makris M, Burroughs AK. Enhanced thrombin generation in patients with cirrhosis-induced coagulopathy. J Thromb Haemost. 2010;8:1994–2000.

21. Premkumar M, Mehtani R, Divyaveer S, Kajal K, Kulkarni AV, Ahmed S, et al. Clinical validation of global coagulation tests to guide blood component transfusions in cirrhosis and ACLF. J Clin Transl Hepatol. 2021;9:210–9.
22. Rout G, Shalimar, Gunjan D, Mahapatra SJ, Kedia S, Garg PK, et al. Thromboelastography-guided blood product transfusion in cirrhosis patients with variceal bleeding: a randomized controlled trial. J Clin Gastroenterol. 2020;54:255–62.
23. O'Leary JG, Greenberg CS, Patton HM, Caldwell SH. AGA clinical practice update: coagulation in cirrhosis. Gastroenterology. 2019;157:34–43.e1.

Chapter 19
Autoimmune Hepatitis

Vaibhav Patil and Dinesh Jothimani

Abstract Autoimmune hepatitis (AIH) is an important cause of chronic and progressive liver disease. Clinical presentation may vary from elevated liver enzymes to jaundice and, rarely, acute liver failure. A combination of elevated liver parameters, a positive autoantibody profile, and increased serum immunoglobulins with compatible liver histology are required for diagnosing AIH. Prompt recognition and treatment improve clinical outcomes. Disease control can be achieved by long-term corticosteroid therapy in tapering doses with azathioprine. Second-line agents are useful in case of intolerance to azathioprine. Patients with AIH should be followed up on a regular basis for disease flares and drug-related adverse reactions. Coexistence of primary biliary cirrhosis or primary sclerosing cholangitis defines overlap syndrome. AIH patients with acute liver failure presentation should be considered for liver transplantation.

Keywords Autoimmune · Immune dysregulation · Interface hepatitis

Key Highlights

Autoimmune hepatitis possesses a heterogeneous clinical presentation, varying from chronic liver disease to a rapid-onset acute presentation.

Diagnosis can be made from positive autoantibodies and elevated serum immunoglobulins.

Liver histopathology is essential for confirmation and treatment guidance.

Corticosteroids with azathioprine remain the cornerstone of AIH treatment.

Liver transplantation should be considered in patients with AIH-related acute liver failure.

V. Patil · D. Jothimani (✉)
Institute of Liver Disease and Transplantation, Dr Rela Institute and Medical Centre, Chennai, Tamil Nadu, India
e-mail: dinesh.jothimani@relainstitute.com

S. Saigal, D. Jothimani (eds.), *Fundamentals of Transplant Hepatology*,
https://doi.org/10.1007/978-981-95-2624-6_19

19.1 Introduction

Autoimmune hepatitis (AIH) is a chronic, progressive disease characterized by the immune-mediated destruction of liver cells. This infection arises from a loss of immune tolerance in genetically susceptible individuals. AIH was first identified as a distinct clinical entity in the 1950s [1]. The presence of autoantibodies, the immunogenic nature of the disease, along with the histopathological features and the overlapping features of AIH with other disease processes like primary biliary cirrhosis, have been recognized for over 7 decades [2]. The response to corticosteroids was established in the 1970s [3]. However, despite this early success, not many advancements have been made in the management of autoimmune hepatitis. This could be attributed to various factors like the limited understanding of the complex disease pathogenesis due to the multifactorial nature of the disease. With a global incidence of 1.28 per 100,000 population, the disease is considered rare. Additionally, there are different modes of onset of the disease. The clinical presentation varies with age of onset, and there is a global variation observed in the presentation of the disease. Some cases do not have the typical antibodies, which are the hallmarks of this disease, further leading to a delay in diagnosis. These complexities and the heterogeneity have limited significant advances in the management of autoimmune hepatitis. Nevertheless, diagnosis of autoimmune hepatitis is associated with significant morbidity and mortality. A long-term study shows a hazard ratio of 2.29 associated with the diagnosis of AIH [4].

19.2 Definition

EASL defines autoimmune hepatitis as "non-resolving chronic liver disease that affects mainly women and is characterized by hypergammaglobulinemia even in the absence of cirrhosis, circulating autoantibodies, association with human leukocyte antigens (HLA) DR3 or DR4, interface hepatitis on liver histology, and a favorable response to immunosuppression" [5].

19.3 Epidemiology

AIH is a relatively rare condition with a global incidence of 1.28 per 100,000 population and a prevalence of 15.65 per 100,000 population. There is a wide variation in the distribution of AIH, with countries with a high human development index, located at high latitudes, and with stable populations showing an increasing prevalence [6]. The incidence of AIH is increasing, with a registry-based study from Denmark reporting a doubling of the incidence of AIH from 1994 to 2012 [7]. Like other autoimmune disorders, there is a higher incidence in females (2.49 vs. 0.90

per 100,000 years). It has a bimodal age of presentation, with peak incidences noted in childhood (10–19 years) and in the elderly (aged more than 65 years).

19.3.1 Genetic Factors

The most convincing genetic associations for AIH have been found with HLA-DR3 and HLA-DR4 alleles. These alleles may increase the risk of AIH by altering immune regulatory pathways [8].

Conversely, certain alleles like DRB11501 and DRB11302 are considered protective, reducing the likelihood of developing AIH. This dichotomy underscores the complex genetic landscape that contributes to AIH pathogenesis [9].

19.3.2 Environmental Triggers

Environmental factors like bacterial, viral infections, food allergens, and vitamin D deficiency play a crucial role in triggering the onset of AIH [9].

Exposure to certain drugs, such as minocycline and nitrofurantoin, has been linked to the development of AIH, possibly through mechanisms of molecular mimicry [8]. Drug-induced AIH represents approximately 9% of all AIH cases and typically manifests with an acute onset [10].

19.4 Pathogenesis

The pathogenesis of autoimmune hepatitis (AIH) involves a complex interplay of immune dysregulation and environmental factors, leading to the destruction of liver cells. Central to this process is the loss of immune tolerance, characterized by the dysfunctional behavior of T-cells and B-cells. Specifically, autoreactive CD4+ T helper cells and CD8+ cytotoxic T-cells become aberrantly activated against hepatocyte antigens, while regulatory T-cells (Tregs), which are crucial for maintaining immune tolerance, often show impaired functionality [11]. Adding to this complexity is the phenomenon of molecular mimicry, where viral or bacterial proteins resembling self-antigens trigger an immune response that mistakenly targets hepatocytes. This can lead to epitope spreading, where the immune system begins attacking additional self-antigens, further exacerbating the disease. The inflammatory environment within the liver is amplified by cytokines and chemokines produced by infiltrating immune cells. Elevated levels of pro-inflammatory cytokines like IFN-γ, TNF-α, and IL-17 enhance the recruitment and activation of additional immune cells, intensifying hepatocyte damage. Moreover, B-cells contribute to AIH pathology by producing autoantibodies such as anti-nuclear antibodies (ANA), smooth muscle antibodies (SMA), and liver-kidney microsome type 1 antibodies (LKM-1). These autoantibodies form immune complexes that activate the complement system, leading to further liver cell damage [11]. These mechanisms underscore the need for a nuanced understanding of AIH's immunopathology to develop targeted therapies that effectively modulate these complex immune responses and reduce liver damage in AIH patients.

19.5 Clinical Manifestations

The clinical presentations of AIH constitute a wide spectrum, from being largely asymptomatic with unexplained elevation in transaminases to presenting with severe acute hepatitis and acute liver failure [11, 12]. The presentations follow two patterns:

1. An insidious onset.
2. An acute onset of AIH or an acute exacerbation of underlying chronic AIH.

The most common clinical phenotype is with non-specific symptoms like weight loss, anorexia, lethargy, fatigue, fluctuating jaundice, and polyarthralgia, with malaise being the most common symptom. Acute onset AIH is seen in 25% of all AIH cases, with acute-on-chronic presentation in one-third of this acute population. A multicenter study by Alijumah found 94% of acute onset AIH had jaundice, followed by fatigue, pruritis, and abdominal pain in 44%, 31%, and 29% patients, respectively [13]. Choudhuri G et al. found AIH contributed to 1.5% of all chronic liver diseases in India, which is relatively lower compared to the Western population [14]. Clinical presentation as chronic liver disease with or without cirrhosis is more than 50% [14]. Cirrhosis at the time of presentation seems to be more common in the younger population. Studies from Asia report a higher incidence of cirrhosis at the time of presentation. Single-center studies from India and Singapore report a 49% and 42% prevalence of cirrhosis at presentation, respectively [15, 16]. The clinical subtypes of AIH are described in Table 19.1.

Type-1 AIH is more common in adults, has a more chronic course, variable relapse rates, variable clinical presentation, and a higher association with other rheumatologic conditions and IBD. Type 2 AIH is characterized by the presence of anti-LKM-1, anti-LC-1, and anti-LKM-3 antibodies. This is more common in children, has a more acute course, and has higher relapse rates, needing longer immunosuppression. Type 3 AIH is similar to type 1 AIH but has a more severe clinical presentation.

Table 19.1 AIH-clinical subtypes

	Type 1 AIH	Type 2 AIH	Type 3 AIH
Age group	90% of all AIH cases Occurs at any age The most common type	10% of all AIH cases Onset in childhood and early adulthood	Similar to AIH-type 1 but rare
HLA associations	HLA DR3/DR4, DR13	HLA-DR3/DR7	HLA DR3/DR4
Autoimmune serology	ANA, SMA, anti-SLA/LP	Anti-LKM1, anti-LC-1	SLA/LP, anti-Ro52
Clinical course	Variable clinical courses and histological	Acute and advanced clinical and histological	Acute, severe presentation.
Relapses	Variable on withdrawal of IS	Common on withdrawal of IS. Frequent treatment failures.	Common
Response	Responsive to treatment	Need high-dose IS with longer maintenance.	Generally refractory
Autoimmune associations	Rheumatological and IBD	Uncommon	Similar to type 1 AIH

19.5.1 *Seronegative AIH*

Seronegative AIH is termed when ANA, SMA, and LKM-1 are absent. These antibodies may manifest later in the course of the disease. The diagnosis is confirmed by the presence of second-line markers like atypical p-ANCA or SLA. The demographics and histopathology findings are similar to classical AIH except for positive serology. They constitute approximately 10% of AIH cases and 14% of cirrhosis cases spuriously labeled as cryptogenic cirrhosis. The clinical presentation is often severe, requiring high-dose immunosuppression for a longer duration. Seronegativity leads to a delay in diagnosis, which allows the progression of the disease. Due to the dynamic nature of serology in seronegative AIH, repeat serology is advisable [17].

19.5.2 *AIH-Variants*

Overlap syndromes are diagnosed when AIH occurs in conjunction with primary biliary cholangitis (PBC) or primary sclerosing cholangitis (PSC). Overlap syndromes occur simultaneously or subsequently. Clinically cholestatic symptoms like pruritus, pale stool, and right hypochondrial pain are common features. The most common overlap is AIH-PBC (12–19%), followed by AIH-PSC (up to 14%) [18]. Elevated alkaline phosphatase (ALP), an increase in GGT in spite of treatment, positive AMA serology, refractoriness to IS, frequent relapses, histology suggestive of bile duct injury or ductopenia, and concomitant IBD in a patient with AIH are some clues that strongly suspect overlap syndrome.

19.5.3 AIH-PBC Overlap

Patients with PBC not responding to treatment with UDCA, with raised IgG levels and the presence of antibodies specific to AIH, must have a liver biopsy to rule out PBC-AIH overlap syndrome.

19.5.4 Paris Criteria

Paris criteria for AIH-PBC overlap suggest, two of the following three criteria should be positive: (1) serum alkaline phosphatase level ≥two-fold the upper limit of normal (ULN) range or serum GGT level ≥ five-fold ULN, (2) presence of anti-mitochondrial antibodies (AMA), and (3) florid bile duct lesions on histological examination and two of the following three features: (1) ALT ≥five-fold ULN, (2) IgG serum levels ≥two-fold ULN or smooth muscle autoantibody positive, and (3) moderate or severe interface hepatitis on histology [18].

Response to IS depends upon AIH activity in overlap syndrome. AIH-PBC overlap is steroid responsive; however, remission occurs in 3–4 years compared to AIH alone (1–2 years), and immunosuppression withdrawal may be considered in these patients, considering the potent adverse effects associated with these agents and the cholestatic nature of their underlying disease.

19.5.5 AIH-PSC

AIH-PSC is more commonly seen in the pediatric age group, with the criteria necessitating the presence of typical features of AIH, absence of AMA, and evidence of large-duct PSC by endoscopic or magnetic resonance cholangiography or evidence of small-duct PSC based on "onion skinning" periductal fibrosis on histology. Response to IS depends upon AIH activity in overlap syndrome. In AIH-PSC, the remission rate is 20–40%, relapses are common, and progression to cirrhosis occurs in 10 years. PBC-PSC, though rare, has the worst prognosis among overlap syndromes [19].

Various clinical manifestations of AIH are shown in Table 19.2.

Table 19.2 Clinical presentations of AIH

Clinical phenotype	Prevalence and features
Asymptomatic/ non-specific symptoms	Insidious onset. Co-incidental detection for evaluation for fatigue, lethargy, malaise, anorexia, weight loss, and arthralgia, two-thirds of AIH constitute this group.
Acute AIH	Histology is characterized by classical AIH histology with centrilobular zone three necrosis without evidence of chronicity. Serology may or may not be positive in the initial stages.
Acute-on-chronic AIH	Histology and clinically clear evidence of underlying cirrhosis. Steroid responsive in delaying progression.
Fulminant	Rare. Clinically, biochemical features of acute liver failure. Needs IV methylprednisolone plasmapheresis. Emergency liver transplantation is required if the patient is refractory to medical therapy in a week's time.
Overlap with cholangiopathies	Predominantly cholestatic clinical and biochemical picture, rapid progression, poorly responsive to IS.

Table 19.3 AIH: associations with other autoimmune conditions

Thyroid dysfunction (10–24%)	Hashimoto's thyroiditis Grave's disease Hypothyroidism Thyroid nodule
Rheumatological (1–5.6%)	Rheumatoid arthritis Systemic sclerosis Systemic lupus erythematosus Mixed connective tissue disorders (MCTD) Sjogren syndrome
Gastrointestinal	Inflammatory bowel disease (8% in AIH, 70% in PSC) Celiac disease (1.6%)
Hematologic	Autoimmune hemolytic anemia

19.5.6 Extra-Hepatic Autoimmune Associations and Their Impact

AIH is associated with other significant autoimmune diseases. The most common are autoimmune thyroid disease and rheumatological diseases like systemic lupus erythematosus (SLE) and connective tissue disorder (CTD). Autoimmune thyroid disorders, including Hashimoto's thyroiditis, Graves' disease, and hypothyroidism, constitute up to 15–20% in AIH and PBC, especially in the 60-year-old and above age group [20]. Sjogren syndrome, connective tissue disorder, SLE, and rheumatoid arthritis are the immune rheumatological associations responsible for limited mobility and toxicities related to therapy [21, 22]. Gut immune diseases like inflammatory bowel disease (especially ulcerative disease, which is strongly associated with PSC, PSC-AIH overlap is up to 70%) and celiac disease are responsible for "leaky gut"-associated autoimmune liver disease relapses [23]. Associations with other autoimmune conditions are described in Table 19.3.

19.6 Diagnosis

Diagnosis in AIH is made using a combination of clinical, serologic, and histologic factors (EASL). The IAIHG group formulated a scoring system in 1993, which was revised in 1999. The revised criteria, though comprehensive with higher sensitivity, are cumbersome and need more information, including response to treatment. However, it may have utility in atypical cases of AIH, particularly AIH occurring with other concurrent liver disorders [24]. Hence, a simplified criterion was proposed by IAIHG in 2008, which is based on a combination of positive findings of autoantibodies, serum IgG levels, and specific histological findings, and a negative viral hepatitis test with scores assigned for each criterion (Table 19.4). This simplified criterion has a sensitivity of 88% and specificity of 97% for diagnosing AIH [25]. It has been postulated that the increase in the incidence of AIH observed over the last two decades could partially be attributed to the utilization of the simplified criteria compared to the cumbersome older criteria of the past.

19.6.1 Autoantibodies

Autoantibody testing is an essential component in the diagnosis of AIH. Indirect immunofluorescence on rodent tissue (liver, kidney, and stomach) is the preferred method of testing, which provides comprehensive testing of most AIH-associated antibodies [26].

Table 19.4 Simplified IAIHG scoring system

Clinical features	Points
ANA or SMA	
>1:40	+1
ANA or SMA >1:80 or LKM1 >1:40 or SLA positive	+2
Serum IgG	
>Upper limit of normal	+1
>1.1 times ULN	+2
Histological findings	
Compatible with AIH	+1
Typical of AIH	+2
Negative: Hepatitis viral serology	+2
Aggregate score without treatment	
Definite AIH	>7
Probable AIH	6

19.6.1.1 ANA

Anti-nuclear antibody, seen in 70% of cases of AIH, is characteristic of type 1 AIH. It's commonly seen in a homogenous pattern. It's also seen in other liver conditions like PBC, PSC, Wilson's disease, viral hepatitis, and DILI.

19.6.1.2 Anti-SMA

Anti-smooth muscle antibody, seen in 85% of AIH, is characteristic of type 1 AIH. It has the advantage of correlation with disease activity. It is also seen in other liver conditions like PBC, PSC, Wilson's disease, viral hepatitis, and DILI.

19.6.1.3 Anti-LKM 1 and Anti-LC1

It is seen in 70% of AIH-type 2 and in 30% of AIH-type 2, respectively. The titer levels of both correlate with disease activity, but it can also be seen in hepatitis C, which needs to be excluded.

19.6.1.4 Anti-SLA

It is seen in 20% of cases of AIH; it indicates a significant disease.

19.6.2 Histopathology (Fig. 19.1)

Liver biopsy is essential to establish a definitive diagnosis of AIH as well as to confirm severity. It is useful to establish a response to treatment where biochemical remission could not be documented and before deciding on immunosuppression withdrawal. The classic histologic features include interface hepatitis, lymphoplasmacytic infiltrates, emperipolesis, and rosette formation [5]. According to the IAIHG simplified criteria, when all of these features are present, it is termed typical AIH; when lymphocyte infiltration is present with some of the above-mentioned features, it is termed "compatible" with the diagnosis of AIH.

19.6.2.1 Portal Inflammation

Portal inflammation is characterized by infiltrates of predominantly lymphocytes, which are seen in the interface (interface hepatitis) with involvement of adjacent parenchyma.

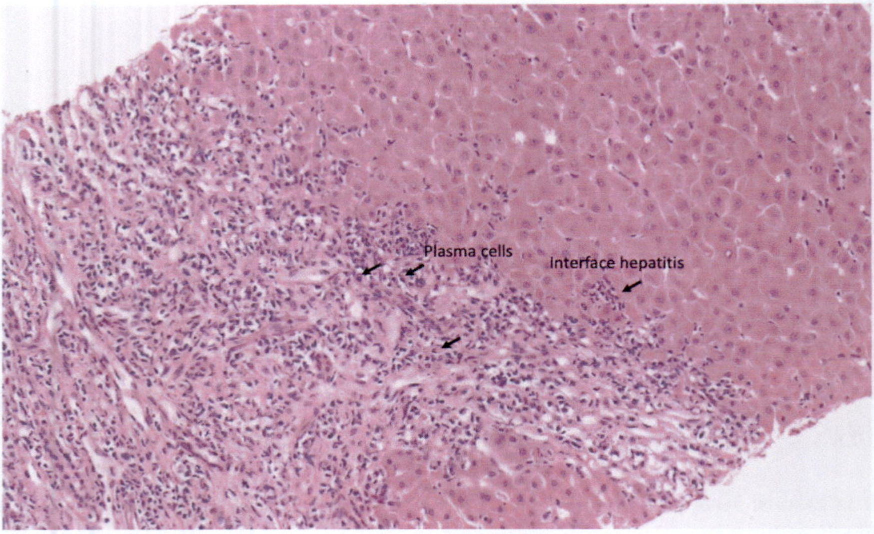

Fig. 19.1 Liver histology of autoimmune hepatitis

19.6.2.2 Emperipolesis

It is a physiological process where the plasma cells or lymphocytes appear engulfed by the hepatocyte. This is needed to maintain the immune tolerance. It is also seen in conditions like AIH, DILI, PBC, etc., where there is a dysregulated immune response.

19.6.2.3 Rosettes

Rosettes are ring-like arrangements of hepatocytes around a central lumen, seen in conditions like AIH, viral-associated hepatitis, etc. They are identified by reticulin stain [27].

Apart from these typical features, there is a wide variation in the histology of autoimmune hepatitis, depending on the presence of overlap syndromes and the mode of onset of AIH (acute onset, insidious onset, or cirrhosis). Various scoring systems (METAVIR, HAI) are used to assess the grades of inflammation and the stages of fibrosis to understand the severity as well as to monitor response to treatment. Histologically, remission is indicated as HAI < 3/18.

19.6.2.4 Histology of Acute AIH

From a histology perspective, a purely acute case of AIH is rare, with most patients labeled as having acute AIH usually showing histological evidence of long-standing chronic disease. The typical finding of acute AIH is centrilobular necrosis without portal inflammation, while portal fibrosis is more typical of chronic AIH [28].

Serologic markers like IgG, IgA titers are also used in the diagnosis and monitoring of the disease. A retrospective multicenter study of AIH patients found that around 10% of patients had normal IgG levels at diagnosis. However, they did not differ in clinical presentation, antibody positivity, or histopathology from those with elevated IgG levels [29].

19.7 Differential Diagnosis

The exclusion of other aetiologies like viral, genetic, drug-induced liver injury, NASH, and alcohol is important in establishing AIH diagnosis (EASL). Table 19.5 shows investigations required for exclusion.

19.8 Treatment of AIH (Table 19.6)

The primary treatment goal of AIH treatment is to achieve

1. Biochemical remission and
2. Histological remission

The normalization of ALT and resolution of necroinflammation on histology are primary targets (EASL). Biochemical remission has been shown to correlate well

Table 19.5 Differential diagnosis for AIH

Differentials for AIH	Investigations to exclude
Chronic hepatitis B, C	Serology for hepatitis B and C
Autoimmune cholangiopathies: PSC, PBC, IgG4 cholangiopathy	MRCP, liver biopsy, IgG4 serology
Alcoholic liver disease	History of alcohol consumption, liver biopsy
Genetic: α-1 antitrypsin deficiency, hemochromatosis, Wilson disease	α-1 antitrypsin level, serum ceruloplasmin, serum ferritin, genetic testing for hemochromatosis and Wilson disease.
Non-alcoholic steatohepatitis	Liver biopsy
Other autoimmune diseases: celiac disease, SLE.	Serology, intestinal biopsy
Drug-induced liver injury: granulomatous, autoimmune.	History of drug consumption, liver biopsy.

Table 19.6 Treatment protocol for AIH in adults

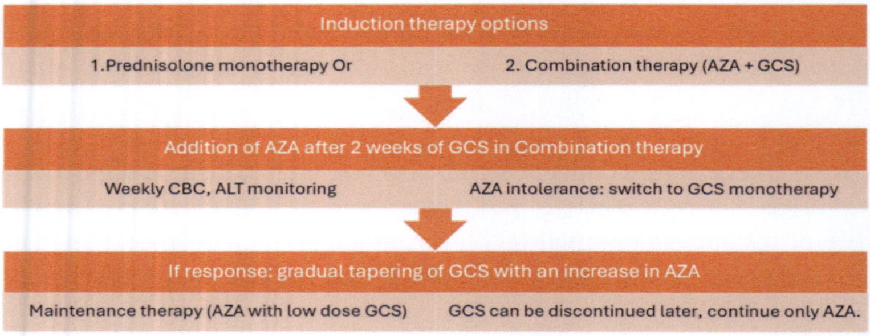

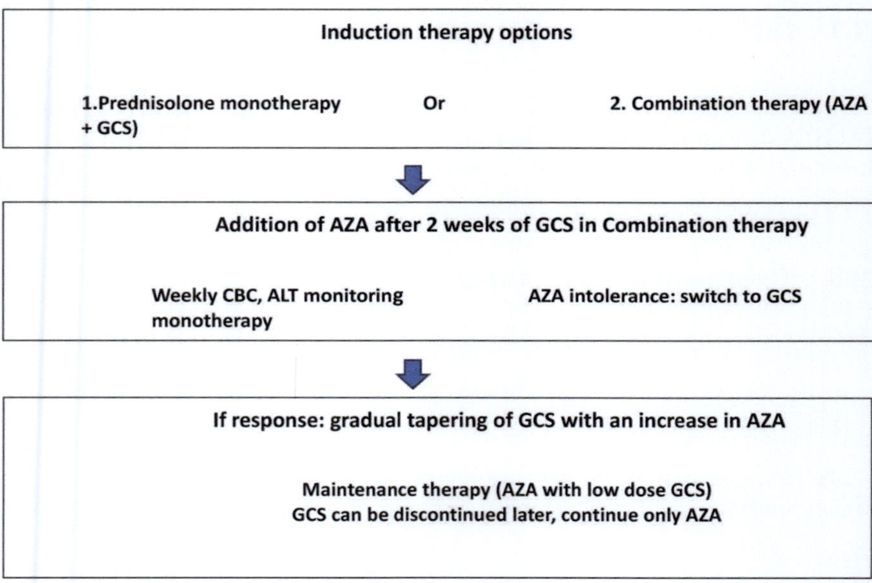

with histological remission. As per EASL guidelines, treatment is recommended for any AIH patient with active disease, especially HAI score > 4/18. For mild cases (ALT<3X UNL, Histology HAI < 4/18, no cirrhosis), induction therapy is optional. However, those not initiated on treatment need 3 monthly ALT surveillances.

The phases of the treatment regime are

1. *Induction phase*, where the aim is to achieve a complete biochemical response.
2. *Maintenance phase*, where the biochemical response is maintained with the lowest possible dose of immunosuppression.

19.8.1 Induction Therapy

The induction regimen is case based. For active disease (HAI > 4/18) or with cirrhosis, induction therapy is required with prednisolone monotherapy or combination therapy (prednisolone and azathioprine) as given in Table 19.6. A systematic review in 2010 based on 11 RCTs showed no difference in monotherapy and combination therapy outcomes in treatment naïve patients (RR: 0.98) [30]. The initial dose of prednisolone should be 0.5–1 mg/kg/day, followed by subsequent tapering. Subsequent addition of azathioprine after 2 weeks has the advantage of discriminating between primary steroid non-response versus azathioprine-induced hepatotoxicity. Azathioprine should be added when bilirubin drops below 6 mg% or generally in 2 weeks post-steroid induction with a 50 mg/day dose and then subsequently increased up to 1–2 mg/kg/day. Close monitoring for hepatoxicity and response to therapy with LFT and for cytopenia with CBC is mandatory.

19.8.2 Maintenance Therapy Post Remission

During tapering of GCS, once biochemical remission is achieved, reduce prednisolone up to 7.5 mg once a day and continue this dose for 3 months, followed by reduction to 5 mg. Simultaneously, the azathioprine dose should be stepped up from 50 mg of initial induction to 100 mg by 25 mg weekly. IS therapy is required for at least 3 years or 2 years following biochemical remission. Liver biopsy is mandatory prior to IS discontinuation [31].

19.9 Treatment Response (IAIHG 2022)

In order to standardize the treatment protocol, IAIHG has proposed a definition of endpoints in the treatment of AIH [32]. Accordingly, complete biochemical response (CBR) entails a decrease in transaminases and IgG to lower than the upper limit of normal, which should be achieved within 6 months. Lack of this CBR is defined as incomplete response or non-response; on the other hand, it is a less than 50% reduction in transaminases within 4 weeks. The possibilities for inadequate normalization or worsening of ALT could be treatment failure, inadequate IS, non-compliance with IS, relapse, drug toxicities, especially azathioprine-induced cholestatic injury or opportunistic infections (CMV, HSV, HEV), overlap syndromes, or misdiagnosis. Causes of persistent liver enzyme elevation are shown in Table 19.7.

Table 19.7 Causes of persistent liver dysfunctions post IS therapy

Possible causes	Diagnosis and treatment
Poor compliance	Ensure compliance, repeat induction therapy with a higher dose, and maintain with a high dose for a long time.
Treatment failure	For fulminant severe cases: higher dose, alternative IS. Likely requires LT. For non-severe cases: addition of alternative IS
Incomplete response	Initial good clinical and biochemical response, but never normalized. Higher IS or additional alternative IS.
Azathioprine-induced hepatotoxicity	6-MMP levels are helpful in predicting DILI. Mostly cholestatic injury or chronic injury in the form of Veno-occlusive disease. Improve with discontinuation or dose reduction.
Relapse	Initial biochemical and histological remission followed by flare in disease activity. Increase in IS (AZA 2 mg/kg/day, prednisolone 30 mg for 1 month, or monotherapy prednisolone 60 mg—slow tapering.
Transition to overlap syndrome	Develop features of two autoimmune liver diseases. Rapid progression, refractory to treatment. Need early LT.

19.9.1 Corticosteroids

Corticosteroids are the established first-line therapy. The initial dose of prednisolone varies according to different guidelines. While EASL recommends a dose of 60 mg/day for steroid monotherapy, some Asian guidelines recommend a reduced dose of 30 mg/day. While it must be borne in mind that higher doses have a higher risk of side effects, meta-analysis has shown that those with acute severe AIH and those with cirrhosis due to AIH respond well to higher doses of steroids.

19.9.2 Azathioprine

AASLD guidelines suggest azathioprine (1–2 mg/kg) in combination with lower doses of prednisolone (30 mg/day) as an induction regimen, which reduces side effects associated with higher doses of steroids. It is the drug of choice for maintenance regimes. Azathioprine is an antimetabolite. Glutathione transferase enzyme (GST) converts it to 6-mercaptopurine (6-MP), the active component. Although effective in most patients, the response varies between individuals, which could partially be attributed to the various genotypes of the GST enzyme [33]. TPMT (thiopurine methyltransferase) converts 6-MP to various inactive metabolites. Genetic variation exists in the level of TMPT. While higher activity of TPMT leads to increased inactive metabolites and reduced efficacy, lower levels are associated with increased side effects. Hence, the efficacy and adverse effects vary depending on the phenotype of enzymes involved in the drug metabolism pathway. Despite these variations, it is not advisable to measure TMPT enzyme activity except during initiation of treatment, as studies have not shown a correlation between TMPT levels and adverse effects. Elevated levels of azathioprine metabolites like 6-MMP (6-Methyl-mercaptopurine) are utilized for supporting the diagnosis of azathioprine-induced hepatotoxicity (EASL). Common adverse effects associated with azathioprine are bone marrow suppression, hepatotoxicity, nausea, vomiting, diarrhea, and pancreatitis. Those not responding to the azathioprine regimen should be started on the next line of therapy only after ensuring the active metabolite level (6-TG) is adequate (6-TG levels above 220 pmol per 8×10^8 red blood cells) and ruling out other coexisting diagnoses. 6-TG levels provide insight into both adequacy of drug dosage and the metabolism of azathioprine. If the 6-TG levels are found to be low, the dose of azathioprine should be optimized and a response should be awaited. Those intolerant to azathioprine can be given a trial of 6-MP (6-Mercaptopurine), the active component, before moving on to other agents [34].

19.9.3 Budesonide

In order to minimize side effects associated with steroids, synthetic steroids such as budesonide were proposed. Though it has been found to have a lower incidence of adverse events and has been effective in milder cases of AIH, studies comparing budesonide and prednisolone for AIH found that budesonide achieved lower rates of CBR (49 vs. 87%) with a longer median time to achieve this (4.9 vs. 3.1 months) [35]. Additionally, budesonide cannot be used in those with cirrhosis due to reduced first-pass hepatic metabolism in those with cirrhosis.

19.9.4 Second-line Agents

Second-line agents are crucial for the 20% of patients who do not respond to first-line agents or who are unable to continue first-line agents due to intolerance. Alternative therapy like 6 MP and mycophenolate mofetil (MMF) needs to be considered, as shown in Table 19.8.

Table 19.8 Second-line agents in the treatment of AIH

Alternative therapy	Dose	Response
Mycophenolate mofetil (MMF)	0.5–3 g/day in divided doses.	Purine antagonist. Alternate IS with maximum experience of use. Refractory cases: complete remission 30–48%, relapse 32%, no response 21%. Conventional IS is an intolerant group: remission 80–88%. Significant reduction in steroid dose requirement [29, 30].
Cyclosporine	2–5 mg/kg/day in daily divided doses.	Calcineurin inhibitor (CNI). Refractory to first-line IS group cases remission 53%. Intolerant to first-line IS remission 67% [31].
Tacrolimus	0.5–3 mg/day BD	CNI. Similar results to cyclosporine [31] with relatively safer [31]
Everolimus	0.25–1 mg BD/day	mTOR inhibitor. Sporadic studies on the use of this new IS [32].

19.9.5 Mycophenolate Mofetil (MMF)

It is a prodrug of the active component mycophenolic acid, which inhibits the enzyme IMPDH essential for purine synthesis. This limits the proliferation of T and B lymphocytes. It has been used in rheumatoid arthritis, IBDs, and as an immunosuppressive agent for organ transplantation. The alternative second-line immunosuppression with which there is the most experience is mycophenolate mofetil, with a remission rate of 48% in the refractory group and complete remission of 80–88% in the first-line intolerant group [36, 37]. Guidelines suggest MMF should be started once a patient has demonstrated non-response or intolerance to azathioprine and 6-MP. A single-center study from India of AIH patients treated with MMF either due to intolerance or refractoriness to first-line agents showed that a biochemical response was observed in 73.6% of patients who were followed up for a median period of 4 years. Adverse effects were noted in 15% of the patients treated with MMF [38]. Meta-analysis of 21 studies using MMF in AIH found a biochemical response rate (BR) of 40.5% in non-responders to first-line agents and a 73.5% biochemical response in those intolerant to first-line agents [39]. A long-term prospective study comparing MMF versus azathioprine, both in combination with steroids, found the MMF group had better CBR at 12 months compared to the azathioprine-based regime (86% vs. 71.8%) while showing a lower incidence of serious adverse effects (3.8% vs. 18.8%) [40].

19.9.6 Third-line Agents

There are not many controlled trials that show the efficacy of the third-line agents. Suggestions in guidelines are based on smaller studies worldwide where dosage and duration have not been standardized. In the article summarizing the evolving therapies in autoimmune hepatitis, a treatment algorithm has been proposed for AIH patients not responding to standard therapy after reviewing the evidence available for each of these third-line agents [41].

19.9.7 Calcineurin Inhibitors

Cyclosporin and tacrolimus are the calcineurin inhibitors widely used. Calcineurin is essential for the production of cytokines, which help in T cell proliferation, and the inhibition of calcineurin results in immunosuppression. They are primarily used as immunosuppressive agents in organ transplant recipients. Analysis of 7 studies (162 adult AIH patients) of patients treated with tacrolimus as a second-line agent either for non-response or intolerance to first-line agents found that CBR was achieved in 74.1% of the patients. They were given tacrolimus ranging from 1 to 8 mg/day [42]. Another multicenter study found CBR was achieved in 94.1% patients who were intolerant to first-line agents and in 56.5% patients with insufficient response [43].

19.9.8 Everolimus

Everolimus belongs to a class of drugs called mTOR (mechanistic target of rapamycin) inhibitors. Everolimus has been used as a third-line agent in a few refractory cases; however, complete remission was not satisfactory. Smaller studies, such as one by Ytting [44], show good biochemical remission in 85% of patients with refractory cases of AIH, allowing reduction of steroid dosage in these patients.

19.9.9 Rituximab

Rituximab is a monoclonal antibody targeting CD20 on the B-cells. It is primarily used in the management of non-Hodgkin's lymphoma, leukemia, and various rheumatological disorders. A multicenter study of 22 patients treated with rituximab found that there was a good, sustained biochemical remission years after treatment with rituximab. There was a reduction of AIH flares with 95% of patients at 1 year and 71% of patients at 2 years remaining flare-free. Lastly, a significant reduction in steroid dose could be achieved in 62% patients [45].

19.9.10 Cyclophosphamide

Cyclophosphamide belongs to a class of drugs called alkylating agents, which work by interfering with cellular DNA and preventing proliferation. Widely used as a chemotherapeutic agent and in other autoimmune disorders, smaller studies have suggested a role in the management of refractory AIH. A systematic review of 7 studies by Xiong et al., where AIH patients were treated with cyclophosphamide either due to refractoriness to first- and second-line agents or as an add-on therapy, found a positive biochemical remission in 92.3% of these patients with no incidence of flares [46].

The acute flare of AIH, treatment failure, or inadequate IS should be treated with either prednisolone 60 mg or azathioprine increased up to 2 mg/kg/day. This dosage is maintained for 1 month with slow tapering.

Acute severe AIH should be treated with IV GCS (>1 mg/kg) as early as possible with close monitoring. Plasmapheresis or IVIg are second-line therapies reserved for refractory cases.

The lack of response in 1 week suggests a significant disease process, which requires early liver transplantation as a curative treatment option [12, 31]. During special situations like pregnancy, the chances of an acute flare are up to 30%, relatively lower due to immune tolerance under the effect of estrogen. IS should be continued only with GCS, with discontinuation of azathioprine due to potential teratogenicity [5]. During breastfeeding, azathioprine can be restarted. In the pediatric age group, treatment of AIH is similar, except that induction therapy requires a higher IS [5]. The complete remission in children with IS is almost 90% in 6-month duration.

19.10 Prognosis

The long-term outcome of treated AIH is considerably good. 93% of AIH patients achieve normalization of ALT within 12 months of treatment. 10–20% of patients progress and require liver transplantation in their lifetime [12]. Post liver transplantation, the 5-year survival for AIH patients is approximately 73%; however, with more effective immunosuppression strategies, the overall survival has improved with a reduction in morbidities like acute cellular rejection (ACR) and antibody-mediated rejection (AMR).

19.11 Liver transplantation

Liver transplantation is indicated as a curative treatment option in decompensated liver cirrhosis, HCC (within criteria), acute-on-chronic liver dysfunction not responding to IS, and fulminant liver failure [12, 31].

19.11.1 Recurrent AIH

Within 1 year post-LT, there is an 8–12% chance of recurrence of AIH, while after 5 years, the chances are 30–65% [47]. Histologically recurrent AIH closely resembles alloimmune rejection; however, classical AIH diagnostic criteria are applicable. Treatment is similar to pre-LT AIH with GCS, azathioprine, and MMF [48]. The progression to cirrhosis occurs in 20% despite adequate IS. However, a new data update is required after everolimus introduction as a promising immunosuppression agent. Aldo Montano et al. showed certain risk factors responsible for recurrence of AIH are active AIH with severe necroinflammation at the time of LT, young age, discontinuation of steroids in the post-LT period, and high IgG level at the time of LT. The preventive strategies include possible disease remission pre-LT with adequate IS and continuation of low-dose GCS post-LT [49].

19.11.2 De Novo AIH

De novo AIH is less common, occurring in the post-LT period in cases with non-AIH as the primary disease. Overall prevalence in adults is <1%, and in the pediatric population, up to 5%. Histological features include severe lymphocytic cholangitis, plasma cell-rich central perivenulitis, and portal microvascular deposition of complement component 4d [50]. The risk factors responsible for de novo AIH are female gender, older donor graft, early withdrawal of GCS, past history of HCV treatment with interferons, and associated other autoimmune disorders.

The algorithmic approach for managing patients with AIH is shown in Fig. 19.2.

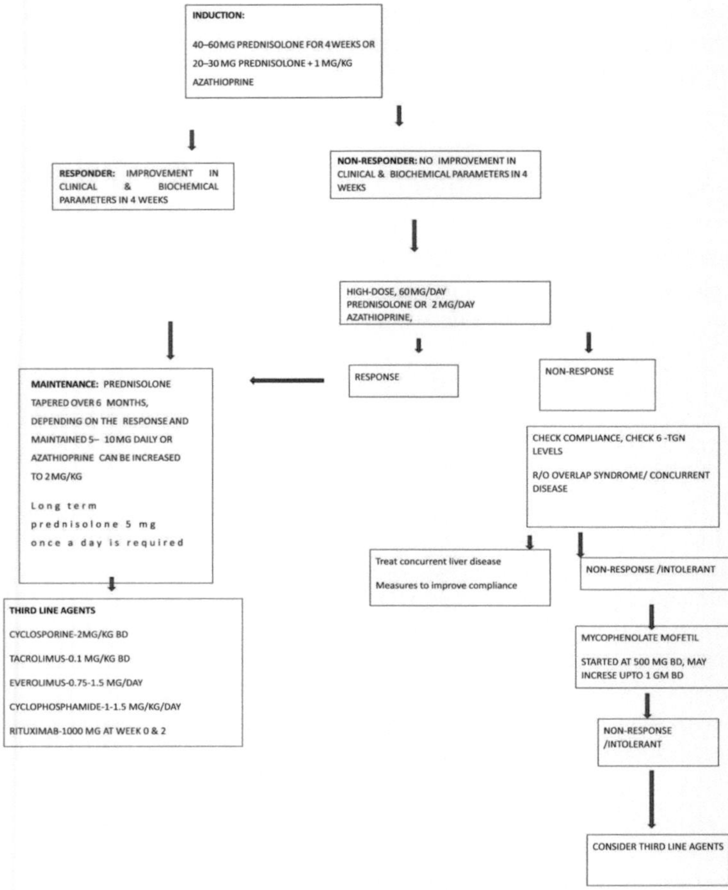

Fig. 19.2 Algorithm for management of autoimmune hepatitis (AIH)

19.12 Conclusion

In conclusion, AIH is a disease of all ages which, though considered to be rare, is increasing in incidence worldwide. It has a wide variation in clinical presentation, severity, and response to treatment. AIH-variants and coexisting autoimmune illnesses of other systems add to the complexity. Most patients respond well to treatment; those not responding to treatment must be considered for the presence of AIH-variants and overlap syndrome or other concurrent liver disease. Second-line agents have been relatively well studied. Controlled trials are needed to assess the role of third-line agents in refractory cases.

References

1. Waldenstrom J. Blutproteine und Nahrungseiweiss. Dtsch Z Verdau Stoffwechselkr. 1950;15:113–9.
2. Doniach D, Walker JG. A unified concept of autoimmune hepatitis. Lancet (London, England) [Internet]. 1969 [cited 2025 Feb 13];293(7599):813–815. Available from: https://pubmed.ncbi.nlm.nih.gov/4180367/.
3. Cook GC, Mulligan R, Sherlock S. Controlled prospective trial of corticosteroid therapy in active chronic hepatitis. Q J Med. 1971;40(158):159–85.
4. Sharma R, Verna EC, Söderling J, Roelstraete B, Hagström H, Ludvigsson JF. Increased mortality risk in autoimmune hepatitis: a nationwide population-based cohort study with histopathology. Clin Gastroenterol Hepatol. 2021;19(12):2636–2647.e13.
5. European Association for the Study of The Liver. EASL clinical practice guidelines: autoimmune hepatitis. J Hepatol. 2015;63(4):971–1004.
6. Hahn JW, Yang HR, Moon JS, Chang JY, Lee K, Kim GA, et al. Global incidence and prevalence of autoimmune hepatitis, 1970–2022: a systematic review and meta-analysis. eClinicalMedicine [Internet]. 2023 Nov 1 [cited 2025 Feb 8];65. Available from: https://www.thelancet.com/journals/eclinm/article/PIIS2589-5370(23)00457-1/fulltext.
7. Grønbæk L, Vilstrup H, Jepsen P. Autoimmune hepatitis in Denmark: incidence, prevalence, prognosis, and causes of death. A nationwide registry-based cohort study. J Hepatol. 2014;60(3):612–7.
8. Wang Q, Yang F, Miao Q, Krawitt EL, Gershwin ME, Ma X. The clinical phenotypes of autoimmune hepatitis: a comprehensive review. J Autoimmun. 2016;66:98–107.
9. Lv T, Li M, Zeng N, Zhang J, Li S, Chen S, et al. Systematic review and meta-analysis on the incidence and prevalence of autoimmune hepatitis in Asian, European, and American population. J Gastroenterol Hepatol. 2019;34(10):1676–84.
10. Björnsson ES, Hoofnagle JH. Categorization of drugs implicated in causing liver injury: critical assessment based on published case reports. Hepatology. 2016;63(2):590–603.
11. Zachou K, Muratori P, Koukoulis GK, Granito A, Gatselis N, Fabbri A, et al. Review article: autoimmune hepatitis—current management and challenges. Aliment Pharmacol Ther. 2013;38(8):887–913.
12. Gleeson D, Heneghan MA. British Society of Gastroenterology. British Society of Gastroenterology (BSG) guidelines for management of autoimmune hepatitis. Gut. 2011;60(12):1611–29.
13. Aljumah AA, Al-Ashgar H, Fallatah H, Albenmousa A. Acute onset autoimmune hepatitis: clinical presentation and treatment outcomes. Ann Hepatol. 2019;18(3):439–44.
14. Choudhuri G, Somani SK, Baba CS, Alexander G. Autoimmune hepatitis in India: profile of an uncommon disease. BMC Gastroenterol. 2005;5:27.
15. Amarapurkar D, Dharod M, Amarapurkar A. Autoimmune hepatitis in India: single tertiary referral centre experience. Trop Gastroenterol. 2015;36(1):36–45.
16. Lee YM, Teo EK, Ng TM, Khor C, Fock KM. Autoimmune hepatitis in Singapore: a rare syndrome affecting middle-aged women. J Gastroenterol Hepatol. 2001;16(12):1384–9.
17. Bhumi SA, Wu GY. Seronegative autoimmune hepatitis. J Clin Transl Hepatol. 2023;11(2):459–65.
18. Chazouillères O, Wendum D, Serfaty L, Montembault S, Rosmorduc O, Poupon R. Primary biliary cirrhosis–autoimmune hepatitis overlap syndrome: clinical features and response to therapy. Hepatology. 1998;28(2):296–301.
19. Czaja AJ. Frequency and nature of the variant syndromes of autoimmune liver disease. Hepatology. 1998;28(2):360–5.
20. Silveira MG, Mendes FD, Diehl NN, Enders FT, Lindor KD. Thyroid dysfunction in primary biliary cirrhosis, primary sclerosing cholangitis and non-alcoholic fatty liver disease. Liver Int. 2009;29(7):1094–100.

21. Gershwin ME, Selmi C, Worman HJ, Gold EB, Watnik M, Utts J, et al. Risk factors and comorbidities in primary biliary cirrhosis: a controlled interview-based study of 1032 patients. Hepatology. 2005;42(5):1194–202.
22. Matsumoto T, Yoshimine T, Shimouchi K, Shiotu H, Kuwabara N, Fukuda Y, et al. The liver in systemic lupus erythematosus: pathologic analysis of 52 cases and review of Japanese autopsy registry data. Hum Pathol. 1992;23(10):1151–8.
23. Weismüller TJ, Trivedi PJ, Bergquist A, Imam M, Lenzen H, Ponsioen CY, et al. Patient age, sex, and inflammatory bowel disease phenotype associate with course of primary sclerosing cholangitis. Gastroenterology. 2017;152(8):1975–1984.e8.
24. Gatselis NK, Zachou K, Papamichalis P, Koukoulis GK, Gabeta S, Dalekos GN, et al. Comparison of simplified score with the revised original score for the diagnosis of autoimmune hepatitis: a new or a complementary diagnostic score? Dig Liver Dis. 2010;42(11):807–12.
25. Hennes EM, Zeniya M, Czaja AJ, Parés A, Dalekos GN, Krawitt EL, et al. Simplified criteria for the diagnosis of autoimmune hepatitis. Hepatology. 2008;48(1):169–76.
26. Terziroli Beretta-Piccoli B, Mieli-Vergani G, Vergani D. Autoimmune hepatitis: serum autoantibodies in clinical practice. Clin Rev Allergy Immunol. 2022;63(2):124–37.
27. Tiniakos DG, Brain JG, Bury YA. Role of histopathology in autoimmune hepatitis. Dig Dis. 2015;33(Suppl. 2):53–64.
28. Immunoserological and histological differences between autoimmune hepatitis with acute presentation and chronic autoimmune hepatitis – Dohmen – 2017 – Hepatology Research – Wiley Online Library [Internet]. [cited 2025 Feb 13]. Available from: https://onlinelibrary.wiley.com/doi/10.1111/hepr.12875.
29. Hartl J, Miquel R, Zachou K, Wong GW, Asghar A, Pape S, et al. Features and outcome of AIH patients without elevation of IgG. JHEP Rep. 2020;2(3):100094.
30. Lamers MMH, van Oijen MGH, Pronk M, Drenth JPH. Treatment options for autoimmune hepatitis: a systematic review of randomized controlled trials. J Hepatol. 2010;53(1):191–8.
31. Manns MP, Czaja AJ, Gorham JD, Krawitt EL, Mieli-Vergani G, Vergani D, et al. Diagnosis and management of autoimmune hepatitis. Hepatology. 2010;51(6):2193–213.
32. Pape S, Snijders RJALM, Gevers TJG, Chazouilleres O, Dalekos GN, Hirschfield GM, et al. Systematic review of response criteria and endpoints in autoimmune hepatitis by the International Autoimmune Hepatitis Group. J Hepatol. 2022;76(4):841–9.
33. Appell ML, Hindorf U, Almer S, Haglund S. Response to azathioprine treatment in autoimmune hepatitis is dependent on glutathione transferase genotypes. Dig Liver Dis. 2025;S1590-8658(24):01151–4.
34. Lohse AW, Sebode M, Jørgensen MH, Ytting H, Karlsen TH, Kelly D, et al. Second-line and third-line therapy for autoimmune hepatitis: a position statement from the European Reference Network on Hepatological Diseases and the International Autoimmune Hepatitis Group. J Hepatol. 2020;73(6):1496–506.
35. Díaz-González Á, Hernández-Guerra M, Pérez-Medrano I, Sapena V, Riveiro-Barciela M, Barreira-Díaz A, et al. Budesonide as first-line treatment in patients with autoimmune hepatitis seems inferior to standard predniso(lo)ne administration. Hepatology. 2023;77(4):1095–105.
36. Sharzehi K, Huang MA, Schreibman IR, Brown KA. Mycophenolate mofetil for the treatment of autoimmune hepatitis in patients refractory or intolerant to conventional therapy. Can J Gastroenterol. 2010;24(10):588–92.
37. Kolev M, Diem S, Diem L, Rodrigues SG, Berzigotti A, Stirnimann G, et al. Mycophenolate mofetil as second line treatment in autoimmune hepatitis – a retrospective single center analysis. J Transl Autoimmun. 2022;5:100172.
38. Jothimani D, Cramp ME, Cross TJS. Role of mycophenolate mofetil for the treatment of autoimmune hepatitis—an observational study. J Clin Exp Hepatol. 2014;4(3):221–5.
39. Abdollahi M, Ekrami NK, Ghojazadeh M, Boezen HM, Somi M, Alizadeh BZ. Tacrolimus and mycophenolate mofetil as second-line treatment in autoimmune hepatitis: is the evidence of sufficient quality to develop recommendations? World J Gastroenterol. 2020;26(38):5896–910.

40. Dalekos GN, Arvaniti P, Gatselis NK, Gabeta S, Samakidou A, Giannoulis G, et al. Long-term results of mycophenolate mofetil vs. azathioprine use in individuals with autoimmune hepatitis. JHEP Rep. 2022;4(12):100601.
41. Jothimani D, Cramp ME, Mitchell JD, Cross TJS. Treatment of autoimmune hepatitis: a review of current and evolving therapies. J Gastroenterol Hepatol. 2011;26(4):619–27.
42. Hanouneh M, Ritchie MM, Ascha M, Ascha MS, Chedid A, Sanguankeo A, et al. A review of the utility of tacrolimus in the management of adults with autoimmune hepatitis. Scand J Gastroenterol. 2019;54(1):76–80.
43. Efe C, Hagström H, Ytting H, Bhanji RA, Müller NF, Wang Q, et al. Efficacy and safety of mycophenolate mofetil and tacrolimus as second-line therapy for patients with autoimmune hepatitis. Clin Gastroenterol Hepatol. 2017;15(12):1950–1956.e1.
44. Ytting H, Larsen FS. Everolimus treatment for patients with autoimmune hepatitis and poor response to standard therapy and drug alternatives in use. Scand J Gastroenterol. 2015;50(8):1025–31.
45. Than NN, Hodson J, Schmidt-Martin D, Taubert R, Wawman RE, Botter M, et al. Efficacy of rituximab in difficult-to-manage autoimmune hepatitis: results from the International Autoimmune Hepatitis Group. JHEP Rep. 2019;1(6):437–45.
46. Xiong A, Li S, Dou X, Yao Y. Cyclophosphamide in refractory autoimmune hepatitis and autoimmune hepatitis coexisting extrahepatic autoimmune disorders. Am J Med Sci. 2024;368(5):446–54.
47. Mack CL, Adams D, Assis DN, Kerkar N, Manns MP, Mayo MJ, et al. Diagnosis and management of autoimmune hepatitis in adults and children: 2019 practice guidance and guidelines from the American Association for the Study of Liver Diseases. Hepatology. 2020;72(2):671–722.
48. Mendes F, Couto CA, Levy C. Recurrent and de novo autoimmune liver diseases. Clin Liver Dis. 2011;15(4):859–78.
49. Montano-Loza AJ, Ronca V, Ebadi M, Hansen BE, Hirschfield G, Elwir S, et al. Risk factors and outcomes associated with recurrent autoimmune hepatitis following liver transplantation. J Hepatol. 2022;77(1):84–97.
50. Demetris AJ, Bellamy C, Hübscher SG, O'Leary J, Randhawa PS, Feng S, et al. 2016 comprehensive update of the Banff Working Group on liver allograft pathology: introduction of antibody-mediated rejection. Am J Transplant. 2016;16(10):2816–35.

Part II
Perioperative Period

Chapter 20
Surgical Anatomy for the Clinicians

Sadhana Shankar and Parthi Srinivasan

Abstract Precise knowledge of anatomy of the liver is fundamental to successful liver transplantation. A thorough understanding of its segmental anatomy and vasculobiliary architecture allows surgeons to take advantage of partial liver allografts for transplantation and also helps minimize complications related to anomalies. The anatomy of the liver is complex and consists of conventional anatomy, based on traditional Couinaud's segments and extra-hepatic vasculature, and segmental-level anatomy, based on detailed branching of major vascular structures and biliary radicles. This chapter aims to provide a brief overview of the conventional and segmental anatomy of the liver with emphasis on its surgical application in liver transplantation.

Keywords Liver anatomy · Segmental anatomy of the liver · Hepatic vein · Portal vein · Hepatic artery · Bile duct · Liver transplantation · Partial liver allograft · Living donor liver transplantation · Split liver transplantation

Key Highlights
1. Thorough knowledge of the functional anatomy of the liver is crucial for liver transplantation using whole and split liver grafts, as well as for living donor liver transplantation.
2. Anatomical planes of the three hepatic veins and the portal vein help split the liver into 8 Couinaud's segments.
3. Each segment of liver receives a 'portal triad' consisting of a portal venous branch, hepatic arterial branch and bile duct radicle, and is drained by a dedicated hepatic vein branch.
4. Anatomical variations in hepatic vasculature and biliary tree are encountered in 50–60% of the population, and understanding these variations helps to minimize surgical complications during liver transplantation.

S. Shankar (✉) · P. Srinivasan
Liver Transplant and Hepato-Pancreatico-Biliary Surgery Unit, Institute of Liver Studies, King's College Hospital NHS Foundation Trust, London, UK
e-mail: sadhushankar@gmail.com

S. Saigal, D. Jothimani (eds.), *Fundamentals of Transplant Hepatology*,
https://doi.org/10.1007/978-981-95-2624-6_20

20.1 Introduction

Comprehensive knowledge of liver anatomy is sine qua non for safe and successful liver transplantation. Precise knowledge of the architecture of the liver, biliary tract, and associated blood vessels helps in reducing complications related to organ retrieval and transplantation. A better understanding of the anatomy of the liver has led to splitting it into partial allografts, which are used in split liver transplantation (SLT) and living donor liver transplantation (LDLT), thereby increasing the donor pool. In recent years, it has also led to technical innovations in liver transplantation such as auxiliary partial orthotopic liver transplantation (APOLT), monosegment liver transplantation, and resection and partial liver segment II-III transplantation with delayed total hepatectomy (RAPID).

Fundamental to the success of liver transplantation is choosing an appropriate liver allograft and avoidance of technical complications in both the donor and recipient, which is largely dependent on the anatomical knowledge and technical acumen of the surgeon. In this context, we aim to describe the surgical anatomy of the liver and biliary tree, with a view to provide a better understanding of its surgical application.

20.2 Embryology

The liver primordium develops as an outpouching from the caudal endoderm of the ventral foregut during the third week of gestation [1–3]. The epithelial cells (hepatoblasts) of the liver primordium give rise to the future liver parenchyma (hepatocytes) and intra-hepatic biliary tree (ductal plates), whereas persistent communication with the foregut forms the gallbladder and extra-hepatic portion of the biliary tree [4]. As the liver primordium rapidly proliferates and expands into right and left lobes, it invaginates into the adjacent septum transversum, the mesenchymal cells of which form the vitelline veins. The portal and hepatic venous channels develop between 4 and 8 weeks of gestation by extensive remodelling of the vitelline veins and show a polar arrangement [5]. The caudal portion of right and left vitelline veins fuses together to form the extra-hepatic portion of the portal vein, thereby creating a single inflow channel. The umbilical vein, which supplies blood to the developing liver from the placenta, joins the left portal vein and the plane of its entrance marks the future umbilical fissure. Initially, much of the blood through the umbilical vein is shunted away from the liver, into the inferior vena cava (IVC), through ductus venosus. After birth, this obliterates to form the ligamentum venosum or Arantius ligament. The cranial portion of vitelline veins forms the three hepatic veins which open into the right cardiac vein, which later develops into inferior vena cava (IVC).

The biliary and arterial systems develop along the framework provided by the already established portal system. According to Couinaud, the embryological liver is supplied by 3 principal arteries, left gastric, common hepatic, and superior mesenteric arteries (SMA) [6]. During foetal development, these three principal arteries fuse at the hilum to form a single artery (common hepatic artery) which predominantly originates from the coeliac trunk. Any of the other arteries may persist to form replaced or accessory left and right hepatic arteries. While the gallbladder and extra-hepatic bile ducts are derived from the foregut, the intra-hepatic bile ducts develop from the ductal plates in the periportal location. Hence, the biliary drainage pattern essentially mimics the portal vasculature.

The hepatocytes and cholangiocytes are endodermal in origin, whereas haematopoietic tissue, Kupffer cells, and interstitial connective tissue originate from the splanchnic mesenchyme of the septum transversum. The ventral mesentery forms the gastrohepatic ligament and the visceral peritoneum of the liver, called Glisson's capsule. Glisson's capsule later involutes into the parenchyma as trabeculae, which support vascular structures and serve as surgical landmarks [7]. The foetal liver develops rapidly and occupies most of the abdominal cavity. It also serves as the main site of haematopoiesis up to the third trimester, after which the bone marrow takes over.

20.3 Topographical Anatomy

The liver weighs about 1200–1500 g and receives blood supply of about 800–1200 ml/min, which is roughly 100 ml/min/100 g of liver tissue [3]. Most of the liver is located in the right upper quadrant of abdomen and is in close contact with the diaphragm and IVC. It is supported in this position by peritoneal reflections which become continuous with Glisson's capsule. This includes the falciform ligament, triangular ligaments, coronary ligaments, and the lesser omentum (Fig. 20.1) [7, 8]. The falciform ligament is a vestige of the ventral mesogastrium and attaches the liver to the anterior abdominal wall. It extends from the umbilicus to the level of hepatic veins and contains the ligamentum teres (obliterated umbilical vein) in its free edge (Fig. 20.1). As the ligamentum teres approaches liver, it runs through a fissure called the umbilical fissure which separates the left lateral segment (LLS) from the rest of the liver. The ligamentum teres is of surgical importance for several reasons. In normal individuals, small paraumbilical veins may run along it; hence, it is always ligated and divided during surgery to prevent bleeding. In patients with portal hypertension, the obliterated umbilical vein can become recanalized, and may cause significant bleeding if injured during transplantation. This recanalization can also shunt blood to systemic circulation through small superficial peri-umbilical veins, producing the characteristic 'caput medusa' in patients with cirrhotic liver disease. Lastly, the falciform ligament is also used to fix the remnant left lobe of liver to the anterior abdominal wall following right hepatectomy in living donors, to avoid rotation of the graft and outflow obstruction.

The triangular and coronary ligaments (Fig. 20.1) attach the superior and posterior surface of liver to the diaphragm. The coronary ligament contains 2 leaves, anterior and posterior. At the level of suprahepatic IVC, the peritoneal reflections

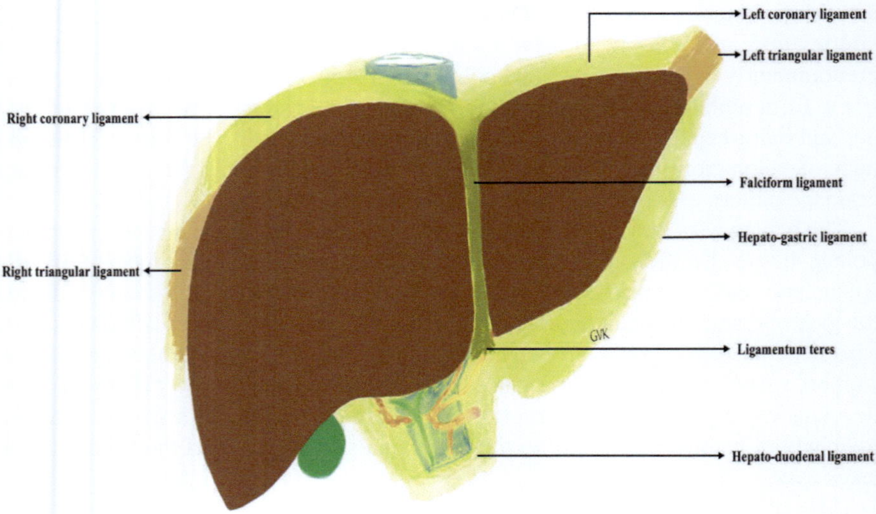

Fig. 20.1 Anterior surface of liver showing various peritoneal attachments

progress laterally to form the anterior leaf of coronary ligament which runs laterally up to the edge of the liver, where it turns to become the posterior leaf. The two leaves are widely separated posteriorly, where the surface of liver lies directly against the diaphragm—the so-called 'bare area of liver'. The right and left triangular ligaments are formed by union of two leaves of the respective coronary ligament. The right coronary ligament fuses with Gerota's fascia around the right kidney to form the hepatorenal ligament. In order to mobilize the liver, it is necessary to divide these ligaments, and as the division approaches midline, the IVC and hepatic veins are in close proximity and at risk; hence, identifying anatomical planes and meticulous dissection is vital.

The lesser omentum extends from the posterior reflection of the left triangular ligament to the lesser curvature of stomach and the proximal 2 cm of duodenum to form the hepatogastric and hepatoduodenal ligaments, respectively (Fig. 20.1). An accessory or replaced left hepatic artery (LHA) usually originates from the left gastric artery and courses through the hepatogastric ligament. Hence, care must be taken to identify and preserve this artery during deceased donor organ retrieval and living donor hepatectomy. The hepatoduodenal ligament contains the porta hepatis and is utilized during the Pringle manoeuvre to occlude the vascular inflow to the liver.

20.4 Segmental Anatomy

Morphologically, the liver is divided into right and left lobes by an imaginary line passing through the centre of gallbladder fossa anteriorly and IVC posteriorly called 'Cantlie's line' [9] (Fig. 20.2). This plane roughly overlies the position of middle hepatic vein (MHV) and is used to delineate the liver into right and left lobes. A better understanding of intra-hepatic vasculature and rapid evolution of hepatic surgery has led to more sophisticated classification of intra-hepatic anatomy. In 1954, Couinaud divided the liver into 8 segments (Fig. 20.2) based on portal vein distribution [6, 10]. The Brisbane 2000 terminology, based on Couinaud's system, is widely accepted and commonly used for describing segmental anatomy of the liver [11]. It describes three orders of division of the liver—first-order division into right and left lobes, second-order division of each lobe into anterior and posterior, or medial and lateral, sections, and third-order division of each section into individual segments or sectors. The hepatic segments are numbered as per the Brisbane 2000 terminology (Fig. 20.2) [11].

The three main hepatic veins travel through the liver in planes called fissures or scissurae (Fig. 20.3). The MHV lies in the main portal fissure (Cantlie's line) which divides the liver into right and left lobes. The left and right portal fissures contain the respective hepatic veins. The right portal fissure subdivides the right lobe into right anterior (segments V and VIII) and right posterior (segments VI and VII) sections. However, in the left lobe, the umbilical fissure (containing the left portal vein) divides the liver into left medial (segments IVA and IVB) and left lateral (segments II and III) sections. The caudate lobe is recognized as segment I of the liver and is an autonomous segment receiving branches from both sides. It also drains independently into the IVC. The portal venous plane serves to delineate the superior from the inferior segments (Fig. 20.3). Each segment of the liver receives a 'portal triad' consisting of a portal venous branch, hepatic arterial branch, and a bile duct radicle, and is drained by a dedicated hepatic vein branch.

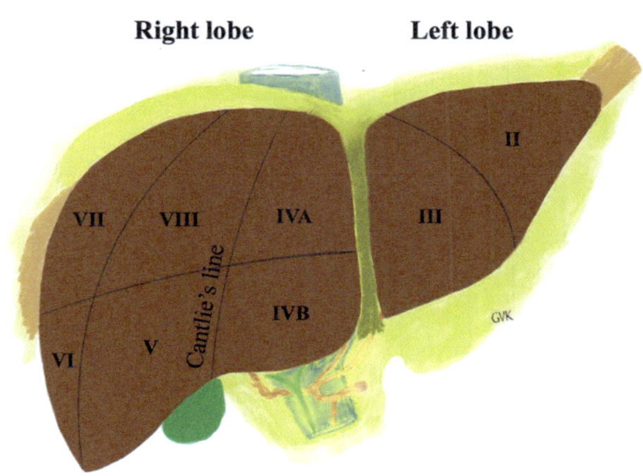

Fig. 20.2 Couinaud's segmental anatomy of the liver

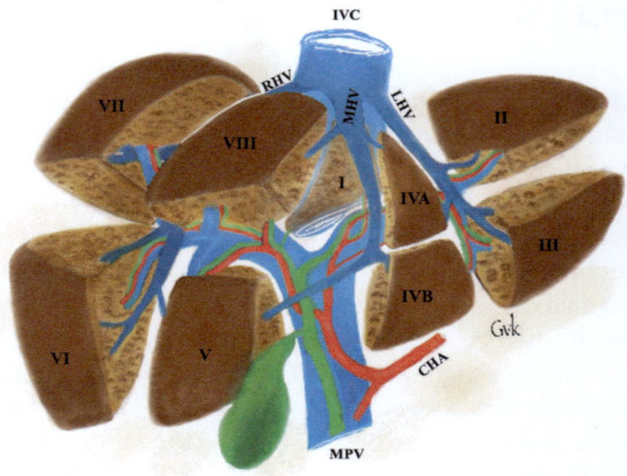

Fig. 20.3 Schematic representation of Couinaud's segments of the liver showing the right, middle, and left portal fissures containing the respective hepatic veins. CHA common hepatic artery, IVC inferior vena cava, LHV left hepatic vein, MHV middle hepatic vein, MPV main portal vein, RHV right hepatic vein

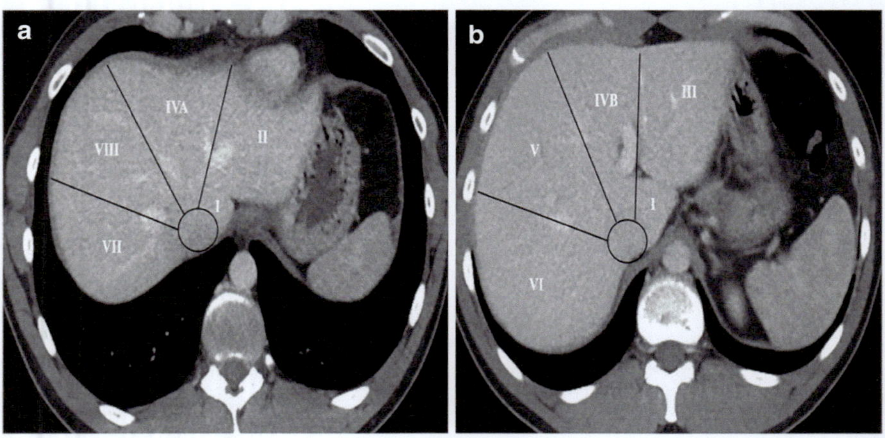

Fig. 20.4 Computed tomography (CT) images showing segments of the liver: black circle represents the position of inferior vena cava, and black lines represent planes of right, middle, and left hepatic veins. (**a**) Superior segments of the liver above the portal plane. (**b**) Inferior segments of the liver seen at the level of left portal vein origin

The functional classification of the liver segments greatly helps in the radiological interpretation of normal and variant anatomy, surgical planning, and assessment of future liver remnant (FLR) (Fig. 20.4). It also permits the use of partial liver grafts in transplantation, derived either from living donors or by splitting a deceased donor liver [12–15]. Knowledge of these anatomical planes also helps in meticulous surgical dissection, thereby minimizing complications such as bile leak.

20.5 Hepatic Vein Anatomy

There are three major hepatic veins which drain directly into the suprahepatic IVC (Fig. 20.5a). The right hepatic vein (RHV) is the largest of them and lies in the fissure between the anterior and posterior sections of the right hemi-liver. A dominant RHV is present in 90% of individuals, and it receives large tributaries from segments V, VI, VII, and VIII [16, 17]. At the level of its termination, it lies almost horizontally and drains independently into the IVC. In 10% of individuals, the right hepatic vein may not be dominant and provides only limited drainage to the posterior segments. This variation occurs in combination with a dominant MHV or with accessory veins which drain segments VI and VII directly into IVC [16–21]. Such accessory veins, called inferior RHV (IRHV), are found in 10–12% individuals, particularly in those with a short, posteriorly located RHV (Fig. 20.5b). In right lobe LDLT grafts, when IRHV of over 5 mm is encountered, they are implanted separately onto the recipient's IVC in order to avoid congestion in the graft.

The middle hepatic vein arises by the confluence of veins draining segments V and IVB (Fig. 20.6). The main trunk of the MHV, as it runs cranially in Cantlie's plane, receives tributaries from segments VIII and IVA. There is considerable variation at the level of its termination into the IVC. In 70–84% of cases, MHV joins the LHV to form a short common trunk just before draining into the IVC [16, 22, 23]. In the remaining cases, there is the absence of a common trunk, and the MHV drains independently into the IVC. The MHV is the most important hepatic vein in hepatobiliary resection and LDLT, as it is often a decisive factor in partial allograft harvesting and utilization [24–30]. Because of its drainage pattern, the MHV is often included in left lobe grafts, to maintain adequate drainage of segment IV, thereby

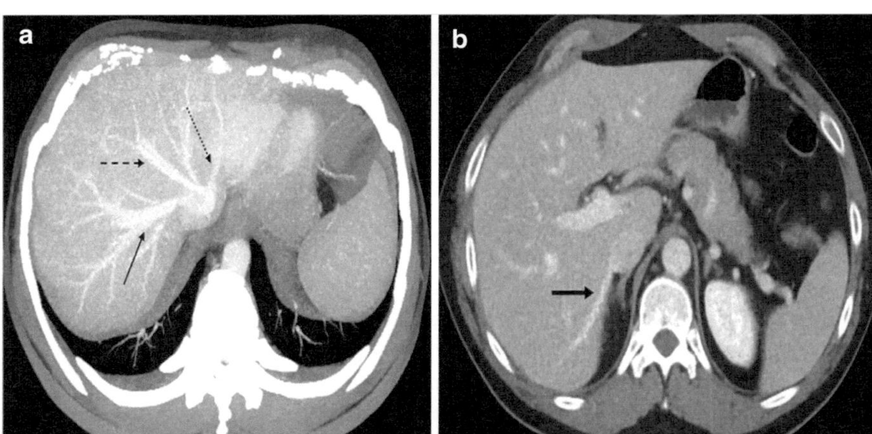

Fig. 20.5 Computed tomography (CT) images showing (**a**) right (solid arrow), middle (dashed arrow), and left (dotted arrow) hepatic veins, and (**b**) inferior right hepatic vein (arrow) draining segment VI into inferior vena cava

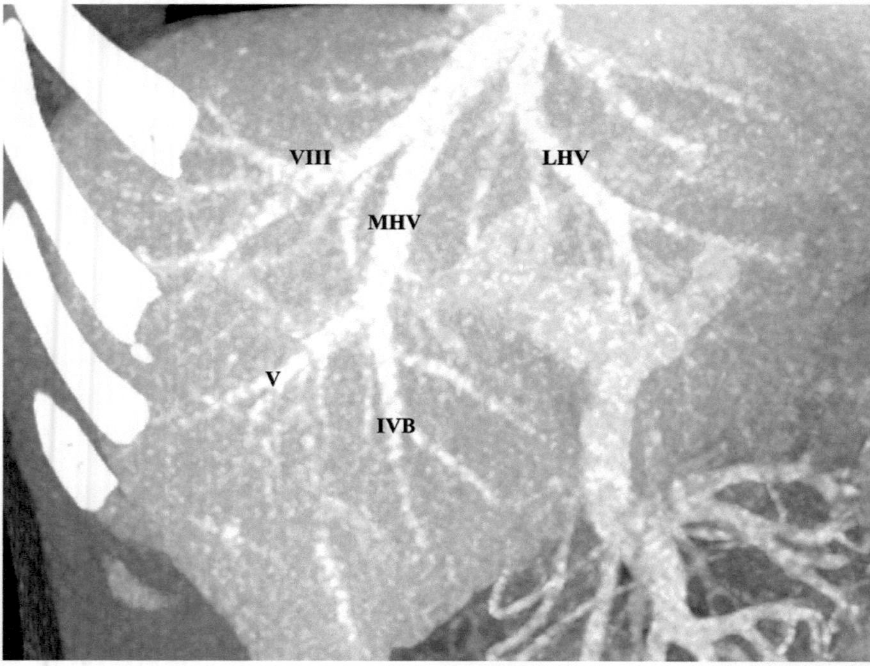

Fig. 20.6 Reconstructed computed tomography (CT) image showing formation of middle hepatic vein (MHV) from segment V and segment IVB veins. Segment VIII tributary is also seen draining into MHV which in turn joins the left hepatic vein (LHV) before draining into the inferior vena cava. LHV left hepatic vein, MHV middle hepatic vein

providing an adequately functioning liver graft [24, 26–30]. On the contrary, MHV is not routinely included in right lobe grafts, and such grafts are particularly prone to venous outflow deficiency, if there are significantly large veins draining segments VIII and V into the MHV. In such cases, the anterior sector outflow requires reconstruction with cadaveric or synthetic extension grafts, prior to implantation, to provide adequate outflow to the anterior sector and to avoid congestion (Fig. 20.7) [24–26, 30].

The left hepatic vein is formed by the confluence of a transverse vein draining segment II and a sagittal vein draining segment III (Fig. 20.8), and shows considerable anatomical variations. In up to two-thirds, segment II and segment III veins join together to form a common trunk which then joins MHV [23, 31–33]. In the remaining cases, segment II and III veins may drain independently into IVC or segment II vein drains into IVC, while segment III vein joins MHV [31]. This drainage pattern of LHV is important while harvesting LLS grafts for paediatric liver transplantation as it may produce 2 outflows in grafts with variant anatomy, which requires unification by venoplasty prior to implantation. In very small children, mapping the LHV tributaries helps in reducing the LLS graft further into a monosegment graft, to overcome size discrepancy between the donor and recipient. A

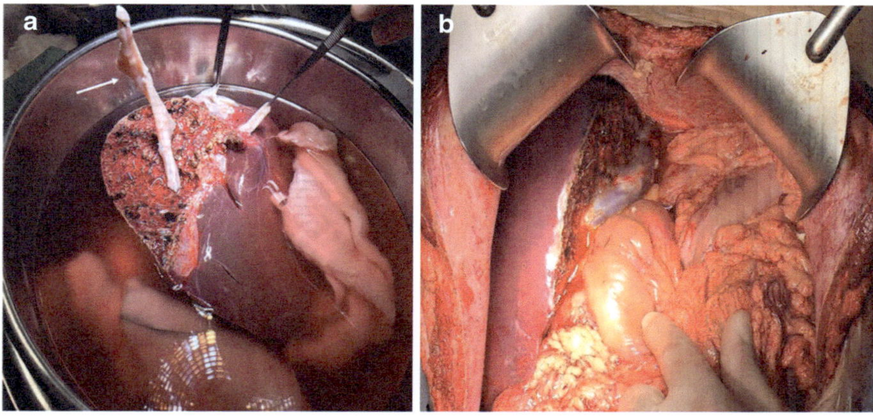

Fig. 20.7 (**a**) Right lobe graft showing segment V outflow reconstruction using cadaveric venous graft (arrow). (**b**) Graft following reperfusion, note the absence of anterior sector congestion

tributary called the umbilical fissural vein (UFV) often drains segments IV and III. It drains into the LHV in 87.5% of cases, whereas in the others, it joins the MHV [34–38].

Rarely, the congenital absence of the IVC is encountered in children with biliary atresia, which poses a unique challenge to paediatric liver transplantation. In such cases, the native hepatic veins open directly into the right atrium and this cuff of confluent hepatic veins can be utilized for implantation of graft. In exceptional situations, a new cava is reconstructed using cadaveric iliac vein which is then used for implantation (Fig. 20.9).

20.6 Portal Vein Anatomy

The main portal vein (MPV) is formed by the confluence of splenic and superior mesenteric veins behind the neck of pancreas (Fig. 20.10). It courses upward towards the hilum of the liver where it divides into the right and left portal veins. The right portal vein (RPV) has a short extra-hepatic course and divides into the right anterior and right posterior sectoral veins. The right anterior portal vein (RAPV) curves forward and runs in a vertical plane, before dividing into ascending and descending branches which supply segments VIII and V, respectively. The right posterior portal vein (RPPV) runs more horizontal and laterally, and, similar to the anterior vein, divides into branches supplying segments VII and VI. The left portal vein (LPV) has a longer extra-hepatic course and consists of two parts: a transverse part lying at the base of segment IV, which curves forward at the base of the umbilical fissure into the vertical part. At the level of this curvature, the LPV gives off the branch to segment II, and as it proceeds further along the umbilical fissure, it gives

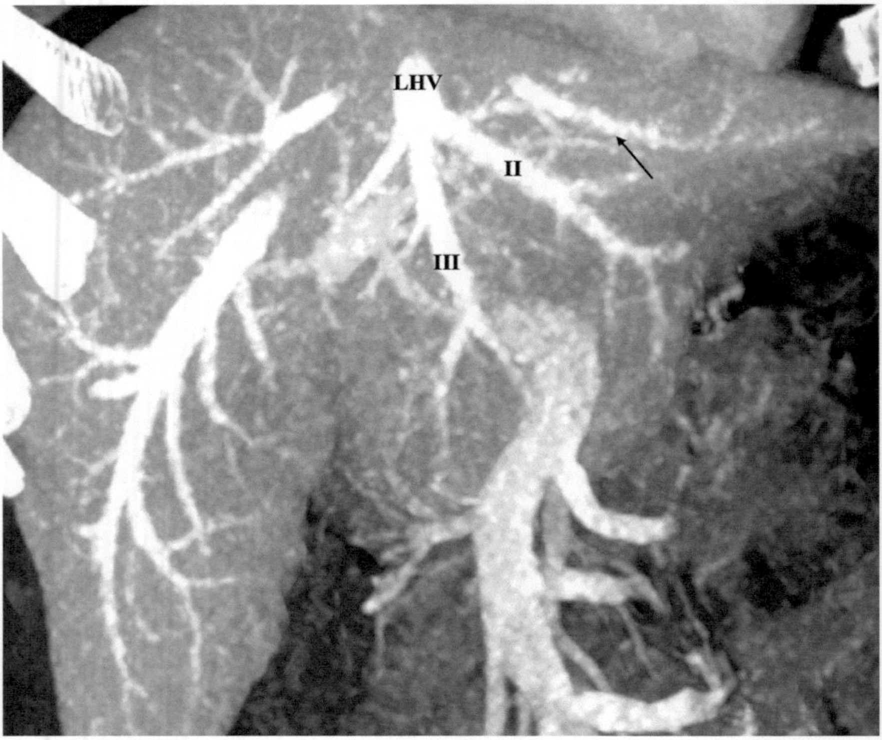

Fig. 20.8 Reconstructed computed tomography (CT) image showing formation of the left hepatic vein (LHV) from segment II and segment III veins. Another subcapsular segment II tributary is also seen at the top (arrow). LHV left hepatic vein

off one or more branches to segment III on the left and to segment IV on the right, before finally terminating by joining the ligamentum teres. The caudate lobe receives individual branches from both right and left portal veins.

Variations in PV anatomy have been described by various authors, but the one described by Nakamura et al. (Fig. 20.11) is the most widely used [39, 40]. The most common pattern is the division of MPV into RPV and LPV; the RPV in turn branches into RAPV and RPPV (type A). A trifurcation of the portal vein (type B) into RAPV, RPPV, and LPV is observed in 10–15% of cases. Other variations include the origin of the RAPV from the LPV (type C), origin of the RPPV from the MPV (type D), and, very rarely, complete absence of the LPV (type E), where a single MPV trunk enters the liver parenchyma to give segmental branches to the right lobe, and then curves to the left to supply the left lobe.

Anatomical knowledge of these variations is important for harvesting reduced liver grafts in LDLT and also for SLT. In right lobe LDLT, the type B and C anatomy produces 2 PV stumps in the graft (Fig. 20.12a, b). This requires reconstruction on the backbench using a cadaveric vein patch or the recipient's portal vein harvested

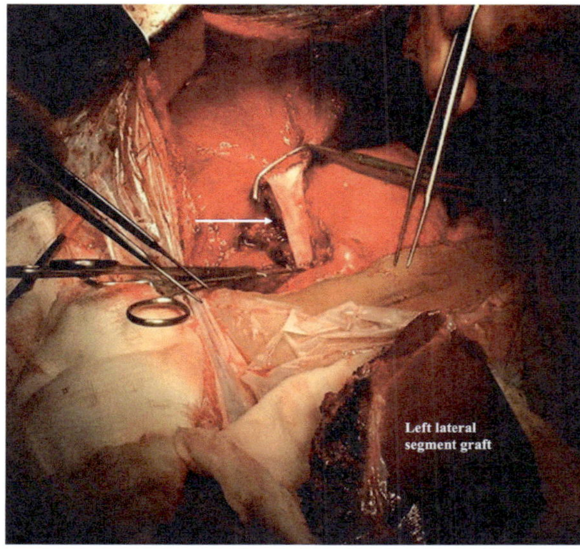

Fig. 20.9 Paediatric recipient with the atretic inferior vena cava requiring caval replacement with cadaveric venous graft (white arrow)

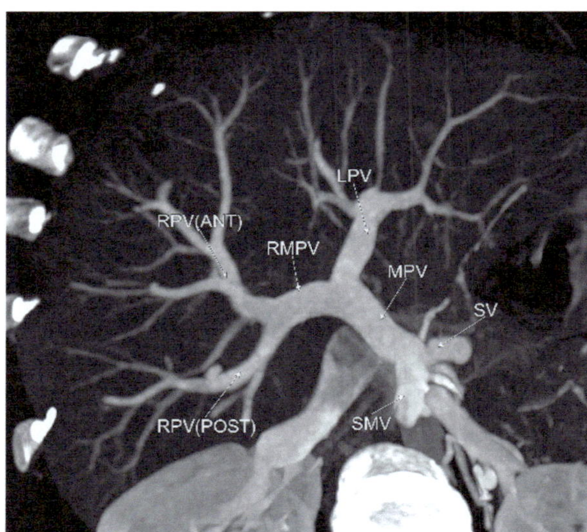

Fig. 20.10 Reconstructed computed tomographic (CT) image showing formation of main portal vein (MPV) from superior mesenteric vein (SMV) and splenic vein (SV). The MPV divides into right main portal vein (RMPV) and left portal vein (LPV). The RMPV in turn divides into anterior (RPV ant) and posterior (RPV post) sectoral branches. LPV left portal vein, MPV main portal vein, RMPV right main portal vein, SMV superior mesenteric vein, SV splenic vein

from the explanted liver [41–43]. Type E PV is an absolute contra-indication to liver donation. In split liver transplantation (SLT), where a deceased donor organ is split into LLS and extended right lobe, division of segment IV PV branches in the umbilical fissure results in ischaemia of segment IV. Whether or not that segment needs to be discarded still remains a matter of debate. An atretic portal vein may be encountered in children with biliary atresia, which may require an interposition or jump graft from the SMV to revascularize the liver graft during transplantation.

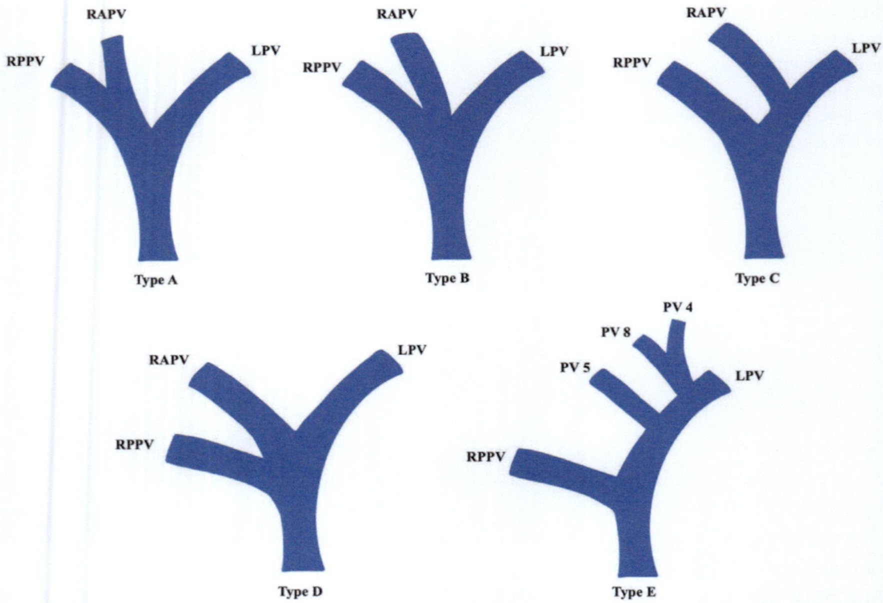

Fig. 20.11 Nakamura classification of the portal venous anatomy. LPV left portal vein, PV portal vein, RAPV right anterior portal vein, RPPV right posterior portal vein

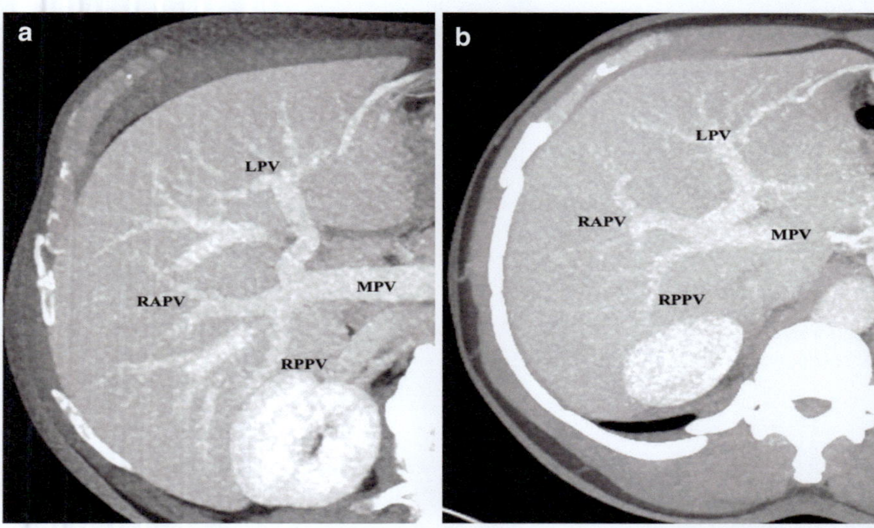

Fig. 20.12 Reconstructed computed tomography (CT) image showing (**a**) type B portal vein and (**b**) type C portal vein both of which produce 2 portal veins in right lobe liver grafts. LPV left portal vein; MPV main portal vein; RAPV right anterior portal vein; RPPV right posterior portal vein

Similarly, portomesenteric thrombosis can occur in cirrhotics, which requires thrombectomy and/or interposition or jump graft from SMV during transplantation. In liver resections for oncological conditions, identification and early ligation of portal vein branches in the hilum help in defining the plane of transection and allow for a more bloodless and oncologically clear resection.

20.7 Hepatic Artery Anatomy

The coeliac axis gives rise to the common hepatic artery (CHA), which in turn gives rise to gastroduodenal (GDA) and right gastric arteries before becoming the proper hepatic artery (Fig. 20.13). This artery then ascends in the porta hepatis between the bile duct superiorly and the MPV inferiorly and in turn divides into left and right hepatic arteries. The left hepatic artery (LHA) extends towards the umbilical fissure and supplies segments II to IV and caudate lobe. Occasionally, segment IV artery, historically called the middle hepatic artery (MHA), may arise from the right hepatic artery (RHA). The RHA commonly courses posterior and lateral to the common hepatic duct (CHD) and often divides extra-hepatically into anterior and posterior branches which supply the right lobe. This typical anatomy is encountered in about 60% of patients. There are numerous variations based on the origin and number of arteries; the most commonly used in practice are those described by Michels and Hiatt et al. (Fig. 20.14) [44, 45].

The commonest variation (25%) is an aberrant (replaced or accessory) LHA that arises from left gastric artery and runs through the hepatogastric ligament to enter

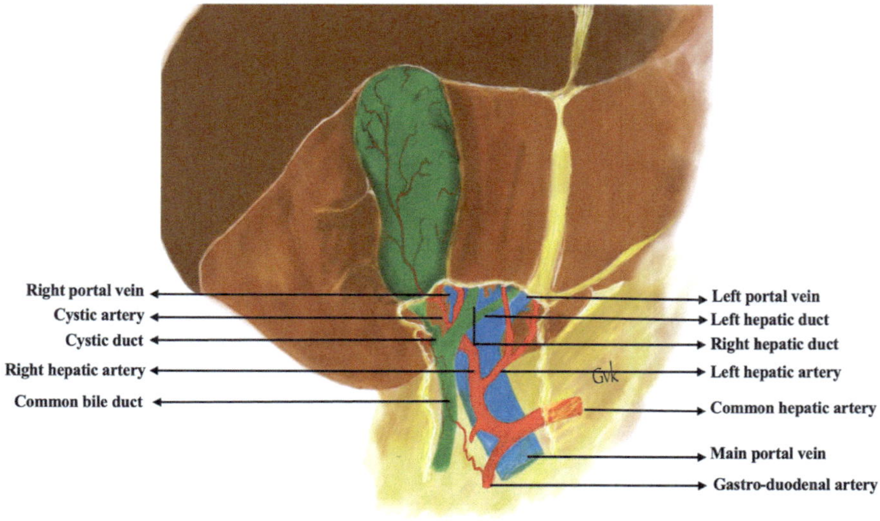

Fig. 20.13 Schematic representation of the anatomy of porta hepatis

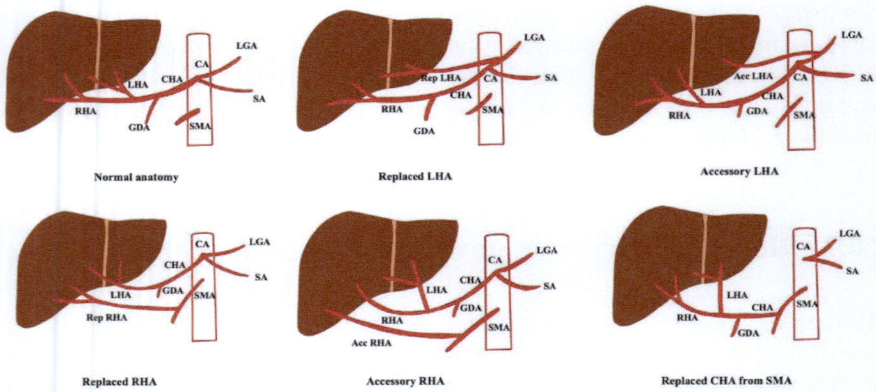

Fig. 20.14 Variations in hepatic arterial anatomy. CA coeliac artery, CHA common hepatic artery, GDA gastroduodenal artery, LGA left gastric artery, LHA left hepatic artery, Rep LHA replaced left hepatic artery, Acc LHA accessory left hepatic artery, RHA right hepatic artery, Rep RHA replaced right hepatic artery, Acc RHA accessory right hepatic artery

the umbilical fissure anterior to the Arantius ligament [44]. If it exclusively supplies the LLS, the artery is called a replaced LHA, and if there is an additional supply from PHA, it becomes an accessory LHA. An aberrant (replaced or accessory) RHA is found in 17% of cases and arises from the superior mesenteric artery [44]. This artery has a more posterior course lying behind the MPV in the porta hepatis, before coursing anterolaterally to enter the liver. In 2.5% of cases, the entire CHA may arise from the SMA, and even more rarely from the LGA or directly from aorta. Variations in PHA anatomy include low division (15%) into RHA and LHA, or early division (5%) where the RHA may pass behind the MPV to reach the hilum [46].

The variations in arterial anatomy are crucial to liver transplantation. Firstly, it is important to recognize the anomalies during multi-organ retrieval in order to avoid iatrogenic injury. The aberrant arteries need to be reconstructed on the back table prior to implantation, in order to avoid complications after transplantation (Fig. 20.15). Secondly, in LDLT and SLT, the presence of variant anatomy can produce more than one artery in the graft. Right lobe grafts can have dual arterial supply if they have an accessory RHA or if there is extra-hepatic bifurcation of the RHA, and the arteries course on either side of the bile duct to enter the right lobe. Similarly, left lobe grafts can have a dual supply if the MHA arises from RHA. LLS grafts with 2 arteries are encountered when there is an accessory LHA. Nevertheless, a decision to reconstruct such dual arteries in the recipient depends upon the size of the larger artery and the presence of pulsatile backflow in the smaller artery upon division, indicating the presence of intra-parenchymal arterial overlap. Such grafts with dual arteries can be implanted by fashioning two separate arterial anastomosis in the recipient or, rarely, by reconstructing using an arterial conduit (recipient's RHA or cadaveric arterial graft) to create a single arterial anastomosis.

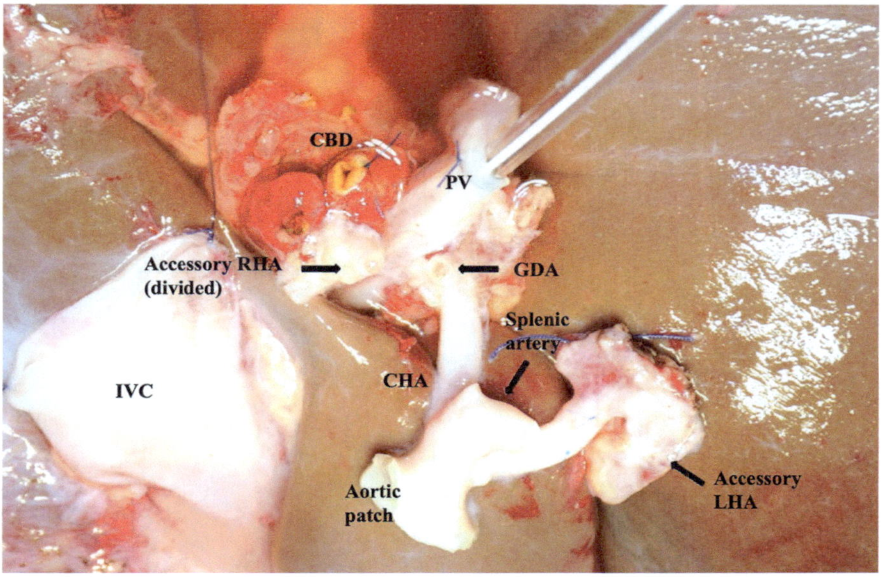

Fig. 20.15 Accessory right and left hepatic arteries found during organ retrieval. CBD common bile duct, CHA common hepatic artery, GDA gastroduodenal artery, IVC inferior vena cava, LHA left hepatic artery, PV portal vein, RHA right hepatic artery

The origin of MHA is of importance in the donor operation of a right lobe LDLT (Fig. 20.16). Preserving MHA while harvesting right lobe graft is crucial, or it may lead to ischaemia of segment IV, compromising the future liver remnant (FLR) in the donor. Similarly, in LLS LDLT/SLT graft, preserving the MHA prevents total ischaemia to segment IV. However, due to persistence of functioning hepatocytes in this relatively ischaemic segment, there may be an increased incidence of bile leaks.

20.8 Biliary Anatomy

The intra-hepatic segmental bile ducts follow a remarkably similar course as the portal inflow due to embryological origin (Fig. 20.17). On the right side, the right hepatic duct (RHD) is formed by the confluence of right anterior sectoral duct (RASD) and right posterior sectoral duct (RPSD). At this confluence, the RPSD curves around the RAPV and the RASD to join it on the left side, producing 'Hjortsjo's crook' [47]. On the left side, the segment II and III ducts join together in the umbilical fissure and this common duct is then joined by the segment IV duct to form the left hepatic duct (LHD). The caudate lobe is unique as it drains by multiple ducts into both the right and left hepatic ducts. The right and left hepatic ducts join together to form the common hepatic duct (CHD). This confluence is extra-hepatic

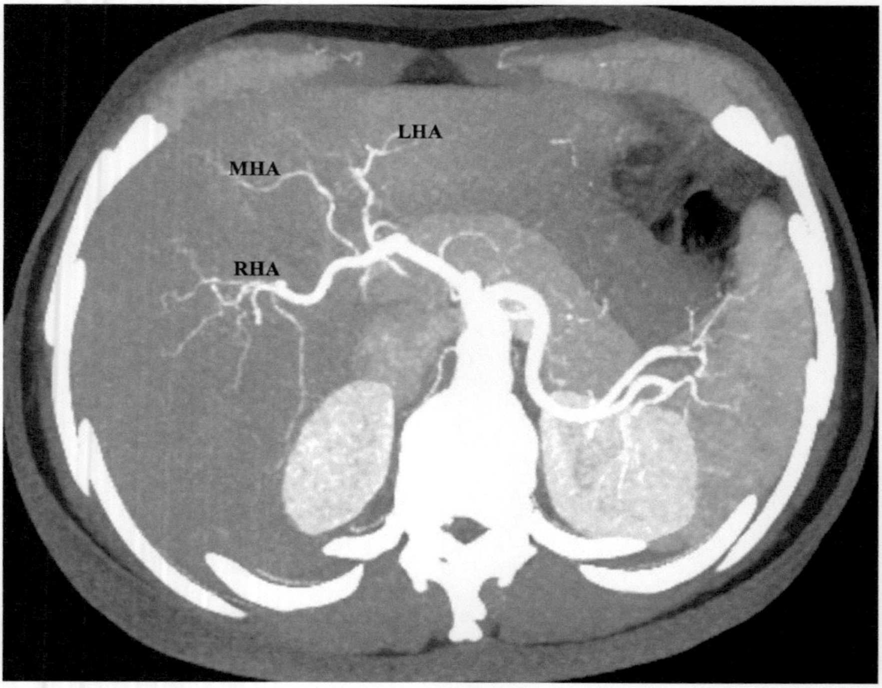

Fig. 20.16 Origin of middle hepatic artery from right hepatic artery. LHA left hepatic artery, MHA middle hepatic artery, RHA right hepatic artery

and is to the right of the hilar fissure overlying the origin of RPV (Fig. 20.13). Thus, the LHD has a longer extra-hepatic course when compared to the right. The CHD as it descends down is joined by the cystic duct from the gallbladder. From henceforth, it becomes the common bile duct (CBD) which then travels through the pancreatic head and joins the main pancreatic duct before opening through the ampulla of Vater into the second part of the duodenum.

Parke et al. described the vascular supply of the extra-hepatic biliary tree [48]. The CBD is supplied by 2 longitudinal arteries that run at 3 and 9 o'clock positions on either side. 60% of the blood supply to these arteries is from the GDA below and 38% from the RHA above. The remaining 2% is non-axial supply arising directly from CHA. At the level of the confluence of the common hepatic duct (CHD), there is a rich plexus of vessels derived from both RHA and LHA. Hence, dissection should be kept to a minimum at this level to minimize the incidence of post-operative ischaemic biliary strictures. Glisson's capsule fuses with the connective tissue around the biliary and vascular structures at the inferior surface of liver to form the 'plate system'. This includes the hilar plate above the confluence of the bile ducts, the cystic plate related to the gallbladder, and the umbilical plate situated above the umbilical portion of the LPV. 'Lowering the hilar plate' is a surgical technique

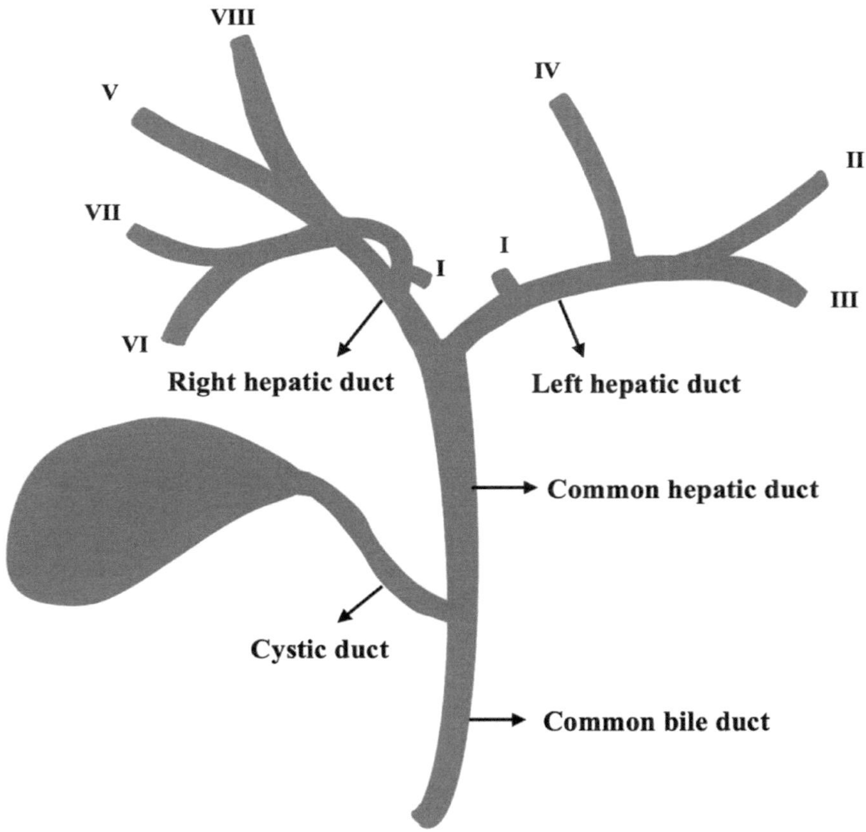

Fig. 20.17 Intra- and extra-hepatic biliary anatomy

where the Glissonian capsule is incised at the base of segment IV. This offers a good exposure of the biliary confluence and LHD during hepatectomy.

Variations in biliary anatomy are very common, and only 50% individuals have a normal anatomy. The commonly used classification systems are those described by Blumgart et al., Huang et al., and Okhubo et al. [49–51]. Smadja and Blumgart [49] have classified biliary variations into six main types (Fig. 20.18). In type A (57%), the anatomy is standard. In type B (12%), there is trifurcation of the CHD into right anterior, right posterior, and left hepatic ducts. In type C (20%), there is an aberrant drainage of the right segmental ducts into the CHD. In type D (6%), there is an aberrant drainage of the right segmental ducts into the LHD. The right posterior duct (21%) is more commonly aberrant than the right anterior duct in both types C and D. In type E (3%), there is the absence of hepatic duct confluence, there being convergence of two or more ducts from either lobe to form the CHD. Finally, in type F (2%), there is an absence of the right hepatic duct with ectopic drainage of

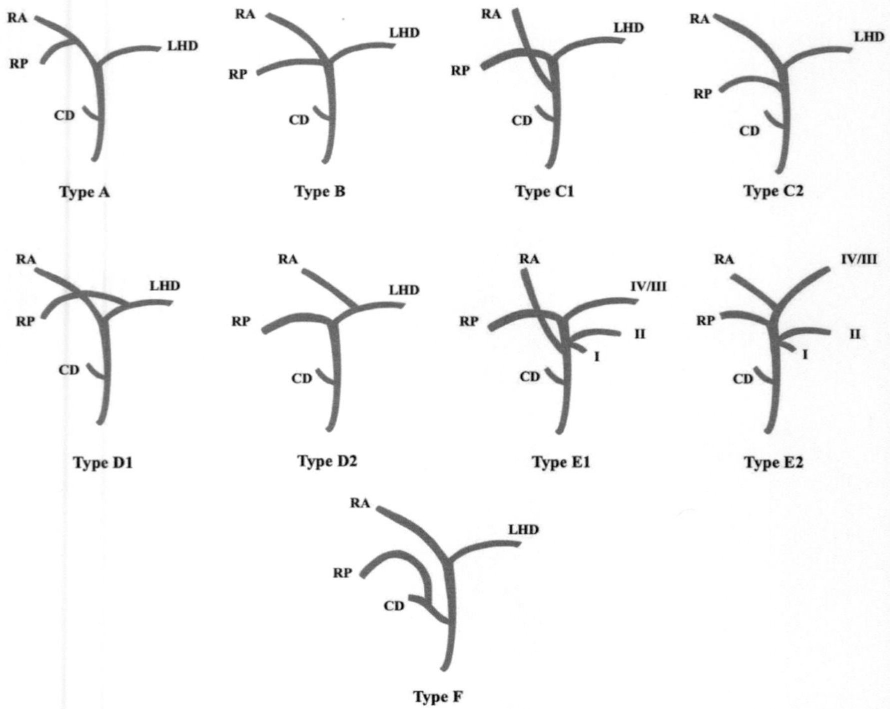

Fig. 20.18 Blumgart's classification of intra-hepatic biliary anatomy. CD cystic duct, LHD left hepatic duct, RA right anterior duct, RP right posterior duct

right posterior duct into the cystic duct. A thorough pre-operative knowledge of biliary anatomy is essential before embarking on donor hepatectomy in LDLT. In right lobe donation, it is crucial to maintain continuity of the donor's biliary tree after dividing the RHD and some centres use intra-operative cholangiography to facilitate safe surgery. Particular care is to be taken while dividing the caudate lobe as failure to ligate transected caudate ducts may lead to troublesome bile leaks. Type B and C anatomy results in two or more ducts in the right lobe graft (Fig. 20.19). If they are close to each other and have an intact hilar plate surrounding them, a single anastomosis can be done. If not, they may require multiple anastomosis in the recipient by using native ducts or with a Roux loop of jejunum. In SLT, while splitting the liver into extended right lobe and left lateral segments, variations in drainage of segment IV duct, if unnoticed, may lead to post-operative bile leak in the right lobe recipient.

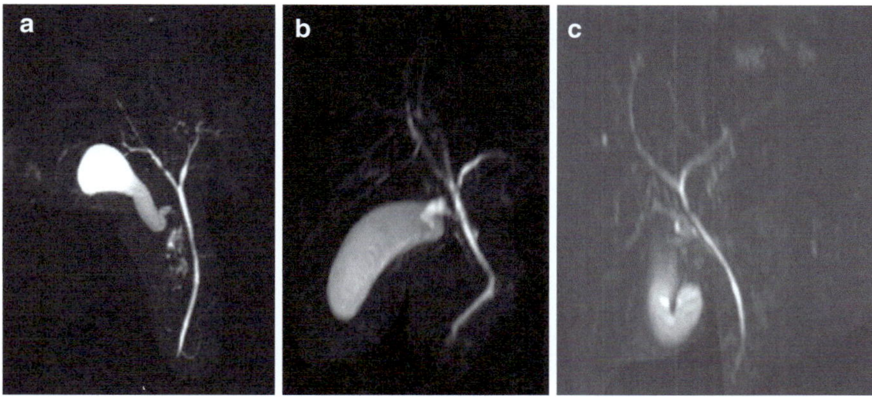

Fig. 20.19 Magnetic resonance cholangiopancreatogram (MRCP) images showing biliary anatomy: (**a**) Type A—normal; (**b**) type B—trifurcation of ducts; (**c**) type C—right posterior duct joining common hepatic duct

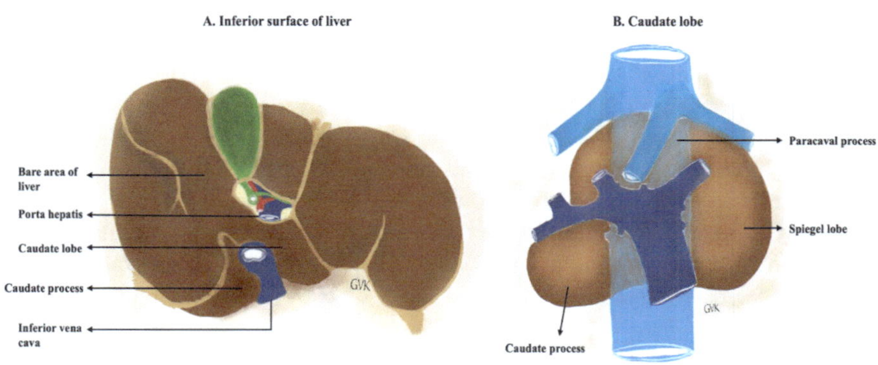

Fig. 20.20 (**a**) Inferior surface of the liver showing the location of the caudate lobe. (**b**) Parts of the caudate lobe

20.9 Anatomy of the Caudate Lobe

The caudate lobe (Fig. 20.20a, b) of the liver (segment I) is divided into three parts: the Spiegel lobe (to the left of IVC), the paracaval portion (anterior to IVC), and the caudate process (to the right of IVC). The vascular inflow to the caudate lobe is predominantly from the left portal pedicle. The caudate and Spiegel processes also receive individual branches from right and left hepatic arteries, respectively. The caudate lobe drains by 1–3 individual veins which open directly into the IVC. In addition, there may be up to 20 small venules attaching the caudate to the retrohepatic IVC. These veins are encountered during mobilization of liver from the retrohepatic cava and have to be carefully ligated to avoid bleeding (Fig. 20.21a, b). In

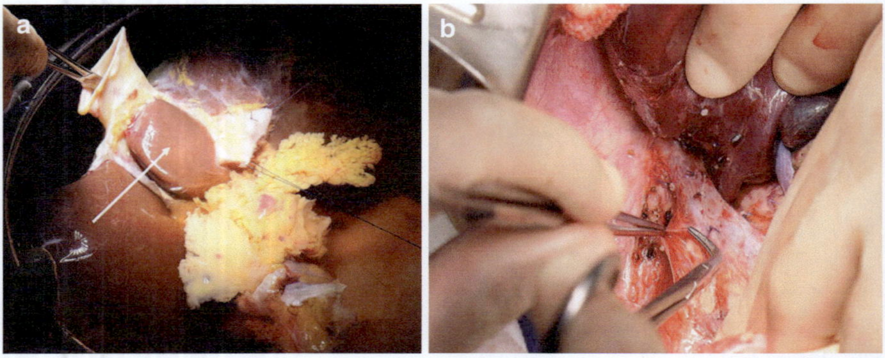

Fig. 20.21 (**a**) Caudate lobe of the liver (arrow). (**b**) Ligation of multiple caudate veins draining into the inferior vena cava during surgery

patients with Budd-Chiari syndrome, compensatory hypertrophy of the caudate is commonly observed due to its unique venous drainage pattern. There are one to three bile ducts draining each part of the caudate lobe. The bile duct from the Spiegel process predominantly drains into LHD, but at times may drain into the RPSD or the biliary confluence. The majority of ducts from the paracaval portion drains into the RPSD, although some may cross to the opposite side to drain into the LHD. Bile leak from divided caudate ducts is a major cause of morbidity in SLT and LDLT [52]. Thus, meticulous identification and suturing of caudate ducts during transection are important to minimize post-operative biliary complications. The caudate lobe may wrap around the IVC which requires careful dissection during explant surgery. Caudate lobectomy is usually undertaken as part of oncological surgeries for tumours involving the caudate lobe or in case of hilar cholangiocarcinoma involving the caudate ducts.

20.10 Partial Liver Allografts

In split liver transplantation, the deceased donor organ is split, either in situ or ex situ, into two grafts for two different recipients [53–56]. In the commonest form of SLT, the liver is split into an extended right lobe graft (segments I, IV, to VIII) for implantation into an adult recipient and a left lateral segment graft (segments II and III) for implantation into a paediatric recipient. In less common cases, the liver is split into right (segments I, V, to VIII) and left (segments II to IV) lobes for implantation into two adult recipients. Similarly, for living liver donation, partial allografts are obtained based on the age and weight of the recipient, and graft recipient weight ratio (GRWR) calculated pre-operatively by volumetric analysis of donor computed tomography scan. The key to successful procurement of partial allografts in either situation is to maintain vascular and biliary supply to both sides of the liver without sabotaging either. Hence, it is imperative to have a thorough knowledge of the surgical anatomy of the hilar structures and the relationship between the middle and right hepatic veins in order to safely execute these procedures and to minimize both donor and recipient post-operative complications.

In SLT, the hilar structures are first evaluated thoroughly to identify the presence of variant anatomy. The technique of splitting the vasculature varies between different centres [53–57]. However, the most common method involves preserving the main trunk of the common hepatic artery with the right lobe graft, by dividing the LHA at the level of its confluence. Similarly, the main trunk of the PV is allocated to the right lobe graft, as the LPV has a longer extra-hepatic course which provides sufficient length for anastomosis to the recipient. The common bile duct is given to the right lobe graft, and the left hepatic duct is sectioned just away from the hilum. The plane of parenchymal transection is just to the right of the umbilical fissure, and transection is done by the Kelly-clysis technique or using a cavitron ultrasonic suction and aspiration (CUSA) device. The LHV is retained with the LLS graft, whereas the RHV and MHV along with the IVC are allocated to the extended right lobe (Figs. 20.22 and 20.23).

In LDLT, the plane of transection for right or left lobe grafts is along the MHV. Controversy exists regarding the allocation of MHV to either graft [58–60].

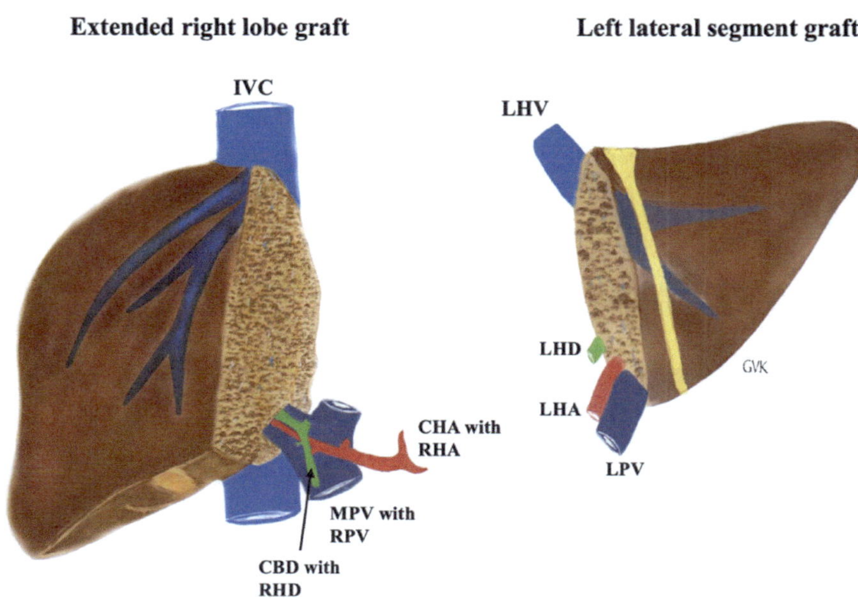

Fig. 20.22 Schematic representation of splitting a whole liver with its vasculature into extended right lobe and left lateral segment grafts. CBD common bile duct, CHA common hepatic artery, IVC inferior vena cava, LHA left hepatic artery, LHD left hepatic duct, LHV left hepatic vein, LPV left portal vein, MPV main portal vein, RHA right hepatic artery, RHD right hepatic duct, RPV right portal vein

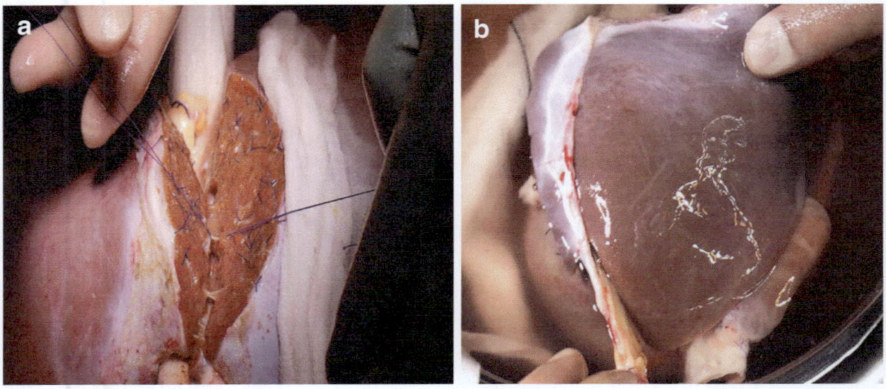

Fig. 20.23 (a) Ex situ splitting of a liver. (b) Left lateral segment graft after split

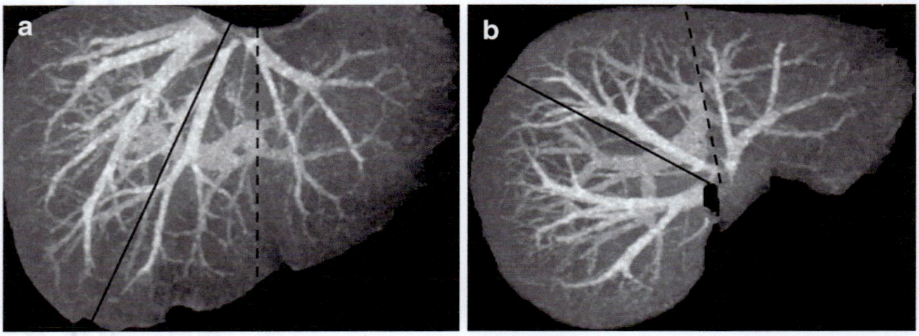

Fig. 20.24 (a) Coronal and (b) axial computed tomography (CT) images showing planes of transection for right/left lobe grafts (solid line) and left lateral segment graft (dotted line)

However, the most common practice is to harvest a right lobe graft without the MHV to ensure adequate drainage of remnant liver, thereby ensuring donor safety. Left lobe grafts, on the other hand, are procured with the MHV. The plane of transection for partial liver allografts from living donors is shown in Fig. 20.24. The partial allograft is then flushed on the backbench with cold preservative solution, and further reconstruction, if needed, is carried out prior to implantation.

In summary, a thorough knowledge of segmental and vasculobiliary anatomy of the liver is indispensable for liver transplantation. Successful application of partial liver allografts in both deceased and living donor liver transplantation mandates a detailed understanding of intra-hepatic anatomy. Vascular supply to the liver is complex with frequent anatomical variations. A precise knowledge and understanding of segmental and vascular anatomy with careful detection of variants can significantly minimize complications and improve outcomes of liver transplantation.

Acknowledgement The authors gratefully acknowledge Dr. Vasanthakumar Gunasekaran, Consultant, Liver Transplant and Hepato-Pancreatico-Biliary Surgeon, Dr. Rela Institute and Medical Centre, Chennai, India, for contributing his original artwork to this chapter.

References

1. Lhuaire M, Tonnelet R, Renard Y, Piardi T, Sommacale D, Duparc F, Braun M, Labrousse M. Developmental anatomy of the liver from computerized three-dimensional reconstructions of four human embryos (from Carnegie stage 14 to 23). Ann Anat. 2015;200:105–13.
2. Jordan H, Kindred J. The liver. In: Jordan H, Kindred J, editors. Textbook of embryology. New York: Appleton-Century; 1942. p. 156–60.
3. Jarnagin WR, editor. Blumgart's surgery of the liver, pancreas and biliary tract E-book. Philadelphia: Elsevier Health Sciences; 2016.
4. Asahina K, Tsai SY, Li P, Ishii M, Maxson RE Jr, Sucov HM, Tsukamoto H. Mesenchymal origin of hepatic stellate cells, submesothelial cells, and perivascular mesenchymal cells during mouse liver development. Hepatology. 2009;49(3):998–1011.
5. Patten BM. Foundations of embryology. New York: Mcgraw hill; 1958.
6. Couinaud C. Surgical anatomy of the liver revisited: embryology. Paris: Couinaud; 1989. p. 11–24.
7. Emond JC, Renz JF. Surgical anatomy of the liver and its application to hepatobiliary surgery and transplantation. In Seminars in liver disease (Vol. 14, No. 02, pp. 158–168). Thieme Medical Publishers, Inc.; 1994.
8. McClusky DA III, Skandalakis LJ, Colborn GL, Skandalakis JE. Hepatic surgery and hepatic surgical anatomy: historical partners in progress. World J Surg. 1997;21:330–42.
9. Cantlie MA. On a new arrangement of the right and left lobes of the liver. Proc Anat Soc Great Britain Ireland. 1898;32:4–9.
10. Couinaud C. Les enveloppes vasculobiliares de foie ou capsule de Glisson. Leur interet dans la chirurgie vesiculaire, les resections hepatiques et l'abord du hile du foie. Lyon Chir. 1954;49:589–615.
11. Strasberg SM, Belghiti J, Clavien PA, Gadzijev E, Garden JO, Lau WY, Makuuchi M, Strong RW. The Brisbane 2000 terminology of liver anatomy and resections. HPB. 2000;2(3):333–9.
12. Renz JF, Yersiz H, Farmer DG, Hisatake GM, Ghobrial RM, Busuttil RW. Changing faces of liver transplantation: partial-liver grafts for adults. J Hepato-Biliary-Pancreat Surg. 2003;10:31–44.
13. Renz JF, Emond JC, Yersiz H, Ascher NL, Busuttil RW. Split-liver transplantation in the United States: outcomes of a national survey. Ann Surg. 2004;239(2):172.
14. Starzl TE, Bell RH, Beart RW, Putnam CW. Hepatic trisegmentectomy and other liver resections. Surg Gynecol Obstet. 1975;141(3):429.
15. Tanaka K, Uemoto S, Tokunaga Y, Fujita S, Sano K, Nishizawa T, Sawada H, Shirahase I, Kim HJ, Yamaoka Y. Surgical techniques and innovations in living related liver transplantation. Ann Surg. 1993;217(1):82.
16. Nakamura S, Tsuzuki T. Surgical anatomy of the hepatic veins and the inferior vena cava. Surg Gynecol Obstet. 1981;152(1):43–50.
17. Busuttil RW, Klintmalm GB. Transplantation of the liver. New York: Elsevier Health Sciences; 2014.
18. Renz J. Normal and variant anatomy of the liver. In National Institutes of Health Workshop on Living-Donor Liver Transplantation, Washington DC, Dec 2000.
19. Cheng YF, Huang TL, Chen CL, Chen TY, Huang CC, Ko SF, Yang BY, Lee TY. Variations of the middle and inferior right hepatic vein: application in hepatectomy. J Clin Ultrasound. 1997;25(4):175–82.

20. Champetier J, Haouari H, Le Bas JF, Létoublon C, Alnaasan I, Farah I. Large inferior right hepatic vein. Clinical implications. Surg Radiol Anat. 1993;15(1):21–9.
21. De Cecchis L, Hribernik M, Ravnik D, Gadžijev EM. Anatomical variations in the pattern of the right hepatic veins: possibilities for type classification. J Anat. 2000;197(3):487–93.
22. Shilal P, Agarwal S, Tuli A, Kakkar S. Variations in the drainage pattern of middle hepatic vein and left hepatic vein in the left lobe of liver. J Clin Diagn Res. 2018;12(9):AC13–7.
23. Hwang S, Lee SG, Choi ST, Moon DB, Ha TY, Lee YJ, Park KM, Kim KH, Ahn CS, Kim KK, Kim YD. Hepatic vein anatomy of the medial segment for living donor liver transplantation using extended right lobe graft. Liver Transpl. 2005;11(4):449–55.
24. Emond JC, Heffron TG, Whitington PF, Broelsch CE. Reconstruction of the hepatic vein in reduced size hepatic transplantation. Surg Gynecol Obstet. 1993;176(1):11–7.
25. Ghobrial RM, Hsieh CB, Lerner S, Winters S, Nissen N, Dawson S, Amersi F, Chen P, Farmer D, Yersiz H, Busuttil RW. Technical challenges of hepatic venous outflow reconstruction in right lobe adult living donor liver transplantation. Liver Transpl. 2001;7(6):551–5.
26. Marcos A, Orloff M, Mieles L, Olzinski AT, Renz JF, Sitzmann JV. Functional venous anatomy for right-lobe grafting and techniques to optimize outflow. Liver Transpl. 2001;7(10):845–52.
27. Faitot F, Vibert E, Salloum C, Gorden DL, Coscas F, Adam R, Castaing D. Importance of conserving middle hepatic vein distal branches for homogeneous regeneration of the left liver after right hepatectomy. HPB. 2012;14(11):746–53.
28. Cronin DC, Millis JM, Siegler M. Transplantation of liver grafts from living donors into adults—too much, too soon. N Engl J Med. 2001;344(21):1633–7.
29. Soejima Y, Shirabe K, Taketomi A, Yoshizumi T, Uchiyama H, Ikegami T, Ninomiya M, Harada N, Ijichi H, Maehara Y. Left lobe living donor liver transplantation in adults. Am J Transplant. 2012;12(7):1877–85.
30. Lee S, Park K, Hwang S, Lee Y, Choi D, Kim K, Koh K, Han S, Choi K, Hwang K, Makuuchi M. Congestion of right liver graft in living donor liver transplantation. Transplantation. 2001;71(6):812–4.
31. Shankar S, Rammohan A, Gunasekaran V, Narasimhan G, Rajalingam R, Palaniappan K, Kanagavelu R, Rajkumar A, Kaliamoorthy I, Rela M. Anatomical variations of left hepatic vein and outflow reconstruction techniques in pediatric living donor liver transplantation. Am J Transplant. 2023;23(6):786–93.
32. Reichert PR, Renz JF, Luiz AD, Rosenthal P, Lim RC, Roberts JP, Ascher NL, Emond JC. Surgical anatomy of the left lateral segment as applied to living-donor and split-liver transplantation: a clinicopathologic study. Ann Surg. 2000;232(5):658–64.
33. Cheng YF, Huang TL, Chen CL, Chen TY, Huang CC, Ko SF, Lee TY. Variations of the left and middle hepatic veins: application in living related hepatic transplantation. J Clin Ultrasound. 1996;24(1):11–6.
34. Neumann JO, Thorn M, Fischer L, Schöbinger M, Heimann T, Radeleff B, Schmidt J, Meinzer HP, Büchler MW, Schemmer P. Branching patterns and drainage territories of the middle hepatic vein in computer-simulated right living-donor hepatectomies. Am J Transplant. 2006;6(6):1407–15.
35. Shankar S, Rammohan A, Rela M, Srinivasan P. Surgical anatomy of segment four of liver and its implications in hepato-biliary surgery and liver transplantation. J Liver Transplant. 2022;6:100076.
36. Tani K, Shindoh J, Akamatsu N, Arita J, Kaneko J, Sakamoto Y, Hasegawa K, Kokudo N. Venous drainage map of the liver for complex hepatobiliary surgery and liver transplantation. HPB. 2016;18(12):1031–8.
37. Honda H, Yanaga K, Onitsuka H, Kaneko K, Murakami J, Masuda K. Ultrasonographic anatomy of veins draining the left lobe of the liver: feasibility of live related transplantation. Acta Radiol. 1991;32(6):479–84.
38. Ortale JR, Bonet C, Prado PF, Mariotto A. Anatomy of the intrahepatic ramification of the intermediate and left hepatic veins in humans. J Morphol Sci. 2017;20(1):0.

39. Nakamura T, Tanaka K, Kiuchi T, Kasahara M, Oike F, Ueda M, Kaihara S, Egawa H, Ozden I, Kobayashi N, Uemoto S. Anatomical variations and surgical strategies in right lobe living donor liver transplantation: lessons from 120 cases 1. Transplantation. 2002;73(12):1896–903.
40. Cheng YF, Huang TL, Chen CL, Sheen-Chen SM, Lui CC, Chen TY, Lee TY. Anatomic dissociation between the intrahepatic bile duct and portal vein: risk factors for left hepatectomy. World J Surg. 1997;21:297–300.
41. Marwan IK, Fawzy AT, Egawa H, Inomata Y, Uemoto S, Asonuma K, Kiuchi T, Hayashi M, Fujita S, Ogura Y, Tanaka K. Innovative techniques for and results of portal vein reconstruction in living-related liver transplantation. Surgery. 1999;125(3):265–70.
42. Sugawara Y, Makuuchi M, Tamura S, Matsui Y, Kaneko J, Hasegawa K, Imamura H, Kokudo N, Motomura N, Takamoto S. Portal vein reconstruction in adult living donor liver transplantation using cryopreserved vein grafts. Liver Transpl. 2006;12(8):1233–6.
43. Lee SG, Hwang S, Kim KH, Ahn CS, Park KM, Lee YJ, Moon DB, Chu CW, Yang HS, Cho SH, Oh KB. Approach to anatomic variations of the graft portal vein in right lobe living-donor liver transplantation. Transplantation. 2003;75(3):S28–32.
44. Michels NA. Newer anatomy of the liver and its variant blood supply and collateral circulation. Am J Surg. 1966;112(3):337–47.
45. Hiatt JR, Gabbay J, Busuttil RW. Surgical anatomy of the hepatic arteries in 1000 cases. Ann Surg. 1994;220(1):50.
46. Launois B, Jamieson GG, Cherqui D, Randone B, Gayet B, Machado MA. The posterior intrahepatic approach in liver surgery. Austin: Landes Bioscience; 2013.
47. Hjortsjö CH. The topography of the intrahepatic duct systems. Cells Tissues Organs. 1950;11(4):599–615.
48. Parke WW. Blood supply of the common bile duct. Surg Gynecol Obstet. 1963;117:47–55.
49. Smadja C. The biliary tract and the anatomy of biliary exposure. In: Surgery of the liver and biliary tract, vol. 1. Edinburgh: Churchill Livingstone; 1988. p. 11–22.
50. Huang TL, Cheng YF, Chen CL, Chen TY, Lee TY. Variants of the bile ducts: clinical application in the potential donor of living-related hepatic transplantation. Transplant Proc. 1996;28(3):1669–70.
51. Ohkubo M, Nagino M, Kamiya J, Yuasa N, Oda K, Arai T, Nishio H, Nimura Y. Surgical anatomy of the bile ducts at the hepatic hilum as applied to living donor liver transplantation. Ann Surg. 2004;239(1):82.
52. Jassem W, Heaton ND, Rela M. Reducing bile leak following segmental liver transplantation: understanding biliary anatomy of the caudate lobe. Am J Transplant. 2008;8(2):271–4.
53. Busuttil RW, Goss JA. Split liver transplantation. Ann Surg. 1999;229(3):313.
54. Rela M, Vougas V, Muiesan P, Vilca-Melendez H, Smyrniotis V, Gibbs P, Karani J, Williams R, Heaton N. Split liver transplantation: King's College Hospital experience. Ann Surg. 1998;227(2):282.
55. Azoulay D, Astarcioglu I, Bismuth H, Castaing D, Majno P, Adam R, Johann M. Split-liver transplantation. The Paul Brousse policy. Ann Surg. 1996;224(6):737.
56. Reyes J, Gerber D, Mazariegos GV, Casavilla A, Sindhi R, Bueno J, Madariaga J, Fung JJ. Split-liver transplantation: a comparison of ex vivo and in situ techniques. J Pediatr Surg. 2000;35(2):283–90.
57. Vagefi PA, Parekh J, Ascher NL, Roberts JP, Freise CE. Outcomes with split liver transplantation in 106 recipients: the University of California, San Francisco, experience from 1993 to 2010. Arch Surg. 2011;146(9):1052–9.
58. Yamaoka Y, Washida M, Honda K, Tanaka K, Mori K, Shimahara Y, Okamoto S, Ueda M, Hayashi M, Tanaka A, Morimoto T. Liver transplantation using a right lobe graft from a living related donor. Transplantation. 1994;57(7):1127–9.
59. Inomata Y, Uemoto S, Asonuma K, Egawa H, Kiuchi T, Fujita S, Hayashi M, Kawashima M, Tanaka K. Right lobe graft in living donor liver transplantation. Transplantation. 2000;69(2):258.
60. Fan ST, Lo CM, Liu CL. Technical refinement in adult-to-adult living donor liver transplantation using right lobe graft. Ann Surg. 2000;231(1):126.

Chapter 21
Donor Selection in Liver Transplantation

Arvinder Singh Soin and Suchet Chaudhary

Abstract The primary sources of liver grafts are deceased donors [donation after brain death (DBD) and donation after cardiac death (DCD)] and living donor liver transplantation (LDLT). Deceased donor livers, particularly those from brain-dead donors, are preferred due to the absence of donor risk, but their scarcity has led to the utilization of marginal or extended criteria grafts. Living donor liver transplantation, especially prevalent in regions like Southeast Asia, addresses organ shortages but poses risks to donors, including complications from partial hepatectomy. In India, LDLT dominates, accounting for 80–85% of transplants, while DBD and DCD donations are gradually increasing. Donor selection involves stringent criteria, including age, liver steatosis, graft-to-recipient weight ratio (GRWR), and anatomical compatibility. Advanced techniques like normothermic machine perfusion (NMP) and hypothermic machine perfusion (HMP) have improved the viability of marginal grafts, particularly from DCD donors. Living donors undergo thorough evaluation to ensure safety, with considerations for liver volume, vascular anatomy, and metabolic health. Ethical concerns, including informed consent and donor autonomy, are paramount. Innovations like ABO-incompatible transplants and paired exchanges have expanded donor pools. Despite advancements, donor selection remains a fine balance between expanding access and ensuring safety, with ongoing research aimed at optimizing outcomes for both donors and recipients.

Keywords Donor selection · Living Donor Liver Transplantation (LDLT) · Deceased Donor (DBD/DCD) · Graft viability · Donor optimization · Machine perfusion (NMP/HMP) · Ethical considerations

A. S. Soin (✉) · S. Chaudhary
Institute of Liver Transplantation and Regenerative Medicine, Medanta The Medicity, Gurugram, Delhi NCR, India
e-mail: absoin@gmail.com

S. Saigal, D. Jothimani (eds.), *Fundamentals of Transplant Hepatology*,
https://doi.org/10.1007/978-981-95-2624-6_21

Key Highlights

Liver transplants use grafts from both deceased and living donors, but living donor procedures are more common in countries like India due to the shortage of deceased donors.

Careful selection of donors—considering age, fat content in the liver, anatomical fit, and overall health—is essential to ensure safe and successful outcomes.

Machine perfusion techniques now allow the safe use of grafts once considered marginal or high-risk.

Ethical oversight is crucial in living donation, where minimizing risk and protecting donor autonomy are top priorities.

Innovations like split-liver surgery and paired exchanges are helping to bridge the gap between organ demand and availability, even as global donation trends continue to shift.

21.1 Introduction

Liver transplantation is a well-established and curative treatment for patients with decompensated liver cirrhosis and acute liver failure. Ideally, the donor is a deceased donor (DBD, Donation after Brain Death), as it involves a complete organ with no risk to the donor. However, the most significant limitation of deceased donor organ transplantation is the unpredictability and scarcity of available organs. Utilizing marginal or extended criteria liver grafts can reduce the risk of mortality for patients on the liver transplant waitlist without affecting patient or graft survival. Many countries now also accept liver grafts from donations after cardiac death (DCD) [1].

While normothermic machine perfusion has advanced the use of DCD donors, DCD remains a less preferred option due to the rigid logistics, unpredictability of the agonal phase, and high probability of complications, such as early allograft dysfunction and non-anastomotic biliary structures [2].

Living donor liver transplantation (LDLT) is a practical solution to these challenges. It expands the donor pool, reducing the morbidity and mortality associated with long waiting lists and ensuring higher survival rates and quality of life [3]. In the eastern part of the globe, particularly in Southeast Asia, LDLT has become routine rather than occasional. However, LDLT has its drawbacks, including the use of a smaller graft compared to a whole organ, associated risks for the donor, and a relatively higher rate of complications. These complications are less frequent with standard anatomy but increase with unconventional anatomy, such as multiple accessory vessels or ducts, presenting unique reconstructive challenges. The operating team must evaluate graft quality and acceptable anatomy to achieve the best possible outcomes.

India has made significant progress since performing its first successful deceased and living donor liver transplants in 1998. Currently, around 2000 liver transplants (LT) are performed annually. Data from the past 3–5 years shows a predominant reliance on living donors, with a smaller contribution from donations after brain

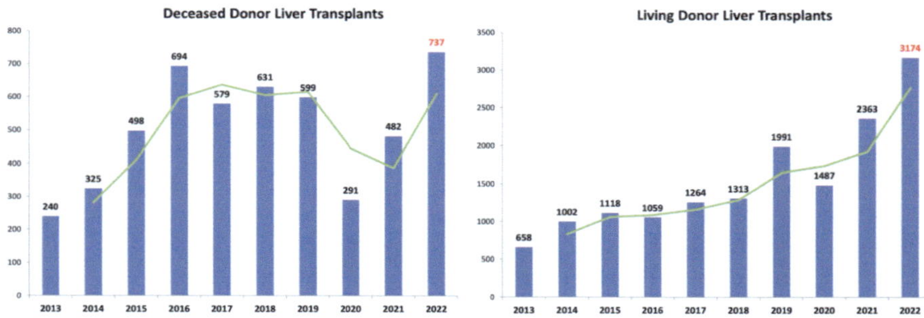

Fig. 21.1 The number of deceased and living donor LTs done from 2013 to 2022 in India [6]

death (DBD) and even fewer from donations after circulatory death (DCD). Approximately 80–85% of liver transplants in India are sourced from living donors due to the limited availability of deceased donors [4]. Although the number of DBD liver transplants is slowly increasing due to growing awareness and improved organ donation frameworks, it remains lower than that of living donors. DCD donations are the least common, hindered by regulatory and ethical challenges as well as logistical complexities [5]. Despite an upward trend in deceased organ donations, living donor liver transplants continue to dominate the transplantation landscape in India (Fig. 21.1). Ongoing efforts aim to boost deceased donation rates through public awareness campaigns and enhancements in organ donation infrastructure.

In recent years, the United Network for Organ Sharing (UNOS) has reported significant trends in liver donations from various sources, reflecting advancements and increased efforts within the organ transplant community. Donation after Brain Death (DBD) has remained a vital source, with over 16,000 in 2023, facilitating 39,679 deceased donor transplants, nearly a 9% increase from the previous year [7]. Donation after Circulatory Death (DCD) has seen remarkable growth, with 4,776 DCD donors in 2022, representing a 14% increase from 2021 [8]. This increase was driven by advancements in perfusion technology and collaborative efforts to enhance DCD organ recovery [9, 10]. Living liver donations have shown variability, with 6466 living donors in 2022, a slight decrease from previous years, though 2019 saw a peak with 7389 living donors. Overall, 2023 was a record year for liver transplants, with 10,660 performed, the highest ever recorded in a single year, reflecting ongoing initiatives to improve equity and patient access to transplants.

21.2 Definitions

21.2.1 Standard Criteria Donor [11]

Standard deceased liver donor: The following criteria are generally accepted by most, but they may differ from center to center:

- The standard organ donor criteria for acceptability also apply to DCD livers.
- The deceased donor is less than age 55.
- The time from withdrawal of support until the heart stops and the donor is declared dead must be less than 30 min.
- The donor liver must be able to be transplanted into the recipient within 8 h of retrieval.
- The donor liver must not have a large amount of fat in the liver cells (<30% is mostly accepted). If in doubt, a biopsy may be done.
- The liver must look healthy after it is flushed with preservation solution before it is removed from the donor.
- The donor liver is free of liver disease, confirmed by biopsy when doubtful.

21.2.2 Marginal/Extended Criteria Liver Donor [12]

Marginal liver grafts included those with any of the following characteristics:

- Liver donor age >70 years
- Livers are discarded regionally and shared nationally
- Livers from HCV-positive donors
- Livers with cold ischemia time >12 h
- Livers from donation after circulatory death donors
- Livers with >30% steatosis
- Livers are split between two recipients

- *DBD (Donation after brain death):* Donation after Brainstem Death (DBD) is possible in patients whose death has been confirmed using neurological criteria (also known as brainstem death or brain death), while the circulatory failure has yet to occur. This diagnosis is only possible in patients who are on mechanical ventilation [13].
- *DCD (Donation after circulatory death):* Donation after circulatory death (DCD) is a pathway to organ donation which can occur when a patient dies from cardiac arrest in the hospital. For a long time, it was also known as "non-heartbeating donation."

21.3 Special Techniques

- *NMN (Normothermic machine perfusion)*: NMP preserves donor livers at body temperature while allowing real-time assessment of function. It improves graft viability, reduces preservation injury, and may extend preservation time, offering better scheduling and broader use of marginal grafts. Studies show improved early outcomes and lower dysfunction rates compared to static cold storage, positioning NMP as a likely future standard [14].

- *HMP (Hypothermic machine perfusion)*: HMP circulates oxygenated cold solution through the liver, offering a dynamic alternative to static cold storage. It reduces ischemic damage and supports cellular health, particularly in high-risk DCD and marginal organs. HMP improves early graft function, limits ischemia-reperfusion injury, and provides viability data before transplantation. Its growing use may help increase the pool of usable livers, though further studies are needed [15].
- *NRP (Normothermic regional perfusion)*: NRP perfuses the liver with warm, oxygenated blood shortly after retrieval, helping maintain normal metabolism and reducing cold injury. It allows for functional assessment pre-transplant and has shown benefits in improving early liver function post-implantation.
- *IFLT (ischemia-free liver transplantation)*: IFLT uses continuous NMP from retrieval through implantation, aiming to eliminate ischemia-reperfusion injury. Initial trials show reduced early dysfunction and better graft outcomes, especially in extended criteria donor organs [16]. Despite some technical challenges and cost considerations, IFLT presents a promising advancement in liver transplantation and could be adapted for other organs. Further randomized controlled trials are underway to confirm these benefits and refine the technique.

21.4 Standard Living Liver Donor

The standard living liver donor should be an 18–55-year-old, willing and healthy family person, should not be overweight or obese, and should preferably have a compatible blood group (either the same blood group as the patient's or blood group "O") [17].

21.5 Making an Unfit Donor Fit

Preparing living liver donors with health concerns—like steatosis, high BMI, liver inflammation, or manageable comorbidities—requires a comprehensive and personalized approach. For those with fatty liver, lifestyle changes such as a low-fat diet and regular exercise are key to reducing liver fat and improving liver health. When lifestyle adjustments aren't enough, medications may be introduced to further optimize the donor's condition.

Overweight donors benefit from structured weight-loss plans that include calorie control, better nutrition, and a consistent exercise routine combining aerobic and strength training. In difficult cases, weight-loss drugs or behavioral support may be added to aid progress.

Liver inflammation must be carefully evaluated and treated at its source, whether due to viral, autoimmune, or other causes. These donors should also avoid alcohol and follow antioxidant-rich diets to support liver recovery, with medications used as needed.

Correctable health issues like diabetes, high blood pressure, or thyroid problems must be well managed through a mix of medications, diet, and exercise, often with specialist input. All donors should receive tailored fitness plans, mental health support, and regular monitoring to ensure they remain safe and surgery-ready, improving outcomes for both donor and recipient.

21.6 Evolving Techniques in Liver Donation: From Open Surgery to Minimally Invasive and Innovative Transplant Strategies

In living liver donation, graft retrieval is typically performed either through traditional open surgery or using minimally invasive techniques like laparoscopy or robotics. As surgical centers gain more experience and confidence with these less invasive methods, they are becoming increasingly popular among donors. The terminology used at most institutions often reflects the surgical approach chosen. With growing evidence supporting their safety and faster recovery, minimally invasive techniques are steadily emerging as a strong alternative to the conventional open method—and may soon become the preferred standard of care.

21.6.1 Open Liver Donation

Open liver donation involves a traditional surgical approach where a portion of the liver is removed through a larger abdominal incision. While more invasive than robotic or laparoscopic methods, it remains the most widely performed technique, especially in complex cases or where minimally invasive tools are not suitable. This method allows for direct access and visibility, which can be crucial for surgical precision and safety. Though recovery may take longer and involve more postoperative discomfort, open donation continues to be a reliable and effective option for liver transplantation.

21.6.2 Minimally Invasive Liver Donation: Robotic and Laparoscopic Approaches

Robotic and laparoscopic surgeries are modern, minimally invasive options for living liver donors. In robotic-assisted donation, the surgeon operates via robotic arms, offering exceptional precision, reduced blood loss, and smaller incisions, which lead to quicker recovery. Similarly, laparoscopic surgery uses small cuts and a camera to guide instruments, minimizing pain and hospital stay. Both techniques provide enhanced safety and faster healing, making them attractive alternatives to traditional open surgery for eligible donors.

21.6.3 Split-Liver Transplantation

In this, a deceased donor's liver is divided (in situ/ex situ) into two separate grafts to be transplanted into two different recipients. Generally, the larger right lobe is given to an adult, while the smaller left lobe is used for a child or a smaller adult. This approach optimizes the use of a single liver, helping to mitigate the shortage of available organs. The procedure demands meticulous surgical planning to ensure that both grafts receive adequate blood supply and function effectively in their respective recipients.

21.6.4 Paired Exchange/Swap LDLT

This is a method in which the incompatible donor-recipient pairs in terms of blood group/graft volume can be matched with other incompatible donor-recipient pairs to achieve a mutually compatible liver transplant.

21.6.5 ABOi Liver Transplantation

In this, a living donor liver graft is transplanted into a recipient with a different blood type. Since the immune system typically reacts against foreign blood types, matching ABO blood types is usually essential for successful organ transplants. In ABO-incompatible transplants, treatments before the procedure are used to eliminate or suppress antibodies that would normally attack the donor organ. This method expands the pool of potential donors and enhances the likelihood of finding a suitable match for patients requiring a transplant.

21.6.6 Domino Liver Transplantation

Domino liver transplantation (DLT) involves transplanting the liver from a patient with metabolic disease into a patient with end-stage liver disease, with the expectation that the recipient will not develop the metabolic syndrome or the recurrent syndrome will have minimal effect.

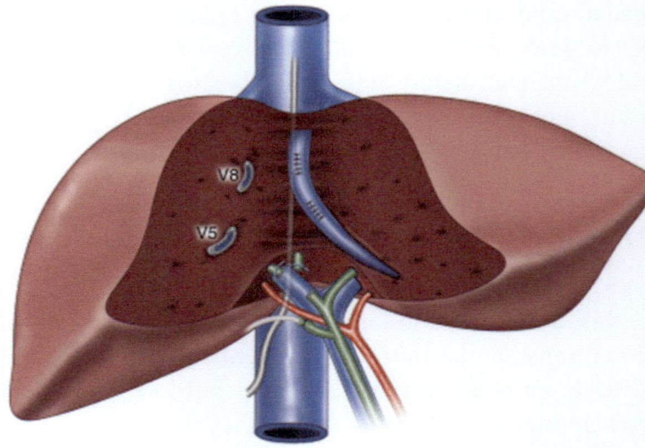

Fig. 21.2 The standard schema of liver transection (right lobe without MHV/ left lobe with MHV) [18]

21.7 Types of Living Donor Liver Grafts

21.7.1 Standard Right Lobe Graft (SRLG)

It includes Segment V, VI, VIII, and IX (which is the entire anatomical right lobe). MHV is typically not included (Figs. 21.2 and 21.3), and no reconstruction is done for the divided segment five veins (S5v) and segment eight veins (S8v). Mostly, the standard right lobe graft is discouraged, as there is compromised SegV and Seg VIII drainage, causing a loss of anterior segment functional liver volume, which is necessary for the function and regeneration of the anterior sector.

21.7.2 Modified Right Lobe Graft (MRLG)

This is a right lobe graft without MHV, and anterior sector venous drainage is reconstructed (Fig. 21.4) with Neo-MHV (cryopreserved/dacron or PTFE vascular grafts are used for the reconstruction) to keep the anterior sector (Seg V & VIII) viable. Cryopreserved vascular grafts are the first choice, considering better long-term patency rates, but the availability of the same is the determining factor.

21.7.3 Right Lobe Graft with Partial/Subtotal MHV

This is the right lobe graft; depending upon the anatomy of MHV, usually the Seg IVb vein is divided, and the graft is harvested with partial or near total MHV while confirming the intact drainage of Seg IVa or the presence of an accessory left vein draining the area.

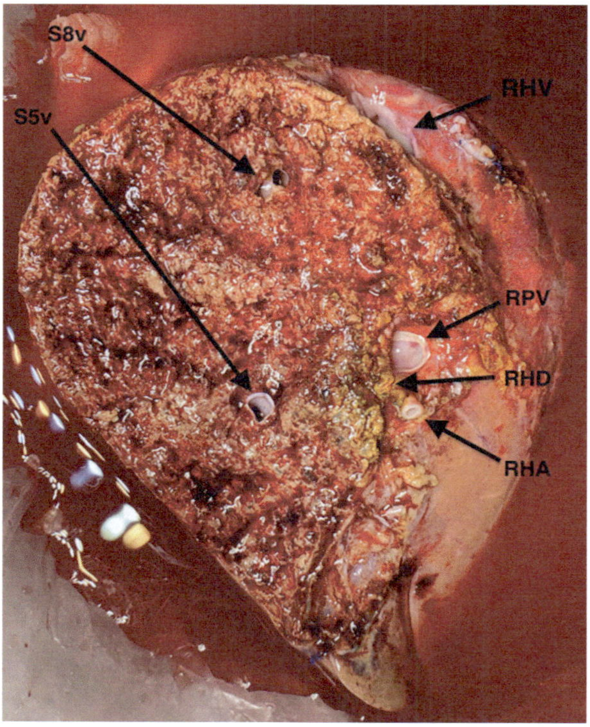

Fig. 21.3 Standard right lobe graft (without MHV reconstruction). RHV Right hepatic vein, RPV right portal vein, RHD right hepatic duct, RHA right hepatic artery, S8v segment 8 vein, S5v segment 5 vein

21.7.4 Left Lobe Graft (LLG)

This includes segments 2–4. It is usually harvested with MHV to maintain the drainage of segment IV (therefore, it doesn't require a complex backbench surgery for venous drainage reconstruction as done in modified right lobe grafts). Caudate may or may not be taken with the LL graft to optimize the GRWR. Figures 21.5, 21.6, and 21.7 show LLG in various aspects.

21.7.5 Left lateral sector graft (LLSG)

This graft includes primarily segments 2 and 3, which are mostly harvested with a sliver of segment 4. The transection phase of the left lateral graft is shown in Fig. 21.8.

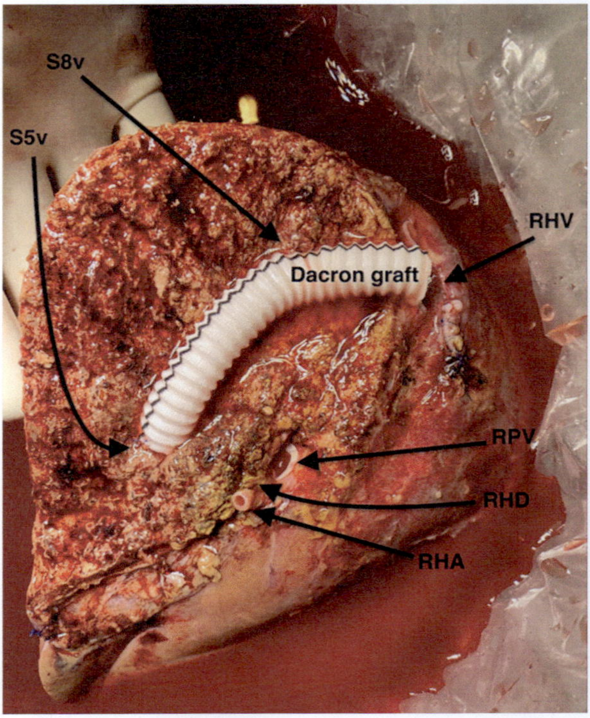

Fig. 21.4 Modified right lobe graft

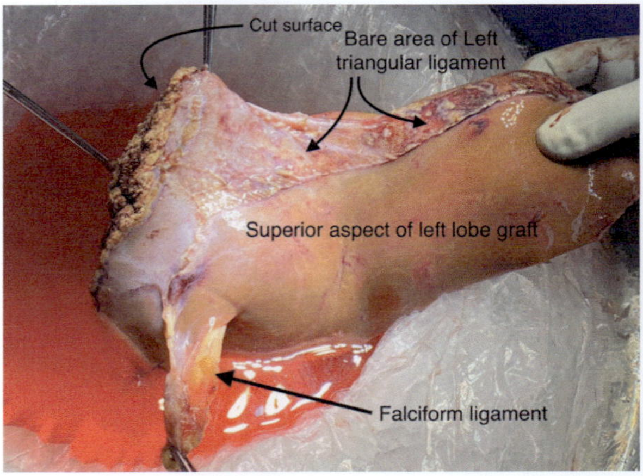

Fig. 21.5 Left lobe graft (superior aspect)

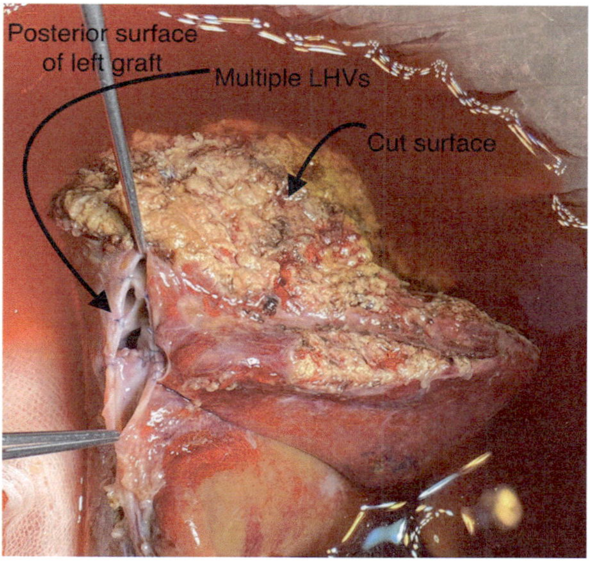

Fig. 21.6 Left lobe graft (postero-superior aspect). LHVs (left hepatic veins)

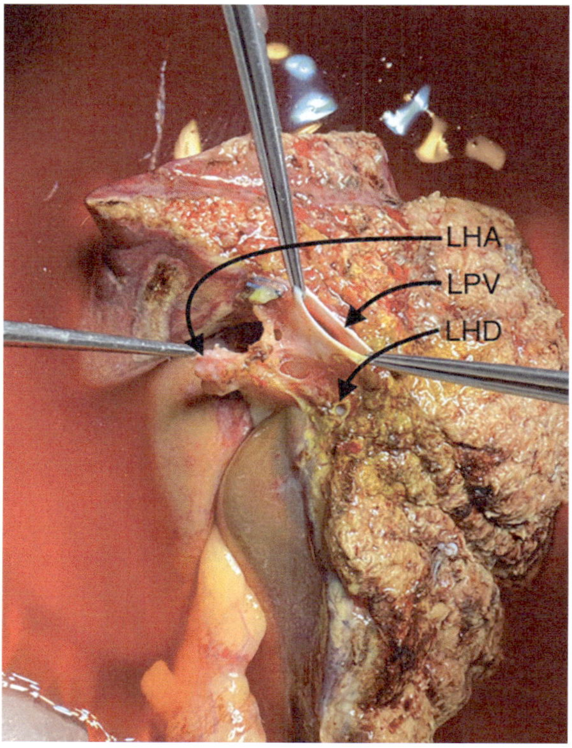

Fig. 21.7 Left lobe graft, showing the hilum. LHA left hepatic artery, LPV left portal vein, LHD left hepatic duct

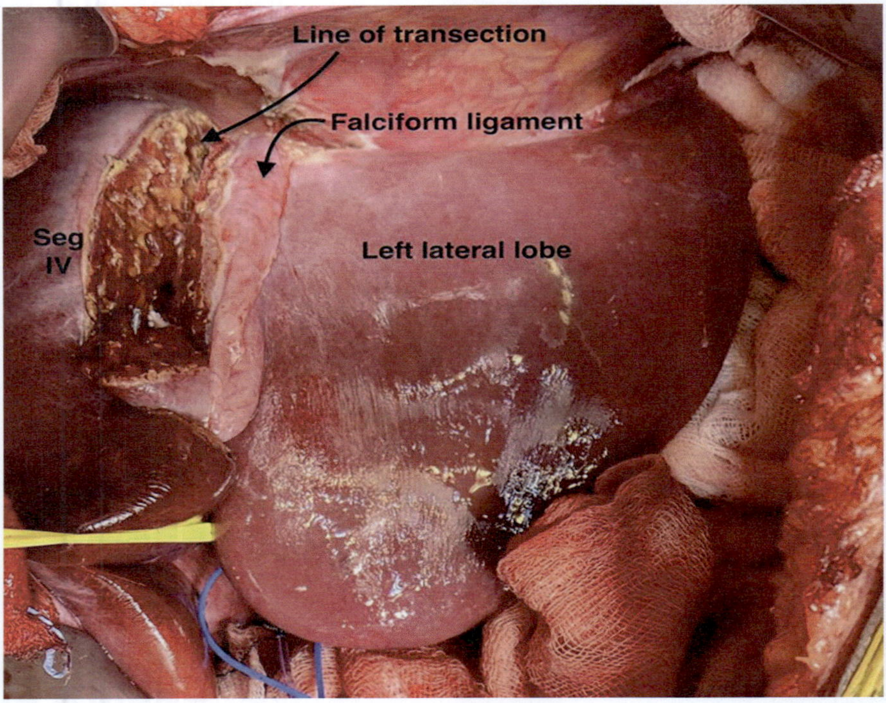

Fig. 21.8 Left lateral section (transection phase)

21.7.6 Uncommon Grafts

- *Reduced graft*: Mostly, LLSG is reduced further for the graft to fit in the recipient or to keep GRWR acceptable. Here the left lateral sector is reduced by reducing Seg-III -III, while the remaining part of Seg-III and Seg-II is kept intact. The lines of transection for graft reduction are shown in Fig. 21.9.
- *Hyper-reduced graft/monosegment graft*: Here, too, LLSG is reduced to an extent to have a nearly monosegment graft. As seen in the picture, the Seg-II is demarcated from Seg-III, which is further reduced to have a hyper-reduced graft. (Fig. 21.10)
- *Posterior sector graft*: It's uncommon to harvest a posterior sector graft. But it can be done when the remnant liver is <30% and the right posterior sector has a favorable anatomy (having a single and separate arterial/portal supply, venous drainage, and duct). The planning and execution of the posterior sector graft are shown in Figs. 21.11, 21.12, 21.13, 21.14, 21.15, and 21.16.

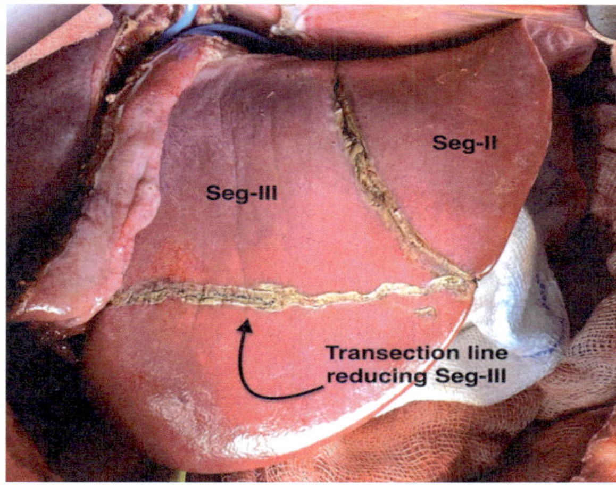

Fig. 21.9 Left lateral sector graft (transection lines marked for graft reduction)

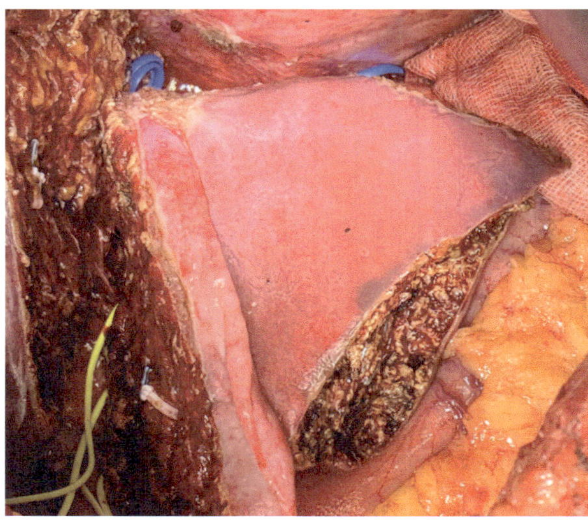

Fig. 21.10 Hyper-reduced graft (Monosegment 3 graft)

21.8 Deceased Donor Selection

We've discussed the characteristics of the ideal deceased donor above. An ideal deceased liver donor is hemodynamically stable (SBP >90) to ensure proper organ perfusion and free of significant hypoxia, acidosis, or hypoglycemia. Viral screening must be negative for HBV, HCV, and HIV, with additional tests for region-specific infections when applicable. Livers with steatosis under 30% are generally acceptable. While older donor age is a known risk factor for graft dysfunction and higher post-transplant mortality, successful outcomes have been reported even with donors in their 90s, provided other health parameters are favorable [19]. Donor age

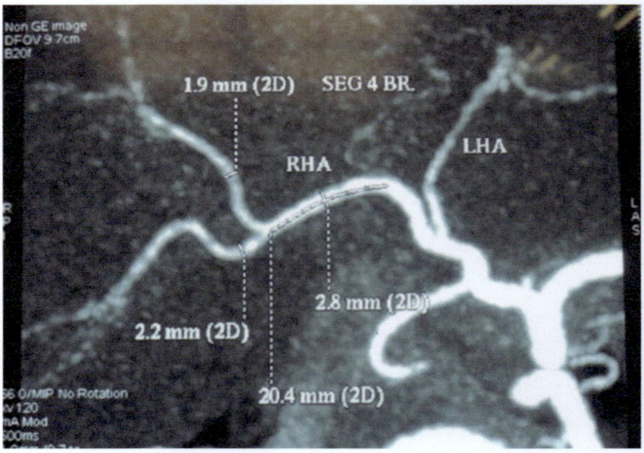

Fig. 21.11 Study of arterial phase (showing a single extrahepatic right posterior artery)

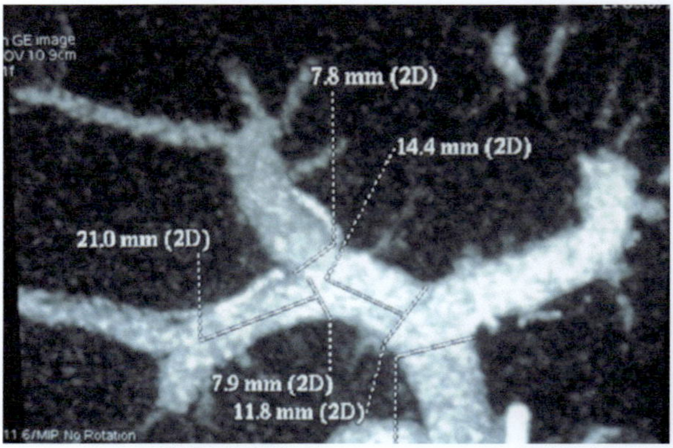

Fig. 21.12 Portal phase study showing a single right posterior portal vein

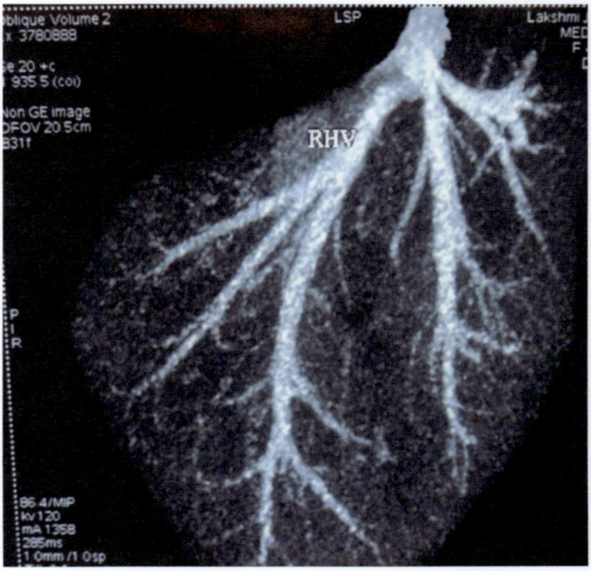

Fig. 21.13 Venous phase study of CT imaging. (showing a compatible single right posterior vein with good drainage of the anterior sector by MHV)

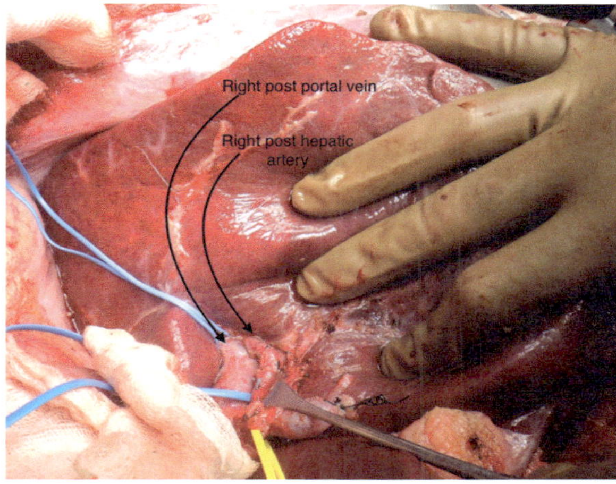

Fig. 21.14 Portal dissection and delineation of right posterior pedicle vessels

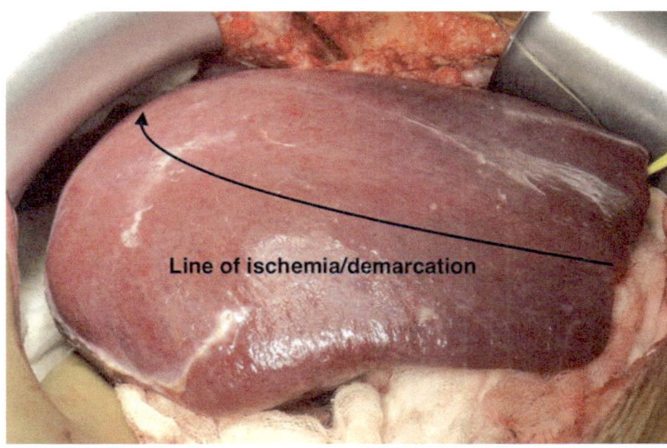

Fig. 21.15 Establishing line of ischemia/transection for the posterior sector

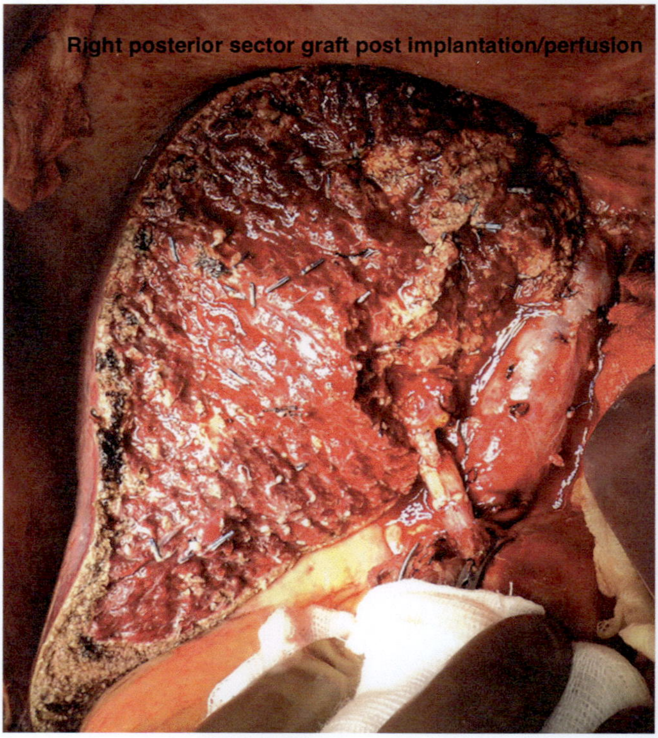

Fig. 21.16 Posterior sector graft after implantation

is discussed separately further in the chapter. The deceased donors are allocated to the highest priority recipients (highest Model for End-Stage Liver Diseases [MELD]/Pediatric End-Stage Liver Disease [PELD]) per the national (NOTTO), state (SOTTO), and regional (ROTTO) regulatory bodies in India [20].

21.8.1 Expanded Criteria for Selection of Deceased Liver Donors

Donors who don't meet standard criteria are often considered under expanded criteria, provided recipient safety and outcomes remain comparable. With the rising number of patients with end-stage liver disease and high mortality on transplant waitlists, there's a growing need to broaden these criteria.

Electrolyte imbalances—especially hypernatremia (Na >160 meq/L)—are linked to poor graft outcomes like early dysfunction or primary nonfunction [21]. High sodium levels may indicate suboptimal donor care, often accompanied by hypovolemia or acidosis. In such cases, delaying procurement until sodium is corrected (preferably <155 meq/L) and hemodynamics improve can enhance graft viability.

As the interval between brain death and organ retrieval lengthens, rising lactate, low bicarbonate, and a widening anion gap may signal metabolic acidosis. This often points to liver dysfunction or unstable donor physiology, requiring prompt intervention to stabilize before graft use [22].

21.8.2 Donation After Circulatory Death (DCD)

DCD refers to organ retrieval after the irreversible cessation of heart and respiratory function, with death formally declared by a physician. Unlike brain-dead donors, DCD donors typically have non-recoverable medical or neurological conditions. Once the family consents, life support is withdrawn in the operating room. Heparin is usually administered prior to extubation to minimize clot formation.

Two important timeframes influence organ viability:

- Total Donor Warm Ischemic Time (tDWIT): From withdrawal of life support to vascular clamping.
- Functional Warm Ischemic Time (fDWIT): Begins when blood pressure or oxygen levels drop significantly (e.g., SBP <80 mmHg or SpO_2 <80%) and ends at cross-clamp [23].

Most centers accept fDWIT <40 min without a significant difference in graft survival [24]. To minimize warm time, a rapid retrieval approach is used. After circulatory arrest and a brief wait, a swift midline incision is made, the aorta is cannulated, and supraceliac clamping is applied. This directs the cold preservation solution to the targeted organs, which are then retrieved once properly cooled and perfused [25].

DCD livers are inherently marginal and must be used cautiously, especially when donor factors like age or fatty liver are present. The phases of withdrawal and procurement are outlined in the table above (Fig. 21.17). Their use in severely ill recipients, such as those with high MELD scores, often leads to poor outcomes. A major limitation remains ischemic cholangiopathy (the Achilles heel of DCD), which still affects 8–12% of DCD grafts, even in top centers [27].

The new open-ended studies should address the impact of novel technologies in DCD procurement and preservation, including normothermic and hypothermic machine perfusion and normothermic regional perfusion. The studies so far have been encouraging using machine perfusion, especially with marginal grafts [28, 29].

21.8.3 The Outline of Deceased Donor Management

The management of a potential organ donor requires meticulous attention to various critical aspects for the optimization of organ function and ensuring the best possible outcomes in organ transplantation. Haemodynamic stability is paramount, necessitating the maintenance of euvolemia with a mean arterial pressure (MAP) of 60–70 mmHg, central venous pressure (CVP) of 6–10 mmHg, and urine output of

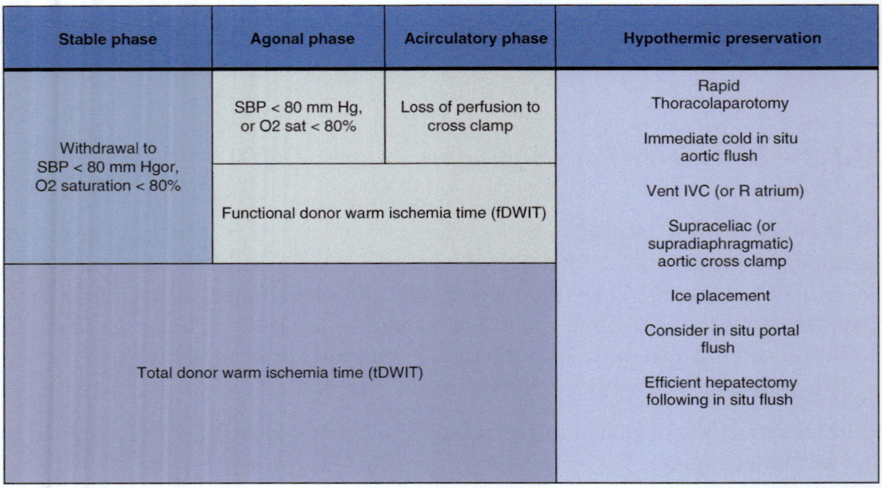

Fig. 21.17 Outline of the phases of DCD donor withdrawal and procurement. DCD (donation after circulatory death) [26]

1–3 ml/kg/h. The left ventricular ejection fraction should exceed 45%, and the cardiac index should be above 2.4 l/min/m^2, with arterial and central venous catheterization for monitoring. Vasoconstrictors should be minimized, favoring vasopressin as the first-line vasopressor, and isotonic crystalloids are recommended for volume replacement. Respiratory management involves a lung-protective ventilatory strategy, targeting PO_2 levels above 10 kPa and maintaining normocapnia, with PEEP set at 5–10 cmH_2O and careful lung recruitment. Pulmonary care should adhere to standard ICU protocols. Metabolic management requires keeping serum sodium levels between 135 and 145 mmol/l and blood glucose below 10 mmol/l, with normothermia and potential use of combined hormone therapy. In the case of Diabetes Insipidus (DI), characterized by large volumes of dilute urine and elevated serum sodium, treatment with DDAVP and vasopressin is essential, with the replacement of volume deficits with 0.45% saline. General care includes ongoing donor management throughout the perioperative period, maintaining hemoglobin levels above 7 g/dl, and treating suspected infections according to ICU protocols, including appropriate sampling for culture and sensitivity. The prevention and management of hypothermia and hyperglycemia is paramount, with possible use of hormonal therapies like vasopressin, glucocorticoids, thyroid hormone, and insulin, although evidence for improved outcomes remains limited [30].

21.9 The Risk of Transmission of Donor-Derived Infections

Donor-derived infections are classified as "expected" or "unexpected." Preoperative screening aims to detect the most expected infections, such as HBV, HCV, HIV, EBV, and CMV. Screening protocols should consider the patient's demographic profile, with a low threshold for additional tests based on history and clinical exam. Unexpected infections occur in less than 1% of solid organ transplants [31]

21.9.1 CMV Infection

Despite effective antivirals, CMV remains common in liver transplant recipients [32]. Prophylaxis protocols vary, as the drugs can cause bone marrow suppression and interact with antibiotics and immunosuppressants. Most centers reserve prophylaxis for high- and intermediate-risk patients. Risk is highest in D+/R− transplants, intermediate in D±/R+, and lowest in D−/R− [33]. High/intermediate-risk patients and those on recent antilymphocyte therapy, potent immunosuppression, or desensitization (e.g., rituximab, bortezomib, or plasmapheresis), require 3–6 months of prophylaxis. Preemptive therapy isn't recommended for low-risk patients [34].

CMV can range from asymptomatic viremia to tissue-invasive disease, with ~70% showing GI symptoms; it may also cause hepatitis and graft injury [35]. Diagnosis may need a biopsy, as viral load is often low [36]. CMV raises the risk of allograft inflammation (3.4×) and fibrosis (1.5×) in HCV-infected patients [37]. Diagnosis is by CMV detection in tissue (via immunohistochemistry, except CNS/retina), with screening by serology and confirmation by NAT/CMV-PCR [33].

21.9.2 HBV Infection

Understanding the potential detrimental effect on liver quality, HBV-positive donors were rejected, and transplants were mostly done with similar seropositivity in recipients; this shrank the donor pool considerably. HBV serology and DNA testing can distinguish between active infection, prior exposure, and vaccination status and can provide insight into disease transmission (Fig. 21.18).

Donors who are HbcAb positive are generally acceptable, whereas HbsAg-positive liver donors are uncommon [38]. These donors require a thorough evaluation of both infection status and liver parenchyma quality. Fibroscan is commonly used to assess fibrosis, but a liver biopsy—especially if Fibroscan is normal—remains the gold standard [39]

The availability of effective antiviral therapy (nucleoside/nucleotide analogues) and long transplant waitlists has led to growing acceptance of such grafts, with post-transplant outcomes comparable to HBV-negative grafts [40–42]. Recipients of

HBsAg	HBV NAT	HBcAb	HBsAb[a]	Interpretation	Risk of donor-derived transmission
+	+	+	+/–	Active HBV Infection	High
+	–	+	+/–	Active HBV Infection	High/medium
–	–	+	+	Recovered with cccDNA in hepatocytes	Organ dependent[b]
–	–	+	–	Recovered with cccDNA in hepatocytes[c]	Organ dependent[b]
–	–	–	+	HBV Vaccinated	No risk
–	–	–	–	No infection, no immunity	No risk

[a]Not usually available for deceased organ donors.

[b]High for liver transplants and typically requires antivirals posttransplant; nonliver patients represents low risk, especially if recipient is vaccinated with detectable HBsAb.

[c]In most cases, this represents recovered with cccDNA in hepatocytes; rarely may reflect false-positive HBcAb, occult chronic infection, resolving acute infection.

Fig. 21.18 Risk of donor-derived HBV infection in liver recipients

these grafts typically require lifelong antiviral therapy (e.g., Entecavir or Tenofovir). They are counseled about long-term risks, including a 20–30% chance of becoming HBsAg-positive and a 10–30% chance of HBV DNA positivity [43].

Early pioneering work by an Italian group showed poor outcomes in patients with HDV co-infection, making it a contraindication. They also observed persistent HBsAg in recipients who were themselves HBsAg-positive, despite HBIg therapy. Most evidence for HBsAg-positive graft use comes from deceased donors. In a single-center Italian study, ten HBsAg-positive livers were transplanted into anti-HBc-positive recipients with no cases of de novo hepatitis B under antiviral prophylaxis [44]. Outcomes in 92 recipients of HBsAg+ livers were reviewed retrospectively by UNOS. Although HBsAg+ livers were more likely to be used in Model for End-Stage Liver Disease (MELD) exception cases, there were no differences in patient or graft survival when compared to recipients of HBsAg– livers [45].

Patients exposed to HBV (positive HbcAb) have covalently closed circular (cccDNA) in the nucleus, which can't be cleared by the host immune response and therefore have lifelong infection. Anti-HBV therapy aims at controlling the viral load as compared to the curative anti-HCV treatment. Donors with negative HbsAg and HBV DNA, having positive HbcAb status, have the potential to transmit infection to the recipient. In non-immune recipients without prophylaxis, the transmission risk is as high as 77%. However, naturally immune recipients (anti-HBs positive) had significantly lower transmission rates (4%), and no transmission was reported in those who were both anti-HBc and anti-HBs positive [46]. Transmission risks also depend on the donor's recent behavior. High-risk donors (e.g., recent IV drug users) can transmit HCV and HBV even after testing, especially during the eclipse period. Nucleic acid testing during this period carries a residual HCV risk of 3%; outside it, the risk falls to 0.32% [47, 48]. Even with normal liver function, HBV-seropositive donors should undergo liver biopsy. Evidence of fibrosis or inflammation warrants rejection, as it affects graft safety and donor regeneration. Donors with active infection (HBeAg or HBV DNA positive) have high transmission rates and are generally avoided [49].

Current guidelines recommend indefinite antiviral prophylaxis for recipients of HbsAg- or anti-HBc-positive grafts, with HBV DNA monitoring every 3 months in the first year and 3–6 months thereafter. Most centers now use nucleos(t)ide monotherapy, phasing out HBIG [50].

21.9.3 HCV Infection

HCV-positive donor organs can be transplanted into HCV-seropositive recipients, ideally with negative HCV RNA and no significant liver fibrosis (biopsy-confirmed). Acute HCV has an 8–11-week antibody window, but PCR detects RNA within one week (99% sensitivity/specificity) [51]. Curative direct-acting antivirals (DAAs) have transformed HCV management, achieving >95% cure rates and reducing HCV-related transplants. Historically poor post-transplant outcomes in HCV are now resolved. Emerging evidence supports using HCV NAT-positive livers in HCV-negative recipients, expanding the donor pool [52]. However, HCV recipients face higher risks of acute cellular rejection (ACR) and graft dysfunction, possibly linked to immunosuppression changes post-SVR. The median donor risk index (DRI) for HCV NAT-positive donors was 1.3 vs. 1.4 in NAT-negative donors [53].

21.9.4 HIV Infection

Since the mid-1990s, the introduction of HAART has significantly reduced HIV-related mortality, transforming it from a fatal disease to a manageable condition. While not curative, HAART enables HIV-positive patients with end-stage liver disease to be considered for transplantation. However, HIV-positive donor organs are used only for HIV-positive recipients, unlike HBV or HCV, where donor use is broader. The serological testing window period is 22 days, but NAT can detect infection 5.6–10.2 days post-exposure, reducing the window to 12 days [54]. Moreover, NAT testing may identify the false seropositive donors too [55].

21.9.5 HIV-HCV Co-infection

HCV infection in HIV-positive individuals shows lower rates of spontaneous HCV RNA clearance, increasing the risk of chronic infection. HIV/HCV co-infection leads to higher rates of acute rejection and faster fibrosis progression than HCV alone, often resulting in graft loss. Outcomes in co-infected patients remain poorer compared to mono-infected individuals, making co-infection a major concern post-LT. Transplanting an HIV-positive graft into an HCV recipient or vice versa yields suboptimal results due to recurrence [56]. Thus, aggressive HCV treatment is essential. In patients with compensated liver disease, pre-transplant HCV therapy may be feasible, while those with severe disease may need to defer DAA therapy until post-transplant. Regular post-transplant monitoring for HCV recurrence is crucial [57].

21.9.6 Septicemia

Deceased donors with positive blood cultures or bacteremia are not uncommon. Controlled sepsis is a relative contraindication, but donors treated appropriately with antibiotics for 48–72 h may still be considered. Donors with undiagnosed fever, encephalitis, or neurological compromise should be excluded [58]. Donors with undiagnosed febrile illness or encephalitis with neurological compromise should be rejected.

21.9.7 Other Donor-Derived Infections

EBV and SARS-CoV-2 Infections EBV is linked to post-transplant lymphoproliferative disorder (PTLD), particularly in seronegative recipients. There is no specific therapy, but high-risk patients are often monitored every 2–4 weeks during the first 6 months post-transplant [59]. SARS-CoV-2 initially disrupted transplant activity, but with evolving protocols and vaccination, even COVID-positive donors (excluding lung donors) are now considered safe [60].

Unexpected Donor-Derived Infections and Viral Hepatitis. Unexpected infections remain a concern. HIV, HBV, and HCV are routinely screened; re-screening is advised near donation time. Vaccination is guided by patient risk and geography [61]. Less commonly screened viruses include HEV, HAV, and HDV. HEV can lead to chronic hepatitis in immunocompromised patients. HAV is self-limiting, and HDV, usually with HBV, rarely transmits via donation [62].

Other Viral Infections: HTLV, Herpesviruses, Arboviruses, and Rabies. HTLV-1 can cause T-cell leukemia, though screening is not universal. HHV-8 is linked to Kaposi's sarcoma and poses a transplant risk. Arboviruses like dengue, Zika, and chikungunya are less documented in donor transmission, though dengue requires attention in endemic areas. Rabies, though rare, is fatal without prophylaxis and must be ruled out in donors with unexplained encephalitis [63, 64].

21.10 Donors with Malignancy

Due to the ongoing organ shortage, evaluating all potential donors, including those with a history of malignancy, is essential. Around 1.7% of deceased donor transplants involve such donors, with 85% having skin, CNS, or genitourinary cancers. The transmission risk is low—only 0.05% of recipients develop donor-derived cancer, especially with careful selection. These organs can still offer lifesaving benefits, as liver function is often preserved [65]. Organs from donors with low-grade CNS malignancies are generally accepted unless risk factors like ventriculoatrial shunting or high-grade tumors are present, which raise transmission rates to 46% [66].

No transmissions have been reported from donors with low-grade renal or prostate cancers. Small prostate cancers (Gleason 3 + 3) with benign follow-up are considered minimal risk; Gleason scores above 6 require more caution [67].

Basal and squamous cell skin cancers pose minimal risk. In select cases with clear staging and long remission, organs from donors with treated melanoma may be considered, though active or aggressive skin cancers (e.g., Kaposi, Merkel cell, melanoma) are unacceptable. High-risk malignancies like breast, colon, or hematologic cancers warrant extreme caution and are only considered in life-threatening cases with full informed consent. Active malignancies, except some CNS and skin cancers, are contraindications [68].

Recipients must be thoroughly counseled on all associated transmission risks and the need for ongoing surveillance.

21.11 Living Donor Safety

Right from initial counseling sessions and the donor workup to the advanced surgical techniques, donor safety is at the core of living donor liver transplantation. The double equipoise is a meaningful concept in evaluating the balance between donor risk and recipient benefit in LDLT, which should be performed only if the donor risk is justified by the acceptable outcome for the recipient [69]. In recent years, the estimates of donor mortality are less than 0.3–0.5% [70] which is comparable to living renal donors [71].

The Donor Risk Index (DRI), introduced by Feng et al. in 2006, is a key tool for predicting liver graft failure risk. It incorporates donor factors like age, cause of death, donation after cardiac death (DCD), and whether the graft is split or partial. It also includes transplant-related factors such as cold ischemia time and transport distance. A higher DRI suggests a higher failure risk, aiding decisions when multiple or high-risk donor options are available.

Feng's study identified seven key donor and graft traits that independently increase the risk of graft failure. Notably, donor age, DCD status, and split/partial grafts are most impactful. Graft failure risk rises with donor age beyond 40, and older donors are increasingly common. Split/partial and DCD grafts have over a 50% higher failure risk than ideal whole grafts. The DRI compares each graft to an ideal donor liver and helps guide decisions by weighing transplant risks against waiting for another organ [72].

21.12 Ethical Concerns and Questions of Potential Donors Need to Be Addressed

We take every precaution to safeguard the donor, ensuring minimal morbidity and mortality, and all potential outcomes are thoroughly discussed. Despite precautions, donor mortality—though rare at 0.15–0.30%—may still occur [73]. Post-donation, most donors report improved satisfaction, self-esteem, and willingness to donate again, with low rates of depression, alcohol abuse, and anxiety. Donors whose recipients died often experienced guilt, with 22% feeling responsible at some point—highlighting the need for ongoing psychosocial support [74, 75].

The questionnaire covers key aspects for potential organ donors—motivation, preparation, and concerns. It helps donors reflect on their reasons, ensuring the decision is voluntary. It also prompts consideration of physical and psychosocial impacts, recovery, lifestyle changes, and possible complications. Financial readiness is addressed, including effects on work and career. Finally, it stresses discussing the decision with family, preparing for unforeseen outcomes, and appointing a proxy decision-maker.

21.13 Living Donor Selection/Acceptability Criteria

These criteria are not strict rules but serve as guidelines for safe donor selection without jeopardizing recipient outcomes. The goal is thorough donor evaluation, emphasizing early exclusion of unfit candidates to allow others to proceed. The process begins with counseling, addressing ethical concerns, ensuring transparency, and keeping the donor informed throughout each stage.

- Age: 18–55 years
- Compatible ABO blood group
- No comorbidities or one well-controlled condition
- BMI <28 kg/m^2
- LAI >5
- GRWR >0.75
- Remnant liver volume >30% of TLV
- Surgically compatible anatomy

Any deviation from these criteria requires multidisciplinary discussion, considering both donor and recipient safety and the feasibility of the transplant.

21.14 Overview of Donor Assessment Protocol

After the initial interview (age: 18–55, blood group compatibility, BMI: 18–28, assessment of comorbidities, prior surgeries—especially upper abdominal—and psychological readiness for major surgery) and detailed physical examination, we proceed with a structured donor workup at the Dept. of Liver Transplantation and Regenerative Medicine at Medanta The Medicity Hospital, Gurugram. This evaluation is carried out in phases:

Phase I—General Screening and Imaging
Includes:

- Blood tests: Blood group, CBC, LFT, RFT, PT/INR/APTT, lipid and thyroid profile, viral markers (HCV, HBsAg, HBcAb, HIV I & II), CMV IgG/IgM, VDRL, RBS, urine routine/microscopy/culture, urine pregnancy test (females), dengue profile, HAV IgM, HEV IgM, and EBV IgM (for pediatric recipients).
- Imaging: Non-contrast CT for liver attenuation, MRI for fat quantification.

Phase II—Liver Volumetry and Anatomy

- Triphasic abdominal CT for liver volume and vascular anatomy.

Phase III—Surgical Fitness and Additional Screening

- Cardiac and respiratory evaluation: ECG, ECHO/TMT (based on age), CXR, PFT.
- Age/gender-based: Mammography (>35 years), carotid Doppler and CT calcium scoring (>50 years), TVS (married females), pelvic USG (unmarried females).
- Biliary anatomy: MRCP.

Phase IV—Multidisciplinary Clearance

- Consults from hepatology, gynecology (females), psychiatry, anesthesia, and cardiology.

  Additional tests are guided by personal or family history (e.g., autoimmune diseases, substance use).

  Donor risks, recovery expectations, and follow-up plans are explained by specialists throughout the process. Informed consent and approval from the legal authorization committee are mandatory.

21.15 Factors Influencing Donor Selection

21.15.1 Age

There has been a notable shift in the age distribution of liver donors, with more elderly donors now being accepted for LDLT due to organ shortages. Various studies have produced mixed results regarding the impact of donor age on liver transplant outcomes. Donor age (Fig. 21.19) is a component of several risk scores, including the Donor Risk Index (DRI), D-MELD, BAR score, and SOFT [76]. Although overall liver function appears to remain stable with age, liver regeneration declines due to reduced cell cycle activity, increased autophagy and apoptosis, smaller liver size, and decreased blood flow. At the cellular level, aging leads to mitochondrial loss (with increased volume), greater hepatocyte polyploidy, and diminished smooth endoplasmic reticulum [77]. In LDLT, donors aged 18 to 55—particularly those without comorbidities—are considered optimal due to better liver quality and regenerative capacity. Chronological age is less critical than physiological status. While there have been cases of successful donations from septuagenarians, most clinicians discourage this due to safety concerns. Ghinolfi et al. analyzed 16 donors over 90 years old, finding no significant difference in 1-year outcomes in matched recipients aged 18–65, provided the grafts had normal liver enzymes and no histological abnormalities [78].

Donor age has been linked to specific complications such as biliary issues and aggressive HCV recurrence. Biliary complications were more common in recipients

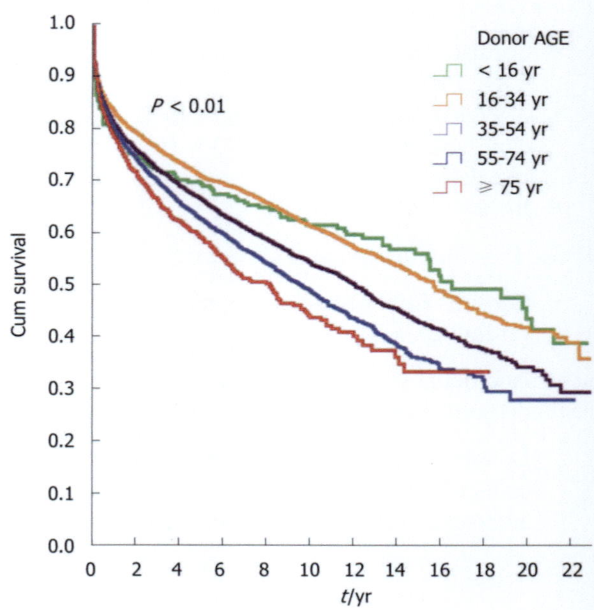

Fig. 21.19 Graft survival depending on donor age. (Source: Spanish Liver Transplant Registry)

of livers from donors >75 years compared to those aged 20–49 (29.6% vs. 13%), though survival was unaffected. In pediatric cases, donors >48 years and recipients with MELD >30 showed a 1.09-fold increase in intrahepatic biliary strictures. Logistic regression identified donor age >60 as an independent predictor of non-ischemic intrahepatic strictures (NAS) (OR = 15.4; 95% CI: 1.42–168.1; $P = 0.024$), likely due to ischemia-reperfusion injury, similar to that in DCD donors. The biliary tract is particularly sensitive to such injury due to lower glutathione expression in hepatocytes [79].

Donor age also adversely affects HCV recurrence. The risk of graft loss increases with donor age brackets of 21–50, 51–60, and >60 years, with age being the strongest predictor in HCV patients. Five-year survival is lower with donors >80 in HCV-positive patients, and donor age influences both fibrosis progression and antiviral treatment outcomes [80].

21.15.2 Blood Group Compatibility

A liver donor should have the same or a compatible blood group. Blood typing and crossmatching are early steps in donor selection, usually addressed during counseling and history. Due to organ shortages, ABO-incompatible (ABOi) liver transplantation has emerged with outcomes comparable to compatible transplants. When no compatible donors are available, paired or swap liver transplants help avoid ABOi LT and expand the donor pool effectively [81].

Who can be the liver donor?

In India, living donor organ donation is generally permitted if a proven relationship exists. Unrelated or altruistic (Good Samaritan) donations are rare and require stringent legal approval.

The Transplantation of Human Organs Act marked a milestone in Indian medicine, modeled after the UK Transplant Act. Its key objectives were:

- Recognizing brain death as legal death.
- Banning the commercial organ trade.
- Defining "near relatives" (parents, siblings, children, spouse) who can donate without special approval.

The law prohibits any monetary exchange between donor and recipient. An unrelated donor must affirm in court that the donation is voluntary and undergo thorough testing. The Authorization Committee verifies compliance. If financial transactions are discovered, both donor and recipient face legal consequences. Organ sales are banned, including to foreigners, and violations attract severe penalties under Indian law [82].

21.15.3 Evaluation of Liver Parenchyma: [Steatosis, Liver Attenuation Index (LAI)]

Hepatic steatosis is the most frequent finding during donor evaluation and the leading cause for donor rejection [83]. Obesity clustering in families, especially when the recipient has MASLD, necessitates careful donor assessment. Steatosis severity significantly affects graft regeneration—<5% fat content offers better outcomes than 5–20%, while severe steatosis increases the risk of ischemia-reperfusion injury, dysfunction, and early mortality [84]. Adults can generally accept <20% macrosteatosis; however, subtracting the fat percentage from GRWR is prudent, especially with marginal donors. In pediatrics, grafts with <30% fat are acceptable if GRWR is >2. Ultrasound often detects steatosis incidentally. CT-based methods like liver-to-spleen attenuation ratio or LAI (difference in Hounsfield Units) are commonly used. Normal liver attenuation is 50–75 HU, and the spleen is 40–60 HU. Another effective modality for fat estimation is spectrophotometry or dual echo Dixon on magnetic resonance spectroscopy (MRS), with a sensitivity of detecting <5% fat of 84% and a specificity of 90%. This can help reduce unnecessary liver biopsies [85]. Magnetic Resonance Proton Density Fat Fraction (MR-PDFF) is increasingly recognized as a standard technique for assessing liver steatosis in living liver donors. MR-PDFF offers accurate, reproducible measurements unaffected by fibrosis, with greater precision than USG or CT, helping avoid unnecessary biopsies. Still, liver biopsy remains the reference standard despite its risks and sampling bias [86].

21.15.4 Liver Attenuation Index (LAI)

Acceptable range: >5
Need for biopsy/weight reduction and/or MR fat estimation: 0–5
Donor to be rejected/need donor's weight reduction: <0 [87]

Limitations of LAI:

Low LAI usually suggests steatosis, but may also indicate:

- Diffuse malignancy
- Non-malignant infiltrative disease (e.g., amyloidosis)

High LAI can result from:

1. Iron overload—Investigate if liver HU >75 (e.g., hemochromatosis, hemosiderosis)
2. Copper deposition—Wilson's disease
3. Glycogen storage disorders
4. Drugs—Amiodarone, gold therapy, historical Thorotrast use (Thorotrast is a suspension that contains thorium dioxide particles, a radioactive material. Historical importance: the substance was used as a radiological contrast in X-ray imaging from the 1930s until the 1950s.)

21.15.5 Adequacy of Liver Volume (Graft-to-Recipient Weight Ratio—GRWR)

In the context of the donor evaluation process, ensuring a graft of optimal volume is always a priority, as it significantly impacts the recipient's outcome. As liver cirrhosis progresses from the compensated to the decompensated stage and/or the waiting time for liver transplantation increases, the metabolic demands of the prospective recipient escalate exponentially. Therefore, ensuring the adequacy of liver volume to support this increased metabolic demand becomes even more critical.

The graft-to-recipient weight ratio (GRWR) is calculated by dividing the graft weight in grams by the recipient's weight in kilograms. This is especially relevant when a partial liver is planned for implantation—commonly seen in living donor transplants, where either the left lateral, left, or right lobe of the liver is harvested. It is also considered in deceased donor liver transplantation when graft splitting is planned.

Standard liver volume (SLV) is determined from large population-based studies and is widely used in many countries. However, such studies are yet to be conducted in India to establish a nationally representative SLV value.

General Schema of Liver Volume:

- Right lobe (segments 5–8), with or without the middle hepatic vein (MHV): 50–70% of total liver volume
- Left lobe (segments 2–4), with or without the caudate lobe: 20–50% of total liver volume
- Left lateral sector (segments 2 and 3): 10–25% of total liver volume

Manual CT volumetry (pencil trace/paintbrush method) is considered the gold standard for preoperative volume assessment (Figs. 21.20 and 21.21). However, various semi-automated (e.g., AW VolumeShare 6 from GE Healthcare, Chicago, Illinois, USA) to fully automated software solutions have been developed, offering similar accuracy. This shift is driven by the time-consuming nature and inter-operator variability associated with manual volumetry.

A contrast-enhanced CT scan of the entire abdomen is performed, and the portal venous phase axial images—where contrast enhancement is maximal—are used for optimal volume assessment. Non-parenchymal anatomical structures such as major vessels (e.g., portal vein, inferior vena cava), large fissures, ligamentum teres, and the gallbladder are excluded from volumetric calculations, as they do not contribute to the liver's metabolic function.

The modified right lobe (without MHV) is most commonly used for adult-to-adult LDLT. In smaller or less sick adults, left lobe grafts (usually with MHV) can be used. Left lateral sector (LLS) grafts are typical for small children and may include the caudate lobe to enhance GRWR. Right posterior sector grafts are rarely used due to higher biliary complication rates [88] (Fig. 21.22).

The middle hepatic vein (MHV) separates the right and left lobes. Caudate lobe volume is measured separately. Graft volumes are often categorized as RL/LL with

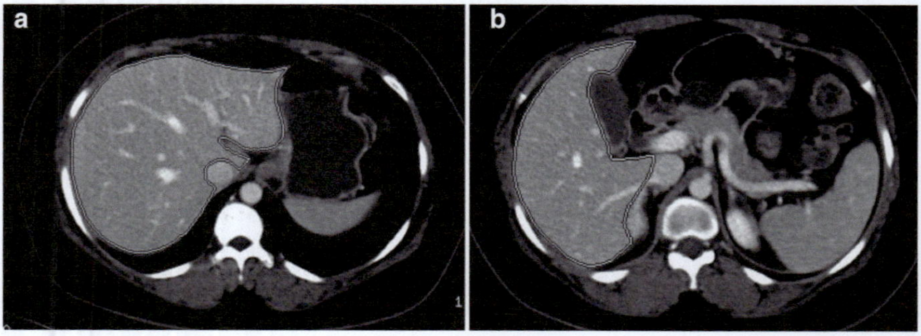

Fig. 21.20 (**a**, **b**) Pencil trace or paintbrush method of volumetry (the liver's outline is traced for every section of imaging; note the exclusion of gall bladder and major vessels)

Fig. 21.21 The software joins the axial sections of liver traced by pencil method/ semi-automated/ automated methods to give total liver volume, and a 3D image is regenerated for further volumetry evaluation

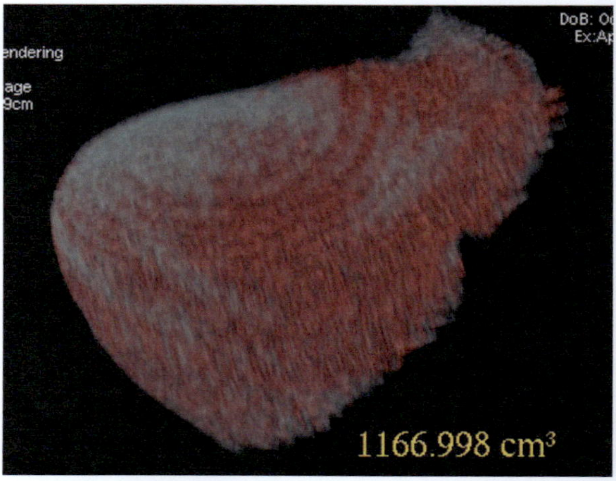

or without MHV. For LLS volume, the transection line extends from the LHV ostium to just right of the falciform ligament. [89]

Traditionally, ideal GRWR has been 1% (e.g., 600 g graft for 60 kg recipient). GRWR ≥0.8 is widely considered the threshold; many centers accept down to 0.75, and some debate that even 0.6 could be the lower safety limit regardless of graft type [90]. Some centers have a tailored approach and consider arterial/portal vein flows and the liver-to-spleen size ratio (as an assessment of the severity of portal hypertension) to decide on adequate graft size. Smaller grafts, mostly of GRWR <0.75, may not meet metabolic needs and increase the risk of early graft dysfunction (EGD) and small-for-size syndrome (SFSS). In such cases, it is safer for less sick recipients and must be thoroughly discussed during informed consent. Small grafts are exposed to high portal flow, leading to portal hyperperfusion and compromised regeneration.

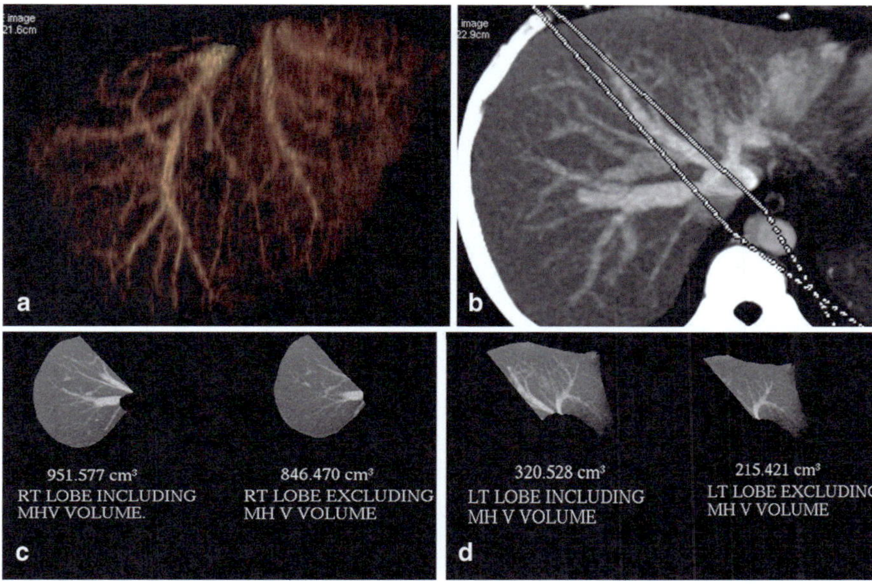

Fig. 21.22 (**a**–**d**) For a conventional right/left lobe requirement. The plane of transection is at MHV, and volumes are calculated including/excluding MHV. Similarly, taking the proposed transection line at RHV or LHV and portal venous branches, various other sectoral or segmental volumes can be calculated as per the requirement. (**a**) Delineating the venous system to assess the completion of the image for 3D rendering. (**b**) Marking the proposed plane of transection (Including/excluding MHV) for volume assessment

The severity of reperfusion injury is inversely related to graft size. Portal inflow modulation and ensuring good outflow can allow safe use of smaller grafts. Careful recipient selection (e.g., low MELD, shorter decompensation duration) makes low GRWR cases more acceptable (the protocol—Fig. 21.23) [91].

When the left lobe provides an adequate graft-to-recipient weight ratio (GRWR >0.75), the patient has a low MELD score, and a left graft is often preferred due to its safety and the absence of remnant liver issues. Additionally, assessing graft volume can be done using graft weight to expected standard liver volume (GW/ESLV). Both GRWR and GW/ESLV should be considered together, as a GW/ESLV of less than 40% indicates a small-for-size graft (SFSG). In cases where a small graft is a concern, especially for overweight or obese patients, dual-lobe liver transplantation may be required to achieve an adequate GRWR [92].

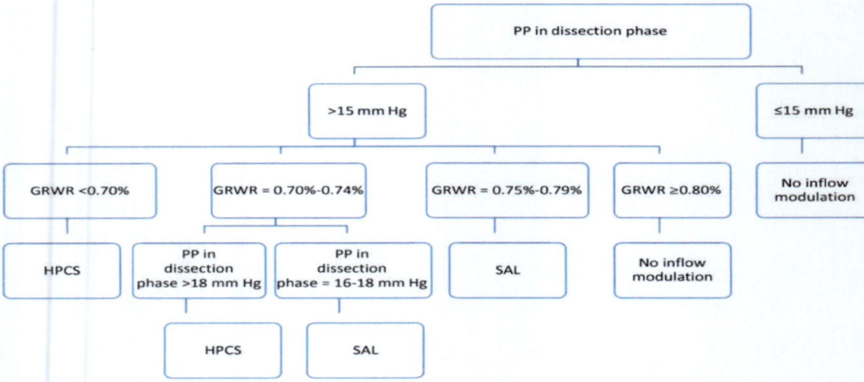

Fig. 21.23 Portal flow modulation protocol

21.16 Donors with Metabolic Syndrome (MS) and Other Comorbidities or Illnesses

At the outset, individuals may present with one or more components of metabolic syndrome (obesity, hypertension, high triglycerides, low HDL, and insulin resistance), warranting thorough evaluation. Although obesity isn't an absolute contraindication for liver donation, high BMI is a concern due to its association with hepatic steatosis. Generally, the acceptable BMI for donors is 18–28 kg/m^2. While some centers accept up to 33, those with a BMI >30 or a BMI >28 with two or more MS components (e.g., large waist circumference, high TG, low HDL, elevated BP, or fasting glucose) require a liver biopsy. Donors can be accepted if macrosteatosis is <20% with no inflammation or fibrosis [87]. Higher BMI also increases risks like sepsis, poor graft regeneration, wound infections, incisional hernia, delayed mobility (raising DVT risk), and pulmonary issues like atelectasis, all of which may prolong hospital stay. Donors with one well-controlled comorbidity (e.g., diabetes, hypertension, asthma, or thyroid disorders) may proceed, while those with two or more require specialist clearance. A history of stroke (CVA) or significant coronary artery disease (CAD) is a contraindication.

Metabolic syndrome components are interlinked; the presence of one increases the risk of others. Liver manifestations range from asymptomatic NAFLD to NASH, fibrosis, or cirrhosis. Reversing metabolic factors is crucial in donor selection. A FibroScan can help avoid a biopsy in some cases. Early NAFLD/NASH may be reversed through lifestyle changes—exercise, reduced carbs/oil, and higher protein intake—to reduce weight and improve muscle mass [93].

Histological types of liver steatosis:

- Microvesicular (1–2 μm, nucleus not displaced): Drug-induced (e.g., steroids, tetracyclines, valproate), Reye's syndrome (aspirin), NSAIDs (nonsteroidal anti-inflammatory drugs), NRTIs (nucleoside reverse transcriptase inhibi-

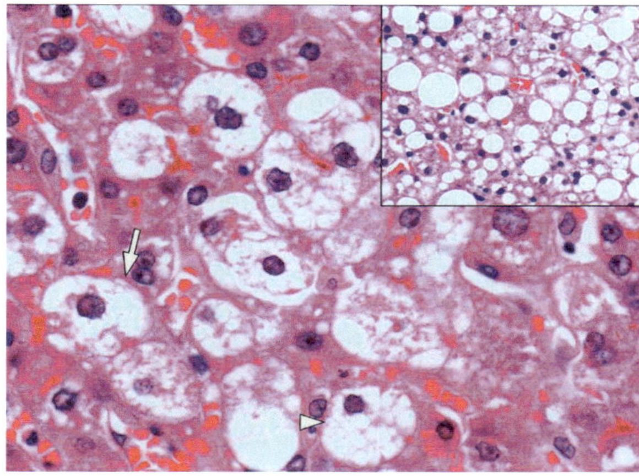

Fig. 21.24 Histopathology of microvesicular steatosis, with foamy hepatocytes (two, annotated by arrows), as opposed to macrovesicular steatosis (insert) [94]

tors), HELLP syndrome, acute fatty liver of pregnancy, LCAT (familial lecithin-cholesterol acyltransferase deficiency), and hepatitis C, etc.

- Macrovesicular (>20 μm, nucleus displaced): Most common; linked to alcohol, obesity, insulin resistance, Hepatitis C (esp. genotype 3), Wilson's disease, lipodystrophy, starvation, and TPN. Also caused by drugs like amiodarone, methotrexate, and steroids (Fig. 21.24).

Grades of steatosis (based on fat content in hepatocytes):

- Grade 0: <5% (healthy)
- Grade 1: 5–33% (mild)
- Grade 2: 34–66% (moderate)
- Grade 3: >66% (severe)

Steatotic grafts pose risks such as ischemia-reperfusion injury, graft dysfunction, and, in severe cases, primary nonfunction. Macrovesicular steatosis is more strongly linked to inflammation and hepatocyte necroapoptosis than microvesicular steatosis. Mild steatosis typically doesn't affect graft regeneration. Grafts with >20% steatosis are usually rejected in LDLT and >30% in DDLT, though normothermic perfusion is increasingly enabling the use of such marginal grafts [95].

21.17 Lowest Acceptable Future Liver Remnant (FLR)

Most of the centers around the world agree on putting a line at 30% as being the minimum safe limit of liver remnant. But in the case of steatotic grafts, the fraction of steatosis must be deduced from the graft volume to have the actual quantification of functioning parenchyma of the remnant.

21.18 Acceptable Level of Transaminases

In healthy adults, the AST to ALT ratio tends to be around 1.15. When it comes to deceased liver donors, transaminase levels that are up to two to three times above the normal upper limit are generally considered acceptable—as long as there's no evidence of systemic sepsis. Curiously, some transplant centers have gone further, using livers with even higher enzyme levels. For example, in a study led by Nasir Farkar, 24 out of 858 patients (about 3%) received grafts from donors whose AST or ALT levels exceeded 500 IU/L. The exact reasons for the elevated enzymes weren't available, but given the pressing need for organs and the critical state of some recipients, the surgical team made the call to proceed [96]. Interestingly, the one-year survival and complication rates in these cases were on par with those of patients who received grafts with normal enzyme levels. So, while high donor enzyme levels often reduce how many livers are actually used, they don't necessarily translate into worse outcomes—especially if the cause is understood and the hemodynamic impact is factored in [97].

The scenario moves a bit when we're talking about living donors. Elevated liver enzymes here are more concerning, as they can affect how well the liver regenerates—something that's vital for both donor safety and recipient recovery. Globally, most centers are comfortable moving forward if AST and ALT levels are below 50 IU/L, assuming the graft-to-recipient weight ratio (GRWR) and the donor's future liver remnant (FLR) are within safe limits—typically over 30%. But when enzyme levels go beyond 50 IU/L, it's important to investigate further. A more thorough evaluation, and sometimes even a liver biopsy, may be needed to rule out any underlying inflammation or liver damage [98].

21.19 When Is a Liver Biopsy Needed?

If imaging doesn't clearly show the quality of the liver—especially when only a marginal remnant is left—a biopsy can help guide donor selection. There are some red flags that raise concern: borderline LAI (+1 to +5), older donors (over 50), high BMI (above 28), small grafts (GRWR <0.75), small remnant liver (<30%), elevated transaminases, metabolic syndrome, or unclear findings on imaging. Most centers would consider a biopsy in these situations [99, 100].

If the biopsy reveals significant fat (>20%), inflammation, or fibrosis, the donor is usually ruled out. These livers don't regenerate well and can lead to serious complications like graft failure, biliary problems, or poor function after transplant—risking both donor and recipient outcomes. Having said that, newer studies suggest that even grafts with moderate fat (30–60%) can work well in low-risk recipients, especially in first transplants with MELD scores <35 [101].

In emergency cases like acute liver failure—especially in children—marginal grafts may still be used. If the left or left lateral lobe gives a safe remnant (60–70%) and no other donor is available, the surgeon may choose to accept the risks to try to save a life.

21.20 Procoagulant Workup

Major liver surgery naturally shifts the body toward a pro-clotting state. That's why it's especially important to screen for hidden clotting risks, particularly when the recipient has Budd-Chiari Syndrome or a known procoagulant condition.

Some people are more prone to clots, especially if they have a history of venous thromboembolism (VTE) or a strong family history. Red flags include clots at a young age (under 50), multiple affected relatives, or clots in unusual spots like the brain or splanchnic veins—these suggest an inherited tendency [102].

Other common risk factors include:

- Obesity (BMI over 28)
- Age over 50
- Women on oral contraceptives (these are usually paused 6–8 weeks before and after surgery)
- Smoking (needs to stop 4–6 weeks before surgery)

Although there are no fixed guidelines for clotting risk assessment in donors, it's pertinent to pay close attention to personal and family history, which is essential. Standard clot prevention is used in all major abdominal surgeries, including liver donation. This typically includes blood thinners like LMWH, compression stockings, pneumatic devices, and encouraging early mobilization post-surgery. Some centers also give a pre-op dose of heparin, though it's not routinely used during the operation itself [103].

21.21 Anatomical Considerations

An ideal liver graft has a single hepatic artery, hepatic duct, portal, and hepatic vein. This is true for approximately 40–50% of grafts, and the rest have some variations [104]. The real question isn't whether the anatomy is perfect—it's whether it's manageable. A donor's liver is considered suitable when the surgical risks linked to variations—like leaks, strictures, or thrombosis—are judged to be low. The focus is always on preserving inflow (via the artery and portal vein) and outflow (through hepatic veins and bile ducts), ensuring the graft functions well and gives the recipient the best chance at recovery.

The recipient's weight and underlying disease influence graft choice. That might mean accepting grafts with multiple arteries, veins, or bile ducts. While these can be reconstructed, smaller vessel or duct sizes and more anastomoses increase the risk of complications.

Ultimately, what's acceptable often comes down to the surgical team's experience, how urgently the transplant is needed, and whether other donor options exist. If a complex anatomy is likely to increase risk, the team should be prepared, and patients and families must be clearly informed as part of the consent process.

21.22 Arterial Inflow

Michel's classification of hepatic arteries (Fig. 21.25).

Type 1: Hepatic trunk arising from CHA
Type 2: Replaced LHA arising from LGA
Type 3: Replaced RHA arising from SMA
Type 4: Replaced LHA and replaced RHA
Type 5: Accessory LHA arising from LGA
Type 6: Accessory RHA arising from SMA
Type 7: Accessory LHA and RHA
Type 8: Replaced RHA and accessory LHA
Type 9: Replaced LHA and accessory RHA
Type 10: Entire hepatic trunk arising from the SMA

Hepatic arterial anatomy is crucial in donor selection in living donor liver transplantation. The presence of multiple arteries/variations in the segment IV artery can complicate both the donor and recipient surgeries. For donors, it increases the technical challenges of hepatectomy, whereas in recipients, these variations necessitate complex vascular reconstructions, which can extend surgery time and elevate the risk of complications such as thrombosis or ischemia times. Any compromise in arterial supply can affect graft function and increase the chance of biliary issues. That's why, when possible, donors with simpler arterial anatomy are preferred.

Experienced centers may accept grafts with up to three arteries, but always with extra caution. The risk of hepatic artery thrombosis is higher when arterial anatomy is atypical—especially if the arteries are narrow. In cases where recipient arterial options are limited, surgeons may perform an arterioplasty during bench surgery to

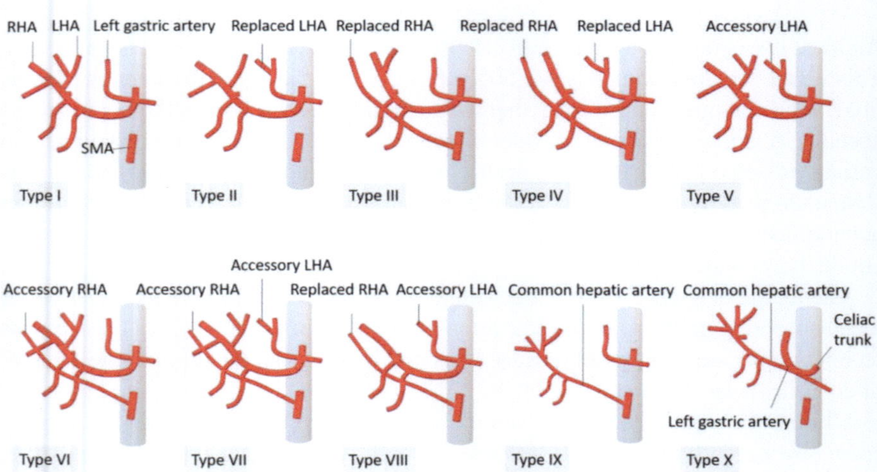

Fig. 21.25 Diagrammatic presentation of the hepatic arterial variations [105]

merge multiple arteries into one for easier implantation. The preferred technique is an end-to-end anastomosis to the recipient's hepatic arteries, depending on vessel size and orientation [106]. Sometimes, if there's a good pulsatile backbleed after anastomosing the main artery, surgeons may choose not to reconstruct small accessory arteries separately [107].

21.23 Portal Venous Inflow (Fig. 21.26)

The main portal vein (MPV) divides into the right (RPV) and the left portal vein (LPV). RPV further divides into the right anterior (RAPV) and right posterior portal veins (RPPV). Approximately 70–80% of patients will have this anatomy; the rest have variations [108]. The most common is a trifurcation, where the MPV splits into RAPV, RPPV, and LPV (Nakamura type B). The next frequent variation is Nakamura type C, where the MPV first divides into the RPPV and a common trunk, which later branches into the RAPV and LPV. In both types, the right lobe ends up with two portal veins. With type B (Fig. 21.27), the veins are close enough to join with a portovenoplasty—sometimes needing a cylindrical graft if the edges aren't wide enough. In type C, however, RAPV and RPPV are farther apart, making direct joining risky. Here, a Y-graft extension is usually needed, as forcing a portovenoplasty can kink the vein and increase the risk of stenosis or thrombosis after surgery [109]. Though portovenoplasty is still possible in type C (Fig. 21.28), it demands careful lumen alignment assessment, and often an interposition or native/cryopreserved portal vein "Y" graft is the safer bet.

When choosing a graft, the autologous portal vein from the recipient offers the best long-term results, followed by cryopreserved veins (portal or iliac) and then synthetic options like Dacron or PTFE [110].

The type D and E variants are not considered suitable for right lobe donation.

Occasionally, the imaging reveals PV crossovers, making a particular volume non-viable, and it should be considered with caution. For example, if a right lobe is planned for donation and a PV crossover runs from right to left, it might make part of the liver left behind non-viable. This can reduce the remnant liver volume, which is especially risky when it's already marginal (30%). Crossovers can also reduce the functional liver parenchyma, affecting GRWR. Each case needs careful, individual assessment.

Classifications		Anatomical variants
Nakamura et al. Type A Normal classical	Cheng et al. Type I	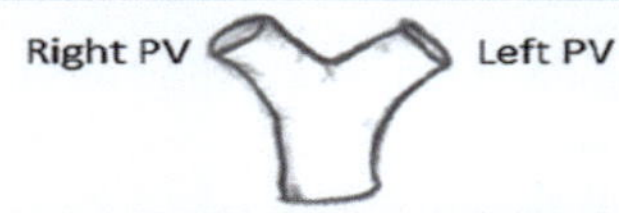
Nakamura et al. Type B Trifurcation	Cheng et al. Type II	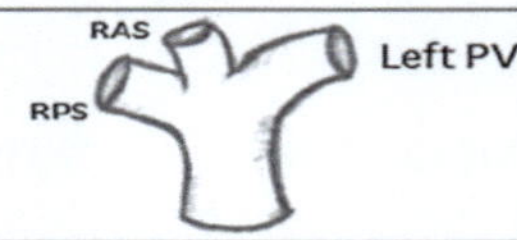
Nakamura et al. Type C	Cheng et al. Type III	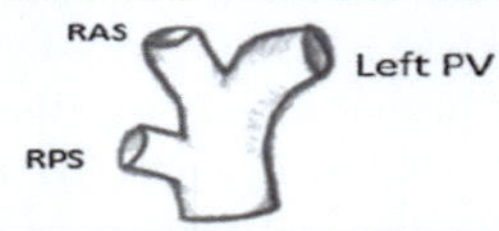
Nakamura et al. Type D	Cheng et al. Type IV	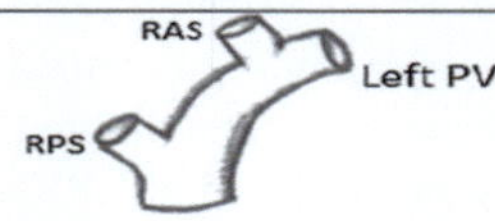
Nakamura et al. Type E	Cheng et al. Type IV (others)	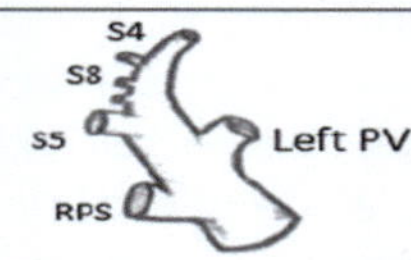

Fig. 21.26 PV anatomical classifications

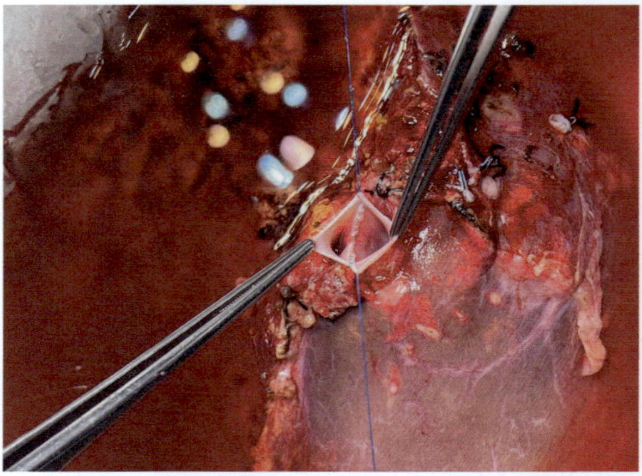

Fig. 21.27 Type B portal vein—after portovenoplasty

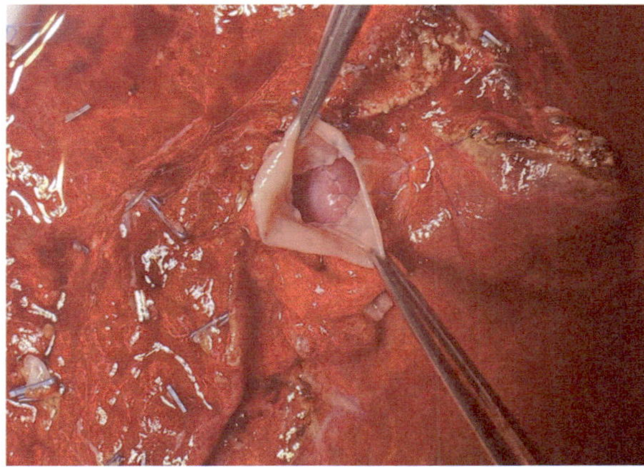

Fig. 21.28 Post PV extension in a Type C PV anatomy (using cryopreserved PV graft)

21.24 Hepatic Venous Outflow

Careful study of hepatic venous outflow (Figs. 21.29, 21.30, and 21.31) of living donors is crucial to minimize venous congestion in both the allograft and the remnant liver. Poor venous drainage may result in reduced functional parenchyma, leading to graft dysfunction and septic complications like infarcts and abscess formation.

The left hepatic vein mainly drains the left lateral segments, while the middle hepatic vein handles Segments IVa, IVb, and the right anterior sector (Segments V and VIII). The right hepatic vein mostly drains the right posterior sector (Segments VI and VII) and also shares some drainage of the right anterior sector. Like much of the liver anatomy, and especially the venous system, the variations are common. The right anterior sector often has dual drainage, with a preference toward the middle hepatic vein. In some cases, a graft with a dominant right hepatic vein may not even need reconstruction of the anterior sector drainage.

The right and left lobes are separated by Cantlie's line, which runs from the IVC to the middle of the gallbladder fossa, following the plane of the middle hepatic vein (MHV). Traditionally, the MHV stays with the left lobe during transection because it's critical for segment 4 regeneration [114]. If a standard right lobe graft is used without reconstructing the anterior sector drainage, it can lead to congestion in the right anterior sector—about 37% of liver volume—effectively reducing the functional graft size and lowering the GRWR.

To address this, we now often use a modified right lobe graft, where the veins from Segments V and VIII are reconstructed with a neo-MHV, using cryopreserved veins (like PV, iliac vein, or IVC) or synthetic grafts (Dacron/PTFE). Venous reconstruction is typically done if the branch is >5 mm, or sometimes >3 mm if multiple veins are involved or if GRWR is marginal [115].

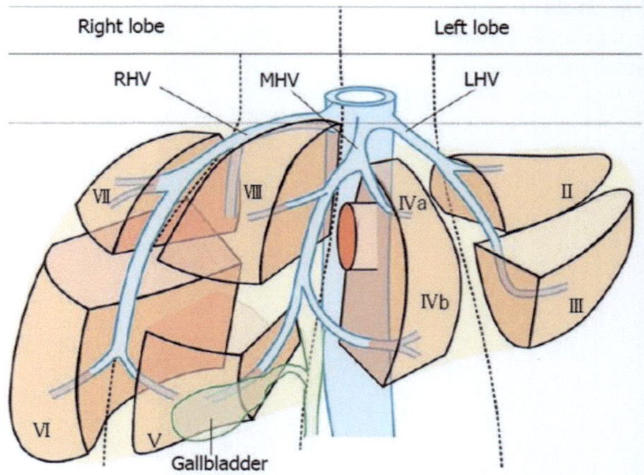

Fig. 21.29 The general schema of venous drainage of the liver: [111]

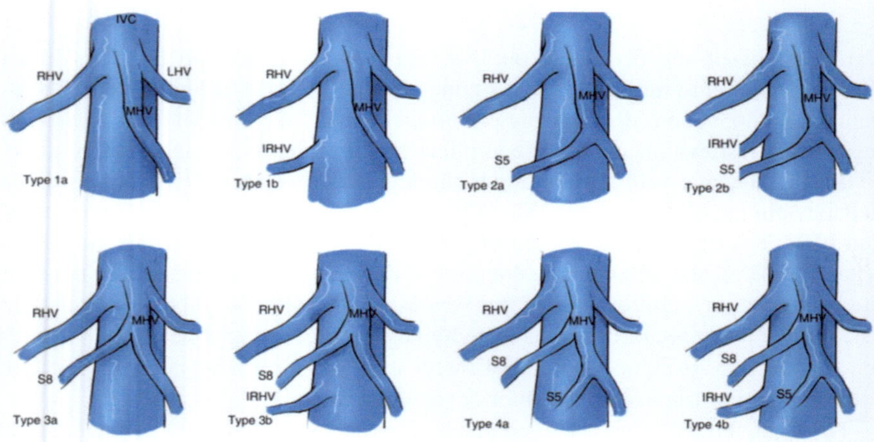

Fig. 21.30 Varotti proposed the variations and incidence of right liver hepatic venous anatomy: [112] • Type 1: Both segment 5 (S5) and segment 8 (S8) veins are missing. If the inferior right hepatic vein (IRHV) is absent, it's called Type 1a (14% of cases); if the IRHV is present, it's Type 1b (8%) • Type 2: S5 vein is present, S8 is absent. Without IRHV, it's Type 2a (20%); with IRHV, Type 2b (9%) • Type 3: S8 vein is present, S5 is missing. Absence of IRHV defines Type 3a (17%), while its presence marks Type 3b (19%) • Type 4: Both S5 and S8 veins are present. If IRHV is absent, it's Type 4a (11%); if present, Type 4b (3%)Abbreviations: IRHV Inferior Right Hepatic Vein, IVC Inferior Vena Cava, LHV Left Hepatic Vein, MHV Middle Hepatic Vein, RHV Right Hepatic Vein

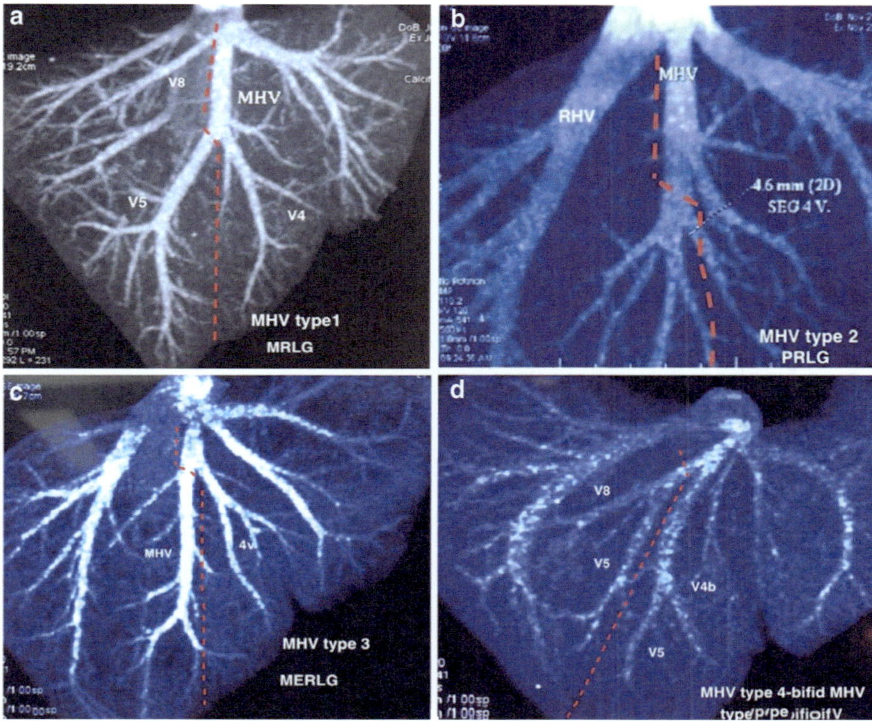

Fig. 21.31 (**a**) Neumann type 1 MHV; (**b**) Neumann type 2 MHV; (**c**) Neumann type 3 MHV; (**d**) Neumann type 4 MHV [113]

Inferior right hepatic veins (IRHV), which mainly drain segments VI and/or VII, are also common findings on donor imaging (Fig. 21.32). Significant IRHVs (>5 mm) may require direct drainage to the IVC, and multiple veins might need a composite "boat graft" reconstruction (Fig. 21.33). Whether to reconstruct them depends on how much liver they drain and the overall GRWR. While multiple inferior veins usually don't affect donor selection in experienced centers, they do increase backbench surgery time. In emergency cases like acute liver failure, longer benching can delay implantation and impact outcomes.

When the remnant liver is adequate (>30%) but the GRWR is low (<0.8), the presence of a prominent accessory left vein draining the medial sector is favorable. After careful anatomical evaluation, the entire MHV can be taken with the right lobe if the left medial sector drainage is assured by the accessory vein. Alternatively, partial MHV harvest (dividing the 4b vein and preserving S4a drainage) or subtotal MHV (here too, the S4b vein is divided, but the MHV is divided proximal to S8v, keeping the drainage of Seg4a intact—this can be done when S4a is draining into MHV distal to S8v) can be taken with the graft. A general plan for taking MRLG (without MHV, partial MHV, and subtotal MHV is presented in Figs. 21.34, 21.35, and 21.36, respectively. The red line depicts the proposed line transection. This attempts to safeguard GRWR while conserving the drainage of the right anterior sector.

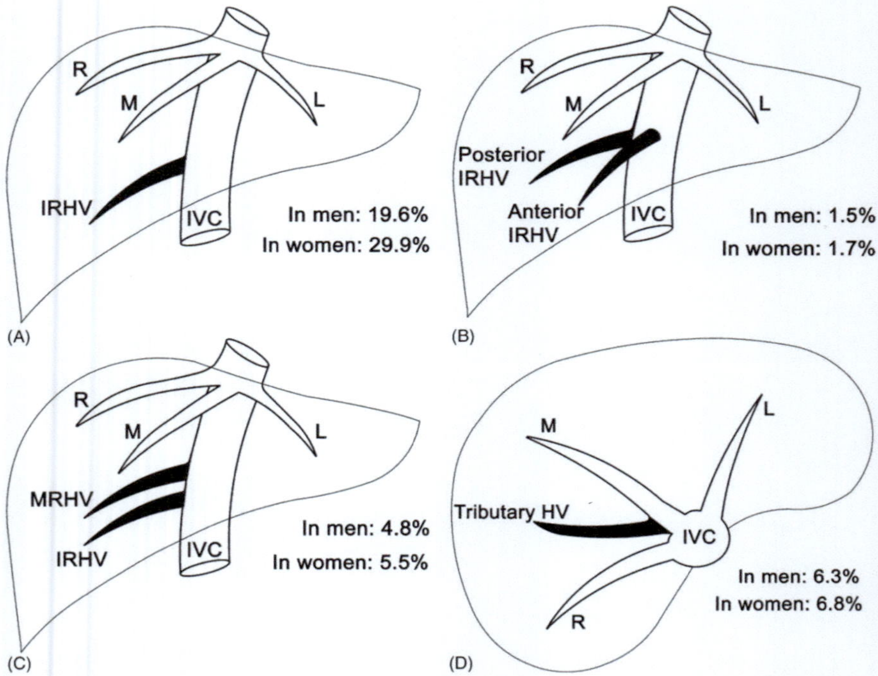

Fig. 21.32 Diagrams of hepatic veins in the coronal (**a–c**) and axial (**d**) plane show normal hepatic vein (HV) anatomy, which comprises three main HVs: the right (R), middle (M), and left (L) hepatic vein. Drawings also depict types and frequency of the inferior right hepatic vein (IRHV), and early tributary hepatic vein in women and men: (**a**) single (type 1) IRHV; (**b**) double IRHVs at the same level (type 2); (**c**) double IRHVs at a different level (type 3); (**d**) tributary HV that drains into the middle HV [116]

Fig. 21.33 Multiple IRHVs reconstruction with boat graft

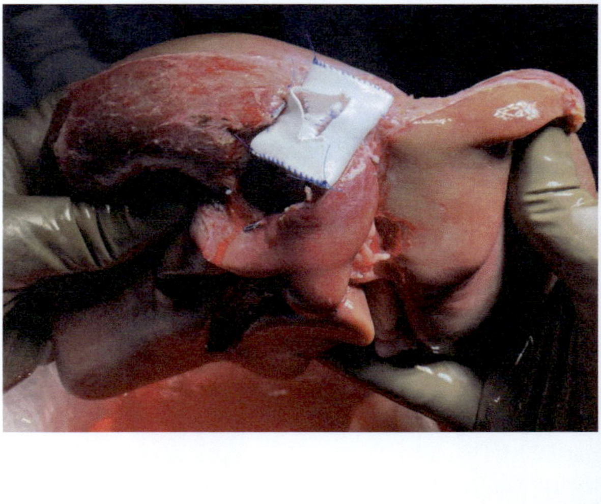

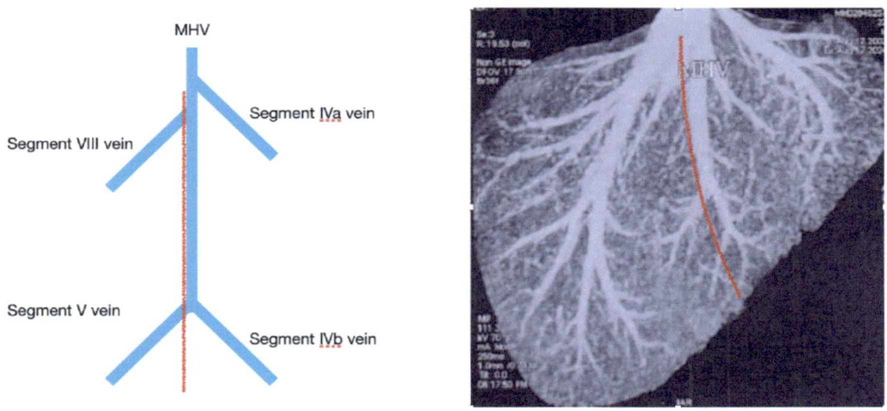

Fig. 21.34 Schema of harvesting RL without MHV

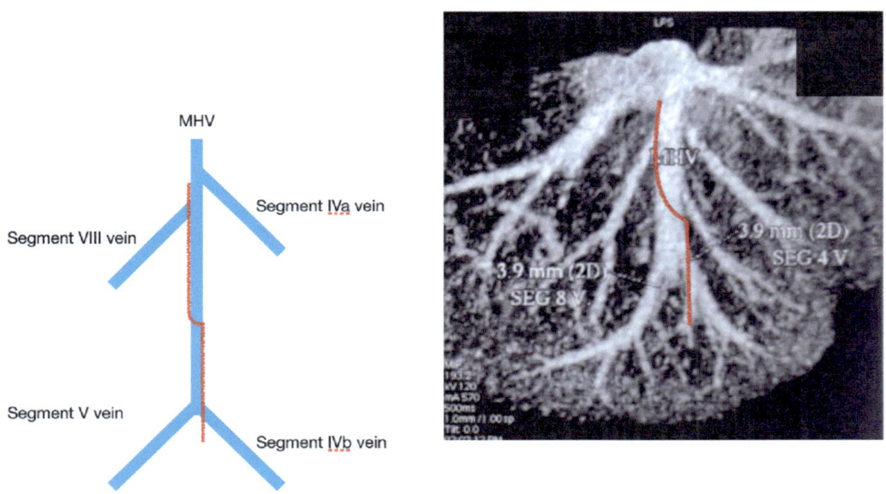

Fig. 21.35 Schema of harvesting RL with partial MHV

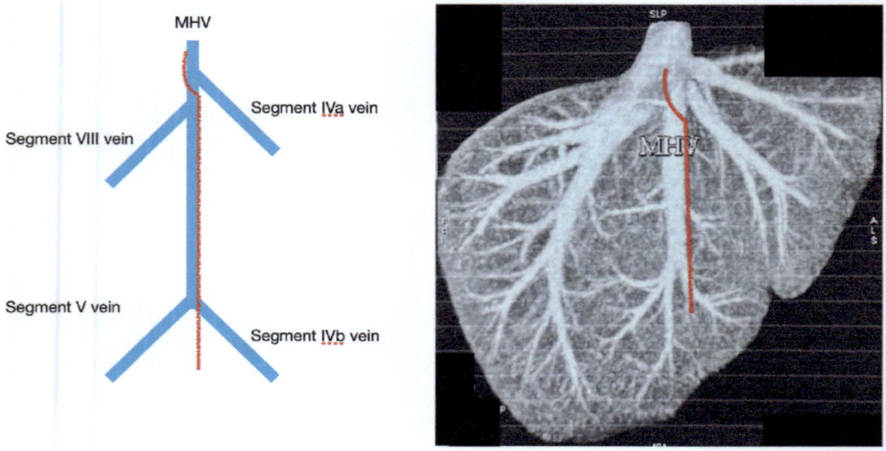

Fig. 21.36 Schema of harvesting RL with subtotal MHV

21.25 Biliary Anatomy

Biliary reconstruction remains the Achilles' heel of liver transplantation, owing to its technical complexity and the serious complications it can cause, from silent bilomas to cholangiolar abscesses and life-threatening sepsis. DDLT has two to three times fewer biliary complications than LDLT, provided the graft quality is sound and other logistics like cold and warm ischemia times are well managed. Also, the fact that an unsplit deceased liver will have a large single bile duct to reconstruct contributes to having fewer biliary complications than LDLT. Split-liver transplant (SLT) is associated with higher biliary and vascular complications as compared to whole liver transplant but didn't show any significant difference in patient and graft survival [118]. SLT and LDLT are similar for biliary complications [119], though LDLT is superior as compared to SLT in terms of allograft and patient survival [120].

In LDLT, most centers assess donor biliary anatomy (Fig. 21.37) with MRCP, as it can influence recipient outcomes. In case of multiple ducts (>2), a choice can be given to identify another donor if feasible. Variations in portal anatomy often coincide with biliary anomalies, seen in 58.3–89.1% of cases [121]. As far as the prevalence of anatomical variations according to Choi classification [122] is concerned, Type 1 is most common (62.7%), followed by Type 3a (16.9%), and Type 3b and Type 2 are close at 7.8% and 8.4% respectively [123].

Typically, duct diameter decreases from the hilum toward the liver periphery. Thus, a greater number of ducts means smaller duct diameters, making biliary reconstruction more complex. Multiple reconstructions raise the risk of postoperative problems like leaks, strictures, and anastomotic narrowing. In general, all ducts are reconstructed except for accessory ducts smaller than 1 mm. However, data from high-volume centers show that even with multiple ducts, early complications and long-term outcomes are comparable [4, 124, 125].

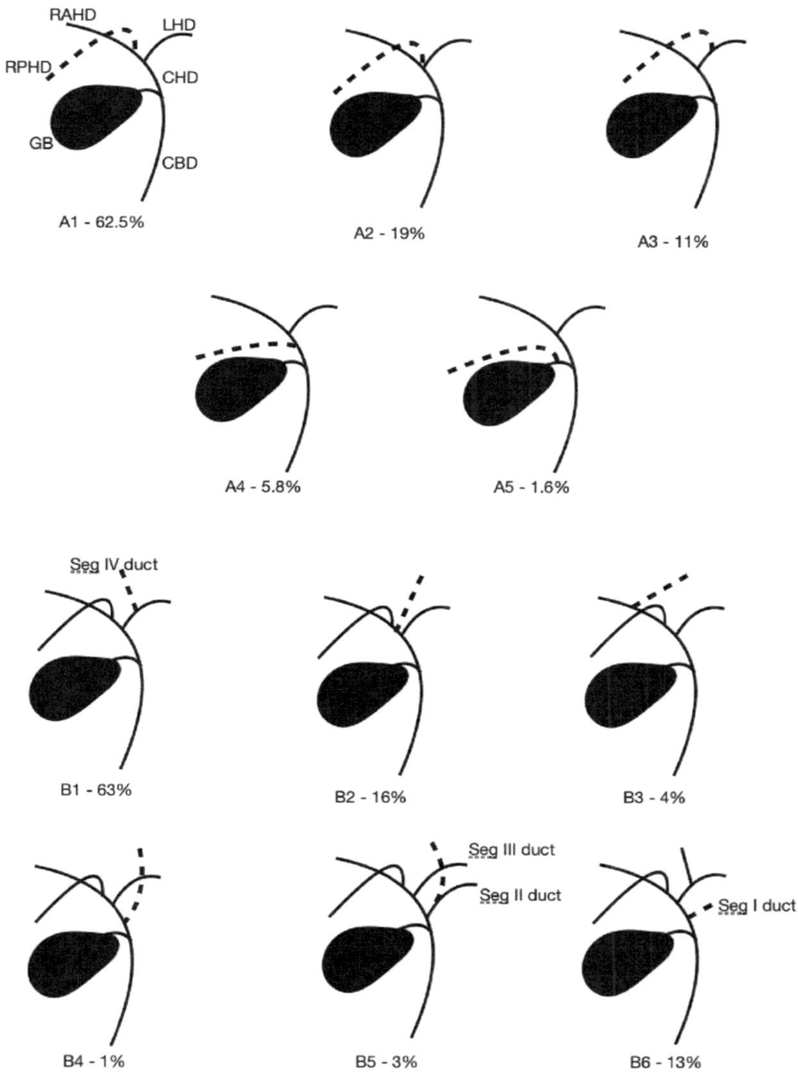

Biliary anatomy

Fig. 21.37 Huang's classification of hepatic duct anatomy [117]

21.26 Conclusion

Choosing a living donor for liver transplantation is a careful, multi-step process, with donor safety placed above all else. In-depth medical, psychological, and social evaluations are mandatory to assess suitability. A key part of this is confirming that the donor's liver is healthy, of appropriate size, and can safely regenerate, with a suitable remnant (at least 30%) to ensure donor safety. Comprehensive imaging evaluation is critical, as any anatomical variation with respect to volume, vascular, and biliary systems can make the operation riskier and threaten donor and recipient outcomes. Therefore, the success of LDLT is firmly based upon meticulous selection, aiming to minimize donor risks while giving the recipient the best possible chance at a healthy life.

Selecting a deceased donor presents its own set of hurdles. Deceased donors—brain-dead or after circulatory death—are often the only hope for patients without a living donor. The liver's quality depends on factors like donor age, medical background, cause of death, and ischemia times. Careful screening based on demography and epidemiology is necessary to avoid transmitting infections or cancers. Although understanding the liver's anatomy is crucial (especially if the liver is to be split), detailed imaging isn't always available, making surgery more unpredictable. Unexpected vascular or biliary variations can complicate or even derail the transplant. The liver must be the right size (especially when the transplant is between an adult and a child) and free of major issues like steatosis, which is more common in deceased donors and can impair graft function. Ethical concerns about fair organ distribution and the use of extended criteria donors bring in another set of complexities. However, DDLT remains a vital option, with careful selection playing a key role in improving patient outcomes, reducing complications, and securing long-term graft success. Moreover, with increasing awareness, government support, and widespread educational campaigns, there is a gradual rise in deceased donor availability.

References

1. Lomero M, Gardiner D, Coll E, Haase-Kromwijk B, Procaccio F, Immer F, et al. Donation after circulatory death today: an updated overview of the European landscape. Transpl Int. 2020;33:76–88.
2. Kalisvaart M, de Haan JE, Polak WG, Metselaar HJ, Wijnhoven BPL, Ijzermans JNM, et al. Comparison of postoperative outcomes between donation after circulatory death and donation after brain death liver transplantation using the comprehensive complication index. Ann Surg. 2017;266:772–8.
3. Abu-Gazala S, Olthoff KM. Status of adult living donor liver transplantation in the United States: Results from the Adult-To-Adult Living Donor Liver Transplantation Cohort Study. Gastroenterol Clin North Am. 2018;47:297.

4. Choudhary NS, Bhangui P, Soin AS. Liver transplant outcomes in India. Clin Liver Dis (Hoboken). 2022;19(1):32–5. https://doi.org/10.1002/cld.1166. PMID: 35106148; PMCID: PMC8785916.
5. Hibi T, Wei Chieh AK, Chi-Yan Chan A, Bhangui P. Current status of liver transplantation in Asia. Int J Surg. 2020;82S:4–8.
6. https://notto.mohfw.gov.in/WriteReadData/Portal/News/814_1_2013_to_2022.pdf.
7. https://unos.org/media-resources/releases/innovations-policy-updates-drive-equity-and-record-organ-transplants-2023/.
8. https://unos.org/news/2022-organ-transplants-again-set-annual-records/.
9. https://unos.org/news/in-focus/2022-heart-transplants-steep-increases-in-transplants-from-dcd-donors/.
10. https://unos.org/news/unos-to-launch-dcd-collaborative/.
11. https://www.bidmc.org/centers-and-departments/transplant-institute/liver-transplant/liver-donor-criteria.
12. Halazun KJ, Quillin RC, Rosenblatt R, et al. Expanding the margins: high volume utilisation of marginal liver grafts among >2000 liver transplants at a single institution. Ann Surg. 2017;266:441.
13. https://www.odt.nhs.uk/deceased-donation/best-practice-guidance/donation-after-brainstem-death.
14. Shen C, Cheng H, Zong T, Zhu H. The role of normothermic machine perfusion (NMP) in the preservation of ex-vivo liver before transplantation: a review. Front Bioeng Biotechnol. 2023;11:1072937.
15. van Rijn R, Schurink IJ, de Vries Y, van den Berg AP, Cortes Cerisuelo M, Darwish Murad S, Erdmann JI, Gilbo N, de Haas RJ, Heaton N, van Hoek B, Huurman VAL, Jochmans I, van Leeuwen OB, de Meijer VE, Monbaliu D, Polak WG, Slangen JJG, Troisi RI, Vanlander A, de Jonge J, Porte RJ, DHOPE-DCD Trial Investigators. Hypothermic machine perfusion in liver transplantation—a randomized trial. N Engl J Med. 2021;384(15):1391–401.
16. Guo Z, Zhao Q, Huang S, Huang C, Wang D, Yang L, Zhang J, Chen M, Wu L, Zhang Z, Zhu Z, Wang L, Zhu C, Zhang Y, Tang Y, Sun C, Xiong W, Shen Y, Chen X, Xu J, Wang T, Ma Y, Hu A, Chen Y, Zhu X, Rong J, Cai C, Gong F, Guan X, Huang W, Ko DS, Li X, Tullius SG, Huang J, Ju W, He X. Ischaemia-free liver transplantation in humans: a first-in-human trial. Lancet Reg Health West Pac. 2021;16:100260.
17. https://www.livertransplantindia.com/liver-donor.
18. Lee SG. Modified right-lobe graft. In: Oniscu GC, Forsythe JLR, Pomfret EA, editors. Transplantation surgery. Springer surgery atlas series. Berlin/Heidelberg: Springer; 2019. https://doi.org/10.1007/978-3-540-73796-4_12.
19. Dasari BV, Mergental H, Isaac JR, Muiesan P, Mirza DF, Perera T. Systematic review and meta-analysis of liver transplantation using grafts from deceased donors aged over 70 years. Clin Transplant. 2017;31(e13139):1–9.
20. https://www.notto.gov.in.
21. Markmann JF, Markmann JW, Markmann DA, Bacquerizo A, Singer J, Holt CD, et al. Preoperative factors associated with outcome and their impact on resource use in 1148 consecutive primary liver transplants. Transplantation. 2001;72:1113–22.
22. Seem DL, Lee I, Umscheid CA, Kuehnert MJ, Service USPH. PHS guideline for reducing human immunodeficiency virus, hepatitis B virus, and hepatitis C virus transmission through organ transplantation. Public Health Rep. 2013;128:247–343.
23. Kalisvaart M, Croome KP, Hernandez-Alejandro R, Pirenne J, Cortés-Cerisuelo M, Miñambres E, et al. Donor warm ischemia time in DCD liver transplantation-working group report from the ILTS DCD, liver preservation, and machine perfusion consensus conference. Transplantation. 2021;105:1156–64.
24. Eden J, Sousa Da Silva R, Cortes-Cerisuelo M, Croome K, De Carlis R, Hessheimer AJ, et al. Utilization of livers donated after circulatory death for transplantation – an international comparison. J Hepatol. 2023;78:1007–16.

25. Reich DJ, Mulligan DC, Abt PL, Pruett TL, Abecassis MM, D'Alessandro A, et al. A.S.o.O.T. Committee. ASTS recommended practice guidelines for controlled donation after cardiac death organ procurement and transplantation. Am J Transplant. 2009;9:2004–11.
26. Barrett M, Sonnenday CJ. CAQ Corner: deceased donor selection and management. Liver Transpl. 2023;29(11):1234–41. https://doi.org/10.1097/LVT.0000000000000242. Epub 2023 Aug 11.
27. Croome KP, Mathur AK, Aqel B, Yang L, Taner T, Heimbach JK, et al. Classification of distinct patterns of ischemic cholangiopathy following DCD liver transplantation: distinct clinical courses and long-term outcomes from a multicenter cohort. Transplantation. 2022;106:1206–14.
28. Friend P, Pollok M. Hypothermic machine perfusion in liver transplantation—a randomised trial and beyond. Transplant Int. 2022;35:10257. https://doi.org/10.3389/ti.2022.10257.
29. Serifis N, Matheson R, Cloonan D, Rickert CG, Markmann JF, Coe TM. Machine perfusion of the liver: a review of clinical trials. Front Surg. 2021;8:625394. https://doi.org/10.3389/fsurg.2021.625394.
30. Conrick-Martin I, Gaffney A, Dwyer R, et al. Intensive Care Society of Ireland—guidelines for management of the potential organ donor (2018—2nd edition). Ir J Med Sci. 2019;188:1111–8. https://doi.org/10.1007/s11845-019-01987-9.
31. Nam H, Nilles KM, Levitsky J, Ison MG. Donor-derived viral infections in liver transplantation. Transplantation. 2018;102(11):1824–36.
32. Razonable RR, Humar A. AST infectious diseases community of practice. cytomegalovirus in solid organ transplantation. Am J Transplant. 2013;13(Suppl 4):93–106.
33. Kotton CN, Kumar D, Caliendo AM, et al. Updated international consensus guidelines on the management of cytomegalovirus in solid-organ transplantation. Transplantation. 2013;96:333–60.
34. Yadav SK, Saigal S, Choudhary NS, Saha S, Kumar N, Soin AS. Cytomegalovirus infection in liver transplant recipients: current approach to diagnosis and management. J Clin Exp Hepatol. 2017;7(2):144–51.
35. Manuel O, Husain S, Kumar D, et al. Assessment of cytomegalovirus-specific cell-mediated immunity for the prediction of cytomegalovirus disease in high-risk solid-organ transplant recipients: a multicenter cohort study. Clin Infect Dis. 2013;56:817–24.
36. Eid AJ, Arthurs SK, Deziel PJ, et al. Clinical predictors of relapse after treatment of primary gastrointestinal cytomegalovirus disease in solid organ transplant recipients. Am J Transplant. 2010;10:157–61.
37. Bosch W, Heckman MG, Pungpapong S, Diehl NN, Shalev JA, Hellinger WC. Association of cytomegalovirus infection and disease with recurrent hepatitis C after liver transplantation. Transplantation. 2012;93(7):723–8.
38. Loggi E, Conti F, Cucchetti A, Ercolani G, Pinna AD, Andreone P. Liver grafts from hepatitis B surface antigen-positive donors: a review of the literature. World J Gastroenterol. 2016;22(35):8010–6.
39. Huprikar S, Danziger-Isakov L, Ahn J, Naugler S, Blumberg E, Avery RK, Koval C, Lease ED, Pillai A, Doucette KE. Solid organ transplantation from hepatitis B virus-positive donors: consensus guidelines for recipient management. Am J Transplant. 2015;15:1162–72.
40. Delman AM, Turner KM, Safdar K, Anwar N, Silski LS, Lee TC, et al. Expanding the donor pool: first use of hepatitis B Virus nat positive solid organ allografts into seronegative recipients. Ann Surg. 2021;274:556–64.
41. Alvaro E, Abradelo M, Fuertes A, et al. Liver transplantation from anti-hepatitis C virus-positive donors: our experience. Transplant Proc. 2012;44:1475–8.
42. Cotter TG, Paul S, Sandıkçı B, Couri T, Bodzin AS, Little EC, et al. Increasing utilisation and excellent initial outcomes following liver transplant of hepatitis C virus (HCV)-viremic donors into HCV-negative recipients: outcomes following liver transplant of HCV-viremic donors. Hepatology. 2019;69:2381–95.

43. Cholongitas E, Papatheodoridis GV, Burroughs AK. Liver grafts from anti-hepatitis B core positive donors: a systematic review. J Hepatol. 2010;52:272–9.
44. Loggi E, Micco L, Ercolani G, et al. Liver transplantation from hepatitis B surface antigen positive donors: A safe way to expand the donor pool. J Hepatol. 2012;56:579–85.
45. Saidi RF, Jabbour N, Shah SA, Li YF, Bozorgzadeh A. Liver transplantation from hepatitis B surface antigen-positive donors. Transplant Proc. 2013;45:279–80.
46. Skagen CL, Jou JH, Said A. Risk of de novo hepatitis in liver recipients from hepatitis-B core antibody-positive grafts—a systematic analysis. Clin Transplant. 2011;25:E243–9.
47. Kucirka LM, Sarathy H, Govindan P, et al. Risk of window period hepatitis-C infection in high infectious risk donors: systematic review and meta-analysis. Am J Transplant. 2011;11:1188–200.
48. Annambhotla PD, Gurbaxani BM, Kuehnert MJ, et al. A model to estimate the probability of human immunodeficiency virus and hepatitis C infection despite negative nucleic acid testing among increased-risk organ donors. Transpl Infect Dis. 2017;19.
49. Gang S, Choi Y, Lee B, et al. Long-term outcomes of liver transplantation using grafts from donors with active hepatitis B virus replication: a multicenter cohort study. Ann Surg Treat Res. 2023;104(4):183–94. https://doi.org/10.4174/astr.2023.104.4.183.
50. Park JS, Gayam V, Pan CQ. Review article: preventing hepatitis B graft infection in hepatitis B patients after liver transplantation: immunoglobulin vs antivirals. Aliment Pharmacol Ther. 2020 Sep;52(6):944–54.
51. Rives CMD, Meka M, Brahmbhatt P, Reddy C. Hepatitis C virus window period causing a false negative screening result despite sensitive screening methods: 840. Am J Gastroenterol. 2015;110:S365.
52. Werbel WA, Durand CM. Pro: use of hepatitis C virus-positive donors should be considered standard of care. Clin Liver Dis. 2018;12(4):100–4.
53. Alghamdi W, Lotfy K, Weernink C, et al. Hepatitis C positive organ transplantation to negative recipients at a multiorgan Canadian transplant centre: ready for prime time. BMC Gastroenterol. 2022;22:34. https://doi.org/10.1186/s12876-022-02107-1.
54. Fishman JA, Grossi PA. Donor-derived infection—the challenge for transplant safety. Nat Rev Nephrol. 2014;10:663–72.
55. Theodoropoulos N, Nowicki MJ, Chinchilla-Reyes C, et al. Deceased organ donor screening for human immunodeficiency virus, hepatitis B, and hepatitis C viruses: discordant serology and nucleic acid testing results. Transpl Infect Dis. 2017.
56. Terrault NA, Roland ME, Schiano T, et al. Outcomes of liver transplant recipients with hepatitis C and human immunodeficiency virus coinfection. Liver Transplant. 2012;18(6):716–26.
57. McCain JD, Chascsa DM. Special considerations in the management of HIV and viral hepatitis coinfections in liver transplantation. Hepat Med. 2022;14:27–36.
58. Feijó MS, Galdino-Vasconcelos MR, Simões V, Atik F, Castro FFS, Ferreira G, Jorge F, Diaz LG, Brizolla de Campos P, Trevizoli N, Cajá G, Ullmann R, Watanabe A. Impact of donor positive blood culture in deceased donor liver transplantation. Transplant Proc. 2020;52(5):1236–42.
59. Allen UD, Preiksaitis JK. Epstein-Barr virus and posttransplant lymphoproliferative disorder in solid organ transplantation. Am J Transplant. 2013;13(Suppl 4):107–20.
60. Agrawal D, Saigal S. Utilization of SARS-COV-2 positive donors and recipients for liver transplantation in the pandemic era – an evidence-based review. J Liver Transplant. 2022;7:100081.
61. Echenique IA, Ison MG. Update on donor-derived infections in liver transplantation. Liver Transpl. 2013;19:575–85.
62. OPTN. Policy 2.0 Deceased Donor Organ Procurement (Policy 2.9). Organ Procurement and Transplant Network (OPTN). Effective Date March 1, 2018. Dated Accessed: March 22, 2018.
63. Kaul DR, Davis JA. AST infectious diseases community of practice. Human T cell lymphotropic virus 1/2 in solid organ transplantation. Am J Transplant. 2013;13(Suppl 4):355–60.

64. Saigal S, Choudhary NS, Saraf N, Kataria S, Mohanka R, Soin AS. Transmission of dengue virus from a donor to a recipient after living donor liver transplantation. Liver Transpl. 2013;19(12):1413–4.
65. Benkö T, Hoyer DP, Saner FH, Treckmann JW, Paul A, Radunz S. Liver transplantation from donors with a history of malignancy: a single-center experience. Transplant Direct. 2017;3(11).
66. Desai R, Collett D, Watson CJ, et al. Estimated risk of cancer transmission from organ donor to graft recipient in a national transplantation registry. Br J Surg. 2014;101:768–74.
67. Montalti R, Rompianesi G, Di Benedetto F, et al. Liver transplantation utilizing grafts from donors with genitourinary cancer detected prior to liver implantation. Transplant Proc. 2009;41:1275–7.
68. Nalesnik MA, Woodle ES, Dimaio JM, et al. Donor-transmitted malignancies in organ transplantation: assessment of clinical risk. Am J Transplant. 2011;11:1140–7.
69. Pomfret EA, Lodge JP, Villamil FG, Siegler M. Should we use living donor grafts for patients with hepatocellular carcinoma? Ethical considerations. Liver Transpl. 2011;17:S128–32.
70. Brige P, Hery G, Chopinet S, Palen A, Azoulay D, Gregoire E. Morbidity and mortality of hepatic right lobe living donors: systematic review and perspectives. J Gastrointestin Liver Dis. 2018;27:169–78.
71. Park JJ, Kim K, Choi JY, Shim SR, Kim JH. Long-term mortality of living kidney donors: a systematic review and meta-analysis. Int Urol Nephrol. 2021;53:1563–81.
72. Feng S, et al. Characteristics associated with liver graft failure: the concept of a donor risk index. Am J Transplant. 6(4):783–90.
73. Ringe B, Strong RW. The dilemma of living liver donor death: to report or not to report? Transplantation. 2008;85:790–3.
74. Ghobrial RM, Freise CE, Trotter JF, Tong L, Ojo AO, Fair JH, et al. Donor morbidity after living donation for liver transplantation. Gastroenterology. 2008;135(2):468–76.
75. DiMartini AF, Dew MA, Butt Z, Simpson MA, Ladner DP, Smith AR, et al. Patterns and predictors of sexual function after liver donation: The adult-to-adult living donor liver transplantation cohort study. Liver Transpl. 2015 May;21(5):670–82.
76. Burroughs AK, Sabin CA, Rolles K, Delvart V, Karam V, Buckels J, O'Grady JG, Castaing D, Klempnauer J, Jamieson N, Neuhaus P, Lerut J, de Ville de Goyet J, Pollard S, Salizzoni M, Rogiers X, Muhlbacher F, Garcia Valdecasas JC, Broelsch C, Jaeck D, Berenguer J, Gonzalez EM, Adam R. 3-month and 12-month mortality after first liver transplant in adults in Europe: predictive models for outcome. Lancet. 2006;367:225–32.
77. Enkhbold C, Morine Y, Utsunomiya T, Imura S, Ikemoto T, Arakawa Y, Saito Y, Yamada S, Ishikawa D, Shimada M. Dysfunction of liver regeneration in aged liver after partial hepatectomy. J Gastroenterol Hepatol. 2015;30:1217–24. https://doi.org/10.1111/jgh.12930. PMID: 25682855.
78. Ghinolfi D, Pezzati D, Rreka E, Balzano E, Catalano G, Coletti L, et al. Simone nonagenarian grafts for liver transplantation. Liver Transpl. 2019;25:1439–44.
79. Cutrin JC, Cantino D, Biasi F, Chiarpotto E, Salizzoni M, Andorno E, Massano G, Lanfranco G, Rizzetto M, Boveris A, Poli G. Reperfusion damage to the bile canaliculi in transplanted human liver. Hepatology. 1996.
80. Selzner N, Renner EL, Selzner M, Adeyi O, Kashfi A, Therapondos G, Girgrah N, Herath C, Levy GA, Lilly L. Antiviral treatment of recurrent hepatitis C after liver transplantation: predictors of response and long-term outcome. Transplantation. 2009;88:1214–21.
81. Soin AS, Raut V, Mohanka R, Rastogi A, Vohra V, et al. Use of ABO-incompatible grafts in living donor liver transplantation—first report from India. Indian J Gastroenterol. 2014;33(1):72–6. https://doi.org/10.1007/s12664-013-0424-0. Epub 2013 Dec 27.
82. https://www.legalserviceindia.com/article/l224-Organ-Transplantation-Law-In-India.html.
83. Crowley H, Lewis WD, Gordon F, et al. Steatosis in donor and transplant liver biopsies. Hum Pathol. 2000;31:1209e13.

84. Imber CJ, St Peter SD, Handa A, et al. Hepatic steatosis and its relationship to transplantation. Liver Transpl. 2002;8:415e23.
85. Krishan S, Jain D, Bathina Y, Kale A, Saraf N, Saigal S, Choudhary N, Baijal SS, Soin A. Non-invasive quantification of hepatic steatosis in living, related liver donors using dual-echo Dixon imaging and single-voxel proton spectroscopy. Clin Radiol. 2016;71(1):58–63.
86. Ratziu V, Charlotte F, Heurtier A, et al. Sampling variability of liver biopsy in nonalcoholic fatty liver disease. Gastroenterology. 2005;128:1898e906.
87. Bhangui P, Sah J, Soin A, et al. Safe use of right lobe live donor livers with up to 20% macrovesicular steatosis without compromising donor safety and recipient outcome. Transplantation. 2020;104(2):308–16.
88. Takagi K, Domagala P, Polak WG, Ijzermans JN, Boehnert MU. Right posterior segment graft for living donor liver transplantation: a systematic review. Transplant Rev. 2019;34(1):100510.
89. Goja S, Yadav SK, Yadav A, Piplani T, Rastogi A, Bhangui P, Saigal S, Soin AS. Accuracy of preoperative CT liver volumetry in living donor hepatectomy and its clinical implications. Hepatobiliary Surg Nutr. 2018;7(3):167–74.
90. Ikegami TMD, Furukawa K, Haruki K, Onda S, Gocho T. Predicted volume or actual weight for graft selection policy in living-donor liver transplantation. Transplantation. 2021;105(4):e43. https://doi.org/10.1097/TP.0000000000003583.
91. Soin AS, Yadav SK, Saha SK, Rastogi A, Bhangui P, Srinivasan T, Saraf N, Choudhary NS, Saigal S, Vohra V. Is portal inflow modulation always necessary for successful utilization of small volume living donor liver grafts? Liver Transpl. 2019;25(12):1811–21. https://doi.org/10.1002/lt.25629. Epub 2019 Oct 1.
92. Kiuchi T, Tanaka K, Ito T, Oike F, Ogura Y, Fujimoto Y, Ogawa K. Small-for-size graft in living donor liver transplantation: How far should we go? Liver Transplant. 2003;9(9):S29–35. https://doi.org/10.1053/jlts.2003.50198.
93. Choudhary NS, Saraf N, Saigal S, Gautam D, Lipi L, Rastogi A, Goja S, Menon PB, Bhangui P, Ramchandra SK, Soin AS. Rapid reversal of liver steatosis with lifestyle modification in highly motivated liver donors. J Clin Exp Hepatol. 2015;5(2):123–6.
94. Liver disease in pregnancy. The Lancet. 2017. Accessed 12 Mar 12, 2017.
95. Cho JY, Suh KS, Kwon CH, Yi NJ, Lee KU. Mild hepatic steatosis is not a major risk factor for hepatectomy and regenerative power is not impaired. Surgery. 2006;139(4):508–15. https://doi.org/10.1016/j.surg.2005.09.007.
96. Fakhar N, Nikeghbalian S, Kazemi K, Shamsayeefar AR, Gholami S, Kasraianfard A, Malek-Hosseini SA. Transplantation of deceased donor livers with elevated levels of serum transaminases at Shiraz Transplant Center. Hepat Mon. 2016;16(10):e40140. https://doi.org/10.5812/hepatmon.40140.
97. Mangus RS, Fridell JA, Kubal CA, Davis JP, Tector AJ. Elevated alanine aminotransferase (ALT) in the deceased donor: impact on early post-transplant liver allograft function. Liver Int. 2015;35:524–31.
98. Soin AS, Chaudhary RJ, Pahari H, Pomfret EA. A worldwide survey of live liver donor selection policies at 24 centers with a combined experience of 19 009 adult living donor liver transplants. Transplantation. 2019;103(2):e39–47.
99. Choudhary NS, Saraf N, Saigal S, Gautam D, Lipi L, Soin AS. Estimation of normal values of serum transaminases based on liver histology in healthy Asian Indians. J Gastroenterol Hepatol. 2015;30(4):763–6.
100. Choudhary NS, Saraf N, Saigal S, Gautam D, Lipi L, Rastogi A, Soin AS. Rapid reversal of liver steatosis with lifestyle modification in highly motivated liver donors. J Clin Exp Hepatol. 2015;5(2):123–6.
101. Steggerda JA, Bloom MB, Noureddin M, Brennan TV, Todo T, Nissen NN, et al. Higher thresholds for the utilisation of steatotic allografts in liver transplantation: analysis from a US national database. PLoS One. 2020;15:e0230995.

102. Kearon C, Akl EA, Ornelas J, et al. Antithrombotic therapy for VTE disease: CHEST guideline and expert panel report. Chest. 2016;149(2):315–52.
103. Connors JM. Thrombophilia testing and venous thrombosis. N Engl J Med. 2017;377(12):1177–87.
104. Nakamura T, Tanaka K, Kiuchi T, Kasahara M, Uemoto S, et al. Anatomical variations and surgical strategies in right lobe living donor liver transplantation: lessons from 120 cases. Transplantation. 2002;73:1896–903.
105. Liao C, Chen M, Yu C, Tsang L, Chen C, Hsu H, Lim W, Chuang Y, Huang P, Cheng Y, Ou H. Non-contrast-enhanced and contrast-enhanced magnetic resonance angiography in living donor liver vascular anatomy. Diagnostics. 2022;12(2):498.
106. Sapisochin G, Goldaracena N, Laurence JM, Levy GA, Grant DR, Cattral MS. Right lobe living-donor hepatectomy-the Toronto approach, tips and tricks. Hepatobiliary Surg Nutr. 2016;5(2):118–26.
107. Sugawara Y, Tamura S, Kaneko J, Iida T, Mihara M, Makuuchi M, et al. Single artery reconstruction in left liver transplantation. Surgery. 2011;149(6):841–5.
108. Covey AM, Brody LA, Getrajdman GI, Sofocleous CT, Brown KT. Incidence, patterns, and clinical relevance of variant portal vein anatomy. AJR Am J Roentgenol. 2004;183:1055–64. https://doi.org/10.2214/ajr.183.4.1831055.
109. Lee SG, Hwang S, Kim KH, Ahn CS, Park KM, Lee YJ, et al. Approach to anatomic variations of the graft portal vein in right lobe living-donor liver transplantation. Transplantation. 2003;75(3 Suppl):S28–32. https://doi.org/10.1097/01.TP.0000047028.97031.66.
110. Sutton TL, Sandoval V, Warner D, Moneta G, Gilbert E, Mayo SC, Politano AD, Maynard E, Sheppard BC, Enestvedt CK. Patency for autologous vein is superior to cadaveric vein in portal-mesenteric venous reconstruction. HPB (Oxford). 2022;24(8):1326–34.
111. Sharma M, Somani P, Rameshbabu CS. Linear endoscopic ultrasound evaluation of hepatic veins. World J Gastrointest Endosc. 2018;10(10):283–93.
112. Varotti G, Gondolesi GE, Goldman J, Wayne M, Florman SS, Schwartz ME, Miller CM, Sukru E. Anatomic variations in right liver living donors1. J Am College Surg. 2004;198(4):577–82.
113. Neumann JO, Thorn M, Fischer L, Schöbinger M, Heimann T, Radeleff B, Schmidt J, Meinzer HP, Büchler MW, Schemmer P. Branching patterns and drainage territories of the middle hepatic vein in computer-simulated right living-donor hepatectomies. Am J Transplant. 2006;6(6):1407–15.
114. Faitot F, Vibert E, Salloum C, Gorden DL, Coscas F, Adam R, et al. Importance of conserving middle hepatic vein distal branches for homogeneous regeneration of the left liver after right hepatectomy. HPB (Oxford). 2012;14(11):746–53.
115. MillerCM DF, HeimbachJK K-SL, LeeSG LJ, et al. The International Liver Transplant Society guideline on living liver donation. Transplantation. 2016;100(6):1238–43.
116. Koc Z, Ulusan S, Oguzkurt L, Tokmak N. Venous variants and anomalies on routine abdominal multi-detector row CT. Eur J Radiol. 2007;61(2):267–78. https://doi.org/10.1016/j.ejrad.2006.09.008. Epub 2006 Oct 17.
117. Huang TL, Cheng YF, Chen CL, Chen TY, Lee TY. Variants of the bile ducts: clinical application in the potential donor of living-related hepatic transplantation. Transplant Proc. 1996;28(3):1669–70.
118. Wan P, Li Q, Zhang J, Xia Q. Right lobe split liver transplantation versus whole liver transplantation in adult recipients: a systematic review and meta-analysis. Liver Transpl. 2015;21(7):928–43.
119. Garzali IU, Akbulut S, Aloun A, Naffa M, Aksoy F. Outcome of split liver transplantation vs living donor liver transplantation: a systematic review and meta-analysis. World J Gastrointest Surg. 2023;15(7):1522–31.
120. Saidi RF, Jabbour N, Li YF, Shah SA, Bozorgzadeh A. Outcomes in partial liver transplantation: deceased donor split-liver vs. live donor liver transplantation. HPB. 2011;13(11):797–801.
121. Takeishi K, Shirabe K, Yoshida Y, et al. Correlation between portal vein anatomy and bile duct variation in 407 living liver donors. Am J Transplant. 2015;15:155–60.

122. Choi JW, Kim TK, Kim KW, et al. Anatomic variation in intrahepatic bile ducts: an analysis of intraoperative cholangiograms in 300 consecutive donors for living donor liver transplantation. Korean J Radiol. 2003;4:85–90.
123. Rastogi A, Gupta AA, Piplani T, Yadav KS, Fysal KV, Bhangui P, Soin AS. Hilar anatomy in 3035 living liver donors: a novel classification for donor surgery and suitability, hepatic surgeries, and hepatobiliary interventions. Transplantation. 2023;108(2):455–63. https://doi.org/10.1097/TP.0000000000004807.
124. Bhangui P, Saha S. The high-end range of biliary reconstruction in living donor liver transplant. Curr Opin Organ Transplant. 2019;24(5):623–30.
125. Tabbal M, Schnickel G, Bruno D, Obeid J, Theodoropoulos I, Kazimi M, Yoshida A, Abouljoud M. Biliary anatomy and reconstruction in living donor liver transplant; impact on short and long-term outcomes: Abstract# D2612. Transplantation. 2014;98:787.

Chapter 22
Living Donor Surgery and Innovations

Ashwin Rammohan and Mohamed Rela

Abstract The development of living donor liver transplantation (LDLT) has primarily been driven by the significant disparity between the number of patients awaiting transplants and the limited availability of deceased donor organs. Despite the complex ethical considerations involved, LDLT remains a technically intricate procedure that should only be undertaken when the potential benefit to the recipient justifies the risk to the donor.

The fundamental objectives of LDLT are to ensure minimal morbidity and nearly zero mortality for the donor while delivering a meaningful survival advantage to the recipient. Achieving these outcomes heavily depends on thorough donor evaluation, which is a critical component of a successful LDLT program.

This chapter outlines the criteria for donor selection and the evaluation process and offers a brief overview of the surgical procedure involved in living liver donation.

Keywords Living donor liver transplantation · Donor selection · Surgery · Outcomes · Innovations

Key Highlights

- Identifying appropriate candidates for living donation in living donor liver transplantation (LDLT) is a complex process that requires a multidisciplinary algorithmic approach. This approach to donor selection and various operative techniques for the different types of liver grafts used in LDLT are presented in this chapter.
- Despite all its advantages, including thorough donor screening, optimization of timing for transplantation, minimal cold ischemia time, and a lowering of the waitlist mortality for the recipient, in LDLT, there always remains the finite risk to the donor, leading to its associated ethical challenges.

A. Rammohan (✉) · M. Rela
Institute of Liver Disease & Transplantation, Rela Institute & Medical Centre, Chennai, India
e-mail: ashwinrammohan@gmail.com

S. Saigal, D. Jothimani (eds.), *Fundamentals of Transplant Hepatology*,
https://doi.org/10.1007/978-981-95-2624-6_22

- Based on the donor considerations and the requirements of the recipient (GRWR, MELD score, body habitus in children, etc.), different types of liver grafts can be procured from the live donor. The paramount consideration here is that of donor safety, especially with regard to the functional liver remnant.

22.1 Introduction

Living donor liver transplantation (LDLT) was developed as a solution to address the growing gap between the increasing number of patients needing liver transplants and the limited availability of deceased donor organs. Despite its ethical complexities and technical challenges, LDLT outcomes have steadily improved over the last decade, in some cases surpassing those of deceased donor liver transplantation (DDLT). The cornerstone of LDLT remains the uncompromising safety of the donor [1].

Beyond the requirement for advanced surgical expertise, success in LDLT also depends on a rigorous donor selection process and a well-structured, validated perioperative protocol. This chapter provides an overview of the criteria for donor eligibility, the evaluation process, and a brief introduction to the donor surgery.

22.2 Ethical Considerations

LDLT is guided by two primary ethical principles: minimizing the risk of harm to the donor and ensuring that the recipient's outcome is not inferior to that of a full graft from a deceased donor [1–3]. However, the procedure inherently challenges the foundational medical ethic of "first, do no harm."

In 2005, an international forum held in Vancouver, Canada, addressed donor safety in living organ transplantation [4]. The resulting guidelines emphasized that LDLT should only proceed if the risk to the donor is justified by a meaningful benefit to the recipient.

Despite the ethical complexities, studies have shown that many liver donors report high levels of personal satisfaction and enhanced self-esteem after donation, with up to 92% stating they would donate again [5, 6]. This positive outlook is largely attributed to comprehensive, multi-stage counseling during the evaluation process, which prepares donors with realistic expectations regarding the surgery, potential complications, and outcomes.

Nevertheless, the ethical debate surrounding living organ donation continues, particularly in weighing donor risk against recipient benefit.

22.3 Donor Evaluation

The evaluation of a potential living liver donor is a critical component of the LDLT process, focused on identifying any factors that may elevate the risk of perioperative complications. This transparent, systematic approach is designed to exclude unsuitable candidates early, while guiding appropriate donors through the subsequent steps toward donation.

Each LDLT program follows a structured and well-defined set of criteria for selecting donor-recipient pairs, and although protocols may vary slightly, the core principles are broadly consistent worldwide. Key elements in selecting an appropriate donor include:

(a) The donation must be genuinely altruistic, with no financial gain or self-interest involved.
(b) The donor must be mentally competent, fully informed of the associated risks, and capable of providing valid consent.
(c) The entire process must be voluntary and free from any form of coercion. Donors must also be clearly informed that they may opt out of the process at any point, even after completing the full evaluation.
(d) The donor must meet all established medical eligibility criteria [7, 8].

Donor assessment involves a comprehensive, multi-stage protocol, including medical and psychological evaluations, as well as detailed imaging studies to analyze liver anatomy. Although there is ongoing discussion about whether the extent of liver resection correlates with donor risk, most centers adopt more stringent criteria for right lobe donation, particularly concerning donor age and the presence of hepatic steatosis [3].

Recipient characteristics must also be considered in the decision-making process. A successful LDLT depends on evaluating both favorable and unfavorable attributes of the donor and recipient together to determine whether the pairing is viable. The table below outlines the donor evaluation protocol used by our team. (Table 22.1).

22.4 Donor Selection Criteria

Blood Group: The blood group criteria for blood transfusion and organ donation, especially the liver, are similar. Therefore, AB group individuals are universal recipients, and those with O group blood are universal donors. It is preferable to choose ABO-identical or ABO-compatible donors. Breaching the ABO blood group barrier is a way to increase donor access, and desensitization protocols have successfully enabled physicians to cross it [9, 10].

Table 22.1 Acceptability criteria for live liver donors

Acceptable donors
Age 18–50 years
ABO-compatible blood group
No comorbidities, or 1 comorbidity such as well-controlled HT
LAI >= +6
BMI <25 kg/m^2
GRWR >0.8
Remnant volume >30% of TLV
Anatomically suitable for donation
To be discussed multidisciplinary team (MDT) meeting—Before accepting for donation
Age >50 years
Comorbidities such as systemic hypertension, bronchial asthma
LAI between −5 to +5
BMI 25–30 kg/m^2
GRWR <0.8 and/or donor liver remnant volume 28–30%
Any unusual anatomic feature

LAI Liver Attenuation Index, *TLV* Total Liver Volume, *BMI* Body Mass Index, *GRWR* Graft-to-Recipient Body Weight Ratio

Relationship: Most governmental bodies across the world stipulate that the prospective donor and recipient be related. There are, however, certain countries like Canada which allow for anonymous altruistic donation [11].

Age: The rate of hepatic regeneration has tremendous implications for both the donor and the recipient. There is a relatively direct correlation between advancing age and a decline in the rate of hepatic regeneration [12, 13]. Donors should strictly be above the age of 18 years. The upper limit, however, varies and is more dependent on their physiological age. Graft volumes are also taken into consideration; it is preferable to avoid a low graft weight to recipient's body weight ratio (GRWR expressed as %), liver from an older donor. Despite reports of successful right lobe donations from septuagenarian live donors, extreme caution must be exercised in selecting elderly donors, and it cannot be recommended as a routine [14].

22.4.1 Weight and Body Mass Index (BMI)

Ideally, living liver donors should have a BMI below 25 kg/m^2. However, if the liver's fat content is under 20%—as measured by the liver attenuation index (LAI)—and the functional liver remnant volume exceeds 35%, this threshold may be relaxed to a BMI of up to 30 kg/m^2 [7, 8, 15, 16].

Research indicates that individuals of Asian descent generally have a higher body fat percentage at a given BMI compared to Western populations. Consequently, a stricter BMI limit of 27.5 kg/m^2 is recommended for potential Asian donors.

In general, a BMI over 30 kg/m^2 is considered a relative contraindication for donation. Nonetheless, in select cases where no other suitable donor is available, individuals with a BMI between 30 and 35 kg/m^2 may still be evaluated. In such scenarios, the donor undergoes a structured diet and exercise program and is reassessed after 6 weeks. For donation to proceed, the BMI should ideally drop below 30 kg/m^2, and the liver steatosis must improve to less than 20%. A liver biopsy is mandatory at the end of this weight reduction period to confirm suitability [7, 17–19].

22.4.2 Comorbidities

An ideal donor is without any comorbidities. Due to its negative influence on liver regeneration, diabetes mellitus remains a contraindication. A single controlled comorbidity, like hypertension, may be considered acceptable. Other, more severe comorbidities like significant renal or cardiorespiratory disease are also considered contraindications to donation. It is, however, advisable to discuss any prospective donor's comorbidity in a multidisciplinary team meeting before making a formal decision. Previous abdominal surgery is not a contraindication to donation, and the indication may be more important than the operation itself.

22.4.3 Steatosis

The liver attenuation index (LAI)—calculated as the difference in attenuation between the liver and spleen on non-contrast CT—is a rapid and convenient method for assessing hepatic steatosis. Ideally, potential donors should have liver fat content below 20%, corresponding to an LAI of $\geq +6$. Steatosis greater than 30% (LAI < -5) is generally considered a contraindication for living donation. When LAI values fall between -5 and $+5$, a liver biopsy may be warranted to obtain a more accurate assessment of fat content.

Recent advancements have improved noninvasive imaging techniques, making them more quantitative. MRI-based fat quantification has demonstrated a strong correlation with histological grading and may serve as a reliable, cost-effective, and widely available tool for evaluating liver fat in the near future [20, 21].

22.4.4 Graft Volumes

Accurate volumetric assessment of the donor liver is essential, with attention to both the graft size and the remaining liver volume in the donor. The Graft-to-Recipient Weight Ratio (GRWR) is commonly used to evaluate whether the graft will be sufficient for the recipient. An ideal GRWR is >0.8. In selected cases, particularly when both donor and recipient profiles are favorable (e.g., young donor, no steatosis, low MELD recipient), a GRWR of 0.7–0.8 may be acceptable. Grafts with GRWR <0.7 are typically unsuitable but may still be used in very select patients with low MELD scores and minimal portal hypertension. In such cases, portal flow modulation may be necessary to prevent small-for-size syndrome [22, 23].

In pediatric recipients, higher GRWR values are usually required. Grafts with GRWR between 1.5 and 3 are considered ideal. If GRWR exceeds 4, or if there is a marked size mismatch—especially in infants under 6 months or weighing less than 5 kg—reduction of the left lateral segment, either anatomical or non-anatomical, may be required [24].

While GRWR is commonly used in Western centers, transplant programs in Japan and Hong Kong often rely on mathematical models to calculate the recipient's Standard Liver Volume (SLV), using formulas based on body weight or body surface area. Most programs consider 30–40% of SLV as the minimum acceptable graft size [2, 17, 25].

22.4.5 Anatomical Suitability

A triphasic CT scan, along with an MRCP, is the most commonly employed modality for evaluating the anatomical suitability of a donor liver. Anatomical anomalies which may complicate the donor or recipient surgery should be carefully identified (Figs. 22.1, 22.2, and 22.3). Certain anatomical variations like a single portal venous supply to the entire liver are an absolute contraindication to donation (Fig. 22.2e).

Due to the shared drainage of segments V, VIII, and IV, one of the biggest dilemmas in LDLT is that of the middle hepatic vein (MHV), and its anatomy holds the key to right lobe (RL) living donation [3, 13, 18, 19]. A detailed study of the hepatic venous anatomy is imperative in deciding whether the MHV is left behind with the donor liver or is partially or totally taken with the graft liver. While there is center-to-center variation in this protocol, there has been a decisive shift toward retaining the MHV with the donor.

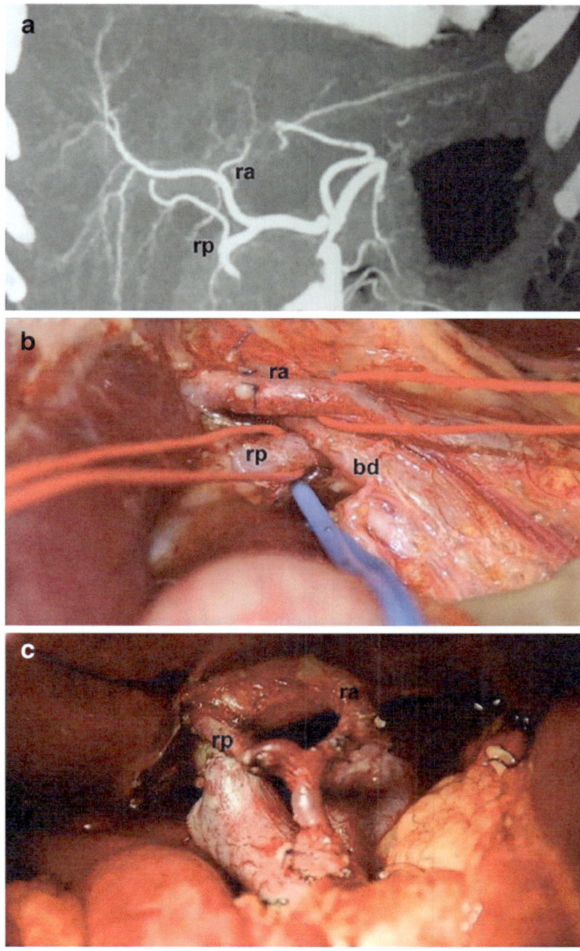

Fig. 22.1 Variation in the Donor's Right Hepatic Artery, which complicates both donor and recipient operation. (**a**) CT scan showing extrahepatic bifurcation of right hepatic artery into its anterior (ra) and posterior (rp) divisions; (**b**) intraoperative view showing the right anterior (ra) and posterior (rp) branches of the right hepatic artery coursing on either side (above and below) the common bile duct (bd). This variation leads to two arteries in a right lobe graft. (**c**) Arteries (ra & rp) reconstructed in the recipient

22.4.6 Donor Evaluation Algorithm

Stage I of the evaluation begins with a comprehensive consultation involving the prospective donor and their family. Donors must also be offered a private discussion to express concerns or ask questions independently. This in-person meeting includes a detailed explanation of the entire evaluation process, the perioperative course, potential complications, and both short- and long-term donor outcomes, ensuring the donor has a realistic understanding of the procedure.

Following the consultation, a clinical examination is performed along with initial laboratory investigations. These include a complete blood count, renal and liver function tests, lipid and thyroid profiles, and immune and viral markers. A non-contrast CT scan is also conducted to assess liver fat content. If a donor is found to

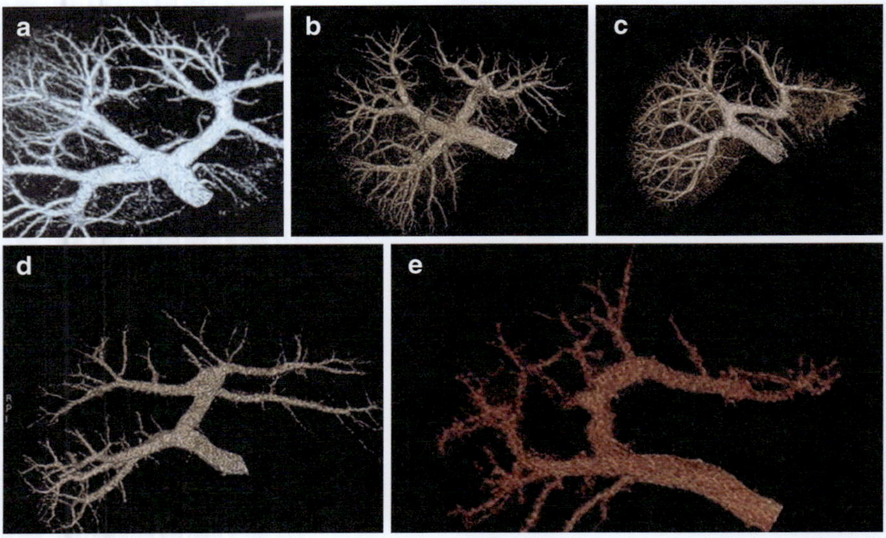

Fig. 22.2 Variations in the Donor's portal venous anatomy which may complicate the donor and recipient operations. (**a**) Type A anatomy with a short stump of the right portal vein. (**b**) Type B anatomy with trifurcation of the main portal vein. (**c**, **d**) Type C, D anatomies with right anterior portal vein arising from the left portal vein. Types B, C, and D will lead to two portal veins in a right lobe liver graft, which will need reconstruction in the recipient. Donor's portal vein stump closures must be done carefully to avoid narrowing the left portal vein. (**e**) Type E: Single portal vein supplying the liver. This anatomical variation is an absolute contraindication to liver donation

be unsuitable due to potentially reversible issues—such as an elevated BMI—they are provided with a structured diet and exercise program. Donors are advised to stop smoking and discontinue oral contraceptives at least 6 weeks before surgery.

Stage II involves a detailed evaluation of liver volume and vascular anatomy using a triphasic CT scan. Based on this imaging, along with considerations such as the donor's functional remnant liver volume, the recipient's expected GRWR, and vascular anatomy, the type of graft is determined.

Cardiac assessment begins with an ECG and echocardiogram. Depending on the findings, further testing with a treadmill test or dobutamine stress echocardiography is carried out. If abnormalities are detected, a coronary angiogram may be performed selectively.

Donors deemed suitable progress to a multidisciplinary evaluation, which includes reviews by a psychiatrist, physician, gynecologist, and anesthesiologist. Additional investigations may be requested if any clinical or laboratory abnormalities are found during the evaluation. Specific tests are conducted to exclude hereditary or familial liver disorders that could negatively impact both donor and recipient outcomes—these include serum copper, ferritin, and autoimmune markers.

It's essential to screen for genetic or regional disorders common in certain populations, such as G6PD deficiency and sickle cell disease in Middle Eastern and

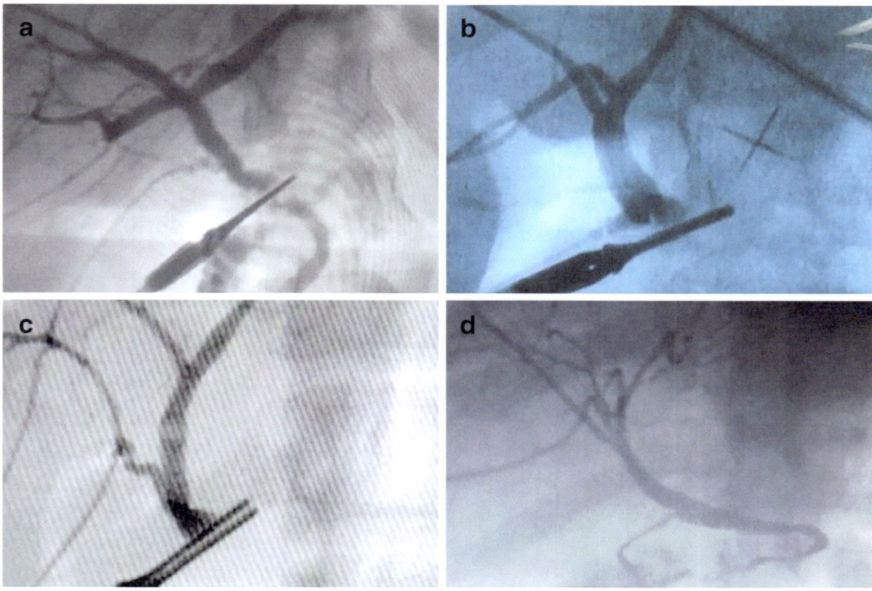

Fig. 22.3 Variations in the Donor's bile duct anatomy, which may make the bile duct reconstruction in the recipient more complex. (**a**) Standard anatomy, however, with a short stump of the right hepatic duct. May lead to two ducts in the graft; (**b**, **c**) Huang A3 and Huang A5 variations, which will lead to two bile ducts in the liver graft; (**d**) complex biliary anatomy, leading to 3 or more ducts in a right lobe graft

African donors, as these conditions could complicate the intraoperative or postoperative course.

22.5 Types of Living Donor Liver Grafts

Based on the donor considerations and the requirements of the recipient (GRWR, MELD score, body habitus in children, etc.), different types of liver grafts can be procured from the live donor. Again, the paramount consideration here is that of donor safety, especially with regard to the functional liver remnant. Three commonly performed living donor operations include 1. Left lateral sectionectomy (LLS), in which the graft consists of segments II and III. 2. Left hepatectomy (LH), in which the graft consists of the whole left lobe, segments I, II, III, and IV. The middle hepatic vein (MHV) is included with the liver graft. Some centers, especially from Japan, procure segment I along with the left lobe. 3. Right hepatectomy (RH), in which the graft consists of the right lobe and segments V, VI, VII, and VIII. Several variations include either including, partially including, or excluding the MHV, depending on the anatomical considerations (discussed previously).

There are other rarer types of grafts which are used in specific situations wherein the above types of hepatectomy could potentially compromise the safety of the donor or the outcomes in the recipient. These include 1. Right Posterior Sectionectomy, in which the graft consists of segments VI and VII. 2. Right Anterior Sectionectomy, wherein the graft consists of segments V and VIII. 3. Monosegmentectomy, in which the grafts consist of either segment II or segment III. This is a type of liver graft used in very small children.

22.6 Operative Approach

Irrespective of the type of grafts, there are three primary approaches to performing the donor hepatectomy in LDLT.

Open Donor Hepatectomy (ODH): Herein, the whole operation is performed via an abdominal incision. The type of surgical incision depends on the need for safe access based on the body habitus, unit protocol, type of liver graft being retrieved, and the surgeon's experience with the operation. Conventionally, most initial donor operations were performed via an incision which included a midline vertical incision and a variable length of transverse rectus muscle-cutting incision in the form of an inverted 'T' or 'hockey stick'. These provided the best possible access to the liver. With evolving experience, most open donor hepatectomy operations are now performed via a midline laparotomy incision or a limited reverse 'L' [26, 27].

Laparoscopic Donor Hepatectomy (LDH): Most complications of this operation are related to the operative wound (hernia, obstruction, wound infection, chronic pain, etc.), and despite increased self-esteem and satisfaction in various quality of life analyses on live donor (LD), the most common grievance is that of the scar [28–31]. Thus, a drive to develop minimally invasive DH (MIDH). A pure laparoscopic approach has been rapidly evolving since the team from France performed the first laparoscopic LLS in 2012 [32]. The laparoscopic approach for LLS has become a standard; however, for the LH/RH, the uptake has been much slower and is largely limited to a few large-volume centers in Asia. As a standard, 4–6 laparoscopic ports are used. Case-control studies and meta-analyses comparing MIDH with ODH observed a significantly reduced intraoperative blood loss, similar or lower donor morbidity, and shortened hospital stay in the MIDH (LDH and RDH) cohort [26, 27, 33–35]. A lower blood loss was explained by the magnified view in MIDH. This allowed for a better dissection and bleeding control. The presence of pneumoperitoneum, with its higher intra-abdominal pressure, reduced low-pressure venous bleeding and allowed for easier control. While the literature has been mixed with regard to the superiority of the MIDH, none of the meta-analyses showed the MIDH to have higher complication rates. Studies from Korea suggest that there could be a higher risk of operative morbidity, including traction injuries, hematomas, and higher postoperative liver enzyme levels at the beginning of the learning curve [36, 37]. There is no report of a donor mortality with MIDH. Postoperative pain scores and morphine requirements were significantly less with MIDH, and so were rates of early wound-related complications. Interestingly, liver-specific morbidity (bile leak, etc.) was also not significant between the two groups (ODH vs. MIDH). Cosmesis, body image, and reduced absenteeism from work were significantly better with MIDH. Long-term outcomes, especially with regard to the incision (keloid, etc.) and quality of life (QOL) analyses, have significantly favored the MIDH [26, 27, 33, 36–38].

Robotic Donor Hepatectomy (RDH): Given its shorter learning curve, the robotic platform has been increasingly utilized to perform the MIDH. The robotic platform has the added benefits of overcoming restrictions in range of motion, physiological tremor, and a limited field of vision. The high-resolution amplified 3D image, tremor filtration, and additional degrees of freedom of instruments allow for meticulous tissue handling, precise dissection, and easier suturing capabilities [35, 39–41]. Literature comparing RDH with ODH shows comparable blood loss, complication rates, and donor recovery times. A series from Taiwan consisting of 13 RDH showed a reduced analgesic requirement and earlier return to work in the RDH group [42]. Another study from Saudi Arabia, consisting of 150 RDH, also showed a significantly lower pain score, blood loss, and in-hospital stay than ODH patients [40]. A series from India highlighted the advantages of the robotic platform and a safe, stepwise approach to adopting MIDH, especially among surgeons who have previously had limited experience with advanced laparoscopic hepatobiliary surgery [41].

22.7 Donor Hospital Stay and Follow-Up

Donors receive five perioperative doses of piperacillin-tazobactam for antibiotic prophylaxis. After extubation in the operating room, they are transferred to the high dependency unit (HDU), where they are closely monitored with serial arterial blood gas and lactate measurements. Donors typically remain in the HDU for 24–48 h and are usually discharged from the hospital by postoperative day five.

Following discharge, they continue under clinic observation for a month, during which they have weekly outpatient follow-up visits. Long-term monitoring is carried out either by the transplant team or the donor's local physician, with routine blood tests performed every 3 months for the first 6 months and annually thereafter.

22.8 Conclusion

Survival outcomes after liver transplantation (LT) have improved significantly, leading to broader indications for the procedure. These advances reflect growing expertise in managing complex liver diseases. The primary objective of living donor liver transplantation (LDLT) remains ensuring minimal donor morbidity and near-zero mortality while maximizing survival benefits for recipients in need.

The ideal liver transplant survivor is one who maintains stable graft function, exhibits normal growth, and avoids complications related to immunosuppression—a standard that clinicians continually strive to achieve. The foundation for this success lies in a structured, protocol-driven, multidisciplinary approach to donor evaluation and selection.

Conflict of Interest & Financial Support Statement The above doctors have no conflicts of interest or financial ties to disclose.

References

1. Miller CM. Ethical dimensions of living donation: experience with living liver donation. Transplant Rev (Orlando). 2008;22(3):206–9.
2. Chen C-L, Cheng Y-F, Yu C-Y, Ou H-Y, Tsang LL-C, Huang T-L, et al. Living donor liver transplantation: the Asian perspective. Transplantation. 2014;97(Suppl 8):S3.
3. Rammohan A, Reddy MS, Narasimhan G, Rajalingam R, Kaliamoorthy I, Krishnan M, et al. Live liver donors: is right still right? World J Surg. 2020;44:2385.
4. Pruett TL, Tibell A, Alabdulkareem A, Bhandari M, Cronin DC, Dew MA, et al. The ethics statement of the Vancouver forum on the live lung, liver, pancreas, and intestine donor. Transplantation. 2006;81(10):1386–7.
5. LaPointe Rudow D, DeLair S, Feeley T, Florman S, Guarrera J, Kinkhabwala M, et al. Longterm impact of living liver donation: a self-report of the donation experience. Liver Transpl. 2019;25(5):724–33.
6. Butt Z, Dew MA, Liu Q, Simpson MA, Smith AR, Zee J, et al. Psychological outcomes of living liver donors from a multicenter prospective study: results from the adult-to-adult living donor liver transplantation cohort Study2 (A2ALL-2). Am J Transplant. 2017;17(5):1267–77.
7. Rela M, Rammohan A. Patient and donor selection in living donor liver transplantation. Dig Med Res. 2020;3. Dig Med Res [Internet]. 2020; Available from: https://dmr.amegroups.org/article/view/6639.
8. Rela M, Rammohan A. Living liver donation in adults. Liver Transplant [Internet]. 2021; 180–9. Available from: https://doi.org/10.1002/9781119634010.ch24.
9. Song G-W, Lee S-G, Hwang S, Kim K-H, Ahn C-S, Moon D-B, et al. ABO-incompatible adult living donor liver transplantation under the desensitization protocol with rituximab. Am J Transplant. 2016 Jan;16(1):157–70.
10. Lee J, Lee JG, Lee JJ, Kim MS, Ju MK, Choi GH, et al. Results of ABO-incompatible liver transplantation using a simplified protocol at a single institution. Transplant Proc. 2015 Apr;47(3):723–6.
11. Goldaracena N, Jung J, Aravinthan AD, Abbey SE, Krause S, Pritlove C, et al. Donor outcomes in anonymous live liver donation. J Hepatol. 2019 Nov;71(5):951–9.
12. Durand F, Levitsky J, Cauchy F, Gilgenkrantz H, Soubrane O, Francoz C. Age and liver transplantation. J Hepatol [Internet]. 2019;70(4):745–58. Available from: https://doi.org/10.1016/j.jhep.2018.12.009.
13. Pomfret EA, Pomposelli JJ, Jenkins RL. Live donor liver transplantation. J Hepatol. 2001;34(4):613–24.
14. Kim SH, Kim YK, Lee SD, Park SJ. Successful living donor liver transplantation between septuagenarians. Am J Transplant. 2015;15(1):274–7. Available from: https://doi.org/10.1111/ajt.13020.
15. Singh SP, Sikri G, Garg MK. Body mass index and obesity: tailoring "cut-off" for an Asian Indian male population. Med J Armed Forces India. 2008;64(4):350–3.

16. WHO EC. Appropriate body-mass index for Asian populations and its implications for policy and intervention strategies. Lancet (London, England). 2004;363(9403):157–63.
17. Lee S-G. A complete treatment of adult living donor liver transplantation: a review of surgical technique and current challenges to expand indication of patients. Am J Transplant. 2015;15(1):17–38.
18. Ghobrial RM, Freise CE, Trotter JF, Tong L, Ojo AO, Fair JH, et al. Donor morbidity after living donation for liver transplantation. Gastroenterology. 2008 Aug;135(2):468–76.
19. Porret PM, Olthoff KM. Current state of living donor liver transplantation. Clin Liver Dis. 2013;2(4):160–4.
20. Caussy C, Reeder SB, Sirlin CB, Loomba R. Noninvasive, quantitative assessment of liver fat by MRI-PDFF as an endpoint in NASH trials. Hepatology. 2018;68(2):763–72.
21. Hutton C, Gyngell ML, Milanesi M, Bagur A, Brady M. Validation of a standardized MRI method for liver fat and T2* quantification. PLoS One. 2018;13(9):e0204175.
22. Emond JC, Goodrich NP, Pomposelli JJ, Baker TB, Humar A, Grant DR, et al. Hepatic hemodynamics and portal flow modulation: the A2ALL experience. Transplantation. 2017;101(10):2375–84.
23. Rammohan A, Govil S, Rela M. Portosystemic shunts for "small for size syndrome" following liver transplantation: a philosopher's stone? World J Surg. 2017;41(1):341–2.
24. Rammohan A, Gunasekaran V, Reddy MS, Rela M. Graft reduction in pediatric liver transplantation: the myth of 4? Am J Transplant. 2018;18:3081–2.
25. Kokudo T, Hasegawa K, Uldry E, Matsuyama Y, Kaneko J, Akamatsu N, et al. A new formula for calculating standard liver volume for living donor liver transplantation without using body weight [Internet]. J Hepatol. 2015;63:848–54. Available from: https://doi.org/10.1016/j.jhep.2015.05.026.
26. Berardi G, Tomassini F, Troisi RI. Comparison between minimally invasive and open living donor hepatectomy: a systematic review and meta-analysis. Liver Transplant [Internet]. 2015 [cited 2021 Feb 7];21(6):738–52. Available from: https://pubmed.ncbi.nlm.nih.gov/25821097/.
27. Li H, Zhang J-B, Chen XL, Fan L, Wang L, Li SH, et al. Different techniques for harvesting grafts for living donor liver transplantation: a systematic review and meta-analysis. World J Gastroenterol. 2017;23:3730–43.
28. Brige P, Hery G, Chopinet S, Palen A, Azoulay D, Gregoire E. Morbidity and mortality of hepatic right lobe living donors: systematic review and perspectives. J Gastrointest Liver Dis [Internet]. 2018 [cited 2021 Feb 7];27(2):169–78. Available from: https://pubmed.ncbi.nlm.nih.gov/29922762/.
29. Rammohan A, Reddy MS, Narasimhan G, Rajalingam R, Kaliamoorthy I, Krishnan M, et al. Live liver donors: is right still right? World J Surg [Internet]. 2020 [cited 2021 Feb 7];44(7):2385–93. Available from: https://pubmed.ncbi.nlm.nih.gov/32140761/.
30. Narasimhan G, Safwan M, Kota V, Reddy MS, Bharathan A, Dabora A, et al. Donor outcomes in living donor liver transplantation-analysis of 275 donors from a single centre in India. Transplantation [Internet]. 2016 [cited 2021 Feb 7];100(6):1251–6. Available from: https://pubmed.ncbi.nlm.nih.gov/27203592/.
31. Sturdevant ML, Zidan A, Broering D. Minimally-invasive donor hepatectomy at the dawn of a decade: can we pick up the pace? Dig Med Res [Internet]. 2020 [cited 2021 Feb 7];3(0):58. Available from: http://dmr.amegroups.com/article/view/6805/html.
32. Soubrane O, Perdigao Cotta F, Scatton O. Pure laparoscopic right hepatectomy in a living donor. Am J Transplant [Internet]. 2013 [cited 2021 Feb 7];13(9):2467–71. Available from: https://pubmed.ncbi.nlm.nih.gov/23865716/.
33. Zhang B, Pan Y, Chen K, Maher H, Chen MY, Zhu HP, et al. Laparoscopy-assisted versus open hepatectomy for live liver donor: systematic review and meta-analysis. Can J Gastroenterol Hepatol. 2017;2017:2956749.
34. Cherqui D, Ciria R, Kwon CHD, Kim KH, Broering D, Wakabayashi G, et al. Expert consensus guidelines on minimally invasive donor hepatectomy for living donor liver transplantation from innovation to implementation: a joint initiative from the International Laparoscopic Liver

Society (ILLS) and the Asian-Pacific Hepato-Pancreat. Ann Surg [Internet]. 2021 [cited 2021 Feb 7];273(1):96–108. Available from: https://pubmed.ncbi.nlm.nih.gov/33332874/.
35. Rammohan A., Rela M. Robotic donor hepatectomy: Are we there yet? http://www.wjgnet.com/ [Internet]. 2021 [cited 2021 Aug 1];13(7):668–77. Available from: https://www.wjgnet.com/1948-9366/full/v13/i7/668.htm.
36. Suh KS, Hong SK, Lee KW, Yi NJ, Kim HS, Ahn SW, et al. Pure laparoscopic living donor hepatectomy: focus on 55 donors undergoing right hepatectomy. Am J Transplant. 2018;18(2):434–43.
37. Hong SK, Lee KW, Choi Y, Kim HS, Ahn SW, Yoon KC, et al. Initial experience with purely laparoscopic living-donor right hepatectomy. Br J Surg [Internet]. 2018 [cited 2021 Feb 8];105(6):751–9. Available from: https://pubmed.ncbi.nlm.nih.gov/29579333/.
38. Broering DC, Zidan A. Advancements in robotic living donor hepatectomy, review of literature and single-center experience [Internet]. Curr Transplant Rep. 2020 [cited 2021 Feb 7]; 7:324–31. Available from: https://link.springer.com/article/10.1007/s40472-020-00311-0.
39. Lincango Naranjo EP, Garces-Delgado E, Siepmann T, Mirow L, Solis-Pazmino P, Alexander-Leon H, et al. Robotic living donor right hepatectomy: a systematic review and meta-analysis. J Clin Med. 2022;11(9):2603.
40. Broering DC, Elsheikh Y, Alnemary Y, Zidan A, Elsarawy A, Saleh Y, et al. Robotic versus open right lobe donor hepatectomy for adult living donor liver transplantation: a propensity score–matched analysis. Liver Transplant. 2020;26(11):1455–64.
41. Rela M, Rajalingam R, Cherukuru R, Palaniappan K, Kumar SA, Kanagavelu R, et al. Experience with establishing a robotic donor hepatectomy program for pediatric liver transplantation. Transplantation. 2023;107:2554.
42. Da CP, Wu CY, Hu RH, Ho CM, Lee PH, Lai HS, et al. Robotic liver donor right hepatectomy: a pure, minimally invasive approach. Liver Transplant. 2016;22(11):1509–18.

Chapter 23
Recipient Surgery in Living Donor Liver Transplant

Subhash Gupta, Rajesh Dey, and Inbaraj Balradja

Abstract This chapter describes how to carry out recipient surgery safely with minimal blood loss in living donor liver transplant. Broadly, the recipient surgery is divided into liver explantation, temporary portocaval shunt creation, harvesting the explant liver's portal vein and umbilical vein, bench work which includes reconstruction of the anterior sector veins of the partial liver graft, and liver graft implantation. Liver explantation is explained in the sequence of operating room requirements, preoperative preparation, incision, left lobe mobilization, right lobe mobilization, retro-hepatic dissection, phrenocaval dissociation, porta dissection, porta division, and explantation. This chapter also briefly explains the need for temporary portocaval shunt creation. Benchwork involves the reconstruction of anterior sector veins and unification of multiple portal veins to create a new middle hepatic vein and single portal inflow, respectively, using either a portal vein graft harvested from the recipient liver or cryopreserved cadaveric vein grafts or synthetic grafts. Implantation involves connecting the graft's hepatic veins and portal vein to the recipient's inferior vena cava and main portal veins. The graft is then given blood flow again through the portal vein (reperfusion). Post-reperfusion, graft hepatic artery is anastomosed to the appropriate recipient hepatic artery. The intraoperative Doppler ultrasound is done to ensure the patency of the anastomosed vessels, followed by anastomosis of the graft bile duct with the recipient bile duct.

Keywords Incision · Recipient hepatectomy · Hemostasis · Temporary portacaval shunt · Benchwork · Portal vein graft · NeoMHV reconstruction · Hepatic · Portal and hepatic artery anastomosis · Bile duct anastomosis · Intraoperative cholangiogram

---

S. Gupta (✉) · I. Balradja
Centre for Liver and Biliary Sciences (CLBS), Max Super Speciality Hospital, Saket, New Delhi, India
e-mail: guptasubash@hotmail.com

R. Dey
Centre for Liver and Biliary Sciences, Max Saket and Vaishali Hospitals, New Delhi, India

S. Saigal, D. Jothimani (eds.), *Fundamentals of Transplant Hepatology*,
https://doi.org/10.1007/978-981-95-2624-6_23

Key Highlights

Liver explantation involves the surgical removal of the diseased liver with minimal blood loss following avascular planes.

Temporary portocaval shunt post-liver explantation helps prevent bowel edema and renal dysfunction.

Native liver right and left portal veins in continuation with the umbilical vein are harvested for use in benching.

Benchwork involves the meticulous reconstruction of segment 5 and segment 8 veins with harvested portal vein or PTFE to create NeoMHV for draining the anterior sector of the graft.

Liver graft implantation involves serial anastomosis of graft hepatic veins, portal vein, hepatic artery, and bile ducts with recipient inferior vena cava, portal vein, right or left hepatic artery, and bile ducts, respectively.

23.1 Operating Room Requirements

The operating room is setup with ECG monitors, temperature probes, cardiac output measurement devices, and equipment for real-time measurement of arterial blood gas, electrolytes, hemoglobin, PT, and thromboelastography and patient temperature regulatory device and positioning devices for head support and limb support. Catheters for rapid infusion of fluids, two arterial lines for monitoring and sampling, and occasionally a Swan-Ganz catheter in a high-risk recipient are positioned.

23.2 Preoperative Preparation

A. The patient is given preoperative medication half an hour before incision. At our center, the antimicrobials in use as per unit protocol are a combination of piperacillin/tazobactam, teicoplanin, and fluconazole. All our patients are given amphotericin B orally 48 h before surgery.
B. An intercostal drainage tube is placed, if there is a pre diagnosed significant pleural effusion
C. A urinary catheter is placed for monitoring urine output.
D. Bair Hugger and warming mattresses are used to prevent hypothermia.
E. Special precaution is taken for the support and care of pressure points such as the heel and scalp. The feet must be supported at 90 degrees flexion to avoid foot drop.

F. The patient is scrubbed with Betadine paint and solution.
G. Three tiers of liver drapes are placed ensuring no fluid seepage occurs thereby prevent cautery burns.
H. Cell saver may occasionally be used in cases where massive bleeding is expected.
I. Dialysis lines may rarely need to be placed in anticipation of the need for intra-operative dialysis support.
J. The instruments include Omni-Tract or Thompson retractors, microvascular surgery set, argon beam coagulator, two cautery machines and handles, two large suction cannulae of which one should be a sump suction, and a small suction cannula. The need for magnification loupe and headlights cannot be overemphasized.

23.3 Incision

A bilateral subcostal incision is given with upper midline extension (Fig. 23.1). The incision extends from the midclavicular line on the left to the anterior axillary line on the right side. The xiphoid process is the limit for upper midline extension. The incision is deepened with diathermy, and the bleeding points are controlled necessary. The umbilical ligament is ligated and divided but can be preserved if there is a large para-umbilical shunt until the time of porta division (Fig. 23.2). The falciform ligament is divided until the loose connective tissue surrounding the hepatic veins is reached. The costal margins are elevated for proper exposure using self-retaining retractors.

23.4 Initial Assessment

For a patient with hepatocellular carcinoma (HCC), an abdominal survey is done to look for any metastatic deposits in the recto-vesical pouch, peritoneum, porta, and liver surface. Any suspicious node in the hepatoduodenal region or along the hepatic artery is sent for frozen section. Usually, the donor surgery is started first prior to the recipient surgery, but in cases of downstaged HCC, recipient surgery is started first to rule out any extrahepatic disease.

23.5 Left Lobe Mobilization

The lesser omentum is divided taking care to preserve any accessory left hepatic artery (Fig. 23.3). The left triangular ligament is divided in the following manner. The surgeon lifts the left lobe from beneath, while the assistant gives a gentle traction on the upper pole of the spleen; a mop is placed beneath the left lobe and the

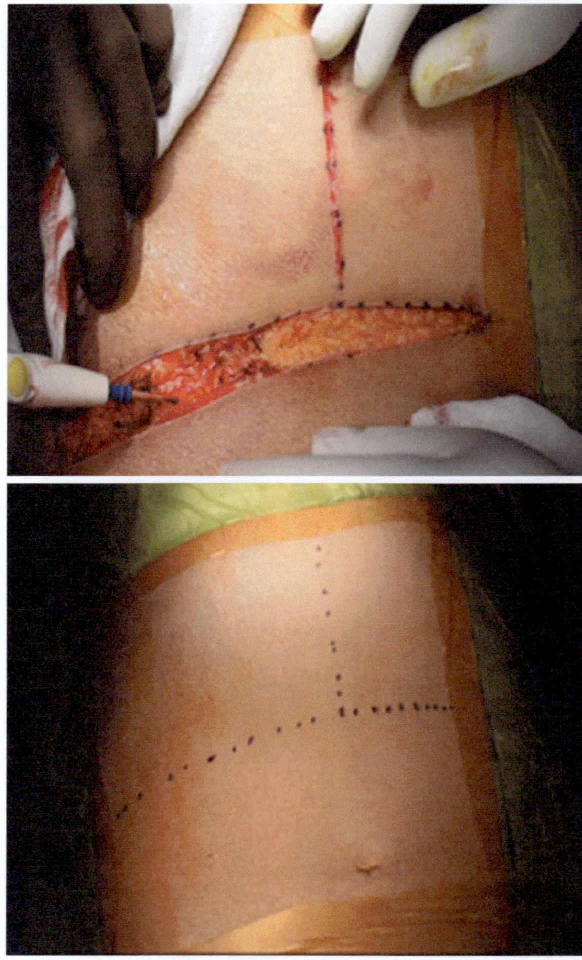

Fig. 23.1 Transverse incision with upper midline extension

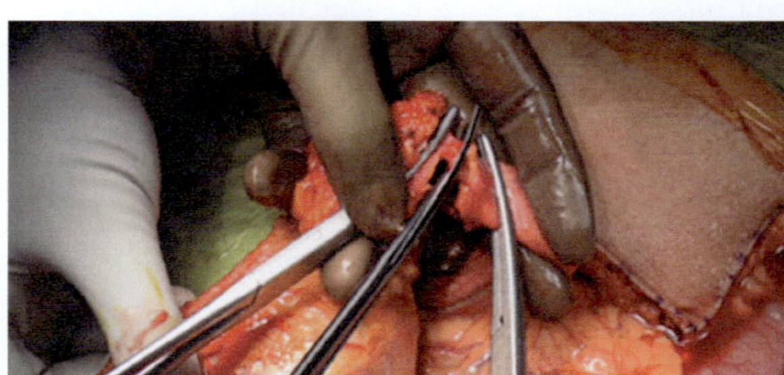

Fig. 23.2 Division of the falciform ligament

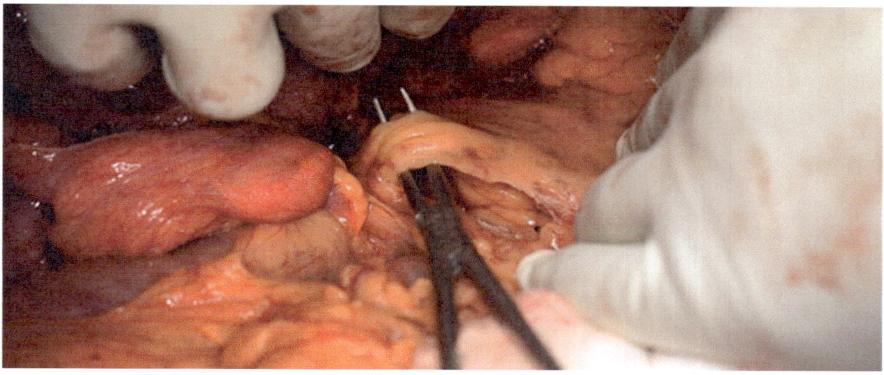

Fig. 23.3 Division of the gastrohepatic ligament and mobilization of the left lobe

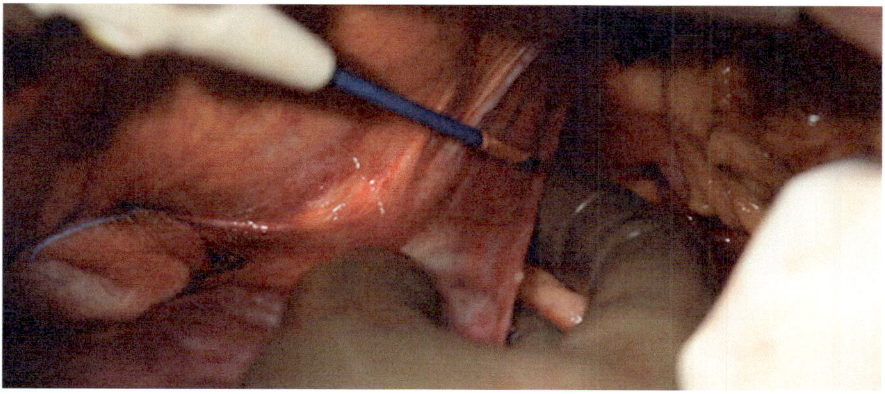

Fig. 23.4 Division of the left triangular ligament

triangular ligament overlying the anterior surface of the stomach and the anterior surface of the upper pole of the spleen. Then, the left triangular ligament is divided from the lateral end (Fig. 23.4). The whole of the ligament is avascular apart from overlying collaterals, which are meticulously cauterized. The lateral end often carries a vessel, which must be ligated and divided. After the division of the lesser

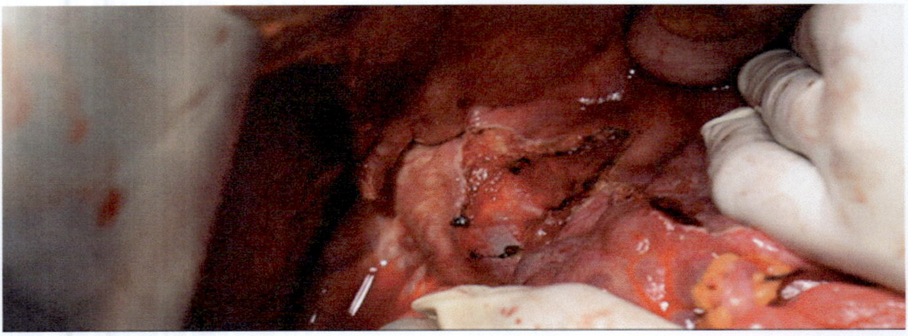

Fig. 23.5 Supra-hepatic dissection to expose the RHV and MHV-LHV confluence

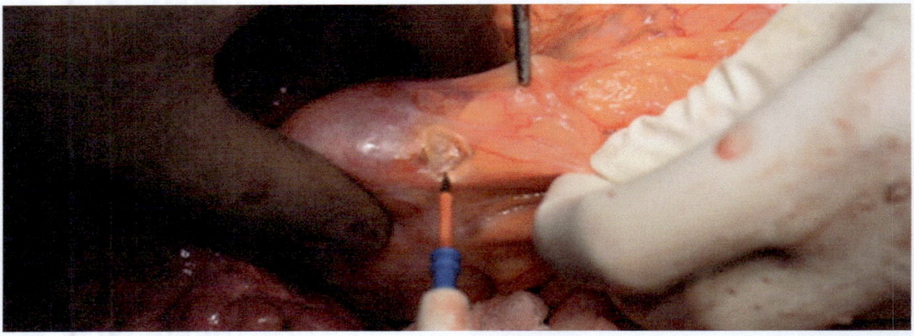

Fig. 23.6 Releasing the adhesion between the gallbladder and omentum

omentum, the Arantius ligament is divided between ties. The peritoneum over the supra-hepatic inferior vena cava is freed, to expose the right hepatic vein (RHV) and middle hepatic vein (MHV)-LHV confluence (Fig. 23.5).

23.6 Right Lobe Mobilization

Initially, the adhesions between the gallbladder and the omentum are released (Fig. 23.6). It starts with the division of the right triangular and coronary ligament (Fig. 23.7). Once the right triangular ligament is divided, the dissection is continued medially dividing the superior and inferior coronary ligament with traction from the assistant to rotate the right lobe medially in the surgical field. The bare area of the liver is exposed, and the retroperitoneal attachments are divided as the right lobe is further retracted medially.

The right adrenal gland must be separated carefully from the right lobe of the liver (Fig. 23.8). Occasionally, the gland is very adherent to the liver in which case it may need to be kept with the right lobe partially. However, staying close to the

Fig. 23.7 Division of the right triangular ligament

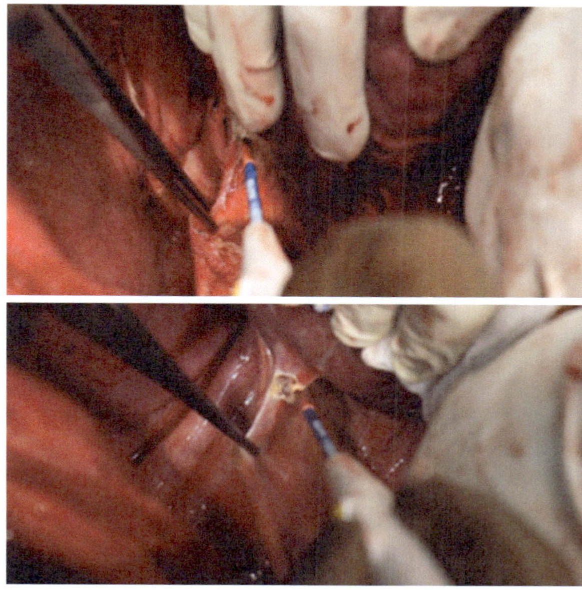

Fig. 23.8 Separation of the right adrenal gland from the liver

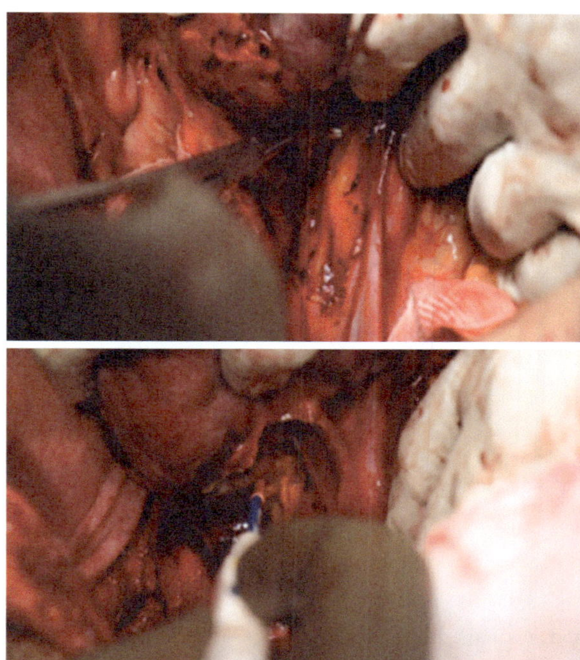

liver capsule, one may be able to separate the adrenal gland from the liver. With the help of saline dissection over the inferior vena cava (IVC), one may be able to open this plane easily. The adrenal vein needs to be identified, ligated, and divided.

Bleeding must be controlled as the surgery progresses to prevent sudden hemodynamic collapse. Bleeding from the liver surface may be controlled by clamping of the porta in cases where the liver has dense vascularized adhesions with the retroperitoneum. It is essential to ensure that dissection proceeds in the plane between liver capsule and peritoneum as deviation from the plane can result in significant bleeding.

23.7 IVC Clearance

As the infra-hepatic vena cava comes into view, the short hepatic veins draining the right lobe and the caudate are then ligated. The peritoneum over the vena-cava inferior to the caudate lobe of the liver is incised and extended circumferentially to loop the cava (Fig. 23.9). Identification and isolation of the infra hepatic cava is an essential step as it provides access for applying a cross clamp in the event of inadvertent significant caval bleeding. The division of short hepatic veins is continued up to the level of the right hepatic vein such that almost the whole of the caval anterior surface is cleared and the right hepatic vein is looped after dividing the hepatocaval ligament (Fig. 23.10).

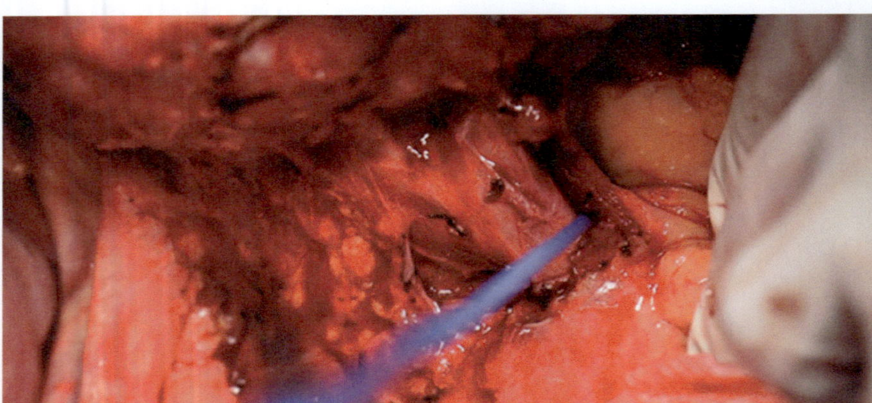

Fig. 23.9 Looping the infra-hepatic vena cava

This is necessary in living donor liver transplant where the piggyback technique of caval preservation is necessary. In cadaveric transplant with caval replacement, this step may not be necessary as once the lower cava is looped, space can be quickly created by blunt dissection so that the supra-hepatic cava can be clamped with a stout clamp prior to rapid hepatectomy.

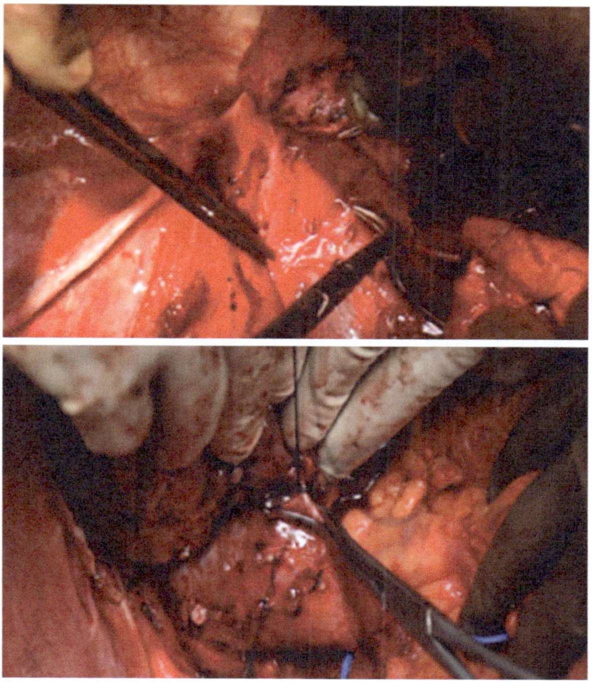

Fig. 23.10 Division of short hepatic veins and inferior hepatic vein (IHV) with exposure of RHV

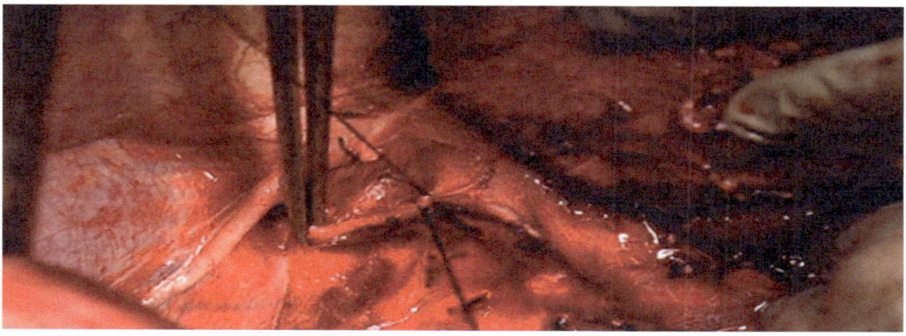

Fig. 23.11 Phrenocaval separation

23.8 Phrenocaval Separation

Ligating the right phrenic veins frees the IVC from diaphragmatic attachment and secures easy application of caval clamp for dividing right hepatic vein prior to liver removal. Further, this maneuver helps in getting a triphasic outflow post-right vein-anastomosis. However, this must be done carefully as the IVC becomes quite thin at this level, particularly in the posterior part. The phrenic veins are doubly ligated prior to division and the stumps are suture transfixed keeping in mind that this site may be a source of potential bleeding (Fig. 23.11).

23.9 Portal Dissection

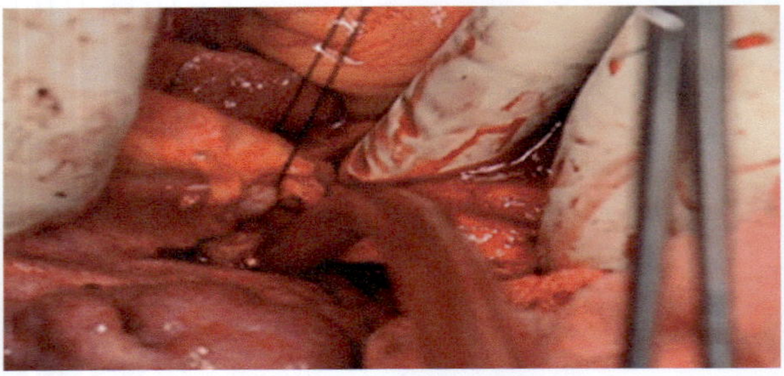

Attention is then turned to the porta where the cystic duct and artery are ligated and divided in the Calot's triangle; the cystic duct stump is kept long (Fig. 23.12). The anterior layer of the peritoneum over the hepatoduodenal ligament is incised with cautery. The left hepatic artery and its segment IV branch are dissected and cleared for around 2 cm, ligated, and divided preferably beyond its branching to prevent arterial dissection of the hepatic artery (Fig. 23.13). The right gastric artery is ligated and divided freeing the left hepatic artery for anastomosis. At the time of dissection, care should be taken to avoid vasospasm and intimal dissection. The main portal vein is looped after incising the peritoneum lateral and posterior to it starting from the right side. The right hepatic artery is dissected and divided distal to its bifurcation close to the bile duct to prevent devascularization of the bile duct (Fig. 23.13).

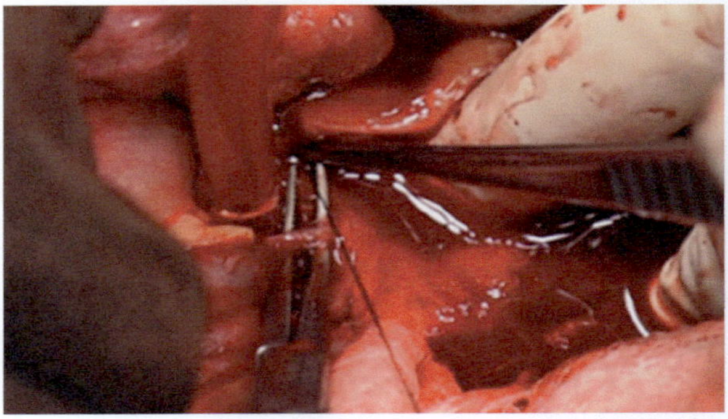

Fig. 23.12 Cystic artery and cystic duct ligation

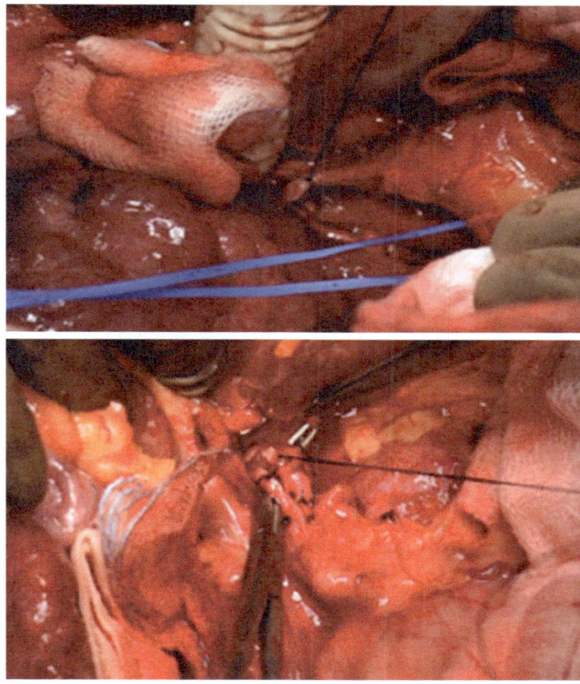

Fig. 23.13 Division of the left hepatic artery and right hepatic artery

23.10 Division of Porta

Once the parenchymal transection has been completed in the donor, the cirrhotic liver in the recipient is removed. In this manner, the anhepatic phase (the period between division of portal vein and reperfusion) can be kept short. In a special circumstance like a fulminant hepatic failure, portal vein thrombosis, or excessive bleeding, the portal vessels are ligated first to remove the liver quickly.

The right and left portal vein branches are identified with corresponding bile duct branches (Fig. 23.14). Adhesions between the bile duct and portal vein are released. Right and left bile ducts are divided using cautery high up in the porta separately so that multiple ducts are obtained in case multiple anastomoses are required during implantation (Fig. 23.14). Periductal vessels in the hilar plate are secured by stitching. The portal vein is lengthened by dividing one or two small branches distally. The portal vein is clamped proximally and distally just below the confluence of the right and left portal vein and divided (Fig. 23.15).

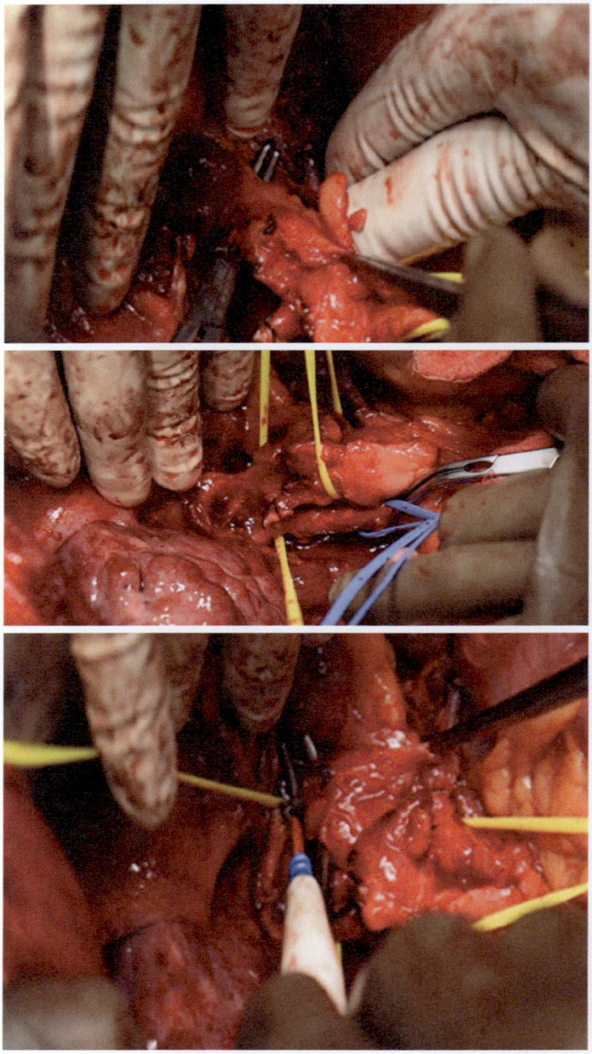

Fig. 23.14 Looping of the common bile duct and the right pedicle separately. Division of the right hepatic duct and left hepatic duct separately with cautery

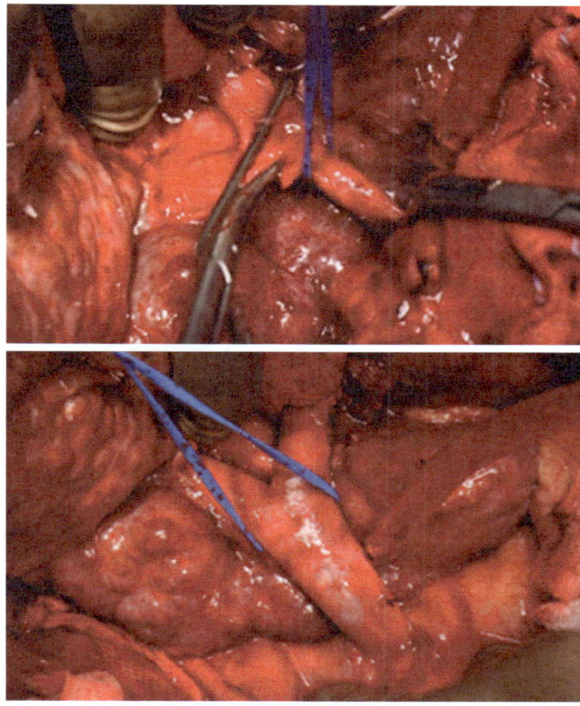

Fig. 23.15 Portal vein extension and division below the confluence

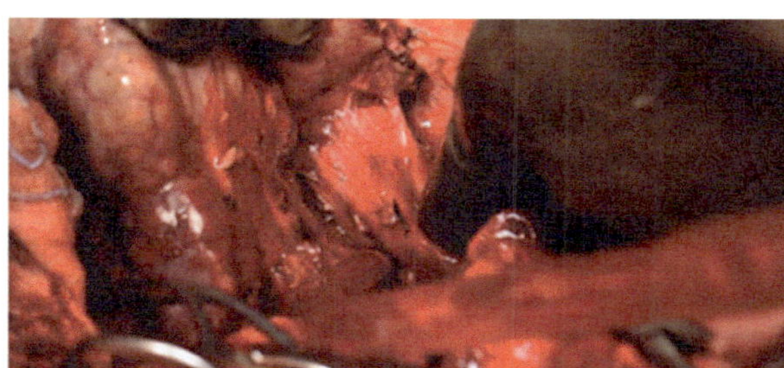

Fig. 23.16 Separating liver from the IVC

23.11 Explantation

The peritoneal layer reflection over the left lateral surface of IVC is divided parallel and close along the length of the IVC until the left hepatic vein (Fig. 23.16). The loose tissue posterior to the cava is gently separated, and the lower cava is freed until the level of renal veins. At this moment, the liver is attached to the IVC only by the hepatic veins. The right hepatic vein is now clamped and divided with a stump of 5 mm in the IVC and closed temporarily with a 4–0 Prolene suture (Fig. 23.17). Middle and left hepatic veins are clamped together and divided into the liver. This leaves a stump of 1–2 cm for MHV implantation (Fig. 23.18).

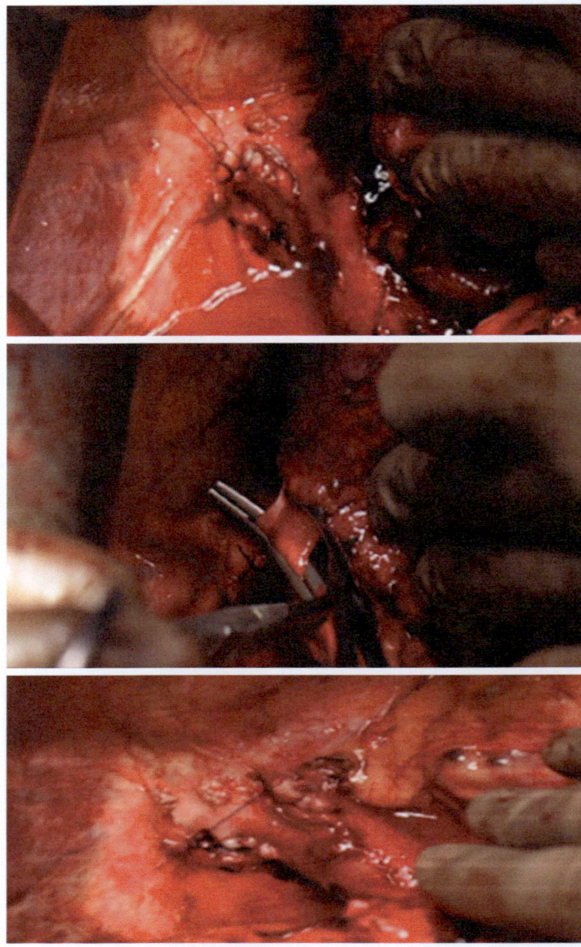

Fig. 23.17 RHV division and temporary closure

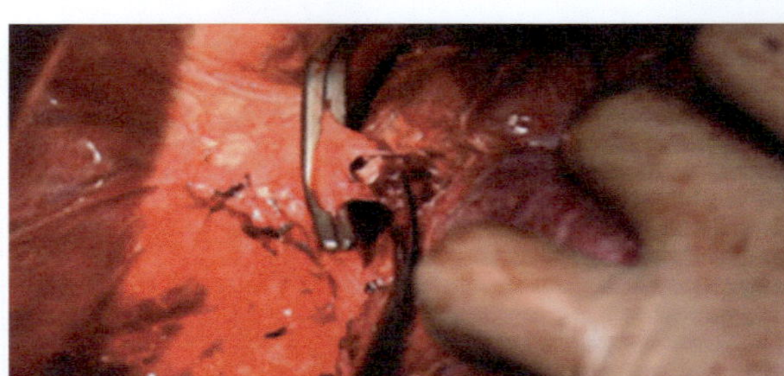

Fig. 23.18 Division of the MHV-LHV and temporary closure

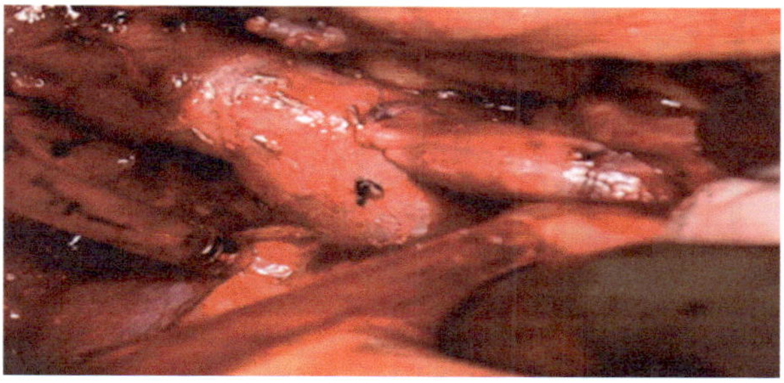

Fig. 23.19 Temporary portocaval shunt

23.11.1 Temporary Portocaval Shunt

A temporary portocaval shunt is made between the porta vein and the IVC to prevent bowel edema, maintain hemodynamic stability and renal function, and reduce blood transfusion (Fig. 23.19).

23.11.2 Hemostasis

Before implantation, an effort is made to achieve hemostasis, especially around the retroperitoneum, retro-hepatic area, and the pericaval region as once the new liver is implanted, this area is hard to visualize and rotating the new liver may jeopardize the newly reconstructed vessels. Hence, it is of prime importance to accomplish appropriate hemostasis before implantation starts. During the anhepatic phase, the use of tranexamic acid may help in the prevention of clot lysis.

23.11.3 Benchwork

Before implantation, the graft must be assessed carefully with a special focus on the V5 and V8 branches, IHVs, and portal vein. Bench surgery while the liver is in ice will facilitate easy anastomosis so that the warm ischemic time is considerably reduced. During bench surgery, the commonest procedure is related to the hepatic vein as usually the right lobe is retrieved without the MHV which is left in the remnant to ensure safe donor outcome. The 5 and 8 segmental branches are then reconstructed to form a new MHV. Similarly, if there are multiple accessory (inferior) hepatic veins, they are joined together to create a common outflow so that the minimal number of anastomoses is needed during the warm ischaemic phase.

23.12 Portal Vein Graft Harvesting from the Explanted Native Liver

The portal vein in the recipient is divided just proximal to the bifurcation so that there is no narrowing in the portal vein graft when it is stitched to make a combined right and left portal vein graft. After the native liver is removed, portal vein and umbilical vein grafts are harvested in the bench (Fig. 23.20). The right anterior, right posterior, and left portal veins with side branches are retrieved for subsequent anastomosis to the MHV tributaries in the donor liver. The dissection plane of PV is continued onto the umbilical vein until a long length of the graft is available. The umbilical vein is then recanalized on the bench by using a mosquito forceps inserted from a segmental branch opening until the constriction at its junction with the portal vein is dilated. Recanalization can also be done in a similar manner from the other end. Occasionally, the junction between the PV and UV cannot be dilated, and in this case, the graft is divided, dilated, and re-anastomosed to obtain an adequate length (Fig. 23.20).

Another popular technique is to use a synthetic (PTFE) or cadaveric grafts for reconstruction of a new MHV.

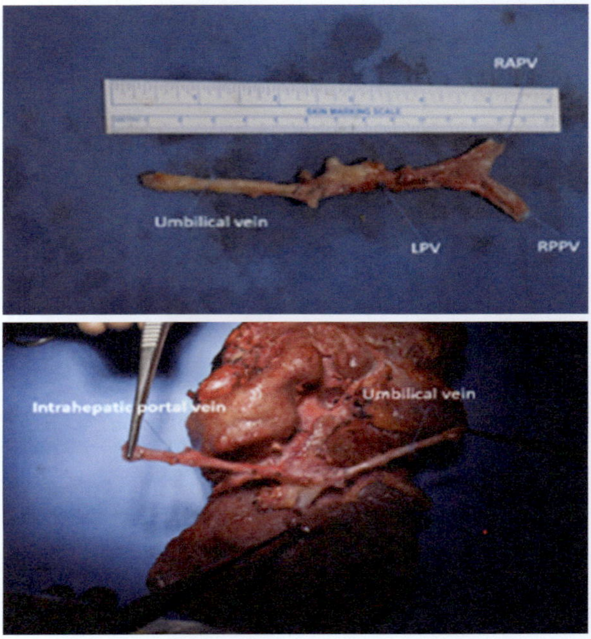

Fig. 23.20 Retrieval of the portal vein with umbilical vein from the explant liver

23.13 MHV Reconstruction

The anastomosis of V5 and V8 is made in the bench. The PV with UV graft is orientated in such a manner that the various tributaries on the graft match the segmental branches of the retrieved graft. V8 is anastomosed first to a branch of the left portal vein graft, then to the farthest V5 vein. For selecting a side branch for V8 reconstruction, the PV&UV graft is placed in the course of MHV in the graft, the side branches are orientated with tributaries in the graft, and a check is made to see that an adequate stump for anastomosis is available. After the first V8 anastomosis, the farthest V5 is anastomosed, and subsequently, the other sizable tributaries are joined to the graft (Fig. 23.21). Commonly, the umbilical end is anastomosed to the MHV stump, but it is quite possible that the lie of the tributaries may be such that the orientation of the graft will need to be reversed and portal vein end will then be joined to the MHV stump. All the anastomoses are made with 6–0 Prolene continuous suture with a growth factor. Patency and leak in the reconstructed MHV are checked by pushing saline in the lumen and marking stitch placed at 12 0'clock for proper alignment during implantation (Fig. 23.22).

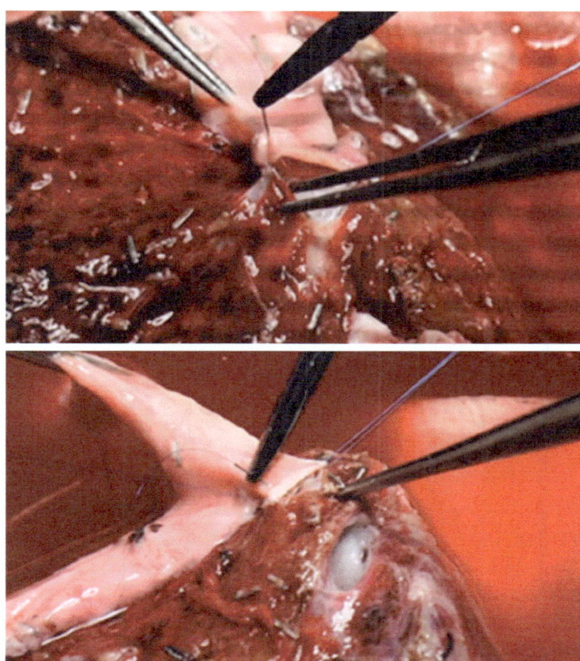

Fig. 23.21 Reconstruction of segment 8 and 5 vein in benching

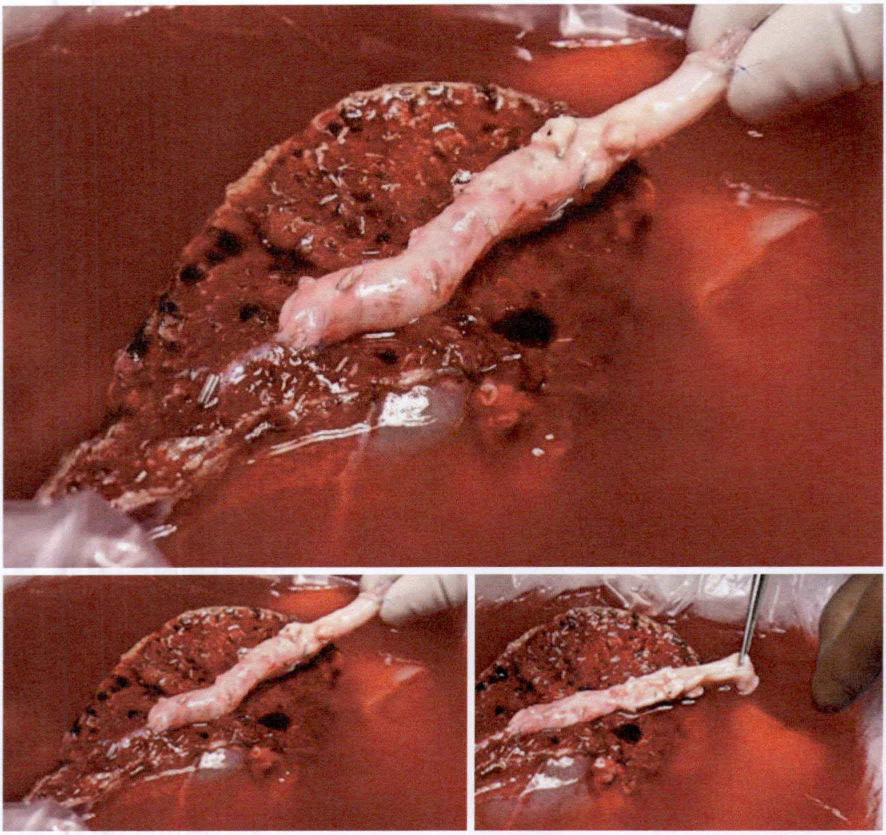

Fig. 23.22 Checking for patency and leak in the reconstructed middle vein and placing marking stitch for correct alignment

23.14 Portal Vein Benching

The portal vein if multiple will need to be anastomosed so that one inflow anastomosis can be carried out. If the cuff is small, hepatic vein can be retrieved from the explant liver and stitched circumferentially to lengthen it (Fig. 23.23). This is particularly helpful as with a short cuff, anastomosis can be particularly difficult. When they are multiple, if they are very close to each other, one wall can be stitched to the adjacent wall of the other branch and then a cuff stitched circumferentially to the combined two veins.

Occasionally, if the branches are far apart, a Y-shaped graft from the explant portal vein together with the right and left portal vein branches is retrieved and the two portal vein branches are joined to each other after ensuring perfect alignment (Fig. 23.24). After each anastomosis is completed, either a growth factor can be left,

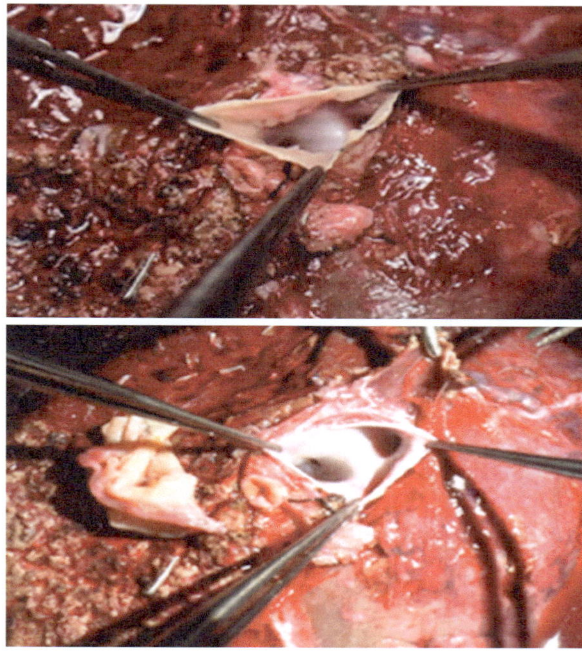

Fig. 23.23 Hepatic vein retrieved from the explant liver stitched circumferentially to lengthen the short cuff of the portal vein

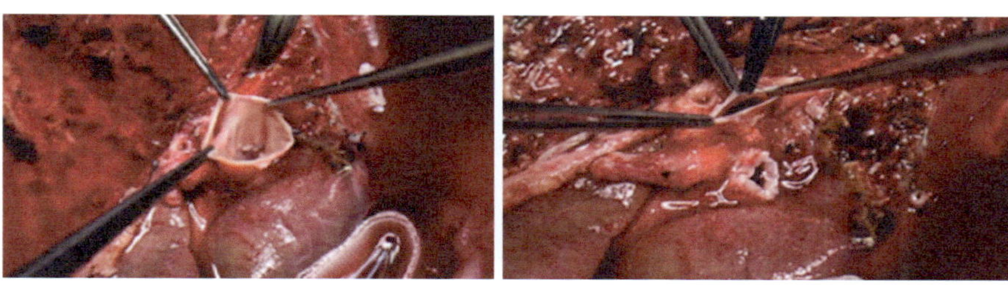

Fig. 23.24 Y-shaped graft used for joining two portal veins

or the anastomosis can be stretched with a large right angle, and then, the knots are tied.

If a Y-shaped graft is not available, a small tubular vein graft may be used for end-to-end anastomosis with each of the portal vein branch. Subsequently, a new opening is made in the center of the graft so that anastomosis can be carried out (Fig. 23.25).

Another option if Y-shaped graft is not available is to place the explant liver hepatic vein patch between the portal vein orifices, and then, a cuff of hepatic vein is stitched circumferentially to enable a single anastomosis in the recipient (Fig. 23.26).

If the graft portal vein is small as compared to the recipient portal vein, a bigger extension vein graft can be stitched to it to ensure size match while anastomosing in the recipient.

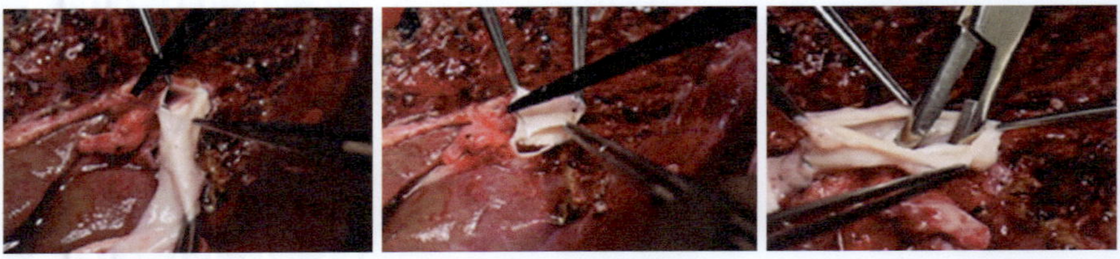

Fig. 23.25 Tubular graft used for joining two portal veins

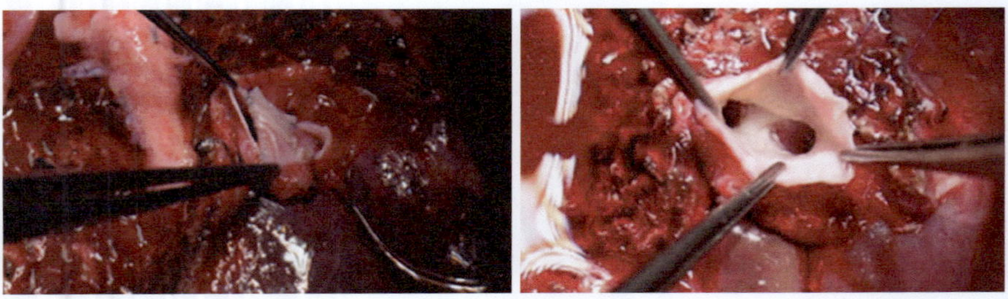

Fig. 23.26 Hepatic vein patch between portal vein orifices with hepatic vein cuff placed circumferentially

23.15 Implantation

Before the start of implantation, hemostasis of the retroperitoneum is checked again. Mobilization of the IVC is checked for ease of reconstruction of IHVs which is often far away from the right hepatic vein. The temporary portocaval shunt is taken down. Any large shunts are identified and ligated after testing for an increase in the portal flow. Orientation and flow in the portal vein are also confirmed.

23.16 Right Hepatic Vein Reconstruction

A side biting vascular clamp is placed around the right hepatic vein stump which may often need to be enlarged. Graft right hepatic vein is anastomosed to recipient right hepatic vein stump. Corner stitches are taken with a 4–0 Prolene suture. Anastomosis starts with a 5–0 Prolene suture from the middle of the posterior layer which is initially continued caudally to the corner stitch. Then, it starts from the middle of the posterior layer to the corners cranially which is continued into the anterior layer, and it is completed with a growth factor (Fig. 23.27). Corner stitches are tied. The Bulldog clamp is placed on the IVC across the anastomosis and the side clamp released.

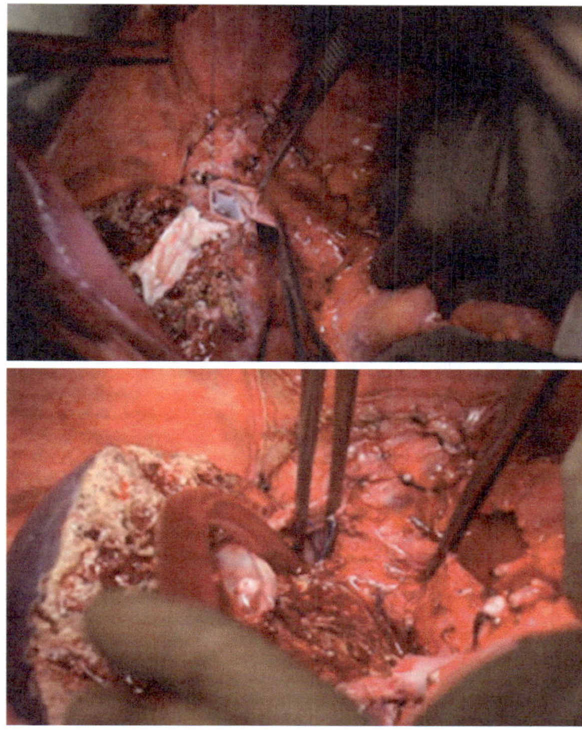

Fig. 23.27 Graft RHV anastomosed to the recipient RHV stump with a growth factor

23.17 IHV Reconstruction

IHVs are considered for anastomosis irrespective of the size if it admits a dilator deep inside. The goal is to decrease the number of anastomosis to decrease the cold ischemia time and warm ischemia time without compromising venous outflow. In cases of difficult implantation such as in big grafts and small retro-hepatic space, multiple hepatic veins can be joined together so that one anastomosis can be done [1]. In general, it is preferable to join all significant IHVs as it also helps in maintaining true orthotopic position as it was in the donor (Fig. 23.28).

23.18 MHV Reconstruction

A side clamp is placed distal to the middle and left hepatic vein stump for anastomosis of the reconstructed MHV (Fig. 23.29). This is usually done with a 5–0 Prolene continuous suture with a growth factor. A Bulldog clamp is placed proximal to the anastomosis and side clamp released. The right hepatic vein and reconstructed

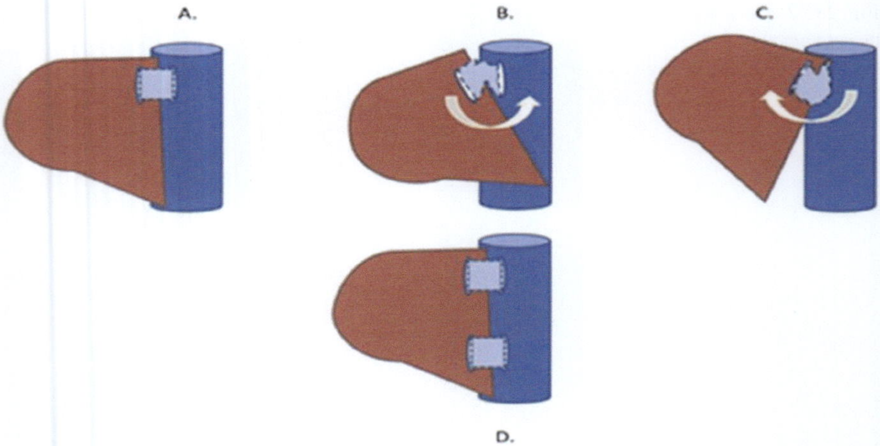

Fig. 23.28 (**a**–**c**) Without IHV reconstruction—graft only fixed at one point; (**d**) with IHV reconstruction—graft fixed at two points—holds graft better in the orthotopic position [2]

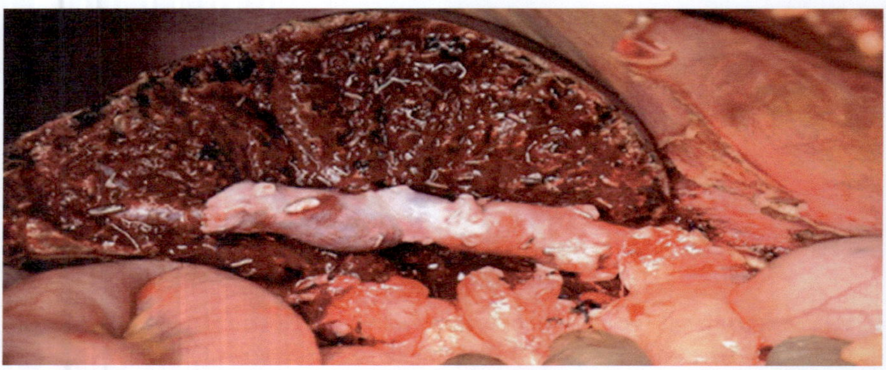

Fig. 23.29 Reconstructed MHV anastomosed to the MHV-LHV stump

MHV can also be joined together in the back bench and anastomosed to the IVC as a single orifice.

23.19 Portal Vein Reconstruction

The orientation of the recipient and graft portal vein is aligned prior to anastomosis with 5–0 Prolene continuous suture with a large growth factor (Fig. 23.30).

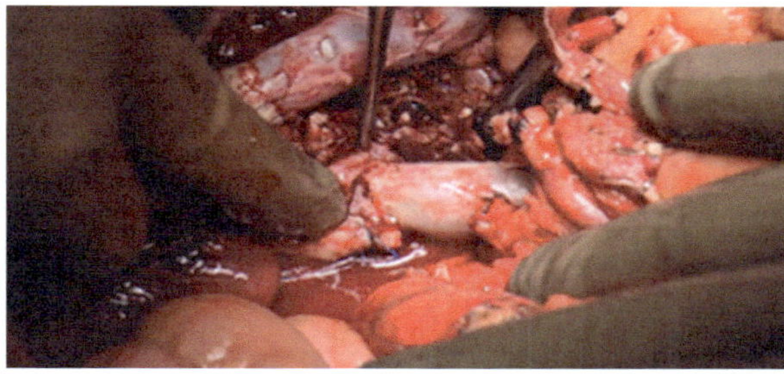

Fig. 23.30 Recipient main portal vein anastomosed to graft right portal vein

23.20 Reperfusion

Clamps are released serially from the right hepatic vein, MHV, IHVs, and portal vein. Major bleeding points after reperfusion are controlled. Growth factors in the portal vein and hepatic vein are inspected to see that they have been taken up completely. If required, additional interrupted sutures are taken in the hepatic vein and portal vein with 6–0 Prolene sutures.

23.21 Hepatic Artery Reconstruction

Backflow in the graft hepatic artery is checked, and the lumen is stretched with a microdilator. The edges are freshened, and a Bulldog clamp is applied with a right-to-left orientation. Preferably, the recipient left hepatic artery is used for anastomosis for reasons of better size matching with the donor artery. The lymph node around the left hepatic artery is removed, and the right gastric artery is ligated and divided so that the reconstructed artery rests on the portal vein. After applying a small metallic Bulldog clamp, the recipient artery is prepared by clearing all adventitial tissues from the intima. The arterial anastomosis is done with 8–0 interrupted Prolene sutures (Fig. 23.31). In case of multiple donor arteries, recipient right and left arteries are anastomosed separately to graft arteries.

23.21.1 Microscope Versus Surgical Loupes

Hepatic artery reconstruction under surgical loupe magnification can be performed expeditiously and yields similar results with the operating microscope [3–7]. The reconstruction with a surgical loupe is faster as compared to the microscope as it can be done without having to set up the microscope [3]. The minimum requirement of hepatic artery reconstruction is a magnification of 3.5× and above [5].

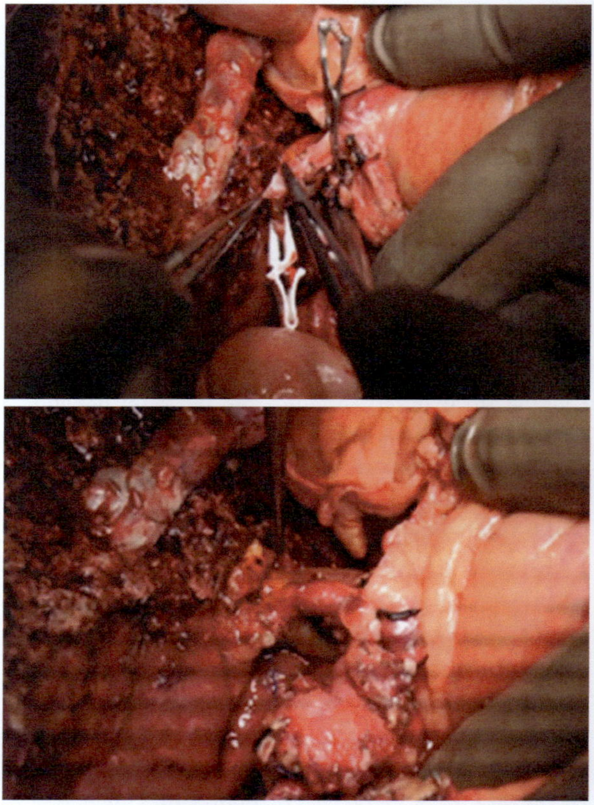

Fig. 23.31 Graft RHA anastomosed to recipient LHA

23.22 Biliary Reconstruction

The number of ducts in the graft is assessed by probing with a dilator or a Watson Cheyne Dissector. The hilar plate small ducts in the graft are sutured with 6 0 polypropylene suture. When the graft duct is single, anastomosis is done to the recipient common hepatic duct after gentle dilatation with a small right angle.

The posterior layer of the bile duct is aligned with the left wall of the duct so that more of the posterior duct is around half the circumference of the bile duct (Fig. 23.32). The anastomosis can be either continuous or interrupted. If interrupted, the knots can be placed both inside and outside depending on personal preference. In case of multiple ducts, if the two ducts are very close to each other, then a single anastomosis can be done. Multiple ducts are joined individually rather than by ductoplasty. The recipient duct should be bigger than the donor duct. If not, Roux-en-Y hepaticojejunostomy may be preferable, or else, the cystic duct and bile duct openings can be made into one prior to anastomosis. The recipient bile duct should be trimmed to avoid redundancy or swan neck deformity. A routine check cholangiogram via the cystic duct is helpful but not an essential part of the reconstruction (Fig. 23.33). Small leaks can be stitched if identified on the cholangiogram.

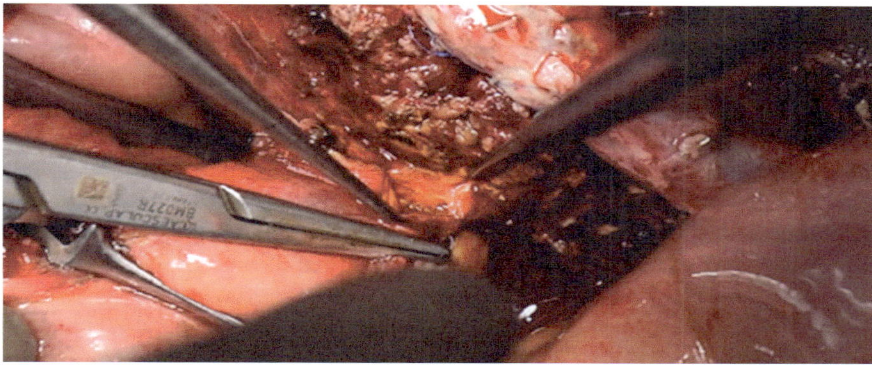

Fig. 23.32 End-to-end bile duct anastomosis with 7–0 interrupted PDS sutures

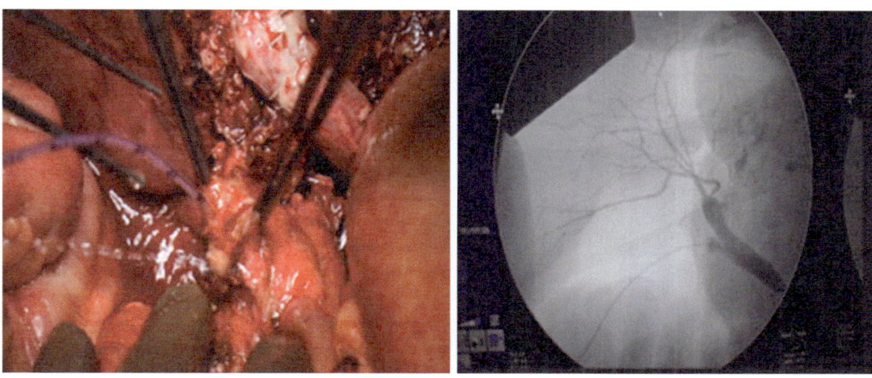

Fig. 23.33 Cystic duct cannulation and intraoperative cholangiogram

Intraoperative Doppler is performed to look for integrity of hepatic veins and portal vein anastomoses. The hepatic vein flows should ideally be triphasic. The portal vein anastomosis is checked for alignment, and the volume flow is measured. The ideal situation would require a portal volume flow of between 150 and 400 ml/100 g of liver tissue. The hepatic artery flow velocity should be greater than 25 ml/min, and the normal hepatic arterial Resistive Index ranges from 0.55 to 0.80 [8, 9].

23.23 Hemostasis and Drain Placement

Post-implantation, thorough hemostasis is attained with special attention in the region of retroperitoneum, pericaval region, phrenic vessels, the cut surface of the liver, and ligated major vessels. Also, the ligated end of the recipient right hepatic artery if present is cross-checked and resutured or clipped. An 22F drain is placed in Morrison's pouch, and it is made sure that the drain does not hit the cut surface of the liver.

23.24 Closure

The abdomen is closed in one layer with the muscle and sheath closed with 1–0 loop Ethilon with alternate stitch being full-thickness and fascial alone to prevent muscle pouting. The subcutaneous tissue with 2–0 Vicryl and the skin are sutured with 3–0 Monocryl subcuticular suturing. The wound is covered with an aseptic dressing.

References

1. Pamecha V, Pattnaik B, Sinha PK, Patil NS, Mohapatra N, Sasturkar SV, Sundararajan VB, Thapar S, Sindwani G, Arora MK. Single orifice outflow reconstruction: refining the venous outflow in modified right lobe live donor liver transplantation. J Gastrointest Surg. 2021;25(8):1962–72. https://doi.org/10.1007/s11605-020-04776-3. Epub 2020 Aug 17.
2. Har B, Balradja I, Sreejith S, Chikkala BR, Dey R, Acharya MR, Pandey Y, Agarwal S, Gupta S, Verma S. The importance of inferior hepatic vein reconstruction in right lobe liver grafts: does it really matter? J Liver Transpl. 2021;3:100025. ISSN 2666-9676.
3. Jwa EK, Kim JD, Choi DL. Comparison of hepatic artery reconstruction using surgical loupe and operating microscope during living donor liver transplantation focusing on the beginner's point. Ann Hepatobiliary Pancreat Surg. 2019;23(2):122–7.
4. Kim JD, Choi DL, Kim TY. A comparison of hepatic artery reconstruction using a surgical loupe and operating microscope during living donor liver transplantation. Transplantation. 2018;102:S901.
5. Tannuri ACA, Monteiro RF, Santos MM, Miyatani HT, Tannuri U. A new simplified technique of arterial reconstruction in pediatric living-donor liver transplantation: a comparison with the classical technique. J Pediatr Surg. 2014;49(10):1518–21.
6. Li P-C, Thorat A, Jeng L-B, Yang H-R, Li M-L, Yeh C-C, et al. Hepatic artery reconstruction in living donor liver transplantation using surgical loupes: achieving low rate of hepatic arterial thrombosis in 741 consecutive recipients-tips and tricks to overcome the poor hepatic arterial flow. Liver Transpl. 2017;23(7):887–98.
7. Guarrera JV, Sinha P, Lobritto SJ, Brown RS, Kinkhabwala M, Emond JC. Microvascular hepatic artery anastomosis in pediatric segmental liver transplantation: microscope vs loupe. Transpl Int. 2004;17(10):585–8.
8. Platt JF, Yutzy GG, Bude RO, Ellis JH, Rubin JM. Use of Doppler sonography for revealing hepatic artery stenosis in liver transplant recipients. AJR Am J Roentgenol. 1997;168:4736.
9. Crossin JD, Muradali D, Wilson SR. US of liver transplants: Normal and abnormal. Radiographics. 2003;23:1093114.

Chapter 24
Recipient Surgery in Deceased Donor Liver Transplantation

S Sreejith, Shaleen Agarwal, and Subhash Gupta

Abstract The recipient surgery in a liver transplantation is one of the most complex procedures which needs good knowledge of the surgical anatomy of the liver with regard to the portal structures and all its variations, especially the arterial anatomy and delicate dissection of the inferior vena cava along with hepatic veins. A good quality preoperative cross-sectional imaging with hepatic protocol is crucial not only to know the vital vascular anatomy and variations but also to assess portal vein thrombus, liver tumors, large portosystemic shunts, and adhesions. In deceased donor liver transplantation (DDLT), the surgical steps involve explant hepatectomy, back-table preparation of the liver allograft or benchwork, and implantation of the graft liver. The importance of proper hemostasis in all the phases of surgery cannot be overemphasized.

Keywords Recipient hepatectomy · Portocaval shunt · Back-bench preparation · Hepatic artery anastomosis · Cavocavostomy · Piggyback technique · Classical technique · Bile duct anastomosis · Reperfusion

Key Highlights

- DDLT is the standard of care worldwide.
- Recipient surgery warrants surgical finesse with proper hemostasis to reduce blood loss and transfusions.
- Early retrohepatic IVC control can be beneficial for rapid explant with cross clamp in case of bleed.
- Porta dissection needs utmost care to avoid injury to inflow especially avoid intimal dissection of the recipient hepatic artery.
- Temporary portocaval shunt is a potential option to reduce bowel edema and maintain hemodynamic stability.
- Piggyback technique and cavocavostomy can avoid cross-clamping.

S. Sreejith (✉) · S. Agarwal · S. Gupta
Centre for Liver and Biliary Sciences (CLBS), Max Super Speciality Hospital, Saket, New Delhi, India
e-mail: drssreejith@gmail.com

S. Saigal, D. Jothimani (eds.), *Fundamentals of Transplant Hepatology*,
https://doi.org/10.1007/978-981-95-2624-6_24

The recipient surgery in a deceased donor liver transplantation (DDLT) is a complex surgical procedure which can broadly be divided into three parts, namely, (a) explant hepatectomy; (b) back-table preparation of the liver allograft or benchwork; and (c) implantation of the graft [1–4].

24.1 Recipient Hepatectomy

The recipient or explant hepatectomy steps can be grouped as follows:

Patient position
Abdominal access
Mobilization of the liver
Dissection of the retrohepatic IVC
Dissection at the porta hepatis
Liver explantation
Preparation of the liver bed for implantation

Patient Position Patient lies supine on the operating table. Gel pads are placed under all pressure points including the occiput, shoulder blades, and the heels.

Abdominal Access A 3-point star ("Mercedes Benz") or an inverted "T" incision is the commonly used skin incision that is used for entry into the abdomen (Fig. 24.1). This is a muscle-cutting incision, and a liberal use of energy device such as a diathermy on coagulation mode is recommended since multiple abdominal wall collaterals are often encountered [2].

Care is taken to achieve proper hemostasis at the cut muscle edges. On entering the abdominal cavity, a thorough inspection and palpation is done to assess the liver, adhesions, and presence of collaterals. In case of malignancy, the presence of any metastatic disease outside the liver would result in abandonment of surgery.

Fig. 24.1 Showing the inverted T-shaped incision which on right lateral side extends to the anterior axillary line

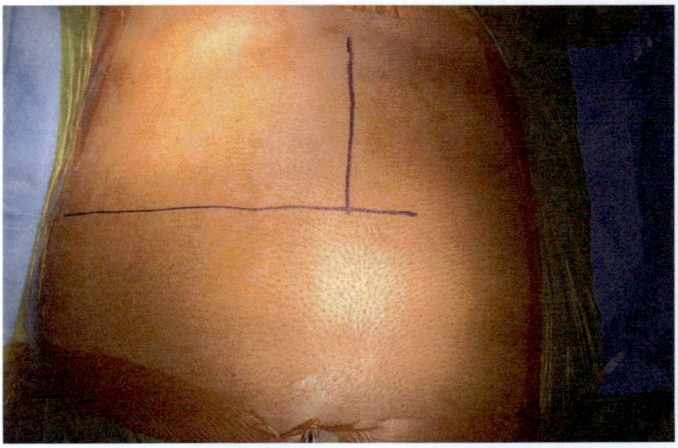

Once the abdomen cavity is entered, the next step is the division of the falciform ligament and the round ligament (ligamentum teres hepatis). The round ligament often contains recanalized paraumbilical veins, and therefore, this structure should be secured with ligatures. The division of the falciform ligament is carried cranially until it divides into the right and left coronary ligaments. The right and left coronary ligaments are also divided in order to expose the bare area of the liver. Once the bare area of the liver is exposed, the junction of the right, middle, and left hepatic veins with the inferior vena cava (IVC) becomes visible. A groove is created between right and middle hepatic vein which helps in subsequent looping of right hepatic vein (RHV) later in surgery. Fixed abdominal wall retractor systems (Omni-Tract or Thompson) are placed in order to get a good exposure of the operative field.

Liver Mobilization The right and left triangular ligaments of the liver are divided using an electrocautery since fine collateral channels are usually present in these otherwise avascular structures. The left half of the gastro-hepatic ligament (lesser omentum) is sharply divided to expose the caudate lobe of the liver. A replaced or accessory left hepatic artery (LHA) is present in the lesser omentum in nearly 13–20% of patients [5, 6]. The lesser omentum should therefore be carefully palpated prior to division in order to avoid injury to this vascular structure which may be an arterial inflow later.

Dissection of the Retrohepatic IVC Once the right triangular ligament is divided, the assistant rotates the right lobe of the liver. This maneuver exposes the right adrenal gland and the retrohepatic cava. The right adrenal gland is adherent to the segment VII of the liver and right border of the IVC, and it has to be dissected off the liver for proper exposure of the IVC. Division of the right adrenal vein is performed during adrenal gland dissection. As one proceeds cranially along the IVC, multiple inferior hepatic veins of varying caliber and short hepatic veins are encountered. These veins should be meticulously divided between ligatures or titanium clips. The larger vein stumps should be transfixed since ligature slippage can lead to torrential bleeding from the IVC. Division of hepatocaval or the "Makuuchi" ligament is required for exposure of extrahepatic portion of the right hepatic vein (RHV). The hepatocaval ligament should be divided between vascular clamps since it invariably contains an inferior hepatic vein that can be source of bleeding if not secured properly. Once this ligament is divided, a tunnel can easily be created between the right and middle hepatic veins and the RHV can be safely looped with a vascular tape. It is advisable at this stage to ligate and divide the right phrenic veins (usually 2–3 in number) that drain into the IVC near the RHV opening. This step helps in obtaining a good length of the RHV stump (Fig. 24.2).

Portal Dissection Having completed the IVC mobilization from the right side, the liver is placed back in its normal anatomical position. Mobilization of the portal structures starts with dissection of Calot's triangle and division of cystic artery and duct between ligatures. No attempt should be made to dissect the cystic plate since it can lead to bleeding from the collaterals coursing through this structure and can be very difficult to control. Dissection of Calot's triangle provides access to the portal triad. The vascularized connective tissue (Glissonian sheath) covering the

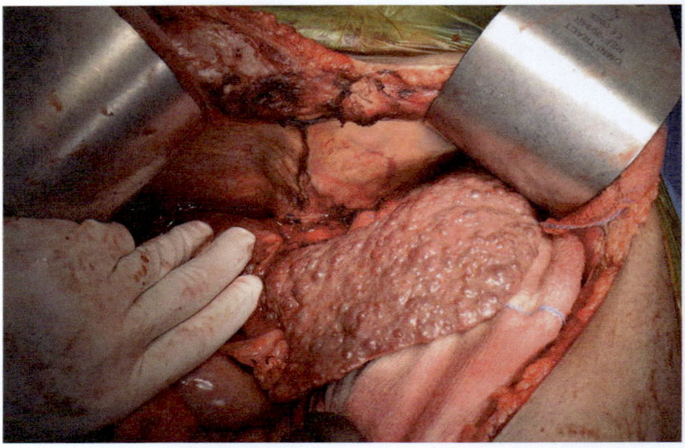

Fig. 24.2 Cirrhotic liver with suprahepatic dissection

portal structures is divided to expose the portal vein, right hepatic artery (RHA), and the common hepatic duct. The main portal vein is dissected and looped; similarly, the RHA is looped preserving the periarterial connective tissue around the artery. There can be a replaced RHA from the superior mesenteric artery (SMA) which should be identified in the preoperative cross-sectional image, and any crude dissection to the right of hepatoduodenal ligament may injure the replaced RHA and cause intimal dissection of the artery. The same procedure is repeated on the left side of the porta hepatis to loop the left hepatic artery (LHA) and the middle hepatic artery (MHA). There can be a replaced LHA from the left gastric artery that must be identified in the preoperative image and dissected and looped properly in the gastrohepatic ligament. Although long lengths of the hepatic arteries may not be required in during a DDLT, it is a good practice to get sufficient lengths on these vessels. The next step is to divide all the three arteries to liver between ligatures. This allows easy looping of the common hepatic duct, which is then transected high up after applying a vascular "bulldog" clamp. This leaves the liver hanging by the portal vein, which is now divided between vascular clamps. This step marks the start of "anhepatic phase," and the time of onset of the anhepatic phase should be noted diligently.

Completion of Explant of the Liver Once the liver has become anhepatic, the only structures holding the liver are the attachments of the caudate lobe to the IVC and the insertion of the 3 hepatic veins into the IVC. Therefore, to remove the liver completely, the caudate lobe is dissected off the IVC by incising the peritoneal reflection along the left border of the caudate lobe and individually ligating and dividing the caudate veins draining into the IVC. The next step is the division of the RHV (already looped) after applying a Satinsky clamp at the RHV-IVC junction. The final step is the division of the common stump of the middle and left hepatic veins (MHV-LHV stump) after applying another Satinsky clamp at the MHV-LHV stump-IVC junction. The cirrhotic liver (specimen) is finally removed from the

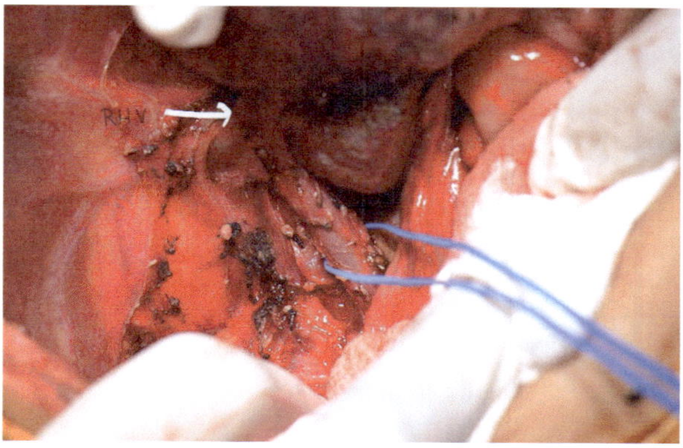

Fig. 24.3 Completion of retrohepatic IVC dissection with looping of IVC and RHV (shown with arrow)

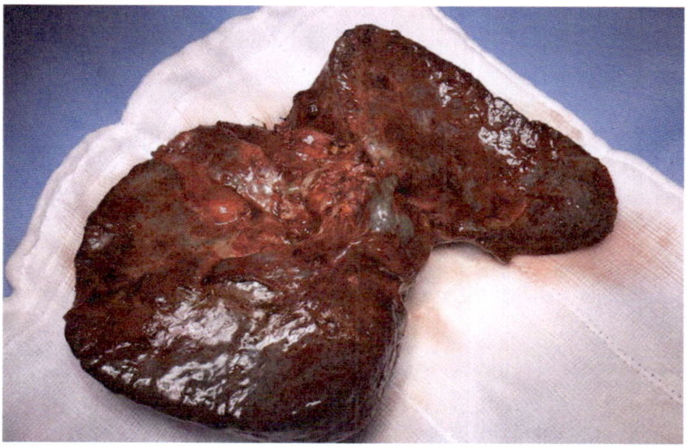

Fig. 24.4 Explant liver

abdominal cavity. The RHV stump and MHV-LHV common stump are secured with a 5-0 Prolene running suture (Figs. 24.3 and 24.4).

24.2 Anhepatic Phase

The anhepatic phase should be as short as possible. It is our practice to perform a temporary end-to-side portocaval shunt using a 5-0 Prolene running suture, until the donor liver is available for implantation. The benefits of a temporary portocaval shunt include avoidance of bowel edema, reduction in oozing from the raw surfaces in the liver bed, and better hemodynamic stability of the recipient during the anhepatic phase. Methyl prednisolone in a dose of 10 mg/kg is administered during the anhepatic phase to reduce the incidence of ischemia/reperfusion injury and early acute allograft rejection.

24.3 Hemostasis and Preparation of the Liver Bed

Preparation of liver bed includes achieving hemostasis from the raw surfaces, preparation of the inflow, outflow vessels, and bile duct for anastomosis to the liver allograft. Portal hypertension can lead to significant blood loss from the raw surfaces created during the explant procedure. Achieving hemostasis is therefore of paramount importance. The retrohepatic and paracaval areas are the common sites of blood loss. Time should be spent to locate each individual bleeding vessel by suturing, ligating, clipping, or using an energy device. It is our practice to suture transfix the short hepatic vein stumps over the IVC and removal of the clips on the IVC so that the clips do not loosen on manipulation during implantation and also for safe application of vascular clamps during implantation. The suprahepatic IVC is freed from the diaphragmatic attachments for safe cross-clamping of the IVC, and a trial clamping must be done to assess the hemodynamics. Also, the hepatic arteries may be prepared for reconstruction if time permits.

24.4 Benchwork

Benchwork or back-table preparation of the liver allograft essentially involves preparing the liver allograft for implantation into the recipient. This includes freeing the liver of all the diaphragmatic muscle and tendinous attachments to the superior surface of the liver, suture ligating the phrenic vein openings into the suprahepatic IVC, and clearing the portal vein, hepatic artery, and bile duct stumps from its surrounding fat and connective tissue. Since we prefer to use the cavocavostomy technique for outflow reconstruction, both the suprahepatic and infrahepatic IVC ends are closed with a running suture of 5-0 polypropylene and a liberal (nearly 10–12 cm) cavotomy is made along the length of the retrohepatic IVC.

24.5 Implantation

If UW solution is used as a preservative fluid, the allograft must be flushed with at least 1 liter of cold normal saline prior to implantation to remove air and prevent potassium-rich preservative fluid from entering the recipient's circulation.

24.6 Reconstruction of Outflow

The implantation process begins with the reconstruction of the vascular outflow. Three techniques are used for this purpose: longitudinal cavocavostomy, piggyback technique, and the classical technique [7–10].

1. *Cavocavostomy*: In this technique, a long (10–12 cm) side-to-side anastomosis is made between the recipient and graft retrohepatic IVC using a running suture of 4-0 polypropylene sutures. This anastomosis can be performed without complete occlusion of recipient IVC, by applying a long side biting vascular clamp. We prefer to use this technique since a long side-to-side anastomosis minimizes the chances of outflow obstruction and involves a single anastomosis for outflow reconstruction (Fig. 24.5).
2. *Piggyback Technique*: This technique was initially described by Sir Roy Calne and popularized by Tzakis. This is a commonly used technique for outflow reconstruction in DDLT. In the classical "piggyback" technique, an end-to-side anastomosis is created between the common funnel made by joining the stumps of recipient RHV, MHV, and LHV and the superior end of the donor suprahepatic IVC using a 4-0 or 5-0 polypropylene running suture [9, 11] (Figs. 24.6 and 24.7). The main advantage of this technique is that cross-clamping of the IVC is avoided leading to better hemodynamic stability in the recipient. After the completion of this anastomosis, the graft is flushed via main portal vein with 1 liter of cold normal saline. The effluent that comes out of the open end of graft infrahepatic IVC is sucked out. Having flushed the graft, the opening of the graft infrahepatic IVC is closed either by using a Prolene running suture or by firing an Endo GIA stapler [12, 13].

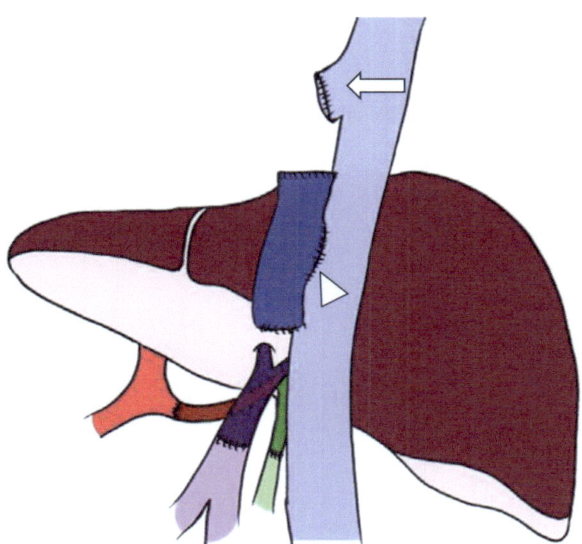

Fig. 24.5 Cavocavostomy technique: here, the stump of the RHV-MHV-LHV orifice in the recipient is closed with 4–0 Polypropylene (white arrow). The donor IVC is closed superiorly and inferiorly with polypropylene, and side-to-side 10- to 12-cm-long cavocaval anastomosis is done (white arrowhead) [12]

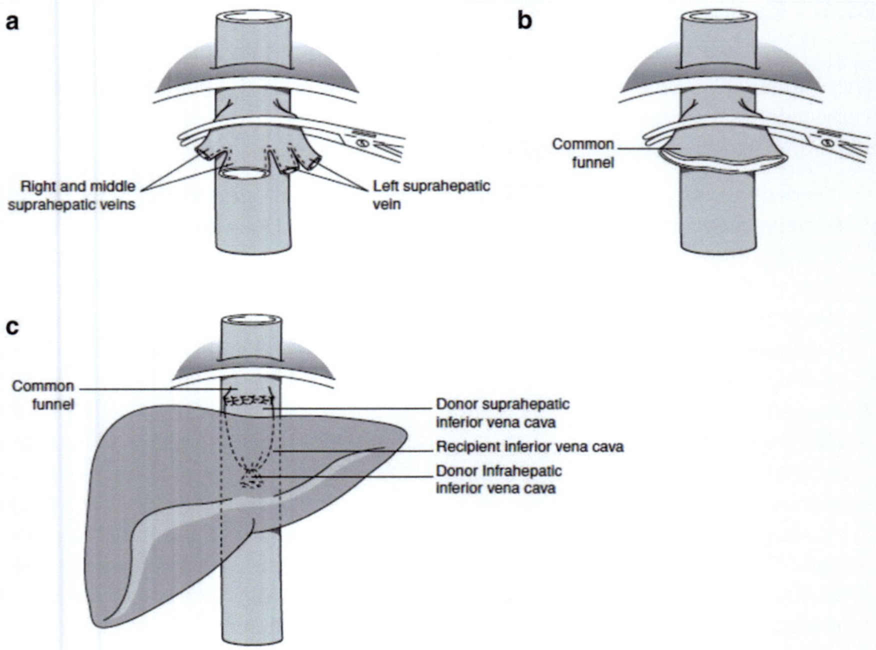

Fig. 24.6 Classical piggyback technique of preserving the IVC by performing an end-to-side cavo-hepatic-venous anastomosis. (**a**) Orifice of RHV-MHV-LHV is seen after removal of the recipient liver. (**b**) Common orifice is created by dividing the intervening septa between individual hepatic veins. (**c**) Finally, an end-to-side cavo-hepatic-venous anastomosis is performed between the end of suprahepatic vena cava of donor and common funnel orifice of recipient hepatic veins; in this technique, cross-clamping of the IVC is avoided [13]

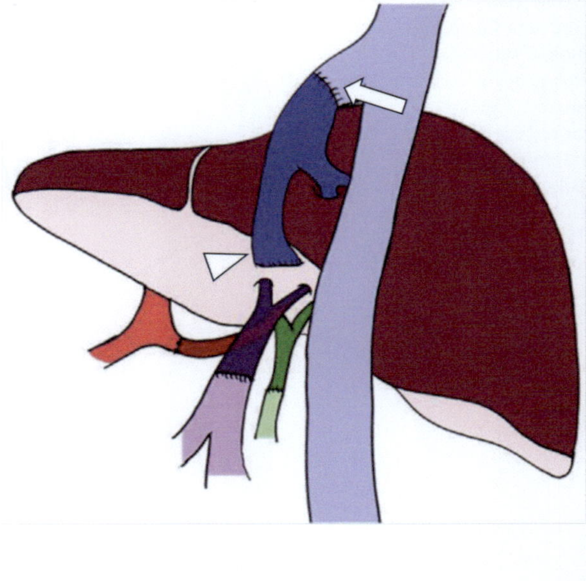

Fig. 24.7 Final appearance of transplanted liver using piggyback technique of outflow anastomosis wherein the common opening of RHV-MHV-LHV orifice is anastomosed with upper end of the donor IVC (white arrow), and the inferior end of the donor IVC is kept open until it drains out the organ perfusion fluid and is subsequently closed with sutures (white arrowhead) [12]

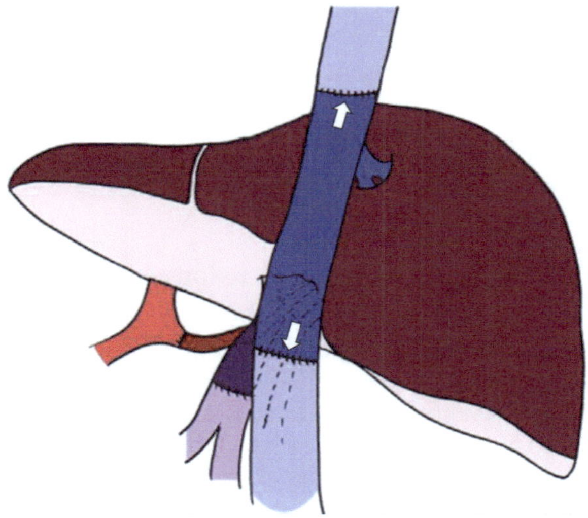

Fig. 24.8 Classical technique of caval replacement with the donor IVC, where a part of recipient IVC is cut and the graft liver with graft IVC is anastomosed in end-to-end manner (arrows) [12]. This technique requires total IVC occlusion

3. *Classical or Caval Replacement Technique*: In this technique, the recipient retrohepatic IVC is replaced by the graft retrohepatic IVC [1]. This method requires cross-clamping of recipient IVC and involves two anastomoses: (a) end-to-end anastomosis between the recipient and donor suprahepatic IVC; and (b) end-to-end anastomosis between the recipient and donor infrahepatic IVC. Cross-clamping of IVC may lead to hemodynamically instability and adversely impact renal function which may be already compromised in some of these patients. Therefore, this technique is used infrequently. The main indication for this technique is when the recipient IVC is stenosed or unhealthy such as in patients with re-do liver transplant, those with Budd-Chiari syndrome, and when the IVC is involved by large hepatocellular carcinoma [14, 15] (Fig. 24.8).

24.7 Reconstruction of Graft Inflow

Reconstruction of graft inflow requires anastomoses between the donor and recipient portal veins and hepatic arteries.

Portal Vein Anastomosis The portal vein anastomosis is performed first and is done in an end-to-end fashion with running 6-0 polypropylene suture. Care should be taken to avoid any redundancy or twisting of the portal vein, and a "growth factor" should be left to allow for expansion of the anastomosis after reperfusion. Few centers perform portal vein anastomosis by posterior layer with continuous sutures and anterior layer with interrupted sutures.

Reperfusion: Having completed the portal vein anastomosis, the vascular clamps on the recipient IVC is released first followed by the clamp on portal vein to allow the portal blood to reperfuse the liver allograft. Following adequate reperfusion, the liver surface turns uniformly pink from a pale brown color. Any major bleeding from the anastomotic sites or from the IVC should be controlled with sutures or clips at this stage.

24.8 Hepatic Artery Anastomosis

Successful hepatic artery reconstruction is crucial for graft function, and a variety of methods have been described. In routine cases, Carrel's patch of donor celiac artery or common hepatic artery is anastomosed end to end to the recipient common hepatic artery or to a branch patch of the bifurcation between the gastroduodenal and the hepatic artery proper using 6-0 or 7-0 polypropylene interrupted or continuous sutures [2, 16].

In donor livers with an accessory RHA, Carrel's patch is fashioned from the superior mesenteric artery (SMA) which is then anastomosed to donor gastroduodenal, left gastric, or splenic artery stump on the back table so that finally only one arterial anastomosis is required to the recipient hepatic artery.

Intraoperative Doppler is performed after the completion of vascular anastomosis. The goal is to look for patency of the arterial and venous anastomoses, and the pattern and volume of blood flow across these anastomoses. The hepatic artery flow velocity should be greater than 25 ml/min and the resistive index between 0.5 and 0.9. The portal vein anastomosis is checked for alignment, and the flow volume is measured. The portal flow volume should be between 150 and 400 ml/100 g of liver tissue. Low portal flow may require modification with ligation of sizable lienorenal shunt or ligation of other sizable collaterals. The flow across the hepatic veins should be hepatofugal and triphasic in pattern [17, 18].

24.9 Restoration of Biliary Continuity

Bile duct anastomosis can either be a duct-to-duct anastomosis between the donor and recipient bile ducts or be a Roux-en-Y hepaticojejunostomy. Before starting the biliary anastomosis, the devascularized gallbladder attached to the liver allograft is dissected off the cystic plate and removed. An end-to-end anastomosis between donor and recipient bile ducts is the preferred technique since it is more physiological. The anastomosis can be performed either in a continuous running fashion or as interrupted sutures using 6-0 Polydioxanone suture. Care must be taken to avoid redundancy of bile ducts since it can lead to bilio-stasis or obstruction and stone formation.

When the recipient bile duct is not suitable for biliary anastomosis due to short length or when it is unhealthy, such as in patients with primary sclerosing cholangitis (PSC), a hepaticojejunostomy is performed for restoration of biliary continuity. A Roux limb of jejunum is passed through a mesocolic window into the supracolic compartment and anastomosed in an end-to-side fashion to the donor bile duct using a 6-0 Polydioxanone suture.

It is advisable to perform a completion cholangiogram after completion of biliary anastomosis to ascertain the patency of the anastomosis and to rule out any leak or narrowing. The cholangiogram is performed via the cystic duct stump or end of a Roux limb in case of a hepaticojejunostomy [2, 3, 19].

24.10 Hemostasis and Drain Placement

Post-implantation, thorough hemostasis is attained with special attention to the region of retroperitoneum, paracaval area, and porta hepatis. A 20–24 Fr abdominal drain is placed in Morrison's pouch and brought out in the right flank.

24.11 Closure

The abdominal wall incision is closed in single layer with the muscle and sheath closed with no. 1 Polydioxanone suture. The subcutaneous tissue is closed with 3-0 polyglyconate suture and the skin is sutured with 3-0 monofilament polyglecaperone subcuticular sutures. The surgical site is covered with a sterile dressing. In case the abdominal closure appears tight, a prosthetic mesh [20] should be used for closure, to prevent the dreaded complication of compartment syndrome, but in general, this situation should be avoided.

References

1. Starzl TE, Marchioro TL, Vonkaulla KN, Hermann G, Brittain RS, Waddell WR. Homotransplantation of the liver in humans. Surg Gynecol Obstet. 1963;117:659–76.
2. Makowka L, Stieber AC, Sher L, Kahn D, Mieles L, Bowman J, Marsh JW, Starzl TE. Surgical technique of orthotopic liver transplantation. Gastroenterol Clin N Am. 1988;17(1):33–51. PMID: 3292430; PMCID: PMC3228369.
3. Lladó L, Figueras J. Techniques of orthotopic liver transplantation. HPB. 2004;6(2):69–75.
4. Busuttil RW. International Liver Transplantation Society 2009 presidential address: The internationalization of liver transplantation: the Internationalization of Liver Transplantation. Liver Transpl. 2010;16(5):558–66.
5. Michels NA. Newer anatomy of the liver and its variant blood supply and collateral circulation. Am J Surg. 1966;112(3):337–47. https://doi.org/10.1016/0002-9610(66)90201-7.

6. Covey AM, Brody LA, Maluccio MA, Getrajdman GI, Brown KT. Variant hepatic arterial anatomy revisited: digital subtraction angiography performed in 600 patients. Radiology. 2002;224(2):542–7.
7. Chen Z, Ju W, Chen C, Wang T, Yu J, Hong X, et al. Application of various surgical techniques in liver transplantation: a retrospective study. Ann Transl Med. 2021;9(17):1367.
8. Mehrabi A, Mood ZA, Fonouni H, et al. A single-center experience of 500 liver transplants using the modified piggyback technique by Belghiti. Liver Transpl. 2009;15(5):466–74.
9. Calne RY, Williams R. Liver transplantation in man. I. Observations on technique and organization in five cases. Br Med J. 1968;4:535–40.
10. Zarrinpar A, Busuttil R. Liver transplantation: past, present and future. Nat Rev Gastroenterol Hepatol. 2013;10:434–40. https://doi.org/10.1038/nrgastro.2013.88.
11. Tzakis A, Todo S, Starzl TE. Orthotopic liver transplantation with preservation of the vena cava. Ann Surg. 1989;210:649–52.
12. Chan T, DeGirolamo K, Chartier-Plante S, Buczkowski AK. Comparison of three caval reconstruction techniques in orthotopic liver transplantation: a retrospective review. North Pac Surg Assoc. 2017;213(5):943–9.
13. Eghtesad B, Hashimoto K, Fung J. The liver transplant procedure. In: Schiff ER, Maddrey WC, Reddy KR, editors. Schiff's diseases of the liver [Internet]. 1st ed. Wiley; 2017 [cited 2024 Mar 26]. p. 1107–26. Available from: https://onlinelibrary.wiley.com/doi/10.1002/9781119251316.ch45
14. Song ATW. Liver transplantation: fifty years of experience. World J Gastroenterol. 2014;20(18):5363.
15. Pravisani R, De Martino M, Mocchegiani F, Melandro F, Patrono D, Lauterio A, et al. Recipient hepatectomy technique may affect oncological outcomes of liver transplantation for hepatocellular carcinoma. Liver Transpl [Internet]. 2024 [cited 2024 Aug 25]. Available from: https://journals.lww.com/10.1097/LVT.0000000000000373
16. Sommacale D, Nagarajan G, Lhuaire M, Dondero F, Pessaux P, Piardi T, et al. Surgical procedures in liver transplant patients: a monocentric retrospective cohort study. Int J Surg. 2017;41:58–64.
17. Okeke RI, Bettag J, Wells R, Wycoff M, Hallcox T, Lok J, et al. Intraoperative Doppler ultrasound for detection of early postoperative vascular complications in orthotopic liver transplants. Cureus [Internet]. 2022 [cited 2024 Mar 26]. Available from: https://www.cureus.com/articles/101287-intraoperative-doppler-ultrasound-for-detection-of-early-postoperative-vascular-complications-in-orthotopic-liver-transplants
18. Sanyal R, Zarzour JG, Ganeshan DM, Bhargava P, Lall CG, Little MD. Postoperative Doppler evaluation of liver transplants. Indian J Radiol Imaging. 2014;24(4):360–6. https://doi.org/10.4103/0971-3026.143898. PMID: 25489129; PMCID: PMC4247505.
19. Jabłonska B. End-to-end ductal anastomosis in biliary reconstruction: indications and limitations. Can J Surg. 2014;57(4):271–7. https://doi.org/10.1503/cjs.016613. PMID: 25078933; PMCID: PMC4119121.
20. Chang E-s, Martino A, Welu A, Nazzal M. Utilization of Vicryl bridging mesh in orthotopic liver transplantation to achieve tension-free abdominal wall closure: a case series. Case Reports Surg. 2020, 2020:4716415, 5 pages. https://doi.org/10.1155/2020/4716415.

Chapter 25
Anesthetic Considerations

Ryan Chadha and Maria A. Estevez

Abstract Optimal outcomes in the perioperative period require a multidisciplinary effort from the surgical, anesthesiology and critical care, and hepatology service teams. In this chapter, we aim to look specifically at the anesthetic considerations for adult liver transplantation. We will discuss the importance of a dedicated liver transplant anesthesia team, basic considerations of intraoperative management, complications that may be encountered, and postoperative considerations.

Keywords Liver transplant anesthesiologists · Transesophageal echocardiography · Post-reperfusion syndrome · Intracardiac thrombus · Early extubation · Opioid sparing analgesia

Key Highlights

1. Dedicated liver transplant anesthesia teams are critical for optimal perioperative outcomes.
2. The anesthesiologist must be prepared for intraoperative critical events, including but not limited to post-reperfusion syndrome and intraoperative cardiac arrest.
3. In recent years, there has been a growing interest in early extubation and innovative approaches to postoperative analgesia.

R. Chadha (✉)
Departments of Anesthesiology and Peri-operative Medicine, Mayo Clinic, Jacksonville, FL, USA
e-mail: Chadha.Ryan@mayo.edu

M. A. Estevez
Mayo Clinic, Jacksonville, FL, USA

S. Saigal, D. Jothimani (eds.), *Fundamentals of Transplant Hepatology*,
https://doi.org/10.1007/978-981-95-2624-6_25

25.1 The Liver Transplant Anesthesia Team

The patient undergoing liver transplantation has complex physiology with multiorgan involvement. As a result, it is critical to have an anesthesia team experienced in the management of these cases for the best possible outcome. Dedicated liver transplant anesthesia teams have been shown to impact mortality, blood product administration, and time under mechanical ventilation [1–3]. The United Network for Organ Sharing (UNOS) in the US has mandated that all certified programs have a director of liver transplant anesthesia with experience in at least 10 cases [4]. In addition, there has been an increasing focus on standardizing the competencies of liver transplant anesthesia teams, including elements of vascular access, complex invasive hemodynamic monitoring like transesophageal echocardiography, and viscoelastic testing [5]. This has also been extended to liver transplant anesthesia fellowship training programs to ensure standardized training pathways for those hoping to enter the field [6, 7]. It is also critical to maintain the quality of the team with continuous audits and involvement in multidisciplinary team engagement [8].

25.2 Intraoperative Considerations

25.2.1 Hemodynamic Monitoring and Management

Liver transplant anesthesiologists have to routinely deal with significant hemodynamic perturbations during the transplant procedure from a variety of pathologies [9]. All patients undergoing transplantation require invasive arterial and central monitoring, although the location and number of arterial lines are center dependent, with no evidence supporting any particular approach [10]. In terms of invasive hemodynamic monitoring, there has been a trend moving away from utilization of pulmonary artery catheters and toward non-invasive cardiac output monitors, most prominently transesophageal echocardiography (TEE). TEE continues to show a good safety profile in liver transplantation, with the presence of varices not being a contraindication for its utilization [11, 12]. Anesthetic maintenance is classically managed with volatile and neuromuscular blockade; however, there is no real benefit difference in the literature when comparing volatile versus total intravenous anesthesia [13].

25.2.2 Blood and Coagulation Management

The liver transplant procedure routinely requires the transfusion of all blood components, including packed red blood cells, fresh frozen plasma, cryoprecipitate, and platelets. The complex nature of the "rebalanced hemostasis" of cirrhotic patients requires an understanding of all elements of the coagulation cascade [14]. This management intraoperatively has been enhanced by viscoelastic testing, such as thromboelastrography and rotational thromboelastometry, which has been shown to reduce the amount of intraoperative products given in numerous studies [15, 16]. Massive transfusion management has also been improved by rapid infusion devices [17, 18]. Cell salvage has been repeatedly shown to be a safe therapy with no evidence of transfer of malignant infection and should be considered for every liver transplant procedure [19]. Finally, there has been increasing literature on the use of blood product concentrates like prothrombin complex concentrates and fibrinogen concentrates and their safety in liver transplantation, although their utilization is very center dependent [20–23]. It is clear that blood and coagulation management is centered and patient specific and requires an individualized approach for each case [24].

25.3 Intraoperative Complications

25.3.1 Post-reperfusion Syndrome

Post-reperfusion syndrome (PRS) has been defined in several studies as a decrease in mean arterial pressure of more than 30% or more in the first 5 min after reperfusion and lasting longer than 1 min [25]. Despite advances in the intraoperative management of these patients, it continues to occur at a relatively steady rate, with the incidence difficult to quantify due to the study type. In addition, it unfortunately has a known association with intraoperative cardiac arrest [26, 27]. Known associations with PRS include increased cold ischemia time, higher Model for End-Stage Liver Disease (MELD), and macrosteatosis [28, 29]. It has been studied whether venting the liver will reduce the incidence of this, with varying success in the literature, and there is potential for machine perfusion to reduce this complication [30, 31]. The anesthesiologist must be aware of risk factors of PRS and be prepared to support the patient appropriately post-reperfusion to avoid a negative perioperative outcome [32–34].

25.3.2 Intracardiac Thrombus

First described in 1989, intracardiac thrombus (ICT) continues to be a devastating complication for anesthesiologists to deal with in the intraoperative arena [34]. Risk factors continue to be unclear, although it appears to be most prominent in the anhepatic and reperfusion phases. It has an estimated incidence of approximately 1.42% and a mortality rate of greater than 40% in recent studies [35]. There has been a significant improvement in detection and management. Some believe that prophylactic heparin prior to clamping the venous outflow may be preventative, although this practice is very center dependent [36]. The use of TEE has enhanced the detection of ICT and reduced the risk of perioperative cardiac arrest [37]. Although the management is unclear, case report-driven management suggests the use of anticoagulation with intravenous heparin and low-dose tissue plasminogen activator, with escalation to extracorporeal support in the setting of cardiac collapse [38]. It is prudent for anesthesiologists to consider at least the availability of TEE and anticoagulants when managing liver transplantation patients intraoperatively [18, 39].

25.3.3 Intraoperative Cardiac Arrest

The incidence of cardiac arrest in orthotopic liver transplantation is significantly higher than in non-cardiac surgery. The first study looked at 1238 patients at a single US center and found a 5.5% incidence of cardiac arrest, with most likely causes being PRS and ICT, with a high MELD model being a risk factor [40]. The next study looked specifically at the Asian population and found a 3.3% incidence in deceased donors and a 1% incidence in living donors, with the causes most likely being PRS and hemorrhage [41]. The most recent study, a 7-center study out of the US, found the incidence to be 3.7%, with risk factors being body mass index (BMI), MELD, PRS, and re-transplant [42]. The use of extracorporeal membrane oxygenation (ECMO) has become of interest to utilize for these patients with cardiac arrest in the perioperative period; however, it has significant logistical and clinical considerations, and overall outcomes are unclear to show a benefit in the literature [43–45].

25.4 Postoperative Considerations

25.4.1 Early Extubation

Early extubation was proven as a feasible concept for liver transplantation in the late 1990s; however, it has been slow to be adopted due to a lack of care team comfort and logistical considerations at many centers [46–48]. However, with the increased promotion of enhanced recovery after surgery worldwide and surgical and perioperative care becoming safer and more streamlined, this is becoming a more common occurrence [49]. It is important to establish risk factors for failure of extubation, which include, depending on the studies assessed, higher MELD, higher blood products transfused, no vasopressors, BMI, cold ischemic time, length of surgery, and Donor Risk Index [50–52]. It is the current recommendation from a recent consensus that all patients should be considered for on-table extubation at the end of the procedure [53]. Fast-track anesthesia is also gaining traction due to limited intensive care capacity, with the liver transplant patient being extubated and going directly to the ward, but again is very center and resource dependent. It also requires significant infrastructure and vast experience with early extubation [54–56].

25.4.2 Analgesia

There is an increasing interest in pain management for this patient population. The classic teaching is that patients with cirrhosis have decreased pain requirements [57]. However, with the change in demographics of liver transplant recipients from hepatitis and alcohol liver disease to metabolic dysfunction-associated liver disease (MASLD), as well as the increasing numbers of patients using opioids and marijuana products preoperatively, it is important to consider alternatives in this patient population [58–60]. It is recommended that opioid-sparing regimens be considered for all patients undergoing liver transplantation [61].

Some previous reports have demonstrated that in selected patients, thoracic epidural analgesia (TEA) can control post-LT pain with reduced postoperative sedation, improved postoperative bowel function, easier expectoration of pulmonary secretions, and early ambulation [62, 63]. During their 10-year experience, Trzebicki et al. used TEA in 67 patients. Of the studied patients, 84% were extubated in the operating room, and 5 cases experienced unsatisfactory analgesia, but no complications were recorded. A recent systematic review and meta-analysis compared the transversus abdominis plane (TAP) block with conventional analgesic regimens for analgesia. Studies comparing 24-h morphine consumption were searched: only two randomized controlled trials and two retrospective studies, involving a total of 160 patients, were included in the analysis. The pooled effect size by the random effects model showed that the TAP group had 27.59 mg (95% CI: 33.47–21.70) lower morphine requirement at 24 h. However, this result is from only two single-center studies, reducing the generalizability of the findings [64, 65].

There is limited literature on the use of non-opioid adjuncts in liver transplant recipients, and it is understandable with the multiorgan effects and metabolism of commonly used drugs like acetaminophen, non-steroidal anti-inflammatories, and ketamine [57]. A 2021 single-center retrospective study by Knorr and colleagues found that a single dose of pregabalin preoperatively reduced opioid requirements in the first 72 h postoperatively [66]. One study evaluated magnesium use as an additional adjunct for pain control postoperatively and found that perioperative use of magnesium sulfate reduced postoperative tramadol requirements and duration of mechanical ventilation [67]. Figure 25.1 summarizes the key intraoperative anesthesia considerations.

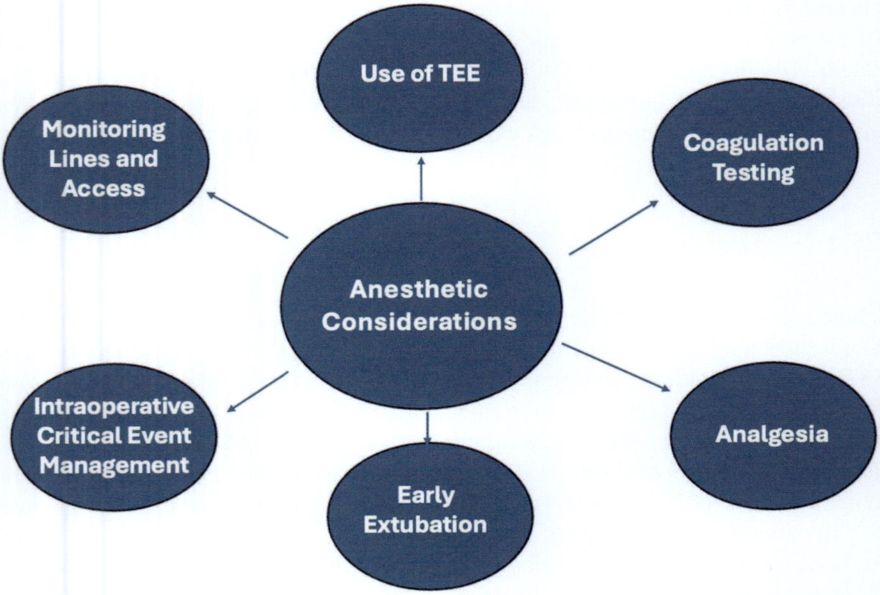

Fig. 25.1 Summary of anesthetic considerations in the intraoperative phase of care

25.5 Conclusion

Considering the complexity of liver transplantation surgery, dedicated and highly experienced transplant anesthesia team should be a part of the program. With recent advances in anesthesia techniques, early extubation, innovative approaches and use of post-operative analgesia are encouraged for quicker recovery.

References

1. Hofer I, et al. Association between anesthesiologist experience and mortality after orthotopic liver transplantation. Liver Transpl. 2015;21(1):89–95.
2. Hevesi ZG, et al. Designated liver transplant anesthesia team reduces blood transfusion, need for mechanical ventilation, and duration of intensive care. Liver Transpl. 2009;15(5):460–5.
3. Mandell SM. Anesthesia for liver transplantation: is this generalist or specialist care? Liver Transpl. 1999;5(4) LWW
4. United Network for Organ Sharing. Attachment I to appendix B of UNOS bylaws. Designated transplant program criteria. http://www.unos.org/wp-content/uploads/unos/Appendix_B_AttachI_XIII.pdf. Published June 28, 2011. Accessed July 25, 2019.
5. Nguyen-Buckley C, et al. International liver transplantation society/society for advancement of transplant anesthesia consensus statement on essential attributes of a liver transplant anesthesiologist. Transplantation. 2023;107(7):1427–33.

6. Chadha RM, et al. Society for the Advancement of Transplant Anesthesia: Liver Transplant Anesthesia Fellowship—White paper advocating measurable proficiency in transplant specialties training. Semin Cardiothorac Vasc Anesth. 2017;21(4) Sage, CA/Los Angeles, CA: SAGE Publications
7. Nguyen-Buckley C, et al. Recommendations from the society for the advancement of transplant anesthesiology: liver transplant anesthesiology fellowship core competencies and milestones. Semin Cardiothorac Vasc Anesth. 2019;23(4) Sage, CA/Los Angeles, CA: SAGE Publications
8. Hendrickse A, et al. Service requirements of liver transplant anesthesia teams: Society for the Advancement of transplant anesthesia recommendations. Liver Transpl. 2020;26(4):582–90.
9. Bezinover D, et al. Hemodynamic instability during liver transplantation in patients with end-stage liver disease: a consensus document from ILTS, LICAGE, and SATA. Transplantation. 2021;105(10):2184–200.
10. Fernandez TMA, et al. What is the optimal anesthetic monitoring regarding immediate and short-term outcomes after liver transplantation?—a systematic review of the literature and expert panel recommendations. Clin Transpl. 2022;36(10):e14643.
11. De Marchi L, et al. Safety and benefit of transesophageal echocardiography in liver transplant surgery: a position paper from the Society for the Advancement of Transplant Anesthesia (SATA). Liver Transpl. 2020;26(8):1019–29.
12. Pai S-L, et al. Complications related to intraoperative transesophageal echocardiography in liver transplantation. Springerplus. 2015;4:1–8.
13. Chadha R, et al. Optimal anesthetic conduct regarding immediate and short-term outcomes after liver transplantation–systematic review of the literature and expert panel recommendations. Clin Transpl. 2022;36(10):e14613.
14. Pillai AA, et al. Coagulopathy and hemostasis management in patients undergoing liver transplantation: defining a dynamic spectrum across phases of care. Liver Transpl. 2022;28(10):1651–63.
15. Bonnet A, Gilquin N, Steer N, et al. The use of a thromboelastometry-based algorithm reduces the need for blood product transfusion during orthotopic liver transplantation: a randomised controlled study. Eur J Anaesthesiol. 2019;36(11):825–33.
16. Roullet S, Freyburger G, Cruc M, et al. Management of bleeding and transfusion during liver transplantation before and after the introduction of a rotational thromboelastometry-based algorithm. Liver Transpl. 2015;21(2):169–79.
17. Schumann R. Intraoperative resource utilization in anesthesia for liver transplantation in the United States: a survey. Anesth Analg. 2003;97(1):21–8.
18. Crouch C, et al. Adult liver transplant anesthesiology practice patterns and resource utilization in the United States: survey results from the society for the advancement of transplant anesthesia. Clin Transpl. 2022;36(1):e14504.
19. Rajendran L, Lenet T, Shorr R, Abou Khalil J, Bertens KA, Balaa FK, Martel G. Should cell salvage be used in liver resection and transplantation? A systematic review and meta-analysis. Ann Surg. 2023;277(3):456.
20. Abuelkasem E, et al. Reduced requirement for prothrombin complex concentrate for the restoration of thrombin generation in plasma from liver transplant recipients. Anesth Analg. 2017;125(2):609–15.
21. Srivastava P, et al. Utility of prothrombin complex concentrate as first-line treatment modality of coagulopathy in patients undergoing liver transplantation: a propensity score-matched study. Clin Transpl. 2018;32(12):e13435.
22. Kirchner C, et al. Coagulation management with factor concentrates in liver transplantation: a single-center experience. Transfusion. 2014;54.10pt2:2760–8.
23. Hartmann M, et al. Safety of coagulation factor concentrates guided by ROTEM™-analyses in liver transplantation: results from 372 procedures. BMC Anesthesiol. 2019;19(1):1–11.
24. Yoon U, et al. Intraoperative transfusion management, antifibrinolytic therapy, coagulation monitoring and the impact on short-term outcomes after liver transplantation—a systematic review of the literature and expert panel recommendations. Clin Transpl. 2022;36(10):e14637.

25. DeMaria S Jr, et al. Prediction, prevention, and treatment of post reperfusion syndrome in adult orthotopic liver transplant patients. Clin Transpl. 2023:e15014.
26. Manning MW, Kumar PA, Maheshwari K, Arora H. Post-reperfusion syndrome in liver transplantation-an overview. J Cardiothorac Vasc Anesth. 2020;34:501–11.
27. Siniscalchi A, Gamberini L, Laici C, et al. Post reperfusion syndrome during liver transplantation: from pathophysiology to therapy and preventive strategies. World J Gastroenterol. 2016;22:1551–69.
28. Bekki Y, Myers B, Wang R, et al. Postreperfusion syndrome in liver transplantation: outcomes, predictors, and application for recipient selection. Clin Transpl. 2022;36(4):e14587.
29. Sahmeddini MA, et al. Risk factors of the post-reperfusion syndrome during orthotopic liver transplantation: a clinical observational study. BMC Anesthesiol. 2022;22(1):89.
30. Kniepeiss D, Zink M, Iberer F, et al. Influence of retrograde flushing via the caval vein on the post-reperfusion syndrome in liver transplantation. Clin Transpl. 2004;18:638–41.
31. van Rijn R, Schurink IJ, de Vries Y, et al. Hypothermic machine perfusion in liver transplantation - a randomized trial. N Engl J Med. 2021;384:1391–401.
32. Siniscalchi A, et al. Post-reperfusion syndrome during orthotopic liver transplantation, which definition best predicts postoperative graft failure and recipient mortality? J Crit Care. 2017;41:156–60.
33. Tokodai K, et al. Association of post-reperfusion syndrome and ischemia-reperfusion injury with acute kidney injury after liver transplantation. Acta Anaesthesiol Scand. 2020;64(6):742–50.
34. Ellis JE, et al. Right heart dysfunction, pulmonary embolism, and paradoxical embolization during liver transplantation: a transesophageal two-dimensional echocardiographic study. Anesth Analg. 1989;68(6):777–82.
35. Kumar N, et al. Intracardiac thrombosis and pulmonary thromboembolism during liver transplantation: a systematic review and meta-analysis. Am J Transplant. 2023;23:1227.
36. Groose MK, et al. Risk factors for intracardiac thrombus during liver transplantation. Liver Transpl. 2019;25(11):1682–9.
37. Fagelman E, et al. Intraoperative intracardiac thrombus in liver transplantation: a 9-year retrospective review focusing on treatment and outcomes. Liver Transpl. 2022;28(10):1603–17.
38. Protin C, et al. Emergent management of intracardiac thrombosis during liver transplantation. Case Rep Transpl. 2016;2016
39. Mandell D, et al. Critical importance of low-dose tissue plasminogen activator policy for treating intraoperative pulmonary thromboembolism during liver transplantation. Semin Cardiothorac Vasc Anesth. 2018;22(4) Sage, CA/Los Angeles, CA: SAGE Publications
40. Matsusaki T, et al. Cardiac arrest during adult liver transplantation: a single institution's experience with 1238 deceased donor transplants. Liver Transpl. 2013;19(11):1262–71.
41. Lee SH, et al. Intra-operative cardiac arrests during liver transplantation–a retrospective review of the first 15 yr in Asian population. Clin Transpl. 2013;27(2):E126–36.
42. Smith NK, et al. Intraoperative cardiac arrest during adult liver transplantation: incidence and risk factor analysis from 7 academic centers in the United States. Anesth Analg. 2021;132(1):130–9.
43. Braun HJ, et al. The utility of ECMO after liver transplantation: experience at a high-volume transplant center and review of the literature. Transplantation. 2019;103(8):1568–73.
44. Reid TD, et al. The role of extracorporeal membrane oxygenation in adult liver transplant patients: a qualitative systematic review of literature. Artif Organs. 2022;46(4):578–96.
45. Hogen R, et al. The evolving role of extra-corporeal membrane oxygenation in liver transplantation. Curr Opin Organ Transplant. 2021;26(3):333.
46. Mandell MS, et al. Reduced use of intensive care after liver transplantation: influence of early extubation. Liver Transpl. 2002;8(8):676–81.
47. Mandell SM, et al. A multicenter evaluation of safety of early extubation in liver transplant recipients. Liver Transpl. 2007;13(11):1557–63.
48. Mandell MS, Lockrem J, Kelley SD. Immediate tracheal extubation after liver transplantation: experience of two transplant centers. Anesth Analg. 1997;84(2):249–53.

49. Pollok JM, Tinguely P, Berenguer M. ERAS4OLT. org collaborative. Enhanced recovery for liver transplantation: recommendations from the 2022 International Liver Transplantation Society consensus conference. Lancet Gastroenterol Hepatol. 2023;8:81–94.
50. Suphathamwit A, et al. Predictive score for immediate extubation after liver transplantation. Clin Transpl. 2021;35(3):e14212.
51. Taner CB, et al. Is a mandatory intensive care unit stay needed after liver transplantation? Feasibility of fast-tracking to the surgical ward after liver transplantation. Liver Transpl. 2012;18(3):361–9.
52. Bulatao IG, et al. Avoiding stay in the intensive care unit after liver transplantation: a score to assign location of care. Am J Transplant. 2014;14(9):2088–96.
53. Tinguely P, et al. The role of early extubation on short-term outcomes after liver transplantation–a systematic review, meta-analysis and expert recommendations. Clin Transpl. 2022;36(10):e14642.
54. Biancofiore G, et al. Fast track in liver transplantation: 5 years' experience. Eur J Anaesthesiol. 2005;22(8):584–90.
55. Rodríguez-Laiz GP, et al. Fast-track liver transplantation: six-year prospective cohort study with an enhanced recovery after surgery (ERAS) protocol. World J Surg. 2021;45:1262–71.
56. Aniskevich S, Pai S-L. Fast track anesthesia for liver transplantation: review of the current practice. World J Hepatol. 2015;7(20):2303.
57. Chadha R, et al. Nonopioid modalities for acute postoperative pain in abdominal transplant recipients. Transplantation. 2020;104(4):694–9.
58. Cron DC, et al. Prevalence and patterns of opioid use before and after liver transplantation. Transplantation. 2021;105(1):100.
59. Fukazawa K, et al. Perioperative opioid use and chronic post-surgical pain after liver transplantation: a single center observational study. J Cardiothorac Vasc Anesth. 2020;34(7):1815–21.
60. Yan K, Forman L. Cannabinoid use among liver transplant recipients. Liver Transpl. 2021;27(11):1623–32.
61. Hogan BJ, et al. Does multimodal perioperative pain management enhance immediate and short-term outcomes after living donor partial hepatectomy? A systematic review of the literature and expert panel recommendations. Clin Transpl. 2022;36(10):e14649.
62. Trzebicki J, Nicinska B, Blaszczyk B, Jureczko L, Kolacz M, Pacholczyk M, et al. Thoracic epidural analgesia in anaesthesia for liver transplantation: the 10-year experience of a single centre. Ann Transplant. 2010;15:35–9.
63. Hausken J, Haugaa H, Hagness M, Line PD, Melum E, Tønnessen TI. Thoracic epidural analgesia for postoperative pain management in liver transplantation: a 10-year study on 685 liver transplant recipients. Transplant Direct. 2021;7:e648.
64. Sharma A, Goel AD, Sharma PP, Vyas V, Agrawal SP. The effect of transversus abdominis plane block for analgesia in patients undergoing liver transplantation: a systematic review and meta-analysis. Turk J Anaesthesiol Reanim. 2019;47:359–66.
65. Assefi M, Trillaud E, Vezinet C, Duceau B, Baron E, Pons S, et al. Subcostal transversus abdominis plane block for postoperative analgesia in liver transplant recipients: a before-and-after study. Reg Anesth Pain Med. 2023;48:342–58.
66. Knorr JP, Barlow A, Reinaker TS, Zaki RF. A single dose of pre-operative pregabalin reduces post-operative opioid use after orthotopic liver transplantation. Clin Transpl. 2021;35:e14319.
67. Gucyetmez B, Atalan HK, Aslan S, Yazar S, Polat KY. Effects of intraoperative magnesium sulfate administration on postoperative tramadol requirement in liver transplantation: a prospective, Double-Blind Study. Transpl Proc. 2016;48:2742–6.

Chapter 26
ABO Incompatible Liver Transplantation

Shekhar Singh Jadaun, Shaleen Agarwal, Shweta A. Singh, Subhash Gupta, and Sanjiv Saigal

Abstract ABO-incompatible living donor liver transplant (ABOi LDLT) is helpful in increasing the donor pool, especially in the countries that predominantly perform living donor liver transplants. With improvements in desensitization protocols and immunosuppression regimes, outcomes of ABO incompatible and compatible liver transplants are comparable. Risk of allograft rejection, biliary complications, and infectious complications are the main reasons for graft dysfunction and mortality in ABOi LDLT recipients. Rituximab and plasmapheresis are the main methods of pretransplant desensitization to decrease the risk of allograft rejection. Postoperative immunosuppression consists mainly of three drugs: tacrolimus, mycophenolate mofetil, and corticosteroids. Post-transplant monitoring of ABO antibody titer should be done for the first 2–4 weeks. Graft rejection is managed by plasmapheresis, steroid pulse, and adjusting the dose of tacrolimus and mycophenolate. Intravenous immunoglobulins and anti-thymocyte globulin are used in steroid refractory rejection. Newer drugs like proteasome inhibitors and complement inhibitors have shown promising results in the management of AMR.

Keywords Liver transplant · ABO incompatible liver transplant · Liver cirrhosis · Living donor related liver transplant

S. S. Jadaun · S. Saigal (✉)
Hepatology and Liver Transplant Medicine, Max Institute of Liver and Gastrointestinal Sciences, Max Super Speciality Hospital, Saket, New Delhi, India
e-mail: sanjivsaigal@hotmail.com

S. Agarwal · S. Gupta
Centre for Liver and Biliary Sciences (CLBS), Max Super Speciality Hospital, Saket, New Delhi, Delhi, India

S. A. Singh
Anesthesia & Critical Care, Centre for Liver and Biliary Sciences, Max Super Specialty Hospital, New Delhi, Delhi, India

S. Saigal, D. Jothimani (eds.), *Fundamentals of Transplant Hepatology*, https://doi.org/10.1007/978-981-95-2624-6_26

Key Highlights

- ABO-incompatible living donor liver transplant (ABOi LDLT) is helpful in increasing the donor pool, especially in the countries that predominantly perform living donor liver transplants.
- With improvements in desensitization protocols and immunosuppression regimes, outcomes of ABO incompatible and compatible liver transplants are comparable.
- Risk of allograft rejection, biliary complications, and infectious complications are the main reasons for graft dysfunction and mortality in ABOi LDLT recipients.
- Rituximab and plasmapheresis are main methods of pretransplant desensitization to decrease the risk of allograft rejection.
- Postoperative immunosuppression consists mainly of three drugs: tacrolimus, mycophenolate mofetil, and corticosteroids.
- Post-transplant monitoring of ABO antibody titer should be done for the first 2–4 weeks.
- Graft rejection is managed by plasmapheresis, steroid pulse, and adjusting the dose of tacrolimus and mycophenolate.
- Intravenous immunoglobulins and antithymocyte globulin are used in steroid refractory rejection.
- Newer drugs like proteasome inhibitors and complement inhibitors have shown promising results in the management of AMR.

26.1 Introduction and Brief History

Living donor-related liver transplant (LDLT) is the predominant form of liver transplant in countries with scarce availability of cadaveric donors. In East and South Asian countries, more than 80% of liver transplants are living donor related. Breaching of the ABO barrier has led to further expansion of donor pools in these countries, and ABOi LDLT constitutes 10–20% of living donor liver transplants [1–3].

Dr. GP Alexandre performed the first successful human ABO incompatible (ABOi) renal transplant in 1985 [4] (Fig. 26.1). However, initial attempts at ABOi liver transplants met with disappointing results. High rates of graft loss and mortality were seen due to hyperacute rejection, antibody-mediated rejection (AMR)-related complications and increased rate of infections in these patients due to immunosuppression [5, 6]. Use of plasmapheresis, splenectomy, and local infusion therapy (LIT) helped in improving results of ABOi LDLT. Introduction of rituximab dramatically reduced the risk of graft rejection in these patients [7–9]. Further improvements in immunosuppression and pretransplant desensitization protocols has led to comparable outcomes of graft and patient survival in ABOi liver transplant and ABO compatible (ABOc) liver transplant [10, 11].

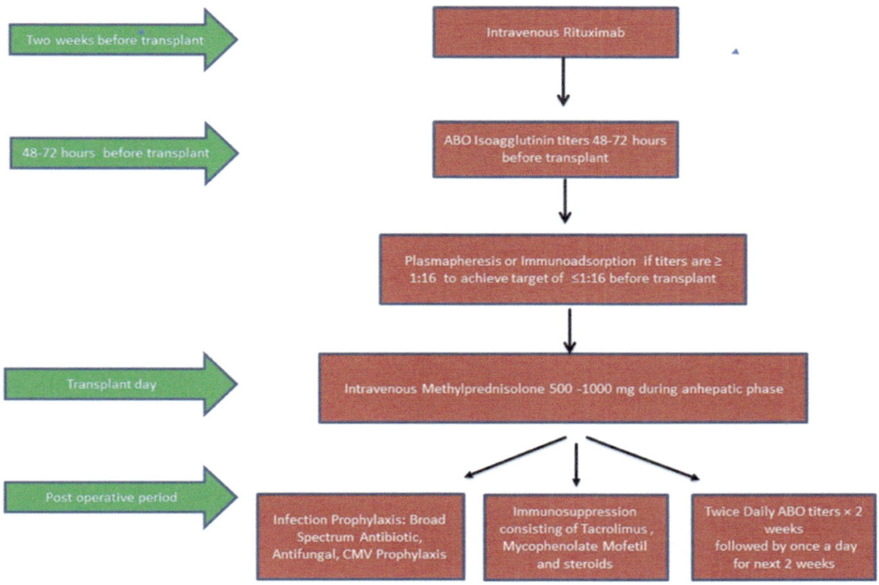

Fig. 26.1 ABO incompatible liver transplantation management protocol. CMV, Cytomegalovirus. (Adapted from Jadaun et al. [23])

26.2 Pathophysiology of Antibody-Mediated Rejection in ABOi Liver Transplant

ABOi liver transplant has the risk of AMR that can manifest as graft dysfunction, rapid graft loss due to hepatic necrosis, and non-anastomotic biliary strictures. ABO antigens are carbohydrate antigens, these antigens are expressed on most of the human tissues in addition to epithelial cells and red blood cells (RBC), which are expressed on a wide variety of human tissues in addition to RBC and endothelium [12, 13]. In liver, these antigens are expressed by RBCs, biliary epithelium, and endothelium in vessels and sinusoids [14]. Antibodies present in recipient blood bind with ABO antigen presents in donor tissue and starts an inflammatory cascade due to complement activation. Recruitment of various inflammatory cells like platelets, neutrophils, and macrophages results in the release of various cytokines and chemokines. These inflammatory cells and cytokines cause vascular endothelium injury and vascular thrombi formation and ultimately result in graft dysfunction. Significant injury to vascular tissues results in parenchymal necrosis and bile ducts ischemia, which may present as biliary strictures, cholestasis, and liver allograft loss [15].

26.3 Pretransplant Management in ABO-Incompatible LDLT

A critical component of ABO-incompatible (ABOi) living donor liver transplantation (LDLT) is pretransplant desensitization, which aims to reduce the risk of antibody-mediated rejection (AMR) and subsequent graft dysfunction. Desensitization lowers the levels of pre-existing ABO antibodies and suppresses B cell activity, thereby limiting further antibody production. Successful removal of anti-A or anti-B antibodies before surgery is a major determinant of post-transplant outcomes. Prior research has shown that elevated perioperative antibody titers significantly increase the risk of biliary injury, graft rejection, and graft loss [16, 17].

26.3.1 Rituximab Therapy

Rituximab, an anti-CD20 chimeric monoclonal antibody, has revolutionized desensitization strategies in ABOi transplantation. Originally introduced in the treatment of lymphomas and autoimmune diseases, its use in transplantation began with kidney transplants by Dr. Tyden and was later applied to liver transplantation by Monterio et al. [7, 18].

Rituximab binds selectively to CD20 receptors present on most mature B lymphocytes (but not on stem cells, pro-B cells, or mature plasma cells). Some activated plasma cells may express CD20. The drug depletes B cells via direct signaling, complement-dependent cytotoxicity (CDCC), and antibody-dependent cellular cytotoxicity (ADCC) [19, 20]. As B cells are crucial for antibody production, cytokine secretion, and antigen presentation, their depletion affects both humoral and cellular immune responses [21, 22].

The standard dose is 375 mg/m^2, administered as a slow IV infusion. A single dose is typically sufficient; multiple doses may increase the risk of infections. Lower doses, such as 200 mg/m^2, have been reported effective, especially in infection-prone patients. For instance, Egawa et al. found that reduced doses did not increase AMR risk [24].

Rituximab is usually administered 2 weeks before transplant, considering its long half-life (around 3 weeks). However, it has also been used 7 days prior or even within 72 h of transplantation in emergencies [10, 25, 26]. To prevent premature drug elimination, plasmapheresis should ideally be avoided within 3 days of rituximab administration. B cell depletion in peripheral blood generally occurs within 48–72 h, with complete depletion taking up to 3 weeks. Rituximab efficacy is monitored by measuring CD19+ cells, with target reduction defined as $<1\%$ of total lymphocytes. A second dose may be considered if depletion is inadequate, although it is rarely needed [15, 27].

Rituximab achieves prolonged depletion of circulating and splenic B and memory B cells, significantly reducing AMR risk, though not eliminating it completely due to residual lymph node B cells [25, 28]. Its use has markedly improved graft survival in ABOi LDLT. A multicenter study from Japan reported AMR rates of 6% in rituximab-treated patients vs. 23% in those not receiving the drug. Other strategies like IVIG, LIT, or splenectomy showed no significant impact [10, 26].

Some studies have explored rituximab monotherapy as a standalone desensitization protocol. For example, Yamamoto et al. found similar survival and AMR rates in patients treated with or without plasmapheresis, with lower infection rates in the monotherapy group [30]. Lee et al. observed similar ABOi-related complications and survival outcomes with or without plasmapheresis, provided antibody titers at transplant were <1:16 [31]. However, more evidence is needed to support monotherapy in patients with high baseline titers, and long-term data on graft survival and biliary complications remain limited. Importantly, rituximab does not negatively affect survival or recurrence risk in patients with HCC [32].

26.3.2 Plasma Exchange (PE) and Immunoadsorption (IA)

Plasmapheresis (plasma exchange) involves removing the patient's plasma to eliminate antibodies, including anti-A and anti-B isoagglutinins, which raise the risk of AMR and graft complications. The risk of these complications increases with higher antibody titers [6, 17]. PE helps reduce these levels, though multiple sessions may be required due to ongoing antibody synthesis [33].

There is no universally defined safe titer before transplant, with acceptable values ranging from <1:8 to <1:64, depending on institutional protocols. If rituximab leads to sufficient B cell depletion and low antibody titers, plasmapheresis may be unnecessary [30, 31]. Typically, a single session of PE reduces IgG and IgM by 50–60%, and additional sessions are tailored to pretransplant titers. Side effects include hypersensitivity, hemodynamic instability, and citrate toxicity [34, 35]. PE may also be used in post-transplant period to treat antibody titer rebound.

Double-filtration plasmapheresis (DFPP) is a modified form of PE that uses separate filters to remove large proteins like immunoglobulins while returning smaller proteins (e.g., albumin, clotting factors) to the patient. DFPP reduces the need for albumin and plasma replacement and is commonly used in Asia, though less so elsewhere [35, 36].

Immunoadsorption (IA) functions similarly to PE but selectively targets and removes ABO antibodies via antigen-specific columns, returning other plasma components to the patient. This selectivity leads to a better safety profile [37]. Although IA is well established in kidney transplantation, its application in liver transplant remains limited [29, 38, 39].

26.4 Intraoperative Period

26.4.1 Splenectomy

The spleen is a major lymphoid organ and a reservoir of plasma cells. It plays an important role in AMR because of antibodies production by plasma cells. Splenectomy can decrease the risk of AMR by eliminating the plasma cell reservoir in the spleen. Before the use of rituximab in liver transplant splenectomy during transplant surgery was the standard practice in ABOi LDLT [16]. With the use of rituximab, splenectomy is not necessary and can also increase the risk of infections in immunocompromised recipients [14, 40, 41]. Rout et al. reported similar ABO isoagglutinin titer, AMR rate, and survival outcomes in patients with and without splenectomy; both groups were given preoperative rituximab [42].

26.5 Post-transplant Management in ABOi LDLT

26.5.1 Target Isoagglutinin Titers (Anti-A/Anti-B Antibodies)

There is currently no universal agreement on the exact anti-A or anti-B antibody levels considered safe for minimizing AMR and associated complications. Different centers use varying cut-offs, with acceptable pre-transplant titers ranging from ≤1:64 to ≤1:8 [5, 43].

In a study involving 381 adult ABOi LDLT recipients, Egawa et al. demonstrated that the risk of AMR increased when pre-transplant titers were ≥1:16 and post-transplant titers reached ≥1:64. Notably, rituximab use was linked to significantly reduced AMR risk in this study [10].

Although many findings suggest a direct correlation between higher preoperative isoagglutinin titers and AMR risk, some research challenges this association, indicating that anti-A/B titers may not reliably predict AMR in liver transplant recipients [6, 44, 45]. Furthermore, non-anastomotic intrahepatic biliary strictures, often linked to AMR, may develop without a corresponding rebound in isoagglutinin titers [46].

26.5.2 Post-transplant Immunosuppression

Immunosuppression in ABOi LDLT typically follows the standard triple-drug regimen, similar to ABO-compatible LDLT protocols. This includes:

1. Steroids
2. Calcineurin inhibitors (CNIs) — Tacrolimus is preferred over cyclosporine.
3. Mycophenolate mofetil (MMF)

Steroids: An initial dose of 500–1000 mg IV methylprednisolone is administered intraoperatively prior to graft perfusion, followed by 100 mg IV on postoperative day 1. The dose is tapered over the first week, after which oral prednisolone is introduced and continued for about 3 months with gradual tapering.

Tacrolimus and MMF: Both are started on postoperative day 1, with tacrolimus trough levels maintained at 10–12 ng/mL during the early post-op period. MMF is dosed at 500–1000 mg/day, with higher doses used in patients with renal impairment to allow for lower tacrolimus dosing [26, 47].

Some clinicians have explored pretransplant initiation of tacrolimus and MMF to reduce rejection risk, but this practice is not widely adopted due to the potential for increased infections post-transplant [48].

Basiliximab, an IL-2 receptor blocker, has been used in cases of renal dysfunction to delay CNI initiation. However, its use in ABOi LDLT is still limited and may be associated with an increased infection risk [49, 50].

26.5.3 Intravenous Immunoglobulin (IVIG)

IVIG, composed mainly of polyclonal IgG derived from healthy donor plasma, is traditionally used in immunodeficiency syndromes and inflammatory conditions like Guillain-Barré syndrome [26].

High-dose IVIG has been applied in cases of steroid-resistant acute rejection in both kidney and liver transplants. In ABOi LDLT, IVIG is primarily utilized for managing post-transplant rebound of ABO antibody titers [2, 51].

IVIG exerts multiple immunomodulatory effects:

1. Suppresses alloreactive T-cell function
2. Inhibits CD19 expression on activated B cells
3. Neutralizes alloantibodies
4. Blocks Fc receptors on phagocytes
5. Inhibits complement activation [16, 52]

Some studies have included IVIG in desensitization protocols. In a simplified approach by Kim et al., 43 patients received IVIG (0.8 g/kg) on postoperative days 1 and 4 after pretransplant rituximab and standard immunosuppression. No AMR cases were observed, although 30% developed biliary strictures [2]. However, the high cost, limited long-term data, and risk of adverse reactions limit routine IVIG use for desensitization.

26.5.4 Local Infusion Therapy (LIT)

Postoperative LIT involves administering agents like gabexate mesylate, methylprednisolone, or prostaglandin E1 into the portal vein or hepatic artery via catheter. LIT aims to suppress the inflammatory response triggered by preformed antibodies interacting with donor antigens, thereby preventing microvascular injury and improving graft survival [15, 16].

A Japanese study showed improved outcomes with LIT in ABOi LDLT patients [14, 16]. However, catheter-related complications—such as bleeding, infection, and thrombosis—are significant, occurring in 16% of hepatic artery and 37% of portal vein infusions [40].

With the advent of rituximab, the utility of LIT has diminished. Song et al. found no difference in AMR incidence or survival between patients who received LIT and those who did not [53]. Furthermore, adverse events led to early discontinuation in many cases [5].

Nonetheless, LIT remains a consideration in emergency ABOi LDLT or DDLT cases where rituximab has insufficient time to deplete B cells effectively [10, 15, 46].

26.6 Management Algorithm for ABO-Incompatible LDLT

26.6.1 Desensitization Protocol

Desensitization begins with rituximab administration approximately 2 weeks prior to transplant surgery. The standard dose is 350 mg, but a reduced dose of 300 mg may be used in patients with acute-on-chronic liver failure or those with prolonged ICU stays, as these patients are more vulnerable to infections.

Response to rituximab is monitored by measuring CD19+ and CD20+ mononuclear cells; a count of <1% is considered an adequate response. Plasmapheresis or immunoadsorption (IA) is performed before surgery to reduce ABO antibody titers to ≤1:16.

Splenectomy, LIT, and IVIG are not routinely included in most center protocols. The anti-IL-2 agent basiliximab is also not routinely used but may be considered in recipients with renal impairment.

26.6.2 Immunosuppression Protocol (Post-transplant)

Recipients receive 500–1000 mg of intravenous methylprednisolone intraoperatively during the anhepatic phase. Post-transplant, immunosuppression follows a standard triple-drug regimen:

- Tacrolimus (target trough: 10–12 ng/mL for 2–3 weeks)
- MMF, typically 500 mg twice daily, increased to 750–1000 mg BID as needed
- Steroids, tapered gradually over 3 months

Some authors recommend starting CNIs and MMF preoperatively, though this is uncommon due to increased infection risk [48].

26.6.3 Antibody Monitoring and Post-transplant Plasmapheresis

- IgG and IgM anti-A/B titers should be measured twice daily for the first 2 weeks, then daily for the next 2 weeks.
- Plasmapheresis is indicated if:

- Titers rise by 2 logs
- Titers reach ≥1:64
- There's an unexplained increase in bilirubin or liver enzymes

Thresholds vary between transplant centers. Protocol liver biopsies are not routinely performed but are indicated in suspected rejection or unexplained liver dysfunction.

26.6.4 Infection Prophylaxis

Due to the high infection risk in ABOi LDLT, patients routinely receive:

- Broad-spectrum antibiotics
- Antifungal prophylaxis
- Pre-emptive cytomegalovirus (CMV) treatment

26.7 Diagnosis and Management of Acute Antibody-Mediated Rejection (AMR)

Despite advances in ABOi LDLT, further refinement is needed—especially in early AMR diagnosis, which is critical for improving graft survival. Identifying biomarkers for early detection before histological damage occurs remains a promising area of research.

26.7.1 Diagnosis of AMR

The reported incidence of AMR in the post-rituximab era is around 5–7% [48]. AMR is suspected when:

- Liver function tests are abnormal
- No vascular, biliary, or mechanical causes are identified
- ABO antibody titers rise post-transplant

Imaging may show portal edema or necrosis early on, and intrahepatic biliary strictures may develop later [54].

Histopathology plays a supportive role but is not definitive. Characteristic features include:

- Endothelial cell injury, swelling, and endothelitis
- C4d complement deposition along the endothelium

Diagnosis is confirmed by:

- Compatible histological findings
- Presence of donor-specific antibodies
- Exclusion of other graft injuries [55, 56]

26.7.2 Treatment of AMR

There is no standardized treatment, making prevention the most effective approach. Avoiding unnecessary blood transfusions before transplant may reduce sensitization risk.

Management Strategies:

1. Mild to Moderate AMR:
    - Plasmapheresis
    - Methylprednisolone pulse therapy
    - Adjustment of tacrolimus and MMF doses
2. Refractory or Severe AMR:
    - Anti-thymocyte globulin (ATG)
    - IVIG
    - Repeat rituximab
3. Experimental or Limited-Use Options:
    - Bortezomib (a proteasome inhibitor)
    - Eculizumab (a complement inhibitor) [57–60]
    - Evidence for these agents is currently limited to small studies.
4. Emerging Therapies:
    - Tocilizumab (IL-6 receptor antagonist)
    - Belatacept (T-cell co-stimulation blocker) [26, 61, 62]

Table 26.1 Newer drugs in ABO incompatible liver transplantation

Drug	Class	Indication
Obinutuzumab	Anti CD20 monoclonal antibody	Pretransplant desensitization
Imlifidase	IgG-degrading enzyme derived from streptococcus pyogenes (IdeS)	Pretransplant desensitization
Tocilizumab	Anti-IL-6 monoclonal antibody	Pretransplant desensitization, chronic AMR, GVHD
Clazzakizumab	IL-6 inhibitors	Acute AMR
Daratumumab	Anti CD-38	Acute AMR
Bortezomib, Carfilzomib	Proteosome inhibitors	Acute AMR
Eculizumab	Compliment inhibitor	Acute AMR
Belimumab, Tabalumab, atacicept	Anti-BAFF monoclonal antibody	Pretransplant desensitization, AMR
Belatacept	Anti-CD80/CD86 monoclonal antibody	Post-transplant immunosuppression

- Obinutuzumab, a next-generation anti-CD20 antibody with more potent B cell depletion than rituximab.

Preliminary results in kidney transplant patients show safety and tolerability, suggesting possible application in ABOi liver transplant [63–65].

Table 26.1 summarizes current and emerging therapies used for AMR prevention and treatment in ABOi liver transplantation.

26.8 ABOi LDLT in Pediatric Population

Studies have reported better outcomes in ABOi LT in children as compared to adults. In a retrospective analysis of the national registry database by Stewart et al., pediatric (<17 years) ABOi DDLT graft survival was similar to ABOc DDLT [66]. Children under 2 years have the best outcomes in pediatric ABOi LDLT and 11 months is the minimum age at which antibody-mediated complications have been reported. Immature immune systems and the resulted decreased risk of AMR are likely the possible reasons for better outcomes in children [17, 67–69]. Mysore et al. devised a new strategy for ABOi DDLT based on pre-transplant ABO antibody titers. Children with pre-transplant titer of ≥1:32 received rituximab and plasmapheresis before transplant, followed by standard triple-drug immunosuppression in the post-transplant period. Children with pre-transplant isoagglutinin titer of <1:16 received only steroids and tacrolimus. Authors reported a 100% graft survival rate over a 3.3-year follow-up. However, in this study, only ten patients underwent ABOi liver transplants [70]. Given the absence of AMR and related complications in children below 1 year, use of rituximab and plasmapheresis is avoided in this group of patients. Anti-AB isoagglutinin titers in small children can be below the pre-transplant target level without any desensitization method because development of these antibodies is age-dependent. Post-transplant immunosuppression protocol usually consisted of a three-drug regime as in adult patients, including CNIs, MMF, and steroids. Use of IVIG has been reported by Markiewicz-Kijewska et al. in children during the post-transplant period for desensitization and in the treatment of severe AMR [71].

26.9 ABOi LT in Emergency Indications

ABOi LT has many challenges in emergency situations like deceased donor LT, acute liver failure, and acute on chronic live failure patients when clinical condition does not allow waiting for a compatible allograft. Risk of severe infections is increased with use of B cells-depleting agents and immunosuppressive regimens in these critically sick patients [26, 72]. Because of limited time available for desensitization protocol, the risk of AMR is also higher in post-transplant period. Although early studies reported suboptimal results in emergency ABOi LT, more recent evidence is encouraging [73, 74]. Dahlgren et al. have reported their successful experience of ABOi LT in DDLT. They developed a protocol in which single dose of rituximab was administered on day 0 before transplant, and PP or IA was started as soon as DDLT was scheduled. IA or PP was also done in post-transplant period on days 2, 5, and 8, regardless of ABO antibody titer levels. Graft and patient survival rates were similar to ABOc control group and only one patient developed AMR [75]. In another study, Shen et al. used Rituximab, IVIG and basiliximab-based protocol in ABOi DDLT with 83% graft survival rates at 3 years [76]. In a small case series of eight patients, Lee et al. used bortezomib, rituximab, and PP in ABOi LDLT for ALF patients. Desensitization protocol took 4.75 days of mean time to prepare these patients. The six-month graft survival rate was 87.5% and one patient developed AMR after 6 months [77]. Published studies on ABOi LDLT in emergency settings are mostly small case series only, and data regarding efficacy and safety is very limited in the present time. Further evidence is needed to establish an effective desensitization protocol in emergency ABOi LDLT.

26.10 Conclusion

ABOi LDLT is now established as an effective, safe method and has resulted in significant expansion of liver donor pools. Current desensitization protocols that include rituximab have shown graft and overall survival almost equivalent to ABOc LDLT. Management of severe AMR and prevention of biliary and infectious complications are the challenges that affect survival outcomes. Regular monitoring of liver allograft function, antibody titers imaging and vigilance for infectious complications are important for optimal outcomes in these patients.

References

1. Goss MB, Rana A. ABO-incompatible liver transplantation: is it a viable option with modern innovation? Clin Liver Dis (Hoboken). 2017;10(5):124–9.
2. Ikegami T, Taketomi A, Soejima Y, Yoshizumi T, Uchiyama H, Harada N, Iguchi T, Hashimoto N, Maehara Y. Rituximab, IVIG, and plasma exchange without graft local infusion treatment: a new protocol in ABO incompatible living donor liver transplantation. Transplantation. 2009;88:303–7.
3. Kawagishi N, Satoh K, Enomoto Y, Akamatsu Y, Sekiguchi S, Fukumori T, Fujimori K, Satomi S. New strategy for ABO-incompatible living donor liver transplantation with anti-CD20 antibody (rituximab) and plasma exchange. Transplant Proc. 2005;37:1205–6.
4. Alexandre GPJ, de Bruyere M, Squifflet JP, Moriau M, Latinne D, Pirson Y. Human ABO-incompatible living donor renal homografts. Neth J Med. 1985;28:231–4.
5. Song GW, Lee SG, Hwang S, et al. ABO-incompatible adult living donor liver transplantation under the desensitization protocol with rituximab. Am J Transplant. 2016;16:157–70.
6. Oh J, Kim JM. Immunologic strategies and outcomes in ABO-incompatible living donor liver transplantation. Clin Mol Hepatol. 2020;26:1–6.
7. Monteiro I, McLoughlin LM, Fisher A, de La Torre AN, Koneru B. Rituximab with plasmapheresis and splenectomy in abo-incompatible liver transplantation. Transplantation. 2003;76:1648–9.
8. Nakamura Y, Matsuno N, Iwamoto H, et al. Successful case of adult ABO-incompatible liver transplantation: beneficial effects of intrahepatic artery infusion therapy: a case report. Transplant Proc. 2004;36:2269–73.
9. Tanabe M, Shimazu M, Wakabayashi G, Hoshino K, Kawachi S, Kadomura T, Seki H, Morikawa Y, Kitajima M. Intraportal infusion therapy as a novel approach to adult ABO-incompatible liver transplantation. Transplantation. 2002;73:1959–61.
10. Egawa H, Teramukai S, Haga H, Tanabe M, Mori A, Ikegami T, Kawagishi N, Ohdan H, Kasahara M, Umeshita K. Impact of rituximab desensitization on blood-type-incompatible adult living donor liver transplantation: a Japanese multicenter study. Am J Transplant. 2014;14:102–14.
11. Farges O, Kalil AN, Samuel D, Saliba F, Arulnaden JL, Debat P, Bismuth A, Castaing D, Bismuth H. The use of ABO-incompatible grafts in liver transplantation: a life-saving procedure in highly selected patients. Transplantation. 1995;59:1124–33.
12. The ABO blood group - Blood Groups and Red Cell Antigens - NCBI Bookshelf. https://www.ncbi.nlm.nih.gov/sites/books/NBK2267/?msclkid=a5865a72cedb11eca29e053e58a41e84. Accessed 8 May 2022.
13. Samuelsson BE, Breimer ME. ABH antigens: some basic aspects. Transplant Proc. 1987;19:4401–7.
14. Tanabe M, Kawachi S, Obara H, Shinoda M, Hibi T, Kitagawa Y, Wakabayashi G, Shimazu M, Kitajima M. Current progress in ABO-incompatible liver transplantation. Eur J Clin Investig. 2010;40:943–9.
15. Egawa H. Challenge to ABO blood type barrier in living donor liver transplantation. Hepatobiliary Pancreat Dis Int. 2020;19:342–8.
16. Kawagishi N, Satomi S. Current aspects of ABO-incompatible liver transplantation. Clin Case Rep Rev. 2016;10.15761/ccrr.1000221
17. Egawa H, Oike F, Buhler L, Shapiro AMJ, Minamiguchi S, Haga H, Uryuhara K, Kiuchi T, Kaihara S, Tanaka K. Impact of recipient age on outcome of ABO-incompatible living-donor liver transplantation. Transplantation. 2004;77:403–11.
18. Tydén G, Kumlien G, Fehrman I. Successful ABO-incompatible kidney transplantations without splenectomy using antigen-specific immunoadsorption and rituximab. Transplantation. 2003;76:730–1.
19. Weiner GJ. Rituximab: mechanism of action. Semin Hematol. 2010;47:115.

20. Sood P, Hariharan S. Anti-CD20 blocker rituximab in kidney transplantation. Transplantation. 2018;102:44–58.
21. Hoffman W, Lakkis FG, Chalasani G. B cells, antibodies, and more. Clin J Am Soc Nephrol. 2016;11:137.
22. von Bergwelt-Baildon M, Schultze JL, Maecker B, Menezes I, Nadler LM, Lapointe R, Thibodeau J, Hwu P. Correspondence re R. Lapointe et al., CD40-stimulated B lymphocytes pulsed with tumor antigens are effective antigen-presenting cells that can generate specific T cells. Cancer res 2003;63:2836-43 (multiple letters). Cancer Res. 2004;64:4055–7.
23. Jadaun SS, Agarwal S, Gupta S, Saigal S. Strategies for ABO incompatible liver transplantation. J Clin Exp Hepatol. 2023;13:698–706.
24. Egawa H, Umeshita K, Uemoto S. Optimal dosage regimen for rituximab in ABO-incompatible living donor liver transplantation. J Hepatobiliary Pancreat Sci. 2017;24:89–94.
25. Egawa H, Ohmori K, Haga H, et al. B-cell surface marker analysis for improvement of rituximab prophylaxis in ABO-incompatible adult living donor liver transplantation. Liver Transpl. 2007;13:579–88.
26. Cheng C-H, Lee C-F, Wang Y-C, Wu T-H, Wu T-J, Chou H-S, Chan K-M, Lee W-C. ABO-incompatible liver transplantation: state of art and future perspectives. Curr Pharm Des. 2020;26:3406–17.
27. Puisset F, White-Koning M, Kamar N, et al. Population pharmacokinetics of rituximab with or without plasmapheresis in kidney patients with antibody-mediated disease. Br J Clin Pharmacol. 2013;76:734–40.
28. Genberg H, Hansson A, Wernerson A, Wennberg L, Tydén G. Pharmacodynamics of rituximab in kidney allotransplantation. Am J Transplant. 2006;6:2418–28.
29. Dahlgren US, Bennet W. ABO-incompatible liver transplantation–a review of the historical background and results. Int Rev Immunol. 2019;38:118–28.
30. Yamamoto H, Uchida K, Kawabata S, Isono K, Miura K, Hayashida S, Oya Y, Sugawara Y, Inomata Y. Feasibility of monotherapy by rituximab without additional desensitization in ABO-incompatible living-donor liver transplantation. Transplantation. 2018;102:97–104.
31. Lee EC, Kim SH, Shim JR, Park SJ. A comparison of desensitization methods: rituximab with/without plasmapheresis in ABO-incompatible living donor liver transplantation. Hepatobiliary Pancreat Dis Int. 2018;17:119–25.
32. Kim SH, Lee EC, Na BG, Park SJ. Impact of ABO-incompatibility on hepatocellular carcinoma recurrence after living donor liver transplantation. Eur J Surg Oncol. 2019;45:180–6.
33. Kozaki K, Egawa H, Ueda M, Oike F, Yoshizawa A, Fukatsu A, Takada Y. The role of apheresis therapy for ABO incompatible living donor liver transplantation: the Kyoto University experience. Ther Apher Dial. 2006;10:441–8.
34. Takahashi K. A new concept of accomodation in ABO-incompatible kidney transplantation. Clin Transpl. 2005;Suppl 19:76–85.
35. Song G-W. ABO Incompatability in liver transplantation. Hanyang Med Rev. 2014;34:202.
36. Thalgahagoda S, Webb NJA, Roberts D, Birch A, Milford DV, Tavakoli A, Shenoy M. Successful ABO incompatible renal transplantation following rituximab and DFPP after failed immunoadsorption. Pediatr Transplant. 2014; https://doi.org/10.1111/PETR.12227.
37. de Weerd AE, van Agteren M, Leebeek FW, Ijzermans JNM, Weimar W, Betjes MGH. ABO-incompatible kidney transplant recipients have a higher bleeding risk after antigen-specific immunoadsorption. Transpl Int. 2015;28:25–33.
38. Genberg H, Kumlien G, Wennberg L, Tyden G. The efficacy of antigen-specific immunoadsorption and rebound of anti-A/B antibodies in ABO-incompatible kidney transplantation. Nephrol Dial Transplant. 2011;26:2394–400.
39. Makroo RN, Agrawal S, Chowdhry M, Kakkar B, Thakur UK. Efficacy of single, extended and goal directed immunoadsorption in ABO incompatible living related donor liver transplantation. Transfus Apher Sci. 2016;55:329–32.
40. Egawa H, Teramukai S, Haga H, Tanabe M, Fukushima M, Shimazu M. Present status of ABO-incompatible living donor liver transplantation in Japan. Hepatology. 2008;47:143–52.

41. Raut V, Uemoto S. Management of ABO-incompatible living-donor liver transplantation: past and present trends. Surg Today. 2011;41:317–22.
42. Raut V, Mori A, Kaido T, et al. Splenectomy does not offer immunological benefits in ABO-incompatible liver transplantation with a preoperative rituximab. Transplantation. 2012;93:99–105.
43. Lee CF, Cheng CH, Wang YC, Soong RS, Wu TH, Chou HS, Wu TJ, Chan KM, Lee CS, Lee WC. Adult living donor liver transplantation across ABO-incompatibility. Medicine. 2015;94:e1796.
44. Shimmura H, Tanabe K, Ishida H, et al. Lack of correlation between results of ABO-incompatible living kidney transplantation and anti-ABO blood type antibody titers under our current immunosuppression. Transplantation. 2005;80:985–8.
45. Skogsberg U, Breimer ME, Friman S, Mjörnstedt L, Mölne J, Olausson M, Rydberg L, Svalander CT, Bäckman L. Adult ABO-incompatible liver transplantation, using A and B donors. Xenotransplantation. 2006;13:154–9.
46. Song GW, Lee SG, Hwang S, et al. Biliary stricture is the only concern in ABO-incompatible adult living donor liver transplantation in the rituximab era. J Hepatol. 2014;61:575–82.
47. Moini M, Schilsky ML, Tichy EM. Review on immunosuppression in liver transplantation. World J Hepatol. 2015;7:1355.
48. Egawa H, Ohdan H, Saito K. Current status of ABO-incompatible liver transplantation. Transplantation. 2023;107:313–25.
49. Lin CC, Chuang FR, Lee CH, Wang CC, Chen YS, Liu YW, Jawan B, Chen CL. The renal-sparing efficacy of basiliximab in adult living donor liver transplantation. Liver Transpl. 2005;11:1258–64.
50. Penninga L, Wettergren A, Wilson CH, Chan AW, Steinbrüchel DA, Gluud C. Antibody induction versus placebo, no induction, or another type of antibody induction for liver transplant recipients. Cochrane Database Syst Rev. 2014; https://doi.org/10.1002/14651858.CD010253.PUB2/MEDIA/CDSR/CD010253/IMAGE_N/NCD010253-CMP-006-02.PNG.
51. Luke PPW, Scantlebury VP, Jordan ML, Vivas CA, Hakala TR, Jain A, Somani A, Fedorek S, Randhawa P, Shapiro R. Reversal of steroid- and anti-lymphocyte antibody-resistant rejection using intravenous immunoglobulin (IVIG) in renal transplant recipients. Transplantation. 2001;72:419–22.
52. Jordan S, Cunningham-Rundles C, McEwanc R. Utility of intravenous immune globulin in kidney transplantation: efficacy, safety, and cost implications. Am J Transplant. 2003;3:653–64.
53. Kim JM, Kwon CHD, Joh JW, Kang ES, Park JB, Lee JH, Kim SJ, Paik SW, Lee SK, Kim DW. ABO-incompatible living donor liver transplantation is suitable in patients without ABO-matched donor. J Hepatol. 2013;59:1215–22.
54. Haga H, Egawa H, Shirase T, Miyagawa A, Sakurai T, Minamiguchi S, Yamabe H, Manabe T, Tanaka K. Periportal edema and necrosis as diagnostic histological features of early humoral rejection in ABO-incompatible liver transplantation. Liver Transpl. 2004;10:16–27.
55. O'Leary JG, Shiller SM, Bellamy C, Nalesnik MA, Kaneku H, Jennings LW, Isse K, Terasaki PI, Klintmalm GB, Demetris AJ. Acute liver allograft antibody-mediated rejection: an inter-institutional study of routine histopathological features. Liver Transpl. 2014;20:1244.
56. Lee M. Antibody-mediated rejection after liver transplant. Gastroenterol Clin N Am. 2017;46:297–309.
57. Lee BT, Fiel MI, Schiano TD. Antibody-mediated rejection of the liver allograft: an update and a clinico-pathological perspective. J Hepatol. 2021;75:1203–16.
58. Montgomery RA, Loupy A, Segev DL. Antibody-mediated rejection: new approaches in prevention and management. Am J Transplant. 2018;18(Suppl 3):3–17.
59. Paterno F, Shiller M, Tillery G, O'Leary JG, Susskind B, Trotter J, Klintmalm GB. Bortezomib for acute antibody-mediated rejection in liver transplantation. Am J Transplant. 2012;12:2526.
60. Tajima T, Hata K, Okajima H, et al. Bortezomib against refractory antibody-mediated rejection after ABO-incompatible living-donor liver transplantation: dramatic effect in acute-phase? Transplant Direct. 2019; https://doi.org/10.1097/TXD.0000000000000932.

61. Choi J, Aubert O, Vo A, et al. Assessment of Tocilizumab (anti-Interleukin-6 receptor monoclonal) as a potential treatment for chronic antibody-mediated rejection and transplant Glomerulopathy in HLA-sensitized renal allograft recipients. Am J Transplant. 2017;17:2381–9.
62. Kirk AD, Guasch A, Xu H, et al. Renal transplantation using Belatacept without maintenance steroids or Calcineurin inhibitors. Am J Transplant. 2014;14:1142.
63. Byrd JC, Flynn JM, Kipps TJ, Boxer M, Kolibaba KS, Carlile DJ, Fingerle-Rowson G, Tyson N, Hirata J, Sharman JP. Randomized phase 2 study of obinutuzumab monotherapy in symptomatic, previously untreated chronic lymphocytic leukemia. Blood. 2016;127:79–86.
64. Marcus R, Davies A, Ando K, et al. Obinutuzumab for the first-line treatment of follicular lymphoma. N Engl J Med. 2017;377:1331–44.
65. Redfield RR, Jordan SC, Busque S, et al. Safety, pharmacokinetics, and pharmacodynamic activity of obinutuzumab, a type 2 anti-CD20 monoclonal antibody for the desensitization of candidates for renal transplant. Am J Transplant. 2019;19:3035–45.
66. Stewart ZA, Locke JE, Montgomery RA, Singer AL, Cameron AM, Segev DL. ABO-incompatible deceased donor liver transplantation in the United States: a national registry analysis. Liver Transpl. 2009;15:883–93.
67. Fong SW, Qaqundah BY, Taylor WF. Developmental patterns of ABO isoagglutinins in normal children correlated with the effects of age, sex, and maternal isoagglutinins. Transfusion (Paris). 1974;14:551–9.
68. Gelas T, McKiernan PJ, Kelly DA, Mayer DA, Mirza DF, Sharif K. ABO-incompatible pediatric liver transplantation in very small recipients: Birmingham's experience. Pediatr Transplant. 2011;15:706–11.
69. Rana A, Kueht ML, Nicholas SK, Jindra PT, Himes RW, Desai MS, Cotton RT, Galvan NTN, O'Mahony CA, Goss JA. Pediatric liver transplantation across the ABO blood group barrier: is it an obstacle in the modern era? J Am Coll Surg. 2016;222:681–9.
70. Mysore KR, Himes RW, Rana A, et al. ABO-incompatible deceased donor pediatric liver transplantation: novel titer-based management protocol and outcomes. Pediatr Transplant. 2018; https://doi.org/10.1111/PETR.13263.
71. Markiewicz-Kijewska M, Kaliciński P, Torres Canizales J, et al. ABO incompatible liver transplantation in children: a 20 year experience from centres in the transplantchild European reference network. Children. 2021; https://doi.org/10.3390/children8090760.
72. Moon DB, Lee SG, Kang WH, et al. Adult living donor liver transplantation for acute-on-chronic liver failure in high–model for end-stage liver disease score patients. Am J Transplant. 2017;17:1833.
73. Mendes M, Ferreira AC, Ferreira A, et al. ABO-incompatible liver transplantation in acute liver failure: a single Portuguese center study. Transplant Proc. 2013;45:1110–5.
74. Yang Y, Xu C, Chen YH, et al. ABO-incompatible liver transplantation for liver failure. Zhonghua Yi Xue Za Zhi. 2007;87:2833–6.
75. Skogsberg Dahlgren U, Herlenius G, Gustafsson B, Mölne J, Rydberg L, Socratous A, Bennet W. Excellent outcome following emergency deceased donor ABO-incompatible liver transplantation using rituximab and antigen specific immunoadsorption. Scand J Gastroenterol. 2022;57:50–9.
76. Shen T, Lin BY, Jia JJ, Wang ZY, Wang L, Ling Q, Geng L, Yan S, Zheng SS. A modified protocol with rituximab and intravenous immunoglobulin in emergent ABO-incompatible liver transplantation for acute liver failure. Hepatobiliary Pancreat Dis Int. 2014;13:395–401.
77. Lee WC, Cheng CH, Lee CF, Hung HC, Lee JC, Wu TH, Wang YC, Wu TJ, Chou HS, Chan KM. Quick preparation of ABO-incompatible living donor liver transplantation for acute liver failure. Clin Transpl. 2022; https://doi.org/10.1111/ctr.14555.

Chapter 27
Combined Liver Kidney Transplant

Gomathy Narasimhan and Jagdish Kanagaraj

Abstract Renal dysfunction is seen very often in patients with liver disease, either secondary to the impact of liver failure or as a direct impact of metabolic syndrome on both organs as it is now the commonest etiology for both liver (MASLD) and renal failure. It is important to identify the etiology of the renal dysfunction, categorize the severity of liver and renal disease, and understand the reversibility of renal dysfunction to decide on the management plan. The fallacy lies in the available markers of renal dysfunction in liver disease; they do not provide a correct assessment of the current condition of renal dysfunction. Guidelines for combined liver and kidney transplant have been developed taking into account this caveat. Once a decision is made to do a dual organ transplant (liver and kidney), the discussion should focus on the timing and sequence of the dual organ transplant, the donor options, and management of the pre- and postoperative periods. This chapter takes a stepwise approach to the assessment and management of patients requiring combined liver and kidney transplantation.

Keywords Combined Liver Kidney Transplant (CLKT) · CLKT allocation · HRS · Primary hyperoxaluria · ADPKD · HVPG

Key Highlights

Renal dysfunction is very common among patients with liver disease and has a significant impact on outcomes after liver transplants.

G. Narasimhan (✉)
Liver and Renal Transplant Surgery, Dr. Rela Institute and Medical Centre, Chennai, India
e-mail: gomathy.narasimhan@relainstitute.com

J. Kanagaraj
Nephrology and Renal Transplantation, Dr. Rela Institute and Medical Centre, Chennai, India

S. Saigal, D. Jothimani (eds.), *Fundamentals of Transplant Hepatology*,
https://doi.org/10.1007/978-981-95-2624-6_27

Categorizing the patients who need a CLKT, especially those with sustained AKI and advanced CKD is still a difficult task, and there are no reliable markers of estimation of severity and reversibility of renal disease.
Several factors in the perioperative period compound the above situation.
Better understanding in terms of timing and management of patients with metabolic disease has evolved, although they are a special cohort, and management in centers with special interest leads to better outcome.
Donor organ quality (DRI) and the recipient's hemodynamic condition at CLKT influence the outcome of CLKT.
Immune suppression has to be tailored in this high-risk cohort.

27.1 Introduction

Combined liver and kidney transplantation (CLKT) is a topic of extensive discussion for several reasons—close association between liver cirrhosis and renal dysfunction, lack of accurate ways to determine reversibility of kidney injury in liver patients, and optimum utilization of the organs in both deceased and live donors. CLKT can be performed either simultaneously or sequentially, with the liver first followed by the kidney a few days, weeks, or months later and hence allows for further discussion on the timing of the transplant(s).

Patients with liver disease very often present with altered renal function, either as a result of the liver disease, as in HRS or AKI (secondary to diuretic intolerance), or as an additional insult on a background of early chronic kidney disease (CKD). In addition, dialysis-dependent chronic kidney disease patients with cirrhosis may also need CLKT. The rise in the incidence of metabolic dysfunction associated steato hepatitis (MASH) is another reason this scenario will be more often seen in the future. Patients with liver cirrhosis had a sevenfold increase in mortality when they had concomitant renal dysfunction, as shown in a systematic review in 2012 [1].

27.2 Impact of Renal Dysfunction in Liver Disease Patients

The model for end stage liver disease (MELD) score was introduced in February 2002 in the US for the allocation of organs. It is calculated using the values of bilirubin, creatinine, and INR.

$$\begin{aligned}\text{MELD} = {} & 3.78 \times \log \text{Se.Bilirubin}(\text{mg}/\text{dl}) + \\ & 11.20 \times \log \text{INR} + \\ & 9.57 \times \log \text{Se.Creatinine}(\text{mg}/\text{dl}) + \\ & 6.43(\text{constant for liver disease etiology})\end{aligned}$$

Renal dysfunction is one of the major determinants of waitlist and post-transplant mortality and hence adequate weightage has been given to renal function in

MELD. As MELD has three components, there could be varying degrees of renal dysfunction among patients with identical MELD scores. Sharma et al. demonstrated that higher S. Cr at similar levels of MELD score was associated with decreased survival benefit across different MELD score categories [2]. Hence better understanding of this cohort and categorizing them enables tailored management in the peri-operative period to produce the optimal outcome.

We can broadly group patients who will be considered for CLKT and discuss the pros and cons in each situation:

27.3 Decompensated Chronic Liver Disease (CLD) with Dialysis-Dependent CKD

This is a straightforward scenario and a clear indication for CLKT. In the case of deceased donor transplantation, the patients will be wait listed for allocation of liver and kidney from the same donor. When live donor transplant is planned, if there are two living donors available to donate, a simultaneous transplant can be planned. A few centres have ventured into two organ retrieval from the same donor, more often sequentially (staggered by a few weeks to months) and very rarely simultaneously, i.e., both organs retrieved and transplanted to the recipient at one surgery [3].

27.4 Decompensated CLD with CKD (Early and Advanced) Not Requiring Dialysis

The peri- and postoperative liver transplant period in a patient has several factors that can potentially jeopardize the renal function (Table 27.1). A combination of these factors and an already compromised kidney as in this group may lead to the need for renal replacement therapy (RRT) post liver transplant. RRT post-transplant is strongly associated with mortality in the early and 1 year period [4]. The renal function at 1 month post-transplant also strongly predicts the long-term renal function [5]. Hence, every effort must be taken to preserve native renal function by adequate fluid balance peri- and post-transplant, avoidance of nephrotoxic drugs, and renal sparing immunosuppression. Criteria have been developed to offer CLKT when an accurate assessment of the stage of CKD is made and is elaborated further on the section on guidelines.

27.5 Patients with Decompensated CLD with Sustained AKI

Accurate assessment of the extent of renal injury and prediction of reversibility of renal injury is the key to decision-making. With the currently available diagnostic modalities, both these prove to be difficult in patients with liver disease. None of the

Table 27.1 Perioperative factors that impact renal function

Pre-operative:
Chronicity of renal disease—HRS, chronic glomerular disease, diuretics, intravascular volume depletion, primary renal disease
Acute kidney injury—severity and duration
Access to transplantation—deceased vs. live—Center expertise
Intraoperative:
Severity of chronic liver disease
Hypotension
Product transfusion
Cold ischemia time
IVC clamp time
Donor organ quality (DRI)
Early postoperative:
Hemodynamic instability/need for inotropes
Graft dysfunction
Infection
Calcineurin inhibitor toxicity
Late postoperative:
Hypertension
Obesity
Diabetes mellitus
Calcineurin inhibitor toxicity

existing markers can accurately predict GFR during AKI due to time lag between renal recovery and reflection of markers in blood. Creatinine is a poor marker in chronic liver disease due to muscle wasting, reduced production of creatinine and malnutrition. Cystatin C, on the other hand, is produced by all nucleated cells and is not affected by liver function, muscle mass, or age [6]. The gold standard for estimation of creatinine clearance has been iothalamate or inulin clearance but is often not available or difficult to perform due to cost or technical complexity. It is important to understand fallacies with existing diagnostic tests that are listed in Table 27.2.

27.6 Patients with CKD (Dialysis Dependant) and Compensated Cirrhosis

The determining factors for CLKT in clinically compensated cirrhosis in dialysis-dependent CKD patients is the presence of portal hypertension and quantification of the risk of decompensation. Both these are predicted accurately by hepatic venous pressure gradient (HVPG). Although portal hypertension can be assessed using other parameters like thrombocytopenia, early varices and presence of ascites (which can be secondary to renal failure also), HVPG is considered the gold standard [7]. A hepatic venous pressure gradient (HVPG) of more than 10 mm Hg signifies clinically significant portal hypertension and qualifies for CLKT listing [8].

Table 27.2 Fallacies of existing diagnostic tests in liver disease

Tests	Challenges
Urine routine	RBC can be present due to coagulopathy Proteinuria—likely to be underestimated in the back drop of low serum albumin from decreased synthetic functions of liver
Se creatinine	Not reliable due to the lower muscle mass, decreased production, and malnutrition
24 h urine protein	Same challenge as above
Renal biopsy	Invasive procedure fraught with risk of bleeding due to coagulopathy Expertise and infrastructure for TJLBx (Transjugular liver biopsy) is limited Will not provide information on the functional HRS component Chronic glomerular disease in liver disease is nearly omnipresent and may be an innocent bystander the majority of the time

27.7 Metabolic and Other Indications

CLKT is indicated when chronic kidney disease is secondary to a genetic defect in the liver (e.g., primary hyperoxaluria, atypical hemolytic uremic syndrome) or a developmental disorder affecting both the liver and kidney: polycystic liver and kidney disease, congenital hepatic fibrosis with autosomal recessive polycystic kidney disease (CHF with ARPKD). The presentation is usually in childhood or early adult life.

27.7.1 Primary Hyperoxlauria (PH1)

An autosomal recessive condition due to AGXT mutation leading to a deficiency of the liver peroxisomal enzyme alanine glyoxylate-aminotransferase (AGT). This results in excessive production of oxalate from the liver. Kidney is the only route for excretion for oxalate, and the ensuing oxaluria leads to the most common presentation with recurrent renal stones and eventually progressing to nephrocalcinosis. As the renal function gradually deteriorates to a GFR of 45 ml/min/1.73 m^2, the renal excretion of oxalate is also compromised, and the ongoing oxalate production results in oxalosis in the blood. The renal function rapidly deteriorates after this point, and the patient becomes dialysis dependent. Lack of thorough analysis of the etiology can land the patients in a renal transplantation and early graft failure due to recurrence of nephrocalcinosis. Combined liver and kidney transplant, either simultaneously or sequentially, is the treatment of choice. As oxalosis leads to significant deposits not only in the kidney but also in several other organs like heart, joints, eyes, bone marrow, etc. Aggressive dialysis (five times a week) is required to optimize the cardiac function prior to transplant and oxalate cardiomyopathy is known to cause sudden death. In the context of deceased donor CLKT, it is usually done simultaneously and maintaining the patient on CRRT intra-operatively and in the initial post-operative period (varies from 48 h to 7 days) has shown to reduce the oxalate burden on the transplanted kidney. The transplanted kidney will be the only route for excretion of the hugely built-up oxalate load with a possibility of oxalate deposition in the graft. Oxaluria post-transplant is present for about 6 months on average, but may prolong for up to 3 years [9]. Hence, the precautionary measures of adequate diuresis and medications like potassium citrate to prevent crystallization of oxalate in the urine are recommended for at least up to a year post CLKT. In living donor, simultaneous transplant is preferred as it has reduced morbidity to the patient with the precondition that the patient is adequately aggressively dialysed. If the patient has a huge oxalate load or when it is the same donor donating liver and kidney (especially if it is right lobe of the liver), sequential liver kidney transplant is performed.

27.7.2 Congenital Hepatic Fibrosis (CHF) with Autosomal Recessive Polycystic Kidney Disease (ARPKD)

Forty percent of patients with this diagnosis will need combined liver and kidney transplant as both organs show derangement. In patients with dialysis-dependent renal failure, significant portal hypertension as evidenced by varices or an episode of cholangitis will be an indication for CLKT even if the liver synthetic function is intact. Cholangitis post-renal transplant has been the main risk factor for mortality when renal transplant alone is performed.

27.7.3 Adult Polycystic Liver and Kidney Disease

This autosomal dominant condition may present with either liver predominant or renal predominant symptoms. Large liver cysts may occupy the entire abdominal cavity and present with heaviness/associated cachexia, occasional infection of the cyst, or hemorrhage into the cysts. Renal presentation may once again be infection or hemorrhage into the cyst or progressive renal dysfunction leading to renal failure and dialysis secondary to the loss of nephron mass. It may be logical to offer CLKT, but if the renal function is absolutely preserved at liver listing, the risk of rapid progression of kidney can be assessed using the PROPKD (predicting renal outcomes in ADPKD) score and CLKT can be offered [10].The PROPKD score: a new algorithm to predict renal survival in autosomal dominant polycystic kidney disease [11].

27.8 Immunological Indications

Liver being a reticuloendothelial organ has a unique advantage of positive and negative selection of immune system. Liver cells mop up preformed antibody, develop anergy of immune cells toward liver antigens, and destroy host immune cells that does not follow the rule. In this process, it reduces graft reactive antibodies and immune cells in circulation. A kidney sharing the same HLA and circulatory system benefits from the immune protective effect of the liver. Drawing on this concept, individuals who are highly sensitized with positive cross match (not relevant to isolated liver transplant but a strong contraindication for isolated renal transplantation) can have good renal allograft outcome if kidney is transplanted after liver transplant [12].

27.9 Guidelines on CLKT

The introduction of the MELD score in February 2002 prioritized patients with renal dysfunction to receive an early liver transplant. This had a significant impact on the allocation of organs, and as per Organ Procurement and Transplant Network (OPTN)/Scientific Registry of Transplant Recipients (SRTR) database report in 2007, the incidence of CLKT tripled from 134 in 2001 to 399 in 2006 in the United States. There was a rising discontent among renal transplant physicians and renal failure patients questioning the possibility of disadvantage to patients on the renal wait list. The debate was between offering a kidney, which may become supernumerary if the native renal function reverses after liver transplant vs. a post-liver transplant patient with renal dysfunction who ends up on long-term dialysis, having lost the opportunity to get a dual organ transplant and as a result left with a poor overall outcome. Lack of accurate predictors of the extent of renal injury and of reversibility has continued to plague this debate to date. Consensus conferences were held in 2006 and 2012 to address this, and later OPTN/ United Network for Organ Sharing (UNOS) adopted a policy in 2016 for allocation of liver and kidney for simultaneous transplant and is detailed below. These policies need to be revisited and modified for a live donor scenario where the discussion is not so much from a utilitarian perspective but from factoring the donor risk involved. In India, the criteria for offering CLKT to a patient are quite variable and follow center-specific criteria. As the majority of transplants in India are live donors, this allows for more subjective decision-making by individual programs.

In 2016, the United States Organ Procurement and Transplant Network (OPTN) and United Network for Organ Sharing (UNOS) approved the policy that formalized the allocation of SLK transplants and has been in practice since August 2017. In accordance with the new UNOS policy, liver transplant candidates who meet one of the following criteria are eligible for SLK allocation:

1. Diagnosis of CKD with a measured or calculated GFR of ≤60 mL/min for more than 90 consecutive days *and* at least one of the following at the time of waiting list registration:
    - ESKD on dialysis
    - Measured or calculated creatinine clearance or GFR ≤30 mL/min

2. Diagnosis of sustained AKI *and* at least one of the following for the last 6 weeks:
   - Dialysis at least once every seven days
   - Measured or calculated creatinine clearance or GFR of ≤25 mL/min documented at least once every seven days
3. Diagnosis of metabolic disease, with an additional diagnosis of at least one of the following:
   - Hyperoxaluria
   - Atypical hemolytic uremic syndrome from mutations in complement factor H or factor I
   - Familial non-neuropathic systemic amyloidosis
   - Methylmalonic aciduria

In addition to the above criteria defining eligibility for SLK, the new policy also includes a *safety-net* component to ensure that a liver transplant patient who is not initially offered SLK but who remains dialysis dependent after liver transplantation would be highly prioritized for subsequent kidney-alone allocation, if both of the following conditions are met:

- The candidate is registered on the kidney waiting list between 60 and 365 days after liver transplantation.
- The candidate is either on chronic dialysis *or* has a measured or calculated creatinine clearance or GFR of ≤20 mL/min.

27.10 Donor Selection and Timing in Combined Liver Kidney Transplant Surgery

Simultaneous—The liver is implanted first, followed by renal implantation, rarely through an intraperitoneal placement but more often through a separate incision and extraperitoneal approach. The outcome of CLKT is significantly affected by the quality of the donor organ. In a deceased donor organ, if the L-DRI (donor risk index) >1.5 and/or the KDRI >1.1, the survival benefit of CLKT is lost [12]. The renal allograft is further jeopardized if the hemodynamic milieu is unfavorable following liver organ reperfusion, which is more likely in marginal donors or in high-risk liver recipients. A fairly new concept has shown possible ways to overcome this situation—delayed implant of the renal allograft after a period of 48–72 h. The renal allograft, in the meantime, is placed on a machine perfusion [13]. This also has had an indirect immunological benefit in patients with high DSA (donor-specific antibody), where the time lag allows for the liver to mop up the antibodies. If the recipient continues to be hemodynamically unstable and not suitable to receive the renal allograft, it can be allocated to another recipient and hence preventing organ wastage too. The same logic can probably be adopted in a live donor scenario when two individual donors are donating the liver and kidney, although the likelihood of significant re-perfusion injury is less common in live donor liver transplantation.

Benefits of combined liver and kidney transplantation:

1. Single surgery, anesthesia, recovery –Less morbidity.
2. Single exposure to induction agents and lower maintenance immunosuppression.
3. CLKT from the same donor has an immunological advantage, as both organs share the same signature of HLA molecules.

Cons of Combined Liver and Kidney Transplantation:

1. Poor utilization of an organ (deceased donor) and risk to the donor (in live donors) in patients where there is reversibility of native renal function post liver transplantation.
2. Higher risk of delayed graft function and, in effect, poor long-term function of renal grafts when CLKT is performed simultaneously due to the hemodynamic instability and re-perfusion injury associated especially with deceased donor transplants.

27.11 Immunosuppression

Optimizing immuno suppression and minimizing calcineurin-induced renal injury is the cornerstone of immune suppression management in liver transplant patients with preoperative renal dysfunction. A renal-sparing regimen with induction (IL 2 or Ab-depleting agents) followed by late introduction of tacrolimus (anywhere from 2 to 5 days) allows for recovery of the kidneys from AKI/HRS.

If a CLKT is performed simultaneously, interleukin Il-2 blockade is often used for induction. T cell depleting agents are used with caution due to the risk of perioperative infections in this high-risk patient population. Subsequent maintenance immune suppression for both organs from the same donor follows the protocol for an isolated liver transplant due to the immunological courtesy extended by the liver. However, if the organs are from two different donors, kidneys will demand higher immunosuppression and follow the rules for an isolated renal transplant, which is usually a triple drug regimen (tacrolimus, MMF, and steroid).

27.12 Conclusion

Genetic conditions such as primary hyperoxaluria warrants CLKT. Patients with chronic liver disease may have coexisting underlying chronic kidney disease and those on long term will dialysis will require CLKT. The challenge remains to identify cirrhotic patients with renal dysfunction but not on dialysis who may benefit from liver alone versus CLKT.

References

1. Fede G.D'Amico G. Arvaniti V.et al.Renal failure and cirrhosis: a systematic review of mortality and prognosis.J Hepatol. 2012;56:810–18.
2. Sharma P, Schaubel DE, Guidinger MK, Merion RM. Effect of pretransplant serum creatinine on the survival benefit of liver transplantation. Liver Transpl. 2009;15(12):1808–13. https://doi.org/lt.21951. PMID: 19938142; PMCID: PMC3356787.
3. Henderson ML, DiBrito SR, Thomas AG, Holscher CM, Shaffer AA, Bowring MG, Purnell TS, Massie AB, Garonzik-Wang JM, Waldram MM, Lentine KL, Segev DL. Landscape of Living Multiorgan Donation in the United States: A Registry-Based Cohort Study. Transplantation. 2018;102(7):1148–55. https://doi.org/10.1097/TP.0000000000002082. PMID: 29952925; PMCID: PMC6029711.
4. Zhipeng W, Wang Yi, Li H, Boxun J, Qinwei Y, Guangming Li, Yingmin M. Development of a nomogram for the prediction of acute kidney injury after liver transplantation: a model based on clinical parameters and postoperative cystatin C level. Annals of Medicine. 2023;55. https://doi.org/10.1080/07853890.2023.2259410.
5. Sanchez EQ, Gonwa TA, Levy MF, Goldstein RM, Mai ML, Hays SR, Melton LB, Saracino G, Klintmalm GB. Preoperative and perioperative predictors of the need for renal replacement therapy after orthotopic liver transplantation. Transplantation. 2004;78(7):1048–54. https://doi.org/10.1097/01.tp.0000137176.95730.5b. PMID: 15480173.
6. https://doi.org/10.1053/j.ajkd.2023.08.013.
7. Bosch J, Abraldes JG, Berzigotti A, García-Pagan JC. The clinical use of HVPG measurements in chronic liver disease. Nat Rev Gastroenterol Hepatol. 2009;6(10):573–82. https://doi.org/10.1038/nrgastro.2009.149. Epub 2009 Sep 1. PMID: 19724251
8. Eason JD, Gonwa TA, Davis CL, Sung RS, Gerber D, Bloom RD. Proceedings of Consensus Conference on Simultaneous Liver Kidney Transplantation (SLK). Am J Transplant. 2008;8(11):2243–51. https://doi.org/10.1111/j.1600-6143.2008.02416.x. Epub 2008 Sep 19. PMID: 18808402.
9. Bergstralh EJ, Monico CG, Lieske JC, Herges RM, Langman CB, Hoppe B, Milliner DS. the IPHR Investigators. Transplantation outcomes in primary hyperoxaluria. https://doi.org/10.1111/j.1600-6143.2010.03271.x.
10. Cornec-Le Gall E, Audrézet MP, Rousseau A, et al. The PROPKD score: a new algorithm to predict renal survival in autosomal dominant polycystic kidney disease (Ref 11: J Am Soc Nephrol. 2016;27(3):942–51. https://doi.org/10.1681/ASN.2015010016. Pubmed: 26150605.
11. Cornec-Le Gall E, Audrézet MP, Rousseau A, Hourmant M, Renaudineau E, Charasse C, Morin MP, Moal MC, Dantal J, Wehbe B, Perrichot R, Frouget T, Vigneau C, Potier J, Jousset P, Guillodo MP, Siohan P, Terki N, Sawadogo T, Legrand D, Menoyo-Calonge V, Benarbia S, Besnier D, Longuet H, Férec C, Le Meur Y. The PROPKD Score: A New Algorithm to Predict Renal Survival in Autosomal Dominant Polycystic Kidney Disease. J Am Soc Nephrol. 2016;27(3):942–51. https://doi.org/10.1681/ASN.2015010016. Epub 2015 Jul 6. PMID: 26150605; PMCID: PMC4769200.
12. Parajuli S, Hidalgo LG, Foley D. Immunology of simultaneous liver and kidney transplants with identification and prevention of rejection. Front Transplant. 2022 Nov 1;1:991546. doi: 10.3389/frtra.2022.991546. PMID: 38994375; PMCID: PMC11235231.
13. Yeh, Hsuan & Chiang, Chun-Cheng & Yen, Tzung-Hai. (2021). Hepatocellular carcinoma in patients with renal dysfunction: Pathophysiology, prognosis, and treatment challenges. World Journal of Gastroenterology. 27. 4104–42. https://doi.org/10.3748/wjg.v27.i26.4104.
14. Lunsford KE, Agopian VG, Yi SG, Nguyen DTM, Graviss EA, Harlander-Locke MP, Saharia A, Kaldas FM, Mobley CM, Zarrinpar A, Hobeika MJ, Veale JL, Podder H, Farmer DG, Knight RJ, Danovitch GM, Gritsch HA, Li XC, Ghobrial RM, Busuttil RW, Gaber AO. Delayed Implantation of Pumped Kidneys Decreases Renal Allograft Futility in Combined Liver-Kidney Transplantation. Transplantation. 2020;104(8):1591–1603. https://doi.org/10.1097/TP.0000000000003040. PMID: 32732836.

Part III
Post Transplantation

Chapter 28
Immediate Postoperative Care

Shweta Mallick, Krishnanunni Nair, and S. Sudhindran

Abstract Optimal postoperative management of liver transplant recipients is a challenging affair and best achieved with the equal involvement of multiple disciplines of transplant medicine. Most practices have evolved over time with a current shift in trend towards enhanced recovery after surgery practices. Most centers practice a protocol-based approach in postoperative management. However, case-by-case alteration is often required, especially while dealing with sick patients with acute-on-chronic liver failure background.

Keywords Liver transplant · Early extubation · Postoperative care · Chronic liver disease · Hemodynamic monitoring · Immunosuppression · Antibiotics · Multi-drug-resistant bacteria · Synbiotics

Key Highlights

- A multidisciplinary, protocolized approach is essential for achieving optimal postoperative outcomes after liver transplantation.
- Invasive blood pressure and central venous pressure monitoring should be routinely used in the immediate postoperative period for prompt diagnosis of hemodynamic dysfunction.
- Restrictive fluid strategy using colloids along with vasopressor support is recommended to maintain hemodynamic stability.
- Early extubation after surgery and early removal of lines and tubes may be considered as it might enhance recovery.
- Short-term universal antibiotic prophylaxis, along with universal or preemptive antifungal and antiviral therapy, may be given based on risk assessment.

S. Mallick · K. Nair · S. Sudhindran (✉)
Department of GI Surgery & Solid Organ Transplantation, Amrita Institute of Medical Sciences, Amrita Vishwavidyapeetham, Kochi, Kerala, India
e-mail: sudhi@aims.amrita.edu

S. Saigal, D. Jothimani (eds.), *Fundamentals of Transplant Hepatology*, https://doi.org/10.1007/978-981-95-2624-6_28

- Viscoelastic testing helps evaluate the balance between bleeding and thrombosis risk and aids in determining the need for coagulation factor replacement.

Introduction: Immediate postoperative care of liver transplant (LT) recipients involves a truly multidisciplinary approach involving various specialties like surgery, hepatology, interventional radiology, anesthesia, and critical care. Postoperative outcomes, furthermore, are significantly influenced by the pre-operative optimization of liver patients, particularly in cases of acute and acute-on-chronic liver failure (ACLF), where survival is contingent upon the timely execution of the transplant. This chapter will examine the critical aspects of immediate postoperative care that must be administered following liver transplantation.

The different aspects of postoperative care will be discussed under the following headings:

1. Hemodynamic monitoring
2. Fluid and electrolyte balance
3. Ventilation and extubation
4. Antimicrobials
5. Nutrition
6. Immunosuppression
7. Analgesia
8. Management of coagulopathy
9. Other supportive management (renal replacement therapy)
10. Doppler ultrasound monitoring of the liver graft

28.1 Hemodynamic Monitoring

Accurate and prompt diagnosis of hemodynamic changes after surgery is crucial, as misdiagnosis or improper treatment can impair graft function, lengthen ICU stays, and increase mortality risk.

As aptly stated by Parekh et al., in liver disease, the management of hemodynamics requires an in-depth understanding of the underlying pathophysiology [1]. End-stage liver disease (ESLD) creates a state of high cardiac output and low systemic vascular resistance, which after a successful transplant, reverses to decreased cardiac output and increased systemic vascular resistance [1]. Invasive hemodynamic monitoring is a real-time assessment of ongoing physiological alterations and is necessary for the immediate period following LT. Monitoring practices differ across various centers between the use of arterial lines, central venous catheters, pulmonary artery catheters (PAC), and transesophageal echocardiography (TEE). At our center, we prefer arterial lines, central venous pressure (CVP) monitoring, and non-invasive continuous cardiac output monitoring. Being invasive in nature with the possibility of complications like ventricular arrhythmias and esophagal perforations, the use of PAC and TEE demands precaution [2, 3]. The exact means of monitoring is probably best left to the choice of individual centers, based on their experiences.

Signs of an adequately functioning liver graft include:

- Hemodynamic stability & ability to wean off inotropes
- Adequate urine output
- Fall in lactate & correction of acidosis
- Patient regaining consciousness
- Normoglycemia

In the presence of a well-functioning liver, denoted by the above-mentioned parameters, de-lining of invasive lines can be carried out preferably by postoperative day (POD) 2, but might differ on a case-to-case basis.

28.2 Fluid & Electrolyte Balance

Most centers prefer either a restrictive fluid management strategy or a goal-directed fluid therapy, administering fluid boluses to attain a CVP of 8–12 mmHg, vasopressors to attain a mean arterial pressure of 65–90 mmHg, and red blood cell transfusions or inotropes to attain a central venous oxygen saturation of at least 70%. Restrictive fluid strategy along with vasopressor support is known to decrease re-intubation rates and ventilator-related complications [4]. It also results in lesser transfusions and related complications [5]. As for the choice of fluid, there is no definitive evidence to prove one better than the other [6]. Colloids, especially albumin, may be preferred by most centers, especially in patients with significant ascites.

Alterations in sodium levels are very common following LT with both hypo- and hypernatremia leading to significant complications. Acute hyponatremia can lead to neurologic impairment and is corrected with an infusion of hypertonic (3%) normal saline [1]. Rapid correction of chronic hyponatremia could lead to drastic complications like osmotic demyelination; hence, one should aim at 1–2 mmol/L of sodium correction for the first 48 h [7]. If correction increases the levels too quickly, hypotonic intravenous fluids like half-normal saline should be started. Hypernatremia occurs less frequently, and it occurs due to loss of free water in this subset of patients who are on regular intake of osmotic laxatives as a prophylaxis against hepatic encephalopathy. Enteral supplementation (oral or via feeding tube) of free water and or hypotonic maintenance fluids serve as a treatment for hypernatremia [1]. It is prudent to avoid hyperosmolar fluids such as branched chain amino acids and L-ornithine L-aspartate in patients with HE. Although parenteral nutrition has low sodium content, being hyperosmolar, its use in hypernatremic patients must be carefully monitored.

Hyperkalemia occurs mainly due to reperfusion injury, renal failure, or massive blood transfusions. The range of management includes the use of insulin with glucose, calcium, sodium bicarbonate, and dialysis if hyperkalemia persists [1].

Another electrolyte abnormality related to blood transfusions is hypocalcemia. Calcium gluconate or calcium chloride can be used for correction [1]. Along with calcium, correction of magnesium too, is vital.

Phosphorous is an integral part of adenosine triphosphate (ATP) or the "cell's battery." Following a transplant, particularly living donor LT (LDLT), phosphorous levels may drop precipitously, indicating regeneration of the liver graft. Correction of phosphorus levels is therefore vital to maintain the requisite supply for ATP buildup.

Adequate glycemic control is important in following LT. Hypoglycemia serves as an indicator for sepsis and graft non-function [8], whereas hyperglycemia increases the risk of liver allograft rejection, surgical site infection (SSI), and increased mortality [9–11]. A modest glucose control in the range of 150–180 mg/dL, using insulin infusion with frequent sugar monitoring, is currently recommended [1].

It is our practice to administer prostaglandin (Alprostadil) infusion for 72 h after transplant. The initial intent was for achieving superior patency of the hepatic artery (HA) by its vasodilatory effect. However, a randomized controlled trial demonstrated only improved renal function with Alprostadil use [12].

28.3 Ventilation and Early Extubation

We extubate our recipients on POD 1 as a protocol once the laboratory parameters and liver Doppler findings corroborate with safe extubation. While some centers practice on-table extubation, there is currently no definite consensus on its role. Patients who are not on high levels of ionotropic support, have been relatively stable intra-operatively and have a low risk for re-exploration or bleeding can be considered for early extubation. Enhanced Recovery After Surgery (ERAS) protocol dictates that every patient undergoing LT should be screened for eligibility for early extubation (<3–8 h) which should be according to scoring systems and institutional protocols [13–15]. In a systematic review, Tinguely et al. found that overall complications, ICU, and hospital stay were lesser in the early extubation cohort (OR = 0.4 (CI 0.2–0.7)), without significantly affecting the mortality or re-admission rates [16]. Whether this protocol applies to all LT candidates uniformly is debatable.

Those requiring prolonged ventilation are usually the sicker pre-operative patients most likely belonging to the ACLF group and are at a higher risk of developing postoperative respiratory complications like acute respiratory distress syndrome (ARDS), pulmonary edema, ventilator-associated pneumonia, transfusion-associated acute lung injury (TRALI), and reperfusion injury. Patients diagnosed with ARDS should be maintained on a low tidal volume ventilation, as recent studies have shown its benefit even in patients without ARDS [17, 18].

28.4 Antimicrobials

The incidence of infectious complications following LT ranges between 50% and 70% [19]. Optimal use of antibiotics should not only address the need for appropriate prophylaxis and treatment but equally importantly, avoid their misuse. The use of inappropriate high-end antibiotics for extended periods in co-morbid, immunocompromised patients increases the risk of infections with multi-drug-resistant organisms [20]. In addition to increased morbidity, longer hospital stays, and additional costs, SSI in transplant patients may be associated with an increased probability of graft loss [21].

28.4.1 Bacterial Infections

Bloodstream infections (BSI) due to Gram-positive cocci may be a result of repeated invasive procedures and quinolone prophylaxis that patients with ESLD are subjected to. However, in India, Gram-negative bacilli are probably the predominant cause of BSI and intra-abdominal infections (as high as 92% compared to GPC—7%) [22, 23].

For prophylaxis, various regimens commonly used for SSI in LT include glycopeptide plus aztreonam, glycopeptide plus quinolone, glycopeptide plus antipseudomonas penicillin, ampicillin plus third-generation cephalosporin, amoxicillin–clavulanic acid plus quinolone, amoxicillin–clavulanic acid, cefazolin, and other antibiotics [24]. We practice the use of broad-spectrum penicillin with a beta-lactam inhibitor (piperacillin + tazobactam) as a prophylactic antibiotic given at incision and continued for a period of 3 days. Specific modifications are made on a case-based approach. Routine cultures (blood, urine, BAL, and intra-abdominal drain fluid) are sent on post-op day 3, and antibiotics are titrated accordingly by many units; however, there is no definitive evidence/recommendation for this practice. With the insurgence of multi-drug-resistant strains of extended-spectrum β-lactamase *E. coli* and carbapenem-resistant *K. pneumoniae*, the antibiotic coverage usually may prove ineffective, and timely tackling of a septic complication using newer antibiotics like ceftazidime avibactam and aztreonam (for metallo beta-lactamase producers) often becomes necessary.

28.4.2 Fungal Infections

Invasive fungal infection, the majority being by Candida (C. non-albicans accounts for 60% of invasive candidiasis, followed by C. albicans in 30%) and Aspergillus, is a serious complication of immunosuppression following LT, and the incidence stands at around 12% as reported by Raghuram et al. [25] Risk factors for invasive fungemia are re-transplantation, bilio-enteric anastomosis, high transfusion requirements, longer operative time, cytomegalovirus (CMV) viremia, and post-transplant dialysis [26]. Azoles act against several Candida species. However, drug interactions, especially with tacrolimus, require careful monitoring of dose, duration, and drug levels. European guidelines recommend oral prophylaxis against Candida species during the initial months after LT as it reduces direct candedimia-related mortality [27].

Aspergillus infection (most often *Aspergillus fumigatus*), although less common, is associated with a higher mortality than Candida (around 60%) [28]. Aspergillus infections have been reported to occur as late as 3 months after LT. Nevertheless, in our experience, invasive aspergillosis appears to occur within the first post-op month more so amongst ACLF patients. Fluconazole is not as potent an antifungal for Aspergillus as it is for Candida. Voriconazole, a triazole antifungal, has shown to be rather efficient as a prophylactic and treatment agent against aspergillosis in LT recipients [29]. In a trial in patients with hematological diseases, voriconazole was found to be more effective and safer than amphotericin B [30]. The intravenous formulation has significantly more toxicity than its oral counterpart due to the associated carrier molecule, cyclodextrin, which accumulates in the kidneys. Although amphotericin B works against Aspergillus, it carries risks of infusion reactions and nephrotoxicity. Caspofungin, an echinocandin, has good activity against both non-albicans Candida and Aspergillus, with a better safety profile [29]. Tacrolimus levels are closely monitored with dose modifications as required for most antifungal drugs, especially for azoles.

There is a general recommendation to use antifungal prophylaxis in high-risk patients with a model for end-stage liver disease (MELD) score above 20, patients needing re-operation (for bleeding or bile leak), on renal replacement therapy, and those receiving steroid pulses and lymphocyte-depleting agents for the treatment of rejection [31]. Our practice is to use IV fluconazole as prophylaxis on the day of transplant and continue the oral formulation once the patient is allowed oral intake. As there is no definite recommendation for the duration of antifungal therapy, we continue it till the abdominal drains are removed. Although there is no evidence backup, it is intuitive that in situ drains may increase the formation of biofilm and consequent fungal colonization; hence, it is preferred that drains are removed as early as possible. Nonetheless, it is imperative to confirm the absence of a bile leak in the drain. A drain fluid bilirubin level more than the serum value is indicative of a bile leak and can perhaps be confirmed by a hepatobiliary iminodiacetic acid scan. In the absence of a bile leak, drains could be removed irrespective of the volume of ascitic fluid. This may be particularly relevant in patients with small-for-size syndrome who have large-volume ascites. This being said, a sound abdominal closure technique is essential to prevent ascites leakage from the surgical wound.

Pre-emptive antifungal treatment involves initiating targeted antifungal therapy based on early evidence of fungal infection, such as colonization, laboratory markers, or imaging, but before clinical disease is fully established. This approach is intermediate between prophylactic treatment (either universal or risk-based) and empiric treatment (which begins after clinical symptoms appear). Therapy is initiated when there is evidence of colonization at multiple sites, positive biomarkers (such as 1,3 B-D glucan for any fungal infection or galactomannan for aspergillus), or radiological suspicion of fungal disease. Commonly used pre-emptive antifungals include echinocandins (anidulafungin, caspofungin, and micafungin) for Candida and voriconazole or liposomal amphotericin B for aspergillus.

Pneumocystis jirovecii is an opportunistic fungal infection that causes pneumonia in immunocompromised patients. Current guidelines, therefore, recommend routine use of co-trimoxazole for 6–12 months [27]. However, we do not follow this practice routinely, as Pneumocystis pneumonia appears to be rare in India.

28.4.3 Viral Infections

CMV can cause a wide range of morbidity following LT and occurs particularly in CMV-seronegative recipients with seropositive donors [32]. The usual period of CMV infection is about 6 weeks after LT. Prophylaxis with valganciclovir (for 3–6 months) is commonly carried out by many centers. A recent randomized controlled trial by Singh et al. compared pre-emptive CMV prophylaxis in seronegative recipients with seropositive donors (900 mg BD valganciclovir upon detection of viremia by polymerase chain reaction (PCR) test up till clearance of viremia in 2 consecutive weekly tests) vs. universal prophylaxis (900 mg OD for 100 days for everyone). They found the preemptive treatment to be more effective in the prevention of CMV disease over 12 months in comparison to prophylactic treatment [33]. Nevertheless, as virtually all our recipients are already CMV IgG positive, we do not use CMV prophylaxis routinely. Upon suspicion of infection, CMV DNA levels are tested, and valganciclovir/ganicilovir is started accordingly.

Of late, the role of synbiotics has been explored in reducing infectious complications in LT recipients. Various trials in both deceased donor LT and LDLT showed favorable results and recommend the use of synbiotic drugs to reduce infectious complications [34, 35]. Some centers were also able to demonstrate a reduction in antibiotic usage with the use of synbiotics [36].

28.5 Nutrition

Patients with ESLD are prone to developing protein energy malnutrition (PEM) as a part of the disease process. It is characterized by sarcopenia (gross muscle wasting and subcutaneous fat loss) and occurs more commonly with a decompensated disease—ascites, HE, portal hypertensive bleeding and those hospitalized for alcoholic liver disease [37, 38]. PEM is a risk factor for morbidity, short- and long-term mortality, and decreased graft survival after LT as it acts as an adjuvant to complications like sepsis, increased blood product usage, prolongation of hospital and ICU stay, delayed physical rehabilitation, and prolonged mechanical ventilation [39].

The European Society for Clinical Nutrition and Metabolism and the European Association for the Study of Liver Disease recommend initiation of normal food and/or enteral nutrition (EN) within 12–24 h. This is reported to be associated with fewer viral infections and better nitrogen retention than parenteral nutrition [40, 41]. In patients in whom EN cannot be initiated early due to prolonged ileus, parenteral nutrition (PN) can be started [13]. Upon comparison, both PN and early EN proved to be equally effective with regard to the maintenance of nutritional state but EN reduced complication rates and costs. Apart from providing optimal nutritional requirements, re-building vitamin and micronutrient supplies is vital in maintaining adequate liver function and improving the outcomes after LT [1].

28.6 Immunosuppression

Our practice is to start with high-dose methylprednisolone as an induction agent at reperfusion, which is tapered over a period of 1 week to oral steroids, which are subsequently used as maintenance immunosuppression. Postoperatively, tacrolimus is started on POD 1 as a bottom-up approach with trough levels monitored every 3 days to reach 5–8 ng/mL. Along with tacrolimus, anti-metabolite agents, either Azoran or Mycophenolate Mofetil, are started provided the platelet count is above 30,000 cells/μL. By the time of discharge, the patient is kept on a triple-drug IS regimen including steroids, tacrolimus, and anti-metabolite. Acute rejection episodes are managed with pulse doses of methylprednisolone. Induction agents like interleukin-2 (IL-2) inhibitors (basiliximab) are given in select scenarios. A randomized trial conducted at our center showed that the steroid-free regimen consisting of basiliximab induction, tacrolimus, and azathioprine, significantly lowered the new onset of post-transplant diabetes, hypertension, and hypertriglyceridemia compared to a steroid-inclusive regimen in live donor liver transplantation [42]. However, the cost of basiliximab precludes its routine use. Our current indication for basiliximab induction includes –

- pre-op creatinine >1.5 mg/dl (so that tacrolimus introduction can be delayed)
- poor pre-operative glycemic control
- history of neurological diseases like a seizure disorder.

With regard to immunosuppression in sepsis, our policy is to follow an a-la-carte approach to the individual patient's needs. In the wake of recent evidence pointing towards the benefit of continuing immunosuppression in the septic setting, we do not withhold immunosuppression, even when the patient is diagnosed with severe sepsis. In the presence of renal dysfunction, tacrolimus is stopped and subsequently restarted once renal function improves. Likewise, anti-metabolite agents are withheld if the patient has leukopenia (total count <3000 cells/mL) and thrombocytopenia (platelets <40,000 cells/μL). If there is septic shock, however, the only immunosuppression given is hydrocortisone in doses of 50–100 mg, eighth hourly which is reverted to the full previous regimen as soon as ionotropic supports can be stopped. Methylprednisolone pulses are given if there is biochemical rejection during recovery [43].

28.7 Analgesia

Liver transplantation is a major surgical procedure, most often being performed by a large reverse-L abdominal incision. Postoperative analgesia after liver transplantation aims to ensure patient comfort, reduce stress, and prevent respiratory complications by maintaining good respiratory effort. This reduces atelectasis risk, enables early mobilization, lowers thromboembolism risk, and enhances recovery. It is crucial to minimize opioid side effects, such as respiratory depression, sedation, ileus, and liver metabolism issues.

There is no single approach that fits all, although multimodal analgesia is recommended. At our center, pain control is usually achieved using fentanyl infusion starting intraoperatively and continued in the postoperative period. Intermittent bolus doses are added as required. This is supplemented with the use of a buprenorphine transdermal patch. We also use Nefopam, a central-acting, non-opioid, nonsteroidal anti-inflammatory drug (NSAID) analgesic, which has been shown to provide adequate pain relief with diminished side effects when used as an adjunct in multimodal postoperative pain management. Acetaminophen can be given at lower doses till the graft functionality is confirmed; however, we usually forgo its use as it can mask febrile episodes.

Epidural analgesia is not preferred given the coagulative instability and risk of bleeding and hypotension associated with epidural analgesia. Some centers use patient-controlled analgesia pumps using longer-acting analgesics [1]. Use of NSAIDs demands caution because of potential renal damage in these patients, as they are already prone to developing renal dysfunction.

28.8 Coagulopathy

Coagulative instability is a characteristic trait of ESLD, and its treatment can often be a challenging feat, as it involves gaining a critical balance between both hypo- and hyper-coagulable states. Standard laboratory tests do not accurately predict the risk of bleeding or thrombosis. Use of viscoelastic tests (VET) like thromboelastography or rotational thromboelastometry has been recommended to guide coagulation correction both intra- and postoperatively. As VETs are performed on whole blood, they accurately reflect the interaction between pro- and anti-coagulants and platelets [44]. The role of VET to guide transfusion in patients with ESLD leading to decreased blood product use has been reported [45, 46]. The use of VET was also recently recommended in the ERAS project performed by the ILTS [47].

Postoperatively, correction of coagulopathy should depend on clinical evidence of bleeding and not merely on laboratory values. The use of fresh frozen plasma (FFP) replenishes coagulation factors; however, the volumes required to achieve adequate correction might be counterproductive to the overall input. Reports suggest that transfusion of six units of FFPs increases the portal pressure by 15 mmHg, which increases the risk of bleeding [48]. FFP transfusion has only a limited effect on correcting factor deficiencies [49]. Overt corrections can, furthermore, lead to fluid overload and transfusion-related complications like pulmonary edema and TRALI. As an alternative to FFP, coagulation factor concentrates are now available. The most commonly used products are prothrombin complex concentrates (PCC), which include factors II, VII, IX, and X. In vitro, PCC has been demonstrated to improve thrombin generation in patients with ESLD significantly better than FFP [50]. However, the fiscal burden associated with factor concentrate use precludes its routine use in the Indian scenario.

It has also been demonstrated that prophylactic fibrinogen administration in LT recipients did not affect transfusion requirements [51]. The ERAS project does not recommend the use of prophylactic antifibrinolytics in LT recipients [46]. They should be used only in the case of fibrinolysis-related clinical bleeding as diagnosed with VET [31].

In view of the lack of definitive evidence, we do not routinely practice the use of anticoagulation to prevent vascular thromboses. The use of aspirin is recommended for thromboprophylaxis to prevent HA thrombosis.

28.9 Renal Insufficiency

Some studies report an incidence of acute kidney injury of around 50%. Acute ischemic tubular necrosis is the most common cause of renal failure post-LT [52]. The usual perioperative factors, which increase the risk of development of renal dysfunction post-op include:

- ACLF
- hepatorenal syndrome
- MELD>21
- hepatitis C
- diabetes mellitus
- intraoperative and postoperative hemodynamic instability
- massive transfusion
- vasopressor infusions
- infections
- frequent radiologic studies
- nephrotoxic drugs (immunosuppressants, analgesics, and antibiotics) [1]

Management usually includes careful fluid management, alterations in doses of drugs causing potential renal harm, and avoidance of further renal insults. Renal replacement therapy is required in 8–17% of post-transplant acute kidney injuries despite supportive care [31]. Renal function using serum creatinine may be less beneficial than using cystatin C, which is found to be more sensitive in picking up renal dysfunction early, although it is more expensive [53].

Tacrolimus should be withheld for the initial period following LT to allow the recovery of renal function [1]. As mentioned earlier, induction agents such as basiliximab may be used in such situations.

Table 28.1 outlines the goals of the key aspects of postoperative management in general and the preferred strategies in each scenario.

28.10 Doppler Ultrasound Monitoring of Graft

Doppler ultrasound positively impacts graft survival, as it allows early pickup of vascular complications following LT. An intraoperative Doppler ultrasound is always performed during LDLT prior to closure. Following that, routine protocol Doppler is performed daily till ICU stay and then once every 2 days for 2 weeks. Any alteration in findings is corroborated with urgent cross-sectional imaging followed by surgical or radiological interventions as indicated. (Table 28.2).

Evaluation of Portal Vein (PV) Typically a normal portal flow is depicted by a non-pulsatile, wavy venous pattern. The average velocity post-LDLT can range between 15 and 400 cm/s. Although there is no definite cut-off value, usually a velocity of <10 cm/sec can point towards a low-flow system with probable shunting of blood to collateral circulation. A high velocity along with high PV pressure of >20 mmHg depicts a high-pressure system, which can lead to hyperperfusion injuries to a hemi-liver graft. Both these scenarios merit consideration of inflow modulation. PV thrombus (PVT) is a complication with dreaded consequences and should be detected early. The absence of flow and color pickup, intraluminal echogenic material, and corresponding areas of infarct on the graft point towards PVT and require immediate action. Doppler ultrasound can also aid identification of stenosis, which can be determined based on pre- and anastomotic caliber and velocities along with flow aliasing (distortion and mixing of forward and reverse flow).

Evaluation of Hepatic Artery (HA) A normal arterial flow is depicted by a biphasic wave pattern, which remains above the baseline in both systole and diastole. The most frequently used parameter for assessment is the resistive index (RI) (peak systolic velocity (PSV)—end diastolic velocity/peak systolic velocity). The normal RI in an LDLT graft ranges between 0.5 and 0.8. An increase in RI above 0.8, dampened PSV, and reversed diastolic flow are ominous signs that portend impending HA thrombosis (HAT). Established HAT can be detected by absent flow and color pick-up with hypo-echoic shadow inside the artery. A decrease in RI (<0.5) denotes poor inflow to the HA and may be due to proximal stenosis or thrombi. Cross-sectional imaging may be warranted in such scenarios, preferably computerized tomography (CT) angiogram.

Table 28.1 Recommended optimum management protocols

Aspect	Desired goals	Preferred strategies
Patient haemodynamics	Early weaning of inotropes. Adequate urine output Fall in lactate Correction of acidosis Patient regaining consciousness Normoglycemia	Arterial line, CVP monitoring and non-invasive continuous cardiac output monitoring Transesophageal echo (in selected cases)
Fluid & electrolyte balance	Restrictive fluid strategy along with vasopressor support to aim for CVP of 8-12 mmHg, MAP of 65 to 90 mmHg, central venous oxygen saturation of at least 70% Maintain sodium, potassium, calcium, phosphorous, magnesium optimally glucose levels between 150–180 mg/dl	Colloids preferred (except starch) Sodium correction at 1–2 mmol/L for the first 48 h For hypernatremia, enteral supplementation of free water, avoidance of hypertonic fluids
Extubation	Early extubation	On table extubation if possible, in hemodynamically stable patients with normal lactate and arterial pH levels and with a low risk for re-exploration If not feasible, consider extubating within 3–8 h after surgery
Antimicrobials	Avoidance of blood stream, surgical site and invasive lines related infections Nosocomial infection CMV infection Opportunistic infections especially Candida, aspergillus and pneumocystis jirovecii infections in high risk patients	Universal prophylactic broad-spectrum antibiotics restricted to 2–3 days Fluconazole as routine antifungal prophylaxis Preemptive antifungal therapy includes Echinocandins for candida non albicans and Voriconazole for aspergillosis CMV prophylaxis, either universal or preemptive
Nutrition	Early EN	Initiation of high calorie high protein diet orally within 12–24 h In patients with prolonged ileus, parenteral nutrition can be started
Analgesia	Effective pain control Prevent respiratory complications Facilitate early mobilization Decrease opioid adverse effects	Multimodal approach Short acting opioids like fentanyl infusion, supplemented with Buprenorphine trans-dermal patch Nefopam, a central-acting, non-opioid, NSAID analgesic Acetaminophen
Coagulopathy	Careful balance between bleeding and prothrombotic states to avoid unnecessary bleeding at the same time mitigating risk of vascular thrombosis	Viscoelastic testing for correction of coagulopathy Coagulation factor concentrates like PCC, are now being recommended although the cost is high

Table 28.2 Doppler assessment in the postoperative period

Graft parameter	Normal	Abnormal
PV	Non-pulsatile, wavy venous pattern Average velocity post-LDLT ranges between 15-400 cm/s	Velocity of <10 cm/sec point towards a low flow system with probable shunting of blood to collateral circulation A high velocity along with high portal vein pressure of >20 mmHg depicts a high-pressure system which can lead to hyperperfusion injuries
HA	Bi-phasic wave pattern which remains above the baseline in both systole and diastole The normal Resitive index (RI) in an LDLT graft ranges between 0.5 and 0.8	An increase in RI above 0.8, dampened peak systolic velocity and reversed diastolic flow can indicate HA thrombosis A decrease in RI (<0.5) denotes poor inflow to the HA and may be due to proximal stenosis or thrombi
HVs	Tri-phasic waveform (w-pattern) corresponding to the cardiac cycle.	Thrombosis presents with low flow and the presence of echogenic thrombus in the lumen, Stenosis is diagnosed with the development of a velocity gradient across the anastomosis (>10 mmHg is considered substantial)

Evaluation of Hepatic Veins (HV) HV flow normally is seen as a tri-phasic waveform (w-pattern) corresponding to the cardiac cycle. Complications like HV thrombosis and stenosis need to be identified in the immediate postoperative period. While the former presents with low flow and the presence of echogenic thrombus in the lumen, the latter complication is typically diagnosed with the development of a velocity gradient across the anastomosis (>10 mmHg is considered substantial) [54].

28.11 Conclusion

A judicious, diligent, round-the-clock, and multidisciplinary team approach is vital in the immediate postoperative care of the LT recipient. Close monitoring of hemodynamic status, ventilatory support, judicious anti-microbials, tailored immunosuppression and enteral nutrition enhances early post-operative recovery.

References

1. Parekh KN, Crowley JC, Liu LL. Postoperative care of the liver transplant recipient. In: Anesthesia and perioperative care for organ transplantation; 2016. p. 365–84. https://doi.org/10.1007/978-1-4939-6377-5_29. PMCID: PMC7120127.
2. Gwak MS, Kim JA, Kim GS, Choi SJ, Ahn H, Lee JJ, et al. Incidence of severe ventricular arrhythmias during pulmonary artery catheterization in liver allograft recipients. Liver Transpl. 2007;13:1451–4.

3. Iriarte F, Riquelme GA, Sorensen P, Pirchi DE, Mihura Irribarra M. Esophageal perforation after transesophageal echocardiography: a case report. Int J Surg Case Rep. 2020;66:21–4. https://doi.org/10.1016/j.ijscr.2019.11.020. Epub 2019 Nov 19. PMID: 31790946; PMCID: PMC6909181.
4. Ponnudurai RN, Koneru B, Akhtar SA, Wachsberg RH, Fisher A, Wilson DJ, de la Torre AN. Vasopressor administration during liver transplant surgery and its effect on endotracheal reintubation rate in the postoperative period: a prospective, randomized, double-blind, placebo-controlled trial. Clin Ther. 2005;27:192–8.
5. Malouf M, Glanville AR. Blood transfusion related adult respiratory distress syndrome. Anaesth Intensive Care. 1993;21:44–9.
6. Morkane CM, Sapisochin G, Mukhtar AM, et al. Perioperative fluid management and outcomes in adult deceased donor liver transplantation—a systematic review of the literature and expert panel recommendations. Clin Transpl. 2022;36:e14651. https://doi.org/10.1111/ctr.14651.
7. Lee J, Kim DK, Lee JW, Oh KH, Oh YK, Na KY, et al. Rapid correction rate of hyponatremia as an independent risk factor for neurological complication following liver transplantation. Tohoku J Exp Med. 2013;229:97–105.
8. Feltracco P, Barbieri S, Galligioni H, Michieletto E, Carollo C, Ori C. Intensive care management of liver transplanted patients. World J Hepatol. 2011;3:61–71.
9. Wallia A, Parikh ND, Molitch ME, Mahler E, Tian L, Huang JJ, et al. Posttransplant hyperglycemia is associated with increased risk of liver allograft rejection. Transplantation. 2010;89:222–6.
10. Park C, Hsu C, Neelakanta G, Nourmand H, Braunfeld M, Wray C, et al. Severe intraoperative hyperglycemia is independently associated with surgical site infection after liver transplantation. Transplantation. 2009;87:1031–6.
11. Ammori JB, Sigakis M, Englesbe MJ, O'Reilly M, Pelletier SJ. Effect of intraoperative hyperglycemia during liver transplantation. J Surg Res. 2007;140:227–33.
12. Bharathan, V.K., Chandran, B., Gopalakrishnan, U., Varghese, C.T., Menon, R.N., Balakrishnan, D., Sudheer, O.V., Dhar, P. And Surendran, S. (2016), Perioperative prostaglandin e1 infusion in living donor liver transplantation: a double-blind, placebo-controlled randomized trial. Liver Transpl, 22: 1067–1074.
13. Brustia R, Monsel A, Skurzak S, Schiffer E, Carrier FM, Patrono D, Kaba A, Detry O, Malbouisson L, Andraus W, Vandenbroucke-Menu F, Biancofiore G, Kaido T, Compagnon P, Uemoto S, Rodriguez Laiz G, De Boer M, Orloff S, Melgar P, Buis C, Zeillemaker-Hoekstra M, Usher H, Reyntjens K, Baird E, Demartines N, Wigmore S, Scatton O. Guidelines for perioperative care for liver transplantation: Enhanced Recovery After Surgery (ERAS). Recommend Transpl. 2022;106(3):552–61. https://doi.org/10.1097/TP.0000000000003808.
14. Skurzak S, Stratta C, Schellino MM, et al. Extubation score in the operating room after liver transplantation. Acta Anaesthesiol Scand. 2010;54:970–8.
15. Bulatao IG, Heckman MG, Rawal B, et al. Avoiding stay in the intensive care unit after liver transplantation: a score to assign location of care. Am J Transplant. 2014;14:2088–96.
16. Tinguely P, Morare N, Ramirez-Del Val A, Berenguer M, Niemann CU, Pollok JM, Raptis DA, Spiro M. Enhanced recovery after surgery programs improve short-term outcomes after liver transplantation-A systematic review and meta-analysis. Clin Transpl. 2021;35:e14453.
17. The Acute Respiratory Distress Syndrome Network. Ventilation with lower tidal volumes as compared with traditional tidal volumes for acute lung injury and the acute respiratory distress syndrome. N Engl J Med. 2000;342:1301–8.
18. Futier E, Constantin JM, Paugam-Burtz C, Pascal J, Eurin M, Neuschwander A, et al. A trial of intraoperative low-tidal-volume ventilation in abdominal surgery. N Engl J Med. 2013;369:428–37.
19. Safdar N, Said A, Lucey MR. The role of selective digestive decontamination for reducing infection in patients undergoing liver transplantation: a systematic review and meta-analysis. Liver Transpl. 2004;10:817–27.
20. Ferrarese A, Zanetto A, Becchetti C, Sciarrone SS, Shalaby S, Germani G, Gambato M, Russo FP, Burra P, Senzolo M. Management of bacterial infection in the liver transplant can-

didate. World J Hepatol. 2018;10(2):222–30. https://doi.org/10.4254/wjh.v10.i2.222. PMID: 29527258; PMCID: PMC5838441.
21. Kim WR, Lake JR, Smith JM, Schladt DP, Skeans MA, Noreen SM, et al. OPTN/SRTR 2017 annual data report: liver. Am J Transplant. 2019;19:184–283. https://doi.org/10.1111/ajt.15276.
22. Kim HK, Park YK, Wang HJ, Kim BW, Shin SY, Lim SK, Choi YH. Epidemiology and clinical features of post-transplant bloodstream infection: an analysis of 222 consecutive liver transplant recipients. Infect Chemother. 2013;45(3):315–24. https://doi.org/10.3947/ic.2013.45.3.315. Epub 2013 Sep 27. PMID: 24396633; PMCID: PMC3848524.
23. Khillan V, Kale P, Pamecha V, Rathor N, Sarin SK. Infections in live donor liver transplant recipients: a study of timeline, aetiology and antimicrobial resistance of bacterial and fungal infections from the developing world. Indian J Med Microbiol. 2017;35:604–6.
24. Vandecasteele E, De Waele J, Vandijck D, Blot S, Vogelaers D, Rogiers X, Van Vlierberghe H, Decruyenaere J, Hoste E. Antimicrobial prophylaxis in liver transplant patients–a multicenter survey endorsed by the European Liver and Intestine Transplant Association. Transpl Int. 2010;23:182–90.
25. Raghuram A, Restrepo A, Safadjou S, Cooley J, Orloff M, Hardy D, Butler S, Koval CE. Invasive fungal infections following liver transplantation: incidence, risk factors, survival, and impact of fluconazole-resistant Candida parapsilosis (2003–2007). Liver Transpl. 2012;18:1100–9.
26. Eschenauer GA, Lam SW, Carver PL. Antifungal prophylaxis in liver transplant recipients. Liver Transpl. 2009;15:842–58. https://doi.org/10.1002/lt.21826.
27. European Association for the Study of the Liver (EASL). EASL clinical practice guidelines: liver transplantation. J Hepatol. 2016;64(2):433–85.
28. Barchiesi F, Mazzocato S, Mazzanti S, Gesuita R, Skrami E, Fiorentini A, et al. Invasive aspergillosis in liver transplant recipients: epidemiology, clinical characteristics, treatment, and outcomes in 116 cases. Liver Transpl. 2015;21(2):204–12.
29. Williams MJ, Hayes PC. Antimicrobial prophylaxis following liver transplantation. In: Neuberger J, Ferguson J, Newsome PN, Lucey MR, editors. Liver transplantation; 2021. https://doi.org/10.1002/9781119634010.ch52.
30. Jenks JD, Hoenigl M. Treatment of Aspergillosis. J Fungi (Basel). 2018;4(3):98. https://doi.org/10.3390/jof4030098. PMID: 30126229; PMCID: PMC6162797.
31. Saner FH, Hoyer DP, Hartmann M, Nowak KM, Bezinover D. The edge of unknown: postoperative critical care in liver transplantation. J Clin Med. 2022;11(14):4036. https://doi.org/10.3390/jcm11144036. PMID: 35887797; PMCID: PMC9322367.
32. Lautenschlager I, Halme L, Hockerstedt K, Krogerus L, Taskinen E. Cytomegalovirus infection of the liver transplant: Virological, histological, immunological, and clinical observations. Transpl Infect Dis. 2006;8:21–30.
33. Singh N, Winston DJ, Razonable RR, Lyon GM, Silveira FP, Wagener MM, Stevens-Ayers T, Edmison B, Boeckh M, Limaye AP. Effect of preemptive therapy vs antiviral prophylaxis on cytomegalovirus disease in seronegative liver transplant recipients with seropositive donors: a randomized clinical trial. JAMA. 2020;323(14):1378–87. https://doi.org/10.1001/jama.2020.3138. PMID: 32286644; PMCID: PMC7157180.
34. Mallick S, Kathirvel M, Nair K, Durairaj MS, Varghese CT, Amma SPT, Dinesh B. A randomized, double-blinded, placebo-controlled trial analyzing the effect of synbiotics on infectious complications following living donor liver transplant—PREPRO trial. J Hepatobiliary Pancreat Sci. 2022;29:1264–73. https://doi.org/10.1002/jhbp.1182.
35. Grąt M, Wronka KM, Lewandowski Z, et al. Effects of continuous use of probiotics before liver transplantation: a randomized, double-blind, placebo-controlled trial. Clin Nutr. 2017;36:1530–9.
36. Zhang Y, Chen J, Wu J, Chalson H, Merigan L, Mitchell A. Probiotic use in preventing postoperative infection in liver transplant patients. Hepatob Surg Nutr. 2013;2(3):142–7. https://doi.org/10.3978/j.issn.2304-3881.2013.06.05. PMID: 24570932; PMCID: PMC3924667.

37. Merli M, Giusto M, Gentili F, Novelli G, Ferretti G, Riggio O, Corradini SG, Siciliano M, Farcomeni A, Attili AF, et al. Nutritional status, its influence on the outcome of patients undergoing liver transplantation. Liver Int. 2010;30:208–14.
38. Stephenson GR, Moretti EW, El-Moalem H, Clavien PA, Tuttle-Newhall JE. Malnutrition in liver transplant patients, preoperative subjective global assessment is predictive of outcome after liver transplantation. Transplantation. 2001;72:666–70.
39. Kaido T, Mori A, Ogura Y, Ogawa K, Hata K, Yoshizawa A, Yagi S, Uemoto S. Pre and perioperative factors affecting infection after living donor liver transplantation. Nutrition. 2012;28:1104–8.
40. Plauth M, Bernal W, Dasarathy S, et al. ESPEN guideline on clinical nutrition in liver disease. Clin Nutr. 2019;38:485–521.
41. European Association for the Study of the Liver. Electronic address: easloffice@easloffice.eu; European Association for the Study of the Liver. EASL Clinical Practice Guidelines on nutrition in chronic liver disease. J Hepatol. 2019;70(1):172–93. https://doi.org/10.1016/j.jhep.2018.06.024. Epub 2018 Aug 23. PMID: 30144956; PMCID: PMC6657019.
42. Kathirvel M, et al. Randomized trial of steroid free immunosuppression with basiliximab induction in adult live donor liver transplantation (LDLT). HPB. 2021;23(5):666–74.
43. Mallick S, Anila KN, Sivaprasadan S, Sudhindran S. Immunosuppression in liver transplant recipients in the setting of sepsis. J Clin Exp Hepatol. 2023;13(4):682–90.
44. Saner FH, Gieseler RK, Akiz H, Canbay A, Gorlinger K. Delicate balance of bleeding and thrombosis in end-stage liver disease and liver transplantation. Digestion. 2013;88:135–44.
45. Kumar M, Ahmad J, Maiwall R, Choudhury A, Bajpai M, Mitra LG, Saluja V, Mohan Agarwal P, Bihari C, Shasthry SM, et al. Thromboelastography-guided blood component use in patients with cirrhosis with Nonvariceal bleeding: a randomized controlled trial. Hepatology. 2020;71:235–46.
46. De Pietri L, Bianchini M, Montalti R, De Maria N, Di Maira T, Begliomini B, Gerunda GE, di Benedetto F, Garcia-Tsao G, Villa E. Thrombelastography-guided blood product use before invasive procedures in cirrhosis with severe coagulopathy: a randomized, controlled trial. Hepatology. 2016;63:566–73.
47. Yoon U, Bartoszko J, Bezinover D, Biancofiore G, Forkin KT, Rahman S, Spiro M, Raptis DA, Kang Y, Group ER. Intraoperative transfusion management, antifibrinolytic therapy, coagulation monitoring and the impact on short-term outcomes after liver transplantation-A systematic review of the literature and expert panel recommendations. Clin Transpl. 2022; https://doi.org/10.1111/ctr.14637.
48. Giannini EG, Stravitz RT, Caldwell SH. Correction of hemostatic abnormalities and portal pressure variations in patients with cirrhosis. Hepatology. 2014;60:1442.
49. Rassi AB, d'Amico EA, Tripodi A, da Rocha TRF, Migita BY, Ferreira CM, Carrilho FJ, Farias AQ. Fresh frozen plasma transfusion in patients with cirrhosis and coagulopathy: effect on conventional coagulation tests and thrombomodulin-modified thrombin generation. J Hepatol. 2020;72:85–94.
50. Kirchner C, Dirkmann D, Treckmann JW, Paul A, Hartmann M, Saner FH, Gorlinger K. Coagulation management with factor concentrates in liver transplantation: a single-center experience. Transfusion. 2014;54(Pt 2):2760–8.
51. Sabate A, Gutierrez R, Beltran J, Mellado P, Blasi A, Acosta F, Costa M, Reyes R, Torres F. Impact of preemptive fibrinogen concentrate on transfusion requirements in liver transplantation: a multicenter, randomized, double-blind, Placebo-Controlled Trial. Am J Transpl. 2016;16:2421–9.
52. Yalavarthy R, Edelstein CL, Teitelbaum I. Acute renal failure and chronic kidney disease following liver transplantation. Hemodial Int. 2007;11(Suppl 3):S7–12.
53. Biancofiore G, Pucci L, Cerutti E, Penno G, Pardini E, Esposito M, et al. Cystatin C as a marker of renal function immediately after liver transplantation. Liver Transpl. 2006;12:285–91.
54. Abdelaziz O, Attia H. Doppler ultrasonography in living donor liver transplantation recipients: intra- and post-operative vascular complications. World J Gastroenterol. 2016;22(27):6145–72.

Chapter 29
The Art of Immunosuppression

Marta Tejedor and Marina Berenguer

Abstract Liver transplantation (LT) has witnessed continuous improvements in outcomes over the past decades; however, long-term survival rates still fall short of those observed in the general population.

Indeed, while increasing the potency of immunosuppressive agents in LT has drastically reduced the rates of steroid-resistant rejection and rejection-related graft loss, an emerging conundrum is the extended exposure of transplant recipients to these powerful agents, driven by both their heightened benefits and the prolonged survival of recipients. This juxtaposition manifests as a double-edged sword, whereby increased immunosuppressive potency combats rejection but exposes recipients to undesirable adverse effects.

Individualizing the selection and titration of immunosuppressive drugs is a critical endeavor aimed at effectively managing alloreactivity while mitigating the burden of toxicities. Although routine laboratory tests fall short in providing a confident diagnosis of allograft rejection, the landscape of biomarkers holds promise. However, these biomarkers are yet to attain the level of validation required for routine clinical use, necessitating the retention of liver biopsy as a guiding tool for clinical decisions.

Understanding the mechanisms of action and adverse effects of commonly used immunosuppressive drugs is pivotal. This review delves into the intricacies of various immunosuppressive regimens for both early and maintenance phases. Achieving the delicate balance between optimal immunosuppression (IS) for rejection prevention

M. Tejedor
Division of GI/Hepatology, University of Iowa Healthcare, Iowa City, United States

M. Berenguer (✉)
Hepatology and Liver Transplantation Unit, Medical Research Institute (IISLaFe)
La Fe University Hospital and University of Valencia, Valencia, Spain

CIBERehd (IISCarlosIII), Madrid, Spain
e-mail: marina.berenguer@uv.es

S. Saigal, D. Jothimani (eds.), *Fundamentals of Transplant Hepatology*,
https://doi.org/10.1007/978-981-95-2624-6_29

and minimizing immunosuppressive-related adverse effects requires the fusion of medical science and clinical expertise. Strategies focused on preserving renal function, averting recurrent or de novo cancer, and recurrent or de novo immune-mediated diseases, as well as tackling metabolic syndrome, are explored in this context.

Keywords Immunosuppression · Calcineurin inhibitors · Tacrolimus · Antimetabolites · Azathioprine · Mycophenolate Mofetil · Everolimus · Sirolimus · Induction immunosuppression

Abbreviations

ABO-I	ABO incompatible
ACLF	Acute-on-Chronic Liver Failure
ACR	Acute cellular rejection
AHT	Arterial hypertension
AIH	Autoimmune hepatitis
ALG	Anti-lymphocyte globulin
AMR	Antibody-mediated rejection
APC	Antigen-presenting cell
ATG	Anti-thymocyte globulin
AZA	Azathioprine
CKD	Chronic kidney disease
Cmax	Highest drug plasma concentration
Cmin	Lowest (trough) drug plasma concentration
CNI	Calcineurin inhibitors
CsA	Cyclosporine
CV	Cardiovascular
CVE	Cardiovascular events
DM	Diabetes mellitus
EC-MPS	Enteric-coated Mycophenolate Sodium formulation
eGFR	Estimated glomerular filtration rate
ELTR	European Liver Transplant Registry
EVR	Everolimus
GFR	Glomerular filtration rate
GI	Gastrointestinal
HCC	Hepatocellular carcinoma
HCV	Hepatitis C virus
HLA	Human leukocyte antigen
HR	Hazard ratio
IL-2	Interleukin 2
IL-2 RA	Monoclonal anti-interleukin-2 receptor antibodies
ILTS	International Liver Transplant Society
IPV	Inter- and intra-patient pharmacokinetic variability

IS	Immunosuppression
IVIG	Intravenous immunoglobulins
LDLT	Living donor liver transplantation
LT	Liver Transplantation
MASLD	Metabolic dysfunction-associated steatotic liver disease
MDRD4	Modification of Diet in Renal Disease (four-variable)
MELD	Model for End-Stage Liver Disease
MHC	Major histocompatibility complex
MMF	Mycophenolate mofetil
MPA	Mycophenolic acid
mTOR	Mammalian target of rapamycin
mTORi	Mammalian target of rapamycin inhibitors
NODAT	New-onset diabetes after transplant
OKT3	Muronomab-CD3
OPTN	Organ Procurement and Transplantation Network
PBC	Primary biliary cholangitis
PSC	Primary sclerosing cholangitis
PTLD	Post-transplant lymphoproliferative disorder
RCT	Randomized controlled trials
RR	Relative risk
SRL	Sirolimus
TAC	Tacrolimus
TCR	T-cell receptor
TDM	Therapeutic drug monitoring
UNOS	United Network for Organ Sharing

Key Highlights

1. Personalizing the selection and dosing of immunosuppressive drugs is essential for effectively controlling alloreactivity and reducing the risk of toxicities.
2. Balancing the efficacy and side effects of immunosuppressive agents while selecting the best combination at each stage—based on factors like the recipient's profile, surgery type, comorbidities, and indications—requires a deep understanding of the drugs to minimize toxicities and preserve effectiveness.
3. Typically, the post-LT immunosuppressive regimen follows an intensive phase during the first 3 months, characterized by high alloreactivity, where the most potent immunosuppressive agents are used, followed by a maintenance phase that introduces protocols for minimizing drug dosages.
4. Currently, Tacrolimus (TAC) combined with mycophenolate mofetil (MMF) ± steroids is the standard immunosuppressive regimen in LT, with non-standard alternatives primarily used as renal-sparing strategies or for oncologic purposes, often involving delayed reduced-dose TAC with antimetabolites or mTOR inhibitors; therapeutic drug monitoring (TDM) is required for calcineurin inhibitors (CNIs) and mTORis; steroid discontinuation is typically aimed for within the first year, though long-term steroids may be necessary for autoim-

mune liver disease recipients or those with recurrent rejection, while simplifying regimens, such as using single daily doses of TAC, can help address nonadherence. Some patients may eventually achieve "tolerance," allowing for successful IS cessation without graft rejection.

29.1 Introduction

Liver transplantation (LT) remains the definitive treatment for end-stage liver disease and hepatocellular carcinoma (HCC). Over the past 50 years, major advances in surgical techniques, perioperative care, and immunosuppressive therapies have significantly improved both graft and patient survival. Data from organizations such as the United Network for Organ Sharing (UNOS), the Organ Procurement and Transplantation Network (OPTN), and the European Liver Transplant Registry (ELTR) show a remarkable improvement in 1-year post-transplant survival—from 62%–66% in 1986–1989 to 89%–92% between 2010 and 2020 [1, 2].

Despite this progress in short-term outcomes, long-term survival has seen more limited improvement. Contributing factors include the cumulative side effects of long-term immunosuppression (IS), increased vulnerability to infections, and post-transplant malignancies [3–7]. Additionally, the typical LT recipient has changed—patients today are generally older, more frail, and have more comorbid conditions. The underlying causes of liver failure have also shifted, moving away from hepatitis C toward alcohol-related liver disease and metabolic dysfunction-associated steatotic liver disease (MASLD), with an expanded scope of oncological indications including cholangiocarcinoma [1, 3, 4, 8, 9].

In this evolving context, managing IS requires a nuanced approach. Selecting the optimal immunosuppressive regimen—both in terms of drug combinations and dosage—requires consideration of multiple factors: recipient characteristics, surgical complexity, comorbidities, and transplant indications. The ultimate goal is to minimize toxicity while maintaining graft protection, a process that demands a deep understanding of the pharmacology and immunology behind each agent.

29.2 Immunology and Liver Transplantation

The liver possesses unique immunological features that render it more resistant to rejection than other transplanted organs, earning it the classification of an immune-privileged organ. As a result, human leukocyte antigen (HLA) matching is not a prerequisite in LT, as it has minimal influence on graft outcomes [10].

This immune privilege is attributed to several factors: the transfer of donor immune cells to the recipient (microchimerism), the secretion of soluble donor (major histocompatibility complex) MHC class I molecules that neutralize circulating antibodies and inhibit T-cell activation, and the liver's inherent resistance to immune-mediated injury due to its large size and regenerative capacity.

Nevertheless, LT recipients still face the risk of immunologic rejection and thus require long-term immunosuppressive therapy, though typically at lower doses compared to other organ transplant recipients. Over time, the immune system may adapt to the graft, reducing its reactivity—a state known as "operational tolerance," where the graft continues to function without ongoing IS and without signs of rejection [10–12].

Rejection of a liver allograft involves both the innate and adaptive immune systems. Mismatches in MHC antigens, coupled with surgical trauma and ischemia-reperfusion injury, initiate this response. Antigen-presenting cells (APCs) from both the donor and the recipient interact with T-cell receptors (TCRs), triggering T-cell activation. This in turn activates multiple intracellular pathways, including the calcium–calcineurin, mitogen-activated protein kinase (MAPK), and protein kinase C–NF-κB signaling cascades, which ultimately contribute to graft rejection.

Immunosuppressive drugs are designed to interfere with these pathways at various levels to prevent or manage rejection.

29.3 Immunosuppressive Agents

Immunosuppressive drugs can be classified into pharmacological (Calcineurin inhibitors—CNIs—including cyclosporine—CsA—and tacrolimus—TAC; antimetabolites, including azathioprine—AZA—and mycophenolate mofetil—MMF; or mammalian target of rapamycin—mTOR inhibitors, including sirolimus—SRL—and everolimus—EVR) and biological agents, each with its distinct mode of action. CNIs inhibit calcineurin, hindering T-cell activation and proliferation. mTORi, by contrast, targets the mTOR complex to prevent signal-3 of T-cell activation, impeding T-cell proliferation. Antimetabolites, exemplified by mycophenolic acid (MPA), curb T-cell replication via reversible inhibition of purine synthesis. Corticosteroids exert their immunomodulatory effects through interactions with antigen-presenting dendritic cells, reduction in CD4+ T-cell numbers, and IL-1-dependent lymphocyte activation. Other biological agents deplete or inhibit T- and B-cell proliferation, thereby suppressing immune responses [13–16] (Fig. 29.1).

In the 1960s, corticosteroids and AZA served as the sole available immunosuppressive agents for LT. Subsequently, the introduction of drugs such as CsA in 1983, TAC in 1994, MMF in 1995, anti-thymocyte globulin (ATG) in 1998, and others revolutionized immunosuppressive efficacy [13–19]. Yet, this progress came at a cost: long-term survivors experienced a mere 1.7% mortality rate due to rejection, whereas IS-linked malignancies (16.4%) and opportunistic infections (10.5%) took precedence as leading causes of death [3, 5–7] (Table 29.1). Potent immunosuppressive agents also contributed to an upsurge in metabolic disorders, cardiovascular events (CVE), and renal dysfunction, culminating in chronic kidney disease (CKD) for a significant proportion of patients surviving beyond 5 years post-LT.

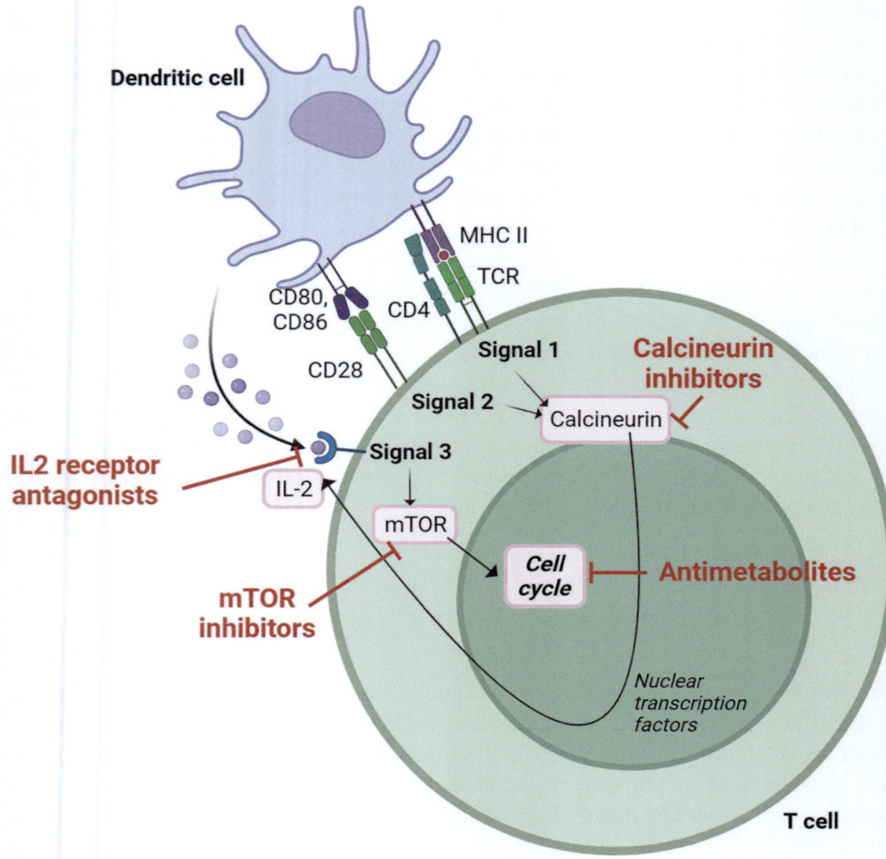

Fig. 29.1 Mechanism of action of several immunosuppressive agents. APCs, such as dendritic cells, present foreign antigens to T-lymphocytes in the MHC. Immunological synapse requires signal 1 (antigen presented in the MHC ligates to TCR) and costimulatory signal 2 (CD80 and CD86 ligates to CD28) to activate several intracellular pathways, including the calcium/calcineurin pathway, which in turn triggers the expression of several cytokines, including interleukin-2 (IL2). IL2 triggers signal 3, able to stimulate cell proliferation via the mTOR pathway. Proliferation of T-cells requires activation of the cell cycle and nucleotide synthesis. Sites of action of the most commonly used anti-rejection medications are marked in the figure. (Modified from Wiesner et al. [106], Montano-Loza et al. [10], and Adams et al. [11])

Table 29.1 Summary of the major immunosuppressants used in liver transplantation

Group	Drug	Dose	Trough levels		Safe in pregnancy	Adverse events	Comment
			Induction	Maintenance			
CNI	TAC	0.1–0.15 mg/kg/d	7–10 ng/ml	4–8 ng/ml	Yes	Nephrotoxicity, neurotoxicity, AHT, DM, DL, hyperkalemia, metabolic acidosis	Prevention of rejection
	CsA	10–15 mg/kg/d	250–300 ng/ml	100–150 ng/ml	If no alternative		
Antimetabolites	MMF	500–1000 mg bd	–	–	No	GI disturbances, myelosuppression, viral infections	Prevention of rejection CNI sparing
	AZA	3-5 mg/kg/d	–	–	Yes		
mTORi	EVR	0.25–0.5 mg bd	No	3–8 ng/ml	No	Proteinuria, DL, poor wound healing, pneumonitis, skin rash, peripheral edema, stomatitis	Prevention of rejection HCC recurrence prevention CNI sparing
	SRL	1 mg/d	No	4–10 ng/ml	No		
Steroids	Prednisone	5 mg–10 mg/kg Followed by a tapering dose	–	–	Yes	Obesity, osteoporosis, Cushing syndrome, mood changes, cataracts	Prevention of rejection Anti-inflammatory
IL2 RA	Basiliximab	20 mg	2 doses (day 0 and day 4 post-LT)	No	No	Hypersensitivity reactions	Prevention of rejection CNI sparing

AHT arterial hypertension, *AZA* azathioprine, *Bd* twice a day, *CNI* calcineurin inhibitors, *CsA* cyclosporine, *DL* dyslipidemia, *DM* diabetes mellitus, *EVR* everolimus, *GI* gastrointestinal, *HCC* hepatocellular carcinoma, *IL2 RA* interleukin-2 receptor antibodies, *MMF* mycophenolate mofetil, *mTORi* mammalian target of rapamycin inhibitor, *SRL* sirolimus, *TAC* tacrolimus

Note: The table provides a general overview and may not include all possible indications and side effects. The specific choice of immunosuppressive agents and monitoring protocols should be tailored to individual patient needs and be guided by the transplant team's expertise and current guidelines

The landscape of immunosuppressive regimens thrives on combination therapy, wielding agents with varying mechanisms to reduce dosages and associated toxicities [13–19]. A pertinent example lies in the realm of CNIs, where strategies like antibody induction and mTOR inhibitor/antimetabolite usage emerge as mechanisms to reduce CNI-related toxicities.

Typically, the journey of post-LT IS traverses an intensive phase during the initial 3 months, marked by high alloreactivity, where the strongest IS is applied, followed by a maintenance phase that witnesses the implementation of minimization protocols (Fig. 29.2).

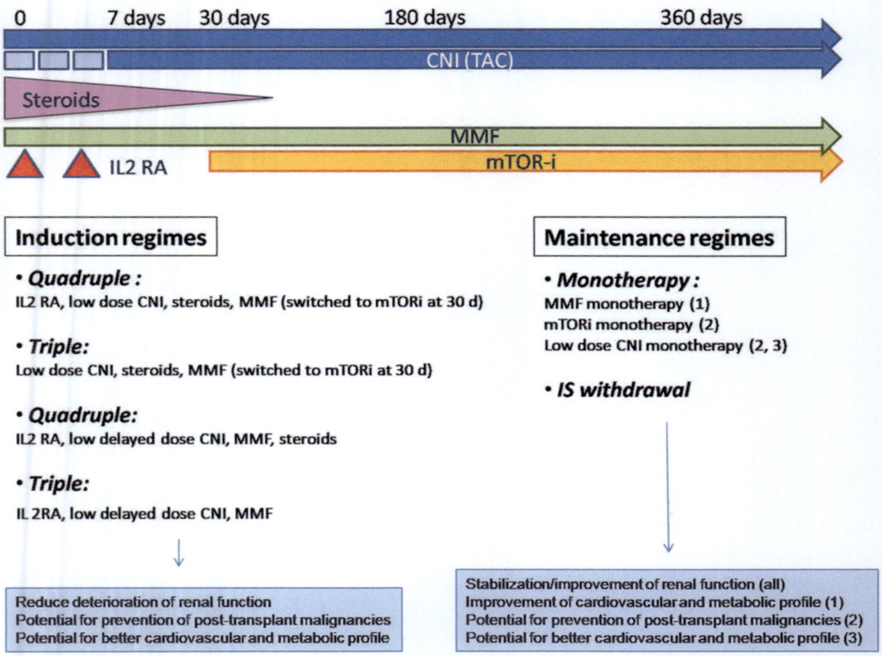

Fig. 29.2 Management of IS following liver transplant (LT). Induction IS is a prophylactic short-term, intense therapy providing additional protection against acute rejection, usually administered immediately after LT. Initial IS pertains to the IS used in the first months post-LT when the risk of rejection is higher. Maintenance treatment is typically a lifelong treatment aimed at preserving the allograft from rejection using a lower effective dose of IS. Advantages of the different approaches are listed in the blue boxes. (Modified from Di Maira et al. [13])

29.3.1 Calcineurin Inhibitors

CNIs block calcineurin, thus inhibiting both T-lymphocyte signal transduction and IL-2 transcription. In particular, TAC binds to the immunophilin FKBP12 (FK506 binding protein), creating a new complex, the FKBP12–FK506 complex that interacts with and inhibits calcineurin.

Oral TAC is slowly absorbed in the gastrointestinal (GI) tract, with a total bioavailability of 20% to 25% (but with variations from 5% to 67%) and the highest blood plasma concentrations (C_{max}) reached after 1–3 h. Taking the drug together with a meal, especially one rich in fat, reduces bioavailability. In the blood, TAC is mainly bound to erythrocytes; only 5% is found in plasma, of which more than 98.8% is bound to plasma proteins [20, 21].

The substance is metabolized in the liver, mainly via CYP3A, and in the intestinal wall. All metabolites found in the circulation are inactive. Biological half-life varies widely due to differences in clearance but is typically around 12 h in LT recipients. It is predominantly eliminated via the feces in the form of its metabolites.

Genetic variations within *CYP3A5* that result in changes to the activity of the CYP3A5 protein can affect concentrations of TAC within the body. In particular, individuals who are homozygous for the G allele at the single-nucleotide polymorphism rs776746 (also known as *CYP3A5* *3/*3) have a non-functional *CYP3A5* protein. The frequency of the G allele varies worldwide, from 4% in some African populations to 80–90% in Caucasian populations. Across many studies, individuals homozygous for the G allele have been shown to have higher concentrations of TAC and require lower doses of the drug, as compared to individuals who are not homozygous for the G allele. The clinical implications of dosing TAC based on *CYP3A5* polymorphism are unclear. While there is evidence to suggest that dosing patients based on rs776746 genotype can result in faster and more frequent achievement of target levels, there is a lack of consistent evidence to demonstrate that it improves clinical outcomes (such as a decreased risk for transplant rejection or drug toxicities), likely due to patients on TAC being subject to therapeutic drug monitoring (TDM) [18–22].

Because TAC is primarily metabolized by the cytochrome P450 system of liver enzymes, it is important to assess potential drug-drug interactions with the many substances that interact with this system and induce or inhibit the system's metabolic activity. For instance, grapefruit and azoles increase tacrolimus plasma concentrations by competing for cytochrome enzymes. Several webpages can be used to assess drug-drug interactions [18–22] (i.e., https://www.uptodate.com/drug-interactions/; https://reference.medscape.com/drug-interactionchecker).

TAC is 100 times more potent than CsA. In several randomized controlled trials (RCTs), TAC-based regimens with or without steroids or MMF generally showed lower rejection rates and improved graft and patient survival compared to CsA, such that currently TAC is considered the standard CNI therapy in LT recipients. In the most recent meta-analysis of 16 RCTs, TAC was superior in terms of patient survival and reducing arterial hypertension (AHT). Yet, new-onset diabetes after transplant (NODAT) was more common in the TAC group [23].

TDM is essential due to the narrow therapeutic index and wide inter- and intra-patient pharmacokinetic variability (IPV) of CNI. Achieving stable trough levels of TAC within the target range is crucial but can be challenging due to various factors, including drug interactions, genetic polymorphisms, or treatment adherence [19, 22]. While measuring trough levels is the most common approach, it may not reflect the actual drug effect. Some authors propose to better establish therapeutic effect and toxicity by calculating IPV, through a simple calculation of a coefficient of variation of immunosuppressive drugs through concentrations (C_{min}) (i.e., by dividing standard deviations of the concentrations by their mean). Patients with higher IPV might have worse outcomes when considering inflammation, graft rejection, and overall patient and graft survival. The mechanism behind this process may be related to the alternation of over- and under-subclinical IS episodes. These episodes could lead to drug toxicity in the first case and to immune activation in the latter case. Consequently, the graft can accumulate lesions progressively, leading to its dysfunction. Most of the studies published on that topic, though, refer to kidney transplantation, and there are only a few inconclusive studies in the LT arena [18–27].

The administration of CNIs, while indispensable, is not devoid of challenges. These agents are associated with nephrotoxicity, neurotoxicity, and metabolic disturbances, warranting vigilant monitoring and dose adjustments [17]. Nephrotoxicity, characterized by impaired renal function, is a significant concern, with up to 40% of patients on TAC experiencing renal dysfunction [28, 29]. Neurotoxicity, including tremors and seizures, was reported in approximately 15–20% of patients on CNIs in initial studies [18]. Metabolic disturbances, such as hyperlipidemia and NODAT, are prevalent in around 30–40% of patients on CNIs [17, 23].

29.3.2 Antimetabolites

MMF is a purine synthesis inhibitor that suppresses lymphocyte proliferation by interfering with the cell cycle, particularly in activated immune cells. MMF is preferred over AZA due to its lower risk of developing non-melanoma skin cancers. It also has minimal drug-drug interactions, making it a favorable option in transplant immunosuppressive regimens.

The duration of MMF therapy varies depending on factors such as the patient's risk of rejection, the broader immunosuppressive strategy in place, and the emergence of adverse effects—most notably gastrointestinal symptoms or bone marrow suppression. TDM is not routinely performed for MMF, and dose adjustments are typically made based on clinical protocols and observed side effects. Whether TDM can improve MMF dosing remains an open question [13–18].

In the first large RCT evaluating MMF in LT, 565 patients were assigned to receive either MMF or AZA alongside cyclosporine (CsA) and corticosteroids. Over a one-year follow-up period, MMF was more effective than AZA in reducing acute rejection within the first 6 months. However, both were similar in preventing graft loss at 1 year, and their safety profiles were comparable [30].

A large U.S. registry analysis involving 11,670 LT recipients showed that patients discharged on triple therapy, including MMF, had better outcomes, including lower risks of mortality (HR = 0.77), graft loss (HR = 0.81), acute rejection (HR = 0.89), and infection-related death (HR = 0.80) [31].

Further supporting MMF's role, a recent prospective RCT demonstrated that combining low-dose tacrolimus (TAC) with MMF led to improved renal function and metabolic outcomes compared to standard-dose TAC alone. The MMF group consistently showed higher glomerular filtration rates (GFR) and fewer episodes of acute rejection ($p = 0.004$) [32].

As a result, MMF use has steadily grown, and today, nearly 80% of LT recipients are discharged on MMF-containing regimens [1].

In terms of adverse effects, both MMF and AZA are associated with gastrointestinal symptoms, hematologic complications, and a higher risk of infections [33]. Gastrointestinal side effects, especially diarrhea, occur in about 25–30% of MMF users and often necessitate dose reduction or discontinuation. To mitigate GI side effects, an enteric-coated formulation of mycophenolate sodium (EC-MPS) has been developed.

However, the benefit of switching from MMF to EC-MPS for improving GI symptoms remains controversial. A recent systematic review of 29 studies—only three of which were considered low risk for bias—found no significant difference in GI-related adverse events or GI-related quality of life between patients on MMF and those switched to EC-MPS. The authors concluded that alternative approaches should be considered before opting for conversion to EC-MPS [34].

Hematologic side effects, such as anemia and leukopenia, occur in 20–25% of patients. Opportunistic infections, particularly viral in nature, affect approximately 10% of MMF users [17, 33].

29.3.3 Steroids

Corticosteroids such as prednisone or methylprednisolone have been a cornerstone of immunosuppressive therapy in LT, yet to minimize the side effects of these drugs, their use has declined with time, such that steroid-sparing protocols either avoiding or minimizing their long-term use are becoming increasingly present in transplant centers. Yet, in a recent Cochrane systematic review ($n = 16$ studies with 1347 participants) assessing steroid avoidance or withdrawal versus steroid-containing IS in LT patients, no statistically significant difference for mortality (Relative Risk (RR) 1.15, 95% CI 0.93–1.44; low-quality evidence), graft loss including death (RR 1.15, 95% CI 0.90–1.46; low-quality evidence), or infection (RR 0.88, 95% CI 0.73–1.05; very low-quality evidence) were detected. Acute rejection and steroid-resistant rejection were statistically significantly more frequent when steroid avoidance or withdrawal was compared with steroid-containing IS (RR 1.33, 95% CI 1.08–1.64;

low-quality evidence; and RR 2.14, 95% CI 1.13–4.02; very low-quality evidence; respectively) [35]. Major side effects of steroids include metabolic side effects (weight gain, increased appetite, fluid retention, development and/or worsening pre-existing diabetes), bone loss with increased risk of osteoporosis and fractures, increased infection risk, and mood and behavioral changes, particularly mood swings, irritability, or sleep disturbances, among others [17]. In the systematic review, DM and AHT were statistically significantly less frequent when steroid avoidance or withdrawal was compared with steroid-containing IS (RR 0.81, 95% CI 0.66–0.99; low-quality evidence; and RR 0.76, 95% CI 0.65–0.90; low-quality evidence) [35]. Currently, steroids are used in patients at increased risk of rejection, such as those undergoing LT for immune-mediated liver disease indications, re-transplantation due to rejection-related indications, or fulminant liver failure, while steroid avoidance or withdrawal may be of benefit in selected patients, especially those at low risk of rejection and high risk of metabolic complications [10–16].

29.3.4 mTOR Inhibitors

mTOR signaling pathway plays a crucial role in regulating APC function and T-cell differentiation, which accounts for its immunomodulatory properties.

Sirolimus (SRL) has not received FDA approval for use in LT due to concerns over hepatic artery thrombosis. However, its immunosuppressive efficacy has led to its off-label use in mTOR inhibitor-based regimens. SRL has a long terminal half-life (48–72 h), allowing for once-daily dosing. However, it is poorly water-soluble, has limited absorption, and a wide volume of distribution, resulting in low bioavailability (\ ~ 14–18%). It is metabolized by CYP3A4, which predisposes it to numerous drug interactions.

Everolimus (EVR) has similar pharmacokinetic limitations, including low bioavailability (\ ~ 20%) and CYP3A4-dependent metabolism. However, its terminal half-life is slightly shorter (26–30 h), necessitating twice-daily dosing [13, 14, 16].

When switching a patient from a CNI to an mTOR inhibitor, careful consideration of pharmacokinetic interactions is required. For example, TAC should only be tapered once EVR levels have reached at least 3 ng/mL, whereas CsA should be reduced immediately upon starting EVR [36, 37].

mTOR inhibitors are primarily used in renal-sparing regimens, especially in patients with existing kidney dysfunction or those at high risk for nephrotoxicity from CNIs (See Kidney Dysfunction section) [36, 37].

Though RCTs have not definitively proven it, mTOR inhibitors may offer oncologic benefits in HCC patients, including reduced tumor recurrence post-transplantation. This is due to the frequent activation of the PI3K/AKT/mTOR pathway in more aggressive forms of HCC (see HCC section) [38].

Additionally, mTOR inhibitors may lower the risk of de novo malignancies post-transplant. They are therefore considered for high-risk groups such as:

- Patients with primary sclerosing cholangitis (PSC) and concurrent inflammatory bowel disease.
- HSV-8 positive patients.
- Recipients with alcoholic cirrhosis, particularly smokers.
- Those receiving grafts from donors with potential malignancy transmission.
  EBV-negative recipients, especially those who become EBV-positive post-LT.

mTOR inhibitors are associated with frequent adverse effects, especially when trough levels are elevated. These include:

- Delayed wound healing or wound dehiscence in \ ~ 15–20% of patients. Due to this, mTOR inhibitors are generally introduced 15–30 days post-transplant, especially in patients with obesity or at higher risk for healing complications.
- Metabolic effects, including hyperlipidemia (both cholesterol and triglycerides), oral ulcers, and stomatitis.
- Interstitial lung disease, particularly when drug levels exceed 8 ng/mL.
- Cardiovascular risk due to hypercholesterolemia, although the actual rate of major CV events (MACE) does not appear significantly higher than with non-mTOR-based regimens.

Hematologic effects such as anemia, leukopenia, and thrombocytopenia occur in up to 10% of patients. If neutropenia ($<1000/mm^3$), leukopenia ($<2000/mm^3$), or thrombocytopenia ($<50{,}000/mm^3$) develops, dose reduction to the minimum effective level is recommended.

Proteinuria is another significant side effect. It may develop or worsen after initiating EVR, and should be monitored regularly. Long-term EVR use has been associated with proteinuria >1 g/day in about 3% of cases. If proteinuria exceeds 800 mg/day, ongoing monitoring is necessary, and EVR should be discontinued if nephrotic range levels are reached. ACE inhibitors or ARBs can be used to offer renal protection.

For mucosal side effects, management includes:

- Preventive strategies (e.g., good oral hygiene, avoiding spicy or acidic foods).
- Topical treatments like steroids, NSAIDs, or anesthetics.

Hyperlipidemia is typically managed with statins or fibrates.

EVR is commonly introduced to reduce TAC exposure, particularly to protect renal function (see Renal Impairment section). A recent systematic review analyzing 8 trials (1570 patients) showed that the use of EVR with reduced CNIs did not increase the risk of rejection, graft loss, or mortality compared to standard CNI regimens. Importantly, renal function improved significantly, with an average increase in eGFR of 5.59 mL/min (95% CI: 2.17–9.01, $p = 0.001$) [39].

However, this benefit came with a higher risk of adverse events (relative risk = 1.22, 95% CI: 1.04–1.42, $p = 0.01$) [39]. Unlike previous analyses, this review did not find a significantly increased infection risk with mTOR-based therapy [40].

29.3.5 Antibody Induction Therapy

Used in the immediate post-transplant period, T-cell specific antibody induction was initially considered in patients at high immunological risk, particularly kidney transplant candidates with previous sensitization, re-transplantation, or a high degree of HLA mismatch, yet its main indication in LT is to preserve perioperative renal function and minimize the need for steroids or high dose CNI allowing the delayed introduction of low TAC doses [10–17]. Muronomab-CD3 (OKT3), an anti-CD3 monoclonal antibody, was among the first used, but its current use is limited due to adverse effects. Basiliximab and daclizumab, anti-interleukin-2 receptor antibodies, are better tolerated and induce less immunogenicity. Daclizumab has been withdrawn from the market after reports of autoimmune encephalitis in Europe [41]. In contrast, ATG and anti-lymphocyte globulin (ALG) are polyclonal antibodies used for the induction and treatment of steroid-resistant rejection. They can cause dose-dependent lymphopenia and suppress T-cells for up to 90 days. Hypersensitivity reactions, including fever, chills, rash, and rarely anaphylaxis, may occur during or after administration of induction agents. In addition, induction therapy can increase the susceptibility to infections, including bacterial, viral, and fungal infections, and the risk of lymphoproliferative disorders and malignancies due to profound IS. Transient decrease in blood cell counts is also commonly observed. The dosage and duration of induction therapy are determined based on the specific induction agent used.

Several meta-analyses have been published to determine the benefits of an antibody induction regimen, particularly to avoid the use of steroids [42, 43]. In a recent meta-analysis updated to include 11 trials involving 1683 patients, the safety and efficacy of T-cell-specific antibodies were compared with steroid induction in LT [43]. The incidence of acute rejection was not significantly different between the antibody and steroid-induction groups (RR 0.85, 95% confidence interval [CI] 0.72, 1.01, $p = 0.06$, I2 = 0%). However, T-cell specific antibody induction significantly reduced the risk of cytomegalovirus infection (RR 0.48, 95% CI 0.33, 0.70, $p = 0.0002$, I2 = 3%), hepatitis C virus (HCV) recurrence (RR 0.89, 95% CI 0.80, 0.99, $p = 0.03$, I2 = 0%), DM (RR 0.41, 95% CI 0.32, 0.54, $P < 0.0001$, I2 = 0%) and AHT (RR 0.71, 95% CI 0.55, 0.90, $P = 0.005$, I2 = 35%). The beneficial effect of steroid avoidance with induction therapy may be relevant for patients at risk of developing CVE, such as those transplanted for MASLD.

29.4 Immunosuppression Strategies

TAC-based IS is the standard approach, though avoiding complete CNI withdrawal early after transplant is essential to prevent rejection. Close monitoring of TAC trough concentrations is crucial for maintaining therapeutic levels and avoiding toxicity. IS protocols often involve combinations to achieve optimal efficacy while

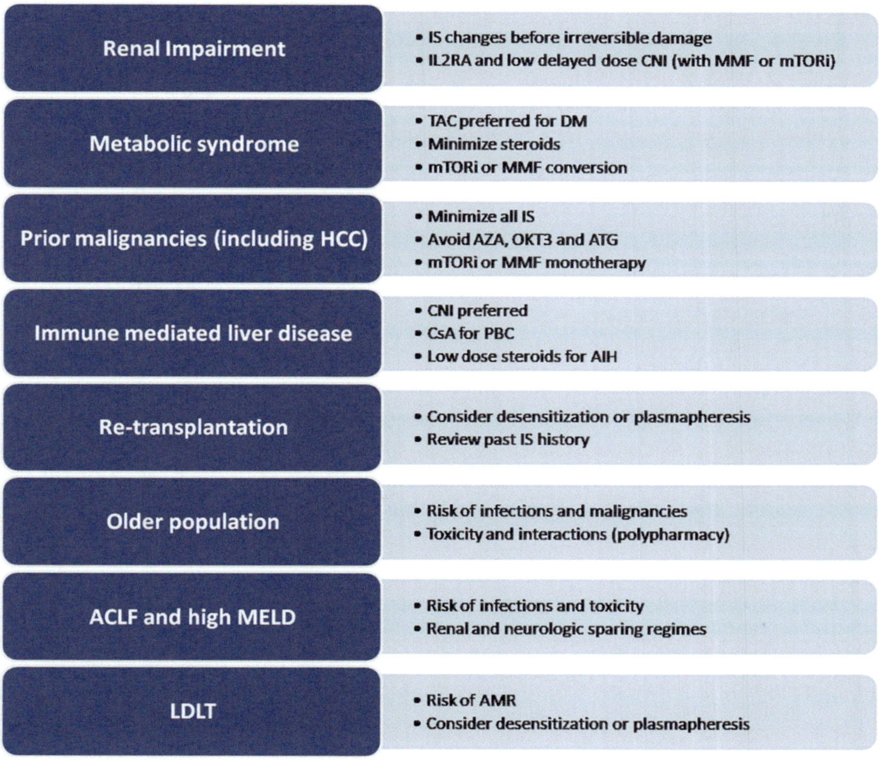

Fig. 29.3 Considerations in special situations. ACLF: acute-on-chronic liver failure. AIH: autoimmune hepatitis. AMR: antibody-mediated rejection. ATG: anti-thymocyte globulin. AZA: azathioprine. CNI: calcineurin inhibitors. CsA: cyclosporine. DM: diabetes mellitus. HCC: hepatocellular carcinoma. IL2 RA: interleukin-2 receptor antibodies. IS: immunosuppression. LDLT: living donation LT. MELD: model for end-stage liver disease. MMF: mycophenolate mofetil. mTORi: mammalian target of rapamycin inhibitor. OKT3: muronomab CD3. PBC: primary biliary cholangitis. TAC: tacrolimus (See text for more details)

minimizing adverse effects. Studies have demonstrated the benefits of these strategies, particularly in terms of preserving renal function and preventing graft rejection [10–16]. Combinations can vary based on factors such as center protocols, patient characteristics, and individual patient needs, considering the patient's overall health, risk factors, immunological status, and potential drug interactions. It is important to note that IS carries the mentioned risks, including increased susceptibility to infections and certain malignancies, enhanced CV risk factors, and kidney dysfunction (Fig. 29.3). Therefore, finding the right balance between preventing rejection and minimizing side effects remains a key challenge in transplantation. Indeed, tailored IS protocols have been developed to minimize side effects and maintain adequate immune suppression while reducing long-term complications. For instance, the initial efforts were made to minimize or avoid long-term steroid use due to associated side effects. In addition, induction agents provide initial intense IS and prevent early acute rejection, allowing the late introduction of TAC at lower doses, thereby minimizing side effects, particularly those related to kidney function.

Caution should be exercised with most recommendations given the low quality of evidence for most outcomes, high risk of bias, and significant heterogeneity of study protocols of the included RCTs, and insufficient information size [44].

29.5 Immunosuppression Monitoring, Rejection Risk, and Adherence

Acute cellular rejection (ACR) was one of the main causes of liver dysfunction after LT, occurring in 30–70% of transplanted patients and potentially leading to allograft failure. The clinical consequences of ACR are different depending on the transplanted organ, and have been shown to be less important in LT. Still, they are related to the degree of rejection, and particularly the time since LT, with late episodes of rejection being associated with higher graft loss than those episodes of ACR occurring within the first 3 months post-LT [10–16, 45].

Accurate diagnosis of ACR is critical to avoid over or under IS, and particularly to differentiate the different potential causes of liver dysfunction. Clinical assessment and histopathological diagnosis of liver samples have been the standard for accurate diagnosis of ACR. Due to the invasive nature of liver biopsy, laboratory tests are commonly used as less invasive methods of monitoring allograft rejection. Still, they are not specific to rejection and are often abnormal in other types of liver dysfunction, such as ischemic/reperfusion injury, cholangitis, and drug toxicity. Despite some advancements in the fields of genomics and proteomics, a specific diagnostic marker that can easily monitor immune status without invasive procedures is still needed [46].

Monitoring IS is crucial for optimizing outcomes and reducing IPV [18, 19, 22]. Regular TDM allows for dose adjustments to maintain drug levels within the therapeutic range, as both sub-therapeutic and supratherapeutic levels can impact transplant outcomes. Target levels of immunosuppressive agents will depend on many factors, including indication, time after transplant, other immunosuppressive agents, and history of rejection or graft function, among others. Typical maintenance target levels for TAC are 5–8 ng/mL, for CsA 75–120 ng/mL, EVR 4–8 ng/mL (all trough whole blood levels). However, even though whole blood levels are a useful guide, sub-therapeutic levels may be consistent with adequate IS, particularly in the long term.

Ensuring patient compliance with prescribed immunosuppressive medications (type, dose, and time) is crucial to prevent rejection and maintain stable graft function, as well as to avoid significant side effects and prolong survival [45]. Unfortunately, nonadherence to immunosuppressive regimens among solid organ transplant recipients ranges from 15% to 55% [47]. Indeed, nonadherence to the immunosuppressive regimen has been cited as a main cause for preventable late acute rejection and allograft loss, suggesting that interventions to improve adherence may improve patient outcomes [48]. There are many risk factors associated with non-compliance, which are particularly evident in pediatric and young adult populations. Other risk factors include concern over side effects, complexity of the drug regimen, affordability, and social factors such as low family cohesion, poor social functioning, poor mental health, and a single-parent family. Detection of non-adherence is difficult, and the risks do not diminish with time. The key issue is to detect non-compliance; this may be suggested by poor attendance at clinics, unexpectedly low trough levels of immunosuppressive agents, and late acute rejection. Looking for a discrepancy between the amount of the drug prescribed and the need is often a useful way to confirm suspicions. Several strategies may be attempted to enhance adherence. Identifying the factors that led to nonadherence and correcting them where possible is the first step. Medication reminder systems, patient counseling, and involvement of support systems are being implemented in many centers [45]. In chronic conditions such as LT, less frequent dosing results in a higher percentage of prescribed doses being taken [49]. A once-daily prolonged-release formulation of TAC has been developed, and according to several studies, conversion from twice-daily to once-daily TAC is well tolerated and is safely and conveniently used in stable patients after LT [50–52]. Besides its potential benefit related to enhanced adherence to therapy, the slower access of once-daily TAC to *CYP3A4* enzyme metabolism may prevent these enzymes from being overwhelmed by a high drug concentration and decreased daily peaks. Avoidance of high peak levels may lead to a lower incidence of CVD, hyperglycemia, and adverse events from CNI therapy. An eight-year long-term follow-up study based on the ELTR was recently published, and the findings were in favor of prolonged-release TAC in terms of graft losses and acute rejections [53].

29.6 Individualized Immunosuppression

Individualized baseline IS regime, both qualitatlively and quantitatively as well as adjustments in IS medications may be warranted in several specific conditions or based on the presence of certain risk factors such as (i) Recipient-specific factors such as advanced age, obesity, diabetes, renal dysfunction, or prior history of malignancy; (ii) High risk or complex cases such as those with high Model for End-Stage Liver Disease (MELD) scores, acute-on-chronic liver failure (ACLF), or HCC; (iii) Allograft-specific factors such as the use of extended criteria donor grafts or donation after circulatory death grafts; (iv) Drug interactions or adverse effects; (iv) Rejection or immunological complications. In these cases, the IS regimen should be tailored to minimize the risks associated with these factors while maintaining adequate IS.

Overall, patients can be categorized into (i) standard, including those at low risk of immune-related complications, such as those with low MELD scores (<25), no history of immune-mediated liver disease or renal dysfunction, and those without an expanded oncologic indication, and (ii) those at high risk, either immunological or oncological.

In the **standard category**, TAC ± MMF ± Steroids is the typical regimen in most transplant centers [1, 2]. However, renal-sparing protocols (induction combined with low-dose and late introduction of TAC, together with either MMF or EVR) are also alternative strategies recommended by some societies [54, 55].

Renal-sparing immunosuppressive strategies include the following options:

- Triple or quadruple regime with use of induction agents in association with antimetabolites and delayed introduction of CNI (within 5–10 days after surgery) ± steroids [56–58];
- EVR-facilitated CNI reduction starting 30 (±5) days after transplantation [36, 37, 59–62] or early (≤10 days) use of EVR to reduce CNI exposure [36, 37].

Most relevant studies based on early EVR use associate reduced TAC and demonstrate significantly improved renal function. The H2304 study investigated de novo use of EVR in 719 LT recipients randomized at 30 ± 5 days post-transplant to reduced TAC + EVR vs standard TAC (±MMF). The adjusted change in eGFR at 12 and 24 months was superior in the reduced TAC + EVR compared with the standard TAC using the Modification of Diet in Renal Disease (four-variable) (MDRD4) formula (difference of 8.5 mL/min/1.73 m^2, $p = 0.002$ and 6.7 mL/min/1.73 m^2; $p < 0.001$ at 12 months and 24 months, respectively) [59, 60]. An extension for up to 3 years post-transplantation in 282 recipients confirmed results with a mean eGFR decreasing from randomization to month 36 by 7.0 ± 31.3 mL/min/1.73 m^2 versus 15.5 ± 22.7 mL/min/1.73 m^2 in the TAC-control group ($p = 0.005$) [61]. Similar results have been achieved in other studies [62–64], and a recent meta-analysis including RCTs of de novo LT in adults receiving EVR with low-dose TAC or TAC discontinuation confirmed that these regimens are associated with renal improvement at 12 months with similar efficacy in terms of mortality and graft rejection [40].

In turn, antibody induction, coupled with MMF and the reduced-dose delayed introduction of TAC, has also been investigated with success in terms of renal dysfunction [56–58]. In the Respect multicenter, prospective, randomized, open-label trial, adult patients with preserved renal function undergoing primary LT were randomized to either: group A (standard-dose TAC [target trough levels >10 ng/mL] and corticosteroids; $n = 183$); group B (MMF 2 g/day, reduced-dose TAC [target trough levels ≤8 ng/mL], and corticosteroids; $n = 170$); group C (daclizumab induction, MMF, reduced-dose TAC delayed until the fifth day post-transplant and corticosteroids, $n = 172$). The eGFR decreased by 23.61, 21.22 and 13.63 mL/min in groups A, B and C, respectively (A vs C, $p = 0.012$; A vs B, $p = 0.199$) and renal dialysis was required less frequently in group C versus group A (4.2% vs. 9.9%; $p = 0.037$), with similar rates of acute rejection as well as similar survival [56].

In summary, two combinations (induction, MMF, steroids with delayed reduced-dose TAC and reduced-dose TAC in combination with early EVR) are associated with less nephrotoxicity than therapy with standard-dose TAC without compromising efficacy or tolerability [13, 15].

Non-standard categories include:

- *Renal Impairment*

CKD develops in the majority of LT patients who survive the first six postoperative months (30–90%) at higher rates than in cardiac and lung transplants [65], requiring renal replacement therapy in 2–5% and with an adverse effect on transplant survival [66]. An extensive prospective study that evaluated the prevalence of CKD through measurement of GFR by iothalamate clearance and the associated mortality in 1211 patients over 25 years reported that after 4 months of LT, 40% of the patients already had CKD stage ≥3, and the risk of death increased when the GFR decreased to values below 30 mL/min/1.73 m^2 or worse. Only 18% of the subjects had normal renal function after 25 years, in contrast to 39% of age-group-matched individuals from the general population [67]. Risk factors predictive of CKD include acute kidney dysfunction early post-transplantation, IS-related nephrotoxicity, as well as pre- and/or post-transplant existing conditions associated with intrinsic renal injury (HCV, MASLD, DM, AHT…). Importantly, an increasing number of patients in need of LT have concomitant renal dysfunction at the time of or soon after LT. The reasons behind this increase are related to changing indications, with a recent increase in MASLD [1–3, 8, 68, 69], and increased severity at transplantation, as a greater number of patients are transplanted in the context of acute kidney injury-hepatorenal syndrome [70].

CNI-induced nephrotoxicity, presumably mediated by renal arteriolar vasoconstriction resulting in reduced glomerular filtration, may be reversible with reduced CNI dose [10–16, 40, 54–64]. While renal function is better preserved with the use of protective renal-sparing immunosuppressive combination, evidence from RCT and retrospective analyses shows that the improvement in renal function is limited if CNI-reducing strategies are postponed until renal function has deteriorated (eGFR <60 mL/min/1.73 m^2) [10–16, 71–73]. In a combined analysis of 2 randomized LT trials evaluating the efficacy and safety of EVR with reduced TAC (EVR + rTAC) versus standard TAC (sTAC) regimen at month 24 ($n = 772$; H2304 [deceased donor, $n = 488$], H2307 [living donor, $n = 284$]), an analysis by CKD stage at randomization showed comparable renal outcomes with EVR + rTAC treatment for patients with CKD stage 4/5, stage 3B, and stage 3A. At the same time, significant benefit was seen in patients with CKD stage 1 and 2 [74]. These findings reiterate the benefit of introducing renal-sparing protocols before irreversible kidney damage has developed.

- *Metabolic syndrome*

Metabolic complications are very frequent in the transplant population due to the toxic profile of several immunosuppressive agents and the increasing prevalence of

MASLD as an LT indication [1–3, 69]. When considering IS in patients with DM, it is important to select medications that have a favorable impact on glycemic control and minimize the risk of worsening diabetes-related complications. TAC is generally preferred over CsA [75], and minimization or avoidance of long-term steroid use is advised [43, 44, 76, 77].

Converting patients from CNI to mTORi or MMF may have a beneficial effect in metabolic syndrome or any of its components [36, 37]. In one study, early conversion to EVR was associated with less weight gain than with TAC 2 years after LT [78].

- *Prior History of Cancer*

Post-transplant malignancy, either de novo or recurrent, is the leading cause of mortality after LT and accounts for 41% of premature deaths in LT recipients [3, 5–7]. Indeed, the risk of cancer is two- to three-fold higher in LT patients compared to the age- and gender-matched general population [79, 80]. After LT, de novo tumors may also be biologically more aggressive, and they are associated with a shorter survival than that observed in the general population [81]. Patients with a prior history of cancer undergoing LT pose a unique challenge, as they require IS to prevent organ rejection while balancing the risk of cancer recurrence [82, 83].

Apart from minimizing overall IS, very few "tailored"immunosuppressive protocols or drug combinations have been evaluated in prospective RCTs aiming to assess the risk of de novo cancer, and none have analyzed specifically the risk of post-transplant recurrence of pre-transplant malignancies [84]. CNIs have intrinsic oncogenic properties. In a large recent multicenter study, a dose-dependent pro-oncogenic effect of TAC in real clinical practice, irrespective of demographic features and concomitant immunosuppressive drugs, was demonstrated [85]. Therefore, CNI minimization, with MMF or mTORi, should be considered in all patients with pre-transplant malignancy in remission [84]. In addition, based on the International Liver Transplant Society (ILTS) recommendations, AZA should be avoided in recipients with pre-transplant non-melanoma skin malignancies. If induction agents are required, monoclonal anti-interleukin-2 receptor antibodies are preferred, as there is no clear association with malignancy or post-transplant lymphoproliferative disorder (PTLD). In contrast, T-cell–depleting agents have been linked to PTLD and other post-transplant malignancies and should be avoided [84]. It is important to highlight that while MMF has been associated with a lower risk of malignancy (with the possible exception of central nervous system cancers), whether this is an intrinsic effect of MMF or simply an indirect benefit of allowing CNI dose reduction has to be elucidated. In addition, while mTORi have immunosuppressive and antitumoral properties, the latter occur at doses markedly higher than those required in transplantation, which likely explains the modest antineoplastic effect in the transplant scenario, which has been demonstrated only in non-melanoma skin cancer in renal transplant recipients.

- *Immune-Mediated Liver Disease*

The current five- and ten-year survival rates post-transplant in autoimmune disease (encompassing AIH, PBC, and PSC) are excellent, at 88% and 78%, respectively

[86, 87]. A key factor in maintaining good outcomes post-LT for these autoimmune conditions is the IS strategy. These patients have increased rates of rejection, and autoimmune conditions can all recur in the graft, ranging from 12% to 60% depending on the population studied, and increasing with time following LT, from 17% to 68% in AIH, 12% to 30% in PBC, and 12% to 60% in PSC. Immunosuppressive regimens are centered on CNI, often combined with low-dose steroids, with or without the addition of antimetabolite therapy. Whether dual vs triple immunosuppressive therapy, CsA versus TAC, or maintenance vs no maintenance steroids lead to better outcomes is still controversial [10, 16, 88–91]. Recommendations based on low evidence data suggest that (i) maintenance steroid use may be helpful to prevent recurrent AIH, (ii) CsA, as opposed to TAC, is associated with lower rates of recurrent PBC but not with higher survival; (iii) Data regarding the impact of the type of IS used on PSC recurrence rate is inconclusive.

- *Hepatocellular Carcinoma*

HCC is an increasing indication for LT in most centers [1–3]. Although LT is the best treatment for patients with localized HCC, recurrence occurs in 6–18% of patients. Several factors, particularly morphological criteria combined with dynamic parameters known prior to LT, modify this risk and, when combined in prediction models, may be used to stratify patients in need of variable surveillance strategies [3, 92]. Additional variables, though, likely explain differences in recurrence rates in patients with the same pre-LT HCC status. One of these variables is possibly IS. The immunosuppressive strategy in patients undergoing LT for HCC can vary depending on individual patient factors, tumor characteristics, and center protocols. The primary goal is to balance the prevention of rejection with minimizing the risk of HCC recurrence. CNI has been shown to be an independent risk factor for the recurrence of HCC by promoting cancer cell proliferation and survival [6, 92]. At the same time, mTORi have been found to have anti-proliferative and anti-angiogenic effects [36, 37].

Overall, and while evidence is low, the results of the different studies and systematic reviews with subsequent meta-analyses suggest that immunosuppressive regimes aimed at reducing TAC levels with mTORi have potential benefits in terms of reducing HCC recurrence rates and improving recurrence-free and overall survival at 1, 3, and 5 years post-transplant [3, 92–99]. The main problems with the data relate to the low quality of the studies, the inherent limitations of observational studies, and the lack of blinding and allocation concealment in the RCTs.

- *Liver Re-transplantation*

Patients undergoing liver re-transplantation may have unique considerations when it comes to IS [10–16, 45]. Several factors may influence the choice and management of immunosuppressive agents in these patients, including sensitization, which can increase the risk of antibody-mediated rejection in subsequent transplants. Specialized protocols, such as desensitization protocols or plasmapheresis, may be considered to reduce antibody levels and minimize the risk of rejection. In addition, patients with prior LT may have received different immunosuppressive regimens and may have experienced complications or side effects associated with those agents. A careful review of the previous immunosuppressive history is essential to guide the selection and adjustment of immunosuppressive agents in re-LT.

- *Older Population*

Due to demographic changes, the number of patients over 65 years of age with indications for LT is rising considerably [1–3]. Older individuals undergoing LT may have age-related changes in immune function and higher susceptibility to infections and malignancies. In turn, these recipients may be more prone to IS-related toxicities, such as CNI-associated nephrotoxicity or steroid-related bone loss. Finally, polypharmacy and the mutual influence of IS and comorbidities need to be considered in the decision-making process [10–16, 45].

- *Acute-on-Chronic Liver Failure (ACLF) or High Model for End-Stage Liver Disease (MELD)*

Transplantation for patients with ACLF≥3 has encouraging results with 1-year survival of 80–90% [100]. These patients with multiple organ failure meet the conditions for serious alterations of drug metabolism and increased toxicity. Similar concerns are present for cirrhotic patients with very high MELD scores, particularly renal dysfunction. Thus, when selecting the most appropriate IS in these cases, consideration should be made to kidney function, neurologic condition, and infectious status. Renal and neurologic sparing protocols may be favored in this setting, but data are lacking [10–16, 101].

- *Sex*

There is limited evidence suggesting that women should receive a different IS protocol compared to men in LT. The available studies primarily focus on evaluating sex-related differences in outcomes rather than specific IS protocols [102, 103]. Overall, the existing literature does not support the notion that women should receive a different regime compared to men. The decision-making process for IS should be based on factors such as patient-specific characteristics, comorbidities, and transplant-related considerations rather than sex alone. Of note, immune-mediated liver diseases and acute liver failure are more often indications for LT in women compared to men, likely impacting the IS strategy [100].

- *Living Donor Liver Transplantation (LDLT)*

Due to organ shortage, LDLT is gradually increasing [1–3], and overall data suggest that there is no specific IS protocol unique to LDLT compared to deceased donor LT. Yet for some patients, ABO-incompatible (ABO-I) LDLT is the only chance for survival. After ABO-I LT, the primary concern is hyperacute and acute antibody-mediated rejection (AMR), especially with an isohemagglutinin titer >1:64. After transplant, blood group incompatibility can result in the activation of complement, resulting in complement-mediated allograft damage. Several desensitization protocols have been described, including pre- and post-transplant plasmapheresis, rituximab, post-transplant induction with ATG, post-transplant intravenous immunoglobulins (IVIG), and specific new agents such as proteasome inhibitor Bortezomib, complement inhibitor Eculizumab, IL-6 receptor antagonist Tocilizumab, T-cell costimulating agent Belatacep, or newer anti-CD20 drug Obinutuzumab [104]. Rituximab, a monoclonal chimeric human-murine anti-CD20 antibody that depletes B cells by complement-dependent cellular cytotoxicity, seems to be the turning point in preventing AMR in ABO-I LT, with significant improvements in outcome since its introduction. In a Japanese nationwide survey, the 3-year survival rates increased from 30% to 80% after the introduction of rituximab [105]. Importantly, since the rituximab era, many centers have attempted to simplify the protocol and avoid splenectomy, local graft infusion, IVIG, and plasmapheresis. Furthermore, repeated administration of rituximab may be unnecessary and may increase the risk of serious infections due to long-term hypoglycemia. Consequently, most centers currently administer a single dose of rituximab (300 or 375 mg/m^2) 2 weeks before surgery.

In conclusion, individualized IS should be based on a thorough evaluation of each patient's unique clinical characteristics, including medical history, comorbidities, risk factors, and specific transplant-related considerations. The decision-making process should involve a multidisciplinary transplant team, including hepatologists, transplant surgeons, pharmacists, and other specialists, to tailor the IS strategy to the individual patient's needs and optimize transplant outcomes.

29.7 Immunotolerance

The liver exhibits intrinsic immune-tolerogenic properties that contribute to a unique propensity toward spontaneous acceptance when transplanted, both in animal models and in humans. Thus, in contrast to what happens after transplantation of other solid organs, several years following LT, a significant subset of patients are capable of maintaining normal allograft function with histological integrity in the absence of immunosuppressive drug treatment. Indeed, under specific conditions, 40% of long-term LT recipients can achieve operational tolerance, with stable graft function and no evidence of rejection after discontinuing IS. Recipient age and the time elapsed since transplantation (preferably >10 years) are the strongest factors associated with successful IS discontinuation. Other factors are: no history of autoimmune liver disease, no recent episodes of rejection, and normal liver histology. Further research is needed to identify reliable predictors of immunotolerance at earlier time points, where discontinuation of immune drugs can actually lead to reduced IS-related toxicities. Refining patient selection criteria and developing strategies to induce and maintain immune-tolerance in a broader population of LT recipients is still an unmet need [10–13].

29.8 Conclusion

LT has cemented its role as the standard of care for end-stage liver failure and HCC. The evolution of IS regimens has bolstered graft and patient survival, but it has also introduced side effects that impact both quality of life and long-term outcomes. Indeed, the heightened potency of immunosuppressive agents has significantly curtailed rates of steroid-resistant rejection and graft loss stemming from rejection, and in fact, a substantial portion of post-LT late mortality is unrelated to graft function, underscoring the pivotal role of potent IS in fostering favorable outcomes both in the early and late phases post-LT. Nonetheless, the benefits derived from more robust immunosuppressive drugs have led to prolonged patient exposure to these agents, culminating in unwanted adverse effects. Balancing the imperative of an ideal immunosuppressive regimen to counteract rejection with the necessity of minimizing adverse events requires a nuanced understanding of medical science and a wealth of clinical experience. Unfortunately, while tailoring IS to the individual is the ultimate goal, the lack of solid data from RCTs and the absence of biomarkers that truly reflect the recipient's immune status hinder real advancements in IS management, and most IS modifications are made downwards in response to drug toxicity or lack of efficacy. Currently, TAC coupled with MMF ± steroids is the standard IS in LT. Non-standard IS alternatives are primarily used as renal-sparing strategies, based on induction therapy with delayed, reduced-dose TAC combined with antimetabolites and/or mTOR inhibitors, or with an oncologic goal, involving the use of reduced CNI and the addition of mTOR inhibitors. TDM is necessary for CNI and mTORis. For many immunosuppressive drugs, there are multiple formulations available. These are only sometimes interchangeable, so a pharmacist's advice should be taken before switching patients from one brand to another. If used, most units aim to discontinue steroids in the first year. However, long-term steroids are usually indicated in those transplanted for autoimmune liver diseases and those with a history of recurrent rejection. As with many chronic conditions, nonadherence is relatively frequent but difficult to detect. Simplifying IS regimes, such as with a single daily dose of TAC, may help deal with this problem. Over time, select patients achieve a state of "tolerance," characterized by successful IS cessation, sustained graft function, and no signs of rejection.

References

1. Kwong AJ, Ebel NH, Kim WR, Lake JR, Smith JM, Schladt DP, Schnellinger EM, Handarova D, Weiss S, Cafarella M, Snyder JJ, Israni AK, Kasiske BL. OPTN/SRTR 2021 annual data report: liver. Am J Transplant. 2023;23(2 Suppl 1):S178–263.
2. Adam R, Karam V, Cailliez V, O Grady JG, Mirza D, Cherqui D, Klempnauer J, Salizzoni M, Pratschke J, Jamieson N, Hidalgo E, Paul A, Andujar RL, Lerut J, Fisher L, Boudjema K, Fondevila C, Soubrane O, Bachellier P, Pinna AD, Berlakovich G, Bennet W, Pinzani M, Schemmer P, Zieniewicz K, Romero CJ, De Simone P, Ericzon BG, Schneeberger S, Wigmore

SJ, Prous JF, Colledan M, Porte RJ, Yilmaz S, Azoulay D, Pirenne J, Line PD, Trunecka P, Navarro F, Lopez AV, De Carlis L, Pena SR, Kochs E, Duvoux C, all the other 126 contributing centers (www.eltr.org) and the European Liver and Intestine Transplant Association (ELITA). 2018 Annual Report of the European Liver Transplant Registry (ELTR)—50-year evolution of liver transplantation. Transpl Int. 2018;31(12):1293–317.
3. Terrault NA, Francoz C, Berenguer M, Charlton M, Heimbach J. Liver transplantation 2023: status report, current and future challenges. Clin Gastroenterol Hepatol. 2023;21(8):2150–66.
4. Adam R, Karam V, Delvart V, O'Grady J, Mirza D, Klempnauer J, Castaing D, Neuhaus P, Jamieson N, Salizzoni M, Pollard S, Lerut J, Paul A, Garcia-Valdecasas JC, Rodríguez FS, Burroughs A, All contributing centers (www.eltr.org); European Liver and Intestine Transplant Association (ELITA). Evolution of indications and results of liver transplantation in Europe. A report from the European Liver Transplant Registry (ELTR). J Hepatol. 2012 Sep;57(3):675–88.
5. Rubín A, Sánchez-Montes C, Aguilera V, Juan FS, Ferrer I, Moya A, Montalva E, Pareja E, López-Andujar R, Prieto M, Berenguer M. Long-term outcome of 'long-term liver transplant survivors'. Transpl Int. 2013;26(7):740–50.
6. Watt KD, Pedersen RA, Kremers WK, Heimbach JK, Charlton MR. Evolution of causes and risk factors for mortality post-liver transplant: results of the NIDDK long-term follow-up study. Am J Transplant. 2010;10(6):1420–7.
7. Åberg F, Gissler M, Karlsen TH, Ericzon BG, Foss A, Rasmussen A, Bennet W, Olausson M, Line PD, Nordin A, Bergquist A, Boberg KM, Castedal M, Pedersen CR, Isoniemi H. Differences in long-term survival among liver transplant recipients and the general population: a population-based Nordic study. Hepatology. 2015;61(2):668–77.
8. Terrault NA, Pageaux GP. A changing landscape of liver transplantation: king HCV is dethroned, ALD and NAFLD take over! J Hepatol. 2018;69(4):767–8.
9. European Association for the Study of the Liver. EASL Clinical Practice Guidelines on acute-on-chronic liver failure. J Hepatol. 2023;79(2):461–91.
10. Montano-Loza AJ, Rodríguez-Perálvarez ML, Pageaux GP, Sanchez-Fueyo A, Feng S. Liver transplantation immunology: immunosuppression, rejection, and immunomodulation. J Hepatol. 2023;78(6):1199–215.
11. Adams DH, Sanchez-Fueyo A, Samuel D. From immunosuppression to tolerance. J Hepatol. 2015;62(1 Suppl):S170–85.
12. Zorzetti N, Lauro A, Khouzam S, Marino IR. Immunosuppression, compliance, and tolerance after orthotopic liver transplantation: state of the art. Exp Clin Transplant. 2022;20(Suppl 1):3–9.
13. Di Maira T, Little EC, Berenguer M. Immunosuppression in liver transplant. Best Pract Res Clin Gastroenterol. 2020;46-47:101681.
14. Panackel C, Mathew JF, Fawas NM, Jacob M. Immunosuppressive drugs in liver transplant: an insight. J Clin Exp Hepatol. 2022;12(6):1557–71.
15. De Martin E, Londoño MC, Emamaullee J, Lerut J, Potts J, Aluvihare V, Spiro M, Raptis DA, McCaughan G, ERAS4OLT.org Working Group. The optimal immunosuppression management to prevent early rejection after liver transplantation: a systematic review of the literature and expert panel recommendations. Clin Transpl. 2022;36(10):e14614.
16. Lerut JP, Gondolesi GE. Immunosuppression in liver and intestinal transplantation. Best Pract Res Clin Gastroenterol. 2021;54–55:101767.
17. Noble J, Terrec F, Malvezzi P, Rostaing L. Adverse effects of immunosuppression after liver transplantation. Best Pract Res Clin Gastroenterol. 2021;54–55:101762.
18. Udomkarnjananun S, Francke MI, De Winter BCM, Mulder MB, Baan CC, Metselaar HJ, den Hoed CM, Hesselink DA. Therapeutic drug monitoring of immunosuppressivedrugs in hepatology and gastroenterology. Best Pract Res Clin Gastroenterol. 2021;54–55:101756.
19. Kourkoumpetis T, Levitsky J. Immunosuppressive drug levels in liver transplant recipients: impact in decision making. Semin Liver Dis. 2019;39(4):414–21.

20. Schutte-Nutgen K, Tholking G, Suwelack B, Reuter S. Tacrolimus -pharmacokinetic considerations for clinicians. Curr Drug Metab. 2018;19(4):342–50.
21. Kirubakaran R, Stocker SL, Hennig S, Day RO, Carland JE. Population pharmacokinetic models of tacrolimus in adult transplant recipients: a systematic review. Clin Pharmacokinet. 2020;59(11):1357–92.
22. Brunet M, van Gelder T, Åsberg A, Haufroid V, Hesselink DA, Langman L, Lemaitre F, Marquet P, Seger C, Shipkova M, Vinks A, Wallemacq P, Wieland E, Woillard JB, Barten MJ, Budde K, Colom H, Dieterlen MT, Elens L, Johnson-Davis KL, Kunicki PK, MacPhee I, Masuda S, Mathew BS, Millán O, Mizuno T, Moes DAR, Monchaud C, Noceti O, Pawinski T, Picard N, van Schaik R, Sommerer C, Vethe NT, de Winter B, Christians U, Bergan S. Therapeutic drug monitoring of tacrolimus-personalized therapy: second consensus report. Ther Drug Monit. 2019;41(3):261–307.
23. Muduma G, Saunders R, Odeyemi I, Pollock RF. Systematic review and meta-analysis of tacrolimus versus Ciclosporin as primary immunosuppression after liver transplant. PLoS One. 2016;11(11):e0160421.
24. Lieber SR, Volk ML. Nonadherence and graft failure in adult liver transplant recipients. Am J Dig Dis. 2012;58:824–34.
25. Christina S, Annunziato RA, Schiano TD, Anand R, Vaidya S, Chuang K, Zack Y, Florman S, Shneider BL, Shemesh E. Medication level variability index predicts rejection, possibly due to nonadherence, in adult liver transplant recipients. Liver Transplant. 2014;20:1168–77.
26. Rayar M, Tron C, Jézéquel C, Beaurepaire JM, Petitcollin A, Houssel-Debry P, Camus C, Verdier MC, Dehlawi A, Lakéhal M, et al. High Intrapatient variability of tacrolimus exposure in the early period after liver transplantation is associated with poorer outcomes. Transplantation. 2018;102:e108–14.
27. Del Bello A, Congy-Jolivet N, Danjoux M, Muscari F, Lavayssière L, Esposito L, Hebral A-L, Bellière J, Kamar N. High tacrolimus intra-patient variability is associated with graft rejection, and de novo donor-specific antibodies occurrence after liver transplantation. World J Gastroenterol. 2018;24:1795–802.
28. Maurel P, Prémaud A, Carrier P, Essig M, Barbier L, Rousseau A, Silvain C, Causse X, Debette-Gratien M, Jacques J, Marquet P, Salamé E, Loustaud-Ratti V. Evaluation of longitudinal exposure to tacrolimus as a risk factor of chronic kidney disease occurrence within the first-year post-liver transplantation. Transplantation. 2021;105(7):1585–94.
29. Durand F, Francoz C, Asrani SK, Khemichian S, Pham TA, Sung RS, Genyk YS, Nadim MK. Acute kidney injury after liver transplantation. Transplantation. 2018;102(10):1636–49.
30. Wiesner R, Rabkin J, Klintmalm G, McDiarmid S, Langnas A, Punch J, McMaster P, Kalayoglu M, Levy G, Freeman R, Bismuth H, Neuhaus P, Mamelok R, Wang W. A randomized double-blind comparative study of mycophenolate mofetil and azathioprine in combination with cyclosporine and corticosteroids in primary liver transplant recipients. Liver Transpl. 2001;7(5):442–50.
31. Wiesner RH, Shorr JS, Steffen BJ, et al. Mycophenolate mofetil combination therapy improves long-term outcomes after liver transplantation in patients with and without hepatitis C. Liver Transpl. 2005;11:750–9.
32. Boudjema K, Camus C, Saliba F, et al. Reduced-dose tacrolimus with mycophenolate mofetil *vs.* standard-dose tacrolimus in liver transplantation: a randomized study. Am J Transplant. 2011;11:965–76.
33. Kaltenborn A, Schrem H. Mycophenolate mofetil in liver transplantation: a review. Ann Transplant. 2013;18:685–96.
34. Gardiner KM, Tett SE, Staatz CE. Is conversion from mycophenolate mofetil to enteric-coated mycophenolate sodium justifiable for gastrointestinal quality of life? Drugs R D. 2018 Dec;18(4):271–82.
35. Fairfield C, Penninga L, Powell J, Harrison EM, Wigmore SJ. Glucocorticosteroid-free versus glucocorticosteroid-containing immunosuppression for liver transplanted patients. Cochrane Database Syst Rev. 2018;4(4):CD007606.

36. Rubín Suárez A, Bilbao Aguirre I, Fernández-Castroagudin J, Pons Miñano JA, Salcedo Plaza M, Varo Pérez E, Prieto Castillo M. Recommendations of everolimus use in liver transplant. Gastroenterol Hepatol. 2017;40(9):629–40.
37. De Simone P, Fagiuoli S, Cescon M, De Carlis L, Tisone G, Volpes R, Cillo U, Consensus Panel. Use of everolimus in liver transplantation: recommendations from a working group. Transplantation. 2017;101(2):239–51.
38. Todeschini L, Cristin L, Martinino A, Mattia A, Agnes S, Giovinazzo F. The role of mTOR inhibitors after liver transplantation for hepatocellular carcinoma. Curr Oncol. 2023;30(6):5574–92.
39. Guan TW, Lin YJ, Ou MY, Chen KB. Efficacy and safety of everolimus treatment on liver transplant recipients: a meta-analysis. Eur J Clin Investig. 2019;49(12):e13179.
40. Lin M, Mittal S, Sahebjam F, Rana A, Sood GK. Everolimus with early withdrawal or reduced-dose calcineurin inhibitors improves renal function in liver transplant recipients: a systematic review and meta-analysis. Clin Transpl. 2017;31(2) https://doi.org/10.1111/ctr.12872.
41. Crins ND, Röver C, Goralczyk AD, Friede T. Interleukin-2 receptor antagonists for pediatric liver transplant recipients: a systematic review and meta-analysis of controlled studies. Pediatr Transplant. 2014;18:839–50.
42. Penninga L, et al. Antibody induction versus placebo, no induction, or another type of antibody induction for liver transplant recipients. Cochrane Database Syst Rev. 2014;2014:010253. 11. Goralczyk AD et al. Interleukin 2 receptor antagonists for liver transplant recipients: a systematic review and meta-analysis of controlled studies. Hepatology. 2011;54:541–54.
43. Jung WS, Kuh JH, Lim L, Yoo HK, Ju JW, Lee HJ, Kim WH. T-cell specific antibody induction versus corticosteroid induction immunosuppression for liver transplant recipients: a meta-analysis. Sci Rep. 2023;13(1):6951.
44. Best LM, Leung J, Freeman SC, Sutton AJ, Cooper NJ, Milne EJ, Cowlin M, Payne A, Walshaw D, Thorburn D, Pavlov CS, Davidson BR, Tsochatzis E, Williams NR, Gurusamy KS. Induction immunosuppression in adults undergoing liver transplantation: a network meta-analysis. Cochrane Database Syst Rev. 2020;(1):1, CD013203.
45. Neuberger JM, Bechstein WO, Kuypers DR, Burra P, Citterio F, De Geest S, Duvoux C, Jardine AG, Kamar N, Krämer BK, Metselaar HJ, Nevens F, Pirenne J, Rodríguez-Perálvarez ML, Samuel D, Schneeberger S, Serón D, Truněcka P, Tisone G, van Gelder T. Practical recommendations for long-term management of modifiable risks in kidney and liver transplant recipients: a guidance report and clinical checklist by the Consensus on Managing Modifiable Risk in Transplantation (COMMIT) Group. Transplantation. 2017;101(4S Suppl 2):S1–S56.
46. Mas VR, Bardhi E, Berenguer M. Circulating MicroRNAs: dynamic markers of liver transplant injury. Transplantation. 2022;106(4):705–6.
47. Kaplan A, Korenjak M, Brown RS Jr. Post-liver transplantation patient experience. J Hepatol. 2023;78(6):1234–44.
48. Mellon L, Doyle F, Hickey A, Ward KD, de Freitas DG, McCormick PA, O'Connell O, Conlon P. Interventions for increasing immunosuppressant medication adherence in solid organ transplant recipients. Cochrane Database Syst Rev. 2022;9(9):CD012854.
49. Bendersky VA, Saha A, Sidoti CN, Ferzola A, Downey M, Ruck JM, Vanterpool KB, Young L, Shegelman A, Segev DL, Levan ML. Factors impacting the medication "adherence landscape" for transplant patients. Clin Transpl. 2023;37(6):e14962.
50. Coilly A, Calmus Y, Chermak F, Dumortier J, Duvoux C, Guillaud O, Houssel-Debry P, Neau-Cransac M, Stocco J. Once-daily prolonged release tacrolimus inliver transplantation: experts' literature review and recommendations. Liver Transpl. 2015;21(10):1312–21.
51. Bzeizi KI, Albenmousa A, Shawkat AM, Ahmed Z, Alabbad S, Al-hamoudi W, Troisi R, Broering D. Efficacy and safety of once daily tacrolimus compared to twice daily tacrolimus after liver transplantation. World J Hepatol. 2021;13(3):375–83.
52. Muduma G, Odeyemi I, Pollock RF. Evaluating the cost-effectiveness ofprolonged-release tacrolimus relative to immediate-release tacrolimus inliver transplant patients based on data from routine clinical practice. Drugs Real World Outcomes. 2016;3:61–8.

53. Adam R, Karam V, Cailliez V, Trunečka P, Samuel D, Tisone G, et al. Improved survival in liver transplant patients receiving prolonged-release tacrolimus-based immunosuppression in the European Liver Transplant Registry (ELTR): an extension study. Transplantation. 2019;103:1844–62.
54. Cillo U, De Carlis L, Del Gaudio M, De Simone P, Fagiuoli S, Lupo F, Tisone G, Volpes R. Immunosuppressive regimens for adult liver transplant recipients in real-life practice: consensus recommendations from an Italian Working Group. Hepatol Int. 2020;14(6):930–43.
55. Charlton M, Levitsky J, Aqel B, O'Grady J, Hemibach J, Rinella M, Fung J, Ghabril M, Thomason R, Burra P, Little EC, Berenguer M, Shaked A, Trotter J, Roberts J, Rodriguez-Davalos M, Rela M, Pomfret E, Heyrend C, Gallegos-Orozco J, Saliba F. International liver transplantation society consensus statement on immunosuppression in liver transplant recipients. Transplantation. 2018;102(5):727–43.
56. Neuberger JM, Mamelok RD, Neuhaus P, Pirenne J, Samuel D, Isoniemi H, Rostaing L, Rimola A, Marshall S, Mayer AD, ReSpECT Study Group. Delayed introduction of reduced-dose tacrolimus, and renal function in liver transplantation: the 'ReSpECT' study. Am J Transplant. 2009;9(2):327–36.
57. Boillot O, Seket B, Dumortier J, Pittau G, Boucaud C, Bouffard Y, Scoazec JY. Thymoglobulin induction in liver transplant recipients with a tacrolimus, mycophenolate mofetil, and steroid immunosuppressive regimen: a five-year randomized prospective study. Liver Transpl. 2009;15(11):1426–34.
58. Otero A, Varo E, de Urbina JO, Martín-Vivaldi R, Cuervas-Mons V, González-Pinto I, Rimola A, Bernardos A, Otero S, Maldonado J, Herrero JI, Barrao E, Domínguez-Granados R. A prospective randomized open study in liver transplant recipients: daclizumab, mycophenolate mofetil, and tacrolimus versus tacrolimus and steroids. Liver Transpl. 2009;15(11):1542–52.
59. De Simone P, Nevens F, De Carlis L, Metselaar HJ, Beckebaum S, Saliba F, et al. Everolimus with reduced tacrolimus improves renal function in de novo liver transplant recipients: a randomized controlled trial. Am J Transplant. 2012;12:3008–200.
60. Saliba F, De Simone P, Nevens F, et al. Renal function at two years in liver transplant patients receiving everolimus: results of a randomized, multicenter study. Am J Transplant. 2013;13:1734–45.
61. Fischer L, Saliba F, Kaiser GM, De Carlis L, Metselaar HJ, De Simone P, et al. Three-year outcomes in de novo liver transplant patients receiving everolimus with reduced tacrolimus: follow-up results from a randomized, multicenter study. Transplantation. 2015;99:1455–62.
62. Sterneck M, Kaiser GM, Heyne N, et al. Everolimus and early calcineurin inhibitor withdrawal: 3-year results from a randomized trial in liver transplantation. Am J Transplant. 2014;14:701–10.
63. Masetti M, Montalti R, Rompianesi G, Codeluppi M, Gerring R, Romano A, et al. Early withdrawal of calcineurin inhibitors and everolimus monotherapy in de novo liver transplant recipients preserves renal function. Am J Transplant. 2010;10:2252–62.
64. Fischer L, Klempnauer J, Beckebaum S, Metselaar HJ, Neuhaus P, Schemmer P, et al. A randomized, controlled study to assess the conversion from calcineurin-inhibitors to everolimus after liver transplantation—PROTECT. Am J Transplant. 2012;12:1855–65.
65. Ojo AO, Held PJ, Port FK, Wolfe RA, Leichtman AB, Young EW, Arndorfer J, Christensen L, Merion RM. Chronic renal failure after transplantation of a nonrenal organ. N Engl J Med. 2003;349:931–40.
66. Charlton MR, Wall WJ, Ojo AO, Ginès P, Textor S, Shihab FS, Marotta P, Cantarovich M, Eason JD, Wiesner RH, Ramsay MA, Garcia-Valdecasas JC, Neuberger JM, Feng S, Davis CL, Gonwa TA, International Liver Transplantation Society Expert Panel. Report of the first international liver transplantation society expert panel consensus conference on renal insufficiency in liver transplantation. Liver Transpl. 2009;15:S1–34.
67. Allen AM, Kim WR, Therneau TM, Larson JJ, Heimbach JK, Rule AD. Chronic kidney disease and associated mortality after liver transplantation—a time-dependent analysis using measured glomerular filtration rate. J Hepatol. 2014;61:286–92.

68. Fussner LA, Charlton MR, Heimbach JK, Fan C, Dierkhising R, Coss E, Watt KD. The impact of gender and NASH on chronic kidney disease before and after liver transplantation. Liver Int. 2014;34:1259–66.
69. Wong RJ, Cheung R, Ahmed A. Nonalcoholic steatohepatitis is the most rapidly growing indication for liver transplantation in patients with hepatocellular carcinoma in the U.S. Hepatology. 2014;59:2188–95.
70. Sharma P, Schaubel DE, Guidinger MK, Goodrich NP, Ojo AO, Merion RM. Impact of MELD-based allocation on end-stage renal disease after liver transplantation. Am J Transplant. 2011;11:2372–8.
71. De Simone P, Metselaar HJ, Fischer L, Dumortier J, Boudjema K, Hardwigsen J, Rostaing L, De Carlis L, Saliba F, Nevens F. Conversion from a calcineurin inhibitor to everolimus therapy in maintenance liver transplant recipients: a prospective, randomized, multicenter trial. Liver Transpl. 2009;15(10):1262–9.
72. Abdelmalek MF, Humar A, Stickel F, Andreone P, Pascher A, Barroso E, et al. Sirolimus conversion regimen versus continued calcineurin inhibitors in liver allograft recipients: a randomized trial. Am J Transplant. 2012;12:694–705.
73. Castroagudin JF, Molina E, Romero R, Otero E, Tome S, Varo E. Improvement of renal function after the switch from a calcineurin inhibitor to everolimus in liver transplant recipients with chronic renal dysfunction. Liver Transpl. 2009;15:1792–7.
74. Lee SG, Jeng LB, Saliba F, Singh Soin A, Lee WC, De Simone P, Nevens F, Suh KS, Fischer L, Jin Joo D, Fung J, Joh JW, Kaido T, Grant D, Meier M, Rauer B, Sips C, Kaneko S, Levy G. Efficacy and safety of everolimus with reduced tacrolimus in liver transplant recipients: 24-month results from the pooled analysis of 2 randomized controlled trials. Transplantation. 2021;105(7):1564–75.
75. Heisel O, Heisel R, Balshaw R, Keown P. New onset diabetes mellitus in patients receiving calcineurin inhibitors: a systematic review and meta-analysis. Am J Transplant. 2004;4(4):583–95.
76. Chaitou AR, Valmiki S, Valmiki M, Zahid M, Aid MA, Fawzy P, Khan S. New-Onset Diabetes Mellitus (NODM) after Liver Transplantation (LT): the ultimate non-diabetogenic immunosuppressive therapy. Cureus. 2022;14(3):e23635.
77. Castedal M, Skoglund C, Axelson C, Bennet W. Steroid-free immunosuppression with low-dose tacrolimus is safe and significantly reduces the incidence of new-onset diabetes mellitus following liver transplantation. Scand J Gastroenterol. 2018;53(6):741–7.
78. Charlton M, Rinella M, Patel D, McCague K, Heimbach J, Watt K. Everolimus is associated with less weight gain than tacrolimus 2 years after liver transplantation: results of a randomized multicenter study. Transplantation. 2017;101(12):2873–82.
79. Collett D, Mumford L, Banner NR, Neuberger J, Watson C. Comparison of the incidence of malignancy in recipients of different types of organ: a UK registry audit. Am J Transplant. 2010;10(8):1889–96.
80. Krynitz B, Edgren G, Lindelöf B, et al. Risk of skin cancer and other malignancies in kidney, liver, heart and lung transplant recipients 1970 to 2008–a Swedish population-based study. Int J Cancer. 2013;132(6):1429–38.
81. Taborelli M, Piselli P, Ettorre GM, et al. Survival after the diagnosis of de novo malignancy in liver transplant recipients. Int J Cancer. 2019;144(2):232–9.
82. Acuna SA, Huang JW, Daly C, Shah PS, Kim SJ, Baxter NN. Outcomes of solid organ transplant recipients with pre-existing malignancies in remission: a systematic review and meta-analysis. Transplantation. 2017;101(3):471–81.
83. Hart A, Pfeiffer RM, Morawski BM, Lynch CF, Zeng Y, Pawlish K, Hurley D, Yu KJ, Engels EA. Mortality among solid organ transplant recipients with a pretransplant cancer diagnosis. Am J Transplant. 2023;23(2):257–64.
84. Salcedo M, Vinaixa C, Javle M, Trapero-Marugán M, Bustamante J, Line PD. Evaluation and management of liver transplant candidates with prior nonhepatic cancer: guidelines from the ILTS/SETH consensus conference. Transplantation. 2022;106(1):e3–e11.

85. Rodríguez-Perálvarez M, Colmenero J, González A, Gastaca M, Curell A, Caballero-Marcos A, Sánchez-Martínez A, Di Maira T, Herrero JI, Almohalla C, Lorente S, Cuadrado-Lavín A, Pascual S, López-Garrido MÁ, González-Grande R, Gómez-Orellana A, Alejandre R, Zamora-Olaya J, Bernal-Bellido C, Chronic Immunosuppression, Cancer Spanish Consortium. Cumulative exposure to tacrolimus and incidence of cancer after liver transplantation. Am J Transplant. 2022;22(6):1671–82.
86. Lee JY, et al. Increased posttransplant mortality for autoimmune hepatitis compared with other autoimmune liver diseases. J Clin Gastroenterol. 2020;54:648–54.
87. Heinemann M, et al. Long-term outcome after living donor liver transplantation compared to donation after brain death in autoimmune liver diseases: experience from the European Liver Transplant Registry. Am J Transplant. 2022;22:626–33.
88. Kelly C, Zen Y, Heneghan MA. Post-transplant immunosuppression in autoimmune liver disease. J Clin Exp Hepatol. 2023;13(2):350–9.
89. Montano-Loza AJ, et al. Risk factors and outcomes associated with recurrent autoimmune hepatitis following liver transplantation. J Hepatol. 2022;77:84–97.
90. Corpechot C, et al. Long-term impact of preventive UDCA therapy after transplantation for primary biliary cholangitis. J Hepatol. 2020;73:559–65.
91. Li X, et al. Risk factors for recurrent primary biliary cirrhosis after liver transplantation: a systematic review and meta-analysis. Dig Liver Dis. 2021;53:309–17.
92. Berenguer M, Burra P, Ghobrial M, Hibi T, Metselaar H, Sapisochin G, Bhoori S, Kwan Man N, Mas V, Ohira M, Sangro B, van der Laan LJW. Posttransplant management of recipients undergoing liver transplantation for hepatocellular carcinoma. Working group report from the ILTS transplant oncology consensus conference. Transplantation. 2020;104(6):1143–9.
93. Liang W, Wang D, Ling X, Kao AA, Kong Y, Shang Y, Guo Z, He X. Sirolimus-based immunosuppression in liver transplantation for hepatocellular carcinoma: a meta-analysis. Liver Transpl. 2012;18(1):62–9.
94. Menon KV, Hakeem AR, Heaton ND. Meta-analysis: recurrence and survival following the use of sirolimus in liver transplantation for hepatocellular carcinoma. Aliment Pharmacol Ther. 2013;37(4):411–9.
95. Cholongitas E, Mamou C, Rodríguez-Castro KI, Burra P. Mammalian target of rapamycin inhibitors are associated with lower rates of hepatocellular carcinoma recurrence after liver transplantation: a systematic review. Transpl Int. 2014;27(10):1039–49.
96. Grigg SE, Sarri GL, Gow PJ, Yeomans ND. Systematic review with meta-analysis: sirolimus- or everolimus-based immunosuppression following liver transplantation for hepatocellular carcinoma. Aliment Pharmacol Ther. 2019;49(10):1260–73.
97. Zhang G, Duan B, Li G. mTORi-based immunosuppression reduces HCC recurrence at the expense of increased adverse side effects: a systematic review and meta-analysis. Clin Transpl. 2022;36(12):e14823.
98. Yan X, Huang S, Yang Y, Lu Z, Li F, Jiang L, Jiang Y, Liu J. Sirolimus or everolimus improves survival after liver transplantation for hepatocellular carcinoma: a systematic review and meta-analysis. Liver Transpl. 2022;28(6):1063–77.
99. ALoun A, Abu-Zeid EED, Garzali IU. Does mtori base immunosuppression offer survival advantage after liver transplantation for hepatocellular carcinoma? Systematic review and meta-analysis of randomized controlled trials. Hepatol Forum. 2023;4(2):82–8.
100. European Association for the Study of the Liver. Electronic address: easloffice@easloffice.eu; European Association for the Study of the Liver. EASL clinical practice guidelines on acute-on-chronic liver failure. J Hepatol. 2023;79(2):461–91.
101. Faitot F, Artzner T, Michard B, Besch C, Schenck M, Herbrecht JE, Janssen Langenstein R, Maestraggi Q, Guillot M, Harlay ML, Castelain V, Addeo P, Ellero B, Woehl-Jaegle ML, Serfaty L, Bachellier P, Schneider F, Strasbourg LIVER Transplantation (SLIVERT) Study Group. Immunosuppression in patients with grade 3 acute-on-chronic liver failure at transplantation: a practice analysis study. Clin Transplant. 2022;36(4):e14580.

102. Melk A, Babitsch B, Borchert-Mörlins B, Claas F, Dipchand AI, et al. Equally interchangeable? How sex and gender affect transplantation. Transplantation. 2019;103(6):1094–110.
103. Sarkar M, Watt KD, Terrault N, Berenguer M. Outcomes in liver transplantation: does sex matter? J Hepatol. 2015;62(4):946–55.
104. Jadaun SS, Agarwal S, Gupta S, Saigal S. Strategies for ABO incompatible liver transplantation. J Clin Exp Hepatol. 2023;13(4):698–706.
105. Egawa H, Teramukai S, Haga H, Tanabe M, Mori A, Ikegami T, et al. Impact of rituximab desensitization on blood-type-incompatible adult living donor liver transplantation: a Japanese multicenter study. Am J Transplant. 2014;14:102–14.
106. Wiesner RH, Fung JJ. Present state of immunosuppressive therapy in liver transplant recipients. Liver Transpl. 2011;17 Suppl 3:S1–9.

Chapter 30
Early Allograft Dysfunction After Liver Transplantation

Dhiraj Agrawal, Subhash Gupta, and Sanjiv Saigal

Abstract Early allograft dysfunction (EAD) is a critical clinical endpoint determining the risk of graft loss associated with various specific donor or recipient risk factors. Importantly, it also acts as an intermediate endpoint in translational studies aiming to identify mechanistic pathways and explore prognostic biomarkers of graft dysfunction or failure. A rising global organ shortage has necessitated using marginal liver organs and liver transplantation in high-acuity recipients, which has proportionately enhanced the risk of EAD. The early recognition of severe EAD is highly relevant and desirable in educating the patients, formulating an effective mitigating strategy, and potentially guiding earlier re-transplantation. This review provides an overview of EAD after LT, discusses current pathophysiology concepts, formulates a management algorithm, and suggests future directions for research.

Keywords Early allograft dysfunction · Primary non-function · Early allograft failure · Small-for-size syndrome · Living donor liver transplantation · Deceased donor liver transplantation

D. Agrawal
Department of Gastroenterology and Hepatology, Continental Hospitals, Financial District, Hyderabad, India

S. Gupta
Centre for Liver and Biliary Sciences (CLBS), Max Super Speciality Hospital, Saket, New Delhi, Delhi, India

S. Saigal (✉)
Hepatology and Liver Transplant Medicine, Max Institute of Liver and Gastrointestinal Sciences, Max Super Speciality Hospital, Saket, New Delhi, India
e-mail: sanjivsaigal@hotmail.com

S. Saigal, D. Jothimani (eds.), *Fundamentals of Transplant Hepatology*,
https://doi.org/10.1007/978-981-95-2624-6_30

Abbreviations

CVP	Central venous pressure
DDLT	Deceased donor liver transplantation
EAD	Early allograft dysfunction
EAF	Early allograft failure
GV	Graft volume
GIM	Graft inflow modification
GRWR	Graft-to-recipient weight ratio
IRI	Ischemia-reperfusion injury
LDLT	Living donor liver transplantation
MELD	Model for end-stage liver disease
PVF	Portal vein flow
PVP	Portal vein Pressure
PGD	Primary graft dysfunction
PNF	Primary non-function
SLV	Standard liver volume
SFSG	small for size graft
SFSS	Small-for-size syndrome

Key Highlights

1. Early allograft dysfunction (EAD) after liver transplantation is a significant clinical problem that negatively impacts graft and patient outcomes.
2. 'EAD after LDLT' is a distinct entity from 'EAD after DDLT'.
3. EAD after LDLT results from a complex interplay of multiple donor, surgery and recipient-related factors.
4. The terms SFSS and EAD are used interchangeably in the literature. SFSS denotes the etiologic diagnosis, while EAD denotes a syndromic diagnosis.
5. EAD and EAF after LDLT represent the two sequential stages where graft dysfunction evolves from a partially reversible stage to an irreversible and life-threatening condition.

30.1 Introduction

Early allograft dysfunction (EAD) following liver transplantation (LT) is a major clinical challenge, with reported incidence rates ranging from 5.3% to 32.3% and graft failure rates between 26.9% and 87.5% [1]. In deceased donor liver transplantation (DDLT), the increasing reliance on extended criteria donors to widen the donor pool has led to a higher risk of both EAD and primary non-function (PNF). Similarly, in living donor liver transplantation (LDLT), the growing global organ shortage has driven the use of grafts with lower

Table 30.1 EAD in LDLT vs DDLT

Parameters	LDLT	DDLT
Incidence	15–30%	DBD 15–30% DCD 60–70%
Size of graft	Partial graft	Complete graft
IRI	Minimal	Significant
CIT	Less	More
Donor graft quality	Good quality	May or may not be of good quality
Onset	Gradual	Sudden
Time of presentation	2nd week	1st week
Pathophysiology	Functional insufficiency	Necro-inflammation
AST/ALT	Not so high	Very high
Severest form	EAF	PNF
Reversibility	EAD—partially reversible	EAD—partially reversible
	EAF—irreversible	PNF—irreversible

graft-to-recipient weight ratios (GRWR <0.8), significant macrosteatosis (>10%), donor age over 50 years, complex vascular or biliary anatomy, and transplantation into high-acuity recipients—factors that collectively elevate the risk of EAD in LDLT.

EAD in LDLT differs from that in DDLT with respect to incidence, underlying mechanisms, and clinical features (as outlined in Table 30.1). In DDLT, EAD typically results from ischemia-reperfusion injury (IRI), particularly when steatotic, older grafts, or those with prolonged cold ischemia time (CIT) undergo reperfusion, leading to extensive hepatic necrosis during the first post-transplant week. Conversely, in LDLT, the graft is generally smaller but functionally sound and transplanted with a shorter CIT, resulting in minimal IRI. However, a complex combination of donor, surgical, and recipient-related factors may still disrupt liver regeneration and contribute to EAD.

30.2 Proposed Classification of Graft Dysfunction After LDLT

EAD is defined as graft insufficiency that may lead to early graft failure or in-hospital mortality within 90 days post-transplant. Allograft dysfunction can be classified as either primary or secondary, depending on the presence or absence of identifiable causes. Secondary graft dysfunction is attributed to technical issues (such as vascular or biliary complications), infections, rejection, drug-induced injury, or recurrence of the original liver disease. In contrast, primary graft dysfunction (PGD) arises from inherent donor or recipient factors without any identifiable complications. Small-for-size syndrome (SFSS) serves as a classic example of PGD.

Early allograft failure (EAF) refers to irreversible graft loss within 90 days of LT, and it can stem from either primary or secondary dysfunction. The 90-day mark is a widely accepted threshold for evaluating graft failure-free survival, as severe EAD typically results in death or the need for re-transplantation within this period. Therefore, EAD and EAF after LDLT represent progressive stages, with EAD being potentially reversible and EAF representing irreversible, life-threatening graft failure.

PNF is a rare but severe form of irreversible graft dysfunction, necessitating re-transplantation or resulting in death within the early postoperative weeks. Delayed graft dysfunction or failure is defined as graft deterioration occurring more than 90 days after LT, usually due to complications like rejection or recurrence of the original liver disease. Figure 30.1 illustrates the newly proposed classification system for graft dysfunction after LDLT by Agrawal and Saigal [1].

EAD after LDLT: A conceptual shift from “small for-size syndrome” to “small-for-flow syndrome”:

EAD in LDLT can be caused by multiple donor, surgery, and recipient-related factors. However, LDLT-EAD is usually due to portal hyperperfusion-related sinusoidal injury in the setting of a small graft leading to “small for-size syndrome” (SFSS) or “portal hyperperfusion syndrome” or “small-for-flow syndrome.” Rapid expansion of LDLT and its intuitive tendency to use smaller liver grafts make SFSS a major clinical problem in LDLT. Although the initial understanding of SFSS focused on identifying an appropriate graft size for safe LDLT, this is a recent paradigm shift suggesting that this phenomenon is a result of portal hyperperfusion and reciprocal arterial ischemia in a small liver graft with a spectrum of susceptibility in the clinical setting [2]. Because SFSS is observed across all graft sizes, differentiating SFSS from LDLT-EAD is difficult. Also there is significant overlap of the causative factors and similar clinical and biochemical features. Thus, the terms SFSS and EAD are used interchangeably in the LDLT literature. However, SFSS denotes the etiologic diagnosis, while EAD denotes a syndromic diagnosis. It may be appropriate to consider SFSS as a subset of EAD.

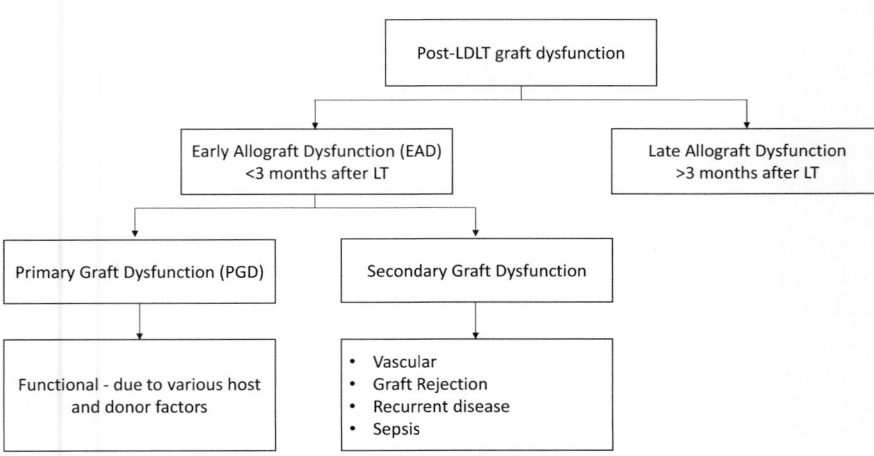

Fig. 30.1 Types of graft dysfunction post-LDLT

30.3 Definition and Grading the Severity of SFSS/EAD After LDLT

Until a recent consensus definition, which recommends using the term SFSS to describe a clinical phenomenon of liver dysfunction using partial liver grafts in LDLT in the absence of specific surgical or nonsurgical causes, it has been referred variously as SFSS, EAD, or PGD. The concept of EAD was first formally proposed in 1998 by Deschenes et al. to identify post-DDLT poor graft function based on a large multicenter population [3]. In contrast, Dahm et al. put forth a slightly different definition in 2005, defining small-for-size dysfunction as dysfunction of a "small" partial liver graft (GRWR <0.8%) during the first postoperative week after the exclusion of other causes [4]. Subsequently, Olthof et al., Ikegami et al., A2ALL, Okamura et al., and Pamecha et al. have proposed definitions of EAD after LDLT [1]. However, to date the 2010's definition of EAD by Olthof et al., is the most followed one [5]. They defined EAD as the presence of 'one or more' of the following laboratory findings: total bilirubin (TB) ≥10 mg/dL on a postoperative day (POD)-7, International normalized ratio (INR) ≥1.6 on POD7, and alanine aminotransferase (ALT) or aspartate aminotransferase (AST) >2000 IU/L within the first 7 days without technical complications [5].

In a recent consensus meeting, a new grading system to stratify the severity of SFSS has been introduced (Table 30.2). SFSS after LDLT is categorized into 3 prognostic grades based on severity: "grade A, pre-SFSS"; "grade B, portal hypertensive phase SFSS"; and "grade C, liver failure phase SFSS" [6]. Grade A-pre-SFSS stage is characterized by T.Bil of >5 mg/dL on day 7 or T.Bil of >5 mg/ dL or ascites output >1 L/d on day 14. Grade B-portal hypertensive phase of SFSS is characterized by T.Bil >10 mg/ dL or INR >1.6 on day 7, or T.Bil >10 mg/dL and ascites >1 L/d on day 14 after LDLT. This form of SFSS can be treated without retransplantation. Grade C-hepatic failure phase of SFSS is characterized by T.Bil >10 mg/dL and INR >1.6 on day 7 or T.Bil >20 mg/dL on day 14. Retransplantation should be considered for grade C SFSS.

Table 30.2 ILTS-iLDLT-LTSI Consensus grading system for small-for-size syndrome

Grade	A (pre-SFSS)	B (portal hypertensive phase—SFSS)	C (liver failure phase—SFSS)
Day7	T.Bil >5 mg/dL	T.Bil >10 mg/dL or INR >1.6	T.Bil >10 mg/dL and INR >1.6
Day14	T.Bil >5 mg/dL or ascites IL/d	T.Bil >10 mg/dL and ascites IL/d	T.Bil >20 mg/dL
Mortality	<9%	9–26%	59–77%
Management	Supportive medical care and pharmacotherapy	Medical care + PIM	Medical care + PIM + retransplantation

30.4 EAD After LDLT: Biochemical and Clinical Markers

In DDLT, EAD is typically identified by markedly elevated aminotransferase levels, ongoing cholestasis, and coagulation abnormalities within the first week post-transplant. In cases of PNF, clinical signs emerge early after surgery and include sharp increases in transaminases (often into the thousands), lack of bile output, severe coagulopathy, metabolic acidosis, and hemodynamic instability—reflecting widespread hepatic necrosis following reperfusion. While EAD is generally reversible, PNF is typically an irreversible, life-threatening condition that requires urgent re-transplantation [7].

In LDLT, EAD tends to develop more gradually during the first postoperative week and presents with persistent cholestasis, coagulation disturbances, and continued ascitic fluid drainage—indicating a temporary functional inadequacy of the regenerating partial graft. SFSS, a key form of PGD, is typically diagnosed within the first 7–14 days after LDLT. Definitions of SFSS have consistently incorporated biochemical markers such as total bilirubin (thresholds: 10 mg/dL, 20 mg/dL) and INR (cutoffs: 1.5, 1.6, 2.0).

Additional predictors of EAD and graft failure include a low postoperative platelet count and delayed platelet recovery, both of which are factored into risk scoring models such as EASE and L-GRAFT. A persistently elevated serum urea level (>100 mg/dL for 5 days) has also been proposed to improve the accuracy of SFSS diagnosis. Furthermore, early elevation of arterial or intragraft lactate concentrations may serve as reliable biomarkers for predicting EAD in LDLT.

Despite identifiable risk factors, approximately 75% of patients with EAD experience graft recovery. However, a subset will progress to graft failure. Clinical features seen in EAD often intensify in EAF and may include hepatic encephalopathy, persistent coagulopathy, hypoglycemia, electrolyte imbalances, metabolic acidosis, lactic acidosis, and reduced urine output due to renal failure. Patients with EAD are at greater risk for infections, multi-organ failure, extended ICU and hospital stays, graft loss, and increased mortality [8]. Delay in recognizing or addressing EAD can allow complications to progress beyond the window of effective re-transplantation, leading to fatal outcomes.

30.5 Risk Factors for EAD After LDLT

EAD after LDLT arises from a complex interaction of donor-related, surgical, and recipient-specific factors, as illustrated in Fig. 30.2. The balance between protective and harmful influences determines whether normal graft regeneration or dysfunction occurs.

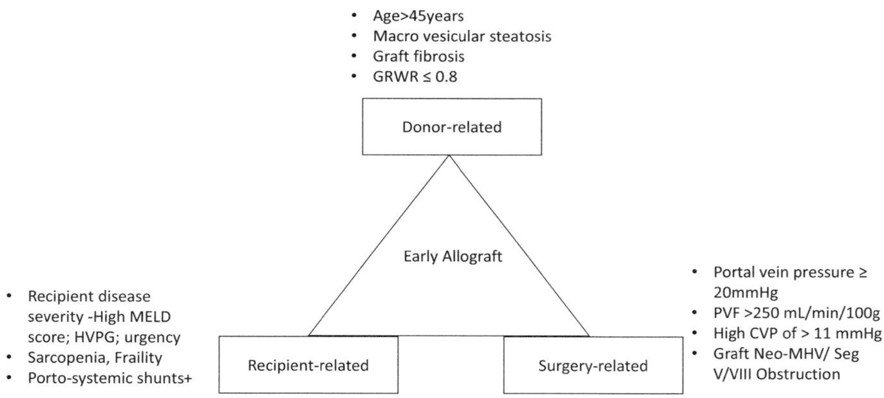

Fig. 30.2 Risk factors for early allograft dysfunction after living donor liver transplantation

30.5.1 Small-for-Size Graft (SFSG)

The GRWR is the most widely used method to determine if the liver graft is adequately sized for the recipient. An alternative metric is graft volume to standard liver volume (GV/SLV). While both methods are valid, liver volumetry—often based on contrast-enhanced CT imaging—can overestimate graft size. This discrepancy between estimated volume and actual intraoperative graft weight may result in transplanting a smaller-than-ideal graft.

Initially described in 1999, grafts with a GRWR <0.8 or GV/SLV <40% are considered small-for-size. In LDLT, such grafts may be insufficient for recipient metabolic needs, leading to SFSS, a concept formally defined in 2005 [4]. Many transplant centers have since established institutional policies regarding the minimum acceptable GRWR. Studies suggest that a GRWR as low as 0.6 or a GV/SLV ≥30% may be acceptable under certain conditions—such as careful patient selection (e.g., low MELD score, non-cirrhotic patients, absence of significant portal hypertension), and in experienced, high-volume centers [9]. However, recipients with high metabolic demand (e.g., acute liver failure, high MELD, sarcopenia, cardiopulmonary or renal compromise) should receive grafts with a GRWR >0.8. Transplantation using grafts with an expected GRWR <0.6 is generally discouraged due to an unacceptably high risk of SFSS, morbidity, and mortality.

30.6 Graft Hemodynamics

Although graft size has long been recognized as a key determinant in SFSS, portal pressure and graft compliance are now considered more accurate predictors of early graft dysfunction in LDLT. A post-reperfusion portal venous pressure (PVP) under

20 mmHg is recommended, with <15 mmHg being optimal [10]. For standard-sized grafts (GRWR ≥0.8%), a portal vein flow (PVF) of <250 mL/min/100 g of liver tissue is ideal to avoid SFSS [11]. When using smaller grafts (GRWR <0.8%), lower PVF targets should be set accordingly.

While PVP and PVF both provide valuable insights, most centers prefer PVP measurement due to its greater reliability, reproducibility, ease of use, and lower cost. Many institutions assess PVP or PVF after graft reperfusion to account for graft compliance and determine the need for portal inflow modulation (PIM). However, some centers base the decision for PIM on pre-implantation hemodynamic measurements during the dissection phase.

Portal hyperperfusion, especially in the presence of compromised venous outflow, may reduce arterial perfusion and hamper regenerative capacity, leading to liver dysfunction. High central venous pressure (CVP) is one example of a non-mechanical factor that can impair hepatic venous drainage, thereby raising PVP and hindering graft recovery. For instance, a post-LDLT CVP >11 mmHg has been associated with hepatic venous outflow (HVO) obstruction, elevating PVP by 45% and delaying graft function restoration [12].

In such scenarios, measuring the hepatic vein–portal gradient (<10 mmHg ideal) may help identify inflow or outflow obstruction as the source of dysfunction. If the portal pressure gradient exceeds 5 mmHg or the hepatic vein/inferior vena cava gradient exceeds 3 mmHg, surgical or interventional radiologic correction should be considered.

There is also evidence that a graft-to-spleen volume ratio (GSVR) <0.95 may predict a PVP >20 mmHg and could be useful in guiding the need for PIM.

30.7 Donor Age

Donor age is a well-established factor influencing outcomes in LDLT. With the growing acceptance of extended criteria donors, the upper age limit for acceptable donors has gradually increased [13]. However, while a precise age cutoff guaranteeing safe outcomes remains unclear, many experts advocate for the use of grafts from donors under 45 years of age [14]. Older donor grafts are more likely to exhibit hepatic steatosis, subclinical inflammation, or fibrosis, which compromises graft resilience. These grafts are more vulnerable to ischemia and shear stress injury from elevated PVP (>15 mmHg), show reduced regenerative potential, and carry a higher risk of SFSS. Additionally, from a donor safety perspective, the minimum future liver remnant (FLR) should be ≥30% in donors under 35 years and ≥35% in donors aged 35 years and above.

30.8 Donor BMI and Graft Quality

The quality of the liver graft is a critical determinant in the development of EAD. Donor obesity is strongly associated with hepatic steatosis. In LDLT, donors are carefully evaluated for steatosis using tools such as the CT liver attenuation index or more advanced techniques like MRI-based proton density fat fraction and MR spectroscopy. In select cases, a liver biopsy is performed. Most transplant centers exclude donors with steatohepatitis or macrosteatosis exceeding 10%, though thresholds as high as 20% may be accepted [15].

Specifically, moderate to severe large-droplet macrovesicular steatosis (≥30%) is a recognized independent risk factor for EAD and PNF due to heightened IRI and impaired graft regeneration [16, 17]. In contrast, microvesicular steatosis is generally considered benign and reversible, and thus not a significant risk for EAD [18]. Moreover, chronic liver fibrosis, being a precursor to cirrhosis, may also contribute to increased susceptibility to EAD.

30.9 Ischemia-Reperfusion Injury

IRI is an inevitable outcome of organ preservation, with reperfusion—not ischemia—being the principal driver of injury and subsequent EAD [19]. Although the liver is relatively tolerant to ischemia, the inflammatory cascade triggered upon reperfusion plays a central role in cellular injury. In LDLT, the shorter CIT associated with partial grafts usually results in less IRI, explaining the lower incidence of EAD and the rarity of PNF in this setting. In contrast, prolonged CIT is a well-documented risk factor for EAD in DDLT [20]. Strategies to mitigate ischemic damage during the preservation phase include minimizing CIT and utilizing various perfusion techniques [21].

Warm ischemia time (WIT) also significantly affects outcomes. Extended WIT—especially exceeding 45 min during complex procedures—is linked to increased PNF risk. To optimize graft and patient survival, keeping WIT below 60 min is generally recommended [22].

30.10 Surgical Techniques

Meticulous surgical technique is essential for achieving optimal graft performance. Although anatomical complexities like multiple hepatic arteries or bile ducts are not directly associated with increased SFSS risk, complications such as hepatic artery thrombosis and biliary strictures can exacerbate graft dysfunction, especially in recipients of low-GRWR grafts.

Minor bile leaks leading to cholestasis require adequate drainage to resolve. Proper venous outflow from all liver segments is equally critical to vascular inflow. Subtle outflow impairments may only be detectable via hepatic portal venous gradient assessments. Of particular concern is middle hepatic vein (MHV) thrombosis, a known cause of graft dysfunction. In right lobe grafts that exclude MHV, ensuring sufficient drainage of the right anterior sector is crucial. This involves reconstructing the MHV tributaries and inferior hepatic veins during the back-table phase using interposition vein grafts.[42]

Maintaining patency of the reconstructed MHV or veins draining segments V and VIII is vital to prevent graft congestion and EAD, particularly in cases of small-for-size grafts. Excessive intraoperative bleeding also negatively impacts graft function. Moreover, minimally invasive donor hepatectomy—though increasingly common—can introduce longer donor warm ischemia, shorter vascular structures, and potentially higher biliary complications. These technical factors can adversely affect both graft quality and the risk of SFSS in recipients.

30.11 Portosystemic Shunt

SPSS are present in about 20–35% of transplant candidates. In LDLT, natural portosystemic shunts can effectively decompress the splanchnic vascular system until the graft regenerates. However, some studies suggest that persistent portosystemic shunt following LDLT may lead to portal steal phenomenon and graft hypoperfusion in the setting of SFSG.[(46)] In all other cases, to prevent portal steal, large SPSS (>10 mm) should ideally be ligated. Conversely, ligating a large collateral vessel during surgery may lead to portal hyperperfusion and the risk of SFSS [23]. Simultaneous measurement of the PVP and/or PVF parameters upon clamping of the SPSS can help identify patients in whom the ligation of SPSS can cause disastrous elevation in the PVP and/or PVF.

30.12 Right Lobe Versus Left Lobe Graft

The initial practice of LDLT utilized smaller left lobe grafts; however, studies have shown a higher percentage of EAD in left lobe vs right lobe graft recipients (34% vs 16%) [8]. Because of these disappointing results, there was a gradual shift to the more routine use of right lobe grafts and eventually either grafts with GRWR >0.8 OR GV/SLV >40% to provide an adequate safety margin in an adult LDLT recipient. Successful mitigation of SFSS after PIM has renewed interest in smaller grafts and left lobe grafts to reduce operative risk in donors without compromising recipient outcomes [24]. Although there is an increasing comfort in using both left and right lobe grafts at most LDLT centers, there is always the risk for the development of small for size syndrome (SFSS) with any partial graft.

30.13 Model for End-Stage Liver Disease (MELD) Score

In the current era of organ shortage, partial grafts are often transplanted into sicker individuals with high MELD scores to prevent waitlist mortality. However, to date, the transplant community is skeptical about the application of LDLT for patients with high MELD scores. Despite high MELD scores in acute liver failure (ALF) patients, PVP may only be mildly or moderately increased and therefore may not increase the risk of SFSS. In comparison to ALF, acute-on-chronic liver failure (ACLF) patients do have high PVP because they have underlying cirrhosis. Additionally, patients with ALF or with ACLF typically present with systemic inflammatory response syndrome and multiorgan failure with or without sepsis, which can be the main driver of SFSS in these patients. In most studies, MELD cutoff of 19 seems to reflect high acuity recipient and is likely to have a higher PVP and does increase the risk for SFSS in combination with a SFSG and other concomitant risk factors. Also, the need to perform transplantation on a sick recipient must be balanced against the risk of EAD post-LDLT.

30.14 Other Recipient-Related Factors

The presence of frailty may have an impact on recipient morbidity and mortality. The high metabolic demand of a frail patient with a reduced functional organ reserve may lead to graft dysfunction. Because graft volume requirements are calculated based on recipients' body weight (BW) and body surface area, in sarcopenic patients the graft size requirements may be underestimated. Non-BW formulas may be more effective such as those utilizing thoraco-abdominal width. ABO-i on its own does not increase the risk of SFSS but can do in combination with other factors such as donor age and recipient acuity. The presence of preoperative renal dysfunction as well as the need for renal replacement therapy (RRT) are additional risk factors for the development of postoperative AKI in patients with SFSS.

30.15 Management of EAD After LDLT

Figure 30.3 summarizes the mitigation strategy to overcome EAD after LDLT. Before considering a diagnosis of SFSS, it is imperative to rule out vascular inflow and outflow technical complications. Doppler ultrasonography (DUS) looking for patency, waveforms, and flow velocities in portal vein, hepatic artery, and hepatic veins, and measurement of hepatic artery resistive index are mandatory for LDLT recipients in the first postoperative week. After vascular complications have been excluded, a sepsis workup and liver biopsy to rule out a rejection are recommended. Recipients with SFSG have a higher risk of sepsis because of bacterial translocation, prolonged ICU stay, and the presence of drains and lines.

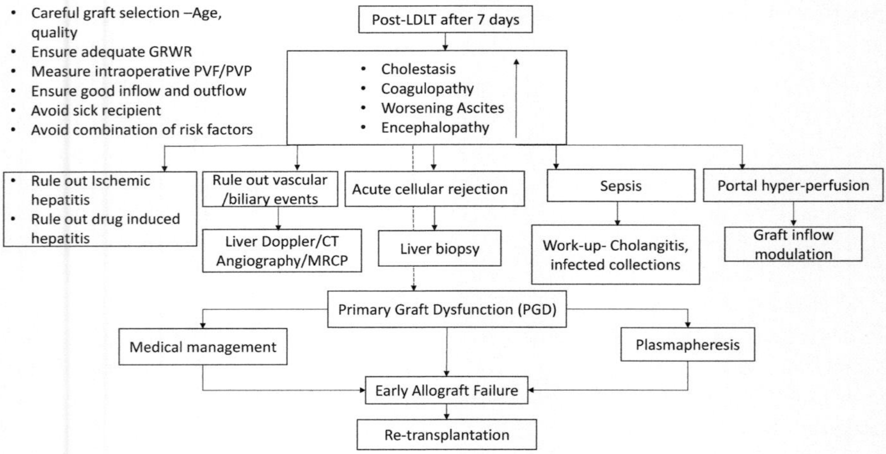

Fig. 30.3 Evaluation and management of early allograft dysfunction post-LDLT

Antibiotic and targeted antifungal prophylaxis is recommended to prevent postoperative bacterial and IFIs, and routine infection surveillance for bacteria, viruses, and fungi should be done. Sub-therapeutic levels of immunosuppression may lead to acute cellular rejection with associated inflammation and increased graft stiffness contributing to graft dysfunction that are especially detrimental to small grafts with limited reserve. Hence, maintaining adequate levels of immunosuppression in recipients with SFSS is recommended in the immediate postoperative period.

Following the exclusion of other causes of graft dysfunction (technical, immunologic, and infectious), the severity of the SFSS guides therapeutic options, with the initial focus on supportive care and pharmacological therapy. When medical management fails or the condition progresses with impending dysfunction or even liver failure, interventional radiology and/or surgical interventions to reduce portal overperfusion should be considered. According to the current literature, up to 20% of all patients with SFSS may require intervention with the risk of graft failure estimated to be about 1–2%, which requires retransplantation [25].

Medical management of SFSS: Medical management of SFSS can be divided into two categories: (A) Supportive care (B) Pharmcotherapy.

Supportive Care: Patients who have developed EAD and EAF after LDLT require intensive medical support to help liver regeneration or to “buy time” while waiting for re-transplantation. The management principles include enhanced recovery protocols, nutrition optimization, management of ascites and fluid balance, metabolic support, on-demand early RRT, mitigating sepsis and hypoglycemia, and correction of an associated coagulopathy.

Within DDLT, a moderately restrictive or “replacement only” fluid strategy has been advocated, particularly during the dissection phase. In LDLT recipients receiving a SFSG, goal-directed fluid therapy, targeting a low CVP threshold of <5 mmHg after reperfusion, has been reported beneficial, as it reduces portal pressure and helps avoid graft congestion and functional outflow obstruction. However, a low MAP during surgery increases the risk of SFSS and mortality posttransplant. Hence, to manage the systemic hemodynamic condition, cardiac output monitoring should be considered. Early RRT can be considered in recipients of SFSG with evidence of renal dysfunction to help avoid graft congestion. Ascites management is one of the key aspects in patients with SFSS. Overall, the approach is focused on diuretic use and sodium restriction for moderate volumes of ascites, whereas large volume paracentesis followed by albumin diuresis would be appropriate for large volume or refractory ascites. In patients with high output ascitic fluid loss via drainage tubes, volume loss should be replaced with 5% albumin to prevent the hypovolemia and renal dysfunction.

30.16 Pharmacotherapy

Pharmacological options, including somatostatin/octreotide/terlipressin can be initiated during the perioperative period and post-LDLT when the index of suspicion for the development of SFSS is high to reduce portal venous flow and PVP in recipients of SFSG.

Somatostatin (SST) and its synthetic analogue, octreotide, induce sinusoidal dilation by inhibiting stellate cell contraction, reduce the parenchymal injury due to microcirculatory shear force, and induce splanchnic vasoconstriction. Similarly, beta blockers can be effective in reducing portal hypertension by both reducing cardiac output via β1 blockade and reducing portal venous flow (PVF) via β2 blockade. An analogue of vasopressin, terlipressin, is activated by endothelial peptidase and acts as a vasopressin receptor agonist, resulting in splanchnic vasoconstriction and reduction in portal flow. Infusions of terlipressin have been used in doses ranging 1–3 μg/kg perioperatively titrated to keep the MAP >65 mm Hg and SVR index <2600 dyn.s/cm^5/m^2. Prostaglandin E1 (PGE1) and prostacyclin (PGI2) are thought to improve hepatic circulation via their vasodilatory properties and prevent congestion of smaller grafts.

Portal inflow modulation (PIM).

When pharmacological portal flow modulators fail in grade B (portal hypertensive phase of SFSS) or the severity of the condition progresses to grade C (impending liver failure), IR/surgical techniques to reduce portal overperfusion via graft inflow modulation (GIM) are recommended. Over the years, several modalities have been developed to reduce the PVP by reducing PVF through modulation of splenic inflow or by diverting the portal flow by creating portosystemic shunts. Of the GIM modalities described, proximal splenic artery ligation/embolization (SAL/SAE), splenectomy, and hemiportocaval shunts (HPCS) are the most commonly performed, and splenic devascularization is preferred in very few centers. Proximal embolization of the splenic artery is the first line PIM modality to mitigate Grade B SFSS (portal hypertensive phase). SAL reduces the PVP along with an increase in the hepatic artery flow. Strikingly proximal SAL is a simple and easily performed procedure with possibly the lowest morbidity compared with other procedures. The splenic component accounts for up to 52% of the PVP and/or total portal blood flow. Hence some of the large volume LDLT centers consider splenectomy as the first modality in reducing portal flow. Although effective, it may be associated with increased morbidity. HPCS diverts >50% of the portal flow away from the graft liver. The large reduction in the PVP may lead to graft hypoperfusion and steal, leading to graft dysfunction, both in the short term and long term after transplant. Failure to respond to SAE or SAL should be managed by transjugular intrahepatic portosystemic shunt, completion of SAE following failed SAL, or re-LT.

30.17 Liver Support Devices

Liver support systems, including molecular adsorbent recirculating systems, bioartificial livers, and therapeutic plasma exchange (TPE), can be used to support patients experiencing EAD, either as a temporary measure before re-transplantation or while awaiting spontaneous graft recovery. TPE enhances liver graft function by removing circulating toxins and replenishing essential plasma proteins normally synthesized by the liver.

One study evaluated the impact of TPE in 50 out of 789 LDLT recipients with severe EAD, reporting a 6-month graft survival rate of 66%. Another study, which followed 107 patients with EAD over 13 years, found that those receiving TPE had 1-month and 1-year survival rates of 82.2% and 53.8%, respectively—compared to 58.3% and 22.2% in the group that did not receive TPE [26]. Despite these promising outcomes, it remains challenging to generalize these findings for routine use in patients with SFSS.

30.18 Re-transplantation

Severe EAD or EAF is often fatal without successful graft recovery or re-transplantation. Most deaths occur within the first 3 months after primary LDLT and are typically related to complications arising from a failing graft, such as sepsis and multi-organ failure. Given the ongoing shortage of donor organs, only a limited number of patients can be rescued through re-transplantation. Currently, no specific criteria exist for prioritizing patients with EAF following LDLT for emergency re-listing.

In cases of Grade A or B SFSS, re-transplantation may be deferred during the initial 2 weeks post-transplant to allow for potential graft regeneration or spontaneous recovery. However, if medical, interventional radiological, or surgical management fails, re-transplantation should be considered. For Grade C SFSS, re-transplantation is generally recommended due to the high risk of irreversible graft failure.

Ethical considerations such as utility and fairness should guide re-transplantation decisions. Caution is advised in offering re-LT to patients with significant renal impairment, escalating vasopressor requirements, or ongoing infections—particularly those involving multidrug-resistant organisms. Early re-transplantation using combinations such as living donor-to-deceased donor (LD-to-DD), living donor-to-living donor (LD-to-LD), or deceased donor-to-living donor (DD-to-LD) is feasible, especially when adequate arterial inflow is ensured in LD-to-LD settings, and the living donor graft volume is >40% of standard liver volume or GRWR $\geq$0.8%.

However, late LD-to-LD re-transplantation is generally discouraged due to technical challenges stemming from graft distortion, adhesions, and vascular collaterals. Since patients needing retransplantation are often more critically ill, it is advisable to use a living donor graft with a GRWR >1.0% when possible. In addition to graft size, factors such as donor age, graft quality, and anatomical complexity should also be considered. Outcomes of re-transplantation for PNF have historically been poor, with high rates of futility [16].

30.19 Conclusions

To minimize the risk of EAD, clinical practice in LT often favors careful recipient selection and refined intraoperative techniques. Nonetheless, successful management of EAD through strategic preoperative planning, advanced surgical methods, and pharmacologic support holds promise for expanding the donor pool and making transplantation accessible to more critically ill patients.

Conflict of Interest Nothing to report.

Financial Support and Sponsorship None.

References

1. Agrawal D, Saigal S. Early allograft dysfunction after living donor liver transplantation-current concepts and future directions. Liver Transplant Off Publ Am Assoc Study Liver Dis Int Liver Transplant Soc. 2023;29(8):871–84.
2. Rela M, Rammohan A, Bhangui P, Emond J. Prediction and management of small-for-size syndrome in living donor liver transplantation: methodology of the ILTS-iLDLT-LTSI consensus conference. Transplantation. 2023;107(10):2098–100. https://doi.org/10.1097/TP.0000000000004768.
3. Deschênes M, Belle SH, Krom RA, Zetterman RK, Lake JR. Early allograft dysfunction after liver transplantation: a definition and predictors of outcome. National Institute of Diabetes and Digestive and Kidney Diseases Liver Transplantation Database. Transplantation. 1998;66(3):302–10. https://doi.org/10.1097/00007890-199808150-00005.
4. Dahm F, Georgiev P, Clavien PA. Small-for-size syndrome after partial liver transplantation: definition, mechanisms of disease and clinical implications. Am J Transplant Off J Am Soc Transplant Am Soc Transpl Surg. 2005;5(11):2605–10. https://doi.org/10.1111/j.1600-6143.2005.01081.x.

5. Olthoff KM, Kulik L, Samstein B, et al. Validation of a current definition of early allograft dysfunction in liver transplant recipients and analysis of risk factors. Liver Transpl. 2010;16(8):943–9. https://doi.org/10.1002/lt.22091.
6. Kow AWC, Liu J, Patel MS, et al. Post living donor liver transplantation small-for-size syndrome: definitions, timelines, biochemical, and clinical factors for diagnosis: guidelines from the ILTS-iLDLT-LTSI consensus conference. Transplantation. 2023;107(10):2226–37. https://doi.org/10.1097/TP.0000000000004770.
7. Masior Ł, Grąt M. Primary nonfunction and early allograft dysfunction after liver transplantation. Dig Dis. 2022;40(6):766–76. https://doi.org/10.1159/000522052.
8. Pomposelli JJ, Goodrich NP, Emond JC, et al. Patterns of early allograft dysfunction in adult live donor liver transplantation: the A2ALL experience. Transplantation. 2016;100(7):1490–9. https://doi.org/10.1097/TP.0000000000001240.
9. Kaido T, Mori A, Ogura Y, et al. Lower limit of the graft-to-recipient weight ratio can be safely reduced to 0.6% in adult-to-adult living donor liver transplantation in combination with portal pressure control. Transplant Proc. 2011;43(6):2391–3. https://doi.org/10.1016/j.transproceed.2011.05.037.
10. Osman AMA, Hosny AA, El-Shazli MA, Uemoto S, Abdelaziz O, Helmy AS. A portal pressure cut-off of 15 versus a cut-off of 20 for prevention of small-for-size syndrome in liver transplantation: a comparative study. Hepatol Res Off J Jpn Soc Hepatol. 2017;47(4) https://doi.org/10.1111/hepr.12727.
11. Pa V, N K, D B, N G. Technical challenges in LDLT - overcoming small for size syndrome and venous outflow reconstruction. Transplant Rev Orlando Fla. 2023;37(1) https://doi.org/10.1016/j.trre.2023.100750.
12. Appukuttan M, Kumar S, Bharathy KGS, Pandey VK, Pamecha V. Impact of functional hepatic venous outflow obstruction on perioperative outcome after living-donor liver transplant. Exp Clin Transplant Off J Middle East Soc Organ Transplant. 2019;17(1):64–73. https://doi.org/10.6002/ect.2017.0138.
13. Pratschke S, Bender A, Boesch F, et al. Association between donor age and risk of graft failure after liver transplantation: an analysis of the Eurotransplant database. Transpl Int Off J Eur Soc Organ Transplant. 2019;32(3):270–9. https://doi.org/10.1111/tri.13357.
14. Durand F, Levitsky J, Cauchy F, Gilgenkrantz H, Soubrane O, Francoz C. Age and liver transplantation. J Hepatol. 2019;70(4):745–58. https://doi.org/10.1016/j.jhep.2018.12.009.
15. Jackson WE, Kaplan A, Saben JL, et al. Practice patterns of the medical evaluation of living liver donors in the United States. Liver Transplant Off Publ Am Assoc Study Liver Dis Int Liver Transplant Soc. 2023;29(2):164–71. https://doi.org/10.1002/lt.26571.
16. Kulik U, Lehner F, Klempnauer J, Borlak J. Primary non-function is frequently associated with fatty liver allografts and high mortality after re-transplantation. Liver Int Off J Int Assoc Study Liver. 2017;37(8):1219–28. https://doi.org/10.1111/liv.13404.
17. Croome KP, Lee DD, Croome S, et al. The impact of postreperfusion syndrome during liver transplantation using livers with significant macrosteatosis. Am J Transplant Off J Am Soc Transplant Am Soc Transpl Surg. 2019;19(9):2550–9. https://doi.org/10.1111/ajt.15330.
18. Croome KP, Lee DD, Croome S, et al. Does donor allograft microsteatosis matter? Comparison of outcomes in liver transplantation with a propensity-matched cohort. Liver Transplant Off Publ Am Assoc Study Liver Dis Int Liver Transplant Soc. 2019;25(10):1533–40. https://doi.org/10.1002/lt.25583.
19. Zhou J, Chen J, Wei Q, Saeb-Parsy K, Xu X. The role of ischemia/reperfusion injury in early hepatic allograft dysfunction. Liver Transpl. 2020;26(8):1034–48. https://doi.org/10.1002/lt.25779.
20. Westerkamp AC, de Boer MT, van den Berg AP, Gouw ASH, Porte RJ. Similar outcome after transplantation of moderate macrovesicular steatotic and nonsteatotic livers when the cold ischemia time is kept very short. Transpl Int Off J Eur Soc Organ Transplant. 2015;28(3):319–29. https://doi.org/10.1111/tri.12504.

21. JM OC, Morgan RD, Knight SR, Morris PJ. The effect of preservation solutions for storage of liver allografts on transplant outcomes: a systematic review and meta-analysis. Ann Surg. 2014;260(1):46–55. https://doi.org/10.1097/SLA.0000000000000402.
22. Kalisvaart M, Schlegel A, Umbro I, et al. The impact of combined warm ischemia time on development of acute kidney injury in donation after circulatory death liver transplantation: stay within the golden hour. Transplantation. 2018;102(5):783–93. https://doi.org/10.1097/TP.0000000000002085.
23. Gomez Gavara C, Bhangui P, Salloum C, et al. Ligation versus no ligation of spontaneous portosystemic shunts during liver transplantation: audit of a prospective series of 66 consecutive patients. Liver Transplant Off Publ Am Assoc Study Liver Dis Int Liver Transplant Soc. 2018;24(4):505–15. https://doi.org/10.1002/lt.24999.
24. Cheng P, Li Z, Fu Z, Jian Q, Deng R, Ma Y. Small-for-size syndrome and graft inflow modulation techniques in liver transplantation. Dig Dis Basel Switz. 2023;41(2):250–8. https://doi.org/10.1159/000525540.
25. Kirchner VA, Shankar S, Victor DW, et al. Management of established small-for-size syndrome in post living donor liver transplantation: medical, radiological, and surgical interventions: guidelines from the ILTS-iLDLT-LTSI consensus conference. Transplantation. 2023;107(10):2238–46. https://doi.org/10.1097/TP.0000000000004771.
26. Choe W, Kwon SW, Kim SS, Hwang S, Song GW, Lee SG. Effects of therapeutic plasma exchange on early allograft dysfunction after liver transplantation. J Clin Apheresis. 2017;32(3):147–53. https://doi.org/10.1002/jca.21472.

Chapter 31
Pathology of Liver Transplantation

Mukul Vij

Abstract Pathologic evaluation of liver allograft biopsies is an essential component of management in patients following orthotopic liver transplantation. Liver allograft biopsy is considered "gold standard" for the diagnosis of T-cell mediated rejection. It is also used to confirm or exclude numerous allograft pathologies, including biliary issues, vascular insults, infection-related complications, and recurrent and de novo liver diseases. This chapter aims to cover all the aspects of liver allograft pathological findings.

Keywords Liver transplant · Pathology · T cell mediated rejection · Chronic rejection · Infections · Recurrent disease

Key Highlights

- Liver allograft biopsy is an important diagnostic tool in the management of patients after liver transplantation (LT).
- Most centers perform allograft biopsies only when there is graft dysfunction, which reveals a wide range of pathologies.
- Biopsy remains the gold standard for the diagnosis of TCMR and chronic rejection.
- Histopathological features together with diffuse immunopositivity of C4d and serum donor-specific antibody (DSA) levels are needed to establish a diagnosis of antibody-mediated rejection (AMR).
- Post-transplant liver biopsy may also highlight other causes of allograft dysfunction, such as infections, biliary and vascular complications, and disease recurrence.

M. Vij (✉)
Department of Pathology, Institute of Liver disease and Transplantation, Dr. Rela Institute and Medical Centre, Chennai, Tamil Nadu, India
e-mail: mukul.vij@relainstitute.com

S. Saigal, D. Jothimani (eds.), *Fundamentals of Transplant Hepatology*,
https://doi.org/10.1007/978-981-95-2624-6_31

Introduction: Liver transplantation (LT) has become an established treatment option for individuals with advanced chronic liver disease, acute liver failure, primary liver cancer, and various inherited and metabolic liver conditions in children [1, 2]. Annually, over 8000 LTs are conducted in the United States and around 3000 in India [3]. The two main surgical approaches to LT are deceased donor liver transplantation (DDLT) and living donor liver transplantation (LDLT). While DDLT is more prevalent in Western countries, LDLT is predominantly performed in transplant centers across Asia [3].

Liver allograft biopsy plays a crucial role in post-transplant patient care, serving as the gold standard for diagnosing T-cell mediated rejection (TCMR). It also aids in identifying or ruling out various causes of graft injury, such as biliary complications, vascular issues, infections, and recurrent liver disease [4]. Typically, liver allograft biopsies are carried out when abnormalities in liver function tests are detected, patients present symptoms like fever or abdominal pain, or imaging results suggest graft dysfunction [5]. Some centers also carry out routine, or protocol, biopsies at predetermined intervals even in the absence of clinical signs of graft problems.

Although LT offers excellent short-term survival outcomes, current focus lies in addressing long-term complications, including disease recurrence, the consequences of prolonged immunosuppression, and newly developed graft-related diseases, which can impact long-term survival [6]. This chapter explores the pre-transplant assessment of donor liver biopsies, the histological characteristics of allograft rejection, and other factors contributing to graft dysfunction. In certain cases, collaboration with transplant clinicians is essential for accurate pathological evaluation.

31.1 Pretransplant Deceased Donor Evaluation

Frozen section histology is done to evaluate livers from cadaveric donors when the transplant team is not clear about the quality of the organ on the basis of clinical and laboratory parameters [7]. Because of the widespread use of LT, there is an increasing need for donor organs, and marginal livers from extended-criteria donors are increasingly being considered for transplantation [8]. Despite the fact that pathological examination is not essential for such organs, pathologists are frequently asked to interpret the frozen sections [9]. Donor liver biopsy can provide useful information regarding the suitability of the organ prior to the LT. These biopsies are performed either at the procurement site or at the recipient hospital. A 1.5 cm^2 subcapsular wedge and/or a 2.0-cm-long Tru-Cut needle biopsy are considered sufficient to report diffuse liver pathologies [8]. Transplant surgeons at our center perform both wedge and needle biopsies. The biopsy should be submitted in

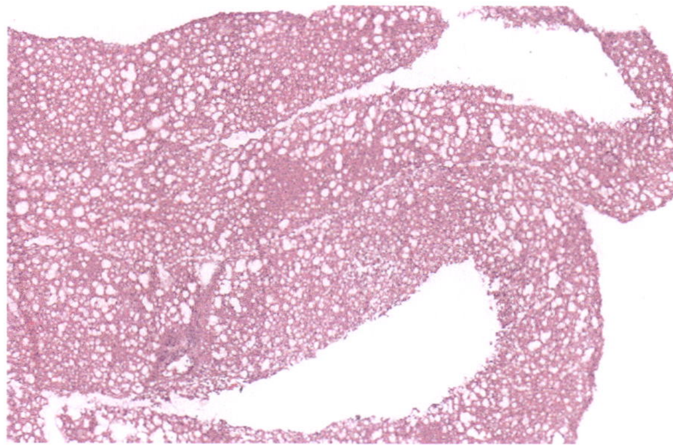

Fig. 31.1 Deceased donor liver frozen section with marked large droplet fat (organ was discarded, H&E)

a sterile container; use of gauze or saline should be avoided because they can introduce artifacts that can lead to incorrect biopsy interpretation [8]. The pathologist's job is to estimate steatosis type and percentage and/or comment on other pathologies like the amount of fibrosis, inflammation, necrosis, granuloma, or any malignancy if identified. The Banff Working Group on Liver Allograft Pathology recently released consensus criteria to report steatosis in frozen sections of potential donor livers [10].

Livers with marked large droplet fat (>60%, Fig. 31.1) are not accepted, as they are associated with severe post-transplant complications like early allograft dysfunction and primary nonfunction in LT recipients [11, 12]. Large droplet fat is defined as a single fat droplet distending the cell, which thus is larger than adjacent non-fatty/minimally fatty hepatocytes, and the nucleus, if present in the section, is displaced to the periphery of the hepatocyte [10]. True microvesicular steatosis is defined as numerous tiny droplets distending and filling hepatocytes and producing a foamy appearance of the cytoplasm, which are generally not seen in donor livers [13]. Smaller droplet fatty change is all fat droplets in a donor liver that are not large droplet fat or "true" microvesicular steatosis. Smaller droplet fatty change is an acute, "short-lived" process and is either a sign of liver injury or repair, and preimplantation donor smaller droplet fatty change has not been found to be a risk factor for early poor graft function and has no impact on long-term graft survival [10, 14]. Mild portal inflammation and/or mild bile ductular reaction in a donor biopsy may be secondary to prolonged intensive treatment and does not appear to have prognostic value for transplant outcome [15]. Livers with bridging fibrosis, centrilobular necrosis (>10%), necrotizing granulomas and malignancies are not utilized for LT [8].

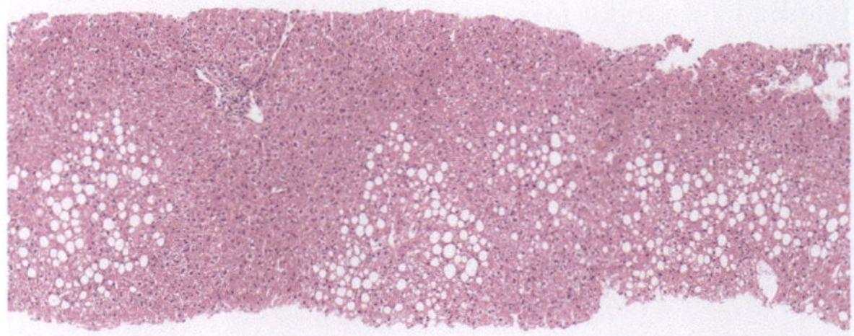

Fig. 31.2 Moderate steatosis (40%) in a living donor liver biopsy (H&E)

31.2 Pretransplant Living Donor Evaluation

A number of transplant centers in Asia perform LDLT due to the non-availability of deceased organs and because of various cultural and socio-economic factors [3]. Good liver quality is essential for both donor and recipient safety. Transplant centers have set protocols to evaluate living donors, and liver biopsies are performed when there are imaging abnormalities or if the body mass index (BMI) of the donor is high (>28 kg/m^2) or the donor has abnormal liver chemistries [16]. Other situations where pre-donation liver biopsy might be performed are donors with a history of significant use of alcohol or positive autoimmune serological tests [17]. The most common abnormality identified in living donor biopsies is macrovesicular steatosis, generally a manifestation of non-alcoholic fatty liver disease (NAFLD) [12]. Study by Minervini et al. reported macrovesicular steatosis in 48.5% of donors, ranging from 5% to 90%; 44 (15.5%) also showed steatohepatitis [18]. As with cadaveric liver grafts, mild degrees of steatosis (<20%) are tolerated, but donors are excluded if macrovesicular steatosis is >25% or 30% (Fig. 31.2) because of the risk to both donor and recipient of compromised liver regeneration [18–20]. Steatohepatitis (Fig. 31.3) is regarded as a contraindication to donation [21]. Living donors with any amount of fibrosis in the liver biopsy are rejected.

Pathologies in the liver allograft: Table 31.1 list causes of liver allograft dysfunction following LT.

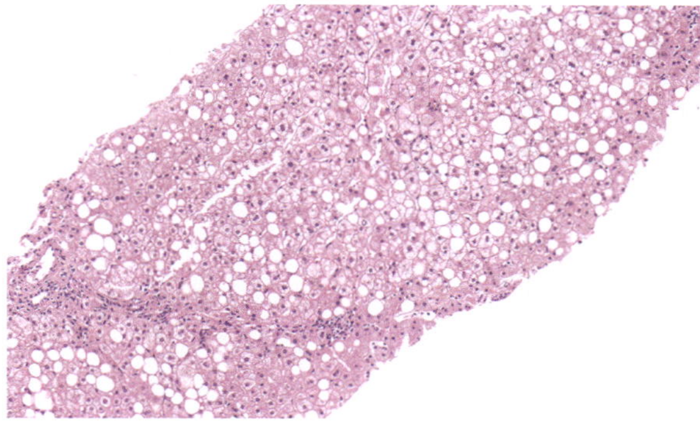

Fig. 31.3 NASH in a living donor liver biopsy (H&E)

Table 31.1 Pathological diagnoses in liver allograft biopsies

Ischemia–Reperfusion or preservation injury
Small-for-size syndrome or portal hyperperfusion injury
Rejection
Antibody-mediated rejection (hyperacute, acute, chronic)
T-cell mediated rejection
Plasma cell-rich rejection
Chronic rejection
Bacterial infections
Opportunistic viral infections
Cytomegalovirus
Herpes simplex virus
Epstein-Barr virus
Severe acute respiratory syndrome coronavirus 2
Arterial thrombosis/stenosis
Venous thrombosis/stenosis
Biliary complications
Recurrent diseases (viral, autoimmune, steatohepatitis)
Recurrent tumors
De novo diseases hepatitis (viral, steatohepatitis)
Idiopathic post-transplant chronic hepatitis
Hepatic structural abnormalities (nodular regenerative hyperplasia, others)

31.3 Ischemia–Reperfusion or Preservation Injury

At the time of organ harvesting and implantation, the liver allograft is subjected to stress and cellular injury, which is termed ischemia–reperfusion or preservation injury [22]. Ischemia–reperfusion injury constitutes a significant source of morbidity and mortality after LT [23]. The pathomechanism of ischemia–reperfusion injury is highly complex and multifactorial and is attributed to warm ischemia, cold ischemia, followed by reperfusion of the liver [13, 24]. Warm ischemia targets hepatocytes and results from poor perfusion of the liver at body temperature [5]. Warm ischemia also affects livers harvested after circulatory (cardiac) death [11]. Cold ischemia damages sinusoidal endothelial cells and results from storage of the liver

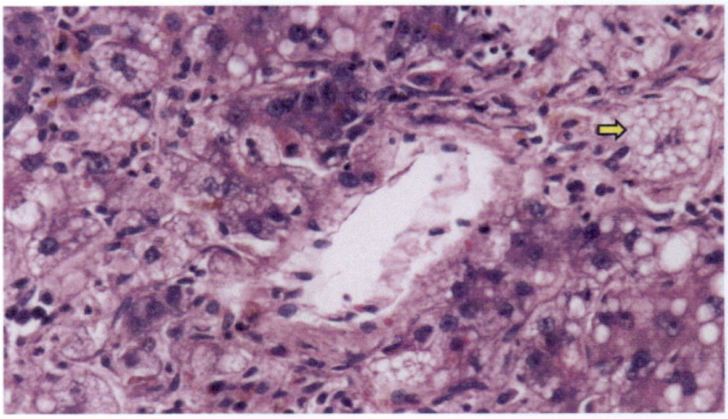

Fig. 31.4 Ischemia–reperfusion injury with centrilobular microvesicular steatosis (arrow) and lobular bilirubinostasis (H&E)

in preservation fluid at cold temperatures [5]. For short-term and long-term graft survival, warm ischemia time of less than 120 min and cold ischemia time of less than 10–12 h are considered optimal [11]. Resumption of blood flow following vascular anastomosis subjects the allograft to reperfusion injury and is the major cause of allograft injury [12]. Ischemia–reperfusion injury causes mitochondrial damage, activation of Kupffer cells and formation of reactive oxygen species, microcirculatory failure, and death of hepatocytes and sinusoidal endothelial cells [22]. Allograft biopsy with mild ischemia–reperfusion injury may show centrilobular hepatocellular swelling, microvesicular steatosis, centrilobular bilirubinostasis, spotty necrosis or apoptosis, polymorph aggregates, and rounding-up of hepatocyte cytoplasm with dissociation from adjacent hepatocytes (Fig. 31.4) [11–13]. Severe injury shows zonal or confluent hepatocyte necrosis, sometimes with bridging necrosis, bile ductular proliferation, cholangiolar cholestasis, and severe neutrophilic exudation.

31.4 Small-for-Size Syndrome or Portal Hyperperfusion Injury

Small-for-size syndrome or portal hyperperfusion injury is a well-recognized clinical syndrome that primarily occurs in LT recipients of reduced size grafts and in those with adequately sized grafts but with severe portal hypertension [25]. It is defined by the presence of prolonged cholestasis, coagulopathy, and ascites within the first postoperative week [26]. If the graft-to-recipient-weight ratio is less than 0.8, a graft is considered “small for size.” [27] The underlying pathogenesis of small-for-size syndrome is not well understood. In the liver graft there is reciprocal regulation between portal vein and hepatic arterial inflow mediated via hepatic arterial buffer response [5, 28]. Increased portal venous flow reduces hepatic arterial flow, whereas decreased portal flow increases hepatic arterial flow. This balance is maintained by a constant release of adenosine, which is a vasodilator among the hepatic arterioles and portal venules. Increased portal flow causes accelerated adenosine washout, resulting in constriction of the hepatic artery and a reduction in

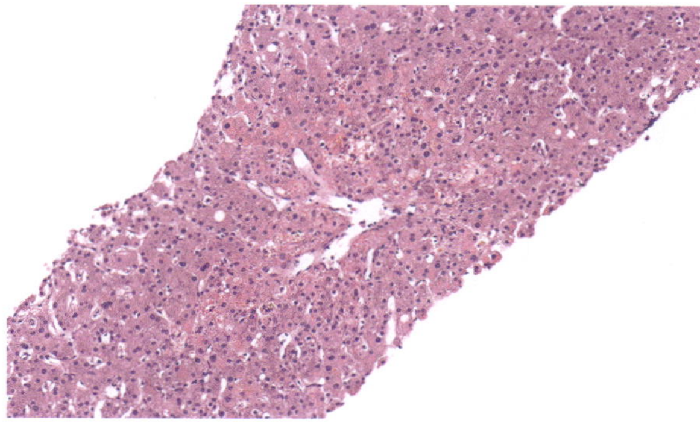

Fig. 31.5 Liver allograft biopsy with lobular bilirubinostasis in a case of small-for-size syndrome

arterial flow. Early pathological findings in the graft include portal vein and periportal sinusoidal endothelial denudation and portal tract hemorrhage, which dissected into the periportal hepatic parenchyma when severe [28]. Hepatocyte ballooning, centrilobular steatosis, and parenchymal bilirubinostasis (Fig. 31.5) are also reported [12]. Poor hepatic arterial flow and vasospasm can lead to functional dearterialization, ischemic cholangitis, and parenchymal infarcts. Late graft sequelae include small portal vein branch thrombosis with occasional luminal obliteration or recanalization, nodular regenerative hyperplasia (NRH), and bile duct strictures [28].

31.5 Antibody-Mediated Rejection

Antibody-mediated rejection (AMR), previously referred to as "humoral" rejection, was initially observed in liver transplants (LT) involving ABO-incompatible (ABO-I) donors and later identified in ABO-compatible (ABO-C) transplants in the presence of lymphocytotoxic or donor-specific antibodies (DSAs) [29]. AMR occurs infrequently in ABO-C grafts due to the liver's unique immunologically privileged status [30, 31]. This immune tolerance is attributed to several features: the liver's dual blood supply (arterial and portal venous), its large parenchymal volume offering extensive endothelial surface area, relatively low expression of HLA class II antigens, the presence of Kupffer cells in the sinusoids that help clear circulating immune complexes, and the organ's robust regenerative capacity.

Though the true incidence of AMR in ABO-C liver transplants is uncertain—largely due to under-recognition—it is believed to affect fewer than 1% of all patients and less than 5% of sensitized individuals [32]. AMR is triggered by preformed or newly developed DSAs that target endothelial antigens, initiating antigen–antibody interactions that damage endothelial cells and activate the complement system [13]. The risk of AMR is influenced by factors such as antibody class, titer, specificity, and timing, as well as the density and distribution of target antigens [29]. Diagnosing AMR has historically been difficult, as updated guidelines and standardized criteria have only recently been introduced [29].

31.5.1 Hyperacute Antibody-Mediated Rejection

Hyperacute AMR of the liver is exceptionally rare and is mostly seen in patients undergoing ABO-I LT [13]. Due to the rapid onset of liver failure and coagulopathy, biopsy is seldom performed in these cases. When affected allografts are removed, they are typically enlarged and exhibit extensive parenchymal hemorrhagic necrosis, polymorphonuclear inflammation, as well as fibrinoid necrosis and thrombosis of blood vessels [4, 12].

31.5.2 Acute Antibody Mediate Rejection in ABO-Compatible Allografts

Acute AMR is usually seen within the first several days/weeks after LT in highly sensitized patients and presents as hyperbilirubinemia, refractory thrombocytopenia, and low serum complement levels [29]. In patients with TCMR not responding to standard corticosteroid therapy, AMR should be considered [30]. A "two-hit" hypothesis has been proposed to describe the acute AMR mechanism [33]. There is an initial insult to the allograft (e.g., TCMR, ischemic insult, ischemia-reperfusion injury, hepatitis) leading to HLA class II upregulation and expression, thus facilitating binding of DSA and activating the classical complement cascade. Liver allograft biopsies in acute AMR show microvascular dilatation, endothelial cell enlargement, hobnailing, and leukocyte sludging/margination involving portal vein branches, portal and peribiliary plexus capillaries, and inlet venules, rarely extending into sinusoids and central veins (Fig. 31.6) [29, 34]. Other findings include portal/periportal edema, periportal necrosis, bile ductular reaction, apoptosis, centrilobular hepatocellular swelling and hepatocanalicular cholestasis, and in severe cases, focal perihilar bile duct necrosis and arterial vasospastic changes. Veno occlusive lesion has also been reported [35]. Arterial endothelitis and mural fibrinoid necrosis are rare but diagnostic of acute AMR when combined with diffuse C4d deposits and DSA.

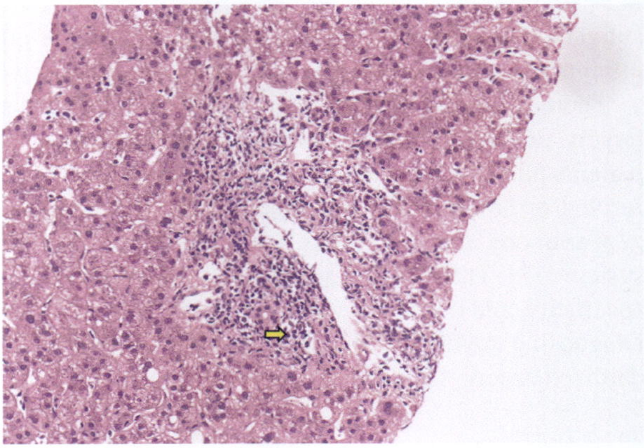

Fig. 31.6 Liver allograft biopsy with microvascular dilatation and leucocyte sludging (arrow) admixed with features of TCMR

Fig. 31.7 Acute AMR in an ABO-I recipient with confluent necrosis (arrow), congestion, and biliary proliferation

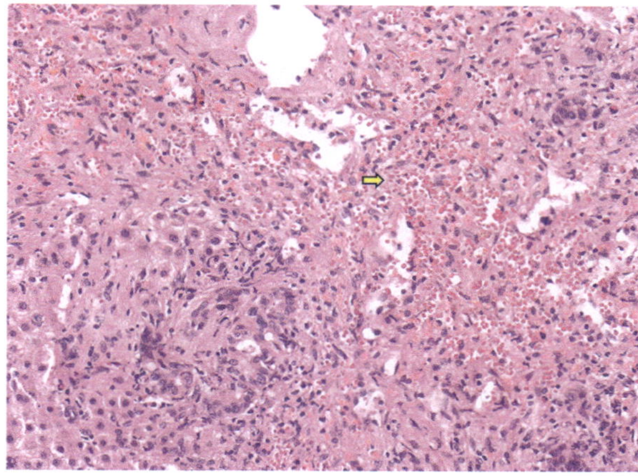

31.5.3 Acute Antibody Mediate Rejection in ABO-Incompatible Allografts

Highly effective desensitizing therapy have markedly reduced the incidence of antibody- AMR in ABO-I LT [36, 37]. Reported biopsy findings include platelet-fibrin thrombi in sinusoidal and portal veins, red blood cell (RBC), and neutrophil sinusoidal sludging, portal hemorrhage, and apoptosis. Biopsy may also demonstrate portal edema, portal microvascular endothelial cell enlargement/hypertrophy, focal fibrin deposition, periportal hepatocyte clusters with necrosis, and congestion (Fig. 31.7) [38, 39]. Fibrinoid necrosis of portal artery branches, neutrophilic inflammation, and cholangitis have also been described. In untreated recipients with high titers, progressive patchy geographic hemorrhagic necrosis occurs. Recipients who survive can develop biliary strictures caused by ischemic cholangiopathy.

31.5.4 C4d Immunohistochemistry

Complement C4d deposition is an indicator of tissue-based complement activation and, in an appropriate pathological context, is a reliable tissue marker of AMR [40, 41]. C4d can be detected by immunohistochemistry (IHC) or immunofluorescence [29]. Demonstration of diffuse linear or granular C4d deposition in portal microvascular endothelial cells is required to establish a diagnosis of definite acute AMR. C4d positivity may also extend into inlet venules or periportal sinusoids. Banff in 2016 proposed the histopathology component (h) score (Table 31.2) and C4d component score (Table 31.3 and Fig. 31.8) to be done on liver biopsy in cases of acute AMR [29]. The criteria for diagnosis of acute antibody-mediated rejection are mentioned in Table 31.4 [29].

Table 31.2 h-(histopathology)-score for acute AMR [29]

1: Portal microvascular endothelial cell enlargement (portal veins, capillaries, and inlet venules) involving a majority of portal tracts with sparse microvasculitis defined as three to four marginated and/or intraluminal monocytes, neutrophils, or eosinophils in the maximally involved capillary with mild dilation
2: Monocytic, eosinophilic, or neutrophilic microvasculitis/capillaritis, defined as at least 5–10 leukocytes marginated and/or intraluminal in the maximally involved capillary, prominent portal, and/or sinusoidal microvascular endothelial cell enlargement involving a majority of portal tracts or sinusoids, with variable portal capillary and inlet venule dilatation and variable portal edema
3: As above, with marked capillary dilatation, marked microvasculitis/capillaritis (10 or more marginated and/or intraluminal leukocytes in the most severely affected vessels), at least focal microvascular disruption with fibrin deposition, and extravasation of red blood cells into the portal stroma and/or space of Disse

Table 31.3 C4d-(immune)-score (formalin-fixed, paraffin-embedded) for acute AMR [29]

0: No C4d deposition in portal microvasculature
2: Minimal (<10% portal tracts) C4d deposition in >50% of the circumference of portal microvascular endothelium (portal veins and capillaries)
3: Focal (10–50% portal tracts) C4d deposition in >50% of the circumference of portal microvascular endothelium (portal veins and capillaries)—usually without extension into periportal sinusoids
4: Diffuse (>50% portal tracts) C4d deposition in >50% of the circumference of portal microvascular endothelia (portal veins and capillaries)—often with extension into inlet venules or periportal sinusoids

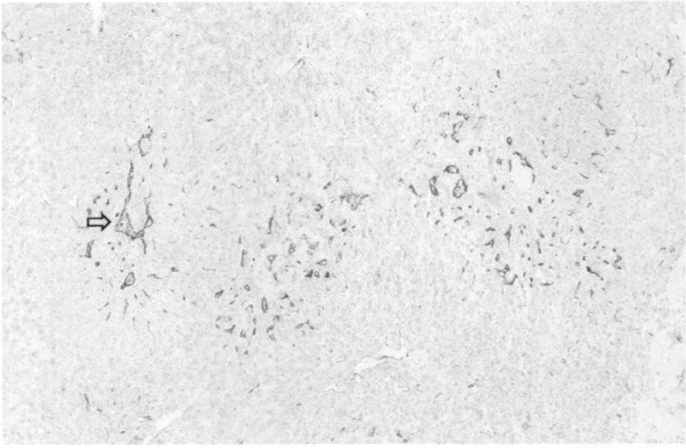

Fig. 31.8 Diffuse C4d deposition (arrow) in portal vessels, inlet venules, and periportal sinusoids in a case of acute AMR in ABO-I LT

Table 31.4 Criteria for diagnosis of acute antibody-mediated rejection [29]

Definite for acute AMR (all four criteria required)	
1.	Portal microvascular endothelial cell hypertrophy; portal capillary and inlet venule dilation; portal microvasculitis (monocytic, eosinophilic, and neutrophilic); portal edema; bile ductular reaction; variable bilirubinostasis; edema and periportal hepatocyte necrosis are more common or prominent in ABO-I grafts; variable active lymphocytic and/or necrotizing arteritis
2.	Positive serum DSA
3.	Diffuse microvascular C4d deposition (C4d score = 3) on frozen or formalin-fixed, paraffin-embedded tissue in ABO-C liver allograft or portal stromal C4d deposition in ABO-I allografts
4.	Reasonable exclusion of other insults that might cause a similar pattern of injury; most patients have C4d scores: 3 + h-score = 5 or 6
Suspicious for AMR (both criteria required)	
1.	Positive serum DSA
2.	Non zero h-score with C4d-score + h-score of 3 or 4
Indeterminate for AMR (requires 1 + 2 and 3 OR 4)	
1.	C4d score + h-score is ≥ 2
2.	DSA not available, equivocal, or negative
3.	C4d staining not available, equivocal, or negative
4.	Coexisting insult might be contributing to the injury

31.5.5 Chronic Antibody-Mediated Rejection

Chronic AMR is a challenging diagnosis due to a lack of specific clinical, biochemical, or pathologic features [42]. Chronic AMR has been believed to occur in approximately 8–15% of recipients who retain or form de novo DSAs against HLA class II molecules (especially DQ) [43, 44]. Evidence in this regard has mostly come from long-term adult and pediatric LT recipients who had protocol liver biopsies or achieved operational tolerance. Histological findings strongly associated with persistent DSA include low-grade portal, periportal, and perivenular lymphoplasmacytic inflammation with low-grade interface and perivenular necro-inflammatory activity [45]. Dense portal collagenization and obliterative portal venopathy have also been reported. The above features, with or without positive C4d immunostaining, are strongly associated with chronic AMR. Consensus criteria for the diagnosis of chronic AMR are listed in Table 31.5 [29].

31.6 T Cell-Mediated Rejection

TCMR, previously referred to as acute cellular rejection (ACR), is the most common cause of allograft dysfunction. TCMR can be categorized as early (occurring <6 months after LT) or late (>6 months after LT) [29]. Most cases occur early and usually resolve with immunosuppressive treatment. The incidence of early TCMR is between 10% and 30% [32]. The classic histologic features (Fig. 31.9) of early

Table 31.5 Consensus criteria for the diagnosis of chronic AMR [29]

1: Histopathological pattern of injury consistent with chronic AMR:
(a) Otherwise, unexplained, and at least mild mononuclear portal and/or perivenular inflammation with interface and/or perivenular necro-inflammatory activity
(b) At least moderate portal/periportal, sinusoidal, and/or perivenular fibrosis
2: Recent circulating anti-HLA DSA in serum samples
3: At least focal C4d-positivity
4: Reasonable exclusion of other insults that might cause a similar pattern of injury
Possible chronic active AMR: As above, but C4d staining is minimal or absent

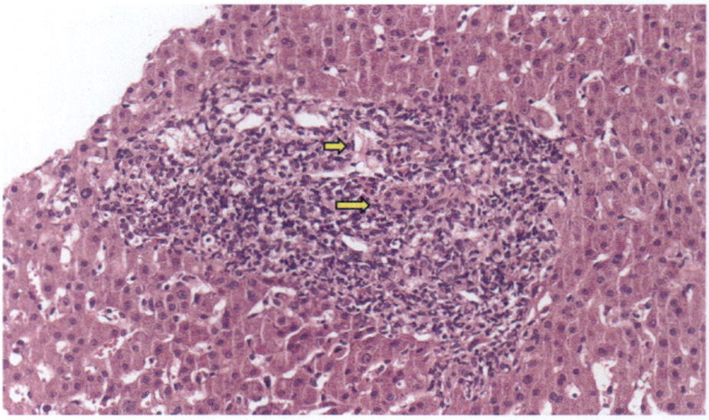

Fig. 31.9 Severe T cell-mediated rejection with marked portal inflammation, ductulitis (large arrow), and portal venulitis (small arrow). Interface activity is also noted

TCMR is (1) portal mixed inflammatory cell infiltrates, (2) bile duct damage, and (3) subendothelial inflammation of portal veins and/or terminal hepatic venules (endotheliitis) [11–13]. At least two of these features should be present for TCMR diagnosis. The portal inflammatory cell infiltrates consist of admixture of lymphocytes, activated or blastic lymphocytes (usually medium or large lymphocytes), macrophages, eosinophils, and neutrophils. Infiltration of bile duct epithelium by lymphocytes (lymphocytic cholangitis) or a mixed population of cells is also noted. Rarely, intraluminal neutrophils mimicking ascending cholangitis may be present. This is accompanied by varying degrees of damage to biliary epithelium manifested as nuclear irregularity, overlapping, and hyperchromasia along with vacuolation of cytoplasm. A mild ductular reaction may be seen. Endotheliitis demonstrating endothelial cell injury and lifting of endothelial cells another feature of rejection and is seen in portal and/or hepatic venules (Fig. 31.10). Endotheliitis of the hepatic arteries may also occur but is exceedingly rare in the smaller arterioles sampled in Tru-Cut biopsies. Recently, isolated "v" lesions (inflammatory, necrotizing, and/or obliterative arteriopathy) have been recognized and associated with impending TCMR and/or chronic AMR [46].

Severity of TCMR is based on the intensity of inflammation and distribution, degree of tissue damage, and direct or indirect signs of vascular/ischemic injury. TCMR is histologically graded in two ways. First is global assessment is graded as indeterminate, mild, moderate, or severe and is based on the severity of portal inflammation and extent of central perivenular inflammation and hepatocyte necrosis/dropout (Table 31.6) [47]. Second is Banff TCMR scoring on a scale of 0–9

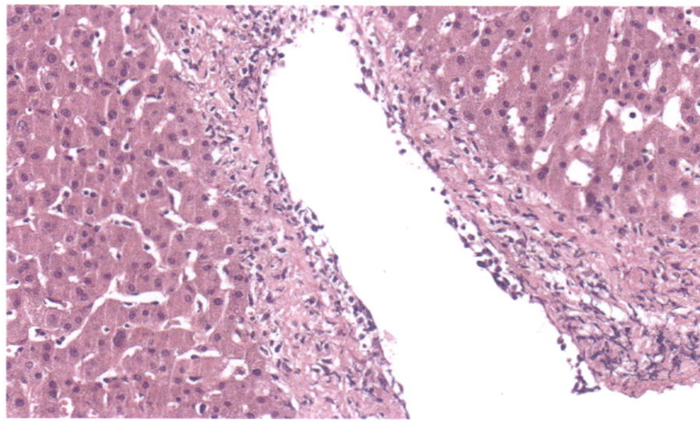

Fig. 31.10 Central vein endothelitis with lifting of endothelium and subendothelial lymphocytic inflammation in a case of severe TCMR (H&E)

Table 31.6 Global assessment of T cell-mediated rejection

Indeterminate: Portal and/or perivenular inflammation related to an alloreactivity, but shows insufficient tissue injury to meet criteria for a diagnosis of mild TCMR
Mild: Rejection-type inflammation in a minority of the portal tracts or perivenular areas that is generally mild and mostly confined within the portal spaces for portal-based rejection and an absence of confluent necrosis/hepatocyte dropout for those presenting with isolated perivenular inflammation
Moderate: Rejection-type inflammation, expanding majority or all of portal tracts and/or focal involvement of perivenular areas with confluent necrosis/hepatocyte dropout
Severe: As above for moderate, with spillover into periportal areas and/or diffuse moderate-to-severe perivenular inflammation that extends into the hepatic parenchyma and is associated with perivenular hepatocyte necrosis

(Table 31.7) [29]. Portal inflammation, bile duct inflammation/damage, and venous inflammation/endotheliitis are semiquantitatively graded as 0 (absent) to 3 (severe). Total score determines whether rejection is indeterminate 1–2, mild 3–4, moderate 5–6, or severe 7–9. Mild TCMR can be treated by optimization of immunosuppressive therapy. Moderate or severe TCMR is more likely to be associated with biochemical signs of graft dysfunction and is treated with pulse steroid therapy.

31.7 Late T-Cell-Mediated Rejection

Late TCMR occurs several months after LT and may show slightly different morphologic features as compared to early TCMR described earlier [48]. Histologically, late TCMR usually resembles chronic hepatitis with monomorphic portal inflammation (Fig. 31.11), low-grade interface activity, patchy lobular activity, and centrizonal necroinflammation, i.e., central perivenulitis [11–13]. Central perivenulitis is characterized by a centrizonal inflammatory cell infiltrate with or without centrilobular hepatocyte injury, necrosis, and dropout. Central perivenulitis may occur in isolation or in association with portal inflammation. Central vein endotheliitisis often not present at this stage. Isolated central perivenulitis is a histologic finding

Table 31.7 Semiquantitative scoring (rejection activity index [RAI])

Score	Parameter	Criteria
1	Portal inflammation	Mostly lymphocytic inflammation in a minority of the portal tracts
2		Mixed inflammatory infiltrate containing lymphocytes with occasional blasts, neutrophils, and eosinophils expanding most or all of the portal tracts
3		Mixed infiltrate containing blasts, macrophages, eosinophils, and/or polymorphs markedly expanding most or all of the portal tracts with inflammatory spillover into the periportal parenchyma
1	Bile duct inflammation and damage	Inflammatory cells involving a minority of the bile ducts and only mild injury to the bile duct epithelium, such as nuclear enlargement of the epithelial cells
2		Inflammatory cells involving most or all of the bile ducts and more than an occasional duct show degenerative changes such as nuclear anisomorphism, disordered polarity, and cytoplasmic vacuolization
3		Inflammatory cells involving most or all of the bile ducts, with most or all of the ducts showing degenerative changes or focal luminal disruption
1	Venous endothelial inflammation	Subendothelial lymphocytic infiltration involving some, but not a majority of the portal and/or hepatic venules
2		Subendothelial infiltration involving most or all of the portal and/or hepatic venules with or without confluent hepatocyte necrosis/dropout involving a minority of perivenular regions
3		Moderate or severe subendothelial infiltration that extends into the perivenular parenchyma and is associated with perivenular hepatocyte necrosis involving a majority of perivenular regions

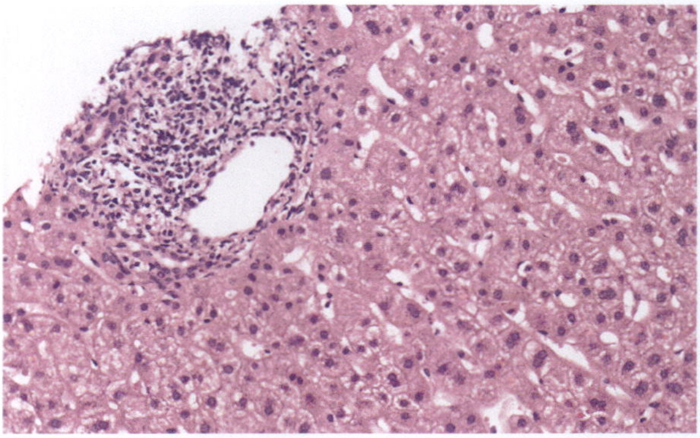

Fig. 31.11 Late T-cell-mediated rejection with monomorphic portal inflammation (H&E)

that may be seen in late TCMR [49]. Late TCMR shows less bile duct injury and portal endotheliitis as compared to early TCMR, and recipients are more likely to be partially response or resistant to increased immunosuppression and may have a higher risk for chronic rejection, fibrosis, and allograft loss [50, 51].

31.8 Plasma Cell–Rich Rejection

Plasma cell-rich rejection, also known as "de novo autoimmune hepatitis," is a type of liver allograft dysfunction that develops in recipients transplanted for etiologies other than autoimmune hepatitis (AIH) [52]. Plasma cell-rich rejection is proposed to be an immune-mediated allograft dysfunction which falls under the spectrum of mixed TCMR/AMR etiology overlapping with autoimmunity in the post-LT setting [29]. This condition was first described in pediatric LT recipients, predominantly in children transplanted for biliary atresia [53]. Subsequently, plasma cell-rich rejection has been recognized in adults patients transplanted for other etiologies [54]. Plasma cell-rich rejection usually responds to standard immunosuppressive therapies; however, in a few cases, it may be a cause of late graft failure and cirrhosis. Several reports indicate the incidence of plasma cell-rich rejection to be 3–5% [55, 56]. It has been reported that these anti-glutathione-s-transferase T1 (GSTT1) antibodies are a risk factor for the development of plasma cell-rich rejection [57]. Histological findings include expanded portal tracts with plasma cell-rich inflammatory cell infiltrates accompanied by prominent interface activity and portal fibrosis (Fig. 31.12). Severe lymphocytic cholangitis is also noted. Lobular inflammation and necrosis, especially plasma cell-rich central perivenulitis, may be seen. Varying degrees of central venular endotheliitis and perivenular fibrosis may be seen. C4d deposits can be demonstrated in the portal microvasculature. Table 31.8 outlines the diagnostic criteria for plasma cell–rich rejection.

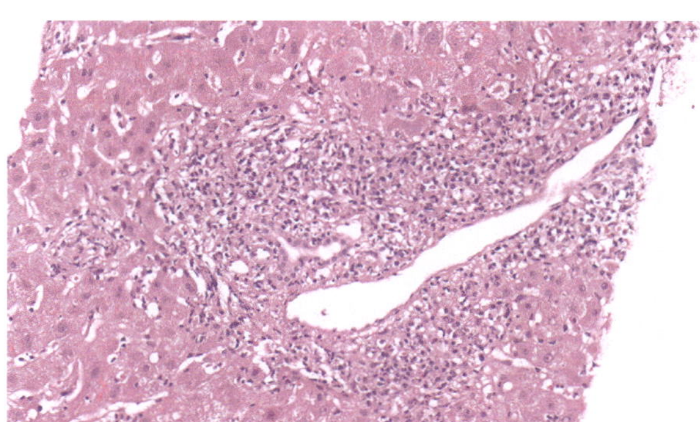

Fig. 31.12 Plasma cell-rich rejection in a liver allograft with severe portal plasma cells (>50%), interface activity, and cholangitis

Table 31.8 Diagnostic criteria for plasma cell-rich rejection [29]

Must fulfill criteria 1 and 3; criterion 2 is desirable, but not absolutely required:
(1) Portal and/or perivenular plasma cells (>30%) with easily identifiable periportal/interface and/or perivenular necro-inflammation usually involving most portal tracts and/or central veins. Histological grading is at least "moderate" with a total RAI score ≥5 because "V score" is usually "3" because of severe perivenular activity, whereas the "portal inflammation" score is usually ≥2
(2) Lymphocytic cholangitis is usually present and a desirable feature, but not absolutely required (bile duct damage secondary to inflammation might be a relatively minor component, but the Banff component score for bile duct injury is usually ≥1)
(3) Original disease other than AIH

31.9 Chronic Rejection

With the advent of improved immunosuppressive therapies, the incidence of chronic rejection has significantly declined, now accounting for the loss of fewer than 2% of liver grafts [58]. Most cases of chronic rejection occur more than 12 months after LT, although some instances have been reported as early as 3 months post-transplant [13]. Known risk factors include autoimmune liver disorders, donor-recipient sex mismatch, prolonged cold ischemia time, suboptimal immunosuppression, recurrent or severe TCMR, untreated or refractory rejection, active cytomegalovirus (CMV) infection, the use of cyclosporine, and older donor age [59–61].

Patients typically present with persistent jaundice, sustained elevation of bilirubin, increased alkaline phosphatase, and elevated transaminases. Chronic rejection is pathologically defined by the loss of small interlobular bile ducts in more than 50% of portal tracts and by the presence of obliterative arteriopathy [48]. The diagnostic criteria are outlined in Table 31.9. Histologically, chronic rejection is categorized into "early" and "late" phases, although no precise timeline distinguishes progression from one to the other [29, 59, 62].

In the early phase, small interlobular bile ducts are infiltrated by lymphocytes, leading to damage of the biliary epithelium. This includes nuclear irregularities, disturbed polarity, nuclear dropout, and cytoplasmic eosinophilia, resulting in ductal atrophy, degeneration, or senescence. At this stage, bile duct loss involves fewer than 50% of portal tracts. Expression of the senescence marker p21 is detectable in the atrophic ducts [63].

In later stages, bile duct loss extends to more than 50% of portal tracts and is typically associated with reduced portal inflammation, producing a characteristic "burnt-out" appearance (Fig. 31.13). The injury predominantly affects small interlobular bile ducts and can be diagnosed via needle biopsy. In most cases, a marked bile ductular reaction is absent unless there is a distal bile duct stricture. Immunohistochemical staining for cytokeratin 7 (CK7) can confirm both bile duct loss and the absence of a ductular reaction. Additional findings may include lobular cholestasis, bile-laden Kupffer cells, and clusters of foamy macrophages. The arteriopathy seen in chronic rejection usually involves medium and large arteries, presenting as lipid-laden foamy macrophages within the intimal layer.

Table 31.9 Pathological features in early and late stages of chronic rejection

Structure	Early chronic rejection (at least two features should be present)	Late chronic rejection (at least two features should be present)
Small bile ducts (<60 μm)	Most ducts show senescence-related changes; loss of bile ducts <50% of portal tracts	Bile duct loss in ≥50% of portal tracts; atrophic changes in residual bile ducts
Hepatic arterioles	Loss of arterioles in <25% of portal tracts	Loss of arterioles in >25% of portal tracts
Terminal hepatic venules and centrizonal hepatocytes	Centrizonal inflammation; centrizonal necrosis and inflammation; and mild perivenular fibrosis	Variable inflammation; focal luminal obliteration; moderate-to severe-(bridging) scarring
Large perihilar hepatic artery branches	Intimal inflammation, focal foam cell collection without luminal narrowing	Intimal foam cells with luminal narrowing; fibrointimal proliferation
Large perihilar bile ducts	Inflammation damage and focal foam cell deposition	Mural fibrosis
Other	Lobular spotty necrosis (so-called "transition" hepatitis)	Accumulation of foam cells in sinusoids; bilirubinostasis

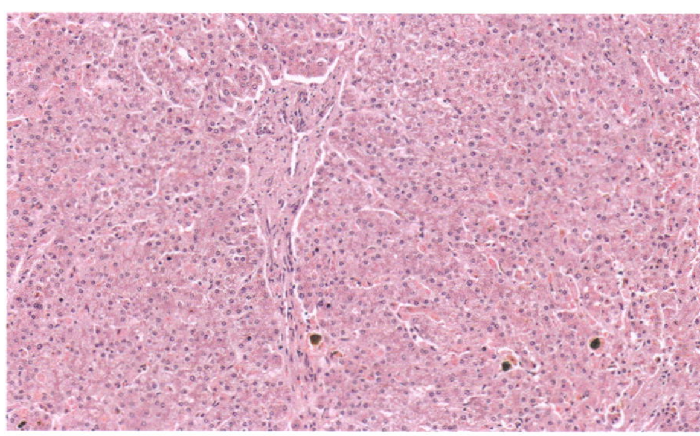

Fig. 31.13 Chronic rejection with duct loss, minimal portal inflammation, and lobular bilirubinostasis

31.10 Infections

Infections are very common and a major cause of morbidity and mortality in LT recipients, particularly in the early post-transplant period [64, 65]. Due to various prophylactic measures along with early diagnosis and treatment, the prevalence of infection as a cause of mortality has declined from >50% before 1980 to <10% in the recent decade. Bacterial infections, fungal infections, and viral infections affect LT recipients [65, 66]. Bacterial infections are the most common in graft recipients; however, direct morphological evidence of bacterial infection in the liver allograft biopsy is not seen. Gram-negative septicemia is associated with a characteristic picture of cholangitis lenta. There is portal expansion with bile ductular reaction and bile plugging at the periphery of portal tracts (Fig. 31.14). Polymorphs are identified in the portal tracts. Lobular bilirubinostasis is also noted.

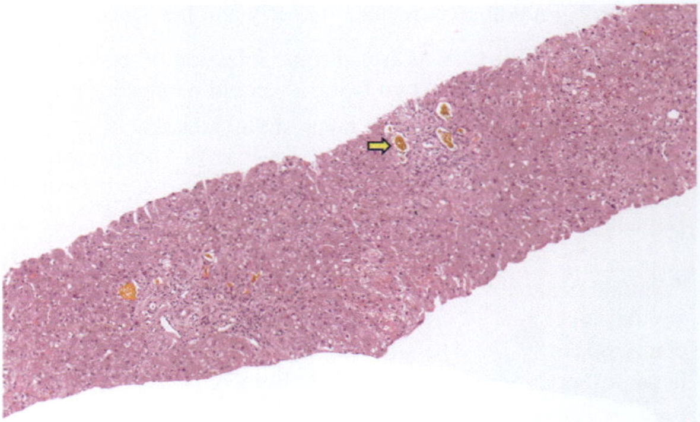

Fig. 31.14 Cholangitis lenta with bile ductular reaction, luminal dilatation, and bile plugging (arrow, H&E)

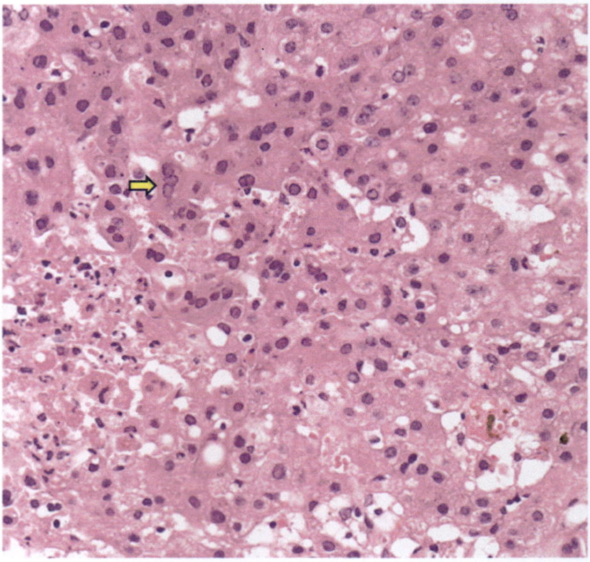

Fig. 31.15 HSV hepatitis with intranuclear inclusions (arrow), multinucleation, and necrosis. Lobular bilirubinostasis is also noted

31.10.1 Opportunistic Viral Infections

Herpes simplex virus (HSV) infection is a rare but very serious complication after LT [66]. It usually presents very early in the postoperative course and may confuse the clinical picture of graft dysfunction and altered liver function tests. HSV hepatitis is infectious disease emergency, with a high mortality rate of 58% [67]. Liver biopsy in HSV hepatitis shows confluent areas of hepatocyte necrosis, glassy amphophilic intranuclear inclusions, and the presence of multinucleated hepatocytes (Fig. 31.15). Mild portal inflammation and lobular bilirubinostasis is also reported. HSV immunostaining is helpful in diagnosis.

There is a marked reduction in CMV infection because of prophylactic antiviral therapy and routine infection monitoring [65, 68]. Reactivation of the latent CMV virus of either donor or recipient origin results in CMV infection. The most important risk factor for CMV infection is donation from a CMV-seropositive donor to a CMV-seronegative recipient [69]. Neutrophil polymorph aggregates (microabscesses) within the liver parenchyma are the most common pathological finding in CMV hepatitis. CMV viral inclusions can be noted in hepatocytes, biliary epithelial cells, endothelial cells, or stromal cells. Basophilic nuclear inclusions separated from the nuclear membrane by a clear halo are noted. Cytoplasmic inclusions are granular and eosinophilic. Immunohistochemical staining can be helpful to identify or confirm the presence of viral inclusions.

31.10.2 Epstein Barr Virus Infection

EBV hepatitis in the allograft is characterized by portal mononuclear inflammation and sinusoidal lymphocytosis in the lobule [70]. Eosinophils and neutrophils are rare. The lymphoid cells may appear larger than mature lymphocytes and atypical. Significant hepatocyte necrosis is not seen. The lymphoid cells in EBV hepatitis predominantly comprise B cells, in contrast to the T cells of other inflammatory diseases [58]. Epstein-Barr encoding region in situ hybridization demonstrates positivity within the infiltrating lymphoid cells.

31.10.3 Severe Acute Respiratory Syndrome Coronavirus 2 Infection

A novel severe acute respiratory syndrome coronavirus 2 (SARS-CoV2), or coronavirus disease 2019 (COVID-19) associated with significant morbidity and mortality, was identified in Wuhan, China, in December 2019 [71]. The COVID-19 pandemic was declared an emergency by the World Health Organization (WHO) in March 2020, and it has significantly impacted many aspects of healthcare, including liver transplant worldwide. SARS-CoV2 infection can occur in liver allograft and biopsies may show portal and lobular inflammation, apoptosis, and rarely vascular thrombi (Fig. 31.16) [71].

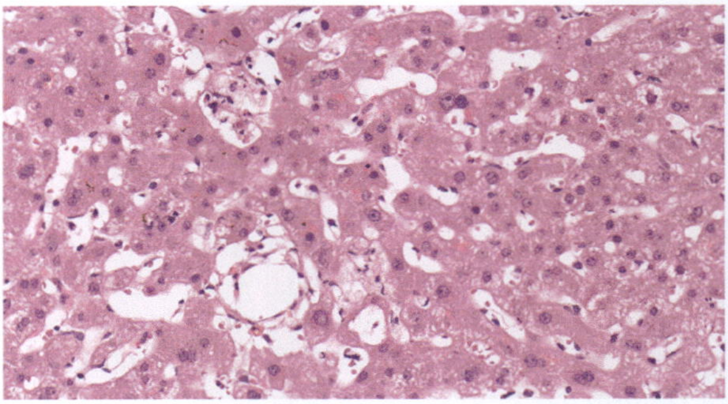

Fig. 31.16 Graft biopsy with lobular disarray, activity, and acute bilirubinostasis in a recipient with SARS-CoV2 infection

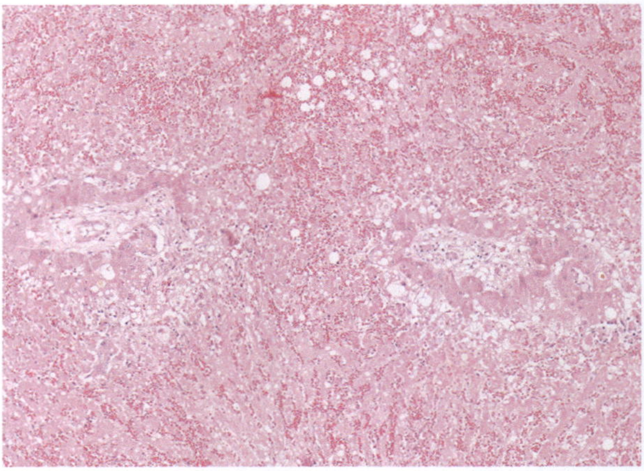

Fig. 31.17 Liver tissue with extensive necrosis and congestion in a case of hepatic artery thrombosis

31.11 Hepatic Artery Thrombosis or Stenosis

Thrombosis, stenosis, or kinking of the hepatic artery may compromise arterial flow. The incidence is reported to be highest in children and reduced size liver grafts because of smaller vessels and size mismatch; however, improved expertise in microvascular anastomotic techniques has remarkably reduced the incidence of hepatic artery thrombosis [72, 73]. Thrombosis occurring early in the posttransplant period causes ischemic parenchymal necrosis (Fig. 31.17). Late slow occurring thrombosis usually results in ischemic bile duct injury, which may resemble primary sclerosing cholangitis (PSC) radiologically. Macroscopically irregular subcapsular pale areas of necrosis that are demarcated from the surrounding parenchyma by a darker border.

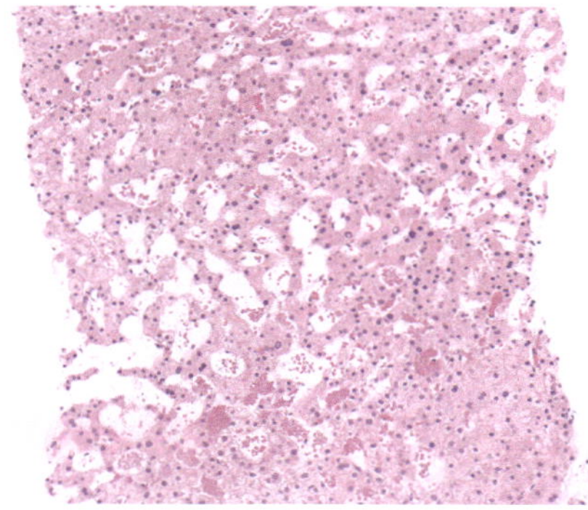

Fig. 31.18 Liver allograft biopsy with sinusoidal dilation, sinusoidal congestion, and hepatocyte atrophy

31.12 Hepatic Venous Outflow Obstruction

Thrombosis of the hepatic vein or anatomical stricture or kinking of the hepatic vein causing venous outflow obstruction is an uncommon complication with an overall frequency of 1% [74]. Pathological diagnosis of venous outflow obstruction in the liver allograft is problematic, because similar changes can also be seen in rejection. Typical findings in such cases include centrilobular sinusoidal dilation, sinusoidal congestion, hepatocyte atrophy, and perivenular hepatocyte dropout (Fig. 31.18).

31.13 Biliary Complications

Biliary complications are a common cause of liver allograft dysfunction and may present as bile leaks (bilioma), strictures, casts, biliary sludge, or stones. Approximately 10–15% in DDLT and 15–30% in LDLT or split-liver transplant recipients develop anastomotic or non-anastomotic biliary complications [75]. Anastomotic complications are usually due to technical issues with the surgery and develop at the site of the surgical anastomosis of the donor bile duct. Nonanastomotic complications are mostly related to vascular and immunological events. Liver allograft biopsies typically show portal expansion with edematous fibroplasia, bile ductular proliferation, neutrophilic inflammation, and cholestasis (Fig. 31.19). Medium- and large bile ducts may show inflammation, ulceration, and necrosis, although such ducts are rarely sampled in biopsy material.

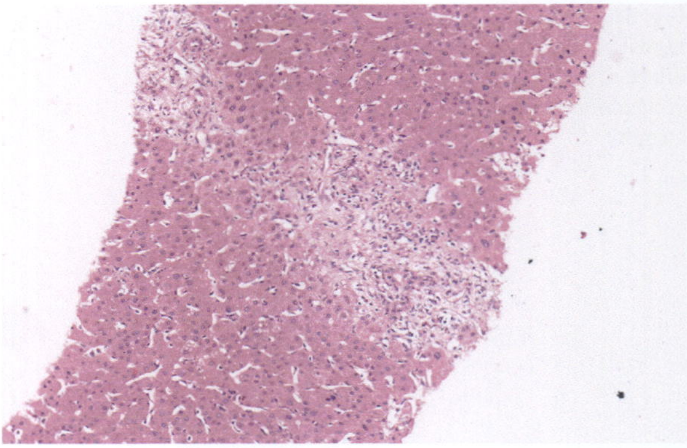

Fig. 31.19 Liver allograft biopsy with features of biliary obstruction. There is portal expansion with edema, bile ductular proliferation, and inflammation (H&E)

31.14 Recurrent Diseases

31.14.1 Recurrent Hepatitis B

Chronic hepatitis B remains a significant global health issue, affecting approximately 296 million individuals, with the highest prevalence in Asia and Africa [76]. Historically, LT for hepatitis B was considered high-risk due to a substantial chance of graft reinfection (approximately 70–80%) and poor post-transplant outcomes, with 2-year survival rates below 50% [65, 77]. Many of these patients developed fibrosing cholestatic hepatitis (FCH), a rapidly progressive and severe liver injury [78].

However, advancements in antiviral therapy—administered both before and after transplantation—and the introduction of hepatitis B immunoglobulin in the postoperative period have markedly improved long-term graft survival [79]. Today, the combination of third-generation nucleos(t)ide analogues with hepatitis B immunoglobulin has reduced the recurrence rate of hepatitis B after orthotopic LT to below 10% [80].

Recurrent hepatitis B is diagnosed by elevated HBV DNA levels, with or without abnormal liver function tests. It tends to follow an aggressive clinical course, featuring rapid fibrosis and severe necroinflammatory activity [81]. Morphologically, recurrent HBV infection in liver allografts presents either as typical patterns resembling those seen in non-transplanted livers (most common) or as less frequent atypical patterns of liver injury.

Typical features in early reinfection include mild lobular disarray and focal cytoplasmic or nuclear staining for HBV core antigen. Mild lobular and portal inflammation may also be present. In later stages, biopsies may show portal expansion with lymphoplasmacytic infiltration, fibrosis, interface activity of varying severity, bile ductular proliferation, disorganized hepatic cell plates, and lobular necrosis (spotty or confluent). Hyperplastic Kupffer cells and classic features like ground-glass hepatocytes or nuclei with a "sanded" appearance can also be observed. HBV surface and core antigens are detectable via IHC.

Less commonly, atypical histological patterns are seen, including steatosis and FCH. FCH is characterized by portal and periportal widening with thin fibrous septa extending into the lobule in a perisinusoidal distribution. This is often accompanied by bile ductular proliferation, which may or may not have a visible lumen. The liver parenchyma typically shows marked hepatocyte ballooning, cholestasis, and positive immunostaining for HBcAg (nuclear and cytoplasmic) and variably for HBsAg [82].

31.14.2 Recurrent Hepatitis C

Recurrence of hepatitis C was universal among LT recipients infected with hepatitis C. Recent availability of highly effective direct-acting antiviral therapy has drastically reduced the burden of hepatitis C recurrence [65]. Making a diagnosis of recurrent hepatitis C requires a liver biopsy. Acute hepatitis C shows lobular inflammation and hepatocellular injury characterized by mononuclear inflammatory infiltrate, foci of necroinflammation, and apoptotic bodies (Fig. 31.20) [5]. Mild lobular disarray and hyperplastic Kupffer cells are also seen. There is mild to moderate portal inflammatory infiltrate that consists predominantly of lymphocytes but may include few eosinophils. Focal endotheliitis, bile duct damage, and ductular reaction may also be seen. It has been suggested that at least 50% of bile ducts or central veins should be involved to establish a diagnosis of TCMR in patients with recurrent hepatitis C [13]. Chronic hepatitis C is morphologically similar to that in the native liver with portal-based lymphocytic inflammation and mild lobular activity (Fig. 31.20). Nodular lymphoid aggregates and lymphoid follicles with germinal centers may also be present. FCH and recurrent hepatitis C with prominent infiltration by plasma cells have also been reported [83, 84].

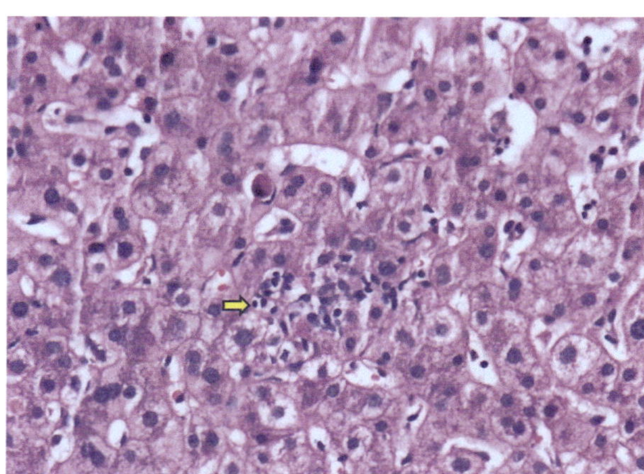

Fig. 31.20 Recurrent hepatitis C with mild lobular activity (arrow) in a graft biopsy

31.14.3 Recurrent Autoimmune Hepatitis

AIH is a chronic progressive inflammatory disease of the liver characterized by hypergammaglobulinemia, the presence of non-organ-specific autoantibodies, and abnormalities in liver chemistry and histology [85]. LT is indicated in patients with AIH who have acute or acute on chronic liver failure, decompensated chronic liver disease, or hepatocellular carcinoma (HCC) [86]. Despite good outcomes post-LT, AIH can develop/recur in the allograft and can cause allograft dysfunction, reduced allograft, and patient survival, and the need for re-transplantation [54, 86]. Post-LT prevalence of recurrent AIH ranges from 17% to 42%, and the frequency of diagnosis is influenced in part by the use of protocol or clinically indicated liver biopsy [53]. Suboptimal immunosuppression, younger age at LT, use of mycophenolate mofetil post-LT, sex mismatch and high IgG pre-LT, severity of disease in the native liver, and possibly HLA phenotype are the risk factors associated with AIH recurrence [12, 87]. Morphological features of recurrent AIH are similar to those in the native liver [54]. Moderate to severe portal inflammation comprising a lymphoplasmacytic cells and variable eosinophils is usually present (Fig. 31.21). There is interface activity and lobular hepatitis accompanied by varying degrees of hepatocellular necrosis, including confluent or bridging necrosis. Rosetting, emperipolesis, and apoptosis may be seen. One may observe focal bile duct injury and endotheliitis. Variable degrees of fibrosis with eventual transition to cirrhosis in patients. Centrilobular necroinflammation without accompanying portal changes may herald recurrent AIH, and the classic portal changes may emerge on sequential biopsies.

31.14.4 Recurrent Primary Sclerosing Cholangitis

Recurrence of PSC post-LT has been documented by multiple studies, and PSC is now the most common disease to recur after LT. Recurrent PSC is reported to occur in 8–27% of patients after a median of 4.7 years [88]. Recurrent PSC increases the

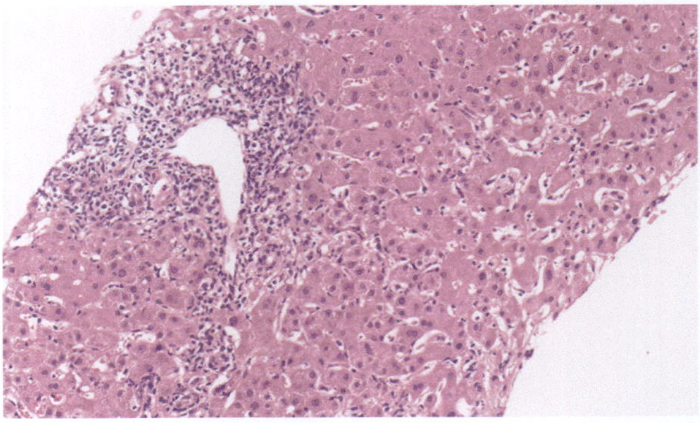

Fig. 31.21 Recurrent AIH with portal inflammation and interface activity in a liver allograft

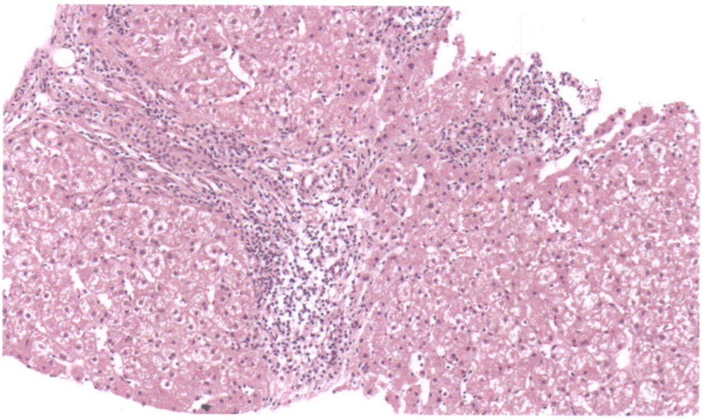

Fig. 31.22 Liver biopsy with portal expansion, mild edema, and inflammation in a recipient with recurrent PSC

risk of graft failure and mortality. Risk factors for recurrent PSC include CMV infection, recipient-donor gender mismatch, male recipient, graft from an extended-criteria donor, high levels of immunosuppression to treat rejection, diagnosis of cholangiocarcinoma, and presence of an intact colon at LT [89]. The diagnosis of recurrent PSC can be challenging because several post-LT complications manifest with biliary strictures. Histological findings in recurrence include portal expansion with bile ductular reaction, mixed inflammation, and biliary fibrosis occurring in the absence of other identifiable causes of biliary tract disease (Fig. 31.22) [5, 58]. Features of chronic cholestasis, including bile duct loss, periportal cellular ballooning with Mallory Denk bodies and copper deposition, are also reported. Periductal concentric fibrosis is infrequent in Tru-Cut graft biopsies.

31.14.5 Recurrent Primary Biliary Cholangitis

Post-transplant outcome for patients with primary biliary cholangitis (PBC) generally good, with 1- and 5-year patient survival rates is between 93–94% and 82–90%, respectively [90, 91]. The median time from LT to diagnosis of recurrent PBC is approximately 5 years [92]. Rates of recurrent PBC increase with time, with 30% prevalence 10 years after LT. The diagnosis of recurrent PBC can be challenging, as anti-AMAs and high IgM may be detectable after LT without pathological findings in the graft [93]. Most patients are asymptomatic at recurrence, and liver chemistries are not abnormal. PBC is most often detected incidentally in protocol graft biopsies, and higher rates of recurrence are therefore observed in centers that obtain protocol biopsies from their long-term liver recipients [86]. Granulomatous destructive cholangitis, the most specific histological sign of recurrent PBC, is often focal and therefore may not be present in Tru-Cut biopsies [58]. Ductular reaction, biliary interface activity, and progressive periportal copper/copper-associated protein deposition are other helpful morphological features. Lymphocytic cholangitis and portal lymphomononuclear inflammation, as well as duct loss, may also be seen, but these can also be seen in chronic rejection and recurrent HCV infection.

31.14.6 Recurrent Non-alcoholic Fatty Liver Disease

NAFLD is one of the most common causes of chronic liver disease worldwide. The estimated worldwide prevalence of NAFLD is around 25%, and that of non-alcoholic steatohepatitis (NASH) ranges between 1.5% and 6.45% currently [94]. NASH has become one of the fastest indications for LT for chronic liver disease and is expected to become the leading indication in the near future [95]. It is well established that liver allograft develops recurrent NAFLD. Persistence of original risk factors for NAFLD related to insulin resistance and the metabolic syndrome, like obesity, hyperinsulinemia, and dyslipidemia, and post-LT immunosuppression, is associated with recurrent NAFLD [96]. Within a few months post-LT, fatty change develops in 45–100% of recipients, and approximately 10–40% of these patients develop NASH, usually mild [12]. Once NASH occurs, 11–14% of patients may develop severe scarring within 5 years after LT [97]. Protocol liver biopsies are suggested in monitoring disease progression in the liver allograft, as around 30% of patients with recurrent NASH in liver biopsy have normal liver enzymes. Current data suggest that recurrent NAFLD does not affect short-term graft and patient survival. Liver biopsy remains the gold standard for establishing a confirmed NAFLD diagnosis as well as to exclude other complications. Pathological findings of fatty liver disease are similar to those reported in the native liver (Fig. 31.23).

31.14.7 Recurrent Alcoholic Liver Disease

Alcoholic liver disease is currently the most common indication for LT in the United States [98]. Moderate or heavy alcohol consumption occurs in up to 13% of LT recipients and is associated with increased risk of allograft loss and patient death [99]. Steatosis and steatohepatitis are the main pathological features of alcohol relapse. More severe recidivism can lead to frank alcoholic steatohepatitis with cellular ballooning, Mallory Denk bodies, inflammation, and fibrosis (Fig. 31.24).

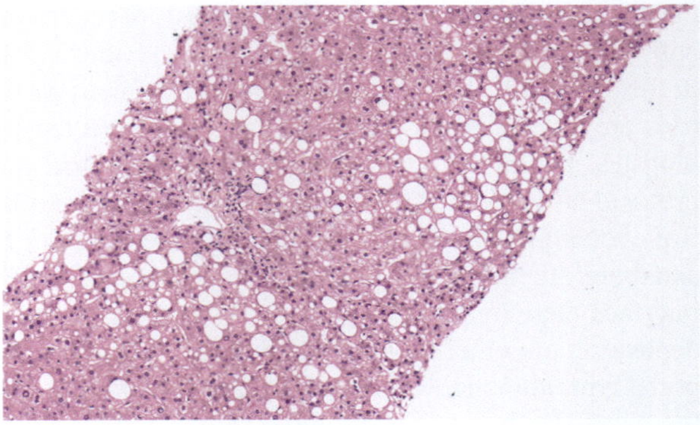

Fig. 31.23 Recurrent NAFLD in an allograft biopsy

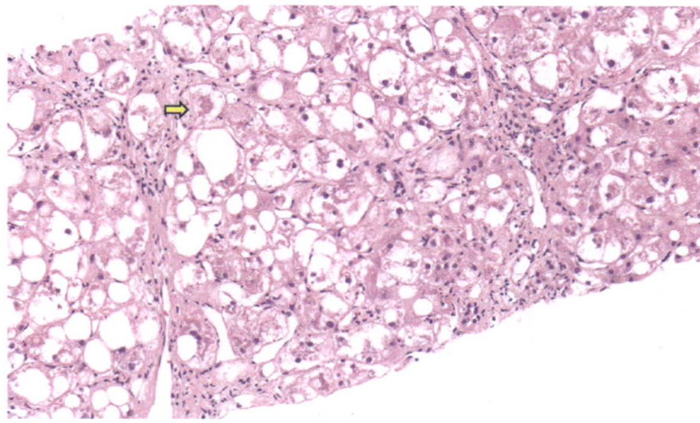

Fig. 31.24 Recurrent alcoholic steatohepatitis with steatosis, prominent cellular ballooning, eosinophilic Mallory Denk bodies (arrow), and fibrosis

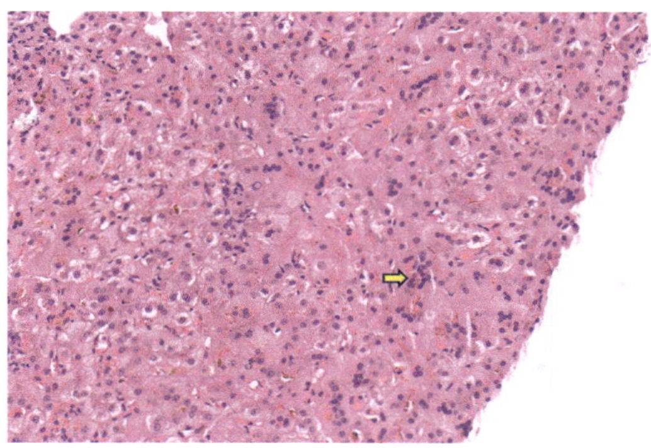

Fig. 31.25 Recurrent BSEP disorder with multinucleate giant cells (arrow) and cholestasis

31.14.8 Recurrent Bile Salt Export Pump Disease

Recurrent bile salt export pump (BSEP) disorder has been reported in patients following liver LT for BSEP defects [100, 101]. Recurrent BSEP disease presents with pruritus, jaundice, and occasionally diarrhea. The pathomechanism of recurrent BSEP disease is suggested to be a form of type II hypersensitivity reaction with the formation of de novo anti-BSEP antibodies that inhibits BSEP transporter activity in the liver allograft. The native liver of these patients lacks BSEP protein, so this can be regarded as an alloimmune antibody-mediated response directed against a foreign canalicular protein in the allograft. Pathologic findings include giant cell hepatitis with cholestasis (Fig. 31.25). Immunohistochemical expression of canalicular BSEP expression may be lost. C4d immunohistochemical or immunofluorescence expression may serve as a surrogate marker for circulating anti-BSEP antibodies. Patients usually respond well to rituximab with or without intravenous immunoglobulins.

Fig. 31.26 Recurrent HCC with moderate cellular differentiation

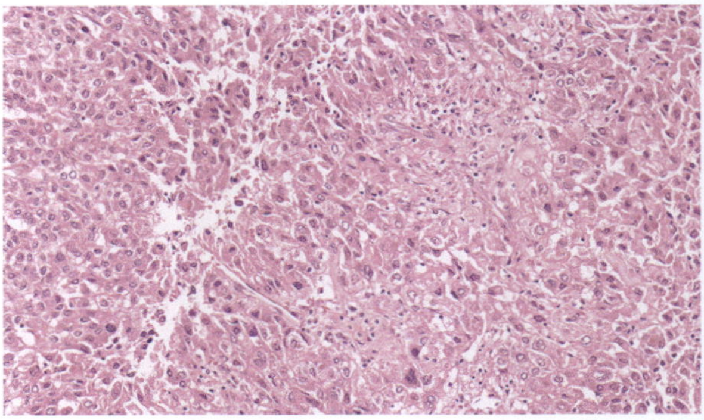

31.14.9 Recurrent Tumors

LT is one of the best treatment modalities for early-stage HCC in cirrhotic patients. However, LT in the setting of HCC is burdened by the risk of tumor recurrence, which affects around 15–20% of the cases, despite the use of restrictive criteria [102]. Post-LT HCC recurrence (Fig. 31.26) is usually associated with poor prognosis and short overall survival [103]. Risk factors for post-transplant HCC recurrence include tumor size, number, tumor histological grade, macroscopic or microscopic vascular invasion, serum alpha-fetoprotein levels, fludeoxyglucose uptake in positron emission tomography scan, response to loco-regional therapy, and post-transplant immunosuppression. For cholangiocarcinoma, the ideal treatment is surgical resection, as earlier studies reported poor outcomes following LT, with recurrence rates as high as 90% and a median survival <1 year [12]. However, recent analyses of post-LT outcomes for intrahepatic cholangiocarcinoma have suggested that transplant may be offered to highly selected patients [104]. Combined hepatocellular-cholangiocarcinoma is also associated with high recurrence post-LT [105].

31.15 De Novo (New Onset) Diseases

The term "*de novo* disease" has been used to describe patients who are transplanted for one type of primary liver disease and subsequently develop features of a different primary liver disease.

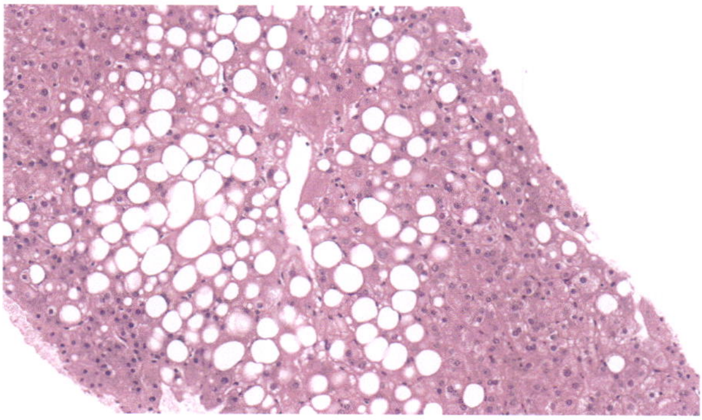

Fig. 31.27 Moderate macrovesicular steatosis in a liver allograft biopsy

31.15.1 De Novo Non-alcohoic Fatty Liver Disease

De novo NAFLD can cause post-transplant complications in patients undergoing LT for indications other than NAFLD [106]. Centers doing protocol allograft biopsies may identify histological features of de novo NAFLD (Fig. 31.27) in patients with normal liver serum chemistries [107]. Some of these cases are thought to develop in patients who underwent LT for "cryptogenic" cirrhosis or had other pretransplant risk factors for fatty liver, so these might be better regarded as recurrent rather than de novo disease [108]. De novo NAFLD has also been reported in patients who underwent LT for familial intrahepatic cholestasis 1 (FIC1) deficiency [109]. FIC1 is coded by the gene ATP8B1, and apart from the liver, it is also strongly expressed in the small intestine and pancreas. LT in FIC1-deficient patients exacerbates diarrhea, which is associated with a high concentration of bile acid in stool. LT leads to restoration of intestinal bile flow and biliary acid secretion, which lead to decompensation of ATP8B1 gene product dysfunction on the intestinal side and may contribute to the development of refractory diarrhea and graft NAFLD [110]. Another possible cause of graft NAFLD is malnutrition secondary to refractory diarrhea and pancreatitis.

31.15.2 De Novo Viral Hepatitis

Hepatitis B and C infections can be transmitted through donor livers, blood transfusions, or, less commonly, from other sources. In liver donors with a prior history of hepatitis B infection—indicated by anti-HBc positivity—reactivation of latent virus may occur due to post-transplant immunosuppression [111]. To prevent de novo hepatitis B infection in these recipients, long-term antiviral prophylaxis is essential. The histological features of de novo hepatitis B (Fig. 31.28) or hepatitis C are comparable to those observed in recurrent infections, as previously described. However, these acquired infections usually follow a milder course, with slower progression to fibrosis or cirrhosis.

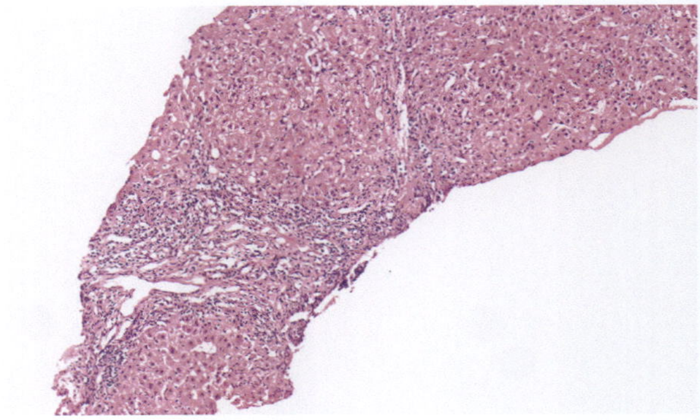

Fig. 31.28 De novo hepatitis B with portal fibrosis and activity (H&E)

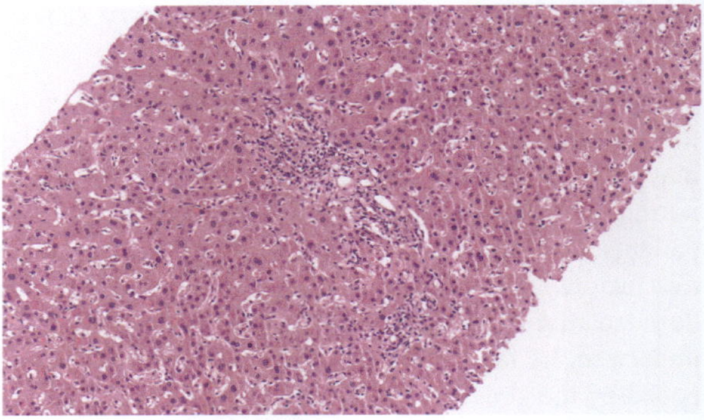

Fig. 31.29 Liver allograft biopsy with portal and lobular inflammation in a patient with hepatitis E infection (H&E)

De novo hepatitis E infection, particularly from genotype 3, is increasingly recognized as a significant cause of liver graft dysfunction [112]. Transmission can occur through undercooked meat—especially pork, venison, and wild boar—as well as through blood products and transplanted organs. PCR testing is valuable in confirming the diagnosis. Given their immunosuppressed state, post-transplant patients are at heightened risk for progression to chronic hepatitis and cirrhosis. On liver biopsy, hepatitis E infection (Fig. 31.29) may be mistaken for rejection or drug-induced liver injury.

31.16 Idiopathic Post-liver Transplant Hepatitis

Idiopathic post-liver transplant hepatitis (IPLTH) is a term used for unexplained portal and/or lobular inflammatory lesions in the liver allograft. It has been reported in 5–85% of adults and 32–97% of children with normal liver chemistries [42]. Clinically, most patients with IPLTH are well with good graft function. Liver serum chemistries may show minor abnormalities, usually a mild elevation in serum transaminases. IPLTH has been variedly called as unexplained hepatitis, nonspecific

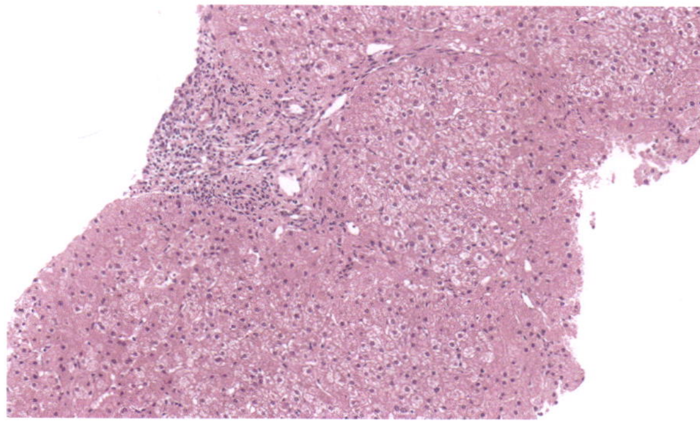

Fig. 31.30 Idiopathic post-transplant chronic hepatitis with mild portal inflammation and mild portal fibrosis (H&E)

portal and/or lobular inflammation, portal/parenchymal mononuclear inflammation, interface hepatitis, and allograft inflammation, leading to an underestimation of its true incidence [6]. Pathological findings frequently observed in IPLTH include predominantly mononuclear (lymphocytes, histiocytes, and some plasma cells) portal inflammatory infiltrate with no significant bile duct injury or portal venulitis and portal fibrosis (Fig. 31.30) [113, 114]. Variable interface activity and/or centrilobular inflammation with spotty to confluent necrosis have also been reported. There is increasing evidence to suggest that many cases of so-called IPLTH probably represent an immune-mediated liver injury, as most patients have auto/allo-antibodies and other uncharacterized serum factors that react with donor hepatocytes and/or bile ducts. Positive antinuclear antibodies and/or anti-smooth muscle antibodies (titers 1:40–1:640) have also been reported in more than 25% of patients with moderate to severe portal inflammation.

31.17 Hepatic Structural Abnormalities

Liver biopsies in 20–30% of post-LT recipients show structural abnormalities. These parenchymal changes include NRH, disarray of liver cell plate, perisinusoidal fibrosis, hepatocellular atrophy, and sinusoidal dilatation/congestion [6, 58]. Possible etiology includes humoral injury, drug-induced injury (azathioprine, tacrolimus), and disturbances in vascular microarchitecture related to liver regeneration in reduced-size allografts. NRH is characterized by diffuse transformation of liver parenchyma into small hyperplastic nodules, usually smaller than 3 mm in diameter, with minimal or no parenchymal fibrosis (Fig. 31.31). NRH is often an incidental finding on protocol biopsies and has no clinical manifestation [115]. Rarely, however, patients may develop signs of portal hypertension and may progress to graft failure, necessitating repeat LT [116].

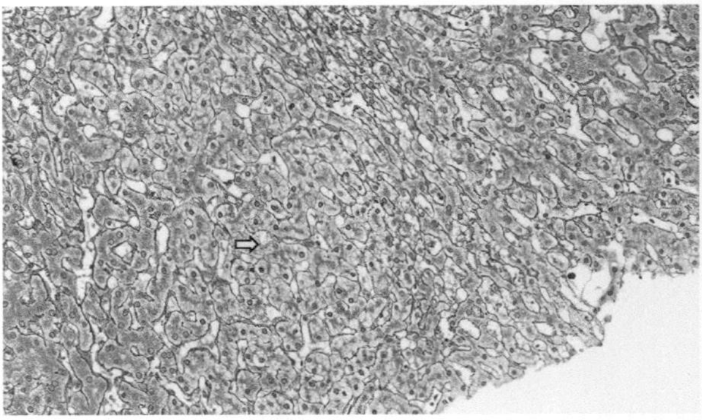

Fig. 31.31 Post-transplant liver biopsy displaying a nodule of hyperplastic hepatocytes (arrow) separated by a zone of compressed cell plates at the periphery (reticulin stain)

References

1. Terrault NA, Francoz C, Berenguer M, Charlton M, Heimbach J. Liver transplantation 2023: status report, current and future challenges. Clin Gastroenterol Hepatol. 2023;21(8):2150–66. https://doi.org/10.1016/j.cgh.2023.04.005. Epub 2023 Apr 20. PMID: 37084928.
2. Menon J, Shanmugam N, Vij M, Rammohan A, Rela M. Liver transplantation in tight junction protein-2 deficiency associated liver disease. Liver Transpl. 2022;28(11):1796–9. https://doi.org/10.1002/lt.26515. Epub 2022 Jun 16. PMID:35615909.
3. Rela M, Rammohan A. Why are there so many liver transplants from living donors in Asia and so few in Europe and the US? J Hepatol. 2021;75(4):975–80. https://doi.org/10.1016/j.jhep.2021.05.036. Epub 2021 Jun 8. PMID: 34111504.
4. Gao ZH. Seeking beyond rejection: an update on the differential diagnosis and a practical approach to liver allograft biopsy interpretation. Adv Anat Pathol. 2009;16(2):97–117. https://doi.org/10.1097/PAP.0b013e31819946aa. PMID: 19550371.
5. Adeyi O, Fischer SE, Guindi M. Liver allograft pathology: approach to interpretation of needle biopsies with clinicopathological correlation. J Clin Pathol. 2010;63(1):47–74. https://doi.org/10.1136/jcp.2009.068254. Epub 2009 Oct 21.PMID: 19847014.
6. Hübscher SG. What is the long-term outcome of the liver allograft? J Hepatol. 2011;55(3):702–17. https://doi.org/10.1016/j.jhep.2011.03.005. Epub 2011 Mar 21. PMID:21426919.
7. Biesterfeld S, Knapp J, Bittinger F, Götte H, Schramm M, Otto G. Frozen section diagnosis in donor liver biopsies: observer variation of semiquantitative and quantitative steatosis assessment. Virchows Arch. 2012;461(2):177–83. https://doi.org/10.1007/s00428-012-1271-6. Epub 2012 Jul 8. PMID:22772768.
8. Melin C, Miick R, Young NA, Ortiz J, Balasubramanian M. Approach tointraoperative consultation for donor liver biopsies. Arch Pathol Lab Med. 2013;137(2):270–4. https://doi.org/10.5858/arpa.2011-0689-RA. PMID: 23368870.
9. Flechtenmacher C, Schirmacher P, Schemmer P. Donor liver histology–a valuable tool in graft selection. Langenbeck's Arch Surg. 2015;400(5):551–7. https://doi.org/10.1007/s00423-015-1298-7. Epub 2015 Mar 26. PMID: 25809015.
10. Neil DAH, Minervini M, Smith ML, Hubscher SG, Brunt EM, Demetris AJ. Banff consensus recommendations for steatosis assessment in donor livers. Hepatology. 2022;75(4):1014–25. https://doi.org/10.1002/hep.32208. Epub 2021 Dec 6. PMID: 34676901; PMCID: PMC9299655.
11. Saxena R, Fiel MI. Pathology of liver transplantation. In: Saxena R, editor. Practical hepatic pathology. A diagnostic approach. 2nd ed; 2017. p. 630–62.

12. Clouston AD, Hübscher SG. Transplantation pathology. In: Burt AD, Ferrell LD, Hubscher SG, editors. Macsween's pathology of the liver. 7th ed. Philadelphia: Elsevier; 2018. p. 881–965.
13. Allende DS, Patil DT, Yerian LM. Pathology of liver, small bowel, and pancreas transplantation. In: Srivastava A, Allende DS, editors. Gastrointestinal and liver pathology. 3rd ed. Elsevier; 2023. p. 657–89.
14. Silva MA, Mirza DF, Murphy N, Richards DA, Reynolds GM, Wigmore SJ, Neil DA. Intrahepatic complement activation, sinusoidal endothelial injury, and lacticacidosis are associated with initial poor function of the liver aftertransplantation. Transplantation. 2008;85(5):718–25. https://doi.org/10.1097/TP.0b013e3181663366. PMID: 18337666.
15. Fiorentino M, Vasuri F, Ravaioli M, Ridolfi L, Grigioni WF, Pinna AD, D'Errico-Grigioni A. Predictive value of frozen-section analysis in the histological assessment of steatosis before liver transplantation. Liver Transpl. 2009;15(12):1821–5. https://doi.org/10.1002/lt.21948. PMID: 19938115.
16. Dorwal P, Gautam D, Sharma D, Singh DR, Raina V. Donor biopsy in living donor liver transplantation: is it still relevant in a developing country? Malays J Pathol. 2015;37(1):39–43. PMID: 25890612.
17. Nadalin S, Malagó M, Valentin-Gamazo C, Testa G, Baba HA, Liu C, Frühauf NR, Schaffer R, Gerken G, Frilling A, Broelsch CE. Preoperative donor liver biopsy for adult living donor liver transplantation: risks and benefits. Liver Transpl. 2005;11(8):980–6. https://doi.org/10.1002/lt.20462. PMID: 16035060.
18. Minervini MI, Ruppert K, Fontes P, Volpes R, Vizzini G, de Vera ME, Gruttadauria S, Miraglia R, Pipitone L, Marsh JW, Marcos A, Gridelli B, Demetris AJ. Liver biopsy findings from healthy potential living liver donors: reasons for disqualification, silent diseases and correlation with liver injury tests. J Hepatol. 2009;50(3):501–10. https://doi.org/10.1016/j.jhep.2008.10.030. Epub 2008 Dec. PMID: 19155086.
19. Lee JY, Kim KM, Lee SG, Yu E, Lim YS, Lee HC, Chung YH, Lee YS, Suh DJ. Prevalence and risk factors of non-alcoholic fatty liver disease in potentialliving liver donors in Korea: a review of 589 consecutive liver biopsies in asingle center. J Hepatol. 2007;47(2):239–44. https://doi.org/10.1016/j.jhep.2007.02.007. Epub 2007 Mar 6. PMID: 17400323.
20. Siriwardana RC, Chan SC, Chok KSH, Lo CM, Fan ST. Effects of donor steatosis on liver biochemistry and significance of body mass index in predicting steatosis. HPB. 2012;14(9):619–24.
21. Lo CM. Evaluating the living donor: expansion by innovation. Hepatol Int. 2016;10(2):242–4. https://doi.org/10.1007/s12072-016-9713-x. Epub 2016 Feb 26. PMID:26916760.
22. Cannistrà M, Ruggiero M, Zullo A, Gallelli G, Serafini S, Maria M, Naso A, Grande R, Serra R, Nardo B. Hepatic ischemia reperfusion injury: a systematic review of literature and the role of current drugs and biomarkers. Int J Surg. 2016;33(Suppl 1):S57–70. https://doi.org/10.1016/j.ijsu.2016.05.050. Epub 2016 May 30.PMID: 27255130.
23. Czigany Z, Lurje I, Schmelzle M, Schöning W, Öllinger R, Raschzok N, Sauer IM, Tacke F, Strnad P, Trautwein C, Neumann UP, Fronek J, Mehrabi A, Pratschke J, Schlegel A, Lurje G. Ischemia-reperfusion injury in marginal liver grafts andthe role of hypothermic machine perfusion: molecular mechanisms and ClinicalImplications. J Clin Med. 2020;9(3):846. https://doi.org/10.3390/jcm9030846. PMID:32244972; PMCID: PMC7141496
24. Jaeschke H. Molecular mechanisms of hepatic ischemia-reperfusion injury and preconditioning. Am J Physiol Gastrointest Liver Physiol. 2003;284(1):G15–26. https://doi.org/10.1152/ajpgi.00342.2002. PMID: 12488232.
25. Hakeem AR, Mathew JS, Aunés CV, Mazzola A, Alconchel F, Yoon YI, Testa G, Selzner N, Sarin SK, Lee KW, Soin A, Pomposelli J, Menon K, Goyal N, Kota V, Abu-Gazala S, Rodriguez-Davalos M, Rajalingam R, Kapoor D, Durand F, Kamath P, Jothimani D, Sudhindran S, Vij V, Yoshizumi T, Egawa H, Lerut J, Broering D, Berenguer M, Cattral M, Clavien PA, Chen CL, Shah S, Zhu ZJ, Ascher N, Bhangui P, Rammohan A, Emond J, Rela M. Preventing small-for-size syndrome in Living Donor liver transplantation: guidelines from

the ILTS-iLDLT-LTSI consensus conference. Transplantation. 2023; https://doi.org/10.1097/TP.0000000000004769. Epub ahead of print. PMID: 37635285.
26. Hernandez-Alejandro R, Sharma H. Small-for-size syndrome in livertransplantation: new horizons to cover with a good launchpad. Liver Transpl. 2016;22(S1):33–6. https://doi.org/10.1002/lt.24513. PMID: 27398648.
27. Rajakumar A, Kaliamoorthy I, Rela M, Mandell MS. Small-for-size syndrome: bridging the gap between liver transplantation and graft recovery. Semin Cardiothorac Vasc Anesth. 2017;21(3):252–61. https://doi.org/10.1177/1089253217699888. Epub 2017 Mar 23. PMID: 28758559.
28. Demetris AJ, Kelly DM, Eghtesad B, Fontes P, Wallis Marsh J, Tom K, Tan HP, Shaw-Stiffel T, Boig L, Novelli P, Planinsic R, Fung JJ, Marcos A. Pathophysiologic observations and histopathologic recognition of the portalhyperperfusion or small-for-size syndrome. Am J Surg Pathol. 2006;30(8):986–93. https://doi.org/10.1097/00000478-200608000-00009. PMID: 16861970.
29. Demetris AJ, Bellamy C, Hübscher SG, O'Leary J, Randhawa PS, Feng S, Neil D, Colvin RB, McCaughan G, Fung JJ, Del Bello A, Reinholt FP, Haga H, Adeyi O, Czaja AJ, Schiano T, Fiel MI, Smith ML, Sebagh M, Tanigawa RY, Yilmaz F, Alexander G, Baiocchi L, Balasubramanian M, Batal I, Bhan AK, Bucuvalas J, Cerski CTS, Charlotte F, de Vera ME, ElMonayeri M, Fontes P, Furth EE, Gouw ASH, Hafezi-Bakhtiari S, Hart J, Honsova E, Ismail W, Itoh T, Jhala NC, Khettry U, Klintmalm GB, Knechtle S, Koshiba T, Kozlowski T, Lassman CR, Lerut J, Levitsky J, Licini L, Liotta R, Mazariegos G, Minervini MI, Misdraji J, Mohanakumar T, Mölne J, Nasser I, Neuberger J, O'Neil M, Pappo O, Petrovic L, Ruiz P, Sağol Ö, Sanchez Fueyo A, Sasatomi E, Shaked A, Shiller M, Shimizu T, Sis B, Sonzogni A, Stevenson HL, Thung SN, Tisone G, Tsamandas AC, Wernerson A, Wu T, Zeevi A, Zen Y. 2016 comprehensive update of the Banff working group on liver AllograftPathology: introduction of antibody-mediated rejection. Am J Transplant. 2016;16(10):2816–35. https://doi.org/10.1111/ajt.13909. Epub 2016 Jul 14. PMID: 27273869.
30. Lee BT, Fiel MI, Schiano TD. Antibody-mediated rejection of the liver allograft: an update and a clinico-pathological perspective. J Hepatol. 2021;75(5):1203–16. https://doi.org/10.1016/j.jhep.2021.07.027. Epub 2021 Jul 31. PMID:34343613.
31. Demetris AJ, Bellamy CO, Gandhi CR, Prost S, Nakanuma Y, Stolz DB. Functional immune anatomy of the liver-as an allograft. Am J Transplant. 2016;16(6):1653–80. https://doi.org/10.1111/ajt.13749. Epub 2016 Mar 21. PMID: 26848550.
32. Charlton M, Levitsky J, Aqel B, O'Grady J, Hemibach J, Rinella M, Fung J, Ghabril M, Thomason R, Burra P, Little EC, Berenguer M, Shaked A, Trotter J, Roberts J, Rodriguez-Davalos M, Rela M, Pomfret E, Heyrend C, Gallegos-Orozco J, Saliba F. International liver transplantation society consensus statement on immunosuppression in liver transplant recipients. Transplantation. 2018;102(5):727–43. https://doi.org/10.1097/TP.0000000000002147. Erratum in: Transplantation. 2019 Jan;103(1):e37. PMID: 29485508.
33. Kim PT, Demetris AJ, O'Leary JG. Prevention and treatment of liver allograft antibody-mediated rejection and the role of the 'two-hit hypothesis'. Curr Opin Organ Transplant. 2016;21(2):209–18. https://doi.org/10.1097/MOT.0000000000000275. PMID: 26918881
34. O'Leary JG, Michelle Shiller S, Bellamy C, Nalesnik MA, Kaneku H, Jennings LW, Isse K, Terasaki PI, Klintmalm GB, Demetris AJ. Acute liver allograftantibody-mediated rejection: an inter-institutional study of significanthistopathological features. Liver Transpl. 2014;20(10):1244–55. https://doi.org/10.1002/lt.23948. PMID: 25045154; PMCID: PMC4412307.
35. Maurice JB, Nwaogu A, Gouda M, Shaw O, Sanchez-Fueyo A, Zen Y. Acute antibody-mediated rejection in liver transplantation: impact and applicabilityof the Banff working group on liver allograft pathology 2016 criteria. Hum Pathol. 2022;127:67–77. https://doi.org/10.1016/j.humpath.2022.06.015. Epub 2022 Jun 18. PMID: 35728694.
36. Puri Y, Rammohan A, Sachan D, Vij M, Rela M. ABO-incompatible living DonorLiver transplant from a blood type A2 donor to a type B recipient: A note of caution. Exp Clin

Transplant. 2022;20(1):100–3. https://doi.org/10.6002/ect.2021.0203. Epub 2021 Oct 19. PMID: 34763633.
37. Kim JM, Kwon CH, Joh JW, Kang ES, Park JB, Lee JH, Kim SJ, Paik SW, Lee SK, Kim DW. ABO-incompatible living donor liver transplantation is suitable inpatients without ABO-matched donor. J Hepatol. 2013;59(6):1215–22. https://doi.org/10.1016/j.jhep.2013.07.035. Epub 2013 Aug 6. PMID: 23928408.
38. Demetris AJ, Jaffe R, Tzakis A, Ramsey G, Todo S, Belle S, Esquivel C, Shapiro R, Markus B, Mroczek E, et al. Antibody-mediated rejection of human orthotopic liver allografts. A study of liver transplantation across ABO blood group barriers. Am J Pathol. 1988;132(3):489–502. PMID: 3046369; PMCID:PMC1880751
39. Haga H, Egawa H, Shirase T, Miyagawa A, Sakurai T, Minamiguchi S, Yamabe H, Manabe T, Tanaka K. Periportal edema and necrosis as diagnostic histologicalfeatures of early humoral rejection in ABO-incompatible liver transplantation. Liver Transpl. 2004;10(1):16–27. https://doi.org/10.1002/lt.20002. PMID: 14755773.
40. Bellamy CO, Herriot MM, Harrison DJ, Bathgate AJ. C4d immunopositivity is uncommon in ABO-compatible liver allografts, but correlates partially with lymphocytotoxic antibody status. Histopathology. 2007;50(6):739–49. https://doi.org/10.1111/j.1365-2559.2007.02677.x. PMID: 17493238.
41. Bellamy CO. Complement C4d immunohistochemistry in the assessment of liver allograft biopsy samples: applications and pitfalls. Liver Transpl. 2011;17(7):747–50. https://doi.org/10.1002/lt.22323. PMID: 21542127.
42. Vij M, Rammohan A, Rela M. Long-term liver allograft fibrosis: a review with emphasis on idiopathic post-transplant hepatitis and chronic antibody mediated rejection. World J Hepatol. 2022;14(8):1541–9. https://doi.org/10.4254/wjh.v14.i8.1541. PMID: 36157865; PMCID: PMC9453462.
43. Del Bello A, Congy-Jolivet N, Muscari F, Lavayssière L, Esposito L, Cardeau-Desangles I, Guitard J, Dörr G, Suc B, Duffas JP, Alric L, Bureau C, Danjoux M, Guilbeau-Frugier C, Blancher A, Rostaing L, Kamar N. Prevalence, incidence and risk factors for donor-specific anti-HLA antibodies in maintenance liver transplant patients. Am J Transplant. 2014;14(4):867–75. https://doi.org/10.1111/ajt.12651. Epub 2014 Mar 1. PMID: 24580771.
44. Kaneku H, O'Leary JG, Banuelos N, Jennings LW, Susskind BM, Klintmalm GB, Terasaki PI. De novo donor-specific HLA antibodies decrease patient and graft survival in liver transplant recipients. Am J Transplant. 2013;13(6):1541–8. https://doi.org/10.1002/ajt.12212. PMID: 23721554; PMCID: PMC4408873.
45. O'Leary JG, Cai J, Freeman R, Banuelos N, Hart B, Johnson M, Jennings LW, Kaneku H, Terasaki PI, Klintmalm GB, Demetris AJ. Proposed diagnostic criteria for chronic antibody-mediated rejection in liver allografts. Am J Transplant. 2016;16(2):603–14. https://doi.org/10.1111/ajt.13476. Epub 2015 Oct 15. PMID: 26469278.
46. Stevenson HL, Prats MM, Isse K, Zeevi A, Avitzur Y, Ng VL, Demetris AJ. Isolated vascular "v" lesions in liver allografts: how to approach this unusual finding. Am J Transplant. 2018;18(6):1534–43. https://doi.org/10.1111/ajt.14708. Epub 2018 Mar 30. PMID: 29464837.
47. Demetris AJ, et al. Banff schema for grading liver allograft rejection: an international consensus document. Hepatology. 1997;25(3):658–63. https://doi.org/10.1002/hep.510250328. PMID: 9049215.
48. Banff Working Group, Demetris AJ, Adeyi O, Bellamy CO, Clouston A, Charlotte F, Czaja A, Daskal I, El-Monayeri MS, Fontes P, Fung J, Gridelli B, Guido M, Haga H, Hart J, Honsova E, Hubscher S, Itoh T, Jhala N, Jungmann P, Khettry U, Lassman C, Ligato S, Lunz JG 3rd, Marcos A, Minervini MI, Mölne J, Nalesnik M, Nasser I, Neil D, Ochoa E, Pappo O, Randhawa P, Reinholt FP, Ruiz P, Sebagh M, Spada M, Sonzogni A, Tsamandas AC, Wernerson A, Wu T, Yilmaz F. Liver biopsyinterpretation for causes of late liver allograft dysfunction. Hepatology. 2006;44(2):489–501. https://doi.org/10.1002/hep.21280. PMID: 16871565.

49. Krasinskas AM, Demetris AJ, Poterucha JJ, Abraham SC. The prevalence and natural history of untreated isolated central perivenulitis in adult allograft livers. Liver Transpl. 2008;14(5):625–32. https://doi.org/10.1002/lt.21404. PMID: 18433038.
50. Ramji A, Yoshida EM, Bain VG, Kneteman NM, Scudamore CH, Ma MM, Steinbrecher UP, Gutfreund KS, Erb SR, Partovi N, Chung SW, Shapiro J, Wong WW. Late acute rejection after liver transplantation: the Western Canada experience. Liver Transpl. 2002;8(10):945–51. https://doi.org/10.1053/jlts.2002.34969. PMID: 12360439.
51. Thurairajah PH, Carbone M, Bridgestock H, Thomas P, Hebbar S, Gunson BK, Shah T, Neuberger J. Late acute liver allograft rejection; a study of its natural history and graft survival in the current era. Transplantation. 2013;95(7):955–9. https://doi.org/10.1097/TP.0b013e3182845f6c. PMID: 23442806.
52. Ozturk NB, Schiano TD, Fiel MI. Histologic and clinical outcomes of patients developing post-liver transplant plasma cell-Rich rejection. Am J Clin Pathol. 2023;160(1):49–57. https://doi.org/10.1093/ajcp/aqad004. PMID: 36883807.
53. Stirnimann G, Ebadi M, Czaja AJ, Montano-Loza AJ. Recurrent and De novo autoimmune hepatitis. Liver Transpl. 2019;25(1):152–66. https://doi.org/10.1002/lt.25375. PMID: 30375180.
54. González IA, Hartley CP, Nalbantoglu I. Recurrent autoimmune hepatitis and De Novo autoimmune hepatitis in the liver allograft. Am J Clin Pathol. 2021;155(3):435–45. https://doi.org/10.1093/ajcp/aqaa147. PMID: 33252121.
55. Sebagh M, Castillo-Rama M, Azoulay D, Coilly A, Delvart V, Allard MA, Dos Santos A, Johanet C, Roque-Afonso AM, Saliba F, Duclos-Vallée JC, Samuel D, Demetris AJ. Histologic findings predictive of a diagnosis of de novo autoimmune hepatitis after liver transplantation in adults. Transplantation. 2013;96(7):670–8. https://doi.org/10.1097/TP.0b013e31829eda7f. PMID: 23982338.
56. Castillo-Rama M, Sebagh M, Sasatomi E, Randhawa P, Isse K, Salgarkar AD, Ruppert K, Humar A, Demetris AJ. “Plasma cell hepatitis” in liver allografts:identification and characterization of an IgG4-rich cohort. Am J Transplant. 2013;13(11):2966–77. https://doi.org/10.1111/ajt.12413. Epub 2013 Sep 6. PMID:24011021.
57. Salcedo M, Rodríguez-Mahou M, Rodríguez-Sainz C, Rincón D, Alvarez E, Vicario JL, Catalina MV, Matilla A, Ripoll C, Clemente G, Bañares R. Risk factors for developing de novo autoimmune hepatitis associated with anti-glutathione S-transferase T1 antibodies after liver transplantation. Liver Transpl. 2009;15(5):530–9. https://doi.org/10.1002/lt.21721. PMID: 19399747.
58. Hübscher SG. Transplantation pathology. Semin Liver Dis. 2009;29(1):74–90. https://doi.org/10.1055/s-0029-1192057. Epub 2009 Feb 23. PMID: 19235661.
59. Demetris A, Adams D, Bellamy C, Blakolmer K, Clouston A, Dhillon AP, Fung J, Gouw A, Gustafsson B, Haga H, Harrison D, Hart J, Hubscher S, Jaffe R, KhettryU LC, Lewin K, Martinez O, Nakazawa Y, Neil D, Pappo O, Parizhskaya M, Randhawa P, Rasoul-Rockenschaub S, Reinholt F, Reynes M, Robert M, Tsamandas A, Wanless I, Wiesner R, Wernerson A, Wrba F, Wyatt J, Yamabe H. Update of the International Banff Schema for Liver Allograft Rejection: working recommendations for the histopathologic staging and reporting of chronic rejection. An international panel. Hepatology. 2000;31(3):792–9. https://doi.org/10.1002/hep.510310337. PMID: 10706577.
60. Blakolmer K, Jain A, Ruppert K, Gray E, Duquesnoy R, Murase N, Starzl TE, Fung JJ, Demetris AJ. Chronic liver allograft rejection in a population treated primarily with tacrolimus as baseline immunosuppression: long-term follow-up and evaluation of features for histopathological staging. Transplantation. 2000;69(11):2330–6. https://doi.org/10.1097/00007890-200006150-00019. PMID: 10868635; PMCID:PMC2967190.
61. Gupta P, Hart J, Cronin D, Kelly S, Millis JM, Brady L. Risk factors for chronic rejection after pediatric liver transplantation. Transplantation. 2001;72(6):1098–102. https://doi.org/10.1097/00007890-200109270-00020. PMID: 11579307.

62. Demetris AJ, Seaberg EC, Batts KP, Ferrell L, Lee RG, Markin R, Detre KM. Chronic liver allograft rejection: a National Institute of Diabetes and Digestive and Kidney Diseases interinstitutional study analyzing the reliability of current criteria and proposal of an expanded definition. National Instituteof Diabetes and Digestive and Kidney Diseases Liver Transplantation Database. Am J Surg Pathol. 1998;22(1):28–39. https://doi.org/10.1097/00000478-199801000-00004. PMID: 9422313
63. Brain JG, Robertson H, Thompson E, Humphreys EH, Gardner A, Booth TA, Jones DE, Afford SC, von Zglinicki T, Burt AD, Kirby JA. Biliary epithelial senescence and plasticity in acute cellular rejection. Am J Transplant. 2013;13(7):1688–702. https://doi.org/10.1111/ajt.12271. Epub 2013 Jun 10. PMID: 23750746;PMCID: PMC3746108.
64. Hernandez Mdel P, Martin P, Simkins J. Infectious complications after liver transplantation. Gastroenterol Hepatol (NY). 2015;11(11):741–53. PMID:27134589; PMCID: PMC4849501.
65. Jothimani D, Venugopal R, Vij M, Rela M. Post liver transplant recurrent and de novo viral infections. Best Pract Res Clin Gastroenterol. 2020;46-47:101689. https://doi.org/10.1016/j.bpg.2020.101689. Epub 2020 Sep 26. PMID:33158469; PMCID: PMC7519014.
66. Reinhold I, Teasca L, Rodriguez ER, Berney T, Mueller NJ, Hilty M, Andermatt R, Saro F, Dutkowski P, Müllhaupt B, van Delden C, Swiss Transplant Cohort Study (STCS). Donor-derived fulminant herpes simplex virus hepatitis after liver transplantation: two cases and review of literature. Transpl Infect Dis. 2023;25(4):e14080. https://doi.org/10.1111/tid.14080. Epub 2023 May 29. PMID: 37247223.
67. Côté-Daigneault J, Carrier FM, Toledano K, Wartelle-Bladu C, Willems B. Herpes simplex hepatitis after liver transplantation: case report and literature review. Transpl Infect Dis. 2014;16(1):130–4. https://doi.org/10.1111/tid.12178. Epub2014 Jan 3. PMID: 24383552.
68. Lautenschlager I. CMV infection, diagnosis and antiviral strategies after liver transplantation. Transpl Int. 2009;22(11):1031–40. https://doi.org/10.1111/j.1432-2277.2009.00907.x. Epub 2009 Jul 10. PMID: 19619175.
69. Bruminhent J, Razonable RR. Management of cytomegalovirus infection and disease in liver transplant recipients. World J Hepatol. 2014;6(6):370–83. https://doi.org/10.4254/wjh.v6.i6.370. PMID: 25018848; PMCID:PMC4081612.
70. Randhawa PS, Markin RS, Starzl TE, Demetris AJ. Epstein-Barr virus-associated syndromes in immunosuppressed liver transplant recipients. Clinical profile and recognition on routine allograft biopsy. Am J Surg Pathol. 1990;14(6):538–47. https://doi.org/10.1097/00000478-199006000-00004. PMID: 2159731; PMCID:PMC2963438
71. Lagana SM, De Michele S, Lee MJ, Emond JC, Griesemer AD, Tulin-Silver SA, Verna EC, Martinez M, Lefkowitch JH. COVID-19 associated hepatitis complicating recent living donor liver transplantation. Arch Pathol Lab Med. 2020; https://doi.org/10.5858/arpa.2020-0186-SA. Epub ahead of print. PMID: 32302212.
72. Mourad MM, Liossis C, Gunson BK, Mergental H, Isaac J, Muiesan P, Mirza DF, Perera MT, Bramhall SR. Etiology and management of hepatic artery thrombosis after adult liver transplantation. Liver Transpl. 2014;20(6):713–23. https://doi.org/10.1002/lt.23874. PMID: 24652787.
73. Jurim O, Csete M, Gelabert HA, Millis JM, Olthoff K, Imagawa D, Shaked A, McDiarmid SV, Busuttil RW. Reduced-size grafts–the solution for hepatic artery thrombosis after pediatric liver transplantation? J Pediatr Surg. 1995;30(1):53–5. https://doi.org/10.1016/0022-3468(95)90609-6. PMID: 7722830.
74. Khorsandi SE, Athale A, Vilca-Melendez H, Jassem W, Prachalias A, Srinivasan P, Rela M, Heaton N. Presentation, diagnosis, and management of early hepaticvenous outflow complications in whole cadaveric liver transplant. Liver Transpl. 2015;21(7):914–21. https://doi.org/10.1002/lt.24154. PMID: 25907399.
75. Daniel K, Said A. Early biliary complications after liver transplantation. Clin Liver Dis (Hoboken). 2017;10(3):63–7. https://doi.org/10.1002/cld.654. PMID:30992762; PMCID: PMC6467113.

76. Sonderup MW, Spearman CW. Global disparities in hepatitis B elimination-A focus on Africa. Viruses. 2022;14(1):82. https://doi.org/10.3390/v14010082. PMID: 35062286; PMCID: PMC8777803.
77. O'Grady JG, Smith HM, Davies SE, Daniels HM, Donaldson PT, Tan KC, Portmann B, Alexander GJ, Williams R. Hepatitis B virus reinfection after orthotopic liver transplantation. Serological and clinical implications. J Hepatol. 1992;14(1):104–11. https://doi.org/10.1016/0168-8278(92)90138-f. PMID: 1737910.
78. Demetris AJ, Todo S, Van Thiel DH, Fung JJ, Iwaki Y, Sysyn G, Ming W, Trager J, Starzl TE. Evolution of hepatitis B virus liver disease after hepatic replacement. Practical and theoretical considerations. Am J Pathol. 1990;137(3):667–76. PMID: 2399936; PMCID: PMC1877527
79. Katz LH, Paul M, Guy DG, Tur-Kaspa R. Prevention of recurrent hepatitis B virus infection after liver transplantation: hepatitis B immunoglobulin, antiviral drugs, or both? Systematic review and meta-analysis. Transpl Infect Dis. 2010;12(4):292–308. https://doi.org/10.1111/j.1399-3062.2009.00470.x. Epub 2009 Nov 24. PMID: 20002355.
80. Burra P, Germani G, Adam R, Karam V, Marzano A, Lampertico P, Salizzoni M, Filipponi F, Klempnauer JL, Castaing D, Kilic M, Carlis LD, Neuhaus P, Yilmaz S, Paul A, Pinna AD, Burroughs AK, Russo FP. Liver transplantation for HBV-related cirrhosis in Europe: an ELTR study on evolution and outcomes. J Hepatol. 2013;58(2):287–96. https://doi.org/10.1016/j.jhep.2012.10.016. Epub 2012 Oct 23. PMID:23099188.
81. Thung SN. Histologic findings in recurrent HBV. Liver Transpl. 2006;12(11 Suppl 2):S50–3. https://doi.org/10.1002/lt.20946. PMID: 17051563.
82. Davies SE, Portmann BC, O'Grady JG, Aldis PM, Chaggar K, Alexander GJ, Williams R. Hepatic histological findings after transplantation for chronic hepatitis B virus infection, including a unique pattern of fibrosing cholestatic hepatitis. Hepatology. 1991;13(1):150–7. PMID: 1988336.
83. Dixon LR, Crawford JM. Early histologic changes in fibrosing cholestatic hepatitis C. Liver Transpl. 2007;13(2):219–26. https://doi.org/10.1002/lt.21011. PMID: 17205558
84. Ward SC, Schiano TD, Thung SN, Fiel MI. Plasma cell hepatitis in hepatitis C virus patients post-liver transplantation: case-control study showing poor outcome and predictive features in the liver explant. Liver Transpl. 2009;15(12):1826–33. https://doi.org/10.1002/lt.21949. PMID: 19938116.
85. Zhang X, Jain D. The many faces and pathologic diagnostic challenges of autoimmune hepatitis. Hum Pathol. 2023;132:114–25. https://doi.org/10.1016/j.humpath.2022.06.019. Epub 2022 Jun 23. PMID: 35753409.
86. Montano-Loza AJ, Bhanji RA, Wasilenko S, Mason AL. Systematic review: recurrent autoimmune liver diseases after liver transplantation. Aliment Pharmacol Ther. 2017;45(4):485–500. https://doi.org/10.1111/apt.13894. Epub 2016 Dec12. PMID: 27957759.
87. Montano-Loza AJ, Ronca V, Ebadi M, Hansen BE, Hirschfield G, Elwir S, Alsaed M, Milkiewicz P, Janik MK, Marschall HU, Burza MA, Efe C, Calışkan AR, Harputluoglu M, Kabaçam G, Terrabuio D, de Quadros Onofrio F, Selzner N, Bonder A, Parés A, Llovet L, Akyıldız M, Arikan C, Manns MP, Taubert R, Weber AL, Schiano TD, Haydel B, Czubkowski P, Socha P, Ołdak N, Akamatsu N, Tanaka A, Levy C, Martin EF, Goel A, Sedki M, Jankowska I, Ikegami T, Rodriguez M, Sterneck M, Weiler-Normann C, Schramm C, Donato MF, Lohse A, Andrade RJ, Patwardhan VR, vanHoek B, Biewenga M, Kremer AE, Ueda Y, Deneau M, Pedersen M, Mayo MJ, FloreaniA BP, Secchi MF, Beretta-Piccoli BT, Sciveres M, Maggiore G, Jafri SM, Debray D, Girard M, Lacaille F, Lytvyak E, Mason AL, Heneghan M, Oo YH, International Autoimmune Hepatitis Group (IAIHG). Risk factors and outcomes associated with recurrent autoimmune hepatitis following liver transplantation. J Hepatol. 2022;77(1):84–97. https://doi.org/10.1016/j.jhep.2022.01.022. Epub 2022 Feb 8. PMID: 35143897.
88. Visseren T, Erler NS, Polak WG, Adam R, Karam V, Vondran FWR, Ericzon BG, Thorburn D, IJzermans JNM, Paul A, van der Heide F, Taimr P, Nemec P, Pirenne J, Romagnoli R,

Metselaar HJ, Darwish Murad S, European Liver and Intestine Transplantation Association (ELITA). Recurrence of primary sclerosing cholangitis after liver transplantation – analysing the European Liver Transplant Registry and beyond. Transpl Int. 2021;34(8):1455–67. https://doi.org/10.1111/tri.13925. Epub 2021 Jun 28. PMID: 34028110; PMCID: PMC8456806

89. Steenstraten IC, Sebib Korkmaz K, Trivedi PJ, Inderson A, van Hoek B, Rodriguez Girondo MDM, Maljaars PWJ. Systematic review with meta-analysis: riskfactors for recurrent primary sclerosing cholangitis after livertransplantation. Aliment Pharmacol Ther. 2019;49(6):636–43. https://doi.org/10.1111/apt.15148. Epub 2019 Feb 10. PMID: 30740723; PMCID: PMC6593422
90. Kashyap R, Safadjou S, Chen R, Mantry P, Sharma R, Patil V, Maloo M, Ryan C, Marroquin C, Barry C, Ramaraju G, Maliakkal B, Orloff M. Living donor and deceased donor liver transplantation for autoimmune and cholestatic liver diseases–an analysis of the UNOS database. J Gastrointest Surg. 2010;14(9):1362–9. https://doi.org/10.1007/s11605-010-1256-1. Epub 2010 Jul 9. PMID:20617395.
91. Montano-Loza AJ, Wasilenko S, Bintner J, Mason AL. Cyclosporine A protects against primary biliary cirrhosis recurrence after liver transplantation. Am J Transplant. 2010;10(4):852–8. https://doi.org/10.1111/j.1600-6143.2009.03006.x. Epub 2010 Feb 3. PMID: 20132169.
92. Carbone M, Mells GF, Alexander GJ, Westbrook RH, Heneghan MA, Sandford RN, Neuberger JM. Calcineurin inhibitors and the IL12A locus influence risk of recurrent primary biliary cirrhosis after liver transplantation. Am J Transplant. 2013;13(4):1110–1. https://doi.org/10.1111/ajt.12132. Epub 2013 Feb 22.PMID: 23433321.
93. Carbone M, Neuberger JM. Autoimmune liver disease, autoimmunity and liver transplantation. J Hepatol. 2014;60(1):210–23. https://doi.org/10.1016/j.jhep.2013.09.020. Epub 2013 Sep 29
94. Jeong SW. Nonalcoholic fatty liver disease: a drug revolution is coming. Diabetes Metab J. 2020;44(5):640–57. https://doi.org/10.4093/dmj.2020.0115. Epub 2020 Oct 21. PMID: 33115209; PMCID: PMC7643594.
95. Taneja S, Roy A. Nonalcoholic steatohepatitis recurrence after liver transplant. Transl Gastroenterol Hepatol. 2020;5:24. https://doi.org/10.21037/tgh.2019.10.12. PMID: 32258528; PMCID: PMC7063497
96. Khullar V, Dolganiuc A, Firpi RJ. Pre-and-post transplant considerations in patients with nonalcoholic fatty liver disease. World J Transplant. 2014;4(2):81–92. https://doi.org/10.5500/wjt.v4.i2.81. PMID: 25032097; PMCID: PMC4094954.
97. Saeed N, Glass L, Sharma P, Shannon C, Sonnenday CJ, Tincopa MA. Incidence and risks for nonalcoholic fatty liver disease and steatohepatitis post-liver transplant: systematic review and meta-analysis. Transplantation. 2019;103(11):e345. https://doi.org/10.1097/TP.0000000000002916. PMID: 31415032.
98. Marroni CA, Fleck AM Jr, Fernandes SA, Galant LH, Mucenic M, de Mattos Meine MH, Mariante-Neto G, Brandão ABM. Liver transplantation and alcoholic liver disease: history, controversies, and considerations. World J Gastroenterol. 2018;24(26):2785–805. https://doi.org/10.3748/wjg.v24.i26.2785. PMID: 30018475; PMCID:PMC6048431.
99. Cotter TG, Odenwald MA, Lieber SR, Rich NE, Im G, Charlton M, Singal AG, Mitchell MC. The practice of retransplantation for recurrent alcohol-associated liver disease in the United States is uncommon with acceptable outcomes. Transplant Direct. 2022;8(3):e1297. https://doi.org/10.1097/TXD.0000000000001297. PMID: 35187219; PMCID: PMC8843372.
100. Patel KR, Harpavat S, Finegold M, Eldin K, Hicks J, Firan M, Keitel V, KubitzR WH. Post-transplant recurrent bile salt export pump disease: a form of antibody-mediated graft dysfunction and utilization of C4d. J Pediatr Gastroenterol Nutr. 2017;65(4):364–9. https://doi.org/10.1097/MPG.0000000000001653. PMID: 28945205.
101. Prusinskas B, Kathemann S, Pilic D, Hegen B, Küster P, Keitel V, Häussinger D, Büscher R, Baba HA, Hoyer PF, Lainka E. Cholestasis after pediatric liver transplantation-recurrence of a progressive familial intrahepatic cholestasis phenotype as a rare differential diagnosis:

a case report. Transplant Proc. 2017;49(7):1628–33. https://doi.org/10.1016/j.transproceed.2017.06.011. PMID: 28838453.
102. Filgueira NA. Hepatocellular carcinoma recurrence after liver transplantation: risk factors, screening and clinical presentation. World J Hepatol. 2019;11(3):261–72. https://doi.org/10.4254/wjh.v11.i3.261. PMID: 30967904; PMCID: PMC6447422.
103. Verna EC, Patel YA, Aggarwal A, Desai AP, Frenette C, Pillai AA, Salgia R, Seetharam A, Sharma P, Sherman C, Tsoulfas G, Yao FY. Liver transplantation for hepatocellular carcinoma: management after the transplant. Am J Transplant. 2020;20(2):333–47. https://doi.org/10.1111/ajt.15697. Epub 2019 Dec 9. PMID: 31710773.
104. Sapisochin G, Ivanics T, Heimbach J. Liver transplantation for intrahepatic cholangiocarcinoma: ready for prime time? Hepatology. 2022;75(2):455–72. https://doi.org/10.1002/hep.32258. Epub 2022 Jan 6. PMID: 34859465.
105. Jaradat D, Bagias G, Lorf T, Tokat Y, Obed A, Oezcelik A. Liver transplantation for combined hepatocellular-cholangiocarcinoma: Outcomes and prognostic factors for mortality. A multicenter analysis. Clin Transplant. 2021;35(2):e14094. https://doi.org/10.1111/ctr.14094. Epub 2021 Jan 15. PMID: 32970878.
106. Losurdo G, Castellaneta A, Rendina M, Carparelli S, Leandro G, Di Leo A. Systematic review with meta-analysis: de novo non-alcoholic fatty liver disease in liver-transplanted patients. Aliment Pharmacol Ther. 2018;47(6):704–14. https://doi.org/10.1111/apt.14521. Epub 2018 Jan 22. PMID: 29359341.
107. Abraham SC, Poterucha JJ, Rosen CB, Demetris AJ, Krasinskas AM. Histologic abnormalities are common in protocol liver allograft biopsies from patients with normal liver function tests. Am J Surg Pathol. 2008;32(7):965–73. https://doi.org/10.1097/PAS.0b013e3181622490. PMID: 18460980.
108. Yalamanchili K, Saadeh S, Klintmalm GB, Jennings LW, Davis GL. Nonalcoholic fatty liver disease after liver transplantation for cryptogenic cirrhosis or nonalcoholic fatty liver disease. Liver Transpl. 2010;16(4):431–9. https://doi.org/10.1002/lt.22004. PMID: 20373454.
109. Shanmugam N, Menon J, Vij M, Rammohan A, Rajalingam R, Rela M. Total internal biliary diversion for post-liver transplant PFIC-1-related allograft injury. J Clin Exp Hepatol. 2022;12(1):212–5. https://doi.org/10.1016/j.jceh.2021.03.008. Epub 2021 Mar 30. PMID: 35068802; PMCID: PMC8766534.
110. Miyagawa-Hayashino A, Egawa H, Yorifuji T, Hasegawa M, Haga H, Tsuruyama T, Wen MC, Sumazaki R, Manabe T, Uemoto S. Allograft steatohepatitis in progressive familial intrahepatic cholestasis type 1 after living donor liver transplantation. Liver Transpl. 2009;15(6):610–8. https://doi.org/10.1002/lt.21686. PMID: 19479804
111. Cholongitas E, Papatheodoridis GV, Burroughs AK. Liver grafts from anti- hepatitis B core positive donors: a systematic review. J Hepatol. 2010;52(2):272–9. https://doi.org/10.1016/j.jhep.2009.11.009. Epub 2010 Jan 19. PMID:20034693.
112. Haagsma EB, van den Berg AP, Porte RJ, Benne CA, Vennema H, Reimerink JH, Koopmans MP. Chronic hepatitis E virus infection in liver transplant recipients. Liver Transpl. 2008;14(4):547–53. https://doi.org/10.1002/lt.21480. PMID: 18383084.
113. Yoshitomi M, Koshiba T, Haga H, Li Y, Zhao X, Cheng D, Miyagawa A, Sakashita H, Tsuruyama T, Ohe H, Ueda M, Okamoto S, Egawa H, Wood K, Sakaguchi S, Manabe T, Tanaka K, Uemoto S. Requirement of protocol biopsy before and after complete cessation of immunosuppression after liver transplantation. Transplantation. 2009;87(4):606–14. https://doi.org/10.1097/TP.0b013e318195a7cb. Erratum in: Transplantation. 2009;87(7):1104. PMID: 19307800.
114. Neil DA, Hübscher SG. Current views on rejection pathology in liver transplantation. Transpl Int. 2010;23(10):971–83. https://doi.org/10.1111/j.1432-2277.2010.01143.x. PMID: 20723179.
115. Sebagh M, Yilmaz F, Kounis I, Saliba F, Feray C, Taupin JL, Cherqui D, Azoulay D, Samuel D, Coilly A, Demetris AJ, Neil D. Evidence for Alloimmune sinusoidal injury in *De Novo*

nodular regenerative hyperplasia after liver transplantation. Transpl Int. 2023;36:11306. https://doi.org/10.3389/ti.2023.11306. PMID: 37565050; PMCID: PMC10409867.

116. Devarbhavi H, Abraham S, Kamath PS. Significance of nodular regenerative hyperplasia occurring de novo following liver transplantation. Liver Transpl. 2007;13(11):1552–6. https://doi.org/10.1002/lt.21142. PMID: 17969192.z

Chapter 32
Liver Allograft Rejection

Vaibhav Patil, Navin Marannan, and Dinesh Jothimani

Abstract The liver is the most immune-privileged organ. The presence of abundant immune cells protects the liver against several disease-causing pathogens and immune-related injury. Coupled with currently available immunosuppression, liver allograft rejection is less common compared to other solid organ transplants. Most rejection episodes occur in the first few weeks to months following LT. T-cell-mediated rejection is the most common type of rejection. Strong suspicion at the time of allograft dysfunction, timely liver biopsy, and treatment improves liver function. Pulsed corticosteroids, upscaling baseline immunosuppression with the addition of mycophenolate mofetil to calcineurin inhibitors, are required to manage rejection episodes. Chronic rejection may lead to allograft failure, usually related to non-compliance with immunosuppressive medications. Donor-specific antibodies may be a useful tool in patients with refractory rejection. A systematic approach to allograft dysfunction is required to manage these patients.

Keywords Liver transplantation · Rejection · Immunology · Corticosteroids · Immunosuppression

Key Highlights

- Post-transplant liver allograft dysfunction should be approached in a systematic way, including liver biopsy in patients with suspected rejection.
- T-cell-mediated rejection (TCMR) may occur in up to 20% of patients; intravenous methyl prednisolone should be administered to patients with moderate to severe TCMR.
- Donor-specific antibodies may be required in patients who do not respond to intravenous corticosteroids to identify antibody-mediated rejection (AMR).

V. Patil · N. Marannan · D. Jothimani (✉)
Institute of Liver Disease and Transplantation, Dr Rela Institute and Medical Centre, Chennai, Tamil Nadu, India
e-mail: dinesh.jothimani@relainstitute.com

S. Saigal, D. Jothimani (eds.), *Fundamentals of Transplant Hepatology*,
https://doi.org/10.1007/978-981-95-2624-6_32

- Non-compliance of immunosuppressive drugs is associated with chronic ductopenic rejection. Addition of m-TOR inhibitors may be useful in patients with early chronic rejection.

32.1 Introduction

The clinical outcome of liver transplantation (LT) has shown a remarkable improvement over the years. The successfulness of LT has been attributed to improvement in various factors, including patient selection, surgical techniques, post-operative care, and more importantly, evolution of immunosuppression. The introduction of CNI drugs has improved long-term graft and patient survival over 75%, in addition to the liver being an immune-privileged organ. The advancement in immunosuppressive regimens over the time played significant contribution to improved outcomes of LT in the last few decades.

Availability of CNI-based immunosuppressive drugs has improved short- and long-term graft and patient survival to over 90% and 80%, respectively.

The introduction of calcineurin inhibitors (CNI) and mTOR inhibitors has provided better control of acute rejections in post-LT period. The incidence of acute cellular rejection (ACR) is 15–20% in the post-LT period and responsiveness to the current immunosuppressive regimen is quite effective. However, there are sparse incidences of difficult-to-treat rejections or steroid resistance rejection, which are real challenges.

32.2 Hepatic Immune Tolerance

The liver has unique anatomical and immunological properties that make it immune tolerant compared to other solid organs. Despite significant antigenic exposure through portal circulation, the liver maintains a balance between immune surveillance and immune clearance [1].

The various factors responsible for the immune-tolerogenic properties of the liver are as follows:

Large surface area: When pathogen-derived products such as lipopolysaccharides pass through the liver, the vast surface area of hepatic sinusoids acts as an immune filter, reducing their concentration 100-fold, thereby enabling the liver to modulate the nature and intensity of the resulting immune response [2].

T cell attenuation: When antigens are presented by non-conventional APC, such as dendritic cells, HSC, hepatocytes, macrophages, liver sinusoidal epithelial cells (LSEC), and B lymphocytes, native T cells are activated but retained within the hepatic circulation independent of lymphoid organs [3]. The eventual clonal expansion of CD8 + T cells is followed by elimination due to a lack of co-stimulation [4]. In addition, hepatocytes engulf and eliminate activated T cells, which is called a "suicidal emporeliosis" [5].

T cell inhibition: LSEC and HSC induce the differentiation of native T cells to Treg (regulatory T) cells [6, 7]. Tregs suppress innate and adaptive immune responses by the expression of inhibitory molecules such as CTLA4, apoptosis of effective cells, and release of inhibitory molecules such as IL10 and TGF beta [8].

T cell exhaustion: T cell exhaustion occurs when T cell receptors are engaged in the absence of costimulatory molecules. This usually occurs after months of repeated antigen exposure leading to progressive hyporeactivity, decreased proliferation, and impaired cytokine production of effector T cells [9].

Microchimerism: The presence of hematopoietic donor-type cells (passenger leukocytes, PL) <1% in the recipient pool is called microchimerism, and more than 1% is called macrochimerism. Macrochimerism is usually observed in BMT and has been associated with tolerance in humans [10]. The donor cells migrate to the recipient's lymphoid cells and prime allospecific T cells to graft antigens.

HLA Expression: Liver has low constitutive expression of HLA Class II molecules [11].

32.3 Types of Liver Allograft Rejection (Table 32.1)

Traditionally, like renal transplantation, rejection was subclassified into hyperacute, acute, and chronic rejection based on the time interval from transplantation.

Table 32.1 Overview: types of liver graft rejection

Types	Mechanism	Duration post-LT
Acute AMR (acute antibody-mediated rejection/hyperacute)	Preformed ABO isoagglutinin or anti-HLA antibodies	Hours to a few days Erratic occurrence Dismal outcome May require re-transplantation
TCMR	Early TCMR: direct alloreactivity by host T cells infiltrating graft allo-specific antigen sites Late TCMR: indirect alloreactivity by host immune cells-internalizing graft antigen and presenting to T cells in host lymph nodes	Generally, a few days to few months. Can arise at any time Early (within 6 months): Good response to IS modulation Late (>6 months): mainly due to non-compliance or early reduction in IS- relatively poor response
AMR (antibody-mediated rejection)	Donor-specific antibody formation (DSA) targeting microvascular endothelium with complement mediated immune complex injury	Anytime Strategies focusing on the removal of DSA: Pulse therapy, plasmapheresis, Rituximab, IVIg
Chronic rejection	Multifactorial immunological: recurrent or inadequately treated TCMR, AMR Non-immunological: metabolic, drug-induced, sepsis, ischemic-reperfusion injury	Early (<6 months) Late (months to years) Extensive fibrosis leads to graft loss Refractory to medical management Re-transplantation is curative

Hyperacute rejection occurs within hours to a few days after transplant due to the presence of preformed antibodies. Currently, this entity is renamed as hyperacute antibody-mediated rejection. Although rarely seen nowadays, in the era of ABO-incompatible (ABO-i) transplantation, the circulating preformed antibodies in the recipient cause graft vessel thrombosis within minutes to hours, resulting in irreversible graft loss. The outcome of such rejection is dismal, necessitating urgent retransplantation [12].

Acute Rejection occurs within weeks to months after transplantation. Acute rejection can be further subclassified into T-cell-mediated (TCMR) or antibody-mediated (AMR).

32.4 T-Cell Mediated Rejection (TCMR)

TCMR (Table 32.2) is the most frequently encountered type of rejection and usually occurs within the first 3 months of transplantation [13]. The incidence of TCMR varies from 10% to 30% to as high as 64%, depending on clinically driven or protocol-driven biopsies [14].

TCMR can be early (<6 months) or late (>6 months). However, considerable overlap does occur and is not strictly time delineated. The pathophysiology and thereby implications of each type vary. Early TCMR is attributed to direct

Table 32.2 Histological diagnosis of TCMR (Rejection Activity Index)

Category	Score
Mixed portal inflammation	1. Lymphocytic predominant inflammatory infiltration 2. Expansion of portal triads with lymphocytic predominant infiltration with occasional blasts and eosinophils 3. Significant expansion of portal triads with inflammatory infiltrate with predominant blasts, eosinophils, spillover of inflammation
Bile ductal injury	1. Mild, occasional bile ductal injury with lymphocytic infiltrate, increased N: C 2. Most of the duct infiltrated with lymphocytic infiltrate with ductal distortion. Ductal epithelium—nuclear polarity disarranged, vacuolization of cytoplasm, degenerative changes 3. In addition to 2, more extensive degenerative changes in the bile duct with focal disruption
Venous endothelial inflammation	1. Subendothelial inflammatory infiltrate in portal/hepatic venules 2. Significant infiltrate noted in the majority of the venules with/without hepatocytic degeneration 3. 2 plus extensive inflammation with peri-venular hepatocytic degeneration

Histological category of TCMR	Histology score RAI
Mild	<4
Moderate	4–6
Severe	>7

Abbreviations N:C-nuclear: cytoplasmic ratio

alloantigen presentation and is generally mild in severity, whereas late TCMR occurs due to indirect alloantigen presentation, resulting in significant injury to the allograft with time. Clinically, late TCMR is often encountered with intentional or unintentional withdrawal of immunosuppressants (IS) [15].

In early TCMR, host T-cells infiltrate directly into the graft MHC-specific alloantigen, causing immune injury to endothelial injury to portal and hepatic venules and bile ductal injury with histologically CD4+/CD3+ T-cell deposition in the portal triad.

In late TCMR, host APCs enter into the graft, internalize the graft antigen, and then present it to local lymph nodal T cells, followed by clonal expansion and then infiltration and injury cycle. This pathogenesis process has more severe injury to the vascular and biliary ductal components and poor responsiveness to conventional T cell depletion strategies to treat this rejection compared to the early type. The diagnosis, severity grading, prognostication, and management strategy are based on histology with rejection activity index (RAI).

32.5 Antibody Mediated Rejection (AMR)

AMR, traditionally referred as humoral rejection, is an uncommon entity in LT with the incidence of less than 1% [16]. Unlike in renal, heart and pancreas transplantation, where AMR is common, liver allografts, on the other hand are resistant to it [17]. AMR was initially recognized in ABO-i LT but later with donor-specific antibodies (DSA) [18, 19]. AMR is usually considered when recipients with suspected TCMR do not respond to standard treatment [20, 47].

AMR can be subclassified into hyperacute (ABO-i LT), acute, and chronic rejection. The presence of DSA and complement C4d staining in biopsies are common in all types and are mandatory for diagnosis. DSA can be preformed or de novo after LT. Considering the rarity, DSA is not screened universally except in the following situations: (i) women with multiple pregnancies, (ii) retransplantation for chronic rejection, and (iii) aggressive minimization of immunosuppression [21].

The pathogenesis of AMR includes “two hit” hypothesis. The first hit is expression of HLA class II molecules secondary to injury like ischemia, reperfusion, or TCMR, and the second hit is DSA binding and classical complement activation [22].

Acute AMR usually occurs within the first few weeks of transplantation. As per the Banff Working Group 2016 criteria, AMR is diagnosed only if the following four criteria are met. (i) endothelial damage—hypertrophy, edema, leucocyte sludge, or capillary dilatation, (ii) presence of DSA in serum, (iii) diffuse microvascular Cd4 staining (especially in portal vein and sinusoidal endothelium), and (iv) exclusion of all other causes [14]. (Table 32.3).

Hyperacute rejection includes all the above in addition to coagulative necrosis of periportal hepatocytes with congestion and hemorrhage [23].

The diagnostic criteria of chronic AMR are not as clearly defined as acute AMR and are often a diagnosis of exclusion. The diagnostic criteria include (i) at least

Table 32.3 Features of acute antibody-mediated rejection

Definitive AMR	All four component are mandatory
1. Histology consistent with AMR	Portal microvascular endothelial hypertrophy, infiltration with monocytes, neutrophils, and eosinophils leading to micro-venulitis, portal edema, ductular reaction-cholestasis, and occasional periportal hepatocytic necrosis
2. Positive serum DSA	
3. C4d positive histology on frozen/ formalin-fixed tissue	Diffuse (C4d score = 3) C4d deposition in microvascular in ABO-compatible LT C4d deposition in the stroma in ABO-i LT
4. Exclusion of other insults causing similar histology	

Table 32.4 C4d staining in liver histology

Score	Histology
1	Portal microvascular endothelial enlargement with sparse microvasculitis
2	Significant endothelial enlargement with monocyte, eosinophils, and neutrophils infiltration causing micro-vasculitis. At least 5–10 leucocytes marginated in portal venules, capillaries
3	2 plus >10 leucocytes marginated in portal capillaries (significant portal inflammation) with focal disruption and extravasation of RBCs in the portal stroma

mild mononuclear portal and or perivenular inflammation with interface hepatitis, often with fibrosis, (ii) presence of circulatory DSA > 3 months, (iii) focal C4d staining (>10% of portal vasculature), and (iv) of exclusion of other causes [14]. However, these features are not specific for chronic AMR, as they can also be seen in recipients with no clinical or biochemical evidence of rejection or with episodes of TCMR [24]. The above findings in the clinical background of improper immunosuppression with persistent circulatory DSA might aid in diagnosis [25, 47].

C4d immunostaining of portal vein and sinusoidal endothelium is most specific for acute AMR [26] whereas portal stromal C4d staining is often seen in hyperacute AMR, TCMR, and CR [14] (Table 32.4).

32.6 Chronic Rejection (CR)

Chronic rejection occurs in less than 5% among recipients of LT, but the incidence increases to 16% in the pediatric population [20]. Although generally occurs after several months to years after transplantation, accelerated cases of CR within 6–12 months have also been reported [14]. Recurrent episodes of inadequately treated TCMR or a single episode of severe AMR result in CR. The graft loss in chronic rejection is irreversible, but early diagnosis holds the key to delaying the natural course of the disease [27].

Table 32.5 Histological features of chronic rejection

Structure	Early chronic rejection (at least 2 required)	Late chronic rejection (at least 2 required)
Small bile ducts	Ductal degeneration with ductopenia <50%	Ductopenia >50%
Portal tract hepatic arterioles	<25% loss	>25% loss
Zone 3 hepatocytes and hepatic venules	Zone 3 hepatocyte inflammation and necrosis Hepatic venule inflammation	Bridging fibrosis (moderate to severe) with variable inflammation Hepatic venular obliteration
Peri-hilar hepatic artery branches	Intimal inflammation with foamy cell deposition	Fibro-intimal obliteration with variable inflammation
Peri-hilar bile duct branches	Inflammation with foamy cell deposition	Mural fibrosis with obliteration
Others	Transition hepatitis 'with spotty hepatic necrosis	Cholestasis, sinusoidal foamy cell deposition

Table 32.6 Fibrosis scoring in chronic liver allograft rejection

Compartmental fibrosis	Score variability
Peri-portal	0 (none) to 3 (portal to portal, portal to central)
Sinusoidal /subsinusoidal	0 (none) to 3 (diffuse, thick, marked)
Peri-venular	0(none) to 3 (central to central, central to portal)

Maximal score 9, minimal score 0

Unlike other types of rejection, the pathogenesis of CR is complex, less clear, and multifactorial. In addition to direct immune-related mechanisms involving TCMR and AMR, the pathophysiology also includes indirect ischemic damage secondary to obliterative arteriopathy and other factors like drugs and cardiovascular and metabolic factors [28]. The hallmark of chronic rejection is significant fibrosis and paucity of inflammation targeting ducts (vanishing duct syndrome), arterioles, and terminal hepatic venules [29].

Chronic rejection can be early CR or late CR based on histological changes and not with respect to the timing of transplantation (Table 32.5). Early CR is characterized by loss of <50% of ducts, perivenular mononuclear infiltrates, and fibrosis, whereas late CR is defined by ductal loss of >50% with progression of perivenular fibrosis to the centrilobular area (Table 32.6) [30]. The presence of duct loss beyond 50% and centrilobular fibrosis has been associated with a high likelihood of graft failure [29].

32.7 Plasma Cell-Rich Rejection

Previously known as de novo autoimmune hepatitis or plasma cell hepatitis, plasma cell-rich rejection (PCRR) was coined by the 2016 Comprehensive Update of the Banff Working Group on Liver *Allograft* Pathology [14]. PCRR is an uncommon cause of late graft dysfunction (>6 months) and occurs in 3–5% recipients, especially among interferon-treated chronic HCV recipients [31].

Table 32.7 Banff diagnostic criteria for PCRR

Criteria	Histological features
Plasma cell infiltration	>30% periportal, perivenular areas infiltrated with plasma cells.
Necro-inflammatory activity	Must be present in periportal, perivenular, and interface areas.
Original disease	Original disease should be other than autoimmune liver disease (AIH)
Lymphocytic cholangitis	Usually present but not mandatory.

The pathophysiology of PCRR is poorly understood and is considered as mixed TCMR and AMR overlapping with autoimmunity in recipients of primary non-autoimmune hepatitis [32]. The risk factors include CNIs, viruses (EBV, CMV, and parvovirus), HCV especially treated with interferon and rejection [14] (Table 32.7).

The diagnostic criteria of PCRR proposed by Banff Working Group 2016 includes (i) portal and/or perivenular plasma cell-rich (estimated >30%) infiltrates with easily recognizable periportal/interface and/or perivenular necroinflammatory activity usually involving a majority of *portal tracts* and/or *central veins*, and (ii) the original disease other than autoimmune hepatitis. The presence of lymphocytic cholangitis often aids in diagnosis although not mandatory [14].

Compared to typical autoimmune hepatitis (AIH), PCRR is characterized by (i) more prevalent and severe lymphocytic cholangitis, (ii) higher IgG4 + plasma cell concentration (>50% vs. 3%), (iii) more aggressive plasma cell-rich perivenulitis, (iv) DSA (60%), (v) portal microvascular C4d deposition, and (vi) coexistent TCMR and CR in 18–24% of cases [14].

32.8 Risk Factors for Allograft Rejection

Recipients with few risk factors are at a high risk for rejection episodes. The younger the age at transplantation, especially pediatric population, HLA DR mismatch, CMV status mismatch, older age of donors, patients with autoimmune etiology, women with previous/multiple pregnancies, prior rejection episodes, and recent change in immunosuppression are considered high risk and hence demand close monitoring [32].

32.9 Non-invasive Diagnosis

The gold standard investigation to diagnose allograft rejection is liver biopsy. Apart from the diagnosis, it also suggests the type of rejection and severity of rejection, based on which further management is planned. However, being an invasive as well as expensive procedure, it is not considered the first-line investigation in routine clinical practice. There are few non-invasive tests, which helps to narrow down the diagnosis.

32.9.1 *Liver Function Test*

The first and foremost test in assessing an allograft function is a liver function test (LFT). Unexplained increase in aminotransferase levels is often the first abnormality that raises the suspicion of rejection. The transaminases, alkaline phosphatase (ALP), and gamma glutamyl transferase are the earliest markers to get elevated in most of the cases of graft dysfunction, followed by total bilirubin.

Postoperative complications often cause non-specific mixed pattern, unlike the hepatic or cholestatic pattern in pretransplant individuals [33]. The liver enzymes alone cannot differentiate between rejection, infection, or biliary obstruction [34]. The rate of rise in enzymes predicts the potential risk to the graft and early intervention [35]. The time period since transplantation, pattern, and rate of rise in enzymes with the appropriate clinical context aid the possible cause of allograft dysfunction.

In the background of noncompliance to IS or inadequate IS levels, transaminases typically rise 5–15× ULN and ALP rises 2–5× ULN in both acute TCMR and acute AMR, whereas a rise in bilirubin occurs only with severe cases. A rise in ALP to 2–5× ULN with or without a rise in bilirubin usually favors chronic TCMR and AMR [35].

32.9.2 *Complete Blood Counts*

Elevated absolute eosinophil counts seem to correlate with episodes of moderate to severe TCMR. These levels also normalize with adequate response to corticosteroids [36]. An algorithm incorporating the progressive rise in bilirubin and eosinophil counts predicted recipients with very high risk (78.3%) of moderate to severe TCMR episodes [37].

32.9.3 *Biomarkers*

A biomarker is a measurable quantity that can evaluate a physiological process, assess, and predict a pathological one. Ideally, it needs to be non-invasive, inexpensive, and easy to perform with a high specificity and sensitivity, and reproducible with validated studies [38]. Neopterin, a catabolic product of purine metabolism, was the first biomarker to be studied in correlation with rejection 40 years ago [39]. Since then, many biomarkers have been studied without promising results.

These biomarkers can be subgrouped as inflammatory (CD 28, CD 38, IL-1 receptor antagonist, IL-2 receptor, IL-6), non-inflammatory (GST, nitric oxide, CA 19-9, nitrate, amyloid protein A), biliary (IL-6, IL-8, IL-2 receptor, ICAM-1,

VCAM-1), transcription factors (miRNA), and genetic (donor-derived cell-free DNA) [34]. The search for an ideal biomarker for rejection still continues and is beyond the scope of this article.

32.9.4 Donor-Specific Antibody (DSA)

DSA are immunoglobulins complementary to polymorphic proteins that are different between the recipient and the graft donor. DSAs are mostly directed against donor human leukocyte antigen proteins. DSAs can be either performed before LT, or they can appear de novo after transplantation [30, 31]. The presence of DSA with mean fluorescence intensity >5000 is a diagnostic criteria for AMR as per Banff Working group [14].

The mere presence of DSAs increases the risk of acute and chronic rejection. As per a metanalysis, the presence of de novo DSA increases the risk of developing acute rejection (OR 6.4) and the risk is more pronounced in the pediatric subgroup (OR 10.2) [40].

32.9.5 Imaging

Ultrasound of graft liver with Doppler is often the first imaging requested in any case of allograft dysfunction to ensure patency of vascular structures and also to rule out biliary causes. A cross-sectional imaging is needed for exclusion of other structural causes responsible for allograft dysfunction. Although imaging does not help in the diagnosis of rejection, it is often the standard of care to rule out other causes before invasive tests like liver biopsy (Table 32.8).

Table 32.8 Differential diagnosis for liver graft rejection

Time from LT	Possible causes	
Within first month	Vascular complications Biliary leak Intra-abdominal sepsis Preservation injuries	Hepatic Artery or Portal Vein thrombosis Venous Outflow obstruction
Up to first year	Infections Biliary Drug toxicity	Intrahepatic abscess, opportunistic infection—CMV, EBV, HSV Persistence/recurrence of hepatitis C Stricture, cholangitis
Beyond first year	Chronic rejection Recurrent disease Steatohepatitis PTLD	AIH, PSC

32.10 Immunosuppression Conversion

To prevent immune-mediated graft injury, immediate post-LT period, induction with immunosuppression is mandatory. CNI tacrolimus-based regimen is standard of treatment accompanied with mycophenolate mofetil and glucocorticoids in the initial postoperate period [41]. There are few challenges related to tacrolimus, like narrow therapeutic window, which requires trough level monitoring, intra- and inter-individual variability of dosages due to CYP3A4 polymorphisms, and drug-drug interactions affecting levels. The desired trough levels for tacrolimus are 7–10 ng/ml for the first month, 4–8 ng/ml for first 1 year, followed by close to 4 ng/ml thereafter [42]. Glucocorticoids need to tapered off over first 2 months. Conversion to cyclosporine is indicated in tacrolimus toxicity cases for a brief period of 3–6 months based on the type of toxicity. Recent RCTs have shown that everolimus, mTOR inhibitor, proven to be effective IS, reducing CNI trough level requirement [43], hence reducing CNI-related toxicity, especially renal impairment. Switching to everolimus-based regimen is done 3–4 months post-LT considering risk-benefit ratio.

32.11 Treatment of Rejection

The treatment, response, and outcomes of rejection vary significantly with the type of rejection. Henceforth, the histology of the graft biopsy not just defines the line of management but also the eventual outcomes [44, 45]. Even when rejection is strongly suspected based on clinical grounds, it is mandatory to look for other potentially reversible causes of allograft dysfunction (refer to Table 32.2 for differential diagnosis) before an invasive biopsy is ordered.

The aggressiveness of management of rejection has also been tailored according to the clinical background, as in the case of autoimmune hepatitis as the primary etiology of liver disease, where treatment should be aggressive even in lower grades of rejection. This is in contrast to liver disease secondary to chronic viral hepatitis where reactivation has to be ruled out precisely before immunosuppression is intensified.

32.11.1 T-Cell Mediated Rejection (TCMR) (Table 32.9)

Once ACR is confirmed by biopsy, the severity of ACR is determined based on RAI. Based on the degree of portal, ductal, and central vein involvement, RAI score is determined, and ACR is subclassified as mild (RAI 3–5), moderate (RAI 6,7), and severe (RAI 8,9).

Table 32.9 Management of mild ACR (TCMR)

- **Optimization of immunosuppression**
- **Increase in dose of CNI/MMF**
- **Increase/addition of GCS.**

a)

Weekly monitoring for response ↓

If responsive-continue maintenance IS.	**No response: Pulse therapy with MPS**

GCS pulse therapy response ↓

If responsive –continue maintenance IS	**No response: review diagnosis & repeat liver biopsy**

32.11.2 Mild TCMR

Once biopsy shows evidence of mild ACR, the dose of mainstay CNI is first increased to maintain trough levels of 8–12 mcg/L for tacrolimus. When the desired trough levels are reached, second immunosuppression is either intensified or changed to Azathioprine and or steroids are added or increased. Majority of the ACR responds to the subtle changes in immunosuppression.

Once the biochemical parameters return to baseline, it is imperative to maintain the current immunosuppression for a few weeks to months and titrated slowly with close monitoring for relapse of rejection episodes. Patients on dual ISs are maintained on three or, at times quadruple drugs based on the response to treatment. Patients on cyclosporine as the mainstay CNI are preferably switched to tacrolimus to prevent recurrence or chronic rejection.

32.11.3 Moderate and Severe TCMR (Table 32.10)

Histological evidence of moderate and severe ACR requires potent immunosuppression with high-dose steroids. The intravenous route helps to attain fast and consistent serum levels and hence is preferred the most. There is no consensus on the ideal form, dose, and duration of steroid use. Although many different protocols are available in literature, intravenous methylprednisolone 10 mg/kg/day, maximum of 1 g/day, for 3 days (usually referred to as pulse therapy) is widely accepted and subsequently scheduled taper to oral prednisolone 20 mg/day over a week once the

Table 32.10 Management of moderate to severe TCMR

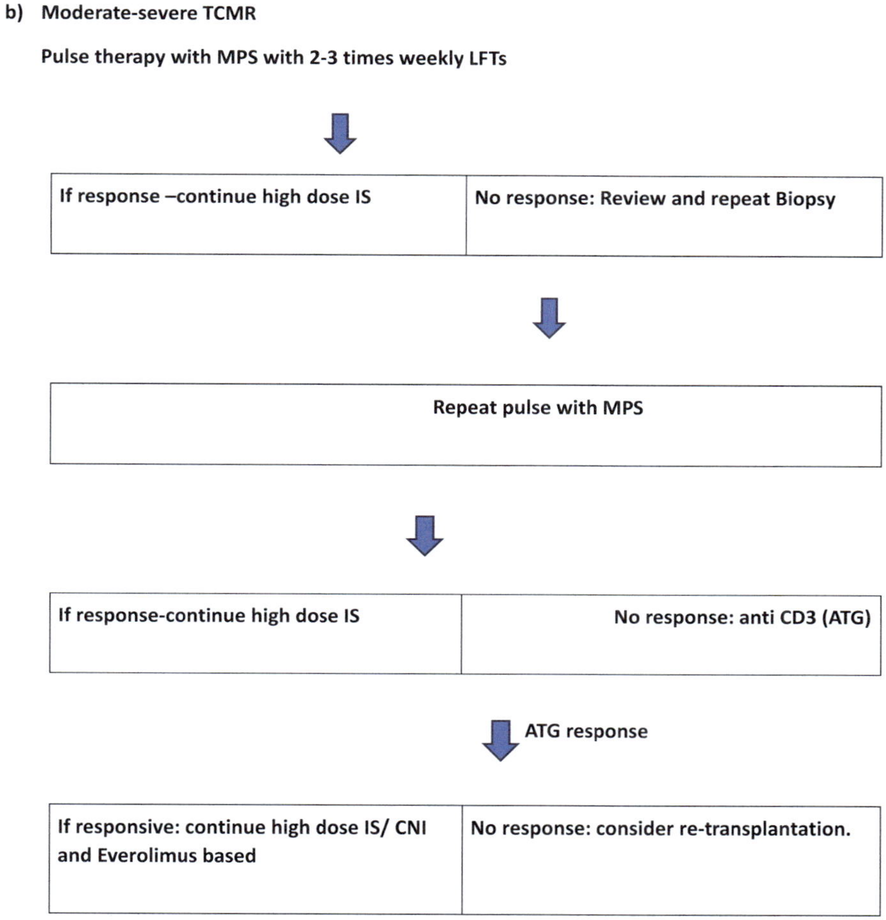

desired response is reached. An alternative to the above protocol is oral prednisolone 200 mg/day for 3 days, followed by gradual tapering of prednisolone to 20 mg/day over a week.

Treatment response: When two of three laboratory parameters (AST or ALT, ALP, and bilirubin) reduce to less than twice the upper limits of normal within the first 2 weeks of treatment, the patient is considered to have responded to treatment, and a repeat biopsy is seldom required to confirm resolution of rejection.

Up to 80% of moderate to severe ACR respond to a single dose of pulse therapy. When the response to steroid pulse therapy is suboptimal, a repeat pulsing with corticosteroids is usually recommended, provided the clinical suspicion of rejection is still high and an alternative cause of allograft dysfunction could not be identified.

32.12 Steroid-Resistant Rejection

When an episode of histologically proven ACR fails to respond to a pulsed dose of corticosteroid therapy, steroid-resistant rejection (SRR) is suspected. This diagnosis ideally requires a repeat allograft biopsy to reconfirm rejection. The repeat biopsy is performed immediately after the first pulse therapy in case of no response or progressive derangement biochemically or after the second dose of pulse therapy in cases of suboptimal response to the first therapy. In the tacrolimus era, the incidence of SRR has reduced by 50% in the first year of transplantation. The incidence of SRR has been reported to be as high as 35% in a few series.

The prognosis of SRR is inferior to steroid-responsive rejection in general. Early identification of SRR is of paramount importance, as it can result in late acute rejection (LAR) and chronic rejection, eventually leading to graft loss. Once SRR is confirmed by histology, the line of management should be changed to any of the following anti T cell targeted therapies, which improve the outcomes by 60–70%.

Anti-thymocyte globulin (ATG) is usually the first-line therapy [45]. These contain a diverse repertoire of antibodies, resulting in varying effectiveness. The usual dose is 1.5 mg/kg/day intravenous over 4 h for 3–7 days and can be extended to 2 weeks based on preparation and clinical response. The common adverse events observed are cytokine release syndrome, neutropenia, and thrombocytopenia, and the dose of ATG can be reduced by 50% during such events.

Monoclonal antibodies cause complement-mediated lysis of lymphoid cells. The commonly used is anti-CD3 antibody which is directed against CD3 component of T-cell receptor, resulting in potent immunosuppression within minutes of administration. They are often used as salvage therapy for steroid-resistant acute rejection or chronic rejection or as an induction agent in high-risk cases. Due to potent immunosuppression, these therapies are associated with a high risk of infection and malignancy.

IL2 receptor antagonists—ILRA (basiliximab)—relatively new class of ISs act by preventing proliferation of T-cells by blocking IL-2 receptor on T cells. RCTs have shown induction regimens with ILRA reduce the incidence of AR compared to standard regimens. Of late, ILRA has been used as an induction agent in high-risk patients to delay the introduction of CNIs or CNI-free regimen and in those requiring early weaning of steroids. Although not often used in SRR, ILRAs have been reasonably successful. Two doses of 20 mg separated by 3–5 days (10 mg if weight < 35 kg) have been the preferred regimen. The median time to respond has been 25–30 days.

In rare cases of poor response to all the above measures, graft irradiation and the use of more potent lymphotoxic drugs are required to salvage the graft or requires retransplantation.

32.13 Late Acute TCMR

Although LAR has similar histological findings to ACR, the degree of necrosis is severe, and similarly, prognosis and response to treatment variy widely. The risk factors for development of LAR are poor compliance to immunosuppression, inadequate dose, underlying primary liver disease, and delayed diagnosis of ACR. The diagnosis of LAR is frequently missed in biopsy and thereby delaying the diagnosis. The management of LAR is similar to ACR. However, only 50% of LAR responds to steroids.

32.14 Chronic Rejection (CR)

CR was traditionally believed to result in end-stage liver disease and can only be managed with re-transplantation. Recent advancements in medicine have changed the context of CR. In general, steroids have no role in chronic rejection, rather increase the risk of infection in the setting of re-transplantation. The usage of tacrolimus has reduced the incidence of CR.

The first step in the management of CR is to optimize the dose of tacrolimus. Patients who were not on tacrolimus at the time of diagnosis of CR (cyclosporine-based regimen) are switched to tacrolimus-based immunosuppression. The dosage of tacrolimus is increased for those who were already on tacrolimus to maintain high optimal trough levels.

The second step is the additional immunosuppression with preferably three or more drugs—mycophenolate mofetil, azathioprine, inhibitors of rapamycin (everolimus, sirolimus) or steroids. The choice of ISs depends on the patient's comorbidities, baseline immunosuppression at the time of diagnosis of CR, and underlying risk factor for CR.

Although the incidence of CR has decreased over the years, re-transplantation is the only treatment for CR when refractory to all the above measures.

32.15 Antibody-Mediated Rejection (AMR)

The major goal of treatment of AMR is the removal or reduction of circulating DSA. Plasmapheresis is the preferred first line of treatment in AMR. With the advent of anti-CD20 antibodies (rituximab) and bortezomib, the outcomes of AMR have improved considerably. Eculizumab, a monoclonal antibody against C5, has also been tried in a few studies with promising results.

Apart from clinical and biochemical response, it is mandatory to repeat the presence of DSA after weeks of treatment. If detected, the need for repeat therapy has to be assessed based on the clinical scenario [45] (Table 32.11).

Table 32.11 Management of AMR

- **AMR (diagnosis: liver histology and donor-specific antibody titers, C4d)**
- **Pulse therapy with MPS & Optimization of Immunosuppression.**

↓

- **If response: continue high dose immunosuppression.**
- **No response: Rituximab (anti-CD20) or IV immunoglobulin G Or plasmapheresis.**

- **If no response: Re transplantation**

32.16 Withdrawal of Immunosuppression

Since liver immune tolerance is significantly better than other solid organs post transplantation, the possibility of complete discontinuation of immunosuppression and post-LT period after which discontinuation is possible, being always fascinating questions. The purpose of discontinuation of IS is to reduce toxicity effects and possible oncogenic potential risk [46]; however, main challenge is the development of graft rejection, which may require treatment with higher immunosuppression or development of alloimmune sensitization leading to development of DSA and eventually graft loss [47]. Based on literature available favorable factors for stable withdrawal or minimization of IS are age of recipient, primary non-autoimmune liver disease etiology, and long duration post LT. Post minimization/discontinuation, close surveillance with liver functions, liver stiffness, de novo development of DSA, and liver biopsy is required to avoid graft loss [48]. RCT done by Shaked et al. showed 13% of recipients could tolerate complete IS withdrawal for a mean period of 2.8 years with the incidence of treatable mild rejections in the withdrawal group was 40% vs. 5.6% in low dose maintenance group recipients [49]. Complete discontinuation is possible only in a few selected post-LT patients.

32.17 Prognosis of Rejection

Unlike other solid organs, the long-term outcomes of acute rejection in LT are relatively superior. A single episode of steroid-responsive acute rejection has similar graft-related outcomes to those who never had rejection. However, repeated episodes of acute rejection affect graft survival in the long term. SRR, even treated, has inferior outcomes compared to steroid-responsive rejection.

Early ACR is not a risk factor for the development of LAR. LAR, unlike ACR, has been associated with increased fibrosis and risk of progression to chronic ductopenic rejection.

The development of chronic rejection is irreversible in general and would warrant a re-transplantation ideally. However, with tacrolimus-based regimens and the addition of everolimus, the graft survival has improved, decreasing the need for re-transplantation [50].

32.18 Conclusion

The understanding of clinical phenotype, histology, and associated immunological pathophysiology guides transplant physicians in managing challenges in the treatment of various rejections in the post-LT period. The tacrolimus-based regimen has a key role in the effective outcome of LT program in terms of prevention as well as therapeutic management of various rejections. The mTOR inhibitor like everolimus is a new hope in various special groups like CKD and HCC and has a vital role to play. The new biologics are a reserve effective modality for the resistant rejection group.

References

1. Egawa H, Ohdan H, Saito K. Current status of ABO-incompatible liver transplantation. Transplantation. 2022; https://doi.org/10.1097/TP.0000000000004250.
2. Dogan N, Husing-Kabar A, Schmidt HH, et al. Acute allograft rejection in liver transplant recipients: incidence, risk factors, treatment success, and impact of graft failure. J Int Med Res. 2018;46(9):3979–90.
3. Demetris AJ, Ruppert K, Dvorchik I, Jain A, Minervini M, Nalesnik MA, et al. Real-time monitoring of acute liver-allograft rejection using the Banff schema. Transplantation. 2002;74:1290–6.
4. Coussement J, Lebeaux D, van Delden C, Guillot H, Freund R, Marbus S, et al. Nocardia infection in solid organ transplant recipients: a Multicenter European Case-control Study. Clin Infect Dis. 2016;63(3):338–45. Epub 2016/04/20
5. O'Leary JG, Kaneku H, Demetris AJ, Marr JD, Shiller SM, Susskind BM, et al. Antibody-mediated rejection as a contributor to previously unexplained early liver allograft loss. Liver Transpl. 2014;20:218–27.
6. Demetris AJ, Bellamy C, Hübscher SG, O'Leary J, Randhawa PS, Feng S, et al. Comprehensive update of the Banff Working Group on liver allograft pathology: introduction of antibody-mediated rejection. Am J Transplant. 2016;16(10):2816–35.
7. Gordon RD, Iwatsuki S, Esquivel CO, Tzakis A, Todo S, Starzl TE. Liver transplantation across ABO blood groups. Surgery. 1986;100:342–8.
8. Doyle HR, Marino IR, Morelli F, et al. Assessing risk in liver transplantation. Special reference to the significance of a positive cytotoxic crossmatch. Ann Surg. 1996;224:168–77.

9. Charlton M, Levitsky J, Agel B, et al. International liver transplantation society consensus statement on immunosuppression in liver transplant recipients. Transplantation. 2018;102(5):727–43.
10. Meszaros M, Dubois V, Congy-Jolivet N, Hamada S, Thevenin C, Faure S, et al. Impact of calcineurin inhibitor-free immunosuppression on de novo donor-specific antibody formation in liver transplant recipients. Liver Int. 2022;42:1132–43.
11. Lee BT, Fiel MI, Schiano TD. Antibody-mediated rejection of the liver allograft: an update and a clinico-pathological perspective. J Hepatol. 2021;75:1203–16.
12. Haga H, Egawa H, Shirase T, et al. Periportal edema and necrosis as diagnostic histological features of early humoral rejection in ABO-incompatible liver transplantation. Liver Transpl. 2004;10(1):16–27.
13. Yamada H, Kondou H, Kimura T, et al. Humoral immunity is involved in the development of pericentral fibrosis after pediatric live donor liver transplantation. Pediatr Transplant. 2012;16(8):858–65.
14. Del Bello A, Congy-Jolivet N, Muscari F, et al. Prevalence, incidence and risk factors for donor-specific anti-HLA antibodies in maintenance liver transplant patients. Am J Transplant. 2014;14(4):867–75.
15. Kozlowski T, Rubinas T, Nickeleit V, et al. Liver allograft antibody-mediated rejection with demonstration of sinusoidal C4d staining and circulating donor-specific antibodies. Liver Transpl. 2011;17:357–68.
16. Angelico R, Sensi B, Manzia TM, Tisone G, Grassi G, Signorello A, et al. Chronic rejection after liver transplantation: opening the Pandora's box. World J Gastroenterol. 2021;27:7771–83.
17. Oguma S, Belle S, Starzl TE, et al. A histometric analysis of chronically rejected human liver allografts: insights into the mechanisms of bile duct loss: direct immunologic and ischemic factors. Hepatology. 1989;9(2):204–9.
18. Blakolmer K, Jain A, Ruppert K, et al. Chronic liver allograft rejection in a population treated primarily with tacrolimus as baseline immunosuppression: long-term follow-up and evaluation of features for histopathological staging. Transplantation. 2000;69(11):2330–6.
19. Neil D, Hubscher SG. Histologic and biochemical changes during the evolution of chronic rejection of liver allografts. Hepatology. 2002;35(3):639–51.
20. Castillo-Rama M, Sebagh M, Sasatomi E, et al. "Plasma cell hepatitis" in liver allografts: identification and characterization of an IgG4-rich cohort. Am J Transplant. 2013;13(11):2966–77.
21. Demetris AJ, Sebagh M. Plasma cell hepatitis in liver allografts: variant of rejection or autoimmune hepatitis? Liver Transpl. 2008;14(6):750–5.
22. Dogan N, Husing-Kabar A, Schmidt HH, et al. Acute allograft rejection in liver transplant recipients: incidence, risk factors, treatment success, and impact on graft failure. J Int Med Res. 2018;46(9):3979–90.
23. Hernandez Mdel P, Martin P, Simkins J. Infectious complications after liver transplantation. Gastroenterol Hepatol (NY). 2015;11:741–53.
24. El Sabagh A, Mohamed IB, Aloor FZ, et al. Current status of biomarkers and molecular diagnostic tools for rejection in liver transplantation: light at the end of the tunnel? J Clin Exp Hepatol. 2023;13(1):139–48.
25. Harding-Theobald E, Kriss M. Evaluation and management of abnormal liver enzymes in the liver transplant recipient: when, why, and what now? Clin Liver Dis (Hoboken). 2023;21(6):178–86.
26. Rodriguez-Peralvarez M, Germani G, Tsochatzis E, Rolando N, Luong TV, Dhillon AP, et al. Predicting severity and clinical course of acute rejection after liver transplantation using blood eosinophil count. Transpl Int. 2012;25:555–63.
27. Rodriguez-Peralvarez M, De Luca L, Crespo G, Rubin A, Marin S, Benlloch S, et al. An objective definition for clinical suspicion of T-cell-mediated rejection after liver transplantation. Clin Transpl. 2017;31:1199.
28. Califf RM. Biomarker definitions and their applications. Exp Biol Med (Maywood). 2018;243:213–21.

29. Margreiter R, Fuchs D, Hausen A, et al. Neopterin as a new biochemical marker for diagnosis of allograft rejection: experience based upon evaluation of 100 consecutive cases. Transplantation. 1983;36:650–3.
30. McCaughan JA, Tinckam KJ. Donor specific HLA antibodies & allograft injury: mechanisms, methods of detection, manifestations and management. Transpl Int. 2018;31:1059–70.
31. Del Bello A, Congy-Jolivet N, Danjoux M, Muscari F, Kamar N. Donor-specific antibodies and liver transplantation. Hum Immunol. 2016;77:1063–70.
32. Beyzaei Z, Geramizadeh B, Bagheri Z, Karimzadeh S, Shojazadeh A. De novo donor specific antibody and long-term outcome after liver transplantation: a systematic review and meta-analysis. Front Immunol. 2020;11:613128.
33. Jenne CN, Kubes P. Immune surveillance by the liver. Nat Immunol. 2013;14(10):996–1006.
34. Levitsky J, Feng S. Tolerance in clinical liver transplantation. Hum Immunol. 2018;79(5):283–7.
35. Adams DH, Sanchez-Fueyo A, Samuel D. From immunosuppression to tolerance. J Hepatol. 2015;62(1 Suppl):S170–85.
36. Olausson M, Mjörnstedt L, Nordén G, et al. Successful combined partial auxiliary liver and kidney transplantation in highly sensitized cross-match positive recipients. Am J Transplant. 2007;7(01):130–6.
37. Sugawara Y, Tamura S, Kaneko J, Togashi J, Makuuchi M, Kokudo N. Positive lymphocytotoxic crossmatch does not adversely affect survival in living donor liver transplantation. Dig Surg. 2009;26(06):482–6.
38. Mastoridis S, Martinez-Llordella M, Sanchez-Fueyo A. Immunotolerance in liver transplantation. Semin Liver Dis. 2017;37(2):95–108.
39. Bowen DG, Zen M, Holz L, Davis T, McCaughan GW, Bertolino P. The site of primary T cell activation is a determinant of the balance between intrahepatic tolerance and immunity. J Clin Invest. 2004;114(05):701–12.
40. Holz LE, Benseler V, Bowen DG, et al. Intrahepatic murine CD8 T-cell activation associates with a distinct phenotype leading to Bim-dependent death. Gastroenterology. 2008;135(03):989–97.
41. Benseler V, Warren A, Vo M, et al. Hepatocyte entry leads to degradation of autoreactive CD8 T cells. Proc Natl Acad Sci USA. 2011;108(40):16735–40.
42. Benten D, Kumaran V, Joseph B, et al. Hepatocyte transplantation activates hepatic stellate cells with beneficial modulation of cell engraftment in the rat. Hepatology. 2005;42(05):1072–81.
43. Jiang G, Yang H-R, Wang L, et al. Hepatic stellate cells preferentially expand allogeneic CD4þ CD25þ FoxP3þ regulatory T cells in an IL-2-dependent manner. Transplantation. 2008;86(11):1492–502.
44. Vignali DAA, Collison LW, Workman CJ. How regulatory T cells work. Nat Rev Immunol. 2008;8(07):523–32.
45. Wherry EJ, Kurachi M. Molecular and cellular insights into T cell exhaustion. Nat Rev Immunol. 2015;15(08):486–99.
46. Strober S. Use of hematopoietic cell transplants to achieve tolerance in patients with solid organ transplants. Blood. 2016;127(12):1539–43.
47. Sriwatanawongsa V, Davies HS, Calne RY. The essential roles of parenchymal tissues and passenger leukocytes in the tolerance induced by liver grafting in rats. Nat Med. 1995;1(05):428–32.
48. Starzl TE, Zinkernagel RM. Transplantation tolerance from a historical perspective. Nat Rev Immunol. 2001;1(03):233–9.
49. Wood K, Sachs DH. Chimerism and transplantation tolerance: cause and effect. Immunol Today. 1996;17(12):584–7.
50. Adams DH, Sanchez-Fueyo A, Samuel D. From immunosuppression to tolerance. J Hepatol. 2015;62:S170–85.

Chapter 33
Role of Interventional Radiology in Liver Transplantation

Shahnawaz Bashir

Abstract Interventional radiology (IR) service has become an essential requirement for any successful liver transplant program. The common complications in the postoperative period are vascular complications (hepatic artery, portal vein, and hepatic vein-related complications) and biliary complications (bile leaks and biliary strictures). IR provides a plethora of procedures for managing these post-liver transplant complications. These include: catheter-directed intra-vascular thrombolysis and stenting for hepatic artery thrombosis, portal vein thrombosis, and hepatic vein thrombosis; covered stents and embolization for pseudoaneurysms and bleeding; and biliary drainage and biliary stents for biliary complications. With refinements in technique and availability of newer hardware, the results of IR procedures continue to improve the patients' outcomes.

Keywords Liver Transplant · Interventional Radiology · Liver transplant complications

Key Highlights

1. Interventional radiology can manage most of the complications, in the early postoperative period as well as the late complications.
2. A dedicated interventional radiology service is essential to a successful liver transplant program.
3. With refinements in technique and availability of newer hardware, the scope of interventional radiology is growing.

S. Bashir (✉)
Interventional Radiology, Max Super Speciality Hospital, Saket, New Delhi, India
e-mail: doctor.kaloo@gmail.com

S. Saigal, D. Jothimani (eds.), *Fundamentals of Transplant Hepatology*,
https://doi.org/10.1007/978-981-95-2624-6_33

33.1 Introduction

Interventional radiology (IR) plays a crucial role in a liver transplant program, providing minimally invasive treatment options. The fact that IR provides a plethora of lifesaving procedures for the management of postoperative complications further exemplifies its role. The role of IR begins much before the liver transplant in chronic liver disease patients in the management of the complication of portal hypertension and management of hepatocellular carcinoma (HCC). IR treatments help a number of patients suffering from HCC to be bridged to liver transplant by helping them to stay within the transplant criteria or by downstaging their disease to fit within the transplant criteria. IR also helps in procedures like hepatic venous pressure gradient (HVPG) measurement, biopsy, percutaneous cholecystostomy drain (PCD), etc. However, in this chapter we will limit our discussion to the role IR plays in the management of complications specific to the liver transplant (LT) recipients.

There are technical differences in the anatomy in living donor liver transplant (LDLT) and dead donor liver transplant (DDLT). Understanding detailed surgical anatomy is critical to recognizing the underlying disease in liver transplant recipients. Reading the operative notes and discussing with the operating surgeon is imperative, as there are individual and institutional differences in technique. Accordingly, review of ultrasound (USG) and cross-sectional imaging studies is important for planning suitable treatment.

The common complications in the perioperative period can be divided into vascular and biliary complications. Vascular complications are further divided into hepatic artery, portal vein, and hepatic vein-related complications. Further, some complications are more commonly seen in the early postoperative period (e.g., hepatic artery thrombosis), while others are more frequently seen in the late post-LT period (e.g., biliary stricture).

1. *Hepatic arterial complications*
   (a) Hepatic artery stenosis (HAS)
   (b) Hepatic artery thrombosis (HAT)
   (c) Hepatic artery pseudoaneurysm
   (d) Splenic artery steal syndrome (SASS)
2. *Portal venous complications*
   (a) Portal vein stenosis (PVS)
   (b) Portal vein thrombosis (PVT)
3. *Hepatic vein outflow complications*
   (a) Hepatic vein stenosis or kinking
   (b) Hepatic vein thrombosis
4. *Biliary complications*
   (a) Bile leak/biloma
   (b) Biliary stricture

33.2 Hepatic Artery Complications

The hepatic artery is the major source of oxygenated blood to the liver. Bile ducts in liver transplant patients are particularly vulnerable to arterial complications and can suffer ischemic bile duct injury, which can later cause biliary strictures or ischemic cholangiopathy [1].

(a) *Hepatic artery stenosis (HAS):* HAS occurs in 4–11% of all liver transplant recipients [2]. HAS is divided into early onset (<30 days after transplant) and late onset (>30 days after transplant). Early-onset HAS can be treated with surgical revision or endovascular options. Late-onset HAS is generally treated by endovascular intervention. HAS may be asymptomatic or present as liver dysfunction or biliary complications. If left untreated, HAS can progress to complete HA occlusion and loss of graft. The diagnosis is often suggested by Doppler ultrasound demonstrating a resistive index (RI) of less than 0.5 with elevated velocities at the anastomosis of the hepatic artery [1]. The diagnosis is often confirmed by CT angiography.

The IR treatment of HAS is usually done by balloon angioplasty with or without stent placement. The balloon-mounted stents are commonly used over 0.014-inch guidewire. Drug-eluting stents are also used by some groups to decrease the risk of restenosis related to intimal hyperplasia. Antiplatelet agents (aspirin with or without clopidogrel) are routinely administered after stent placement in the hepatic artery.

Complication rates for endovascular treatment are low (<5%), with dissection being the most commonly encountered complication. A 2012 meta-analysis compared the effectiveness of angioplasty to that of stent placement in HAS and found both to be efficacious, with comparable patency and requirements for reintervention [3]. A retrospective comparative single-institution study showed a higher 1-year patency rate with stent placement than with angioplasty alone (93.8% vs. 73.5%) [4]. Another large study also showed a strong trend toward improved patency with stent placement versus with angioplasty [5].

(b) *Hepatic artery thrombosis (HAT):* HAT is a feared complication after LT, which can rapidly cause graft loss. The estimated prevalence of HAT is 4.8–9% [6]. The diagnosis is often made on routine Doppler, even before the clinical signs and symptoms appear. CT angiography is used to confirm the diagnosis. Treatment options include surgical revision, endovascular revascularization, and re-transplantation. In the very early post-LT period (up to 3 or 7 days), surgical thrombectomy is preferred. Subsequently, IR techniques are preferred to re-establish the HA blood flow.

The IR treatment usually begins with femoral artery access and a celiac axis angiogram to confirm the diagnosis. This is followed by microcatheter placement in the hepatic artery proper and catheter-directed thrombolysis using intra-arterial infusion of tissue plasminogen activator (t-PA) (Fig. 33.1). If the initial t-PA bolus is unable to restore the blood flow, t-PA boluses are repeated a few times, and subsequently a continuous infusion of t-PA is given (doses

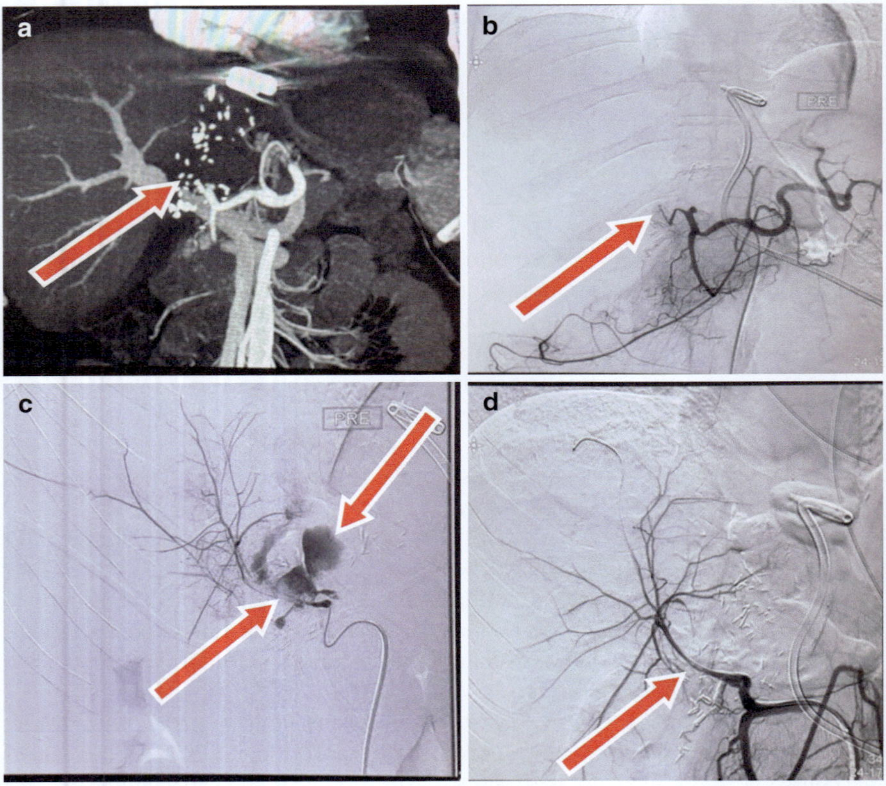

Fig. 33.1 (**a**) Coronal CECT image of a 38-year-old female on POD 30 showing HAT. (**b**) DSA of the same patient. (**c**) After initial thrombolysis the HA flow was restored, but there was active contrast extravasation from a previously obscure pseudoaneurysm. (**d**) HA angio after covered stent placement shows no more extravasation

ranging from 0.25 to 2.0 mg/h). If the infusion is continued overnight, check that the angiogram is done the following day. Generally, this should clear any thrombus in the hepatic artery. In resistant cases when the thrombus fails to dissolve or there is a dissection flap or stenosis underlying the HAT, early stent placement can be done to restore HA blood flow, with subsequent t-PA infusion if needed. IR techniques have shown mixed results for treatment of HAT, with much lower patency rates compared with those for HAS. This is partly explained by the heterogeneity of the causes of HAT, which could be related to difficult surgical anastomosis; size mismatch between the donor and recipient artery; time from the onset of HAT and the diagnosis; and the heterogeneity in the techniques used. Failure to treat HAT will lead to ischemic biliary injury and require re-transplant.

Most studies reporting endovascular treatments for HA thrombosis have small sample sizes. In a review of 69 patients (63 DDLT cases) included in 16 studies, thrombolysis was successful in 47 (68%) patients, and 29 (62%) of the 47 patients underwent additional balloon angioplasty and/or stent placement [7]. In comparison, in another study of 26 patients, the recanalization and major complication rates were merely 46% and 42%, respectively [8]. There were no statistical differences between patients with successful and unsuccessful recanalization with respect to the survival rates, need for surgical revascularization, re-transplantation rates, ischemic biliary complications, or procedural complications.

Late onset HAT may be the result of the progression of HAS to HAT. This is usually a gradual process and sometimes may be slow enough to allow for collateral formation. In this case, if enough collateralization has occurred, HAT may not need any treatment.

(c) *Hepatic artery pseudoaneurysm:* HA pseudoaneurysm has an estimated prevalence of 0.3–2.6% in liver transplant recipients and commonly occurs at the anastomotic site [1]. Risk factors include bacteraemia, bile leak, abdominal infection, and iatrogenic interventions. Rupture of an HA pseudoaneurysm can be devastating; therefore, urgent surgical or endovascular treatment is required. In the early post-transplant period, surgical therapy is the first choice because maintenance of HA flow and management of coexisting infection are important [9].

Endovascular treatments include covered stent placement or embolization. Embolization is effective in achieving haemostasis; however, selective embolization of a pseudoaneurysm while preserving HA flow is almost impossible.

Covered stent placement may be a good option to treat a pseudoaneurysm while preserving the HA inflow. However, the small diameter and tortuous course of the HA, especially in LDLT, makes stent placement challenging.

Sometimes thrombosis may occur in an HA with an existing pseudoaneurysm, and thus the pseudoaneurysm may be missed at the initial imaging (Fig. 33.1c and d). In such cases when thrombolysis is done, the existing pseudoaneurysm gets revealed, which starts fresh bleeding as the thrombus dissolves. These cases usually require urgent stent graft placement to cover the diseased segment of the hepatic artery. If stent placement is not feasible, embolization or surgical repair should be attempted to achieve haemostasis.

Non-anastomotic intrahepatic pseudoaneurysms involving the hepatic artery branches can also occur in LT recipients. These are generally secondary to iatrogenic injury, such as liver biopsy or biliary drainage procedure. These are treated by embolization using coils or liquid embolic agents.

(d) *Splenic artery steal syndrome (SASS):* SASS (also called nonocclusive hepatic artery hypoperfusion syndrome) can be seen in up to 4% of transplant patients [1]. The pathophysiology of SASS has been debated. Initially thought to be due to preferential flow to an enlarged splenic artery "stealing" from the transplant hepatic artery, it is now theorized to be due to portal vein hyperperfusion. This syndrome may be a significant cause of graft ischemia after transplantation, and its most common presentation is elevated liver enzymes. The combination of graft dysfunction, poor hepatic artery perfusion without structural obstruction,

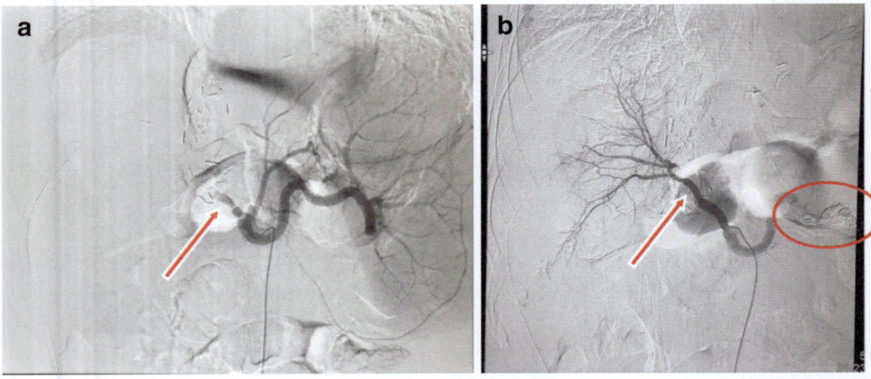

Fig. 33.2 (**a**) DSA in a 48-year old male on POD 1 after LDLT shows non-opacification of HA and early opacification of splenic artery and parenchyma. (**b**) Angio after splenic artery coil embolization shows excellent HA flow

and increased flow in the portal vein is diagnostic for SASS. The diagnosis is often suggested by poor HA signal on Doppler with high resistive index (RI > 0.80). During angiography the contrast injection in the celiac axis preferentially fills the splenic artery with poor or no discernible contrast going into the HA (Fig. 33.2). IR treatment for SASS is by proximal SAE, usually by coils or vascular plug placement. SAE increases HA flow and decreases portal hyperperfusion [9].

33.3 Portal Vein Complications

Portal vein complications are a significant but uncommon cause of morbidity and mortality in LT recipients. The portal vein complications are more frequently seen in paediatric LT and LDLT than DDLT. Common complications include PVT and PVS.

(a) *Portal vein stenosis (PVS):* Portal vein stenosis (PVS) occurs in less than 1–2% of adult DDLT cases, 2–3% of adult LDLT cases, and 8–14% of paediatric LDLT cases [9]. Technical factors, such as a tight suture line, discrepancy in PV size, tension or torsion of the PV, a redundant PV, or the use of a bypass graft, can contribute to early PVS. Furthermore, in the later period, intimal hyperplasia or fibrosis around the anastomosis may induce PVS.

PVS is usually a delayed complication, and the majority of PVS cases encountered are asymptomatic and discovered at surveillance USG. The presentation is usually insidious, with ascites, liver dysfunction, and hypersplenism. The diagnosis is further confirmed by contrast CT or MRI, which also provides information about the presence of any major portosystemic shunts,

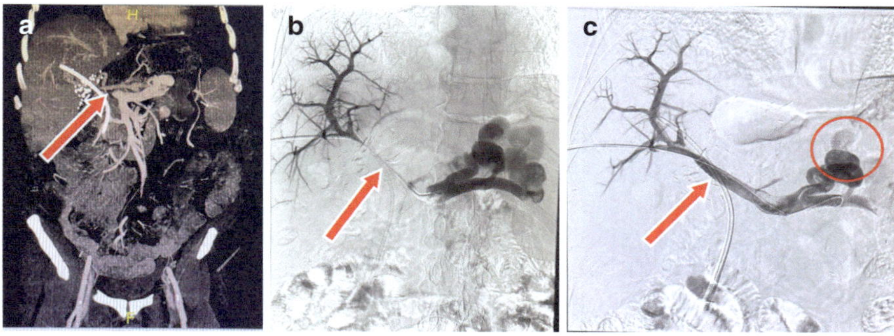

Fig. 33.3 (**a**) Coronal CECT image of a 55-year-old male 5 months after LDLT shows abrupt cutoff and non-opacification of main PV. (**b**) Portovenogram showing complete stenosis of the main PV. (**c**) Portovenogram after stent placement showing excellent hepatopetal blood flow (note significant reduction in the lieno-renal shunt)

which may need to be embolized to divert blood flow towards portal circulation (Fig. 33.3).

Treatment is undertaken in symptomatic patients or those with a high-grade stenosis thought to be at risk for progression to PVT. Interventional techniques, including balloon angioplasty and stent placement, have recently been accepted as the initial treatment of choice [9].

The access to PV can be achieved by anyone of the below methods:

(a) Percutaneous transhepatic access
(b) Trans-jugular access
(c) Percutaneous trans-splenic access
(d) Meso-colic vein access

Each access method has advantages and disadvantages. The access choice depends on variables including preoperative PV status, interval from LDLT, coagulation profile, location and degree of the stenosis, status of the intrahepatic PV and splenic vein, and the operator's preference. In our experience transhepatic access is easy and gives better control over the hardware due to its short length. However, transhepatic access should be performed carefully, and the target should be a peripheral PV branch under ultrasonography and/or fluoroscopy to reduce the risk of complications.

The IR procedure begins by measuring the pressure gradient across the stenosis. In general, a pressure gradient above 4 mm Hg is considered hemodynamically significant; however, reported cut-offs range from 3 to 8 mm Hg [10]. The treatment involves balloon dilatation of the stenotic segment and repeating the pressure measurements.

If the balloon dilation fails to reduce the pressure gradient, a stent is placed across the stenosis (Fig. 33.3c). The other indications for stent placement are elastic recoiling or recurrent PVS after balloon angioplasty or PVS early after LT. Post-stenting patients are often started on anticoagulants, like subcutaneous injections of LMWH, which are followed by oral warfarin or newer directly acting oral anticoagulants. These patients are monitored in follow-up by regularly periodic Doppler ultrasound for any recurrence of stenosis or occurrence of thrombus. In case of recurrence, the balloon dilation can be repeated, or additional stents can be placed.

A recent study compared angioplasty to stent placement in PVS patients and found that the 5-year patency rate for angioplasty alone was 82% but 100% in the stent group [11]. However, stents have several potential drawbacks, including in-stent restenosis, thrombosis, stent fractures, interference with PV anastomosis during re-transplantation, and functional stenosis of the stent in children as they grow [9].

(b) *Portal vein thrombosis (PVT):* PVT can occur in the perioperative period (<72 hours from transplant), early (<30 days), or late (>30 days). PVT in the early post-LT period (<30 days) can rapidly lead to graft dysfunction, whereas PVT later may lead to ascites and persistent portal hypertension. The prevalence of PVT in adult whole-liver grafts is estimated between 1.0% and 2.6% [12]. Risk factors include pre-transplant PVT, small PV diameter, splenectomy, use of interposition grafts for PV reconstruction, large portosystemic collateral vessels, and PVS [9].

There are no established guidelines for the management of early PVT post LT. Conventionally surgery has been employed for revascularization of PV in the early post-PT period because of its clinical urgency and the risk of bleeding during thrombolysis. IR techniques are commonly reserved for late PVT. Recently IR techniques have also been used even in early PVT with decent outcomes.

Therapeutic options for PVT range from systemic anticoagulation to interventional radiological (IR) treatment to surgical revision to re-transplantation. The IR options presented in the literature include thrombolysis, portal vein angioplasty, stent placement, and shunt occlusion if present.

The commonly used IR strategy is catheter-directed thrombolysis by using t-PA infusion (Fig. 33.4). Direct PV catheterization is preferred because most

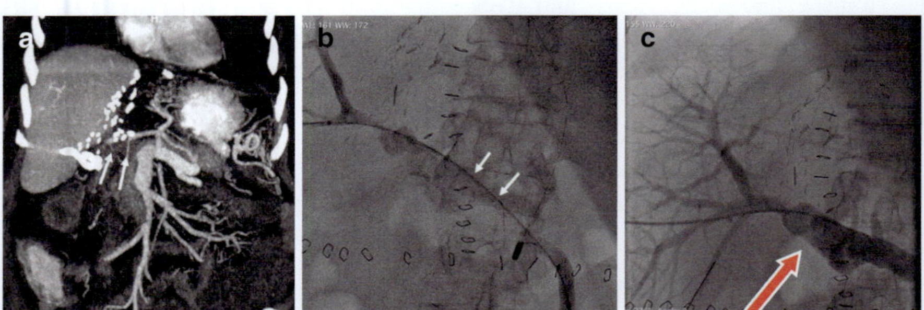

Fig. 33.4 (**a**) Coronal CECT images of a 63-year-old female post LDLT on day 17 show complete thrombosis of the portal vein. (**b**) Catheter in the portal vein shows barely any flow. (**c**) After thrombolysis, the flow is restored in the PV and its branches

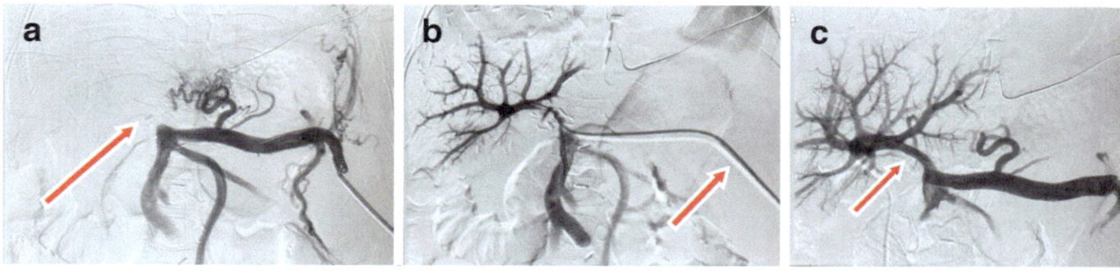

Fig. 33.5 (**a**) DSA images of a 3.5-year-old female on POD 14 who underwent re-transplant for HAT. Complete non-visualization of the PV and its branches suggestive of PVT. (**b**) DSA after balloon dilation shows improved flow with residual filling defects in PV (note trans-splenic catheter access). (**c**) After PV stenting, excellent PV flow is seen

cases of PVT have underlying PV anastomotic abnormalities such as anastomotic stenosis, kinking, or size mismatch. Besides thrombolytic infusion, mechanical thrombectomy, thrombus aspiration or balloon angioplasty, and clot maceration can be done. Use of aspiration or mechanical thrombectomy devices can reduce the total dose of the thrombolytic agent and procedural time but increase the total cost of the procedure.

Indications for stent placement are persistent thrombus after overnight infusion of t-PA, stenosis, or kinks (Fig. 33.5). In adults SEMS are commonly used; however, in paediatric cases balloon-mounted stents are often used for their short length, accurate placement, and possibility to overdilate the stent when the child grows.

Data are limited on endovascular treatment of PVT, with several adult case reports in the literature; the technical success rate ranges from 55% to 70% [10, 13], with little data on long-term efficacy.

A common scenario in patients with PVT is the simultaneous presence of patent large porto-systemic shunts, siphoning off porto-mesenteric blood flow away from MPV. These shunts are simultaneously embolized during the IR procedure to augment flow in the MPV. We found the IR technique safe and effective in embolizing these shunts with coils or vascular plugs [14].

(c) *Large porto-systemic shunts:* The diversion of the PV flow through these veins may cause hypoperfusion-induced graft failure or PVT. There is general agreement that hepatofugal collateral veins should be closed to avoid PV stealing [9]. Large persistent porto-systemic shunts can result in portal hypoperfusion, leading to graft dysfunction, PVT, or encephalopathy. These shunts are generally ligated during the transplant surgery. However, some shunts may be missed or left unligated during the surgery. These shunts sometimes divert "too much" blood away from the portal circulation. In such cases these shunts can be closed by percutaneous embolization. The choice of access would depend on the anatomical details of these shunts. For example, lieno-renal shunts are commonly accessed retrogradely from the renal vein. Vascular plugs or coils may be used to occlude these shunts (Fig. 33.6).

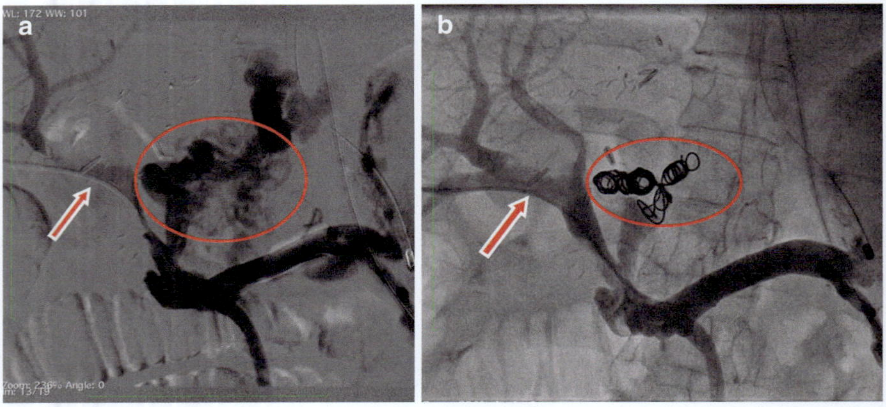

Fig. 33.6 (**a**) DSA images in a 47-year-old female on POD 12 after LDLT showing poor PV flow (arrow) and large coronary vein shunt (circle) (**b**) Coils in the coronary vein shunt. Note the improved flow in PV (arrow)

33.4 Hepatic Vein Outflow Complications

The hepatic vein complications are another uncommon but significant cause of graft dysfunction in LT recipients. The prevalence of hepatic vein outflow complications in orthotopic liver transplants is between 1% and 6% [15]. Early complications will often be related to surgical technique, such as a tight anastomosis or twisted allograft causing vascular kinking. The common HV complications are anastomotic site stenosis and HV thrombosis.

(a) *HV stenosis:* HV stenosis is more commonly seen in LDLT than DDLT, where individual HVs are anastomosed to inferior vena cava (IVC) [1]. The risk factors are discrepancies in the HV size, a tight suture line, twisting or kinking, and multiple anastomoses in the early post-transplant period [9]. Patients may present with large-volume ascites and abnormal liver function tests. Diagnosis may be difficult, but loss of phasicity in the hepatic veins at Doppler USG can suggest a stenosis.

    HV catheterization is mostly achieved from a jugular or femoral vein approach (Fig. 33.7). A direct puncture by percutaneous transhepatic approach is reserved for cases with severely tight stenosis. Diagnosis is confirmed by measuring the pressure gradient between HV and IVC. The definition of a significant gradient is controversial, with a threshold between 3 and 10 mm Hg [1].

    Balloon angioplasty is the first choice for the treatment of HV stenosis and offers a high technical success rate. However, elastic recoiling or recurrence is common, and some patients may require multiple sessions of balloon dilatation or stent placement. After balloon dilatation the pressure measurements are repeated. If the pressure gradient fails to decrease due to

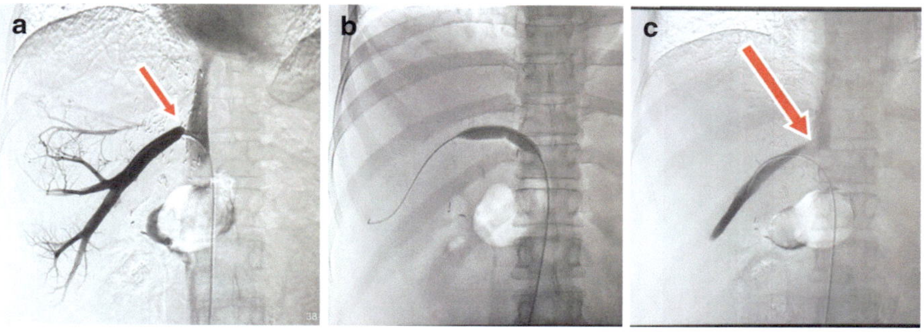

Fig. 33.7 (**a**) Hepatic venogram in a 34-year-old female on POD 43 shows anastomotic site narrowing with contrast opacification of the branches of the HV and refluxing of contrast into a smaller HV superiorly. (**b**) Balloon dilation of HV anastomotic site. (**c**) Contrast injection with non-filling of branches of HV suggestive of brisk wash out of contrast into IVC

the nature of the outflow obstruct, for example, kinking or elastic recoiling, stent placement is considered. Stent placement is also effective for managing recurrent stenosis after balloon angioplasty. For stent placement, the length of a stent protruding toward the IVC should be as short as possible to avoid potential IVC stenosis or interference with the re-transplantation in the future.

With balloon dilatation alone for hepatic vein interventions, recurrence is seen in up to 55% of patients [16]. Improved patency of up to 92% may be achieved with the use of stents during primary treatment [1].

There is no consensus regarding whether short HVs (i.e., the right inferior HV or the middle HV tributaries) should be revascularized during right lobe LDLT. However, several authors assumed that revascularization of these HVs might be necessary to avoid small-for-size graft syndrome and to facilitate the restoration of liver function [9].

(b) *Acute HV thrombosis:* Thrombosis of HVs can cause acute onset of symptoms. The primary cause of thrombosis is often underlying HV stenosis. HV thrombosis is common in reconstructed middle HV (neo-MHV). When there are multiple outflow veins, thrombosis in some of the veins may remain asymptomatic. However, when a major HV is thrombosed, the patients present with liver dysfunction similar to small-for-size syndrome. Diagnosis is made by Doppler USG. Contrast CT or MRI can provide further information, including features of congestion in the form of poor enhancement in the territory of the liver parenchyma drained by the thrombosed vein (Fig. 33.8).

Treatment is often thrombolysis, endovascular clot aspiration, balloon dilatation, and stent placement. The stent selection and placement should be meticulous such that it does not jail the ostia of the other hepatic veins and does not protrude into the IVC more than a few millimetres.

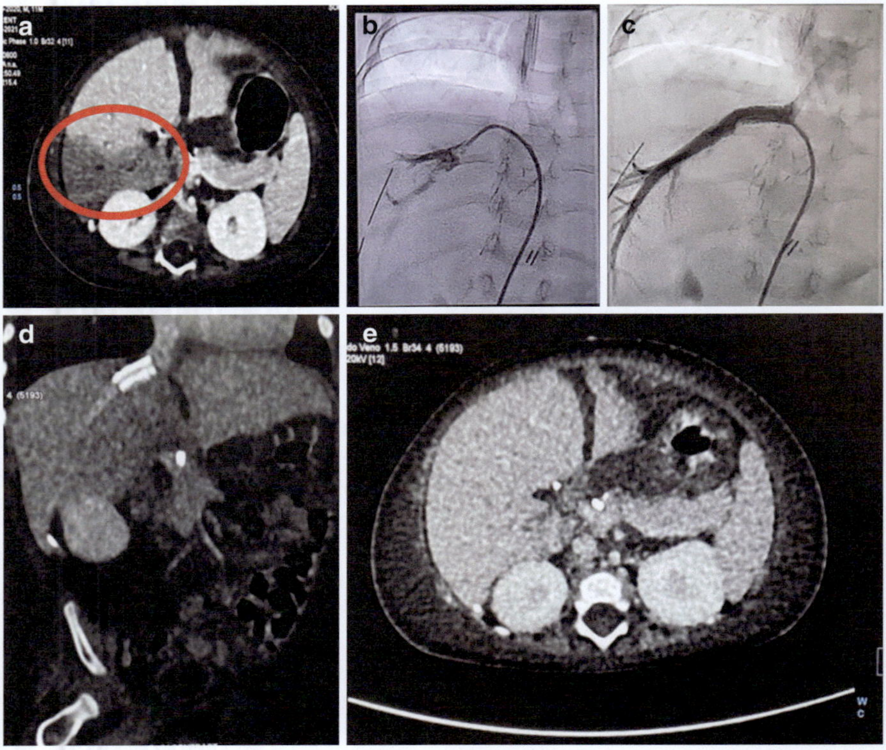

Fig. 33.8 (**a**) Axial CT image shows poor contrast enhancement of the posterior sector of liver graft in a 13-month-old male baby on POD 18 who underwent a domino transplant. (**b**) Venogram shows filling defects in the RHV suggestive of thrombosis (**c**) Venogram after HV stent placement shows satisfactory RHV flow. (**d**) Coronal CT image shows stent position in RHV. (**e**) Axial CT image after 1 month of follow-up shows normal liver enhancement including posterior sector

33.5 Biliary Complications

Biliary complications are seen in nearly all liver surgeries and are not exclusive to LT; however, biliary complications are the commonest complication of LT. Prevalence of biliary complications after liver transplant is between 5% and 45%, with higher prevalence in LDLT [17]. The various complications include bile leaks, bilomas, and biliary strictures.

A. *Bile leaks:* The incidence of bile leak is between 7.8% and 9.5% in LT recipients [18]. Sources of leaks include the biliary anastomosis, cystic duct, or cut surface of the liver. Management consists of percutaneous drainage of the bilomas. This is often done under USG guidance using a 10 or 12F pigtail catheter placed over a guidewire. Bilomas can sometimes be multiple or multiseptated. These require more than one PCD or upsizing of the drain size. Bilomas sometimes continue

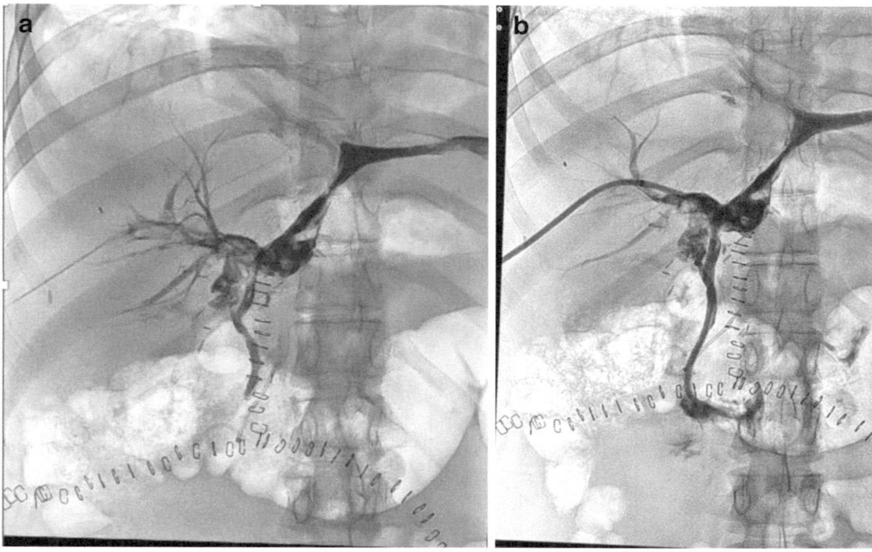

Fig. 33.9 (**a**) PTC in a LDLT recipient shows bile leak at the hilum. (**b**) PTBD catheter placement across the leak with catheter tip in the second part of deudenum

to drain for days to weeks. Bilomas may also get infected, and the initial drain output can be purulent, which becomes clear and golden in colour over the next few days as the fresh bile starts coming out.

The PCD is removed when the bile stops leaking. This can happen spontaneously or may require biliary stenting to divert the bile leak. Biliary stenting can be done via ERCP or via PTBD (Fig. 33.9). Although endoscopic therapy with bile diversion is the first choice of treatment, percutaneous treatment is a valuable alternative for treating bile leaks resistant to or inaccessible by endoscopic methods [19].

B. *Biliary stricture:* In a systemic review, the incidence of BS was 12% and 19% among DDLT and LDLT recipients ($p < 0.001$), respectively [18]. Strictures result in bile duct obstruction and upstream duct dilatation and commonly present as pruritus, jaundice, and recurrent fever (cholangitis). Biliary strictures usually involve anastomotic sites, which are localized short-segment strictures. Non-anastomotic site strictures are multifocal or long-segment and are difficult to treat. Risk factors for non-anastomotic site strictures include HAS or HAT, chronic rejection, prolonged ischemia time, or recurrent disease in patients with underlying primary sclerosing cholangitis.

PTBD is indicated in cases with hepatico-jejunostomy stricture (bilioenteric anastomosis), single duct-to-duct anastomosis with failed ERCP, and multiple duct-to-duct anastomosis in which ERCP may fail to cannulate all the systems. Two or more PTBDs are sometimes required, especially in right lobe LDLT because of the separated anterior and posterior bile ducts associ-

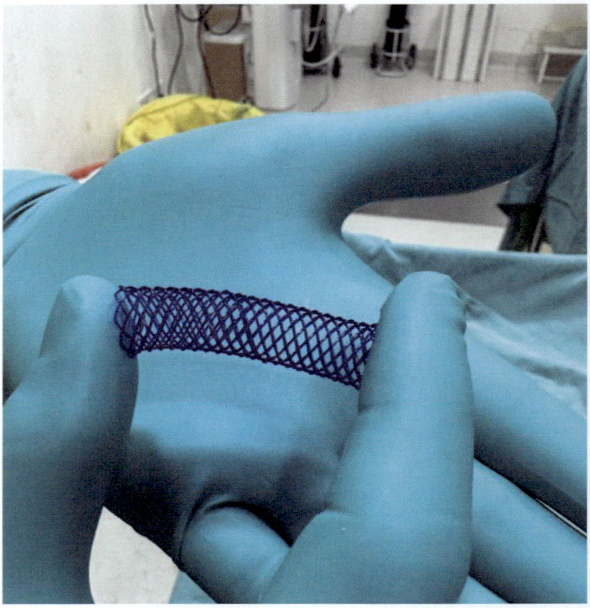

Fig. 33.10 Ella SX biodegradable stent

ated with a short donor extrahepatic bile duct and a high incidence of multiple ductal openings. Multiple ductal openings have been reported in 22–56% of living-donor liver grafts [9]. IHBR dilatation in LT recipient patients with biliary strictures is often mild compared to IHBR dilatation in biliary strictures in native livers. Lesser dilatation of IHBR can lead to difficulty in performing PTBD. Often a micro puncture set (like NEFF set, Cook Medical, USA) is required to cannulate such small ducts. Once crossed, the stricture can be treated with balloon dilation and placement of a biliary catheter across the stenosis. BS treatment protocols are highly controversial and institute-specific. Catheter exchanges and upsizing are often required over many months for long-term successful treatment. One study that used such a protocol achieved patency of 84% at 1 year, 78% at 2 years, and 74% at 5 years. That study included liver transplant strictures and other benign biliary strictures [20].

Recently, biodegradable stents have been used for biliary stricture treatment (Fig. 33.10). The advantage is that repeated hospitalizations can be avoided. Preliminary results are encouraging, suggesting patency rates equal to the conventional long-term repeated catheter placement. Dopazo et al. [21] used a biodegradable biliary stent for treating 16 anastomotic strictures after liver transplantation and reported technical and clinical success rates of 100% and 81%, respectively, during a median follow-up of 18 months.

33.6 Conclusion

Outcomes of LT have continued to improve, in part owing to the use of IR techniques to treat post-transplant complications. The complications may involve the hepatic arteries, portal vein, hepatic veins, and biliary system. Minimally invasive IR techniques can help manage most of these post-transplant complications with excellent results. With refinements in hardware, the results of IR treatments will further improve, and in the future, IR may play a greater role in the management of LT complications.

References

1. Naidu SG, Alzubaidi SJ, Patel IJ, Iwuchukwu C, Zurcher KS, Malik DG, Knuttinen MG, Kriegshauser JS, Wallace AL, Katariya NN, Mathur AK, Oklu R. Interventional radiology management of adult liver transplant complications. Radiographics. 2022;42(6):1705–23. https://doi.org/10.1148/rg.220011. PMID: 36190864.
2. da Silva RF, Raphe R, Felício HC, et al. Prevalence, treat-ment, and outcomes of the hepatic artery stenosis after liver transplantation. Transplant Proc. 2008;40(3):805–7.
3. Rostambeigi N, Hunter D, Duval S, Chinnakotla S, Golzarian J. Stent placement versus angioplasty for hepatic artery stenosis after liver transplant: a meta-analysis of case series. Eur Radiol. 2013;23(5):1323–34.
4. Magand N, Coronado JL, Drevon H, et al. Primary angioplasty or stenting for hepatic artery stenosis treatment after liver transplantation. Clin Transpl. 2019;33(12):e13729.
5. Le L, Terral W, Zea N, et al. Primary stent placement for hepatic artery stenosis after liver transplantation. J Vasc Surg. 2015;62(3):704–9.
6. Sugi MD, Albadawi H, Knuttinen G, et al. Transplant artery thrombosis and outcomes. Cardiovasc Diagn Ther. 2017;7(suppl 3):S219–27.
7. Singhal A, Stokes K, Sebastian A, Wright HI, Kohli V. Endovascular treatment of hepatic artery thrombosis following liver transplantation. Transpl Int. 2010;23:245–56.
8. Kogut MJ, Shin DS, Padia SA, Johnson GE, Hippe DS, Valji K. Intra-arterial thrombolysis for hepatic artery thrombosis following liver transplantation. J Vasc Interv Radiol. 2015;26:1317–22.
9. Ko GY, Sung KB, Gwon DI. The application of interventional radiology in living-donor liver transplantation. Korean J Radiol. 2021;22(7):1110–23. https://doi.org/10.3348/kjr.2020.0718. Epub 2021 Mar 9. PMID: 33739630; PMCID: PMC8236365.
10. Saad WE. Portal interventions in liver transplant recipients. Semin Intervent Radiol. 2012;29(2):99–104.
11. Kim KS, Kim JM, Lee JS, Choi GS, Cho JW, Lee SK. Stent insertion and balloon angioplasty for portal vein stenosis after liver transplantation: long-term follow-up results. Diagn Interv Radiol. 2019;25(3):231–7.
12. Khalaf H. Vascular complications after deceased and living donor liver transplantation: a single-center experience. Transplant Proc. 2010;42(3):865–70.
13. Bashir S, Gupta S. Early portal vein thrombosis after living donor liver transplant: interventional radiology may be the answer [abstract]. Arab J Intervent Radiol. 2019;03(03):S16–7. https://doi.org/10.1055/s-0041-1730562.
14. Vijayashanker A, Chikkala BR, Ghimire R, Nidoni R, Acharya MR, Pandey Y, Dey R, Kaloo SB, Agarwal S, Gupta S. Do natural portosystemic shunts need to be compulsorily ligated in living donor liver transplantation? J Clin Exp Hepatol. 2022;12(1):29–36.

https://doi.org/10.1016/j.jceh.2021.04.009. Epub 2021 Apr 24. PMID: 35068782; PMCID: PMC8766688.
15. Darcy MD. Management of venous outflow complications after liver transplantation. Tech Vasc Interv Radiol. 2007;10(3):240–5.
16. Pandhi MB, Lipnik AJ, Niemeyer MM. Endovascular treatment of hepatic venous outflow obstruction after liver transplant. Dig Dis Interv. 2019;3(4):277–86.
17. Lee HW, Shah NH, Lee SK. An update on endoscopic management of post–liver transplant biliary complications. Clin Endosc. 2017;50(5):451–63.
18. Akamatsu N, Sugawara Y, Hashimoto D. Biliary reconstruction, its complications and management of biliary complications after adult liver transplantation: a systematic review of the incidence, risk factors and outcome. Transpl Int. 2011;24:379–92.
19. Kim JH, Ko GY, Sung KB, Yoon HK, Gwon DI, Kim KR, et al. Bile leak following living donor liver transplantation: clinical efficacy of percutaneous transhepatic treatment. Liver Transpl. 2008;14:1142–9.
20. DePietro DM, Shlansky-Goldberg RD, Soulen MC, et al. Long-term outcomes of a benign biliary stricture protocol. J Vasc Interv Radiol. 2015;26(7):1032–9.
21. Dopazo C, Diez I, Quintero J, Curell A, González-Junyent C, Caralt M, et al. Role of biodegradable stents as part of treatment of biliary strictures after pediatric and adult liver transplantation: an observational single-center study. J Vasc Interv Radiol. 2018;29:899–904.

Chapter 34
Role of Endotherapy in the Treatment of Post–Liver Transplant Biliary Complications

Kalpana Acharya and Vikas Singla

Abstract Of all the complications post–liver transplant (LT), biliary complications account for a major morbidity, roughly estimated to be around 10 to 30%. These complications are encountered more frequently in patients of a living-donor LT compared to a deceased-donor LT. Notable complications encountered commonly include biliary strictures, bile leakage or biloma, biliary stones, and sphincter of Oddi dysfunction, while hemobilia, bile casts, and retained foreign bodies account for minor events post-transplantation. Endotherapy has been evolving rapidly and has come a long way in mitigating these complications. With advancement in endoscopic techniques and refinement of the procedure, the outcome and the success rate have been consistently reaching up to 80%. With regard to ductal reconstruction, conventional endoscopic retrograde cholangiopancreatography (ERCP) remains the preferred initial treatment; however, in endoscopically challenging cases like Roux-en-y reconstruction or complex hilar strictures, percutaneous transhepatic cholangiography becomes the preferred modality. Novelities in the endoscopy methods such as the rendezvous technique, peroral cholangioscopy, and magnetic compression anastomosis, coupled with advancements in stent design and structure, have largely improved the outcome of endoscopic management. This chapter aims to concisely discuss the current state of endoscopic treatment of post–LT biliary complications and enlist both the existing and the emerging techniques.

Keywords Endotherapy · Liver Transplantation · Anastomotic Stricture · Cholangitis · Endoscopic Retrograde Cholangiography

---

K. Acharya · V. Singla (✉)
Department of Gastroenterology, Max Super Specialty Hospital, Saket, New Delhi, India
e-mail: singlavikas1979@gmail.com

S. Saigal, D. Jothimani (eds.), *Fundamentals of Transplant Hepatology*,
https://doi.org/10.1007/978-981-95-2624-6_34

Key Highlights

Biliary complications can occur in 10–30% of liver transplant (LT) patients, characterized by bile leak, biliary strictures, and bilioma, with slightly higher prevalence in living donor liver transplant (LDLT) recipients.

Post-transplant biliary strictures are usually anastomotic; however, non-anastomotic strictures can occur due to diffuse ischemic injury to the bile ducts as seen in hepatic artery thrombosis, chronic rejection, and ABO-incompatible liver transplantation.

Biliary stricture should be diagnosed based on clinical suspicion, biochemical parameters, and imaging modalities such as abdominal ultrasound and an MRCP.

Patients with biliary anastomotic stricture require intervention through an endoscopic approach as the first-line therapy or occasionally percutaneous approach and uncommonly surgical correction.

34.1 Introduction

Liver transplant (LT) is an effective treatment for the management of end-stage liver disease with 1-, 3-, and 5-year survival rates of 91.8%, 83.8%, and 76.1%, respectively [1]. Biliary complications continue to pose a significant threat to the success of liver transplantation. Biliary leak and stricture are the most common complications and can occur not only in the immediate postoperative period but also during longer follow-up and may affect graft function and survival. These complications are caused by multitudes of underlying factors such as surgical technique, rejection episodes, disease recurrence, vascular issues, and infections contributing to biliary complications. Endotherapy plays an important role in the management of post-transplant biliary complications with percutaneous transhepatic biliary drainage (PTBD) or surgery reserved as rescue techniques. Biliary complications are more likely to occur after living donor liver transplant (LDLT) with a reported incidence of ~15–30% than deceased donor liver transplantation, which affects 10–15% of patients [2]. Table 34.1 summarizes various types of biliary complications.

Table 34.1 Biliary complications post–liver transplantation

Biliary adverse event	Timing of presentation	Incidence	Clinical pointers	Endoscopic management
Bile leak/ Bilioma	Early to late	7.1% to 11.8% [3, 4]	Fever Bilious drainage from the drain Pain abdomen Deranged liver function tests	Sphincterotomy and/ or stenting Percutaneous transhepatic biliary drainage
Anastomotic stricture	Early to late	6.6% to 12.3% [5, 6]	Icterus Cholestatic pattern of liver function tests Abdominal pain Asymptomatic	Balloon dilatation or stenting Multiple plastic stenting/FCSEMS
Non-anastomotic stricture	Late	10% to 16% [7]	Abdominal pain, jaundice Derangement of liver function test with cholestatic pattern Asymptomatic	Balloon dilatation or stenting Multiple plastic stenting/FCSEMS Retransplant
Biliary stones	Early to late	3% to 6% [8, 9]	Abdominal pain Jaundice Cholestatic liver function test	ERCP with stenting
Sphincter of Oddi dysfunction	Early to late	2% to 3.5%	Abdominal pain Cholestatic liver injury	ERCP with sphincterotomy
Vanishing bile duct	Early to late	Data scarce	Jaundice Fatigue	Retransplant Spontaneous resolution (quite rare)

34.2 Risk Factor for Biliary Complications (Table 34.2)

Various donor- and recipient-related predisposing factors for biliary complications have been explained [10–17]. A transplanted liver from a living donor or from a cardiac death donor, older age of donor, high BMI, graft steatosis >25% have been related to a higher chance of biliary complications.

Recipient-related factors include primary disease such as primary sclerosing cholangitis.

Vascular events such as thrombosis or stenosis of the hepatic artery increase the risk of biliary complications. Donor–recipient size mismatch and ischemic/reperfusion injury are the other causes leading to biliary complications.

Another way of establishing the risks for biliary complication post–liver transplantation includes stratifying into preoperative, operative, and postoperative risks. Among the preoperative risks, advancing age and poor synthetic function of liver in the recipient are identified as risk factors for developing biliary strictures. LDLT has higher risks than deceased donor liver transplant (DDLT)

Table 34.2 Risk factors for post-transplant biliary strictures

Presurgical risks	Surgical risks	Postsurgical risks
LDLT has more risk than DDLT. Age: Advanced age of donor and recipient. Donor–recipient bile duct mismatch Blood group incompatibility Steatosis of more than 25% in the transplanted liverPrimary sclerosing cholangitis as an indication for liver transplantation	Ischemia: Long warm and cold time Cold storage and preservative solution Extensive periductal tissue dissection during procurement of the graft Type of anastomosis, duct to duct vs. hepaticojejeunostomy Tension at the anastomotic site Vascular injury of peribiliary plexus Prolonged use of electrocautery for control of hemorrhage during surgery Subsequent transplant Experience of the surgeon	Bile leakage in the postoperative period. Chronic B and T cell–mediated rejection Type of immunosuppression Infections of graft like cytomegalovirus (CMV) Vascular catastrophe like hepatic artery thrombosis or stenosis

(19% vs. 12%; $p < 0.0001$) [5]. The plausible explanations of this cause are a smaller duct size in LDLT and more challenging anastomosis between donor and recipient and the devascularization due to hilar dissection. Various operative risks factors that have been studied include prolonged ischemia time (warm and cold), lack of standardization in graft preservation methods, variations of biliary reconstruction techniques, and lack of experience of the surgeon.

One such published series of 640 orthoptic liver transplants showed that the biliary adverse events reduced from 23% to 5% ($p = 0.003$) over 6-year follow-up period due to better experience of the transplant team [18]. Regarding the type of anastomosis, a meta-analysis, which included 1286 cases, reported a lower rate of biliary strictures in patients with hepaticojejunostomy as compared with duct-to-duct reconstruction (OR 0.448; $p < 0.001$). [19] However, duct-to-duct anastomosis eases the endoscopic access to the biliary tree and preserves the sphincter of Oddi, thereby theoretically avoiding the reflux of duodenal contents into the bile duct [20]. At present, the use of T-tube for biliary reconstruction remains controversial. Most transplant centers hesitantly use it because of the fear of developing cholangitis in the postoperative period. The incidence of biliary strictures following OLT was reported to be lower when biliary reconstruction was performed.

Using a splinting T-tube (9.7% vs. 12.5%) [5] a subsequent meta-analysis showed that biliary strictures occurred significantly less frequently when a T-tube was utilized (odds ratio of 0.49 for the group with T-tube reconstruction vs. the other group) [20] mostly preventing occurrence of strictures later in the post–OLT course [21]

34.3 Endoscopic Management of Specific Complications

Biliary strictures are of two types: anastomotic strictures (AS) and non-anastomotic strictures (NAS). AS account for 80% of all strictures and NAS account for about 20%. AS occur more commonly after LDLT than DDLT because LDLT anastomoses are made between multiple small peripheral bile ducts. AS that occur early after transplantation, within 3 months, are often due to surgical issues [22], whereas late AS beyond 3 months are primarily because of ischemia with poor healing.

In a systematic evaluation of 61 studies including over 14, 000 liver transplants, the total incidence of biliary stricture was 13%, and occurred in 19% and 12% of patients with LDLT and DDLT, respectively [5]. Early strictures occurring within 2 months following transplantation are frequently associated with surgical techniques, while late-stage strictures are typically the result of vascular complications such as thrombosis [23]. Biliary strictures develop in around 20% of patients with postoperative bile leakage [18].

34.3.1 Anastomotic Strictures

Anastomotic strictures are short-segment localized strictures with narrowing at the site of anastomosis between the donor and recipient bile ducts. Anastomotic strictures account for 86% of all biliary strictures after LT and cumulative risk increases with time [24]. The cumulative incidence of AS increases with time (6.6% at 1 year and 12.3% at 10 year) [24]. Strictures that occur early within 2 months of transplantation are by and large related to technical problems during surgery, whereas late strictures are mainly due to vascular insufficiency, ischemia, and fibrosis [24].

Anastomotic stricture may either present with jaundice, cholangitis, or abdominal pain or may be asymptomatic with deranged liver function test or imaging evidence of biliary obstruction. Though transabdominal ultrasound is frequently the first radiological test carried out, it has low sensitivity, ranging from 30% to 70% [25]. Ultrasonography (USG) Doppler is particularly helpful in diagnosing hepatic artery thrombosis or stenosis [26]. The absence of bile duct dilation should not prevent further investigation if suspicion is high for a biliary tract complication. Magnetic resonance cholangio-pancreato-graphy (MRCP) is the most sensitive radiological technique for evaluating biliary strictures [26]. MRCP has gained wide recognition and acceptance given the noninvasive nature of the technique and its ability to map and gauge the entire biliary tree and even demonstrate ducts upstream from a tight stricture. Therefore, it is quite helpful for hilar and intrahepatic anastomotic strictures. MRCP has a sensitivity of 93–96% and specificity of 90–94% for diagnosing biliary obstruction [26]. The main disadvantage of MRCP is poor sensitivity when looking for minor leaks, sludges, and small stones (<5 mm) [27].

Computed tomography has a low accuracy in the range of 40% for diagnosing biliary strictures [26]. However, if there is suspicion of hepatic artery stenosis or

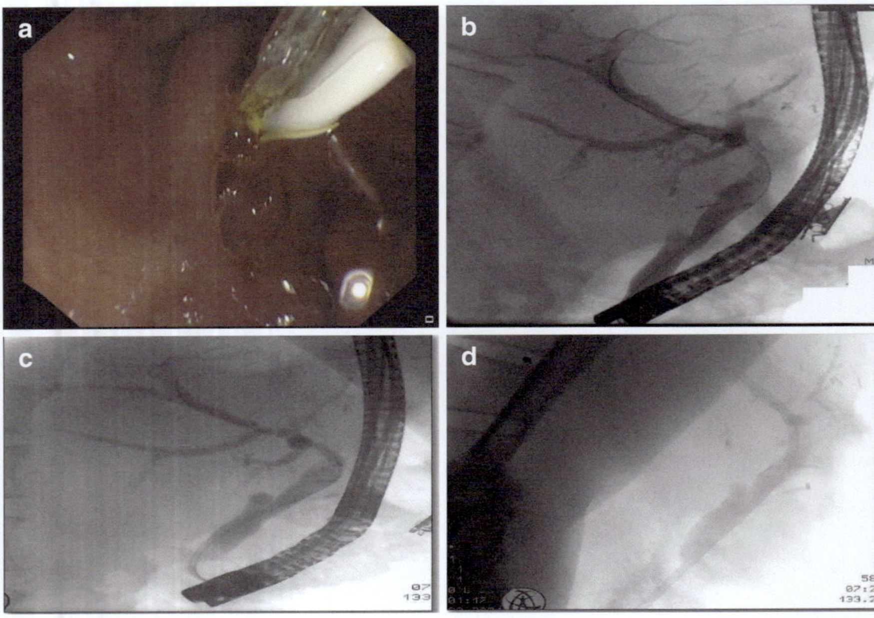

Fig. 34.1 (**a**) Endoscopic image showing CRE balloon inside the papilla. (**b**) Cholangiogram shows anastomotic stricture after LDLT. (**c**) Stricture on balloon occluded cholangiogram with a balloon dilatation of 4 mm. (**d**) Single plastic stent deployed across the stricture

occlusion in Doppler ultrasound, computed tomography remains as the modality of choice for pretreatment confirmation and on confirmation of this vascular catastrophe angiographic intervention should be performed immediately to establish hepatic artery flow [26]. Though endoscopic retrograde cholangiography (ERC) is the gold standard for confirmation for diagnosis of biliary strictures, because of associated complications, this procedure is reserved for therapeutic purposes only. Because of lesser use of T-tube placement during biliary reconstruction, T-tube cholangiogram is no longer available in most patients for evaluation of biliary tree [26].

- *Endoscopic management* (Fig. 34.1)

Objective of endotherapy: Resolution of stricture, improved bile flow through the constricted/narrowed segment, and resolution of obstruction-related symptoms and laboratory abnormalities (such as jaundice, cholangitis, and increased liver enzymes) are the objectives of endoscopic therapy with ERCP [28]. Anastomotic strictures are usually small and unifocal and can be managed with endotherapy by the placement of either plastic or metal stents [28].

Although the management of biliary strictures require multidisciplinary approach, endoscopic therapy is the first line of treatment in patients with duct to duct anastomosis. Endotherapy includes biliary sphincterotomy, balloon dilatation of strictures, basket and balloon extraction of stones, sludge, and casts, and deployment of single or multiple side-by-side plastic stent or fully covered SEMS. Many patients with Roux-en-Y hepaticojejunostomy can also be treated endoscopically with enteroscopy and percutaneous transhepatic cholangiography (PTC) being mostly reserved as salvage measure [29].

Initially, balloon dilatation (BD) was used alone. However, because of the high rate of recurrent stricture formation, biliary stenting is combined with balloon dilatation [8, 24, 30]. In a comparative study, combination therapy of BD plus stenting was more effective than dilatation alone [30, 31]. Most patients will require multiple sessions of ERCP every 3 months, with stenting and dilation for 1–2 years. Typically, a guidewire is placed across the stricture, dilated with 6- to 8-mm balloons and then one or multiple 7 to 11.5 Fr plastic stents are placed. Plastic stents should be exchanged every 3 months to avoid occlusion and thereby prevent cholangitis.

A review of 440 patients with AS treated with plastic stents showed that the resolution rate was 85%. The rate of recurrence of stricture depends on the duration of stenting. Less than 12 months of stenting had a 78% stricture resolution rate, while >12 months with a stent [32] had a 97% resolution rate [32]. In a study by Costamagna et al., balloon dilation, followed by deployment of an increasing number of 10 Fr stents and repetition of ERCP every 3 months with stent stacking, could be used until complete resolution of the stricture on fluoroscopy. This study showed 80–95% success, with 20–35% recurrence [33]. With the available literature, the usual practice remains deploying a progressive number of plastic stents (8.5, 10, or 11.5 Fr in size) to calibrate the stricture until its complete resolution. After the first ERCP, repeat examination with insertion of an increasing number of stents every 3 months to reduce the chance of stent blockage is done until there is a complete resolution of the stricture. Patients with LDLT often require more number of endoscopic sessions with the placement of smaller caliber (7 or 8.5 Fr) stents due to the small size of bile duct [34]. In a study by Tabibian et al., a group of 83 patients was studied. Of these patients, 63 AS were treated successfully, and a total of 8 stents were used, with an average of 2.5 stents per ERCP and a median of three to five sessions of ERCP needed per patient [35]. Long-term follow-up data from Tringali et al. [39], on the multiple plastic stenting, showed stricture resolution in 98% of patients with AS in the per protocol analysis and in 89% of the patients in the intention-to-treat analysis [36]. Recurrence of stricture was seen only in 6% of the patients during a median follow-up of 2.9 years and these patients were treated with same method [37]. Frequent ERCP sessions come with the risks of radiation exposure and costs. To mitigate these limitations, various methods have been advocated:

1. Multiple plastic stenting with stent exchange, only in cases of biliary obstruction or cholangitis [36]
2. Placement of a new stent alongside the previously placed stent [38, 39]
3. Placement of fully covered self-expanding metal stent (FcSEMS) [39]

Temporary placement of FcSEMS has been the latest alternative to multiple plastic stents. FcSEMS is composed of stainless steel or nitinol [37]. It is prudent to confirm the etiology, size, and location of the stricture. When the etiology of stricture is indeterminate, the size is smaller than 5 mm, or there is an

Table 34.3 RCTs: comparing multiple plastic stents and FcSEMSs placement

Author	Year	Number of patients	Median number of ERCPs performed per patient: FCSEMS vs. MPS arm	Stricture resolution in FCSEMS vs. MPS arm	Stricture recurrence in FCSEMS vs. MPS arm	Complications in FCSEMS vs. MPS arm	Cost effective
Kaffes et al. [41]	2014	20	2 vs. 4.5 ($p = 0.0001$)	100% vs. 80% (p = not significant)		10% vs. 50% ($p = 0.051$)	FCSEMS
Tal et al. [42]	2017	48	2 vs. 4 ($p < 0.001$)	95.8% vs. 100% ($p = 1$)	20.8% vs. 21.7% (p = not specified)	Not evaluated	Not evaluated
Martins et al. [43]	2018	59	2 vs. 5 (p = not specified)	96.5% vs. 83.3% ($p < 0.01$)	32% vs. 0%	23.3 vs. 6.4 ($p < 0.01$)	FCSEMS

intrahepatic location of stricture, the placement of FcSEMS should be avoided. At present, 8- and 10-mm diameter FcSEMS are used. The 8-mm stents should be used if duct size is 5–7 mm, and 10-mm self-expanding metal stent (SEMS) should be used if >8 mm [40]. While deploying the FcSEMS, it should be ensured that the proximal end of the stent should remain distal to the bifurcation to avoid obstructing of bile flow from one lobe of the liver to the common bile duct (CBD). Migration is the most common drawback associated with FcSEMS. Leaving the long part of stent into the duodenum, avoiding dilatation prior to stent placement, and keeping the FcSEMS in the center of stricture are some important strategies to reduce the migration risks. Three randomized trials comparing multiple plastic stenting with FcSEMSs' placement have been summarized in (Table 34.3) [40–43]. Overall, the three studies randomized patients to multiple plastic stents (MPS) and FcSEMS group. The number of endoscopic sessions was significantly higher in the multi-stenting technique group. Martins et al. [43] found higher stricture recurrence rate in case of SEMS group.

In a systematic review of 200 patients, comparing the two different stenting groups, FcSEMS group had stricture resolution rates between 80% and 95% when the stent was left in place for 3 months or longer [32]. In contrast, the stricture resolution varied from 94% to 100% for patients treated with plastic stents. In another meta-analysis with four RCTs, 213 patients showed that temporary insertion of either MPS or a covered SEMS for the treatment of strictures provided similar results (ORs [95%CIs] for stricture resolution, recurrence, and adverse events, respectively: 1.07 [0.97–1.18], 0.88 [0.48–1.63], and 1.16 [0.71–1.88]) [213]. Fewer ERCPs were required with covered SEMS (mean difference − 1.71, 95%CI − 2.34 to −1.09) [44]. Cost -analysis of the strategy showed that the SEMS approach is more cost-effective than the multi-stenting technique.

The actual duration for placement of FCSEMS is not well known; however, a meta-analysis comprising 37 studies, 1677 patients showed that the median duration of stenting was 4.4 month. Another meta-analysis comprising 22 studies with 1298 patients showed a lower stricture recurrence with 6 and 3 months [45] of stenting. The superiority of FcSEMS cannot be established over multiple plastic stents with the available data. A well-designed multicenter randomized trial needs to be conducted to frame a more meaningful and definitive conclusion.

In patients of Roux-en-Y reconstruction (4–17%) with anastomotic stricture, single- or double-balloon enteroscopy can be used to treat the stricture. Wang et al. [44, 46] demonstrated cannulation in 12 of 13 patients and a successful intervention rate of 90% when using single-balloon enteroscopy. In another study by Shah et al., of a total of 129 patients who underwent enteroscopy and a subsequent ERCP, 92 patients (71%) had a successful enteroscopy (single- or double-balloon enteroscopy, or over-tube enteroscopy); these patients had successful treatment of anastomotic strictures [44].

– *Endpoint of endotherapy*

No definite criteria for endoscopic success have been laid out; however, symptomatic and/or biochemical improvement, imaging showing resolution of stricture, and the absence of recurrence of cholestasis are acceptable endpoints [47]. These patients' anastomotic stricture should be in lifelong follow-up monitoring for clinical, biochemical, and radiological evidence of stricture recurrence.

34.3.2 Non Anastomotic Stricture (NAS)

NAS are also called ischemic strictures [48]. NAS are at a distance of more than 1 cm from the reconstruction site. NAS are frequently intrahepatic and are usually associated with the biliary casts or stones. Hepatic artery thrombosis is a contributory factor in nearly 50% of patients [48]. NAS are associated with graft loss of up to 60% [7]. They typically present at a median of 6 months post-transplantation. Long-term studies have demonstrated an increase in the incidence of NAS from 10% at 1 year to almost double of ~16% at 10 years of transplantation [49]. Because of multifocal involvement of small ducts and location at intrahepatic ducts, ERCP interventions are challenging in patients with NAS, and re-transplantation is often required.

Endoscopic treatments of NAS include papillotomy, guidewire placement, dilatation with 4- to 6-mm balloon, and plastic stenting. The most commonly used stents are of size 7–10 Fr and are replaced regularly at monthly interval for nearly 6 to 12 months. NAS are usually resistant to treatment and often need prolonged therapy with a cure rate of only 50% [7, 50]. In a study by Graziadei et al., 19 patients with NAS were treated with balloon dilatation (BD) followed by multiple plastic stents. Overall, a median of 7 ERCPs was performed per patient involving four sessions of BDs and 3 stents placed per session. No patient showed complete resolution of the stricture, 7 patients (36.8%) had no response at all, and 8 patients (42.1%) had complete resolution of symptoms with slight abnormalities of LFT [51].

Patients with intrahepatic small ducts NAS, percutaneous transhepatic choalangiography may be an alternative. NAS resulting from thrombosis of hepatic artery should be managed with immediate revascularization or redo transplantation. An early repeat transplantation should also be reserved in the cases where there is evidence of diffuse disease in smaller intrahepatic ducts.

Refractory strictures have been treated with myriad of therapies including magnetic compression anastomosis (MCA) and steroid injection through cholangioscope followed by balloon dilatation. A novel through-the-scope magnet has demonstrated an 86% cure rate for refractory strictures. Injection of steroid at the stricture site through the cholangioscopy and then dilating with balloon was reported as safe, durable and effective therapy, for refractory anastomotic strictures [52]. Paclitaxel-eluting balloons have also been evaluated at for treating refractory strictures. Possible hypothesis behind using paclitaxel being its antifibrotic properties which help to prevent fibrosis near the stricture [53].

34.4 Peroral Cholangioscopy

Single-operator peroral cholangioscopy allows direct visualization inside the bile duct and further evaluation of the stricture. Once visualization and inspection of bile duct is achieved, a guidewire can be secured through the tight stricture and this facilitates therapeutic interventions. Success rate with this method has been nearly 81% based on one study [54]. Furthermore, direct visualization of the bile duct allows for better delineation and characterization of stricture either from erythema, edema, or ulceration to navigate endoscopic therapy and predict resolution of stricture. Strictures formed from edema respond better to endoscopic therapy compared to ulcerated strictures. Tissue inside the duct can be obtained under direct visualization. A course of antibiotics should be given to prevent bacteremia due to water irrigation of bile duct [55]. In a study by Domingo et al., patients of AS displaying mild erythema showed earlier resolution of stricture as compared to the group of AS showing ulcers and friability (457 vs. 167 days, $p = 0.02$).

- *Bile leak* (Fig. 34.2)

Bile leaks can be classified as early or late leaks with 4 weeks as cut-off period and can occur either at site of anastomosis or other sites [56]. Early leaks usually occur at the site of reconstruction. Early bile leaks (<4 weeks) arises due to surgery. Ischemic injury at the anastomotic site, excess tension, prolonged dissection of the bile duct, and the excessive cautery use in stopping of hemorrhage of bile duct increases the chance of leak in postoperative period. Choledochocholedochostomy has lower risks of bile leakage as compared to choledochojejunostomy [57]. Late bile leaks arise after 4 weeks and are usually related to premature T-tube removals leading to formation of fistula at the T-tube site. Pain after removal of the tube may be suggestive of a bile leak, evolving to

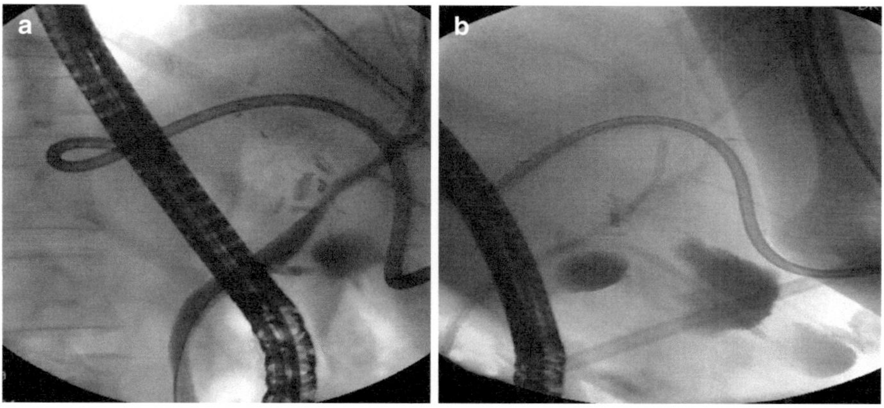

Fig. 34.2 (**a**) Cholangiogram showing bile leak at mid CBD level. (**b**) Plastic stent being deployed across the leak

biliary peritonitis. In patients with biliary anastomosis over T-tube, minor bile duct leaks can be picked up with a T-tube cholangiogram.

Thrombosis of hepatic artery can also lead to ischemic necrosis of bile duct in postoperative period, leading to strictures or leak. Bile leak can be silent but usually presents with pain in abdomen, rise in temperature, nausea, and anorexia. USG abdomen coupled with Doppler examination remains the initial investigation in identifying collections and hepatic artery thrombosis. MRCP has higher sensitivity for detection of biliary leak, stricture, and collections.

Treatment of bile leak consists of diverting the bile flow away from the site of leak. If a T-tube is in place, bile flow will be diverted and it results in closure of the leak in one third to one half of patients within the first 24 hours [58].

In leaks after duct-to-duct anastomosis, endotherapy is the first line of treatment. Papillotomy alone is sufficient for minor leaks, but stents are often placed for 2 to 3 months to bridge the site of leak and providing conduit for healing the biliary tree. A longer duration stent may be required in the setting of high-dose immunosuppression and prolonged leakage. FcSEMS can be considered in the setting of non-healing and large leaks [59]. Treatment by ERCP with plastic stent has resolved early bile leaks in 90–95% of cases [60]. Recent studies have described the use of endoscopic ultrasound (EUS)-guided antegrade drainage approaches [61]. Percutaneous transhepatic biliary drainage (PTBD) can be a rescue measure if the site of leak cannot be negotiated during ERCP. The overall success with ERCP for managing the bile leak is reported to be from 80% to 90% [62]. For leaks after Roux-en-Y hepaticojejunostomy, percutaneous drainage is often required. Enteroscopy-guided biliary intervention, if available, can be used as an alternative.

- *Biliary stones casts and sludges* (Fig. 34.3)

Bile duct stones and casts are seen in about 3–6% of patients clinically manifesting as abdominal pain and abnormal liver function tests. Bile duct filling defects

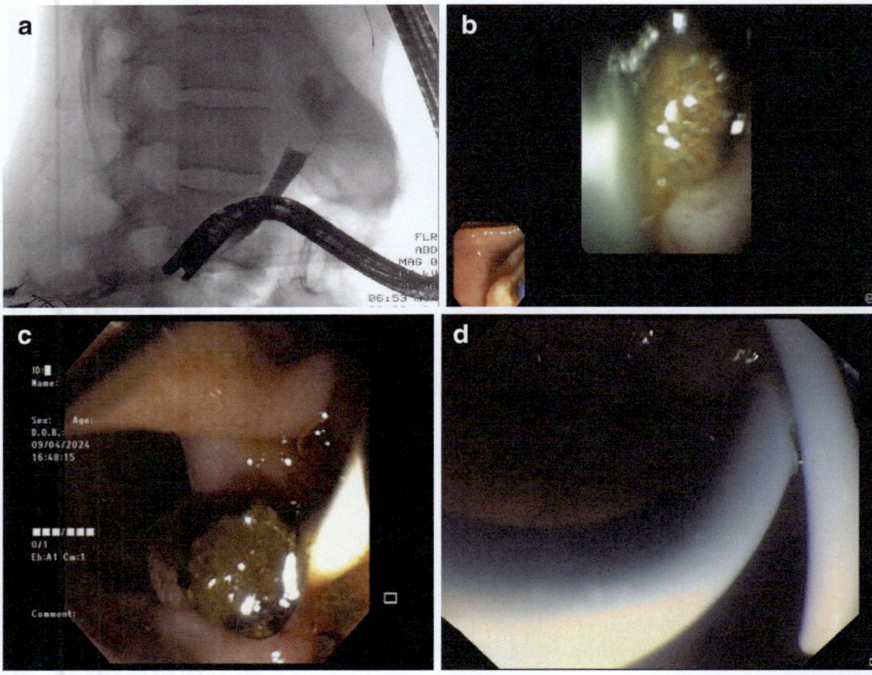

Fig. 34.3 (**a**) Cholangiogram showing a large filling defect at the junction of upper to mid CBD. (**b**) Spyglass cholangioscopy directly visualizing the stone. (**c**) Removal of stone in duodenum. (**d**) Partial clearance of stone in the patient, mild narrowing at lower CBD, and placement of two plastic stents

arise due to sludges, stone migrated stents, casts, or clots [63–65]. Sphincterotomy followed by balloon extraction or basket clearance of stones is usually successful in these cases. ERCP is successful in 90–100% of patients for clearance of stones [66]. There was a 17% recurrence rate of an obstructing stone within 6 months of removal of the initial stone, in one study. In another study, two sessions were required in 24% of patients, and 3 or more sessions were required in 17% of patients [61, 67]. In many cases stones might coexist with strictures complicating the scenarios. In such circumstances, delayed stone clearance following stent placement, the use of peroral cholangioscopy, endoscopic hydraulic lithotripsy, and laser lithotripsy should be utilized for attempting stone clearance.

In cases of altered anatomy, enteroscopy-guided ERCP can be performed. In patients with coagulopathy, balloon dilatation reduces the risk of bleeding during ERCP. Balloon dilation of papilla should be avoided in patients of distal biliary strictures due to risk of perforation.

34.5 Conclusion (Fig. 34.4)

Biliary adverse events quite often complicate liver transplantation with an overall incidence of 10–30% [68]. Suspicion for biliary complication should be kept in the setting of fever, jaundice, pain abdomen and cholestatic liver function tests. Initial work up should include USG abdomen including Doppler study, followed by MRCP. When MRCP is inconclusive, ERCP is to be attempted albeit primarily with

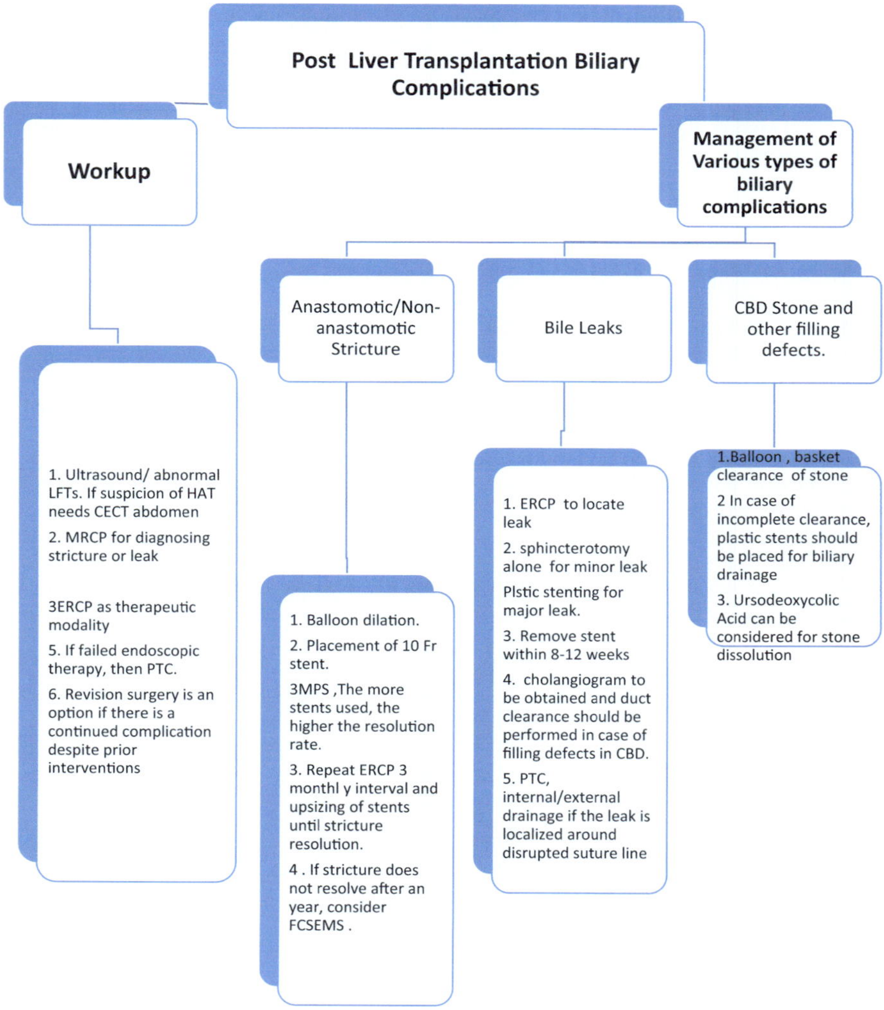

Fig. 34.4 Flow diagram depicting post–liver transplantation biliary complications and algorithmic approach for management

therapeutic intent. Strictures are best treated with combined balloon dilation and stenting. Most patients will require 3–5 sessions of ERCPs, with multiple plastic or FcSEMS exchanged for at least one year duration before stricture resolution. In case of a bile leak papillotomy with or without stenting needs to be performed [69]. Prompt recognition and aggressive treatment have shown to reduce morbidity, mortality, and graft survival after liver transplantation.

The American Society for Gastrointestinal Endoscopy guideline on management of post–liver transplant biliary strictures 2023 highlights ERCP as the initial therapy of choice for biliary complication in post–liver transplant period. FcSEMS is the preferred stenting technique for the strictures not involving intrahepatic ducts. Pre-procedural MRCP should be obtained to confirm and delineate stricture location and morphology. Antibiotics to be given to all transplant patients heading for ERCP.

References

1. Israni AK, Zaun D, Rosendale JD, Schaffhausen C, McKinney W, Snyder JJ. OPTN/SRTR 2019 annual data report: deceased organ donors. Am J Transplant. 2021;21(Suppl 2):521–58.
2. Hampe T, Dogan A, Encke J, et al. Biliary complications after liver transplantation. Clin Transpl. 2006;20(Suppl 17):93–6.
3. Riediger C, Müller MW, Michalski CW, et al. T-tube or no T-tube in the reconstruction of the biliary tract during orthotopic liver transplantation: systematic review and meta-analysis. Liver Transpl. 2010;16(6):705–17.
4. Wojcicki M, Milkiewicz P, Silva M. Biliary tract complications after liver transplantation: a review. Dig Surg. 2008;25(4):245–57.
5. Akamatsu N, Sugawara Y, Hashimoto D. Biliary reconstruction, its complications and management of biliary complications after adult liver transplantation: a systematic review of the incidence, risk factors and outcome. Transpl Int. 2011;24(4):379–92.
6. Daniel K, Said A. Early biliary complications after liver transplantation. Clin Liver Dis (Hoboken). 2017;10(3):63–7.
7. Guichelaar MM, Benson JT, Malinchoc M, Krom RA, Wiesner RH, Charlton MR. Risk factors for and clinical course of non-anastomotic biliary strictures after liver transplantation. Am J Transplant. 2003;3(7):885–90.
8. Rerknimitr R, Sherman S, Fogel EL, et al. Biliary tract complications after orthotopic liver transplantation with choledochocholedochostomy anastomosis: endoscopic findings and results of therapy. Gastrointest Endosc. 2002;55(2):224–31.
9. Sheng R, Ramirez CB, Zajko AB, Campbell WL. Biliary stones and sludge in liver transplant patients: a 13-year experience. Radiology. 1996;198(1):243–7.
10. Seehofer D, Eurich D, Veltzke-Schlieker W, Neuhaus P. Biliary complications after liver transplantation: old problems and new challenges. Am J Transplant. 2013;13(2):253–65.
11. Thuluvath PJ, Pfau PR, Kimmey MB, Ginsberg GG. Biliary complications after liver transplantation: the role of endoscopy. Endoscopy. 2005;37(9):857–63.
12. Larghi A, Tringali A, Rimbaş M, et al. Endoscopic management of Benign Biliary strictures after liver transplantation. Liver Transpl. 2019;25(2):323–35.
13. Brunner SM, Junger H, Ruemmele P, et al. Bile duct damage after cold storage of deceased donor livers predicts biliary complications after liver transplantation. J Hepatol. 2013;58(6):1133–9.
14. Baccarani U, Isola M, Adani GL, et al. Steatosis of the hepatic graft as a risk factor for post-transplant biliary complications. Clin Transpl. 2010;24(5):631–5.

15. Wan P, Yu X, Xia Q. Operative outcomes of adult living donor liver transplantation and deceased donor liver transplantation: a systematic review and meta-analysis. Liver Transpl. 2014;20(4):425–36.
16. Zimmerman MA, Baker T, Goodrich NP, et al. Development, management, and resolution of biliary complications after living and deceased donor liver transplantation: a report from the adult-to-adult living donor liver transplantation cohort study consortium. Liver Transpl. 2013;19(3):259–67.
17. Greif F, Bronsther OL, Van Thiel DH, et al. The incidence, timing, and management of biliary tract complications after orthotopic liver transplantation. Ann Surg. 1994;219(1):40–5.
18. Rammohan A, Govil S, Vargese J, Kota V, Reddy MS, Rela M. Changing pattern of biliary complications in an evolving liver transplant unit. Liver Transpl. 2017;23(4):478–86.
19. Chok KS, Lo CM. Prevention and management of biliary anastomotic stricture in right-lobe living-donor liver transplantation. J Gastroenterol Hepatol. 2014;29(10):1756–63.
20. Sun N, Zhang J, Li X, Zhang C, Zhou X, Zhang C. Biliary tract reconstruction with or without T-tube in orthotopic liver transplantation: a systematic review and meta-analysis. Expert Rev Gastroenterol Hepatol. 2015;9(4):529–38.
21. Sotiropoulos GC, Sgourakis G, Radtke A, et al. Orthotopic liver transplantation: T-tube or not T-tube? Systematic review and meta-analysis of results. Transplantation. 2009;87(11):1672–80.
22. Chang JH, Lee I, Choi MG, Han SW. Current diagnosis and treatment of benign biliary strictures after living donor liver transplantation. World J Gastroenterol. 2016;22(4):1593–606.
23. Atwal T, Pastrana M, Sandhu B. Post-liver transplant biliary complications. J Clin Exp Hepatol. 2012;2(1):81–5.
24. Verdonk RC, Buis CI, Porte RJ, et al. Anastomotic biliary strictures after liver transplantation: causes and consequences. Liver Transpl. 2006;12(5):726–35.
25. Altman A, Zangan SM. Benign biliary strictures. Semin Intervent Radiol. 2016;33(4):297–306.
26. Boraschi P, Donati F, Pacciardi F, Ghinolfi D, Falaschi F. Biliary complications after liver transplantation: assessment with MR cholangiopancreatography and MR imaging at 3T device. Eur J Radiol. 2018;106:46–55.
27. Macías-Gómez C, Dumonceau JM. Endoscopic management of biliary complications after liver transplantation: an evidence-based review. World J Gastrointest Endosc. 2015;7(6):606–16.
28. Boeva I, Karagyozov PI, Tishkov I. Post-liver transplant biliary complications: current knowledge and therapeutic advances. World J Hepatol. 2021;13(1):66–79.
29. Saleem A, Baron TH. Successful endoscopic treatment of biliary cast syndrome in an orthotopic liver transplant patient with a roux-en-Y anastomosis via balloon enteroscopy. Liver Transpl. 2010;16(4):527–9.
30. Morelli J, Mulcahy HE, Willner IR, Cunningham JT, Draganov P. Long-term outcomes for patients with post-liver transplant anastomotic biliary strictures treated by endoscopic stent placement. Gastrointest Endosc. 2003;58(3):374–9.
31. Alazmi WM, Fogel EL, Watkins JL, et al. Recurrence rate of anastomotic biliary strictures in patients who have had previous successful endoscopic therapy for anastomotic narrowing after orthotopic liver transplantation. Endoscopy. 2006;38(6):571–4.
32. Kao D, Zepeda-Gomez S, Tandon P, Bain VG. Managing the post-liver transplantation anastomotic biliary stricture: multiple plastic versus metal stents: a systematic review. Gastrointest Endosc. 2013;77(5):679–91.
33. Costamagna G, Pandolfi M, Mutignani M, Spada C, Perri V. Long-term results of endoscopic management of postoperative bile duct strictures with increasing numbers of stents. Gastrointest Endosc. 2001;54(2):162–8.
34. Arain MA, Attam R, Freeman ML. Advances in endoscopic management of biliary tract complications after liver transplantation. Liver Transpl. 2013;19(5):482–98.
35. Tabibian JH, Asham EH, Han S, et al. Endoscopic treatment of postorthotopic liver transplantation anastomotic biliary strictures with maximal stent therapy (with video). Gastrointest Endosc. 2010;71(3):505–12.

36. Tringali A, Barbaro F, Pizzicannella M, et al. Endoscopic management with multiple plastic stents of anastomotic biliary stricture following liver transplantation: long-term results. Endoscopy. 2016;48(6):546–51.
37. Girotra M, Soota K, Klair JS, Dang SM, Aduli F. Endoscopic management of post-liver transplant biliary complications. World J Gastrointest Endosc. 2015;7(5):446–59.
38. Barakat MT, Huang RJ, Thosani NC, Choudhary A, Girotra M, Banerjee S. Liver transplant-related anastomotic biliary strictures: a novel, rapid, safe, radiation-sparing, and cost-effective management approach. Gastrointest Endosc. 2018;87(2):501–8.
39. Sauer P, Chahoud F, Gotthardt D, et al. Temporary placement of fully covered self-expandable metal stents in biliary complications after liver transplantation. Endoscopy. 2012;44(5):536–8.
40. Coté GA, Slivka A, Tarnasky P, et al. Effect of covered metallic stents compared with plastic stents on benign biliary stricture resolution: a randomized clinical trial. JAMA. 2016;315(12):1250–7.
41. Kaffes A, Griffin S, Vaughan R, et al. A randomized trial of a fully covered self-expandable metallic stent versus plastic stents in anastomotic biliary strictures after liver transplantation. Ther Adv Gastroenterol. 2014;7(2):64–71.
42. Tal AO, Finkelmeier F, Filmann N, et al. Multiple plastic stents versus covered metal stent for treatment of anastomotic biliary strictures after liver transplantation: a prospective, randomized, multicenter trial. Gastrointest Endosc. 2017;86(6):1038–45.
43. Martins FP, De Paulo GA, Contini MLC, Ferrari AP. Metal versus plastic stents for anastomotic biliary strictures after liver transplantation: a randomized controlled trial. Gastrointest Endosc. 2018;87(1):131.e1–.e13.
44. Shah RJ, Smolkin M, Yen R, et al. A multicenter, U.S. experience of single-balloon, double-balloon, and rotational overtube-assisted enteroscopy ERCP in patients with surgically altered pancreaticobiliary anatomy (with video). Gastrointest Endosc. 2013;77(4):593–600.
45. Khan MA, Baron TH, Kamal F, et al. Efficacy of self-expandable metal stents in management of benign biliary strictures and comparison with multiple plastic stents: a meta-analysis. Endoscopy. 2017;49(7):682–94.
46. Wang AY, Sauer BG, Behm BW, et al. Single-balloon enteroscopy effectively enables diagnostic and therapeutic retrograde cholangiography in patients with surgically altered anatomy. Gastrointest Endosc. 2010;71(3):641–9.
47. Buxbaum JL, Biggins SW, Bagatelos KC, Ostroff JW. Predictors of endoscopic treatment outcomes in the management of biliary problems after liver transplantation at a high-volume academic center. Gastrointest Endosc. 2011;73(1):37–44.
48. Egawa H, Inomata Y, Uemoto S, et al. Biliary anastomotic complications in 400 living related liver transplantations. World J Surg. 2001;25(10):1300–7.
49. Colonna JO, 2nd, Shaked A, Gomes AS, et al. Biliary strictures complicating liver transplantation. Incidence, pathogenesis, management, and outcome. Ann Surg. 1992;216(3):344–50; discussion 50–2.
50. Buis CI, Verdonk RC, Van der Jagt EJ, et al. Nonanastomotic biliary strictures after liver transplantation, part 1: radiological features and risk factors for early vs. late presentation. Liver Transpl. 2007;13(5):708–18.
51. Graziadei IW, Schwaighofer H, Koch R, et al. Long-term outcome of endoscopic treatment of biliary strictures after liver transplantation. Liver Transpl. 2006;12(5):718–25.
52. Jang SI, Cho JH, Lee DK. Magnetic compression anastomosis for the treatment of post-transplant biliary stricture. Clin Endosc. 2020;53(3):266–75.
53. Hüsing A, Reinecke H, Cicinnati VR, et al. Paclitaxel-eluting balloon dilation of biliary anastomotic stricture after liver transplantation. World J Gastroenterol. 2015;21(3):977–81.
54. Shin M, Joh JW. Advances in endoscopic management of biliary complications after living donor liver transplantation: comprehensive review of the literature. World J Gastroenterol. 2016;22(27):6173–91.
55. Balderramo D, Sendino O, Miquel R, et al. Prospective evaluation of single-operator peroral cholangioscopy in liver transplant recipients requiring an evaluation of the biliary tract. Liver Transpl. 2013;19(2):199–206.

56. Thuluvath PJ, Atassi T, Lee J. An endoscopic approach to biliary complications following orthotopic liver transplantation. Liver Int. 2003;23(3):156–62.
57. Kasahara M, Egawa H, Takada Y, et al. Biliary reconstruction in right lobe living-donor liver transplantation: comparison of different techniques in 321 recipients. Ann Surg. 2006;243(4):559–66.
58. Wang SH, Lin PY, Wang JY, Lin HC, Hsieh CE, Chen YL. Predictors of biliary leakage after T-tube removal in living donor liver transplantation recipients. Transplant Proc. 2015;47(8):2488–92.
59. Phillips MS, Bonatti H, Sauer BG, et al. Elevated stricture rate following the use of fully covered self-expandable metal biliary stents for biliary leaks following liver transplantation. Endoscopy. 2011;43(6):512–7.
60. Morelli J, Mulcahy HE, Willner IR, et al. Endoscopic treatment of post-liver transplantation biliary leaks with stent placement across the leak site. Gastrointest Endosc. 2001;54(4):471–5.
61. Lisotti A, Caponi A, Gibiino G, Muratori R. Safety and efficacy of extracorporeal shock-wave lithotripsy in the management of biliary stones after orthotopic liver transplantation. Dig Liver Dis. 2015;47(9):817–8.
62. Polese L, Cillo U, Brolese A, et al. Endoscopic treatment of bile duct complications after orthotopic liver transplantation. Transplant Proc. 2007;39(6):1942–4.
63. Gor NV, Levy RM, Ahn J, Kogan D, Dodson SF, Cohen SM. Biliary cast syndrome following liver transplantation: predictive factors and clinical outcomes. Liver Transpl. 2008;14(10):1466–72.
64. Spier BJ, Pfau PR, Lorenze KR, Knechtle SJ, Said A. Risk factors and outcomes in post-liver transplantation bile duct stones and casts: a case-control study. Liver Transpl. 2008;14(10):1461–5.
65. Eminler AT, Parlak E, Koksal AS, Toka B, Uslan MI. Endoscopic treatment of biliary stones in patients with liver transplantation. Surg Endosc. 2017;31(3):1327–35.
66. Maheshwari A, Maley W, Li Z, Thuluvath PJ. Biliary complications and outcomes of liver transplantation from donors after cardiac death. Liver Transpl. 2007;13(12):1645–53.
67. Lisotti A, Fusaroli P, Caletti G. Role of endoscopy in the conservative management of biliary complications after deceased donor liver transplantation. World J Hepatol. 2015;7(30):2927–32.
68. Jadaun SS, Nekarakanti PK, Bhatia S, Kumar M, Singh P, Singla V, Singh SA, Agarwal S, Saigal S, Gupta S. Post-living donor liver transplant biliary strictures: prevalence, predictors, and long-term outcomes in a retrospective study. Clin Transplant Res. 2025;39:55–65.
69. Londoño MC, Balderramo D, Cárdenas A. Management of biliary complications after orthotopic liver transplantation: the role of endoscopy. World J Gastroenterol. 2008;14(4):493–7.

Chapter 35
Post–Liver Transplant Viral Infections (Non-hepatotropic)

Dinesh Jothimani and Radhika Venugopal

Abstract Survival rates after liver transplantation have significantly improved due to advancements in surgical techniques, perioperative care, and the use of effective immunosuppressive regimens. However, de novo or recurrent viral infections following liver transplantation (LT) remain a major cause of allograft dysfunction and can severely impact graft and patient survival if left untreated. The introduction of potent antiviral therapies has markedly enhanced posttransplant outcomes.

Chronic de novo hepatitis E virus (HEV) infection is now increasingly recognized as a contributor to liver graft dysfunction. Without treatment, chronic HEV infection can progress to liver fibrosis and eventual allograft failure. Similarly, the reactivation of cytomegalovirus (CMV) and Epstein-Barr virus (EBV) can result in systemic illness posttransplant.

In the context of the COVID-19 pandemic, liver transplant recipients are particularly susceptible to SARS-CoV-2 infection. Most affected patients require hospitalization, and mortality among this group is estimated to be around 20%.

Timely detection of allograft dysfunction and accurate identification of the underlying viral cause are critical in managing de novo or recurrent posttransplant infections. Adjusting immunosuppressive therapy plays a key role in mitigating allograft injury. Early initiation of high-potency antiviral treatment is essential for achieving viral control or clearance.

Keywords Infection · Post–liver transplantation · Immunosuppression · CMV · EBV · COVID-19 · Hepatitis E

Key Highlights

- Cytomegalovirus (CMV) is the most common viral infection post–liver transplantation and occurs mostly in the first 3 months.

D. Jothimani (✉) · R. Venugopal
Institute of Liver Disease and Transplantation, Dr Rela Institute and Medical Centre, Chennai, Tamil Nadu, India
e-mail: dinesh.jothimani@relainstitute.com

S. Saigal, D. Jothimani (eds.), *Fundamentals of Transplant Hepatology*,
https://doi.org/10.1007/978-981-95-2624-6_35

- CMV infection may vary from asymptomatic allograft dysfunction to severe systemic illnesses.
- Mycophenolate mofetil (MMF) increases the risk of posttransplant CMV infection.
- COVID-19 is associated with 20% mortality.
- Posttransplant chronic hepatitis E infection may lead to graft fibrosis.
- About 90% of posttransplant lymphoproliferative disorder is associated with Epstein-Barr virus (EBV) infection.

35.1 Introduction

The 1- and 5-year survival rates following liver transplantation (LT) have significantly improved, now reaching approximately 90% and 70%, respectively. These advancements are largely attributed to improvements in surgical techniques, perioperative care, and effective immunosuppression strategies. However, as transplant indications broaden and patient selection becomes increasingly complex, these factors may influence posttransplant outcomes.

Maintaining optimal immunosuppression is crucial to strike a balance between preventing rejection and minimizing infection risk during the posttransplant period. In the past, recurrent viral infections posed a major challenge, often resulting in severe graft dysfunction, graft loss, and patient mortality.

Due to the need for long-term immunosuppression, LT recipients face a heightened risk of developing de novo viral infections—defined as new viral illnesses in individuals without prior exposure. These infections can be acquired from environmental sources or may be donor-derived at the time of transplantation. In addition, patients transplanted for viral hepatitis remain at considerable risk for reactivation of latent viruses, leading to disease recurrence.

Both de novo and recurrent viral hepatitis can inflict significant damage on the liver allograft, negatively impacting both graft and patient survival. A deeper understanding of the progression of viral hepatitis in LT recipients, alongside advances in antiviral therapy, has markedly improved long-term outcomes for these patients.

In this chapter, we focus on the prevalence, natural history, and clinical management of cytomegalovirus (CMV), hepatitis E virus (HEV), HSV, EBV, SARS-CoV-2, and parvovirus in LT recipients.

35.2 Cytomegalovirus Infection

Cytomegalovirus is part of Betaherpesvirinae subfamily and is an ubiquitous large DNA virus. CMV causes asymptomatic illness affecting 60–100% of population by adulthood. Being a herpes family, CMV causes latent infection affecting blood cells particularly myeloid lineage.

CMV is the most common viral infection in posttransplant patients, particularly in the first 3 months following liver transplantation, in correspondence with higher

Table 35.1 CMV disease clinical presentation

Viral-like syndrome	Tissue-invasive disease	Indirect effects
Fever	Gastritis	Acute rejection
Malaise	Esophagitis	Chronic rejection
Neutropenia	Enteritis	Opportunistic infections—bacterial, fungal, and viral
Thrombocytopenia	Colitis	EBV/PTLD
	Hepatitis	Diabetes mellitus—new onset
	Pneumonitis	Vascular endothelial damage and thrombosis
	Retinitis	HCV recurrence

EBV Epstein Barr virus, *PTLD* posttransplant lymphoproliferative disorders

immunosuppression [1]. CMV infection may manifest as any of the following three clinical scenarios in the immunocompromised setting [2]. First, de novo CMV infection is characterized by primary CMV infection in a CMV seronegative recipient when the donor is seropositive. Second, CMV may reactivate following prior exposure to CMV; and third, CMV disease is characterized by the presence of CMV viremia along with clinical manifestations. CMV serology performed in donor and recipient during pretransplant evaluation may guide risk assessment. The highest risk (45–65%) of CMV is for recipients with no previous CMV exposure receiving liver from a CMV-positive donor (D+/R−).

Seropositive recipients receiving a seronegative or seropositive donor (D−/R+ or D+/R+) carry a moderate risk (8–20%). Seronegative recipients receiving seronegative donors (D−/R−) has the lowest risk (1–2%) of CMV, either via blood transfusion or as a primary infection [3–5].

Majority of patients with CMV infection are asymptomatic. Patients with CMV disease may present with fever, malaise in 60% of patients, and features of bone marrow suppression such as neutropenia and thrombocytopenia. Gastrointestinal symptoms are observed in 70% of tissue-invasive CMV disease [6]. In liver transplant recipients, CMV causes allograft dysfunction by direct toxicity, potentiating the risk of acute cellular rejection by upregulation of alloantigens and vascular complications such as hepatic artery and portal venous thrombosis (Table 35.1) [7].

35.3 Diagnosis of CMV

Clinicians require a high index of suspicion for CMV in liver recipients in the first 3 months following transplantation when presented with allograft dysfunction, sudden onset of neutropenia, or occasional febrile illness. Serology testing of CMV IgM and CMV IgG is less useful in the posttransplant setting due to suboptimal immune response in the presence of immunosuppression [8]. Patients should undergo CMV DNA quantitative polymerase chain reaction (PCR) for early detection of the illness. The severity of the infection is proportional to the level of CMV

DNA in the blood. The level of CMV DNA determines the risk and severity of the disease [9].

CMV DNA is often negative in patients with tissue-invasive CMV, which requires histological corroboration in patients with clinical symptoms. Such cases require concomitant immunohistochemical testing for pp65 antigen is useful in diagnosis [10].

The reference standard set by the World Health Organization (WHO) for assessing CMV DNA analysis is recommended and should be carried out. A rise of CMV titre by a factor 3 (>0.5 log copies/mL) within 1 week is an indication for initiation of treatment [11].

A weekly PCR-based testing is necessary in case of preemptive treatment strategy. Monthly testing for CMV DNA PCR followed by test every 3 months is recommended for patients on antiviral therapy in their first year.

35.4 Post Liver Transplant CMV Preventive Strategies

There are two main therapeutic strategies for managing CMV infection following liver transplantation: preemptive therapy and prophylactic treatment, with particular emphasis during the first month after transplant. The choice between these approaches is guided by a risk-benefit assessment, considering potential drug-related toxicities and the likelihood of CMV disease, which is largely influenced by the donor and recipient CMV serostatus.

In high-risk patients—specifically those with CMV-positive donors and CMV-negative recipients (D+/R−)—current guidelines recommend antiviral prophylaxis for 3 months [12]. A recent multicenter randomized trial involving 205 CMV-negative recipients of CMV-positive livers compared preemptive therapy using valganciclovir (VGCV) 900 mg twice daily (until two consecutive negative CMV DNA tests a week apart) with 100-day antiviral prophylaxis. The study found that CMV disease with end-organ involvement occurred in 9% of patients in the preemptive group versus 19% in the prophylaxis group at 12 months posttransplant. However, the rates of allograft rejection (28% vs. 25%), graft loss (2% vs. 2%), and opportunistic infections (25% vs. 27%) were similar between both strategies [13]. These findings suggest that preemptive therapy with VGCV may also be a viable option for high-risk individuals.

Preemptive therapy involves weekly monitoring of CMV DNA levels during the first 3 months after transplantation and initiating treatment when viral replication reaches a defined threshold—thus aiming to prevent progression to CMV disease. According to Onor et al., the incidence of viremia was significantly higher in the preemptive group (50%) compared to 4.9% in the prophylaxis group, although clinical outcomes were comparable between the two [14].

Valganciclovir is the preferred agent for prophylaxis, administered at a dose of 900 mg/day orally for 3–6 months in high-risk recipients and for 3 months in moderate-risk recipients, with dose adjustments based on renal function.

Intravenous ganciclovir may be given at 5 mg/kg per day. Both drugs are associated with hematologic toxicities, which may limit the duration of therapy or require dose modifications. Despite the need for ongoing drug monitoring, universal prophylaxis is considered more cost-effective and does not require intensive surveillance [15].

35.4.1 *Treatment of CMV Disease*

DNA polymerase inhibitor such as ganciclovir 3–5 mg twice daily (intravenous) or oral valganciclovir 900 mg twice daily is the recommended treatment for CMV disease. The intravenous route is preferred for life-threatening CMV infection. These drugs are excreted through the kidneys and hence regular monitoring of renal function is recommended for nephrotoxicity. In addition, although no direct drug interaction is documented with calcineurin inhibitor (CNI), patients should be observed for nephrotoxicity.

Figure 35.1 illustrates the approach to CMV infection in post–liver transplant patients.

Foscarnet is a viral DNA polymerase inhibitor used as a second-line agent in patients, particularly in those with Ganciclovir resistance (UL 97). Cidofovir has been tried in difficult-to-treat CMV cases. Both these drugs have been used off-label in posttransplant setting.

Leflunomide, used as immunosuppressive in rheumatoid arthritis, is also tried in gancyclovir-resistant CMV infection with mixed results. Letermovir is a recently approved drug for stem cell recipients which is devoid of myelosuppression and minimal drug-to-drug interactions, not subjected to UL97 and UL54 mediated resistance. It is yet to be approved for use in post-LT patients [16]. Treatment should be continued till two samples are negative for CMV DNA 1 week apart. Table 35.2 illustrates the antiviral therapy in the treatment of CMV disease.

Late-onset CMV disease occurs after completion of prophylaxis. Especially in (R−/D+) recipients, its incidence is 25% which when compared to 8.3% in preemptive treatment 3–6 months reduces the advantage of universal prophylaxis. Some studies report mitigation of this by extending the prophylaxis to 200 days, but data are insufficient [17]. Hence, surveillance after prophylaxis needs to be advocated as an alternative when prolonged drug exposure is not warranted and especially in high-risk individuals.

35.4.2 *CMV and Immunosuppressive Drugs*

Main stay of posttransplant immunosuppressive therapy are CNI inhibitors. They possess renal and neurotoxic side effects along with risk of cancer. A combination of CNIs, antimetabolites, and steroids is used to minimize CNI-induced toxicities.

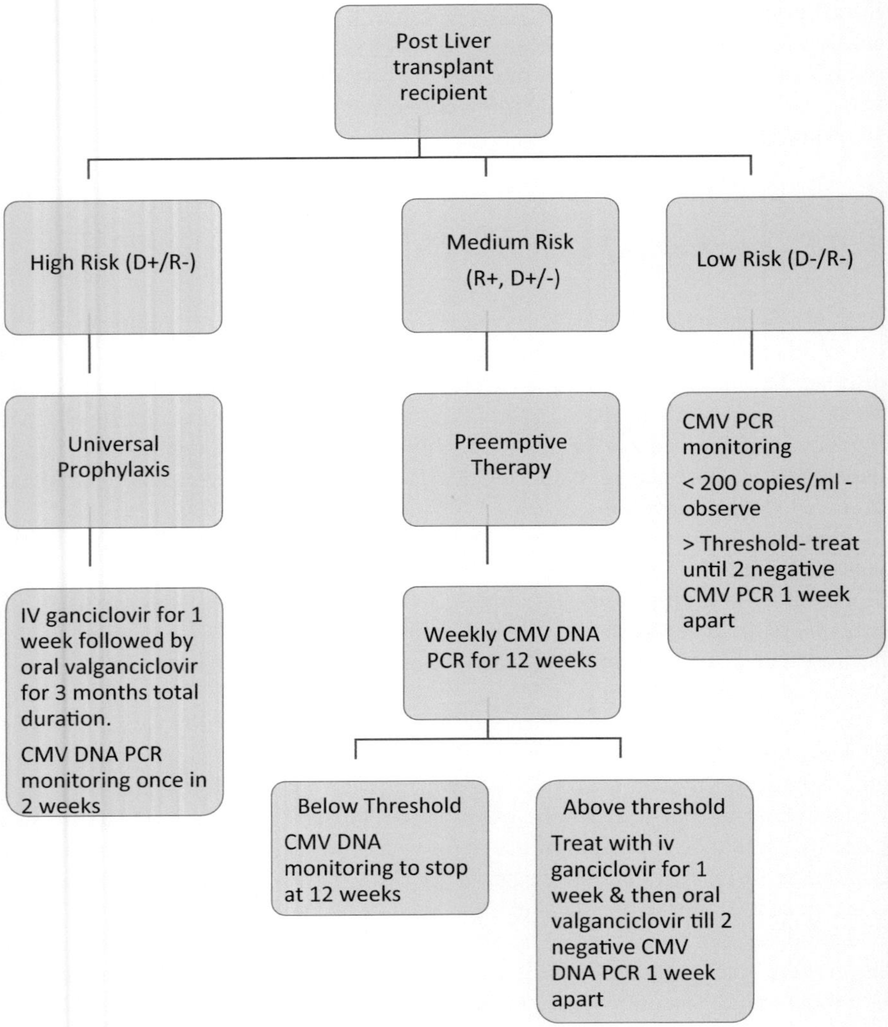

Fig. 35.1 Approach to CMV prophylaxis post–liver transplant patients

However, the antimetabolite mycophenolate mofetil (MMF) increases the severity of CMV infection. Whereas Everolimus, an mTOR inhibitor, has virostatic effects on CMV [18]. Therefore, in patients with CMV disease, MMF is to be stopped and low trough level of tacrolimus is to be maintained. Moreover, immunosuppressive therapy in CMV infection needs to be tailored based on individual patient's needs.

Persistence of CMV DNA beyond 6 weeks despite antiviral therapy indicates drug resistance which entails resistance testing for pUL-97 and UL54 genes. Resistance mutation occurs in both genes for ganciclovir and only in UL54 for cidofovir and foscarnet [19].

Table 35.2 Antiviral drugs for cytomegalovirus infection

Drug	Prophylaxis	Treatment	Toxicity
Ganciclovir	5 mg/kg IV once daily Or 1 gm thrice daily oral	5 mg/kg IV twice daily	Nephrotoxicity Bone marrow suppression Poor oral bioavailability
Valganciclovir	900 mg oral once daily	900 mg oral twice daily	Bone marrow suppression Leucopenia
Foscarnet	Not recommended	60 mg/kg IV thrice daily Or 90 mg/kg IV twice daily	Second-line drug Nephrotoxicity
Cidofovir	Not recommended	5 mg/kg IV once weekly for 2 weeks followed by once in every 2 weeks	Third-line drug Nephrotoxicity

35.5 Epstein-Barr Virus (EBV)

Epstein-Barr virus (EBV), also referred to as human herpes virus 4 (HHV-4), is a DNA virus that belongs to the Herpesvirus family. EBV is typically acquired during childhood, with around 90% of adults testing seropositive. Acute de novo EBV infections are generally self-limiting and resolve with supportive care. Once acquired, the virus remains latent in B lymphocytes and can reactivate during periods of immunosuppression [20].

Reactivation of EBV is linked to a decrease in cytotoxic T-cell activity. After liver transplantation, immunosuppressive therapy impairs memory T-cell function, which can lead to unchecked EBV-driven B-cell proliferation in up to 10% of transplant recipients. While this is often asymptomatic, in some cases the proliferation becomes uncontrolled, leading to clonal transformation of EBV-infected B cells and the development of posttransplant lymphoproliferative disorders (PTLD). The incidence of PTLD is approximately 4.7% in pediatric recipients and 1% in adults [21, 22].

PTLD most commonly arises within the first year following transplantation, and roughly 90% of cases are associated with EBV infection. A large analysis from the Scientific Registry of Transplant Recipients (SRTR) identified PTLD in 383 of 40,437 liver transplant recipients (0.95%). The study highlighted recipient EBV seronegativity as a major risk factor for PTLD, with an adjusted hazard ratio (HR) of 3.49 ($p < 0.0001$) [23].

In pediatric transplant recipients, PTLD is frequently attributed to the activation of residual donor-derived B lymphocytes that persist after graft engraftment.

EBV serostatus is routinely determined by serological assays, EBV viral capsid antigen (VCA), early antigen (EA), and Epstein-Barr Nuclear Antigen (EBNA) (Table 35.3) [24]. These are useful only in pretransplant setting and become obsolete after immunosuppression. EBV DNA viral load monitoring is needed in these circumstances for surveillance of reactivation.

Table 35.3 EBV-specific markers and interpretation

	EBV-negative status	Primary infection	Past infection	Reactivated infection
VCA IgM	Negative	Positive	Negative	Negative
VCA IgG	Negative	Positive	Positive	Positive
EA IgG	Negative	Negative	Negative	Positive
EBNA IgG	Negative	Negative	Positive	Positive
EBNA IgM	Negative	Positive	Negative	Positive

VCA viral capsid antigen, *EA* early antigen, *EBNA* Epstein-Barr nuclear antigen

According to WHO, PTLD has been classified in to early, polymorphic, monomorphic. and classic Hodgkin's lymphoma types. Early PTLD is always associated with EBV and further subclassified into infectious mononucleosis-like PTLD, plasmacytic, and florid follicular PTLD that are more commonly associated with EBV infections. Early PTLD is characterized by abnormal B-cell production due to reactive hyperplasia but there is no formation of tumor cells. Monomorphic PTLD is the most common representing 50% of cases, with a clinical presentation of a diffuse large B-cell lymphoma. The classic Hodgkins-like PTLD is also associated with EBV [25]. Chronic low grade fever, night sweats, anorexia and weight loss (B symptoms) occur in classical lymphomas in LT recipients. PTLD features a bimodal clinical distribution, with an early disease occurring within 12 months following transplantation affecting liver allograft and a "delayed" presenting as Hodgkin's lymphoma. High EBV viral load is associated with the severity of PTLD and therefore serial monitoring of EBV DNA level is recommended in these patients. Investigations include PET-CT and tissue histology. There are no definitive established treatments for PTLD. A preemptive reduction of immunosuppressive medications has BEEN shown to regress PTLD with reduction of EBV DNA. Rituximab, an anti-CD20 monoclonal antibody, may be required every week for a 4-week duration in patients who do not respond to the initial immunosuppression reduction [26]. Patients with aggressive tumor often requires cytotoxic chemotherapy as used in other lymphomas. Localized lesions can be surgically removed or can be given radiation therapy. EBV-specific cytotoxic T lymphocytes are being used as immunotherapy but cumbersome and expensive. One-year survival with PTLD is 56.5% in adult LT recipients. Hepatic, neurological, bone marrow involvement are associated with poor prognosis [27]. Figure 35.2 illustrates the approach to the management of PTLD.

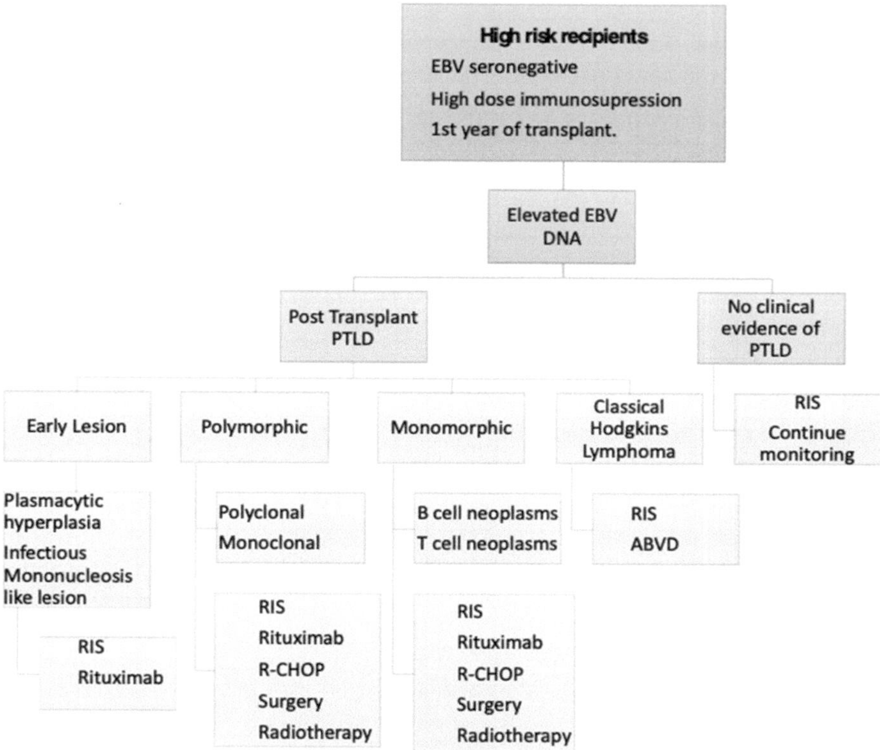

Fig. 35.2 Management of post-transplant PTLD. RIS reduction in immunosuppression, R-CHOP Rituximab combined cyclophosphamide/doxorubicin/vincristine/prednisolone, ABVD adriamycin/bleomycin/vinblastine/dacarbazine

35.6 COVID-19

35.6.1 COVID-19 and Liver Involvement

COVID-19 pandemic was caused by a novel coronavirus strain known as SARS-CoV-2, which shares approximately 80% genetic similarity with the earlier SARS-CoV virus. SARS-CoV-2 is a single-stranded positive-sense RNA virus from the *Betacoronavirus* genus and is considered a chimeric strain of bat-derived coronaviruses. The outbreak originated in December 2019 from a seafood market in Wuhan, China, initially as a zoonotic transmission. It quickly evolved into a global pandemic due to human-to-human transmission through respiratory droplets, with the World Health Organization declaring it a pandemic on March 11, 2020 [28].

The virus enters host cells via the Angiotension converting enzyme 2 (ACE2) receptor, which it targets using a receptor-binding domain structurally similar to that of SARS-CoV. ACE2 receptors are abundantly expressed in alveolar type II cells in the lungs, and to a lesser extent in bronchial epithelium. Beyond the lungs, ACE2 is also present in the stratified epithelium of the oral and esophageal mucosa, enterocytes of the small intestine and colon, liver cells, cardiac myocytes, vascular endothelium, and smooth muscle cells [29]. Notably, SARS-CoV-2 exhibits a 10–20-fold greater binding affinity for ACE2 receptors than SARS-CoV.

Clinical manifestations of COVID-19 vary widely—from mild respiratory or gastrointestinal symptoms to interstitial pneumonia, acute respiratory distress syndrome (ARDS), and diffuse thromboembolic complications, which may lead to multiorgan failure and death. Case fatality rates show geographical variation and range from 5.65% to 15% [30].

35.6.2 Liver Involvement in SARS-CoV-2 Infection (Fig. 35.3)

Hepatic involvement has been observed in 14% to 53% of COVID-19 patients, especially those with severe illness [31]. ACE2 is highly expressed in cholangiocytes (59.7%) and vascular endothelial cells, though only about 2% of hepatocytes express ACE2, with no detectable expression in sinusoidal endothelial cells.

A multicenter study involving 50 COVID-19 patients with cirrhosis found that 97% required hospitalization and 71% needed respiratory support. The proportion of patients with a MELD score > 15 increased from 13% to 26% ($p = 0.037$), and 28% developed acute-on-chronic liver failure (ACLF). The 30-day mortality rate was 34% [32]. SARS-CoV-2 has been linked with increased mortality among patients experiencing decompensation [33].

The APASL COVID-19 Liver Injury Spectrum Study (APCOLIS), which included 228 patients (43 with cirrhosis), reported hepatic decompensation in 9% and ACLF in 11.6% of cases. A Child-Pugh score greater than 9 was associated with significantly higher mortality (ROC 0.94, HR 19.2). In patients with decompensated cirrhosis, mortality was 33%, compared to 16.3% in those with compensated cirrhosis [34].

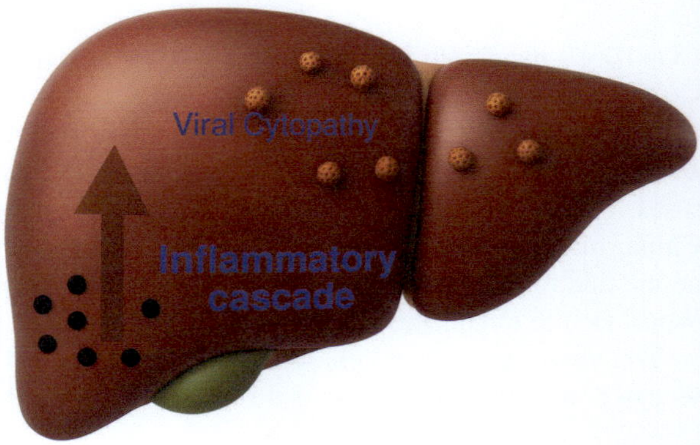

Fig. 35.3 Liver injury in SARS-CoV-2 infection

A survey from the European Liver Transplant Registry reported a crude COVID-19 incidence of 1.05% (ranging from 0.5% to 20%) among patients on the liver transplant waiting list, with a crude death rate of 18%. Among post-transplant patients, the incidence was 0.34% (0.1% to 4.8%), with a death rate of 15% [35].

35.7 COVID-19 and Liver Transplantation

Liver transplant (LT) recipients are at increased risk of contracting SARS-CoV-2 due to their immunosuppressed state and the presence of coexisting medical conditions. In an early study involving 90 solid organ transplant recipients with COVID-19, 76% required hospitalization, and the mortality rate was 18% [36].

A study by Donato et al. in Italy reported a COVID-19 incidence of 1.25% among 640 post-LT patients, with the majority experiencing only mild illness [37]. Becchetti et al. found that symptoms in LT recipients closely resembled those in the general population, with fever (79%), cough (55%), and gastrointestinal complaints (33%) being most common. Common comorbidities included hypertension (56%) and diabetes (37%). Acute respiratory distress syndrome (ARDS) developed in 19% of cases, and the case fatality rate ranged from 12% to 17% [38].

An interim analysis from the COVID-Hep registry reported a 23% mortality rate among 39 LT recipients, noting that mortality was not associated with the time elapsed since transplantation or the type of immunosuppressive therapy [39]. Similarly, data from the Spanish Society for Liver Transplantation involving 111 LT recipients revealed that 86.5% required hospitalization, 19.8% needed respiratory support, and 10.8% were admitted to the ICU. Mycophenolate mofetil (MMF) was found to be an independent risk factor for severe COVID-19, whereas tacrolimus appeared to confer a protective effect. Mild elevations in liver enzymes occurred in 14.7% of patients, with only 2.7% showing signs of graft dysfunction. Overall mortality in this group was 18% [40].

A large international multicenter analysis comparing 151 LT recipients with 627 patients with chronic liver disease found that the LT group had significantly higher rates of ICU admission (28% vs. 8%, $p < 0.0001$) and mechanical ventilation (20% vs. 5%, $p < 0.0001$). Interestingly, mortality was lower in LT recipients (19% vs. 27%, $p = 0.046$), as confirmed by a propensity-matched analysis [41].

35.8 Drug-Related Liver Injury in COVID-19 Treatment

Several medications used to treat COVID-19 have been associated with hepatotoxicity and drug interactions. Although initially recommended, remdesivir failed to demonstrate clinical benefit in a randomized controlled trial and was linked to drug-induced liver injury (DILI) in 10–13% of patients, which could compromise allograft function in LT recipients. Similarly, lopinavir-ritonavir can inhibit cytochrome P450 enzymes, significantly affecting calcineurin inhibitor (CNI) drug levels in post-LT patients.

35.8.1 Clinical Recommendations

COVID-19 illness is not a major clinical problem these days. LT has to be temporarily delayed by a week in those who develop COVID-19. In post transplant patients, expert consensus and international guidelines advise against discontinuing immunosuppressive therapy—particularly CNIs—during COVID-19 illness. However, MMF may be reduced or temporarily withheld, especially in patients with severe lymphopenia or coexisting bacterial or fungal infections.

35.9 Hepatitis E

35.9.1 Hepatitis E Virus (HEV) and Liver Transplantation

HEV is a single-stranded RNA virus, classified into four genotypes. Genotypes 1 and 2 are transmitted via the fecal–oral route and typically cause a self-limiting illness, primarily in Asian and African regions. In contrast, genotypes 3 and 4 are zoonotic, acquired through the consumption of undercooked meat from swine, wild boars, deer, camels, or their milk, and have recently emerged in Western countries [42]. Post–liver transplantation (LT), hepatitis E—mainly genotypes 3 and 4—is increasingly recognized as a cause of chronic graft dysfunction.

A US-based surveillance study found a 22% HEV seroprevalence among blood donors, suggesting the possibility of transfusion-related transmission [43]. In a study by Koning et al., 42% of patients who had undergone LT for hepatitis C showed HEV seropositivity, though none experienced HEV reactivation, possibly due to the protective effect of pegylated interferon used in HCV treatment [44].

35.9.2 Posttransplant HEV Infection

The clinical presentation of acute hepatitis E in LT recipients is similar to that in the general population. Chronic HEV infection, however, has been reported primarily in Europe and is defined as the persistence of detectable HEV RNA or IgM in the blood for at least six months in transplant recipients [45].

Investigations into causes of graft dysfunction have identified chronic HEV infection in LT recipients, with viral RNA detected in blood or stool for durations ranging from 10 to 24 months. The exact prevalence of HEV among LT patients is not well established. Retrospective analyses of stored serum samples have shown HEV RNA or IgG seroprevalence ranging between 1% and 16% [46].

In one study, 12.9% of patients evaluated for transplantation had anti-HEV IgG antibodies pre-LT, and about one-third of these seroconverted posttransplant [47]. Despite the overall lower prevalence of HEV exposure in transplant recipients compared to the general population, the immunosuppressed state leads to a high rate of chronic infection—estimated at 50–65%—which can result in significant fibrosis and graft failure. Most cases represent de novo chronic infections, though rare donor-derived cases have been confirmed through phylogenetic sequencing of HEV RNA in stored donor tissue.

35.9.3 Clinical and Histological Features of Chronic HEV

Chronic HEV infection is often characterized by a moderate elevation of ALT (100–300 IU/L), distinguishing it from acute viral hepatitis. Histologically, liver biopsies may show portal fibrosis, variable portal inflammation, interface hepatitis, and—in severe cases—lobular inflammation and progressive fibrosis.

A European multicenter study identified tacrolimus as an independent risk factor for chronic HEV infection (OR 1.87, $p = 0.04$), though further research is needed to clarify the role of various immunosuppressants in disease progression [48]. Chronic HEV in post-LT patients can lead to allograft dysfunction, chronic liver disease, cirrhosis, and death.

35.9.4 Diagnosis and Treatment

Diagnosing HEV posttransplant can be challenging due to inconsistencies in the sensitivity of HEV IgM assays. HEV RNA quantification is more reliable but not widely accessible, and assay variability further complicates diagnosis.

Treatment focuses on reducing allograft injury. Similar to other posttransplant viral infections, lowering immunosuppressive therapy may help reduce HEV RNA levels. While no standard treatment exists, ribavirin has shown effectiveness in managing post-LT chronic HEV, with a reported clearance rate of 78% [49]. However, approximately 20% of patients remain viremic, risking disease progression.

In vitro studies have suggested that sofosbuvir may inhibit genotype 3 HEV replication and could serve as an adjunct to ribavirin. Yet, a phase II study involving nine posttransplant patients with chronic HEV who received sofosbuvir (400 mg daily for 24 weeks) showed no virological clearance. Interestingly, those on MMF (but not mTOR inhibitors) exhibited greater viral suppression [50].

35.10 Herpes Virus

35.10.1 Herpes Simplex Virus (HSV)

Herpes simplex virus types 1 and 2 (HSV-1 and HSV-2) belong to the Alpha Herpesvirus subfamily within the Herpesviridae family. Humans are the exclusive reservoir for HSV. With widespread global prevalence, most adults become seropositive by their fifth decade. In liver transplant (LT) recipients, HSV infection typically arises from reactivation of latent virus, though de novo or donor-derived infections may also occur [51].

Most post-LT HSV infections involve mucocutaneous lesions, with 85% affecting the orolabial region, followed by anogenital areas. These lesions are often mild and localized to the posterior pharynx, oral cavity, chin, or neck. Anogenital involvement includes the penile shaft and glans in males, and vulva, labia, or vaginal introitus in females [52]. A study on HSV infection after LT reported that 91% of cases were confined to localized disease, whereas 9% progressed to fatal disseminated infection [53].

HSV esophagitis can be difficult to differentiate from other causes like Candida or CMV. Concurrent orolabial lesions may aid in diagnosis. HSV pneumonitis in LT recipients is associated with significant morbidity and mortality. Antiviral prophylaxis in the first post-transplant month can reduce the risk of infection or reactivation. Acyclovir is the first-line treatment, with alternatives including valacyclovir and ganciclovir. Mucocutaneous infections are generally treated for 7–14 days, while visceral disease requires extended antiviral therapy [54].

35.10.2 Varicella Zoster Virus (VZV)

VZV, the causative agent of chickenpox, lies dormant in dorsal root ganglia and can reactivate under immunosuppression, resulting in herpes zoster. This reactivation presents as a painful, vesicular rash typically restricted to a single dermatome. The incidence is about 3% within the first year post-LT and rises to 14% and 18% by the fifth and tenth years, respectively [55].

In a study of 209 LT recipients, 12% developed zoster at a median of 23 months posttransplant [56]. Post-herpetic neuralgia developed in roughly one-third of affected individuals. Management includes reducing immunosuppression, especially temporarily discontinuing antimetabolites like azathioprine or mycophenolate mofetil. Antivirals such as acyclovir, valacyclovir, and ganciclovir are effective and should be administered for at least 2 weeks, often in conjunction with analgesics like gabapentin.

35.10.3 Human Herpes Virus 6 (HHV-6)

HHV-6 belongs to the Beta Herpesviridae subfamily under the *Roseolovirus* genus and includes two variants: HHV-6A and HHV-6B, with the latter responsible for most human infections. Most people are asymptomatically exposed to HHV-6 during childhood, with 90–95% of adults being seropositive. The viral DNA can integrate into the host genome and remain dormant in mononuclear cells [57].

Reactivation commonly occurs posttransplantation, although donor-derived transmission or blood product-related transmission have been reported [58]. The incidence post-LT ranges from 14% to 82%, most commonly within 2–8 weeks. Cases have been noted as early as 10 days and as late as 5 years posttransplant [59]. In a study of 51 LT patients, HHV-6B reactivation was observed in 21.5%, with fever and abdominal pain in a few cases. Ganciclovir prophylaxis for CMV appears to reduce reactivation risk.

Most HHV-6 reactivations are asymptomatic with low viral loads and do not require treatment. Symptomatic cases may present with fever, skin rash, and elevated liver enzymes.

Liver histology can resemble acute cellular rejection, with portal lymphocytic infiltration and periportal necrosis [57]. In a study of 170 LT patients with graft hepatitis, intrahepatic HHV-6 DNA and antigenemia were linked to poorer graft outcomes [60].

Rarely, HHV-6 causes encephalitis, particularly 4–6 weeks posttransplant. HHV-6A, which is neurotropic, can be detected in plasma and CSF. MRI often shows signal abnormalities in the amygdala and hippocampus. Other presentations include colitis or co-infection with CMV [61].

In one study of 45 LT recipients, 51.1% had CMV and 26.7% had HHV-6 infections [62]. HHV-6 was associated with a higher incidence of opportunistic, fungal, and mycobacterial infections [63]. Donor livers positive for HLA-DR15 were more prone to HHV-6 infection and graft rejection. Due to the cell-associated nature of HHV-6, PCR detection rates are low in plasma (33%) and whole blood (19%) [64].

Histologically, high viral load is associated with severe periportal inflammation and necrosis; low viral load correlates with lobular inflammation and mild portal activity. Liver biopsy remains the diagnostic gold standard. HHV-6 IgM appears 2–4 weeks post-primary infection, while IgG titres rise fourfold within 4–6 weeks.

Treatment options include ganciclovir and valganciclovir. In ganciclovir-resistant cases, cidofovir can be used, though its nephrotoxicity requires careful monitoring. Foscarnet is the most selective inhibitor of HHV-6 and is preferred in anemic patients [65].

In summary, although HHV-6 reactivation post-LT is relatively rare, it is linked with increased risk of graft failure, mortality, hepatitis C progression, and CMV disease. Treatment with CMV-targeted antivirals—ganciclovir, cidofovir, and foscarnet—can be effective.

35.11 Conclusion

Post–liver transplant viral infections pose a significant threat to graft function. Prompt recognition, accurate diagnosis, and a structured approach to management are crucial to preserving graft health. Emerging viruses like SARS-CoV-2 should also be considered in differential diagnoses. Over the past decade, advances in immunosuppression protocols and the availability of high-potency antiviral medications with strong resistance barriers have greatly improved outcomes. These developments have translated into better long-term graft and patient survival.

References

1. Razonable RR, Emery VC. 11th annual meeting of the IHMF (International Herpes Management Forum). Management of CMV infection and disease in transplant patients. 27-29 February 2004. Herpes. 2004;11(3):77–86. PMID: 15960905.
2. European Association for the Study of the Liver. Electronic address: easloffice@easloffice.eu. EASL clinical practice guidelines: liver transplantation. J Hepatol. 2016;64(2):433–85. https://doi.org/10.1016/j.jhep.2015.10.006. Epub 2015 Nov 17. PMID: 26597456.
3. Gane E, Saliba F, Valdecasas GJ, O'Grady J, Pescovitz MD, Lyman S, Robinson CA. Randomised trial of efficacy and safety of oral ganciclovir in the prevention of cytomegalovirus disease in liver-transplant recipients. The Oral Ganciclovir International Transplantation Study Group [corrected]. Lancet. 1997;350(9093):1729–33. https://doi.org/10.1016/s0140-6736(97)05535-9. Erratum in: Lancet 1998;351(9100):454. PMID: 9413463.
4. Razonable RR, van Cruijsen H, Brown RA, Wilson JA, Harmsen WS, Wiesner RH, Smith TF, Paya CV. Dynamics of cytomegalovirus replication during preemptive therapy with oral ganciclovir. J Infect Dis. 2003;187(11):1801–8. https://doi.org/10.1086/375194. Epub 2003 May 9. PMID: 12751039.
5. Singh N, Wannstedt C, Keyes L, Wagener MM, Cacciarelli TV. Who among cytomegalovirus-seropositive liver transplant recipients is at risk for cytomegalovirus infection? Liver Transpl. 2005;11(6):700–4. https://doi.org/10.1002/lt.20417. PMID: 15915496.
6. Paya CV, Hermans PE, Wiesner RH, Ludwig J, Smith TF, Rakela J, Krom RA. Cytomegalovirus hepatitis in liver transplantation: prospective analysis of 93 consecutive orthotopic liver transplantations. J Infect Dis. 1989;160(5):752–8. https://doi.org/10.1093/infdis/160.5.752. PMID: 2553824.
7. Jothimani D, Venugopal R, Vij M, Rela M. Post liver transplant recurrent and de novo viral infections. Best Pract Res Clin Gastroenterol. 2020;46–47:101689. https://doi.org/10.1016/j.bpg.2020.101689. Epub 2020 Sep 26. PMID: 33158469; PMCID: PMC7519014.
8. Pastacaldi S, Teixeira R, Montalto P, Rolles K, Burroughs AK. Hepatic artery thrombosis after orthotopic liver transplantation: a review of nonsurgical causes. Liver Transpl. 2001;7(2):75–81. https://doi.org/10.1053/jlts.2001.22040. PMID: 11172388.
9. Razonable RR, Humar A. AST Infectious Diseases Community of Practice. Cytomegalovirus in solid organ transplantation. Am J Transplant. 2013;13(Suppl 4):93–106. https://doi.org/10.1111/ajt.12103. PMID: 23465003.
10. Sun HY, Cacciarelli TV, Wagener MM, Singh N. Preemptive therapy for cytomegalovirus based on real-time measurement of viral load in liver transplant recipients. Transpl Immunol. 2010;23(4):166–9. https://doi.org/10.1016/j.trim.2010.06.013. Epub 2010 Jul 4. PMID: 20609386.

11. Breda G, Almeida B, Carstensen S, Bonfim CM, Nogueira MB, Vidal LR, Almeida SM, Raboni SM. Human cytomegalovirus detection by real-time PCR and pp65-antigen test in hematopoietic stem cell transplant recipients: a challenge in low and middle-income countries. Pathog Glob Health. 2013;107(6):312–9. https://doi.org/10.1179/2047773213Y.0000000114. PMID: 24188241; PMCID: PMC4001611.
12. Kotton CN, Kumar D, Caliendo AM, Huprikar S, Chou S, Danziger-Isakov L, Humar A. The Transplantation Society International CMV Consensus Group. The third international consensus guidelines on the management of cytomegalovirus in solid-organ transplantation. Transplantation. 2018;102(6):900–31. https://doi.org/10.1097/TP.0000000000002191. PMID: 29596116.
13. Singh N, Winston DJ, Razonable RR, Lyon GM, Silveira FP, Wagener MM, Stevens-Ayers T, Edmison B, Boeckh M, Limaye AP. Effect of preemptive therapy vs antiviral prophylaxis on cytomegalovirus disease in seronegative liver transplant recipients with seropositive donors: a randomized clinical trial. JAMA. 2020;323(14):1378–87. https://doi.org/10.1001/jama.2020.3138. PMID: 32286644; PMCID: PMC7157180.
14. Onor IO, Todd SB, Meredith E, Perez SD, Mehta AK, Marshall Lyon G, Knechtle SJ, Hanish SI. Evaluation of clinical outcomes of prophylactic versus preemptive cytomegalovirus strategy in liver transplant recipients. Transpl Int. 2013;26(6):592–600. https://doi.org/10.1111/tri.12101. Epub 2013 Apr 16. PMID: 23590709.
15. Yadav SK, Saigal S, Choudhary NS, Saha S, Kumar N, Soin AS. Cytomegalovirus infection in liver transplant recipients: current approach to diagnosis and management. J Clin Exp Hepatol. 2017;7(2):144–51. https://doi.org/10.1016/j.jceh.2017.05.011. Epub 2017 May 22. PMID: 28663679; PMCID: PMC5478971.
16. Ligat G, Cazal R, Hantz S, Alain S. The human cytomegalovirus terminase complex as an antiviral target: a close-up view. FEMS Microbiol Rev. 2018;42(2):137–45. https://doi.org/10.1093/femsre/fuy004. PMID: 29361041; PMCID: PMC5972660.
17. Humar A, Lebranchu Y, Vincenti F, Blumberg EA, Punch JD, Limaye AP, Abramowicz D, Jardine AG, Voulgari AT, Ives J, Hauser IA, Peeters P. The efficacy and safety of 200 days valganciclovir cytomegalovirus prophylaxis in high-risk kidney transplant recipients. Am J Transplant. 2010;10(5):1228–37. https://doi.org/10.1111/j.1600-6143.2010.03074.x. Epub 2010 Mar 26. PMID: 20353469.
18. Herzer K, Strassburg CP, Braun F, Engelmann C, Guba M, Lehner F, Nadalin S, Pascher A, Scherer MN, Schnitzbauer AA, Zimmermann T, Nashan B, Sterneck M. Selection and use of immunosuppressive therapies after liver transplantation: current German practice. Clin Transplant. 2016;30(5):487–501. https://doi.org/10.1111/ctr.12708. Epub 2016 Mar 31. PMID: 26855333.
19. Lurain NS, Chou S. Antiviral drug resistance of human cytomegalovirus. Clin Microbiol Rev. 2010;23(4):689–712. https://doi.org/10.1128/CMR.00009-10. PMID: 20930070; PMCID: PMC2952978.
20. Straus SE, Cohen JI, Tosato G, Meier J. NIH conference. Epstein-Barr virus infections: biology, pathogenesis, and management. Ann Intern Med. 1993;118(1):45–58. https://doi.org/10.7326/0003-4819-118-1-199301010-00009. PMID: 8380053.
21. Kamdar KY, Rooney CM, Heslop HE. Posttransplant lymphoproliferative disease following liver transplantation. Curr Opin Organ Transplant. 2011;16(3):274–80. https://doi.org/10.1097/MOT.0b013e3283465715. PMID: 21467936; PMCID: PMC3167800.
22. Burra P, Buda A, Livi U, Rigotti P, Zanus G, Calabrese F, Caforio A, Menin C, Canova D, Farinati F, Luciana Aversa SM. Occurrence of post-transplant lymphoproliferative disorders among over thousand adult recipients: any role for hepatitis C infection? Eur J Gastroenterol Hepatol. 2006;18(10):1065–70. https://doi.org/10.1097/01.meg.0000231752.50587.ae. PMID: 16957512.
23. Dharnidharka VR, Lamb KE, Gregg JA, Meier-Kriesche HU. Associations between EBV serostatus and organ transplant type in PTLD risk: an analysis of the SRTR National Registry Data in the United States. Am J Transplant. 2012;12(4):976–83. https://doi.org/10.1111/j.1600-6143.2011.03893.x. Epub 2012 Jan 6. PMID: 22226225.

24. Parker A, Bowles K, Bradley JA, Emery V, Featherstone C, Gupte G, Marcus R, Parameshwar J, Ramsay A, Newstead C. Haemato-oncology Task Force of the British Committee for Standards in Haematology and British Transplantation Society. Diagnosis of post-transplant lymphoproliferative disorder in solid organ transplant recipients - BCSH and BTS Guidelines. Br J Haematol. 2010;149(5):675–92. https://doi.org/10.1111/j.1365-2141.2010.08161.x. Epub 2010 Apr 16. PMID: 20408847.
25. Swerdlow SH. World Health Organization. WHO classification of tumours of haematopoietic and lymphoid tissues. 4th ed. Lyon, France: International Agency for Research on Cancer; 2008.
26. Allen UD, Preiksaitis JK. AST Infectious Diseases Community of Practice. Epstein-Barr virus and posttransplant lymphoproliferative disorder in solid organ transplantation. Am J Transplant. 2013;13(Suppl 4):107–20. https://doi.org/10.1111/ajt.12104. PMID: 23465004.
27. Zimmermann H, Trappe RU. Therapeutic options in post-transplant lymphoproliferative disorders. Ther Adv Hematol. 2011;2(6):393–407. https://doi.org/10.1177/2040620711412417. PMID: 23556105; PMCID: PMC3573421.
28. World Health Organization. Situation report - 120; Coronavirus disease 2019 (COVID-19). 2020. www.who.int.
29. Chai X, Hu L, Zhang Y, Han W, Lu Z, Ke A. Specific ACE2 expression in cholangiocytes may cause liver damage after 2019-nCoV infection. BioRxiv. 2020.
30. Benvenuto D, Giovanetti M, Ciccozzi A, Spoto S, Angeletti S, Ciccozzi M. The 2019-new coronavirus epidemic: Evidence for virus evolution. J Med Virol. 2020;92(4):455–59. https://doi.org/10.1002/jmv.25688. Epub 2020 Feb 7. PMID: 31994738; PMCID: PMC7166400.
31. Jothimani D, Venugopal R, Abedin MF, Kaliamoorthy I, Rela M. COVID-19 and the liver. J Hepatol. 2020;73(5):1231–40. https://doi.org/10.1016/j.jhep.2020.06.006. Epub 2020 Jun 15. PMID: 32553666; PMCID: PMC7295524.
32. Iavarone M, D'Ambrosio R, Soria A, Triolo M, Pugliese N, Del Poggio P, Perricone G, Massironi S, Spinetti A, Buscarini E, Viganò M, Carriero C, Fagiuoli S, Aghemo A, Belli LS, Lucà M, Pedaci M, Rimondi A, Rumi MG, Invernizzi P, Bonfanti P, Lampertico P. High rates of 30-day mortality in patients with cirrhosis and COVID-19. J Hepatol. 2020;73(5):1063–71. https://doi.org/10.1016/j.jhep.2020.06.001. Epub 2020 Jun 9. PMID: 32526252; PMCID: PMC7280108.
33. Rela M, Patil V, Narasimhan G, Jothimani D. COVID-19 in decompensated cirrhosis. Hepatol Int 2020. https://doi.org/10.1007/s12072-020-10092-4.
34. Sarin SK, Choudhury A, Lau GK, et al. Pre-existing liver disease is associated with poor outcome in patients with SARS CoV2 infection; the APCOLIS Study (APASL COVID-19 Liver Injury Spectrum Study) [published online ahead of print, 2020 Jul 4]. Hepatol Int. 2020:1e11. https://doi.org/10.1007/s12072-020-10072-8.
35. Polak WG, Fondevila C, Karam V, Adam R, Baumann U, Germani G, Nadalin S, Taimr P, Toso C, Troisi RI, Zieniewicz K, Belli LS, Duvoux C. Impact of COVID-19 on liver transplantation in Europe: alert from an early survey of European Liver and Intestine Transplantation Association and European Liver Transplant Registry. Transpl Int. 2020;33(10):1244–52. https://doi.org/10.1111/tri.13680. Epub 2020 Aug 13. PMID: 32609908; PMCID: PMC7361228.
36. Pereira MR, Mohan S, Cohen DJ, Husain SA, Dube GK, Ratner LE, Arcasoy S, Aversa MM, Benvenuto LJ, Dadhania DM, Kapur S, Dove LM, Brown RS Jr, Rosenblatt RE, Samstein B, Uriel N, Farr MA, Satlin M, Small CB, Walsh TJ, Kodiyanplakkal RP, Miko BA, Aaron JG, Tsapepas DS, Emond JC, Verna EC. COVID-19 in solid organ transplant recipients: Initial report from the US epicenter. Am J Transplant. 2020;20(7):1800–08. https://doi.org/10.1111/ajt.15941. Epub 2020 May 10. PMID: 32330343; PMCID: PMC7264777.
37. Donato MF, et al. Clin Gastroenterol Hepatol. 2020;S1542-3565(20)30538–3. https://doi.org/10.1016/j.cgh.2020.04.041.
38. Becchetti C, Zambelli MF, Pasulo L COVID-LT group, et al. COVID-19 in an international European liver transplant recipient cohort. Gut. 2020;69:1832e40.
39. Bhoori S, Rossi RE, Citterio D, Mazzaferro V. COVID-19 in long-term liver transplant patients: preliminary experience from an Italian transplant centre in Lombardy. Lancet

Gastroenterol Hepatol. 2020;5(6):532–33. https://doi.org/10.1016/S2468-1253(20)30116-3. Epub 2020 Apr 9. PMID: 32278366; PMCID: PMC7146678.
40. Tejedor-Tejada J, Fuentes-Valenzuela E, Alonso-Martin C, Almohalla-Alvarez C, Garcia-Pajares F. COVID-19 and short- and medium-term outcomes in liver transplant patients: a spanish single-center case series. J Clin Exp Hepatol. 2022;12(2):689–95. https://doi.org/10.1016/j.jceh.2021.05.009. Epub 2021 May 31. PMID: 34092967; PMCID: PMC8166038.
41. Webb GJ, Moon AM, Barnes E, Barritt AS, Marjot T. Determining risk factors for mortality in liver transplant patients with COVID-19. Lancet Gastroenterol Hepatol. 2020;5(7):643–4. https://doi.org/10.1016/S2468-1253(20)30125-4. Epub 2020 Apr 25. PMID: 32339474; PMCID: PMC7182520.
42. Lee GH, Tan BH, Teo EC, Lim SG, Dan YY, Wee A, Aw PP, Zhu Y, Hibberd ML, Tan CK, Purdy MA, Teo CG. Chronic Infection With Camelid Hepatitis E Virus in a Liver Transplant Recipient Who Regularly Consumes Camel Meat and Milk. Gastroenterology. 2016;150(2):355–7.e3. https://doi.org/10.1053/j.gastro.2015.10.048. Epub 2015 Nov 6. PMID: 26551551.
43. Meng XJ, Wiseman B, Elvinger F, Guenette DK, Toth TE, Engle RE, Emerson SU, Purcell RH. Prevalence of antibodies to hepatitis E virus in veterinarians working with swine and in normal blood donors in the United States and other countries. J Clin Microbiol. 2002;40:117e22.
44. Koning L, Charlton MR, Pas SD, Heimbach JK, Osterhaus AD, Watt KD, Janssen HL, de Knegt RJ, van der Eijk AA. Prevalence and clinical consequences of Hepatitis E in patients who underwent liver transplantation for chronic Hepatitis C in the United States. BMC Infect Dis. 2015;15:371. https://doi.org/10.1186/s12879-015-1103-9. PMID: 26328802; PMCID: PMC4557757.
45. Kamar N, Selves J, Mansuy JM, Ouezzani L, Péron JM, Guitard J, Cointault O, Esposito L, Abravanel F, Danjoux M, Durand D, Vinel JP, Izopet J, Rostaing L. Hepatitis E virus and chronic hepatitis in organ-transplant recipients. N Engl J Med. 2008;358(8):811–7. https://doi.org/10.1056/NEJMoa0706992. PMID: 18287603.
46. Haagsma EB, Niesters HG, van den Berg AP, Riezebos-Brilman A, Porte RJ, Vennema H, Reimerink JH, Koopmans MP. Prevalence of hepatitis E virus infection in liver transplant recipients. Liver Transpl. 2009;15(10):1225–8. https://doi.org/10.1002/lt.21819. PMID: 19790147.
47. Legrand-Abravanel F, Kamar N, Sandres-Saune K, Lhomme S, Mansuy JM, Muscari F, Sallusto F, Rostaing L, Izopet J. Hepatitis E virus infection without reactivation in solid-organ transplant recipients, France. Emerg Infect Dis. 2011;17(1):30–7. https://doi.org/10.3201/eid1701.100527. PMID: 21192851; PMCID: PMC3298369.
48. Kamar N, Garrouste C, Haagsma EB, Garrigue V, Pischke S, Chauvet C, Dumortier J, Cannesson A, Cassuto-Viguier E, Thervet E, Conti F, Lebray P, Dalton HR, Santella R, Kanaan N, Essig M, Mousson C, Radenne S, Roque-Afonso AM, Izopet J, Rostaing L. Factors associated with chronic hepatitis in patients with hepatitis E virus infection who have received solid organ transplants. Gastroenterology. 2011;140(5):1481–9. https://doi.org/10.1053/j.gastro.2011.02.050. Epub 2011 Feb 24. PMID: 21354150.
49. Kamar N, Izopet J, Tripon S, Bismuth M, Hillaire S, Dumortier J, Radenne S, Coilly A, Garrigue V, D'Alteroche L, Buchler M, Couzi L, Lebray P, Dharancy S, Minello A, Hourmant M, Roque-Afonso AM, Abravanel F, Pol S, Rostaing L, Mallet V. Ribavirin for chronic hepatitis E virus infection in transplant recipients. N Engl J Med. 2014;370(12):1111–20. https://doi.org/10.1056/NEJMoa1215246. PMID: 24645943.
50. Cornberg M, Pischke S, Müller T, Behrendt P, Piecha F, Benckert J, Todt D, Steinmann E, Papkalla A, von Karpowitz M, Koch A, Lohse A, Hardtke S, Manns MP, Wedemeyer H. Sofosbuvir monotherapy fails to achieve HEV RNA elimination in patients with chronic hepatitis E - The HepNet SofE pilot study. J Hepatol. 2020;73(3):696–99. https://doi.org/10.1016/j.jhep.2020.05.020. Epub 2020 Jul 2. PMID: 32624195.
51. Singh N, Dummer JS, Kusne S, Breinig MK, Armstrong JA, Makowka L, Starzl TE, Ho M. Infections with cytomegalovirus and other herpesviruses in 121 liver transplant recipi-

ents: transmission by donated organ and the effect of OKT3 antibodies. J Infect Dis. 1988;158(1):124–31. https://doi.org/10.1093/infdis/158.1.124. PMID: 2839576; PMCID: PMC2976493.
52. Gnann JW. Herpes simplex virus and varicella-zoster virus infections in hematopoietic stem cell or solid organ transplantation. In: Bowden RA, Ljungman P, Paya CV, editors. Transplant infections. 2nd ed. Philadelphia: Lippincott, Williams, and Wilkins; 2003. p. 350e66.
53. Kusne S, Dummer JS, Singh N, Iwatsuki S, Makowka L, Esquivel C, Tzakis AG, Starzl TE, Ho M. Infections after liver transplantation. An analysis of 101 consecutive cases. Medicine (Baltimore). 1988;67(2):132–43. https://doi.org/10.1097/00005792-198803000-00006. PMID: 3280944; PMCID: PMC2979316.
54. Wilck MB, Zuckerman RA. AST Infectious Diseases Community of Practice. Herpes simplex virus in solid organ transplantation. Am J Transplant. 2013;13(Suppl 4):121–7. https://doi.org/10.1111/ajt.12105. PMID: 23465005.
55. Hamaguchi Y, Mori A, Uemura T, Ogawa K, Fujimoto Y, Okajima H, Kaido T, Uemoto S. Incidence and risk factors for herpes zoster in patients undergoing liver transplantation. Transpl Infect Dis. 2015;17(5):671–8. https://doi.org/10.1111/tid.12425. Epub 2015 Sep 21. PMID: 26201686.
56. Herrero JI, Quiroga J, Sangro B, Pardo F, Rotellar F, Alvarez-Cienfuegos J, Prieto J. Herpes zoster after liver transplantation: incidence, risk factors, and complications. Liver Transpl. 2004;10(9):1140–3. https://doi.org/10.1002/lt.20219. PMID: 15350004.
57. Feldstein AE, Razonable RR, Boyce TG, Freese DK, El-Youssef M, Perrault J, Paya CV, Ishitani MB. Prevalence and clinical significance of human herpesviruses 6 and 7 active infection in pediatric liver transplant patients. Pediatr Transplant. 2003;7(2):125–9. https://doi.org/10.1034/j.1399-3046.2003.00028.x. PMID: 12654053.
58. Emery VC, Clark DA. HHV-6A, 6B, and 7: persistence in the population, epidemiology and transmission. In: Arvin A, Campadelli-Fiume G, Mocarski E, et al., editors. Human herpesviruses: biology, therapy, and immunoprophylaxis. Cambridge: Cambridge University Press; 2007. Chapter 49. Available from: https://www.ncbi.nlm.nih.gov/books/NBK47441/.
59. Lautenschlager I, Höckerstedt K, Linnavuori K, Taskinen E. Human herpesvirus-6 infection after liver transplantation. Clin Infect Dis. 1998;26(3):702–7. https://doi.org/10.1086/514592. PMID: 9524848.
60. Pischke S, Gösling J, Engelmann I, Schlue J, Wölk B, Jäckel E, Meyer-Heithuis C, Lehmann U, Strassburg CP, Barg-Hock H, Becker T, Manns MP, Schulz T, Wedemeyer H, Heim A. High intrahepatic HHV-6 virus loads but neither CMV nor EBV are associated with decreased graft survival after diagnosis of graft hepatitis. J Hepatol. 2012;56(5):1063–69. https://doi.org/10.1016/j.jhep.2011.12.017. Epub 2012 Jan 13. PMID: 22245897.
61. Revest M, Minjolle S, Veyer D, Lagathu G, Michelet C, Colimon R. Detection of HHV-6 in over a thousand samples: new types of infection revealed by an analysis of positive results. J Clin Virol. 2011;51(1):20–4. https://doi.org/10.1016/j.jcv.2011.02.001. Epub 2011 Mar 3. PMID: 21376662.
62. Härmä M, Höckerstedt K, Lyytikäinen O, Lautenschlager I. HHV-6 and HHV-7 antigenemia related to CMV infection after liver transplantation. J Med Virol. 2006;78(6):800–5. https://doi.org/10.1002/jmv.20626. PMID: 16628583.
63. Rogers J, Rohal S, Carrigan DR, Kusne S, Knox KK, Gayowski T, Wagener MM, Fung JJ, Singh N. Human herpesvirus-6 in liver transplant recipients: role in pathogenesis of fungal infections, neurologic complications, and outcome. Transplantation. 2000;69(12):2566–73. https://doi.org/10.1097/00007890-200006270-00016. PMID: 10910278.
64. Guardia AC, Stucchi RS, Milan A, Costa SC, Boin Ide F. Human herpesvirus-6 and cytomegalovirus DNA in liver donor biopsies and their correlation with HLA matches and acute cellular rejection. Braz J Infect Dis. 2014;18(2):220–4. https://doi.org/10.1016/j.bjid.2013.07.007. Epub 2013 Nov 22. PMID: 24275367; PMCID: PMC9427445.
65. Pritchett JC, Naesens L, Montoya J. Treating HHV-6 infections. In: Flamand L, Lautenschlager I, Krueger G, Ablashi D, editors. Human herpesviruses HHV- 6A, HHV-6B & HHV-7: diagnosis and clinical management. 3rd ed. Oxford, UK: Elsevier; 2014:311–20.

Chapter 36
Post–Liver Transplant Viral Infections (Hepatitis B and C)

James Fung

Abstract Recurrence of viral hepatitis B and C after liver transplantation is a universal phenomenon for patients who are viremic at the time of transplant in the absence of antiviral therapy. Prior to the availability of effective antiviral strategies, liver transplantation for patients with chronic viral hepatitis B and C infection was associated with poor outcomes due to graft loss from recurrence of hepatitis. Fortunately, with current antiviral agents, graft loss and mortality due to recurrence of viral hepatitis have become exceedingly rare. For chronic hepatitis B, third-generation nucleos(t)ide analogues (NA) are highly effective in the prevention of hepatitis recurrence, with minimal risk of viral resistance and reactivation. However, as transplantation does not completely eradicate hepatitis B infection, lifelong antiviral prophylaxis is required. In the past decade, there has also been a decline in the use of hepatitis B immune globulin (HBIG), due to the effectiveness of current oral NAs. For hepatitis C, highly effective all-oral pan-genotypic direct antiviral agents (DAAs) have significantly simplified antiviral treatment, resulting in these patients having one of the best post-transplant outcomes amongst liver diseases. The decision to treat before or after liver transplantation will depend on individual cases, and both can achieve high rates of sustained virological response.

Keywords Hepatitis B · Hepatitis C · Antiviral · Prophylaxis · Directing acting antivirals

J. Fung (✉)
Department of Medicine, The University of Hong Kong, Pok Fu Lam, Hong Kong SAR

The Liver Transplant Center, Queen Mary Hospital, Pok Fu Lam, Hong Kong SAR

State Key Laboratory Of Liver Research, The University of Hong Kong, Pok Fu Lam, Hong Kong SAR
e-mail:jfunggastro@gmail.com

S. Saigal, D. Jothimani (eds.), *Fundamentals of Transplant Hepatology*,
https://doi.org/10.1007/978-981-95-2624-6_36

Key Highlights

- Third-generation nucleos(t)ide analogues are highly effective in preventing reactivation of hepatitis B after liver transplantation with or without the use of hepatitis B immune globulin, and should be given long term.
- The availability of direct-acting antivirals allows an opportunity to treat decompensated cirrhosis on the liver transplant waiting list. The decision to treat should be individualized.
- Direct-acting antivirals are safe and effective after liver transplantation, with high rates of sustained virological response, and should be given pre-emptively early after transplant for those who remain viremic after transplant.
- The effectiveness of post–liver transplant antiviral strategies has enabled the use of both hepatitis B– and C–positive donors.

36.1 Introduction

Chronic hepatitis B virus (HBV) and hepatitis C virus (HCV) infection remains a global burden and is one of the leading indications for liver transplantation (LT) in areas where infection is still endemic. The natural history of chronic HBV and HCV infection is similar to other chronic liver diseases, where untreated inflammation of the liver can lead to fibrosis and its progression to cirrhosis [1]. Complications may include decompensation and symptoms arising from underlying portal hypertension, and the development of hepatocellular carcinoma (HCC), where LT is often the only curative option for eligible patients. In addition, patients with chronic hepatitis B (CHB) may develop severe flares of hepatitis leading to acute-on-chronic liver failure (ACLF), which is another major indication for LT in these patients.

For patients who are viremic at the time of transplant, re-infection of the allograft is universal. Recurrence of infection after LT can lead to rapid graft failure if untreated, and in fact, was deemed a contraindication during a period where there was no adequate antiviral prophylaxis. Fortunately, highly effective antiviral therapies against hepatitis B virus (HBV) and hepatitis C virus (HCV) are currently available to prevent recurrence and reactivation of disease after LT. As a result, graft loss and mortality related to HBV and HCV reactivation after LT are now uncommon, and likely due to non-compliance or omission of antiviral drugs rather than prophylaxis failure.

36.2 Hepatitis B

Despite the availability of universal vaccination in many parts of the world, CHB remains a major global health burden, affecting 292 million people, with an annual death rate of 0.8 million [2]. Therefore, CHB remains a leading liver disease aetiology for LT in many regions where HBV infection remains at endemic levels [3]. The most common indications for LT in CHB include decompensated cirrhosis, HCC and HBV-induced ACLF secondary to severe flares [4].

In the absence of antiviral prophylaxis, CHB was regarded as a contraindication to LT due to rapid recurrence of HBV infection with a cumulative rate of over 90% without antiviral therapy [5, 6]. For those with recurrence, severe flares leading to graft loss and death may occur, accounting for the poor short-term survival [7–9]. There are two major types of treatment for CHB, namely oral nucleos(t)ide analogues (NAs) and interferon, although the latter is contraindicated for patients with advanced liver disease, and plays no role in the prevention of HBV reactivation after LT. Hepatitis B immune globulin (HBIG), often used for post-exposure prophylaxis, is also used for prophylaxis after LT for CHB patients.

36.2.1 Hepatitis B Immunoglobulin

The introduction of HBIG was the first major milestone in antiviral prophylaxis against HBV recurrence after LT for CHB [10]. This is a form of passive immunoprophylaxis whereby protection is conferred by parenteral administration of immunoglobulins prepared from pooled plasma donors. Although it is not clearly understood how HBIG prevents recurrent hepatitis, it is believed that the immunoglobulins may form immune complexes to have a neutralizing effect, and may also prevent viral entry into the hepatocytes [11].

Early studies using HBIG monotherapy have shown that for it to be effective, long-term administration is required, as short-term treatment only delays the recurrence of hepatitis [12, 13]. The antibody level which is deemed protective is unknown, although the arbitrary titre of >100 U/L is often used. To maintain this protective level, HBIG can be administered according to antibody levels or as a fixed-dose regimen at regular intervals. HBIG monotherapy is associated with up to 30% recurrence rate, with higher doses were associated with even lower rates of recurrence [14–16]. The development of the escape mutation G145R of the S protein may reduce binding to anti-HBs, thereby increasing the chance of recurrence [17–19]. As monoprophylaxis, HBIG is inadequate to completely prevent reactivation of HBV after LT, requiring high doses to maintain its efficacy. Other limitations associated with HBIG use include the need for parenteral administration at regular intervals and its high cost.

36.2.2 Oral Nucleos(t)ide Analogues

The second major milestone was the approval of NAs for the treatment of CHB. Lamivudine (LAM), a reverse transcriptase inhibitor, was the first NA to be approved in 1998. The major limitation of LAM therapy was the high resistance rate, occurring in up to 70% after 8 years of treatment in non-transplant patients [20]. Once resistance occurs, virological rebound may occur, with subsequent biochemical relapse with severe hepatitis leading to graft loss if untreated [21]. The reported efficacy of LAM monotherapy showed a highly variable recurrence rate of <5% to 50% after LT [22–25]. The huge disparity likely stems from the difference in the definition of HBV recurrence and the viral load at the time of LT.

Given that both HBIG and LAM were suboptimal as monotherapy, with an approximate 70% efficacy each, these two agents were combined and became the most widely adopted regimen at the time, with an efficacy of over 95% in the prevention of recurrence after LT [26–28]. Although much higher doses were used initially, later studies have demonstrated that using a lower dose of HBIG was also effective as part of a combination regimen [29, 30].

When adefovir disoproxil (ADV), a nucleotide analogue, was approved in 2003, this was an important development as it was shown to be effective against both wildtype and LAM-resistant HBV, and was widely used as rescue therapy for the latter [31–34]. Furthermore, a combination of LAM and ADV without HBIG was shown to be effective, and provided early evidence that an HBIG-free regimen can be associated with minimal risk of recurrence after LT [35–37]. However, ADV is associated with significant nephrotoxicity, and has been replaced by other more potent nucleotide analogues including tenofovir disoproxil fumarate (TDF) and tenofovir alafenamide (TAF).

The current first-line antiviral therapy for CHB includes entecavir (ETV), TDF and TAF, approved in 2005, 2008 and 2016 respectively. These third-generation NAs are highly potent with high barrier to resistance. ETV has been shown to be highly effective as monotherapy with minimal risk of HBV reactivation after LT, and high rates (>90%) of HBsAg seroclearance with almost universal viral suppression even without the use of HBIG [38]. Moreover, the use of ETV monotherapy was associated with excellent long-term outcome with a 9-year survival of 85%, a HBsAg seroclearance rate of over 90% and 100% viral suppression, without any deaths directly related to HBV reactivation [39]. For those with prior LAM-resistant HBV, and in keeping with the previous results with ADV, third-generation NAs alone without HBIG were also effective in preventing reactivation [40].

Prior to the availability of these potent NAs, the viral load at the time of transplantation was also a significant factor for post-LT outcomes, with higher levels associated with poorer outcomes and higher rates of reactivation [6, 41]. This is not surprising as HBIG alone is unlikely to prevent re-infection in highly viremic patients, and higher viral loads have been correlated with the development of resistance to LAM. In fact, patients with evidence of high viral loads may not have been considered good candidates for LT previously. Severe flares leading to ACLF have become a common indication for LT in CHB patients, and the majority will have high viral load on presentation which may not be lowered significantly given the short window period for LT even with NA treatment. With current NAs, the viral load at the time of LT has not been shown to be associated with poor outcome, and in fact, a significant proportion of the patients had high viral loads at the time of LT in these studies [39].

36.2.2.1 Shifting Paradigm of HBIG Use

With the availability of third-generation NAs, and with data showing excellent long-term outcomes, there has been a worldwide shift in paradigm of HBV prophylaxis after LT in using less HBIG [3]. The trend had started initially with LAM with the transition from using high-dose to low-dose HBIG. The use of HBIG-free regimens has only been made possible with third-generation NAs, and many centres have adopted limited duration and peri-operative HBIG regimens only. As all CHB patients should already be on a third-generation NA at the time of LT, the choice of NA after LT is likely a continuation of their existing treatment. The type of NA used will also be dependent on underlying patient and viral factors, including previous resistance, and the presence of renal impairment, bone disorders and HCC. One approach is to stratify patients according to their virological risk to determine whether HBIG should be used and for how long it should be given [42]. Through this approach, significant cost saving can be achieved by abandoning the use of life-long HBIG administration [43].

There have been many studies, meta-analyses and systematic reviews comparing NAs alone with NAs in combination with HBIG. Most of the older studies have shown combination prophylaxis to be better than NA monotherapy, largely due to the inclusion of studies using LAM [44–47]. In a more recent systematic review on studies using high-potency NAs, the addition of HBIG did not translate to better long-term outcomes with regards to HBV recurrence or overall survival [48].

36.2.2.2 Goal of HBV Prophylaxis

LT does not offer a sterilizing cure for chronic HBV infection, and this is likely due to the extra-hepatic reservoirs that persist even with removal of the diseased liver [49, 50]. HBV can be present in peripheral blood mononuclear cells (PBMCs) and can serve as a viral reservoir contributing to chronic infection. In these instances, viral replication likely occurs at very low levels with detection of HBV mRNA sequences and cccDNA [51–54]. Other extra-hepatic organs which may harbour HBV include the kidneys, spleen, thyroid and lymph nodes [55–57]. Therefore, antiviral prophylaxis per se does not prevent recurrence as the virus has never been eradicated. There is the noble intention of preventing the allograft from becoming infected with HBV. However, studies have shown that the re-infection of the allograft occurs early on post-LT despite the use of prophylaxis including HBIG, even in patients without evidence of re-infection using conventional serological assays, including HBsAg and HBV DNA [58].

In addition, the use of qualitative HBsAg in the serum as a surrogate marker of re-infection of the liver is relatively insensitive, and easily masked by exogenous

HBIG administration, especially as levels will be at extremely low levels after removal of the infected liver where the bulk of the HBV reservoir resides as cccDNA. It is important to note that re-infection of the graft probably occurs early on after LT, and that biomarkers that are not affected by exogenous HBIG, including hepatitis B core-related antigen (HBcrAg) and intrahepatic cccDNA, remain detectable [59–61]. Therefore, to define re-infection based on HBsAg positivity is likely inadequate, as HBsAg may still be negative in these instances, which may exist at very low levels below the level of detectability by conventional qualitative assays. Hence, the goal of antiviral prophylaxis after LT in fact may be to prevent reactivation of HBV activity rather than to prevent re-infection. Prevention of re-infection only occurs at the level of the uninfected graft and not the chronically infected host.

36.2.3 HBsAg− and Anti-HBc+ Recipients

Anti-HBc positivity may indicate prior exposure or infection from HBV, and the potential to harbour occult HBV infection (OBI) [62]. The risk of reactivation after LT is likely low, due to the fact that the main reservoir of occult infection is removed at the time of transplant. However, the risk is not negligible, as reactivation has been shown to occur in these instances, and may be due to extra-hepatic sources [63]. Without prophylaxis, the risk of HBV reactivation and HBsAg seroconversion in a recipient with isolated anti-HBc+ and HBV-naive liver is uncommon. The guidelines on the prevention of HBV reactivation in OBI patients receiving immunosuppression are applied to non–liver transplant patients with their native liver, and no guidelines have been devised for anti-HBc+ recipients receiving HBV-naïve livers [64]. Despite the low risk, some LT centres still prefer to prescribe oral antiviral therapy long term as prophylaxis as recipients will be maintained on lifelong immunosuppression.

36.2.4 Anti-HBc+ Donors

In areas where organ donation is low and CHB infection remains high, anti-HBc+ donors serve as an important group to expand the donor pool. There is potential for occult HBV infection inside the livers of anti-HBc donors, with a risk of de novo HBV infection in non-hep B recipients, with up to as high as 75% transmission risk [65–67]. The risk may also be dependent on the recipient's immune status, being lowest for anti-HBs+ recipients and highest for those who are negative for both anti-HBc and anti-HBs.

There have been variable outcomes demonstrated on the use of anti-HBc+ grafts, with varying antiviral prophylaxis strategies adopted by different LT centres [68–71]. The recommendation is that these recipients should be treated with an NA, and it should be started as soon as possible after transplant, and HBIG is not required

[72, 73]. Although LAM has been widely used in many of the studies, the use of ETV, TDF or TAF will have the lowest risk of resistance and virological breakthrough with long-term use. In a study of over 100 HBsAg− recipients receiving anti-HBc+ grafts, NA monotherapy prophylaxis was associated with a 2.8% risk of de novo HBV, all occurring in patients on LAM, and none with patients treated with ETV, highlighting the importance of using a third-generation NA even in this setting [74].

36.2.4.1 HBsAg+ Donors

The significant shortage of liver organs coupled with the increasing demand for LT has led to the increasing use of HBsAg+ grafts in some LT centres [75]. The overall patient and graft survival has been shown to be comparable with HBsAg− grafts [75–78]. Transmission of HBV is universal, with de novo infection in non-HBV recipients even with antiviral prophylaxis. In these instances, HBIG is of no use, and to prevent reactivation, recipients of such grafts will require lifelong antiviral prophylaxis with a third-generation NA. In addition, the graft will be at a lifelong risk of developing HCC, and long-term surveillance is required.

The antiviral strategies for HBV in post–liver transplant recipients are shown in Table 36.1, with the proposed algorithm shown in Fig. 36.1.

Table 36.1 Antiviral strategies for hepatitis B and C after liver transplantation

Hepatitis B	**Treatment**	**Duration**
HBsAg+ recipient	Entecavir *or* Tenofovir disoproxil fumarate *or* Tenofovir alafenamide	Lifelong
	+/− Hepatitis B immune globulin	Variable
HBsAg- recipient		
HBsAg+ or anti-HBc positive grafts	Entecavir *or* Tenofovir disoproxil fumarate *or* Tenofovir alafenamide	Lifelong
Anti-HBc+ recipient	Entecavir *or* Tenofovir disoproxil fumarate *or* Tenofovir alafenamide	Lifelong
HBsAg−, anti-HBc− graft and anti-HBc− recipient	None	
Hepatitis C	**Treatment**	**Duration**
Non-cirrhotic/compensated Child-Pugh A graft cirrhosis	Sofosbuvir + velpatasvir *or* Glecaprevir + pibrentasvir	12 weeks 12 weeks
With prior failed DAA treatment	Sofosbuvir + velpatasvir + voxilaprevir	12 weeks
Decompensated Child-Pugh B/C graft cirrhosis	Sofosbuvir + velpatasvir + ribavirin *or* Sofosbuvir + velpatasvir	12 weeks 24 weeks

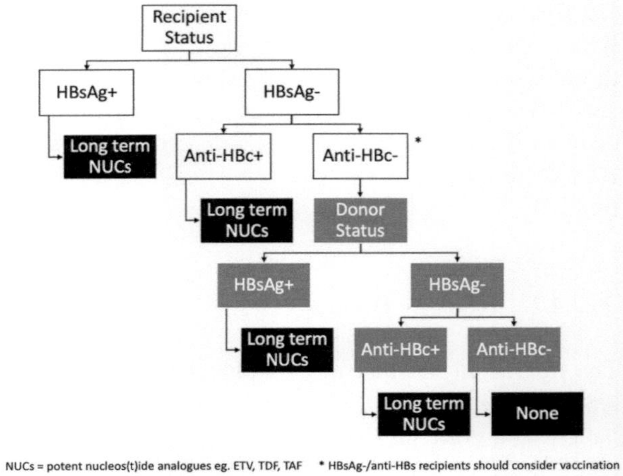

Fig. 36.1 Proposed algorithm for antiviral therapy against hepatitis B virus after liver transplantation

36.3 Chronic Hepatitis C

The approval of all-oral pangenotypic direct antiviral agents (DAAs) has altered the landscape of liver transplantation in many parts of the world. Only less than a decade ago, chronic hepatitis C (CHC) was still one of the leading primary liver disease indications for LT. In 2023, with DAAs being widely available, HCV has now become an uncommon indication for LT [79]. In addition, the post-LT outcomes have improved drastically.

Recurrence of HCV infection is universal if the patient is viremic at the time of LT, and rare if HCV is eradicated prior to LT [80]. It has been shown that graft re-infection occurs likely at the time of reperfusion, and that liver injury is already evident as early as within 2 weeks after LT [81]. By 3 months after transplant, most will have histological features of acute hepatitis and up to 80% may have chronic hepatitis by 1 year [82]. Unlike non-transplant patients where cirrhosis has a slow and indolent course taking decades to occur, the disease progression is accelerated after LT, with up to 20% developing cirrhosis by 5 years post-LT [83, 84]. The accelerated course after LT is due to multiple factors, including donor, recipient and virological factors. Donor factors include age, graft steatosis, presence of donor-specific alloantibodies and the use of organs from HCV+, living and cardiac death donors. Underlying diabetes and metabolic syndrome, female gender and co-infection with HIV in the recipient may also affect the progression of disease after LT. Other contributing factors include ischemic-perfusion injury and the use of immunosuppression, in particular, with high-dose steroid [85, 86].

The most dreaded complication of recurrent HCV is the development of fibrosing cholestatic hepatitis (FCH), which may affect ~5% of patients after LT [87]. FCH is characterized by rapid portal fibrosis and cholestasis, leading to liver failure and graft loss within 1–2 years after LT, with a high mortality and the need for re-LT. Fortunately, FCH is rarely observed nowadays with DAA treatment.

36.3.1 Pre-Direct Acting Antivirals (DAA) Era

Prior to the availability of DAAs, pegylated (peg) interferon (IFN) in combination with ribavirin was the mainstay of treatment for HCV patients. For patients with decompensated cirrhosis, treatment was limited as IFN-based therapies were contraindicated with the risk of further exacerbation of the underlying liver dysfunction. Therefore, for these patients, LT was the only treatment option for eligible patients, and antiviral therapy could only be offered afterwards. However, peg-IFN remains poorly tolerated after LT with multiple adverse effects. Furthermore, the immunomodulatory action of IFN may theoretically increase the risk of graft rejection [88]. Many patients with significant portal hypertension and splenomegaly will have residual hypersplenism after LT, with ongoing pancytopenia precluding adequate dosing of Peg-IFN. Moreover, anaemia is common after LT and may preclude the use of RBV. These factors, in addition to the immunosuppressive therapy, may contribute to the low sustained virological response (SVR) rates of around 30% that is typically observed in this group of patients [89]. Fortunately, IFN-based therapies are now remnants of the past and have been largely replaced by DAAs.

36.3.2 Direct-Acting Antivirals

The HCV genome encodes three structural proteins and seven non-structural (NS) proteins, of which three are important for viral replication (NS3/4A, NS5A. NS5B) [90]. The latter are targets for DAAs, forming the three major groups of DAAs. The protease inhibitors target NS3, and include boceprevir, telaprevir, simeprevir, paritaprevir, grazoprevir and voxilaprevir. The NS5A inhibitors include daclatasvir, ledipasvir, ombitasvir, elbasvir and velpatasvir. The polymerase inhibitor targets NS5B and includes sofosbuvir and dasabuvir.

The first DAAs, boceprevir and telaprevir, were approved in 2011. Both were protease inhibitors and had to be combined with peg-IFN. Although the SVR rates were increased by 20–30%, the same adverse effects and limitations associated with IFN-based therapies persisted [91, 92]. In addition, both are substrates and inhibitors of the CYP3A4 and CYP3A5 pathways, with a significant effect on the metabolism of immunosuppression drugs commonly used in LT [93–95]. One of the most important milestone was the approval of sofosbuvir (SOF) in 2013, paving the way for an all-oral DAA regimen. In 2014, fixed-dose combinations including SOF/ledipasvir (LED) and ombitasvir/paritaprevir/ritonavir/dasabuvir were approved, and elbasvir(EBR)/grazoprevir(GZR) was approved in 2016. In the same year, the pangenotypic all-oral regimen SOF/VEL was approved, followed by glecaprevir/pibrentasvir (GLE/PIB) a year later. The combination of SOF/VEL/VOX for retreatment was also approved in 2017. Within a decade, the paradigm of HCV treatment has been completely overturned. Some of these regimens combined the different DAAs into a single fixed-dose tablet, further simplifying the treatment and reducing the pill burden.

The advent of pan-genotypic all-oral DAAs has revolutionized HCV outcomes in LT patients, from being associated with poor outcomes relative to other liver disease aetiologies (such as chronic hepatitis B) to become perhaps one of the most favourable outcomes after transplant. The effectiveness of these DAAs has also expanded the donor pool through the use of HCV-positive grafts. To prevent recurrence of HCV after LT, treatment can be considered while awaiting LT, or after transplant.

36.3.2.1 Pre-transplant Treatment

Direct-acting antivirals enable treatment of HCV for decompensated cirrhosis prior to LT with high efficacy. Once HCV is eradicated and the patient is rendered non-viremic at the time of LT, there should be no recurrence [69]. This may also improve liver function significantly and may obviate the need for LT. Improvements in MELD score were associated with delisting, and patients with MELD score < 16 were more likely to be delisted, whereas those with MELD score > 20 were unlikely [96]. Similarly, the risk of disease progression can be reduced with DAA-induced SVR in patients with Child–Pugh–Turcotte (CPT) A cirrhosis, but not in CPT B/C [97]. The recommendation was to treat those with CPT B and/or MELD score <20 on the waiting list without refractory portal hypertensive symptoms, and not treat those with MELD >30 or expected to undergo LT within 3 months [98].

Several additional factors need to be taken into consideration. First, the SVR rates may be lower for patients with decompensated cirrhosis, in particular, those with underlying HCC [99, 100]. Although there was an initial controversy regarding DAA therapy associated with HCC recurrence, subsequent studies, including those undergoing LT, did not show any increase in risk [101, 102]. Second, the reduction in MELD score may unintentionally place the transplant candidate at a disadvantage through lower prioritization, even though the symptoms of portal hypertension may not be completely resolved, and the improvements may not be sufficient to avoid liver-related deaths or delisting [103]. In regions where HCV-positive donors are used, eradication prior to LT may also render them ineligible for these grafts if they are destined for HCV-positive recipients only.

The current recommended treatment for patients with decompensated cirrhosis who are RBV-eligible include SOF/VEL + weight-based RBV for 12 weeks, with an overall SVR rate of >90% [104]. For non-GT 2/3, SOF/LED + RBV may be considered, with a similar SVR rate [105, 106]. For those who are ineligible for RBV, treatment duration is extended to 24 weeks. Similarly, for those with prior SOF or NS5A inhibitor-based treatment failure, treatment should be extended to 24 weeks.

36.3.2.2 Post-LT Treatment

After LT, antiviral treatment can be given pre-emptively early after transplant, to prevent active hepatitis from occurring, or be given at the time of established hepatitis with biochemical and histological confirmation. With the high SVR rates and low side effect profile, it would be prudent to treat once the patient is clinically stable after LT before the onset of graft dysfunction [107]. This will prevent any long-term damage to the allograft, and may also prevent unnecessary investigations. Furthermore, early treatment will prevent the development of extrahepatic complications, and fibrosing cholestatic hepatitis with liver decompensation, which may limit the choice of DAAs regimens to those without a protease inhibitor.

The current recommendation for those without decompensated grafts is 12 weeks of DAAs with either GLE/PIB or SOF/VEL, with an overall SVR rate of >95% [108, 109]. For non-GT 2,3, SOF/LED can also be considered. Once decompensation occurs, the use of a protease inhibitor is usually contraindicated. For these patients, the addition of RBV to SOF/VEL and consideration of treatment to 24 weeks is recommended. The antiviral strategies for HCV after liver transplant are shown in Table 36.1.

36.3.3 Drug–Drug Interactions

It is important to be aware of and to monitor for potential drug–drug interactions (DDI) with the current DAA treatments where the latter can act as a substrate or as enzyme inducers/inhibitors. DDIs can result in alterations in the pharmacodynamic or pharmacokinetic effects or concentrations of the drugs. The use of SOF with amiodarone may trigger severe/fatal bradycardia, and this combination must be avoided [110]. The use of antibiotics such as moxifloxacin or clarithromycin together with a protease inhibitor may lead to QT-interval prolongation. Therefore, it is important to exercise precaution when using protease inhibitors together with proarrhythmic medications. Gastric pH may also affect the solubility of some DAAs including LED and VEL, with higher pH associated with lower solubility. For LED, PPI and H2-anatagnoist should be avoided, and for VEL, PPI should be avoided, or taken 4 hours prior.

All patients will receive immunosuppression after LT, and significant DDIs have been shown to occur between these agents and DAAs. Co-administration of the older regimen of ombitasvir/paritaprevir/ritonavir/dasabuvir with calcineurin inhibitors (CNI) can lead to a dramatic increase in drug levels of the latter, with up to a 57-fold increase of tacrolimus AUC, requiring significant dose reduction down to 0.5 mg every 1–2 weeks [111]. Fortunately, the present-generation DAAs have far fewer DDIs with CNIs than the earlier DAA regimens. The CNI of choice after LT is tacrolimus, and no dose adjustment is required for SOF/LED, SOF/VEL, SOF/VEL/VOX, GLE/PIB or EBR/GZR regimens. Cyclosporine, which is less commonly used, may increase the AUC of some DAAs, including VOX, GLE, GZR and EBR, and co-administration of these DAAs with cyclosporine is not recommended.

36.4 Conclusion

There has been a significant impact of antiviral therapies on LT for both CHB and CHC-infected patients over the last few decades. Chronic viral hepatitis has been steadily declining as an indication for LT, and the reduction is more pronounced for CHC. In the Western world, fatty liver and alcoholic liver diseases have surpassed CHC as the leading indications for LT. The World Health Organization Global Hepatitis Strategy aims to reduce new hepatitis infections by 90% and deaths by 65% by 2030 and have no doubt contributed to the changes observed at regional levels where policies have been implemented to achieve this goal.

For CHB, the use of NAs has led to a reduction in decompensated cirrhosis. However, as it does not eliminate the risk of HCC, and patients are living longer with effective antiviral treatment, there has been a rising trend in HCC as an indication. The goal of antiviral prophylaxis in CHB patients after LT is to prevent reactivation of HBV with virological breakthrough and subsequent graft hepatitis and damage. Current evidence suggests that graft re-infection occurs early during the post-transplant period. The use of third-generation NAs is highly effective in preventing HBV reactivation, with a shifting trend away from using long-term HBIG. Due to the increasing discrepancy between the liver donor pool and the number of patients needing LT, the use of anti-HBc+ donors have become routine in many centres. More recently, HBsAg+ donors have also been considered in order to expand the donor pool. With third-generation NAs, there has been a transition from using HBsAg-negativity as a benchmark for outcome success of antiviral prophylaxis in preventing HBV in the allograft, to transplanting a liver full of intrahepatic HBV and where the patient will likely remain HBsAg after LT.

For CHC, the current all-oral pan-genotypic DAAs have altered the landscape of HCV treatment in LT recipients, whereby re-transplantation for recurrent HCV infection with graft failure has become exceedingly rare. There is also an opportunity to treat decompensated cirrhosis for those on the waiting list, and the decision to treat should be individualized, considering the expected short-term survival, MELD score, expected time on the waiting list and clinical benefits. After LT, those patients who are viremic should receive early DAA treatment once stable, and careful attention must be taken to avoid any potentially harmful DDIs. Similar to HBV, the availability of highly effective antiviral therapies has enabled the use of HCV+ donors to expand the donor pool.

References

1. Seto WK, Lo YR, Pawlotsky JM, Yuen MF. Chronic hepatitis B virus infection. Lancet. 2018;392(10161):2313–24.
2. Razavi H. Global epidemiology of viral hepatitis. Gastroenterol Clin N Am. 2020;49(2):179–89.

3. Fung J, Mak LY, Chan A, Wong T, Dai WC, Sin SL, et al. Trends in liver transplantation for chronic hepatitis B in an era of highly potent antiviral therapies. Liver Transplant. 2021;27(1):134–9.
4. Fung J, Lai CL, Yuen MF. Management of chronic hepatitis B in severe liver disease. World J Gastroenterol. 2014;20(43):16053–61.
5. O'Grady JG, Smith HM, Davies SE, Daniels HM, Donaldson PT, Tan KC, et al. Hepatitis B virus reinfection after orthotopic liver transplantation. Serological and clinical implications. J Hepatol. 1992;14(1):104–11.
6. Samuel D, Muller R, Alexander G, Fassati L, Ducot B, Benhamou JP, et al. Liver transplantation in European patients with the hepatitis B surface antigen. N Engl J Med. 1993;329(25):1842–7.
7. Demetris AJ, Todo S, Van Thiel DH, Fung JJ, Iwaki Y, Sysyn G, et al. Evolution of hepatitis B virus liver disease after hepatic replacement. Practical and theoretical considerations. Am J Pathol. 1990;137(3):667–76.
8. Poterucha JJ, Wiesner RH. Liver transplantation and hepatitis B. Ann Intern Med. 1997;126(10):805–7.
9. Demetris AJ, Jaffe R, Sheahan DG, Burnham J, Spero J, Iwatsuki S, et al. Recurrent hepatitis B in liver allograft recipients. Differentiation between viral hepatitis B and rejection. Am J Pathol. 1986;125(1):161–72.
10. Samuel D, Bismuth A, Mathieu D, Arulnaden JL, Reynes M, Benhamou JP, et al. Passive immunoprophylaxis after liver transplantation in HBsAg-positive patients. Lancet. 1991;337(8745):813–5.
11. Shouval D, Samuel D. Hepatitis B immune globulin to prevent hepatitis B virus graft reinfection following liver transplantation: a concise review. Hepatology. 2000;32(6):1189–95.
12. Lauchart W, Muller R, Pichlmayr R. Long-term immunoprophylaxis of hepatitis B virus reinfection in recipients of human liver allografts. Transplant Proc. 1987;19(5):4051–3.
13. Lauchart W, Muller R, Pichlmayr R. Immunoprophylaxis of hepatitis B virus reinfection in recipients of human liver allografts. Transplant Proc. 1987;19(1 Pt 3):2387–9.
14. Terrault NA, Zhou S, Combs C, Hahn JA, Lake JR, Roberts JP, et al. Prophylaxis in liver transplant recipients using a fixed dosing schedule of hepatitis B immunoglobulin. Hepatology. 1996;24(6):1327–33.
15. McGory RW, Ishitani MB, Oliveira WM, Stevenson WC, McCullough CS, Dickson RC, et al. Improved outcome of orthotopic liver transplantation for chronic hepatitis B cirrhosis with aggressive passive immunization. Transplantation. 1996;61(9):1358–64.
16. McGory R, Ishitani M, Oliveira W, Stevenson W, McCullough C, Pruett T. Hepatitis B immune globulin dose requirements following orthotopic liver transplantation for chronic hepatitis B cirrhosis. Transplant Proc. 1996;28(3):1687–8.
17. Brind A, Jiang J, Samuel D, Gigou M, Feray C, Brechot C, et al. Evidence for selection of hepatitis B mutants after liver transplantation through peripheral blood mononuclear cell infection. J Hepatol. 1997;26(2):228–35.
18. Terrault NA, Zhou S, McCory RW, Pruett TL, Lake JR, Roberts JP, et al. Incidence and clinical consequences of surface and polymerase gene mutations in liver transplant recipients on hepatitis B immunoglobulin. Hepatology. 1998;28(2):555–61.
19. Ghany MG, Ayola B, Villamil FG, Gish RG, Rojter S, Vierling JM, et al. Hepatitis B virus S mutants in liver transplant recipients who were reinfected despite hepatitis B immune globulin prophylaxis. Hepatology. 1998;27(1):213–22.
20. Yuen MF, Seto WK, Chow DH, Tsui K, Wong DK, Ngai V, et al. Long-term lamivudine therapy reduces the risk of long-term complications of chronic hepatitis B infection even in patients without advanced disease. Antivir Ther. 2007;12(8):1295–303.
21. Chan HL, Chui AK, Lau WY, Chan FK, Hui AY, Rao AR, et al. Outcome of lamivudine resistant hepatitis B virus mutant post-liver transplantation on lamivudine monoprophylaxis. Clin Transpl. 2004;18(3):295–300.

22. Mutimer D, Pillay D, Dragon E, Tang H, Ahmed M, O'Donnell K, et al. High pre-treatment serum hepatitis B virus titre predicts failure of lamivudine prophylaxis and graft re-infection after liver transplantation. J Hepatol. 1999;30(4):715–21.
23. Perrillo RP, Wright T, Rakela J, Levy G, Schiff E, Gish R, et al. A multicenter United States-Canadian trial to assess lamivudine monotherapy before and after liver transplantation for chronic hepatitis B. Hepatology. 2001;33(2):424–32.
24. Lo CM, Cheung ST, Lai CL, Liu CL, Ng IO, Yuen MF, et al. Liver transplantation in Asian patients with chronic hepatitis B using lamivudine prophylaxis. Ann Surg. 2001;233(2):276–81.
25. Chen J, Yi L, Jia JD, Ma H, You H. Hepatitis B immunoglobulins and/or lamivudine for preventing hepatitis B recurrence after liver transplantation: a systematic review. J Gastroenterol Hepatol. 2010;25(5):872–9.
26. Markowitz JS, Martin P, Conrad AJ, Markmann JF, Seu P, Yersiz H, et al. Prophylaxis against hepatitis B recurrence following liver transplantation using combination lamivudine and hepatitis B immune globulin. Hepatology. 1998;28(2):585–9.
27. Han SH, Martin P, Edelstein M, Hu R, Kunder G, Holt C, et al. Conversion from intravenous to intramuscular hepatitis B immune globulin in combination with lamivudine is safe and cost-effective in patients receiving long-term prophylaxis to prevent hepatitis B recurrence after liver transplantation. Liver Transplant. 2003;9(2):182–7.
28. Han SH, Ofman J, Holt C, King K, Kunder G, Chen P, et al. An efficacy and cost-effectiveness analysis of combination hepatitis B immune globulin and lamivudine to prevent recurrent hepatitis B after orthotopic liver transplantation compared with hepatitis B immune globulin monotherapy. Liver Transplant. 2000;6(6):741–8.
29. Gane EJ, Angus PW, Strasser S, Crawford DH, Ring J, Jeffrey GP, et al. Lamivudine plus low-dose hepatitis B immunoglobulin to prevent recurrent hepatitis B following liver transplantation. Gastroenterology. 2007;132(3):931–7.
30. Angus PW, McCaughan GW, Gane EJ, Crawford DH, Harley H. Combination low-dose hepatitis B immune globulin and lamivudine therapy provides effective prophylaxis against posttransplantation hepatitis B. Liver Transplant. 2000;6(4):429–33.
31. Lampertico P, Vigano M, Manenti E, Iavarone M, Lunghi G, Colombo M. Adefovir rapidly suppresses hepatitis B in HBeAg-negative patients developing genotypic resistance to lamivudine. Hepatology. 2005;42(6):1414–9.
32. Lo CM, Liu CL, Lau GK, Chan SC, Ng IO, Fan ST. Liver transplantation for chronic hepatitis B with lamivudine-resistant YMDD mutant using add-on adefovir dipivoxil plus lamivudine. Liver Transplant. 2005;11(7):807–13.
33. Wai CT, Prabhakaran K, Wee A, Lee YM, Dan YY, Sutedja DS, et al. Adefovir dipivoxil as the rescue therapy for lamivudine-resistant hepatitis B post liver transplant. Transplant Proc. 2004;36(8):2313–4.
34. Limquiaco JL, Wong J, Wong VW, Wong GL, Tse CH, Chan HY, et al. Lamivudine monoprophylaxis and adefovir salvage for liver transplantation in chronic hepatitis B: a seven-year follow-up study. J Med Virol. 2009;81(2):224–9.
35. Angus PW, Patterson SJ, Strasser SI, McCaughan GW, Gane E. A randomized study of adefovir dipivoxil in place of HBIG in combination with lamivudine as post-liver transplantation hepatitis B prophylaxis. Hepatology. 2008;48(5):1460–6.
36. Neff GW, Kemmer N, Kaiser TE, Zacharias VC, Alonzo M, Thomas M, et al. Combination therapy in liver transplant recipients with hepatitis B virus without hepatitis B immune globulin. Dig Dis Sci. 2007;52(10):2497–500.
37. Gane EJ, Patterson S, Strasser SI, McCaughan GW, Angus PW. Combination of lamivudine and adefovir without hepatitis B immune globulin is safe and effective prophylaxis against hepatitis B virus recurrence in hepatitis B surface antigen-positive liver transplant candidates. Liver Transplant. 2013;19(3):268–74.

38. Fung J, Cheung C, Chan SC, Yuen MF, Chok KS, Sharr W, et al. Entecavir monotherapy is effective in suppressing hepatitis B virus after liver transplantation. Gastroenterology. 2011;141(4):1212–9.
39. Fung J, Wong T, Chok K, Chan A, Cheung TT, Dai J, et al. Long term outcomes of Entecavir monotherapy for chronic hepatitis B after liver transplantation: results up to 8 years. Hepatology. 2017;66:1036.
40. Fung J, Wong T, Chok K, Chan A, Sin SL, Cheung TT, et al. Oral nucleos(t)ide analogs alone after liver transplantation in chronic hepatitis B with preexisting rt204 mutation. Transplantation. 2017;101:2391.
41. Marzano A, Gaia S, Ghisetti V, Carenzi S, Premoli A, Debernardi-Venon W, et al. Viral load at the time of liver transplantation and risk of hepatitis B virus recurrence. Liver Transplant. 2005;11(4):402–9.
42. Duvoux C, Belli LS, Fung J, Angelico M, Buti M, Coilly A, et al. 2020 position statement and recommendations of the European Liver and Intestine Transplantation Association (ELITA): management of hepatitis B virus-related infection before and after liver transplantation. Aliment Pharmacol Ther. 2021;54(5):583–605.
43. Cortesi PA, Vigano R, Conti S, Lenci I, Volpes R, Martini S, et al. Economic impact of European liver and intestine transplantation association (ELITA) recommendations for hepatitis B prophylaxis after liver transplantation. Transplant Int. 2023;36:10954.
44. Loomba R, Rowley AK, Wesley R, Smith KG, Liang TJ, Pucino F, et al. Hepatitis B immunoglobulin and Lamivudine improve hepatitis B-related outcomes after liver transplantation: meta-analysis. Clin Gastroenterol Hepatol. 2008;6(6):696–700.
45. Rao W, Wu X, Xiu D. Lamivudine or lamivudine combined with hepatitis B immunoglobulin in prophylaxis of hepatitis B recurrence after liver transplantation: a meta-analysis. Transplant Int. 2009;22(4):387–94.
46. Katz LH, Paul M, Guy DG, Tur-Kaspa R. Prevention of recurrent hepatitis B virus infection after liver transplantation: hepatitis B immunoglobulin, antiviral drugs, or both? Systematic review and meta-analysis. Transplant Infect Dis. 2010;12(4):292–308.
47. Wang P, Tam N, Wang H, Zheng H, Chen P, Wu L, et al. Is hepatitis B immunoglobulin necessary in prophylaxis of hepatitis B recurrence after liver transplantation? A meta-analysis. PLoS One. 2014;9(8):e104480.
48. Sheng LP, Zhang JC, Zhong ZQ, Sheng XH, Ren J, Wang GQ. High-potency nucleos(t)ide analogues alone or plus immunoglobulin for HBV prophylaxis after liver transplantation: a meta-analysis. Hepatol Int. 2023;17(5):1113–24.
49. Fung J. Management of chronic hepatitis B before and after liver transplantation. World J Hepatol. 2015;7(10):1421–6.
50. Ciesek S, Helfritz FA, Lehmann U, Becker T, Strassburg CP, Neipp M, et al. Persistence of occult hepatitis B after removal of the hepatitis B virus-infected liver. J Infect Dis. 2008;197(3):355–60.
51. Stoll-Becker S, Repp R, Glebe D, Schaefer S, Kreuder J, Kann M, et al. Transcription of hepatitis B virus in peripheral blood mononuclear cells from persistently infected patients. J Virol. 1997;71(7):5399–407.
52. Lu L, Zhang HY, Yueng YH, Cheung KF, Luk JM, Wang FS, et al. Intracellular levels of hepatitis B virus DNA and pregenomic RNA in peripheral blood mononuclear cells of chronically infected patients. J Viral Hepat. 2009;16(2):104–12.
53. Umeda M, Marusawa H, Seno H, Katsurada A, Nabeshima M, Egawa H, et al. Hepatitis B virus infection in lymphatic tissues in inactive hepatitis B carriers. J Hepatol. 2005;42(6):806–12.
54. Yan Q, Lan YH, Huang YX, Fan RS, Liu L, Song SP, et al. Hepatitis B virus replication is upregulated in proliferated peripheral blood lymphocytes. Mol Med Rep. 2016;13(4):3581–7.
55. Jin Y, Gao H, Chen H, Wang J, Chen M, Li G, et al. Identification and impact of hepatitis B virus DNA and antigens in pancreatic cancer tissues and adjacent non-cancerous tissues. Cancer Lett. 2013;335(2):447–54.

56. Lai KN, Ho RT, Tam JS, Lai FM. Detection of hepatitis B virus DNA and RNA in kidneys of HBV related glomerulonephritis. Kidney Int. 1996;50(6):1965–77.
57. Gao S, Duan ZP, Chen Y, van der Meer F, Lee SS, Osiowy C, et al. Compartmental HBV evolution and replication in liver and extrahepatic sites after nucleos/tide analogue therapy in chronic hepatitis B carriers. J Clin Virol. 2017;94:8–14.
58. Villeret F, Lebosse F, Radenne S, Samuel D, Roche B, Mabrut JY, et al. Early intrahepatic recurrence of HBV infection in liver transplant recipients despite antiviral prophylaxis. JHEP Rep. 2023;5(6):100728.
59. Hussain M, Soldevila-Pico C, Emre S, Luketic V, Lok AS. Presence of intrahepatic (total and ccc) HBV DNA is not predictive of HBV recurrence after liver transplantation. Liver Transplant. 2007;13(8):1137–44.
60. Yasunaka T, Takaki A, Yagi T, Iwasaki Y, Sadamori H, Koike K, et al. Serum hepatitis B virus DNA before liver transplantation correlates with HBV reinfection rate even under successful low-dose hepatitis B immunoglobulin prophylaxis. Hepatol Int. 2011;5:918.
61. Matsuzaki T, Tatsuki I, Otani M, Akiyama M, Ozawa E, Miuma S, et al. Significance of hepatitis B virus core-related antigen and covalently closed circular DNA levels as markers of hepatitis B virus re-infection after liver transplantation. J Gastroenterol Hepatol. 2013;28(7):1217–22.
62. Raimondo G, Locarnini S, Pollicino T, Levrero M, Zoulim F, Lok AS, et al. Update of the statements on biology and clinical impact of occult hepatitis B virus infection. J Hepatol. 2019;71(2):397–408.
63. Chazouilleres O, Mamish D, Kim M, Carey K, Ferrell L, Roberts JP, et al. "Occult" hepatitis B virus as source of infection in liver transplant recipients. Lancet. 1994;343(8890):142–6.
64. Lau G, Yu ML, Wong G, Thompson A, Ghazinian H, Hou JL, et al. APASL clinical practice guideline on hepatitis B reactivation related to the use of immunosuppressive therapy. Hepatol Int. 2021;15(5):1031–48.
65. Skagen CL, Jou JH, Said A. Risk of de novo hepatitis in liver recipients from hepatitis-B core antibody-positive grafts – a systematic analysis. Clin Transpl. 2011;25(3):E243–9.
66. Prieto M, Gomez MD, Berenguer M, Cordoba J, Rayon JM, Pastor M, et al. De novo hepatitis B after liver transplantation from hepatitis B core antibody-positive donors in an area with high prevalence of anti-HBc positivity in the donor population. Liver Transplant. 2001;7(1):51–8.
67. Cholongitas E, Papatheodoridis GV, Burroughs AK. Liver grafts from anti-hepatitis B core positive donors: a systematic review. J Hepatol. 2010;52(2):272–9.
68. Perrillo R. Hepatitis B virus prevention strategies for antibody to hepatitis B core antigen-positive liver donation: a survey of North American, European, and Asian-Pacific transplant programs. Liver Transplant. 2009;15(2):223–32.
69. Forns X, Garcia-Retortillo M, Serrano T, Feliu A, Suarez F, de la Mata M, et al. Antiviral therapy of patients with decompensated cirrhosis to prevent recurrence of hepatitis C after liver transplantation. J Hepatol. 2003;39(3):389–96.
70. Chang MS, Olsen SK, Pichardo EM, Stiles JB, Rosenthal-Cogan L, Brubaker WD, et al. Prevention of de novo hepatitis B in recipients of core antibody-positive livers with lamivudine and other nucleos(t)ides: a 12-year experience. Transplantation. 2013;95(7):960–5.
71. Saab S, Waterman B, Chi AC, Tong MJ. Comparison of different immunoprophylaxis regimens after liver transplantation with hepatitis B core antibody-positive donors: a systematic review. Liver Transplant. 2010;16(3):300–7.
72. European Association for the Study of the Liver. Electronic address eee, European Association for the Study of the L. EASL 2017 clinical practice guidelines on the management of hepatitis B virus infection. J Hepatol. 2017;67(2):370–98.
73. Terrault NA, Lok ASF, McMahon BJ, Chang KM, Hwang JP, Jonas MM, et al. Update on prevention, diagnosis, and treatment of chronic hepatitis B: AASLD 2018 hepatitis B guidance. Hepatology. 2018;67(4):1560–99.

74. Wong TC, Fung JY, Cui TY, Lam AH, Dai JW, Chan AC, et al. Liver transplantation using hepatitis B core positive grafts with antiviral monotherapy prophylaxis. J Hepatol. 2019;70(6):1114–22.
75. Ali SE, Vutien P, Bonham CA, Landis C, Kwo P, Esquivel C, et al. Use and outcomes of hepatitis B virus-positive grafts in orthotopic liver transplantation in the United States from 1999 to 2021. Liver Transplant. 2023;29(1):80–90.
76. Delman AM, Turner KM, Safdar K, Anwar N, Silski LS, Lee TC, et al. Expanding the donor pool: first use of hepatitis B virus nat positive solid organ allografts into seronegative recipients. Ann Surg. 2021;274(4):556–64.
77. Wei L, Chen D, Zhang B, Zhao Y, Liu B, Shi H, et al. Long-term outcome and recurrence of hepatitis B virus following liver transplantation from hepatitis B surface antigen-positive donors in a Chinese population. J Viral Hepat. 2018;25(12):1576–81.
78. Yu S, Cen C, Zhang X, Cheng L, Xia W, Jia J, et al. Utilization of hepatitis B virus surface antigen positive grafts in liver transplantation: a matched study based on a national registry cohort. J Gastroenterol Hepatol. 2022;37(6):1052–9.
79. Terrault NA, Pageaux GP. A changing landscape of liver transplantation: King HCV is dethroned, ALD and NAFLD take over! J Hepatol. 2018;69(4):767–8.
80. Wright TL, Donegan E, Hsu HH, Ferrell L, Lake JR, Kim M, et al. Recurrent and acquired hepatitis C viral infection in liver transplant recipients. Gastroenterology. 1992;103(1):317–22.
81. Garcia-Retortillo M, Forns X, Feliu A, Moitinho E, Costa J, Navasa M, et al. Hepatitis C virus kinetics during and immediately after liver transplantation. Hepatology. 2002;35(3):680–7.
82. Burra P, De Martin E, Zanetto A, Senzolo M, Russo FP, Zanus G, et al. Hepatitis C virus and liver transplantation: where do we stand? Transplant Int. 2016;29(2):135–52.
83. Berenguer M, Ferrell L, Watson J, Prieto M, Kim M, Rayon M, et al. HCV-related fibrosis progression following liver transplantation: increase in recent years. J Hepatol. 2000;32(4):673–84.
84. Gane EJ, Portmann BC, Naoumov NV, Smith HM, Underhill JA, Donaldson PT, et al. Long-term outcome of hepatitis C infection after liver transplantation. N Engl J Med. 1996;334(13):815–20.
85. Samonakis DN, Germani G, Burroughs AK. Immunosuppression and HCV recurrence after liver transplantation. J Hepatol. 2012;56(4):973–83.
86. Berenguer M, Aguilera V, Prieto M, San Juan F, Rayon JM, Benlloch S, et al. Significant improvement in the outcome of HCV-infected transplant recipients by avoiding rapid steroid tapering and potent induction immunosuppression. J Hepatol. 2006;44(4):717–22.
87. Verna EC, Abdelmessih R, Salomao MA, Lefkowitch J, Moreira RK, Brown RS Jr. Cholestatic hepatitis C following liver transplantation: an outcome-based histological definition, clinical predictors, and prognosis. Liver Transplant. 2013;19(1):78–88.
88. Selzner N, Guindi M, Renner EL, Berenguer M. Immune-mediated complications of the graft in interferon-treated hepatitis C positive liver transplant recipients. J Hepatol. 2011;55(1):207–17.
89. Gane EJ, Agarwal K. Directly acting antivirals (DAAs) for the treatment of chronic hepatitis C virus infection in liver transplant patients: "a flood of opportunity". Am J Transplant. 2014;14(5):994–1002.
90. Gu M, Rice CM. Structures of hepatitis C virus nonstructural proteins required for replicase assembly and function. Curr Opin Virol. 2013;3(2):129–36.
91. Verna EC, Saxena V, Burton JR Jr, O'Leary JG, Dodge JL, Stravitz RT, et al. Telaprevir- and Boceprevir-based triple therapy for hepatitis C in liver transplant recipients with advanced recurrent disease: a multicenter study. Transplantation. 2015;99(8):1644–51.
92. Saab S, Manne V, Bau S, Reynolds JA, Allen R, Goldstein L, et al. Boceprevir in liver transplant recipients. Liver Int. 2015;35(1):192–7.
93. Hulskotte E, Gupta S, Xuan F, van Zutven M, O'Mara E, Feng HP, et al. Pharmacokinetic interaction between the hepatitis C virus protease inhibitor boceprevir and cyclosporine and tacrolimus in healthy volunteers. Hepatology. 2012;56(5):1622–30.

94. Garg V, van Heeswijk R, Lee JE, Alves K, Nadkarni P, Luo X. Effect of telaprevir on the pharmacokinetics of cyclosporine and tacrolimus. Hepatology. 2011;54(1):20–7.
95. O'Leary JG, McKenna GJ, Klintmalm GB, Davis GL. Effect of telaprevir on the pharmacokinetics of sirolimus in liver transplant recipients. Liver Transplant. 2013;19(4):463–5.
96. Belli LS, Berenguer M, Cortesi PA, Strazzabosco M, Rockenschaub SR, Martini S, et al. Delisting of liver transplant candidates with chronic hepatitis C after viral eradication: a European study. J Hepatol. 2016;65(3):524–31.
97. Krassenburg LAP, Maan R, Ramji A, Manns MP, Cornberg M, Wedemeyer H, et al. Clinical outcomes following DAA therapy in patients with HCV-related cirrhosis depend on disease severity. J Hepatol. 2021;74(5):1053–63.
98. Terrault NA, McCaughan GW, Curry MP, Gane E, Fagiuoli S, Fung JYY, et al. International liver transplantation society consensus statement on hepatitis C management in liver transplant candidates. Transplantation. 2017;101(5):945–55.
99. Beste LA, Green PK, Berry K, Kogut MJ, Allison SK, Ioannou GN. Effectiveness of hepatitis C antiviral treatment in a USA cohort of veteran patients with hepatocellular carcinoma. J Hepatol. 2017;67(1):32–9.
100. Prenner SB, VanWagner LB, Flamm SL, Salem R, Lewandowski RJ, Kulik L. Hepatocellular carcinoma decreases the chance of successful hepatitis C virus therapy with direct-acting antivirals. J Hepatol. 2017;66(6):1173–81.
101. Reig M, Marino Z, Perello C, Inarrairaegui M, Ribeiro A, Lens S, et al. Unexpected high rate of early tumor recurrence in patients with HCV-related HCC undergoing interferon-free therapy. J Hepatol. 2016;65(4):719–26.
102. Tse CS, Yang JD, Mousa OY, Nelson KM, Pungpapong S, Keaveny A, et al. Direct-acting antiviral therapy in liver transplant patients with hepatocellular carcinoma and hepatitis C. Transplant Direct. 2021;7(1):e635.
103. Bittermann T, Reddy KR. In the era of direct-acting antivirals, liver transplant delisting due to clinical improvement for hepatitis C remains infrequent. Clin Gastroenterol Hepatol. 2021;19(11):2389–97 e2.
104. Curry MP, O'Leary JG, Bzowej N, Muir AJ, Korenblat KM, Fenkel JM, et al. Sofosbuvir and velpatasvir for HCV in patients with decompensated cirrhosis. N Engl J Med. 2015;373(27):2618–28.
105. Charlton M, Everson GT, Flamm SL, Kumar P, Landis C, Brown RS Jr, et al. Ledipasvir and sofosbuvir plus ribavirin for treatment of HCV infection in patients with advanced liver disease. Gastroenterology. 2015;149(3):649–59.
106. Manns M, Samuel D, Gane EJ, Mutimer D, McCaughan G, Buti M, et al. Ledipasvir and sofosbuvir plus ribavirin in patients with genotype 1 or 4 hepatitis C virus infection and advanced liver disease: a multicentre, open-label, randomised, phase 2 trial. Lancet Infect Dis. 2016;16(6):685–97.
107. Terrault NA, Berenguer M, Strasser SI, Gadano A, Lilly L, Samuel D, et al. International liver transplantation society consensus statement on hepatitis C management in liver transplant recipients. Transplantation. 2017;101(5):956–67.
108. Reau N, Kwo PY, Rhee S, Brown RS Jr, Agarwal K, Angus P, et al. Glecaprevir/Pibrentasvir treatment in liver or kidney transplant patients with hepatitis C virus infection. Hepatology. 2018;68(4):1298–307.
109. Agarwal K, Castells L, Mullhaupt B, Rosenberg WMC, McNabb B, Arterburn S, et al. Sofosbuvir/velpatasvir for 12 weeks in genotype 1-4 HCV-infected liver transplant recipients. J Hepatol. 2018;69(3):603–7.
110. Back DJ, Burger DM. Interaction between amiodarone and sofosbuvir-based treatment for hepatitis C virus infection: potential mechanisms and lessons to be learned. Gastroenterology. 2015;149(6):1315–7.
111. Badri PS, Parikh A, Coakley EP, Ding B, Awni WM, Dutta S, et al. Pharmacokinetics of tacrolimus and cyclosporine in liver transplant recipients receiving 3 direct-acting antivirals as treatment for hepatitis C infection. Ther Drug Monit. 2016;38(5):640–5.

Chapter 37
De Novo and Recurrent Metabolic Dysfunction Associated Steatotic Liver Disease

Laxmi Parsa and Sanjaya K. Satapathy

Abstract Metabolic Dysfunction Associated Steatotic Liver Disease (MASLD) encompasses hepatic steatosis, steatohepatitis (MASH), and cirrhosis and is one of the two leading causes of liver transplantation globally. The recurrence and emergence of MASLD following transplantation is an increasing concern, with significant progression to fibrosis and cirrhosis widely documented. MASLD is linked to higher mortality rates due to cardiovascular disease, non-hepatic cancers, and graft cirrhosis. Early diagnosis through non-invasive fibrosis tests, alongside strategies to modify existing risk factors, is essential for management, as there is currently no optimal medical therapy available for post-transplant patients. Further research into the pathogenesis, natural progression, metabolic risk factors, and the impact of immunosuppressive medications on MASLD is needed to improve the management of post-transplant patients.

Keywords Metabolic Dysfunction Associated Liver Disease (MASLD) · Liver transplantation · Hepatic steatosis · Metabolic Dysfunction Associated Steatohepatitis (MASH) · Cirrhosis · Obesity · De novo MASLD · Cardiovascular disease · Metabolic syndrome · Weight loss

Key Highlights

- MASLD, including Metabolic Dysfunction Associated Steatohepatitis (MASH) and cirrhosis, is now a leading cause of liver transplantation globally.
- Recurrence and de novo MASLD post-transplantation are increasing, with progression to fibrosis and cirrhosis well documented.

L. Parsa
University of Tennessee College of Medicine, Chattanooga, TN, USA
e-mail: lparsa@uthsc.edu

S. K. Satapathy (✉)
Division of Hepatology, Department of Medicine, North Shore University Hospital/Northwell Health, Manhasset, NY, USA
e-mail: ssatapat@northwell.edu

S. Saigal, D. Jothimani (eds.), *Fundamentals of Transplant Hepatology*,
https://doi.org/10.1007/978-981-95-2624-6_37

- MASLD is linked to higher mortality rates, primarily due to cardiovascular disease, non-hepatic cancers, and graft cirrhosis.
- Risk factors such as obesity, metabolic syndrome, diabetes, and immunosuppressive therapy play a key role in disease progression.
- Insulin resistance, lipotoxicity, and inflammation drive MASLD progression in both pre- and post-transplant settings.
- Genetic polymorphisms (e.g., PNPLA3, TM6SF2, MBOAT7) contribute to disease susceptibility, while others (HSD17B13, CIDEB) offer protective effects.
- No optimal medical therapy currently exists for post-transplant MASLD.
- Management relies on early diagnosis via non-invasive fibrosis tests, lifestyle modifications (weight loss, exercise), and potential pharmacologic options like GLP-1RAs, SGLT-2 inhibitors, and resmetirom.
- Further studies are required to understand MASLD progression post-transplant, the role of immunosuppressive medications, and novel therapeutic approaches.
- A multidisciplinary approach involving hepatologists, endocrinologists, and transplant specialists is essential for optimizing post-transplant outcomes.

37.1 Introduction

Metabolic Dysfunction Associated Steatotic Liver Disease (MASLD) is characterized by the presence of macrovesicular steatosis in more than 5% of hepatocytes, without any other identifiable cause, and with an average alcohol consumption of less than 20 g/day for women and less than 30 g/day for men. The global prevalence of MASLD is rising rapidly, leading to increased rates of cirrhosis and hepatocellular carcinoma (HCC). In women, MASLD has surpassed alcohol as the leading cause of liver transplantation, and it is also competing with alcohol as the leading cause in men in the United States [1, 2]. By 2030, the overall estimated prevalence of MASLD in individuals over 15 years of age in the USA is projected to reach 33.5%, with a prevalence of 25–30% in the general population, though this may vary based on geographic location, race, or ethnicity [1, 3, 4]. The global epidemic of obesity and related metabolic conditions, such as central obesity, diabetes, dyslipidemia, and hypertension, is further exacerbating the burden of MASLD [3, 5]. By 2030, the incidence of advanced hepatic fibrosis, cirrhosis, hepatocellular carcinoma, and related mortality is expected to double or triple [1, 6]. Recurrent and de novo MASLD have been recognized as complications after liver transplantation [7–9]. The pathogenesis is influenced by obesity and metabolic comorbidities, which are further aggravated by immunosuppressive medications such as tacrolimus, cyclosporine, and corticosteroids [7–10].

37.2 MASLD and Liver Transplantation

The Third National Health and Nutrition Examination Survey (NHANES III) reported a 19% prevalence of MASLD among adults in the USA, although various studies have provided a range of estimates from 17% to 50% [1, 11, 12]. The overall prevalence of MASH among adults is estimated to be 3–5%, with approximately 20% of MASLD patients having significant MASH with fibrosis greater than F3 [13]. Estes et al. estimated that 25.8% of the general population had MASLD in 2015, with projections suggesting an increase to 33.5% among those aged over 15 years and 28.4% across all ages by 2030 [1]. It was also estimated that 27% of MASLD cases would progress to MASH, with 29% of these cases advancing to severe MASH (F3-F4) [1]. The prevalence and incidence of decompensated cirrhosis are predicted to increase by 180% and 168%, respectively, from 2015 to 2030 [1]. Surveillance, Epidemiology, and End Results (SEER) studies reported that the rates of HCC attributable to MASLD ranged from 13.3% to 20.3% between 2004 and 2009 [14]. The cumulative incidence of HCC is projected to increase 2–3 fold, reaching 135,000 cases between 2015 and 2030 [1].

The Global Burden of Disease (GBD) study indicates a worsening burden of MASLD globally, with a significant rise expected in Asia, the Middle East, and North Africa [15, 16]. A large meta-analysis estimated a pooled global prevalence of MASLD at 30.9%, based on data from 1989 to 2020, with the highest rates observed in the Middle East and North Africa at 42.6% [15, 17].

A study based on the United States Scientific Registry of Transplant Recipients showed that MASH is the most common indication for liver transplantation in individuals over 65 years of age and in females [18, 19]. The proportion of elderly candidates listed for transplantation due to MASH increased from 13% (2002–2005) to 39% (2018–2020) [19]. MASLD is also rapidly becoming the most common cause of liver transplantation, nearly matching the rates of alcohol-related liver disease in the USA and Europe [20, 21]. Liver transplant recipients with MASLD as the indication are typically elderly, obese with higher BMI, male, and more likely to have HCC [22].

P

37.3 Pathogenesis of MASLD in Pre- and Post-Transplant Patients

The pathogenesis of MASLD arises from the complex interplay of various factors that regulate the metabolism of free fatty acids, diacylglycerols, cholesterol, and phospholipids within the liver. Central to this process is insulin resistance and metabolic disease [23]. When there is an excess of energy from carbohydrates such as glucose, fructose, and sucrose, along with saturated fats, fat accumulates in hepatocytes in the form of triglycerides through a process known as de novo lipogenesis

[24–27]. Insulin resistance plays a critical role by affecting lipogenesis in the liver, adipose tissue, and muscles [26]. It also leads to increased lipolysis, releasing free fatty acids from adipose tissue, which is closely associated with the progression of MASLD [25, 28]. Additionally, inadequate clearance and synthesis of very low-density lipoproteins (VLDL) contribute to triglyceride accumulation in the liver [29–31].

Several retrospective studies, including large meta-analyses, have identified metabolic abnormalities such as increased BMI, post-transplant hypertriglyceridemia, metabolic syndrome, steroid use, diabetes, and sirolimus-based immunosuppression as significant risk factors for post-transplant hepatic steatosis (HS), all of which promote insulin resistance [9, 10, 32, 33]. Furthermore, serum levels of leptin and adiponectin, which regulate steatosis, are often impaired in the post-liver transplant (LT) period, further contributing to steatosis [34]. Insulin resistance also results in inadequate suppression of gluconeogenesis, reduced glycogen synthesis, and increased triglyceride production. Elevated circulating levels of free fatty acids can trigger the overexpression of inflammatory markers such as TNF-alpha and IL-6 and lead to endoplasmic reticulum stress. Although the precise mechanism of fibrosis progression in post-LT patients remains unclear, the activation of hepatic stellate cells, upregulation of pro-inflammatory cytokines, and increased leptin levels are implicated [35–39].

There is considerable variation in the factors that contribute to the development and progression of MASLD in both pre- and post-transplant patients [40, 41]. Notably, several genetic polymorphisms have been identified as playing a role in the pathogenesis and progression of MASLD. For instance, polymorphisms in PNPLA3, TM6SF2, and MBOAT7 have been shown to impair the lipolysis of triglycerides, cholesterol metabolism, and phospholipid metabolism, respectively, which can lead to more advanced MASLD [42–44]. Conversely, loss-of-function mutations in Hydroxysteroid 17-beta Dehydrogenase 13 (HSD17B13) and Cell Death Inducing DFFA Like Effector B (CIDEB) have been shown to offer some protection against more severe forms of MASLD [45, 46].

The lipotoxic injury resulting from fat accumulation eventually activates hepatic stellate cells, macrophages, and inflammatory cytokines such as IL-6, TNF-alpha, and leptin, which can induce fibrosis and drive the progression of the disease [47–49]. The presence of PNPLA3 variants in either the donor or recipient, or in both, as well as the presence of TM6SF2 variants in the donor, has been shown to increase the risk of post-LT HS [10, 50]. Conversely, a variant in superoxide dismutase-2 in the donor has been found to have a protective effect [51], while variants in adiponectin in the recipients have been associated with an increased risk of post-LT HS [52].

37.4 Recurrent and De Novo MASLD

MASLD can manifest either as a recurrence or as a de novo disease after LT [8, 9, 53]. When MASLD is diagnosed after transplantation without prior evidence of HS, it is termed "de novo" MASLD. This condition has the potential to progress to cirrhosis, leading to complications that can negatively impact the graft.

The reported prevalence of HS, whether recurrent or de novo, in the post-LT period varies significantly. A recent large meta-analysis and systematic review by Silva AS et al., which included 40 studies with a total of 6979 post-transplant patients, found that the prevalence of fatty liver in the post-LT period ranged from 12% to 88%, with a global weighted prevalence of 39.76% [10]. This study also reported a pooled prevalence of recurrent hepatic steatosis at 52.47% (95% CI: 40.27–64.64) and de novo steatosis at 31.67% (95% CI: 23.85–39.53), based on 29 studies that separately estimated both recurrent and de novo HS [10]. Additionally, the study found that patients transplanted for MASLD-associated cirrhosis had a greater than five-fold increased risk of HS, followed by a greater than 2.5-fold increase for those with alcohol-associated liver disease, compared to other underlying liver disease etiologies [10]. Similarly, a meta-analysis by Saeed et al. reported incidence rates for de novo graft steatosis at 1, 3, and 5 years post-LT as 67%, 40%, and 78%, respectively, with de novo graft steatohepatitis rates at 13%, 16%, and 17% [9].

Interestingly, only a few studies have reported a linear time-dependent increase in the prevalence of post-LT HS [54, 55], with some instances of HS developing as early as 3 weeks post-transplant [10, 56]. The prevalence of significant fibrosis and cirrhosis post-LT also varies depending on the study [57–60]. Prior reports indicate that significant fibrosis developed in 13.99% of cases (range: 7.62–20.31%) [10]. Notably, only two studies reported the prevalence of cirrhosis post-LT as 1.8% [61] and 13% [40, 62], although the majority of studies did not report post-LT cirrhosis secondary to MASLD [10]. Recurrent MASLD is characterized by earlier onset and more rapid progression to fibrosis compared to de novo occurrence [63].

The risk of post-LT HS is associated with pre-LT metabolic factors such as higher BMI, obesity, type II diabetes mellitus (DM), and hypertension, but not with dyslipidemia. Donor factors like living donor status, donor age, or sex were not found to be associated with post-LT HS. Although donor BMI was slightly higher in cases of post-LT HS, donor obesity or overweight did not particularly show an increased risk [10]. Rapid weight gain in the post-LT period, higher BMI, and abdominal obesity were strongly associated with post-LT HS, as well as metabolic diseases like type II DM with poor glycemic control, hypertension, and dyslipidemia [10].

Immunosuppressive therapy also significantly affects the components of metabolic syndrome. Corticosteroids exacerbate insulin resistance, mammalian target of Rapamycin (mTOR) inhibitors worsen dyslipidemia, and calcineurin inhibitors (CNI) induce new-onset DM, renal disease, and hypertension [64–66]. Some studies have shown benefits from weight loss attributed to the combined use of mTOR inhibitors and low-dose tacrolimus [67, 68]. However, a large meta-analysis found that only sirolimus was associated with post-LT HS [10].

37.5 Donor Risk Factors

Graft steatosis has been identified as a significant risk factor for post-LT HS [69, 70]. Moreover, steatosis can lead to microcirculatory and cellular changes in the liver graft, potentially causing hepatic necrosis and impaired regeneration, particularly in grafts with more than 60% steatosis. Severe graft steatosis is also associated with an increased risk of graft failure and impaired graft function due to ischemia-reperfusion injury. A systematic review highlighted that grafts with over 60% steatosis have a high risk of poor functioning, and grafts with more than 30% steatosis show decreased survival rates [71–74]. While donor livers with microvesicular steatosis have been associated with delayed postoperative recovery, this condition has not been shown to contribute to graft failure or loss [72, 75]. Interestingly, recent studies indicate that long-term outcomes are not adversely affected and that steatosis can be reversed. However, macrosteatosis can impact post-reperfusion syndrome, initial graft function, and early post-transplant outcomes, especially when donor steatosis is reliably estimated [69, 70, 76, 77].

37.6 Recipient Risk Factors

Pre-LT characteristics such as abdominal obesity, high BMI, dyslipidemia, and diabetes are significant risk factors for developing post-LT steatosis [40, 62]. In the post-LT period, rapid weight gain, abdominal obesity, and components of metabolic syndrome—such as diabetes with poor glycemic control, hypertriglyceridemia, and arterial hypertension—are also major risk factors for post-LT steatosis [10, 62]. While immunosuppressive therapies, including steroids and calcineurin inhibitors, can exacerbate diabetes, hypertension, and dyslipidemia, mTOR inhibitors like sirolimus have been particularly associated with worsening post-LT steatosis [10]. Additionally, MASLD and Cryptogenic Cirrhosis (CC) as indications for transplantation are linked to a significant risk of both recurrent and de novo HS [10, 40].

37.7 Outcomes of LT for MASLD Cirrhosis

Multiple studies, including several large meta-analyses and systematic reviews, have demonstrated excellent outcomes in terms of overall and graft survival for patients receiving LTs for MASLD, with survival rates ranging between 85–90% at 1 year and 70–80% at 5 years post-transplant [10, 78, 79]. A large meta-analysis involving 15 studies with a total of 119,237 LT recipients reported a prevalence of MASH as the indication for transplant at 20.2% (95% CI: 12.9–30.2) [79]. The overall survival rates between MASH and non-MASH (such as alcohol, HCV, and autoimmune) LT recipients were found to be similar (HR, 0.91 [0.76–1.1]; $p = 0.34$) [79]. Additionally, there was no significant difference in graft survival between these groups (HR, 0.95 [0.88–1.03]; $p = 0.20$). The all-cause mortality rates at 1, 5, and 10 years post-transplant were 12.5%, 24.4%, and 37.9%, respectively [79]. Interestingly, while sepsis posed a non-significant risk for mortality in the MASH group, cardiovascular-related events (OR 1.38 [0.621–3.06]; $p = 0.37$) and malignancy (OR 0.57 [0.26–1.26]; $p = 0.14$) did not show a significantly higher risk of mortality compared to non-MASH LT recipients [79].

However, previous studies have reported significant cardiovascular mortality in LT recipients with MASH as the underlying disease [22, 80]. One study, evaluating 938 liver transplant recipients for MASH from 1997 to 2017 across seven transplant centers, showed excellent survival rates of 93%, 88%, 83%, 69%, and 46% at 1, 3, 5, 10, and 15 years, respectively [81]. The most common causes of mortality in this study included infection (19%), cardiovascular disease (18%), cancer (17%), and liver-related causes. Factors such as age over 65 years, end-stage renal disease, and the use of non-calcineurin inhibitor-based regimens were associated with increased mortality [81]. Interestingly, statin use in the post-LT period was found to have a favorable impact on survival [81].

37.8 Management of MASLD in Post-LT Patients

There are currently no randomized controlled trials specifically addressing treatment options for MASLD in the post-LT setting. Management strategies primarily focus on lifestyle modifications and the adjustment of risk factors, early diagnosis and detection of advanced fibrosis through non-invasive tests and protocol biopsies, and the treatment of associated metabolic comorbidities. A multidisciplinary approach is essential for effectively managing MASLD in the context of transplantation.

37.8.1 Weight Loss and Dietary Modifications

A modest weight loss of 3–5% can lead to improvements in HS, but a minimum of 10% weight loss is necessary to improve steatohepatitis and slow fibrosis progression [6, 82, 83]. However, sustaining such weight loss remains challenging, even with structured interventions over a year, emphasizing the need for a multidisciplinary approach that includes a psychologist, dietitian, and family support [84–88]. Dietary modifications, such as caloric restriction, low-carbohydrate and low-saturated-fat diets, intermittent fasting, and the Mediterranean diet, can benefit cardiovascular health and reduce HS [89–91]. Additionally, coffee consumption is recommended based on findings from meta-analyses and epidemiological studies, which suggest it may decrease the risk of MASLD [6, 92].

37.8.2 Exercise

Moderate exercise, performed at least 5 times per week for a total of 150 minutes, or an increase in activity level by 60 min per week, can lead to improvements in MASLD. However, more vigorous or high-intensity exercise is required to achieve improvements in fibrosis [93, 94]. Post-transplant patients may face limitations in their exercise capacity due to associated comorbidities, making it essential to develop an individualized exercise plan aimed at increasing physical activity as much as possible [6, 94].

37.8.3 Bariatric Surgery

Bariatric surgery is generally indicated for the treatment of obesity in individuals with a BMI greater than 40 kg/m^2 or a BMI greater than 35 kg/m^2 when accompanied by comorbidities such as diabetes, uncontrolled hypertension, or severe osteoarthritis. MASLD or MASH is also recognized as an acceptable indication for bariatric surgery. However, patients with advanced fibrosis or cirrhosis are typically excluded from these procedures due to the risk of perioperative complications and the potential for decompensation of cirrhosis [95]. Bariatric surgery, when resulting in significant weight loss, has been shown to lead to the resolution of MASH, improvements in fibrosis scores, and the resolution of comorbidities such as diabetes and cardiovascular disease [95–97].

Although bariatric surgery is not generally recommended as a therapeutic option for patients with compensated MASH cirrhosis, it can be considered in carefully selected patients [6]. Restrictive surgeries, such as sleeve gastrectomy, rather than malabsorptive surgeries, can be considered in high-volume centers in conjunction with LT [6]. A study published by the Mayo Clinic [98] included 13 patients who underwent simultaneous LT and sleeve gastrectomy with over 3 years of follow-up, compared to 36 patients who underwent LT alone. In the LT and sleeve gastrectomy cohort, 29.4% of patients maintained more than 10% weight loss, compared to 100% of those in the LT alone cohort ($p < 0.0001$) [98]. The LT and sleeve gastrectomy group also experienced a significantly higher percentage of weight loss (34.8% ± 17.3% vs. 13.3% ± 3.9%; $p < 0.001$). Additionally, this group showed a lower prevalence of hypertension, insulin resistance, and HS and reduced requirements for antihypertensive and lipid-lowering medications [98].

Another case series [99] investigated the safety and efficacy of bariatric surgery in post-LT patients. Twelve morbidly obese patients were matched with 36 non-LT controls and followed for 2 years. While the non-LT patients experienced significant weight loss (53.7% vs. 45.2%; $p < 0.001$), both groups saw similar resolution of comorbidities. Bariatric surgery did not necessitate changes to immunosuppressive medications, and no liver-related complications were observed in the post-LT group [99]. Another small case series [100] involving two morbidly obese patients with recurrent and de novo MASLD post-LT who underwent sleeve gastrectomy reported a mean reduction in body weight of 31.98 kg, a decrease in BMI of 10.2 kg/m^2, and improvements in steatosis and fibrosis scores (0.34 and 0.05, respectively) [100].

Although large studies specifically addressing the impact of bariatric surgery on post-LT recurrent or de novo MASLD are lacking, several case series have reported favorable outcomes. Malabsorptive surgeries, such as gastric bypass, pose potential challenges, including the risk of malabsorption of immunosuppressive medications and difficulty with endoscopic access to bile ducts when needed.

37.8.4 Medical Management

There are currently no specific randomized trials investigating the use of medications for the treatment of MASLD in post-LT patients. However, the same pharmacotherapy used in the non-LT population may be considered, with careful selection and adjustment of agents on a case-by-case basis.

37.8.4.1 Vitamin E

In the PIVENS trial, Vitamin E at a dose of 800 IU was studied in non-diabetic patients over 96 weeks, comparing its effects to placebo and pioglitazone. The trial demonstrated that Vitamin E significantly improved MASH histology compared to placebo [101]. A subsequent meta-analysis further supported the benefits of Vitamin E, showing improvements in serum aminotransferase levels, as well as biopsy findings, including reductions in steatosis, inflammation, and hepatocyte ballooning [102]. Additionally, Vitamin E was shown to enhance transplant-free survival and reduce hepatic decompensation in patients with MASH and advanced fibrosis [103]. However, there have been conflicting reports and concerns regarding the use of Vitamin E, particularly in relation to an increased risk of prostate cancer, bleeding, and hemorrhagic stroke [103, 104].

37.8.4.2 Thiazolidinediones

Pioglitazone can be used in patients with or without diabetes and has been shown to achieve a greater than 2-point reduction in the NAS score for MASH, along with some improvement in fibrosis. Although Pioglitazone did not meet the primary endpoint of a >2-point reduction in NAS score in the PIVENS trial, a subsequent

18-month study demonstrated its benefit in reducing the NAS score by 2 points and improving fibrosis [101, 105]. However, potential side effects such as weight gain, worsening of congestive heart failure, and an increased risk of osteoporosis in post-menopausal women need to be carefully considered [106]. Given these risks, especially the potential for rapid weight gain, pioglitazone may not be an ideal option for treating post-LT MASLD.

37.8.4.3 GLP-1RAs

Several GLP-1 receptor agonists (GLP-1RAs) are approved for the treatment of diabetes and have shown considerable benefits in improving lipid profiles, promoting weight loss, and enhancing cardiovascular outcomes. Although none of these agents are currently approved for the treatment of MASH, liraglutide and semaglutide have demonstrated the ability to improve HS, resolve MASH, and decrease fibrosis progression [107, 108]. Additionally, tirzepatide has been shown to significantly reduce hepatic fat content and promote weight loss [109]. However, potential side effects such as upper gastrointestinal symptoms, gallstones due to rapid weight loss, and pancreatitis should be carefully considered when using these medications.

37.8.4.4 SGLT-2i

SGLT-2 inhibitors are approved for the treatment of type 2 DM and are known to cause mild weight loss, as well as provide cardiac and renal protection [110]. A few small studies have shown that these agents may improve HS, but their impact on MASH histology has not been well studied or clearly established [111, 112].

37.8.4.5 Metformin and Ursodeoxycholic Acid (UDCA)

Metformin and UDCA have been extensively studied in the treatment of MASLD, but no significant improvement in liver histology was observed [113, 114]. Similarly, studies on polyunsaturated fatty acids and ezetimibe did not demonstrate any benefit in the management of MASLD.

37.8.4.6 Resmetirom

Resmetirom, a selective thyroid hormone receptor-β (THR-β) agonist, has emerged as a promising therapeutic agent in the management of Metabolic Associated Steatohepatitis (MASH). It functions by targeting the liver's THR-β, which plays a crucial role in regulating lipid metabolism, reducing HS, inflammation, and fibrosis—key pathological features of MASH. Clinical trials have demonstrated that resmetirom effectively decreases liver fat content, improves liver histology, and shows potential in reversing the progression of fibrosis [115]. These findings make resmetirom a valuable option for patients with MASH, particularly those who do not achieve sufficient results through lifestyle modifications alone. However, its utility in the post-LT setting remains to be fully explored, and further research is needed to determine its safety and efficacy in this specific patient population. The development and approval of resmetirom mark a significant advancement in the treatment of MASH, offering hope for improved outcomes in this challenging and increasingly prevalent liver disease [116].

37.9 Conclusion

MASLD has increasingly become the leading indication for LT in the United States and is rapidly rising in prevalence worldwide. Post-transplant recurrence and de novo occurrence of MASLD are becoming more common and present significant challenges. Current management strategies focus on addressing insulin resistance and the metabolic syndrome associated with MASLD in the post-LT period. However, further studies are needed to better understand the natural history and pathophysiology of post-LT MASLD and to develop specific treatment strategies for this growing problem.

References

1. Estes C, Razavi H, Loomba R, Younossi Z, Sanyal AJ. Modeling the epidemic of nonalcoholic fatty liver disease demonstrates an exponential increase in burden of disease. Hepatology. 2018;67(1):123–33.
2. Le P, Chaitoff A, Rothberg MB, McCullough A, Gupta NM, Alkhouri N. Population-based trends in prevalence of nonalcoholic fatty liver disease in US adults with type 2 diabetes. Clin Gastroenterol Hepatol. 2019;17(11):2377–8.
3. Younossi ZM, Koenig AB, Abdelatif D, Fazel Y, Henry L, Wymer M. Global epidemiology of nonalcoholic fatty liver disease-meta-analytic assessment of prevalence, incidence, and outcomes. Hepatology. 2016;64(1):73–84.
4. Henry L, Paik J, Younossi ZM. Review article: the epidemiologic burden of non-alcoholic fatty liver disease across the world. Aliment Pharmacol Ther. 2022;56(6):942–56.
5. Sayiner M, Koenig A, Henry L, Younossi ZM. Epidemiology of nonalcoholic fatty liver disease and nonalcoholic Steatohepatitis in the United States and the rest of the world. Clin Liver Dis. 2016;20(2):205–14.
6. Rinella ME, Neuschwander-Tetri BA, Siddiqui MS, Abdelmalek MF, Caldwell S, Barb D, et al. AASLD practice guidance on the clinical assessment and management of nonalcoholic fatty liver disease. Hepatology. 2023;77(5):1797–835.
7. Haddad EM, McAlister VC, Renouf E, Malthaner R, Kjaer MS, Gluud LL. Cyclosporin versus tacrolimus for liver transplanted patients. Cochrane Database Syst Rev. 2006;2006(4):CD005161.

8. Losurdo G, Castellaneta A, Rendina M, Carparelli S, Leandro G, Di Leo A. Systematic review with meta-analysis: de novo non-alcoholic fatty liver disease in liver-transplanted patients. Aliment Pharmacol Ther. 2018;47(6):704–14.
9. Saeed N, Glass L, Sharma P, Shannon C, Sonnenday CJ, Tincopa MA. Incidence and risks for nonalcoholic fatty liver disease and Steatohepatitis post-liver transplant: systematic review and meta-analysis. Transplantation. 2019;103(11):e345–e54.
10. Silva AC, Nogueira P, Machado MV. Hepatic steatosis after liver transplantation: a systematic review and meta-analysis. Liver Transpl. 2023;29(4):431–48.
11. Lazo M, Hernaez R, Eberhardt MS, Bonekamp S, Kamel I, Guallar E, et al. Prevalence of nonalcoholic fatty liver disease in the United States: the third National Health and nutrition examination survey, 1988–1994. Am J Epidemiol. 2013;178(1):38–45.
12. Rinella ME. Nonalcoholic fatty liver disease: a systematic review. JAMA. 2015;313(22):2263–73.
13. Williams CD, Stengel J, Asike MI, Torres DM, Shaw J, Contreras M, et al. Prevalence of nonalcoholic fatty liver disease and nonalcoholic steatohepatitis among a largely middle-aged population utilizing ultrasound and liver biopsy: a prospective study. Gastroenterology. 2011;140(1):124–31.
14. Altekruse SF, Henley SJ, Cucinelli JE, McGlynn KA. Changing hepatocellular carcinoma incidence and liver cancer mortality rates in the United States. Am J Gastroenterol. 2014;109(4):542–53.
15. Paik JM, Golabi P, Younossi Y, Mishra A, Younossi ZM. Changes in the global burden of chronic liver diseases from 2012 to 2017: the growing impact of NAFLD. Hepatology. 2020;72(5):1605–16.
16. Golabi P, Isakov V, Younossi ZM. Nonalcoholic fatty liver disease: disease burden and disease awareness. Clin Liver Dis. 2023;27(2):173–86.
17. Golabi P, Paik JM, AlQahtani S, Younossi Y, Tuncer G, Younossi ZM. Burden of non-alcoholic fatty liver disease in Asia, the Middle East and North Africa: data from global burden of disease 2009–2019. J Hepatol. 2021;75(4):795–809.
18. Noureddin M, Vipani A, Bresee C, Todo T, Kim IK, Alkhouri N, et al. NASH leading cause of liver transplant in women: updated analysis of indications for liver transplant and ethnic and gender variances. Am J Gastroenterol. 2018;113(11):1649–59.
19. Stepanova M, Kabbara K, Mohess D, Verma M, Roche-Green A, AlQahtani S, et al. Nonalcoholic steatohepatitis is the most common indication for liver transplantation among the elderly: data from the United States scientific registry of transplant recipients. Hepatol Commun. 2022;6(7):1506–15.
20. Wong RJ, Singal AK. Trends in liver disease etiology among adults awaiting liver transplantation in the United States, 2014–2019. JAMA Netw Open. 2020;3(2):e1920294.
21. Younossi ZM, Stepanova M, Ong J, Trimble G, AlQahtani S, Younossi I, et al. Nonalcoholic steatohepatitis is the most rapidly increasing indication for liver transplantation in the United States. Clin Gastroenterol Hepatol. 2021;19(3):580–9 e5.
22. Haldar D, Kern B, Hodson J, Armstrong MJ, Adam R, Berlakovich G, et al. Outcomes of liver transplantation for non-alcoholic steatohepatitis: a European Liver Transplant Registry study. J Hepatol. 2019;71(2):313–22.
23. Kahn CR, Wang G, Lee KY. Altered adipose tissue and adipocyte function in the pathogenesis of metabolic syndrome. J Clin Invest. 2019;129(10):3990–4000.
24. Donnelly KL, Smith CI, Schwarzenberg SJ, Jessurun J, Boldt MD, Parks EJ. Sources of fatty acids stored in liver and secreted via lipoproteins in patients with nonalcoholic fatty liver disease. J Clin Invest. 2005;115(5):1343–51.
25. Hardy T, Oakley F, Anstee QM, Day CP. Nonalcoholic fatty liver disease: pathogenesis and disease spectrum. Annu Rev Pathol. 2016;11:451–96.
26. Bril F, Barb D, Portillo-Sanchez P, Biernacki D, Lomonaco R, Suman A, et al. Metabolic and histological implications of intrahepatic triglyceride content in nonalcoholic fatty liver disease. Hepatology. 2017;65(4):1132–44.

27. Sanders FWB, Acharjee A, Walker C, Marney L, Roberts LD, Imamura F, et al. Hepatic steatosis risk is partly driven by increased de novo lipogenesis following carbohydrate consumption. Genome Biol. 2018;19(1):79.
28. Cusi K. Role of obesity and lipotoxicity in the development of nonalcoholic steatohepatitis: pathophysiology and clinical implications. Gastroenterology. 2012;142(4):711–25 e6.
29. Fabbrini E, Mohammed BS, Magkos F, Korenblat KM, Patterson BW, Klein S. Alterations in adipose tissue and hepatic lipid kinetics in obese men and women with nonalcoholic fatty liver disease. Gastroenterology. 2008;134(2):424–31.
30. Fujita K, Nozaki Y, Wada K, Yoneda M, Fujimoto Y, Fujitake M, et al. Dysfunctional very-low-density lipoprotein synthesis and release is a key factor in nonalcoholic steatohepatitis pathogenesis. Hepatology. 2009;50(3):772–80.
31. Fabbrini E, Sullivan S, Klein S. Obesity and nonalcoholic fatty liver disease: biochemical, metabolic, and clinical implications. Hepatology. 2010;51(2):679–89.
32. El Atrache MM, Abouljoud MS, Divine G, Yoshida A, Kim DY, Kazimi MM, et al. Recurrence of non-alcoholic steatohepatitis and cryptogenic cirrhosis following orthotopic liver transplantation in the context of the metabolic syndrome. Clin Transpl. 2012;26(5):E505–12.
33. Galvin Z, Rajakumar R, Chen E, Adeyi O, Selzner M, Grant D, et al. Predictors of de novo nonalcoholic fatty liver disease after liver transplantation and associated fibrosis. Liver Transpl. 2019;25(1):56–67.
34. Man K, Zhao Y, Xu A, Lo CM, Lam KS, Ng KT, et al. Fat-derived hormone adiponectin combined with FTY720 significantly improves small-for-size fatty liver graft survival. Am J Transplant. 2006;6(3):467–76.
35. Trevisani F, Caraceni P, Simoncini M, Micati M, Domenicali M, Dazzani F, et al. Evidence of oxidative imbalance in long-term liver transplant patients. Dig Liver Dis. 2002;34(4):279–84.
36. Angulo P, Alba LM, Petrovic LM, Adams LA, Lindor KD, Jensen MD. Leptin, insulin resistance, and liver fibrosis in human nonalcoholic fatty liver disease. J Hepatol. 2004;41(6):943–9.
37. Satapathy SK, Nair S, Vanatta JM. Nonalcoholic fatty liver disease following liver transplantation. Hepatol Int. 2013;7(2):400–12.
38. Asrih M, Jornayvaz FR. Metabolic syndrome and nonalcoholic fatty liver disease: is insulin resistance the link? Mol Cell Endocrinol. 2015;418(Pt 1):55–65.
39. Han MAT, Olivo R, Choi CJ, Pyrsopoulos N. De novo and recurrence of metabolic dysfunction-associated fatty liver disease after liver transplantation. World J Hepatol. 2021;13(12):1991–2004.
40. Cotter TG, Charlton M. Nonalcoholic steatohepatitis after liver transplantation. Liver Transpl. 2020;26(1):141–59.
41. Cotter TG, Rinella M. Nonalcoholic fatty liver disease 2020: the state of the disease. Gastroenterology. 2020;158(7):1851–64.
42. Wang Y, Liu Y, Zhang G, Zhang M, Zhu K, Wang Y, et al. Complete mitochondrial genome of Cladosporium zixishanense sp. nov. YFCC 8620 isolated from the spider in Yunnan, southwestern China. Mitochondrial DNA B Resour. 2019;5(1):210–1.
43. Longo M, Meroni M, Paolini E, Erconi V, Carli F, Fortunato F, et al. TM6SF2/PNPLA3/MBOAT7 loss-of-function genetic variants impact on NAFLD development and progression both in patients and in in vitro models. Cell Mol Gastroenterol Hepatol. 2022;13(3):759–88.
44. Luo F, Oldoni F, Das A. TM6SF2: a novel genetic player in nonalcoholic fatty liver and cardiovascular disease. Hepatol Commun. 2022;6(3):448–60.
45. Abul-Husn NS, Cheng X, Li AH, Xin Y, Schurmann C, Stevis P, et al. A protein-truncating HSD17B13 variant and protection from chronic liver disease. N Engl J Med. 2018;378(12):1096–106.
46. Rutledge SM, Soper ER, Ma N, Pejaver V, Friedman SL, Branch AD, et al. Association of HSD17B13 and PNPLA3 with liver enzymes and fibrosis in Hispanic/Latino individuals of diverse genetic ancestries. Clin Gastroenterol Hepatol. 2023;21:2578.

47. Dhar D, Baglieri J, Kisseleva T, Brenner DA. Mechanisms of liver fibrosis and its role in liver cancer. Exp Biol Med (Maywood). 2020;245(2):96–108.
48. Berumen J, Baglieri J, Kisseleva T, Mekeel K. Liver fibrosis: pathophysiology and clinical implications. WIREs Mech Dis. 2021;13(1):e1499.
49. Kisseleva T, Brenner D. Molecular and cellular mechanisms of liver fibrosis and its regression. Nat Rev Gastroenterol Hepatol. 2021;18(3):151–66.
50. Mikova I, Neroldova M, Hubacek JA, Dlouha D, Jirsa M, Honsova E, et al. Donor PNPLA3 and TM6SF2 variant alleles confer additive risks for graft steatosis after liver transplantation. Transplantation. 2020;104(3):526–34.
51. Satapathy SK, Tran QT, Kovalic AJ, Bontha SV, Jiang Y, Kedia S, et al. Clinical and genetic risk factors of recurrent nonalcoholic fatty liver disease after liver transplantation. Clin Transl Gastroenterol. 2021;12(2):e00302.
52. John BV, Aiken T, Garber A, Thomas D, Lopez R, Patil D, et al. Recipient but not donor adiponectin polymorphisms are associated with early posttransplant hepatic steatosis in patients transplanted for non-nonalcoholic fatty liver disease indications. Exp Clin Transplant. 2018;16(4):439–45.
53. Andrade A, Cotrim HP, Bittencourt PL, Almeida CG, Sorte N. Nonalcoholic steatohepatitis in posttransplantation liver: review article. Rev Assoc Med Bras (1992). 2018;64(2):187–94.
54. Hejlova I, Honsova E, Sticova E, Lanska V, Hucl T, Spicak J, et al. Prevalence and risk factors of steatosis after liver transplantation and patient outcomes. Liver Transpl. 2016;22(5):644–55.
55. Dobrindt EM, Allex L, Saipbaev A, Ollinger R, Schoning W, Pratschke J, et al. Association between obesity after liver transplantation and steatosis, inflammation, and fibrosis of the graft. Clin Transpl. 2020;34(12):e14093.
56. Kim WR, Poterucha JJ, Porayko MK, Dickson ER, Steers JL, Wiesner RH. Recurrence of nonalcoholic steatohepatitis following liver transplantation. Transplantation. 1996;62(12):1802–5.
57. Bhagat V, Mindikoglu AL, Nudo CG, Schiff ER, Tzakis A, Regev A. Outcomes of liver transplantation in patients with cirrhosis due to nonalcoholic steatohepatitis versus patients with cirrhosis due to alcoholic liver disease. Liver Transpl. 2009;15(12):1814–20.
58. Malik SM, Devera ME, Fontes P, Shaikh O, Sasatomi E, Ahmad J. Recurrent disease following liver transplantation for nonalcoholic steatohepatitis cirrhosis. Liver Transpl. 2009;15(12):1843–51.
59. Malik SM, deVera ME, Fontes P, Shaikh O, Ahmad J. Outcome after liver transplantation for NASH cirrhosis. Am J Transplant. 2009;9(4):782–93.
60. Miyaaki H, Miuma S, Taura N, Shibata H, Sasaki R, Soyama A, et al. Risk factors and clinical course for liver steatosis or nonalcoholic steatohepatitis after living donor liver transplantation. Transplantation. 2019;103(1):109–12.
61. Kakar S, Dugum M, Cabello R, Humar A, Ahmad J, Malik SM. Incidence of recurrent NASH-related allograft cirrhosis. Dig Dis Sci. 2019;64(5):1356–63.
62. Charlton MR, Burns JM, Pedersen RA, Watt KD, Heimbach JK, Dierkhising RA. Frequency and outcomes of liver transplantation for nonalcoholic steatohepatitis in the United States. Gastroenterology. 2011;141(4):1249–53.
63. Vallin M, Guillaud O, Boillot O, Hervieu V, Scoazec JY, Dumortier J. Recurrent or de novo nonalcoholic fatty liver disease after liver transplantation: natural history based on liver biopsy analysis. Liver Transpl. 2014;20(9):1064–71.
64. Farkas SA, Schnitzbauer AA, Kirchner G, Obed A, Banas B, Schlitt HJ. Calcineurin inhibitor minimization protocols in liver transplantation. Transpl Int. 2009;22(1):49–60.
65. Watt KD. Metabolic syndrome: is immunosuppression to blame? Liver Transpl. 2011;17(Suppl 3):S38–42.
66. Becchetti C, Ferrarese A, Zeni N, Russo FP, Senzolo M, Gambato M, et al. A prospective longitudinal assessment of de novo metabolic syndrome after liver transplantation. Clin Transpl. 2022;36(2):e14532.

67. Charlton M, Rinella M, Patel D, McCague K, Heimbach J, Watt K. Everolimus is associated with less weight gain than tacrolimus 2 years after liver transplantation: results of a randomized multicenter study. Transplantation. 2017;101(12):2873–82.
68. Shalaby S, Battistella S, Zanetto A, Bizzaro D, Germani G, Paolo Russo F, et al. Changings and challenges in liver transplantation for nonalcoholic fatty liver disease/steatohepatitis. Clin Liver Dis. 2023;27(2):225–37.
69. Zhang QY, Zhang QF, Zhang DZ. The impact of steatosis on the outcome of liver transplantation: a meta-analysis. Biomed Res Int. 2019;2019:3962785.
70. Hartog H, Hann A, Perera M. Primary nonfunction of the liver allograft. Transplantation. 2022;106(1):117–28.
71. Spitzer AL, Lao OB, Dick AA, Bakthavatsalam R, Halldorson JB, Yeh MM, et al. The biopsied donor liver: incorporating macrosteatosis into high-risk donor assessment. Liver Transpl. 2010;16(7):874–84.
72. Chu MJ, Dare AJ, Phillips AR, Bartlett AS. Donor hepatic steatosis and outcome after liver transplantation: a systematic review. J Gastrointest Surg. 2015;19(9):1713–24.
73. Patel YA, Berg CL, Moylan CA. Nonalcoholic fatty liver disease: key considerations before and after liver transplantation. Dig Dis Sci. 2016;61(5):1406–16.
74. Mikolasevic I, Milic S, Filipec-Kanizaj T. Fatty liver allografts are associated with primary graft non-function and high mortality after transplantation. Liver Int. 2017;37(8):1113–5.
75. Andert A, Ulmer TF, Schoning W, Kroy D, Hein M, Alizai PH, et al. Grade of donor liver microvesicular steatosis does not affect the postoperative outcome after liver transplantation. Hepatobiliary Pancreat Dis Int. 2017;16(6):617–23.
76. Croome KP, Lee DD, Croome S, Chadha R, Livingston D, Abader P, et al. The impact of postreperfusion syndrome during liver transplantation using livers with significant macrosteatosis. Am J Transplant. 2019;19(9):2550–9.
77. Croome KP, Lee DD, Croome S, Nakhleh RE, Abader Sedki Senada P, Livingston D, et al. Does donor allograft microsteatosis matter? Comparison of outcomes in liver transplantation with a propensity-matched cohort. Liver Transpl. 2019;25(10):1533–40.
78. Mikolasevic I, Filipec-Kanizaj T, Mijic M, Jakopcic I, Milic S, Hrstic I, et al. Nonalcoholic fatty liver disease and liver transplantation – where do we stand? World J Gastroenterol. 2018;24(14):1491–506.
79. Yong JN, Lim WH, Ng CH, Tan DJH, Xiao J, Tay PWL, et al. Outcomes of nonalcoholic steatohepatitis after liver transplantation: an updated meta-analysis and systematic review. Clin Gastroenterol Hepatol. 2023;21(1):45–54 e6.
80. Afzali A, Berry K, Ioannou GN. Excellent posttransplant survival for patients with nonalcoholic steatohepatitis in the United States. Liver Transpl. 2012;18(1):29–37.
81. Rinella ME, Satapathy SK, Brandman D, Smith C, Elwir S, Xia J, et al. Factors impacting survival in those transplanted for NASH cirrhosis: data from the NailNASH Consortium. Clin Gastroenterol Hepatol. 2023;21(2):445–55 e2.
82. Vilar-Gomez E, Martinez-Perez Y, Calzadilla-Bertot L, Torres-Gonzalez A, Gra-Oramas B, Gonzalez-Fabian L, et al. Weight loss through lifestyle modification significantly reduces features of nonalcoholic steatohepatitis. Gastroenterology. 2015;149(2):367–78 e5; quiz e14–5.
83. Koutoukidis DA, Astbury NM, Tudor KE, Morris E, Henry JA, Noreik M, et al. Association of Weight Loss Interventions with changes in biomarkers of nonalcoholic fatty liver disease: a systematic review and meta-analysis. JAMA Intern Med. 2019;179(9):1262–71.
84. Lowe MR, Miller-Kovach K, Phelan S. Weight-loss maintenance in overweight individuals one to five years following successful completion of a commercial weight loss program. Int J Obes Relat Metab Disord. 2001;25(3):325–31.
85. Thoma C, Day CP, Trenell MI. Lifestyle interventions for the treatment of non-alcoholic fatty liver disease in adults: a systematic review. J Hepatol. 2012;56(1):255–66.
86. Postrach E, Aspalter R, Elbelt U, Koller M, Longin R, Schulzke JD, et al. Determinants of successful weight loss after using a commercial web-based weight reduction program for six months: cohort study. J Med Internet Res. 2013;15(10):e219.

87. Stewart KE, Haller DL, Sargeant C, Levenson JL, Puri P, Sanyal AJ. Readiness for behaviour change in non-alcoholic fatty liver disease: implications for multidisciplinary care models. Liver Int. 2015;35(3):936–43.
88. Malespin MH, Barritt AS, Watkins SE, Schoen C, Tincopa MA, Corbin KD, et al. Weight loss and weight regain in usual clinical practice: results from the TARGET-NASH observational cohort. Clin Gastroenterol Hepatol. 2022;20(10):2393–5 e4.
89. Kawaguchi T, Charlton M, Kawaguchi A, Yamamura S, Nakano D, Tsutsumi T, et al. Effects of Mediterranean diet in patients with nonalcoholic fatty liver disease: a systematic review, meta-analysis, and meta-regression analysis of randomized controlled trials. Semin Liver Dis. 2021;41(3):225–34.
90. Kouvari M, Boutari C, Chrysohoou C, Fragkopoulou E, Antonopoulou S, Tousoulis D, et al. Mediterranean diet is inversely associated with steatosis and fibrosis and decreases ten-year diabetes and cardiovascular risk in NAFLD subjects: results from the ATTICA prospective cohort study. Clin Nutr. 2021;40(5):3314–24.
91. George ES, Reddy A, Nicoll AJ, Ryan MC, Itsiopoulos C, Abbott G, et al. Impact of a Mediterranean diet on hepatic and metabolic outcomes in non-alcoholic fatty liver disease: the MEDINA randomised controlled trial. Liver Int. 2022;42(6):1308–22.
92. Chen YP, Lu FB, Hu YB, Xu LM, Zheng MH, Hu ED. A systematic review and a dose-response meta-analysis of coffee dose and nonalcoholic fatty liver disease. Clin Nutr. 2019;38(6):2552–7.
93. Johnson NA, Sachinwalla T, Walton DW, Smith K, Armstrong A, Thompson MW, et al. Aerobic exercise training reduces hepatic and visceral lipids in obese individuals without weight loss. Hepatology. 2009;50(4):1105–12.
94. Kistler KD, Brunt EM, Clark JM, Diehl AM, Sallis JF, Schwimmer JB, et al. Physical activity recommendations, exercise intensity, and histological severity of nonalcoholic fatty liver disease. Am J Gastroenterol. 2011;106(3):460–8; quiz 9.
95. Mechanick JI, Apovian C, Brethauer S, Garvey WT, Joffe AM, Kim J, et al. Clinical practice guidelines for the perioperative nutrition, metabolic, and nonsurgical support of patients undergoing bariatric procedures – 2019 update: cosponsored by American Association of Clinical Endocrinologists/American College of Endocrinology, the Obesity Society, American Society for Metabolic & Bariatric Surgery, Obesity Medicine Association, and American Society of Anesthesiologists. Surg Obes Relat Dis. 2020;16(2):175–247.
96. Wiggins T, Guidozzi N, Welbourn R, Ahmed AR, Markar SR. Association of bariatric surgery with all-cause mortality and incidence of obesity-related disease at a population level: a systematic review and meta-analysis. PLoS Med. 2020;17(7):e1003206.
97. Mazzini GS, Augustin T, Noria S, Romero-Marrero C, Li N, Hameed B, et al. ASMBS position statement on the impact of metabolic and bariatric surgery on nonalcoholic steatohepatitis. Surg Obes Relat Dis. 2022;18(3):314–25.
98. Zamora-Valdes D, Watt KD, Kellogg TA, Poterucha JJ, Di Cecco SR, Francisco-Ziller NM, et al. Long-term outcomes of patients undergoing simultaneous liver transplantation and sleeve gastrectomy. Hepatology. 2018;68(2):485–95.
99. Tsamalaidze L, Stauffer JA, Arasi LC, Villacreses DE, Franco JSS, Bowers S, et al. Laparoscopic sleeve gastrectomy for morbid obesity in patients after orthotopic liver transplant: a matched case-control study. Obes Surg. 2018;28(2):444–50.
100. Ayloo S, Guss C, Pentakota SR, Hanna J, Molinari M. Minimally invasive sleeve gastrectomy as a surgical treatment for nonalcoholic fatty liver disease in liver transplant recipients. Transplant Proc. 2020;52(1):276–83.
101. Sanyal AJ, Chalasani N, Kowdley KV, McCullough A, Diehl AM, Bass NM, et al. Pioglitazone, vitamin E, or placebo for nonalcoholic steatohepatitis. N Engl J Med. 2010;362(18):1675–85.
102. Sato K, Gosho M, Yamamoto T, Kobayashi Y, Ishii N, Ohashi T, et al. Vitamin E has a beneficial effect on nonalcoholic fatty liver disease: a meta-analysis of randomized controlled trials. Nutrition. 2015;31(7–8):923–30.

103. Vilar-Gomez E, Vuppalanchi R, Gawrieh S, Ghabril M, Saxena R, Cummings OW, et al. Vitamin E improves transplant-free survival and hepatic decompensation among patients with nonalcoholic steatohepatitis and advanced fibrosis. Hepatology. 2020;71(2):495–509.
104. Neuhouser ML, Barnett MJ, Kristal AR, Ambrosone CB, King IB, Thornquist M, et al. Dietary supplement use and prostate cancer risk in the Carotene and Retinol Efficacy Trial. Cancer Epidemiol Biomarkers Prev. 2009;18(8):2202–6.
105. Cusi K, Orsak B, Bril F, Lomonaco R, Hecht J, Ortiz-Lopez C, et al. Long-term pioglitazone treatment for patients with nonalcoholic steatohepatitis and prediabetes or type 2 diabetes mellitus: a randomized trial. Ann Intern Med. 2016;165(5):305–15.
106. Viscoli CM, Inzucchi SE, Young LH, Insogna KL, Conwit R, Furie KL, et al. Pioglitazone and risk for bone fracture: safety data from a randomized clinical trial. J Clin Endocrinol Metab. 2017;102(3):914–22.
107. Armstrong MJ, Gaunt P, Aithal GP, Barton D, Hull D, Parker R, et al. Liraglutide safety and efficacy in patients with non-alcoholic steatohepatitis (LEAN): a multicentre, double-blind, randomised, placebo-controlled phase 2 study. Lancet. 2016;387(10019):679–90.
108. Newsome PN, Buchholtz K, Cusi K, Linder M, Okanoue T, Ratziu V, et al. A placebo-controlled trial of subcutaneous semaglutide in nonalcoholic steatohepatitis. N Engl J Med. 2021;384(12):1113–24.
109. Jastreboff AM, Aronne LJ, Ahmad NN, Wharton S, Connery L, Alves B, et al. Tirzepatide once weekly for the treatment of obesity. N Engl J Med. 2022;387(3):205–16.
110. Tahrani AA, Barnett AH, Bailey CJ. SGLT inhibitors in management of diabetes. Lancet Diabetes Endocrinol. 2013;1(2):140–51.
111. Cusi K. Time to include nonalcoholic steatohepatitis in the management of patients with Type 2 diabetes. Diabetes Care. 2020;43(2):275–9.
112. Cusi K. A diabetologist's perspective of non-alcoholic steatohepatitis (NASH): knowledge gaps and future directions. Liver Int. 2020;40(Suppl 1):82–8.
113. Dufour JF, Oneta CM, Gonvers JJ, Bihl F, Cerny A, Cereda JM, et al. Randomized placebo-controlled trial of ursodeoxycholic acid with vitamin e in nonalcoholic steatohepatitis. Clin Gastroenterol Hepatol. 2006;4(12):1537–43.
114. Loomba R, Lutchman G, Kleiner DE, Ricks M, Feld JJ, Borg BB, et al. Clinical trial: pilot study of metformin for the treatment of non-alcoholic steatohepatitis. Aliment Pharmacol Ther. 2009;29(2):172–82.
115. Harrison SA, Bashir MR, Guy CD, Zhou R, Moylan CA, Frias JP, Alkhouri N, Bansal MB, Baum S, Neuschwander-Tetri BA, Taub R, Moussa SE. Resmetirom (MGL-3196) for the treatment of non-alcoholic steatohepatitis: a multicentre, randomised, double-blind, placebo-controlled, phase 2 trial. Lancet. 2019;394(10213):2012–24.
116. Friedman SL, Neuschwander-Tetri BA, Rinella M, Sanyal AJ. Mechanisms of NAFLD development and therapeutic strategies. Nat Med. 2018;24(7):908–22.

Chapter 38
Long-Term Complications of Immunosuppression

Rohit Mehtani, Jaya Agarwal, and Sanjiv Saigal

Abstract With the advent of effective immunosuppression, short-term outcomes after liver transplant (LT) have improved drastically, while long-term outcomes remain static at around 75% at 5 years. This is predominantly linked to complications related to immunosuppressive drugs, which could be drug-specific, class-specific, or generic. The backbone of immunosuppression post-LT, calcineurin inhibitors (cyclosporine and tacrolimus) are associated with most of the complications, including renal dysfunction, post-transplant diabetes mellitus (PTDM), and metabolic syndrome (MS). Development of diabetes, osteoporosis, and metabolic syndrome post-LT has been linked to the cumulative steroid dose. Infections post-LT and de novo malignancies (DNMs) are linked to the overall cumulative immunosuppression. These complications increase the healthcare costs, long-term morbidity and mortality, and hamper the quality of life of LT recipients. Thus, it is imperative that transplant physicians are made aware of the long-term risks of immunosuppression and strategies to mitigate these complications by keeping the immunosuppression at the lowest level while simultaneously preventing allograft rejection. This chapter provides clinicians with an updated, comprehensive review of the long-term complications of immunosuppression post-LT, associated risk factors, and ways to minimize these complications.

R. Mehtani
Department of Hepatology, Amrita School of Medicine, Amrita Vishwa Vidyapeetham, Faridabad, Haryana, India

J. Agarwal
Department of HPB Surgery and Solid Organ Transplant, Amrita School of Medicine, Amrita Vishwa Vidyapeetham, Faridabad, Haryana, India

S. Saigal (✉)
Hepatology and Liver Transplant Medicine, Max Institute of Liver and Gastrointestinal Sciences, Max Super Speciality Hospital, Saket, New Delhi, India
e-mail: sanjivsaigal@hotmail.com

S. Saigal, D. Jothimani (eds.), *Fundamentals of Transplant Hepatology*,
https://doi.org/10.1007/978-981-95-2624-6_38

Keywords Immunosuppression minimization · Post-transplant diabetes mellitus · De novo malignancies · Liver transplantation · Metabolic syndrome · MASLD · Fatty liver

Abbreviations

ACE	Angiotensin converting enzyme
AKI	Acute kidney injury
ARBs	Angiotensin receptor blockers
ATP	Adult treatment panel
BMI	Body mass index
BP	Blood pressure
CKD	Chronic kidney disease
CMV	Cytomegalovirus
CNIs	Calcineurin inhibitors
CT	Computed tomography
DEXA	Dual-energy X-ray absorptiometry
DM	Diabetes mellitus
DNA	Deoxyribonucleic acid
DNMs	De novo malignancies
EBV	Epstein-barr virus
GFR	Glomerular filtration rate
GLP-1	Glucagon-like peptide 1
HCC	Hepatocellular carcinoma
HRS	Hepatorenal syndrome
IBD	Inflammatory bowel diseases
IL2	Interleukin 2
ILTS	International liver transplant society
LDL	Low-density lipoprotein
LT	Liver Transplant
MASH	Metabolic dysfunction associated steatohepatitis
MASLD	Metabolic dysfunction associated steatotic liver
MDR	Multi-drug resistant
MELD	Model for end-stage liver disease
MMF	Mycophenolate mofetil
MS	Metabolic syndrome
mTOR	mammalian target of rapamycin
NAFLD	Non-alcoholic fatty liver disease
NASH	Non-alcoholic steatohepatitis

NODAT	New-onset diabetes after transplant
OGTT	Oral glucose tolerance test
PSC	Primary sclerosing cholangitis
PTDM	Post-transplant diabetes mellitus
PTLD	Post-transplant lymphoproliferative disorder
RRT	Renal replacement therapy
SGLT-2	Sodium-glucose co-transporter 2
UNOS	United Network for Organ Sharing

Key Highlights

- Long-term survival of liver transplant recipients has improved significantly with the availability of CNI-based immunosuppressive medication.
- Long-term management of liver transplant recipients should focus on addressing metabolic risk factors and immunosuppression-related complications.
- Chronic kidney disease may occur in up to one-third of patients following liver transplantation over a 10-year period.
- Denovo and recurrent NASH/MASH occur in a significantly higher proportion of recipients due to the increased prevalence of one or more components of metabolic syndrome in the post-transplant period.
- Over 30% liver transplant recipients may develop diabetes mellitus, 50% may develop dyslipidemia, 30% may develop obesity, and 70% can develop hypertension.
- Improvement in long-term survival post-liver transplant has led to an increase in the risk of de novo malignancies, necessitating a need for rigorous surveillance and cancer screening protocols in these patients.

38.1 Introduction

Improvements in critical care, better recipient and donor selection, refined surgical techniques, and optimized immunosuppressive protocols have collectively enhanced outcomes following liver transplantation (LT). Despite these advances, medical or non-surgical complications remain the leading causes of morbidity and mortality

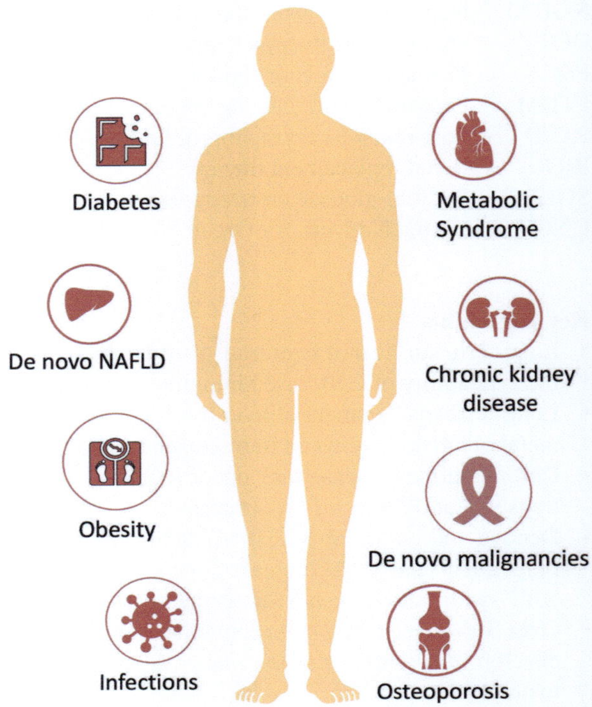

Fig. 38.1 Long-term complications of immunosuppression in the liver transplant recipient (NAFLD non-alcoholic fatty liver disease)

beyond the first year post-transplant [1]. Many of these complications stem from the long-term use of immunosuppressive drugs, which may result in:

- General adverse effects (e.g., infections and cancer),
- Class-specific effects (e.g., kidney injury from calcineurin inhibitors),
- Or drug-specific toxicities [2].

Since most LT recipients require lifelong immunosuppression, the goal is to maintain the lowest effective dose to prevent rejection while minimizing side effects [3]. This chapter provides a comprehensive overview of long-term complications associated with immunosuppression post-LT, and offers practical guidance for minimizing these risks (see Fig. 38.1).

38.2 Renal Dysfunction After Liver Transplantation

38.2.1 *Burden of Disease*

Renal impairment is frequently observed in patients who survive beyond 6 months post-LT [4, 5]. Data from the Scientific Registry of Transplant Recipients (SRTR) show that the 5-year cumulative incidence of chronic kidney disease (CKD) following LT is around 18%—a rate higher than that seen in heart or lung transplant recipients [4].

A 25-year follow-up study from the Mayo Clinic, involving over 1200 LT recipients, revealed:

- 9% of patients eventually required kidney transplantation.
- 21% had a GFR < 60 mL/min/1.73 m^2, and 18% had a GFR < 30 mL/min/1.73 m^2.
- Only 18% of LT recipients maintained normal renal function, compared to 39% in age-matched controls [6].

Recipients of deceased donor liver transplants (DDLT) were 2.5 times more likely to develop CKD than those who underwent living donor liver transplantation (LDLT) [7]. CKD is associated with reduced graft and patient survival [6, 8], and annually, 2–5% of patients progress to end-stage renal disease (ESRD), requiring renal replacement therapy (RRT) [9].

38.2.2 *Risk Factors and Preventive Strategies*

Regular monitoring of kidney function post-LT is crucial. This includes:

- Estimating or calculating GFR, and
- Evaluating for proteinuria at least once per year [10].

Preventive measures are best understood by dividing them into three phases:

1. Pre-transplant:
    - Hepatorenal syndrome (HRS) is a key risk factor. Early treatment with albumin and terlipressin can lower the risk of CKD and RRT post-LT [12].
    - Non-alcoholic steatohepatitis (NASH), now renamed as metabolic dysfunction associated steatohepatitis (MASH) as an LT indication is also linked to higher post-transplant CKD risk [13–15].
2. Perioperative:
    - Risk factors include hemodynamic instability, ischemia-reperfusion injury, and nephrotoxic medications [11].

3. Post-transplant:

   - The primary cause of renal dysfunction is calcineurin inhibitor (CNI)-induced nephrotoxicity, compounded by diabetes and hypertension [11, 16].

38.2.3 CNI Nephrotoxicity

CNI-associated kidney damage can be categorized into:

- Early (within 1 year):

Caused mainly by vasoconstriction of renal arterioles, this is functional and potentially reversible with dose reduction [9, 17].

Use of anti-thymocyte globulin (ATG) induction, CNI minimization, and maintaining stable liver graft function helps reduce early renal injury [18].

Serum creatinine at 4 weeks post-LT is predictive of CKD risk over 5 years [19]. However, the need for RRT in the immediate post-op period does not necessarily predict long-term kidney damage, underscoring the importance of early AKI management [18].

- Late (>1 year):
  - Primarily structural damage due to chronic tubulointerstitial fibrosis, often worsened by post-transplant metabolic syndrome (MS) [20].

38.2.4 Strategies to Preserve Renal Function

- CNI-sparing regimens are key to preventing renal damage:
  - In patients with pre-existing renal dysfunction, delaying CNI initiation using induction agents like IL-2 receptor blockers (e.g., basiliximab, daclizumab) leads to improved renal outcomes [5, 21, 22].
  - Belatacept is not routinely used due to an observed increase in mortality [23].
- Mycophenolate mofetil (MMF):
  - When introduced early, MMF allows for lower CNI dosing without compromising graft function [24].
  - Early MMF initiation prevents post-op GFR decline [25].
- Everolimus, an mTOR inhibitor:
  - Provides renal protection for up to 5 years post-transplant [26–29].
  - Must be introduced after 4 weeks due to risk of hepatic artery thrombosis and impaired wound healing [27, 28].

- As monotherapy, it improves GFR but has higher risks of infection, hyperlipidemia, leukopenia, and treatment discontinuation [27].
- Sirolimus, another mTOR inhibitor, is no longer favored due to higher rates of rejection, sepsis, and mortality [30, 31].

• Timing Matters:

- Late introduction (after 1 year) of MMF or everolimus offers limited benefit, as damage is more structural [32].
- However, if MMF is introduced later along with a >50% CNI dose reduction, GFR can improve without compromising graft function [33–36].
- Complete CNI withdrawal increases the risk of rejection and offers minimal renal benefit and is not recommended [36, 37].

• Current Best Practice:

- Early MMF initiation (immediately post-LT), and/or
- Everolimus introduction after 4 weeks in high-risk patients.

These approaches offer optimal renal protection [38].

• In cases where end-stage renal disease develops despite these strategies, renal transplantation should be considered, as it provides better survival outcomes compared to long-term RRT [39–41].

38.3 Metabolic Syndrome (MS) Post-LT

Metabolic syndrome has been defined by the Adult Treatment Panel III (ATP III) [42] as "a combination of any 3 out of 5 of the following—hypertension (BP ≥ 130/85 mm Hg or taking antihypertensives), obesity (abdominal waist circumference > 102 cm for men and 90 cm for women), diabetes mellitus (fasting blood glucose > 100 mg/dL or on treatment), raised triglycerides (≥150 mg/dL), and low HDL (<40 mg/dL for men and <50 mg/dL for women)." MS occurs in about 40–60% of patients after LT when diagnosed as per the ATPIII criteria. Its incidence post-LT is rising as the number of transplants for NASH-related cirrhosis is increasing [43, 44]. Those who develop MS are at a higher risk of cardiovascular events but without an increase in all-cause mortality [45].

38.3.1 Obesity

Obesity is becoming rampant in patients with cirrhosis awaiting LT. In the United States, the numbers have reached more than 30% [46]. There is conflicting data regarding the effect of obesity on post-LT mortality. While some studies report an increased post-transplant mortality in obese patients [47, 48], the United Network for Organ Sharing (UNOS) database highlights the presence of an obesity paradox. A better post-LT survival was noted in overweight and class I obese patients than in patients with a normal BMI [49]. Most recipients have a rapid weight gain of up to 5 kg in the first year after LT and 10 kg over the next 3 years [50]. Multiple factors are involved in the increase in weight after LT, with reversal of the catabolic state and corticosteroid use having a major contribution. The incidence of post-LT obesity is also increased in elderly recipients ≥50 years and those who were obese before transplant [50, 51].

Although adherence is poor, lifestyle interventions, including dietary modifications and exercise, are the stepping stones for prevention and management of post-LT obesity [52]. A randomized controlled trial comparing the combination of exercise and dietary counselling with standard of care led to increased effort tolerance in the combination group, without an appreciable difference in post-LT weight [52]. There is limited evidence regarding the use of anti-obesity drugs after LT due to concerns of significant drug interactions. Orlistat for 6 months led to a decrease in waist circumference post-LT, but about 50% needed modification of the tacrolimus dose [53]. Semaglutide, a glucagon-like peptide 1 (GLP-1) analogue, has emerged as a panacea for weight loss [54] and is increasingly being considered for use in NASH [55]. However, it has not been used in the post-LT period. Lack of any major interactions with immunosuppressive medications makes it an ideal candidate for further studies. Patients with severe obesity (Class II with comorbidities or Class III) are ideal candidates for bariatric surgery [56]; however, the timing of surgery in LT recipients is a topic of debate [57]. The preferred approach is laparoscopic sleeve gastrectomy, as it does not affect absorption of immunosuppressive drugs and preserves access to the biliary tree in case postoperative biliary interventions are warranted [58]. Pre-LT bariatric surgery has been performed in patients with a low MELD score but was shown to have a mortality rate of about 16% [59]. The first report of pre-LT bariatric surgery from India comes from 2013. The recipient first underwent a sleeve gastrectomy, which allowed weight loss from 160 kg to 102 kg over 6 months, and subsequently underwent live donor LT [60]. Sleeve gastrectomy was also associated with good weight loss in a cohort of patients with CTP-A cirrhosis and portal hypertension, without any major complications [61]. Patients with a high MELD score and severe obesity can safely undergo bariatric surgery at the time of LT [62]. This strategy offers multiple advantages, like single anesthesia exposure, increased post-LT weight loss, lower insulin resistance, and a reduced antihypertensive drug requirement post-LT [63]. Endoscopic placement of an intragastric balloon in obese patients awaiting LT has also helped in achieving adequate weight loss, making LDLT safe and possible [64]. Bariatric surgery post-transplant has good outcomes [65]; however, it is technically difficult and associated with increased postoperative mortality and even the occasional need for a redo surgery [66].

Table 38.1 Risk factors for post-transplant diabetes mellitus (PTDM)

General factors	Transplant specific factors	Donor factors
Old age	High cumulative dose of steroids	Elderly donor (>60 years)
Males	Tacrolimus use (more than cyclosporine) in high dose	Fatty grafts
Overweight and obesity	Infection with CMV	Cadaveric graft
Family history of diabetes	Chronic hepatitis C	Long cold ischemia time (>9 hours)
Impaired fasting glucose before transplant	Prolonged ICU stay post-LT (>15 days)	
	Increased blood sugars first 4 weeks after LT	

CMV Cytomegalovirus, *ICU* intensive care unit, *LT* liver transplant

38.3.2 Post-Transplant Diabetes Mellitus (PTDM)

Post-transplant diabetes mellitus (PTDM) affects approximately 30% of liver transplant (LT) recipients [67]. Previously referred to as new-onset diabetes after transplant (NODAT), the term has been updated to PTDM following a recent consensus [67].

PTDM is diagnosed at least 45 days after liver transplantation [68] using one or more of the following criteria:

- Fasting blood glucose ≥126 mg/dL on at least two occasions,
- Random blood glucose >200 mg/dL with classic symptoms,
- 2-hour glucose >200 mg/dL following an oral glucose tolerance test (OGTT), HbA1C > 6.5% [67, 68].

38.3.2.1 Risk Factors

The development of PTDM may result from recipient-specific factors or general risk factors common to the broader population [51, 69, 70]—summarized in Table 38.1.

Both pre-existing donor diabetes and recipient diabetes prior to transplant are independently associated with worse graft and patient outcomes post-LT [71]. PTDM is also linked to:

- Postoperative renal dysfunction [72]
- Bacterial infections [72]
- Late-onset hepatic artery thrombosis [73]
- Increased risk of acute or chronic graft rejection [73, 74]

38.3.2.2 Management of PTDM

Management strategies are largely aligned with general diabetes care but must be personalized due to the complexity of transplant patients. Over one-third of LT recipients experience poor glycemic control, necessitating a tailored approach [75].

Monitoring & Targets:

- HbA1C testing is recommended at 3–6 months, again at 12 months, and then annually [76].
- Target HbA1C should be maintained at <7%.
- Annual screening for proteinuria and retinopathy is advised [76].

Treatment Strategy:

Management should follow a stepwise approach:

1. Lifestyle modifications (diet and exercise) for all patients,
2. Oral hypoglycemic agents, and
3. Insulin therapy if needed.

Immunosuppressive adjustments are crucial:

- Minimization of calcineurin inhibitors (CNIs),
- Tapering or stopping steroids, ideally by 3 months post-LT [68].

38.3.2.3 Pharmacologic Options

- Metformin:
  First-line agent; promotes weight loss, offers cardiovascular benefits, and is generally safe post-LT [77].
- Sulfonylureas:
  Effective but metabolized in the liver, posing potential for drug interactions with immunosuppressants.
- Thiazolidinediones (e.g., pioglitazone):
  Considered safe after LT and may help improve hepatic steatosis [77].
- DPP-4 Inhibitors (e.g., linagliptin, sitagliptin) and
  GLP-1 Receptor Agonists (e.g., semaglutide, liraglutide):
  These are well-tolerated in post-LT patients and generally do not cause significant drug interactions. However, they may delay gastric emptying, potentially affecting the absorption of other medications.
- SGLT-2 Inhibitors (e.g., dapagliflozin, empagliflozin):
  These drugs offer cardiovascular and renal benefits but are not routinely used post-LT due to concerns over fungal urinary tract infections [76].
  However, positive safety data from kidney transplant recipients [78–81] suggest potential for future use in LT populations.

38.3.3 Dyslipidemia

About one-half of LT recipients develop hyperlipidemia [82], which is a risk factor for increased cardiovascular morbidity and mortality [83]. Development of dyslipidemia post-LT is often related to CNI [84] and mTOR inhibitor [76] use. Among the CNIs, cyclosporine has a more atherogenic profile than tacrolimus. Cyclosporine inhibits hepatic bile acid 26-hydroxylase, leading to impaired bile acid synthesis from cholesterol. This, in turn, decreases the transport of cholesterol into bile [84]. Additionally, it binds to low-density lipoprotein (LDL) cholesterol receptor increasing the blood levels of LDL [84].

Similar to HBA1C monitoring, the ILTS recommends monitoring of fasting lipid profile 3–6 months after LT, followed by once at 1 year and then annually [76]. Treatment of dyslipidemia in the general population is guided by various cardiovascular risk assessment scores [85] available online; however, these lack validation in LT recipients. All LT recipients with persistent dyslipidemia despite adequate lifestyle measures need pharmacotherapy. The goals of treatment should be LDL cholesterol levels less than 100 mg/dL and triglyceride levels below 250 mg/dL [76]. Despite their metabolism by cytochrome P450, statins are safe post-LT, and they are considered the first-line drugs for dyslipidemia management. However, there is concern for drug interactions with CNIs. Hence, CNI drug monitoring should be done more frequently in patients on statins. A hydrophilic statin such as pravastatin or fluvastatin is preferred as the first choice. Low doses of lipophilic statins such as simvastatin 20 mg/day or atorvastatin 10 mg/day may also be initiated with gradual titration of dose based on response [39, 82]. Add-on therapy with ezetimibe is recommended if LDL cholesterol does not reach target levels with statins alone [86]. Patients with persistently high LDL cholesterol should be switched to tacrolimus from cyclosporine or everolimus if feasible [87]. Isolated hypertriglyceridemia post-LT warrants a different management approach. Most patients would respond to omega-3 fish oil 1000 mg twice a day, which can be titrated up to 4000 mg per day [76, 88]. There is a risk of an increase in LDL cholesterol with omega-3 supplementation, necessitating a dose reduction. Fibric acid derivatives like clofibrate, fenofibrate, etc., are also effective for hypertriglyceridemia. They should be best used in isolation, as their combination with statins increases the risk of rhabdomyolysis.

38.3.4 Hypertension After Liver Transplantation

Elevated blood pressure (BP) is observed in nearly 70% of liver transplant (LT) recipients [43, 89, 90]. The rise in BP is often multifactorial, with major contributors being calcineurin inhibitor (CNI)-induced renal vasoconstriction and the mineralocorticoid effects of corticosteroids. Among CNIs, cyclosporine is more likely to cause hypertension than tacrolimus, especially during the first year post-transplant [91]. Despite treatment, about one-third of patients experience poor BP control after LT [92].

Since well-managed hypertension correlates with lower mortality, it is essential for clinicians to prioritize BP control in post-transplant care [93]. The International Liver Transplantation Society (ILTS) recommends regular BP monitoring—every 3–6 months after discharge, and annually thereafter [76]. The target BP is below 130/80 mm Hg.

Lifestyle modifications—such as regular exercise, reducing dietary salt, and avoiding alcohol and tobacco—are foundational. Immunosuppression strategies should aim to minimize CNI doses and discontinue steroids by 3 months post-transplant, when possible.

38.3.4.1 Pharmacological Management

- Calcium channel blockers (amlodipine, felodipine) are preferred for post-LT hypertension, as they counteract CNI-induced vasoconstriction [76].
- Nifedipine and non-dihydropyridine CCBs (e.g., verapamil, diltiazem) are not recommended due to CYP450-mediated increases in CNI levels [50].
- ACE inhibitors and ARBs are generally avoided in the early post-transplant period due to low renin activity but can be beneficial in patients with CKD or diabetes in the later stages [76].
- Cardio-selective beta blockers (e.g., atenolol, metoprolol, bisoprolol) are safe and serve as effective second-line agents with minimal interaction with CNIs [50].
- Diuretics (thiazides and loop diuretics) are generally not preferred due to risks of electrolyte imbalances and renal dysfunction.

38.4 Recurrent and De Novo MASLD Post-liver Transplantation

Globally, metabolic dysfunction associated steatohepatitis (MASLD) affects up to 30% of the population [94] and is now the third leading cause of liver transplantation in the USA [50]. The prevalence is even higher in India [95].

- Recurrent MASLD (rMASLD) occurs when a patient transplanted for MASLD-related cirrhosis redevelops hepatic steatosis after LT [96].
- Prevalence of rMASLD may reach 70%, with biopsy-confirmed MASH found in about 25% of these cases. Around 18% develop fibrosis, and approximately 2% progress to cirrhosis [97, 98].
- Indian data report rMASH in up to 33% of LT recipients with steatosis, all of whom showed fibrosis on liver biopsy [99].

Table 38.2 Risk factors for de novo malignancies (DNMs) post-transplant

DNMs	Modifiable risk factors	Unmodifiable risk factors
Skin cancer	Alcohol abuse Smoking Excessive sun exposure Azathioprine use	Alcohol-associated liver disease Primary sclerosing cholangitis Light skin color Age more than 40 years at the time of LT
Post-transplant lymphoproliferative disorder	Use of induction agent Donor/recipient EBV mismatch High cumulative immunosuppression	Chronic hepatitis C Seronegative for EBV before LT Young age (<18 years) or elderly (>50 years) at LT
Lung cancer	Smoking Alcohol use	Alcohol-associated liver disease
Colorectal cancer	Obesity Alcohol and smoking Tobacco use	Primary sclerosing cholangitis (with or without IBD) Diabetes Non-alcoholic steatohepatitis
Stomach cancer	Alcohol use Smoking EBV and/or H. Pylori infection	East Asians Autoimmune liver disease Male gender Age more than 40 years at LT
Upper aerodigestive tract (oral cavity, pharynx, larynx, esophagus)	Human papillomavirus Smoking Alcohol use Tobacco chewing	ALD Barrett's esophagus
Cervical	Human papillomavirus	Cervical dysplasia

EBV Epstein-Barr Virus, *IBD* Inflammatory bowel disease, *LT* liver transplant

38.4.1 Risk Factors

- Metabolic syndrome and its components (obesity, diabetes, hypertension, and dyslipidemia) are primary drivers of both recurrent and de novo MASLD [100, 101].
- The PNPLA3 genetic variant in recipients raises rMASLD risk by 13-fold [102].
- Cumulative steroid exposure is another important contributor [103].
- Compared to de novo MASLD, rMASLD tends to be earlier in onset, more aggressive, and often irreversible [101].

38.4.2 Diagnosis

- Abdominal ultrasound may detect steatosis in patients with elevated liver enzymes but has limited accuracy.
- Transient elastography is commonly used in the general population but not validated in post-LT patients [104].
- MRI provides superior detection, with ~90% sensitivity and specificity, outperforming both CT and ultrasound [105].
- Non-invasive fibrosis markers (e.g., APRI, FIB-4, MR elastography) lack validation in this population [106].
- Liver biopsy remains the gold standard, as it can assess both steatosis and fibrosis and rule out other causes like rejection or drug-induced liver injury [107].

38.4.3 Management

- Early identification and control of modifiable risk factors—including diabetes, hypertension, dyslipidemia, and post-transplant weight gain—are essential [100, 101].
- Once these comorbidities are established, aggressive management becomes necessary.
- Currently, no pharmacological agent is approved specifically for managing MASLD in the post-transplant setting due to a lack of robust evidence [104].

38.5 De Novo Malignancies (DNMs) Following Transplantation (LT)

As long-term survival after liver transplantation improves, the incidence of de novo malignancies (DNMs) in transplant recipients has also risen. Compared to the general population, individuals who undergo LT are twice as likely to develop solid organ cancers and up to 30 times more likely to develop hematologic malignancies [108, 109]. The risk of DNMs increases with time after transplantation, peaking between 6 and 10 years post-LT [108]. Patients transplanted for alcoholic cirrhosis may face a higher risk of developing post-transplant cancers [110]. DNMs represent the leading cause of death during the second decade following LT [111, 112].

In Western countries, skin cancers constitute about 40% of DNMs, making them the most prevalent post-transplant malignancies [113, 114]. Non-melanoma skin cancers, such as squamous cell carcinoma and basal cell carcinoma, are most common, followed by melanoma and Kaposi sarcoma. Post-transplant lymphoproliferative disorder (PTLD) is the second most frequent DNM, occurring in 1–3% of adult recipients [115]. PTLD can range from indolent forms like plasmacytic hyperplasia to aggressive lymphomas and may be associated with Epstein-Barr virus (EBV) [116]. It typically arises within the first year after transplantation and carries high mortality [115].

Other cancers observed post-LT include colorectal, lung, prostate, and gastric cancers [117, 118]. However, in the Indian population, skin cancer and PTLD are rare [119]. Instead, oropharyngeal cancers are the most common, followed by lung cancer [119]. Generally, transplant recipients experience poorer cancer-specific survival rates compared to the general population [120], possibly due to more aggressive tumors induced by chronic immunosuppression [121] and suboptimal oncologic treatment because of concerns over graft rejection [122].

Risk factors for DNMs may be general—such as alcohol use and smoking [123, 124]—or malignancy-specific [125] (Table 38.2). Calcineurin inhibitors (CNIs), known for their pro-oncogenic properties, contribute to increased cancer risk, especially at higher concentrations [126]. Immunosuppression-related insulin resistance and oncogenic viral infections or reactivations are also linked to DNM development [127, 128].

Prevention strategies should target modifiable risk factors, promoting healthy lifestyle habits such as smoking and alcohol cessation and weight management [125]. Reducing CNI use and transitioning to mTOR inhibitors has been shown to lower DNM risk [129].

Cancer screening post-LT aims at early diagnosis to improve outcomes and generally follows population-based guidelines with a few LT-specific adaptations. Patients should be informed about their heightened cancer risk. Skin cancer risk can be reduced by minimizing sun exposure and undergoing yearly dermatologic evaluations [125].

EBV-seronegative recipients are more susceptible to PTLD and may benefit from regular EBV DNA monitoring and antiviral treatment when viral titers rise [125]. Immunosuppression reduction remains the cornerstone of PTLD treatment, achieving a response in up to 90% of cases. Additional therapies, including chemotherapy with or without rituximab, may be necessary for refractory cases. Surgery is an option for localized disease [130].

Smokers or those who quit within the last 15 years with a history of over 20 pack-years should receive annual low-dose chest CT scans to screen for lung cancer [125]. Patients with inflammatory bowel disease (IBD) require yearly colonoscopies with random biopsies. Individuals with primary sclerosing cholangitis (PSC) without IBD should undergo colonoscopy every 3–5 years. Furthermore, LT recipients over 50 with a history of MASH or hepatocellular carcinoma (HCC) should have colonoscopies every 5 years [125].

Treatment of DNMs after LT should be personalized and planned through multidisciplinary discussions involving transplant hepatologists, medical and radiation oncologists, and surgical oncologists. Immune checkpoint inhibitors pose a significant risk of graft rejection, loss, and mortality and are best avoided [125]. Radiation therapy, however, is considered safe and may be used with curative, neoadjuvant, or palliative intent [125].

38.6 Infections Following Liver Transplantation (LT)

Infections are a frequent and significant cause of illness and death after LT. Nearly 80% of LT recipients experience some form of infection over time, with bacterial infections being the most prevalent, accounting for about 70% of all cases [131]. Viral infections occur in approximately 20% of patients, while fungal infections affect around 8% [131].

Post-transplant infections may arise as new infections, reactivations of latent infections, donor-derived infections, or those acquired in a hospital setting. The likelihood of developing an infection depends on both the level of immunosuppression and the extent of exposure to pathogens [132]. More than 80% of infections occur within the first 6 months after transplantation, although infections may also develop later [131].

In the immediate postoperative period, nosocomial infections are most common and are often caused by multidrug-resistant (MDR) organisms, largely due to extensive antibiotic use around the time of surgery [133, 134]. Between one and 6 months post-transplant, the risk of viral and fungal infections increases due to heightened immunosuppression [133]. Early cytomegalovirus (CMV) infection—within 90 days of LT—is associated with a greater risk of acute cellular rejection, extended ICU stays, concurrent bacterial and fungal infections, and higher 90-day mortality rates [135].

After 6 months, community-acquired infections become more prevalent, depending on the recipient's immunosuppressive state [133]. Though less common, infections like aspergillosis, cryptococcosis, and pneumocystis jirovecii pneumonia may also occur during this late post-transplant period [136, 137]. Among viral infections, CMV (late-onset) and herpes zoster are most frequently observed beyond 1 year after transplantation. Late-onset CMV infection is particularly concerning, with an incidence of about 26% within 2 years [138, 139]. Recipients of ABO-incompatible grafts are at an even higher risk for CMV, likely due to the increased immunosuppression required [140].

CMV may manifest as systemic CMV disease or tissue-invasive CMV. The more common presentation is CMV disease—typically involving fever and bone marrow suppression—accounting for over 60% of post-LT CMV cases [141]. The gastrointestinal tract is the most frequently affected site in tissue-invasive disease, though CMV hepatitis, pneumonitis, and retinitis may also occur [142]. Treatment usually involves intravenous ganciclovir or oral valganciclovir.

Herpes zoster affects roughly 12% of recipients, usually appearing around 23 months after transplantation [143]. Most cases present as localized dermatomal zoster, while disseminated forms are rare [143, 144]. Early treatment with antiviral agents such as acyclovir, valacyclovir, or famciclovir is essential for better outcomes.

38.7 Osteoporosis

Patients with cirrhosis develop hepatic osteodystrophy due to low bone mineral density. Indian patients with cirrhosis have an alarmingly high prevalence of hepatic osteodystrophy, seen in 83% of patients [145]. Those with already pre-existing osteoporosis at the time of LT are at a heightened risk of post-LT fragility fractures. This is compounded by the fact that there is a steady decrease in bone mineral density within the first 3 to 6 months after transplant before returning to baseline levels. Patients with cholestatic liver diseases, alcohol and smoking abuse, hypogonadism, and pre-LT osteopenia/osteoporosis are at increased risk of post-LT osteoporosis [146, 147]. The risk of osteoporotic fractures is as high as 14% and 21% at 1 and 2 years post-LT, respectively [146, 147]. Thus, it is important that all LT recipients be evaluated for osteoporosis by dual-energy X-ray absorptiometry (DEXA). The fracture risk assessment tool (FRAX) is being increasingly used in Indian patients with cirrhosis and may be considered as a part of pre-transplant evaluation [145].

The management is based on principles similar to those used for the general population. Cessation of alcohol and smoking must be emphasized along with an increase in physical activity. LT recipients should compulsorily receive 1500 mg of elemental calcium along with 800 IU of vitamin D daily. Bisphosphonate use within 12 months of LT in patients with confirmed osteoporosis on DEXA helps in improving bone mineral density [148].

38.8 Therapeutic Drug Monitoring and Complications Post-transplant

As described before, cumulative immunosuppression is linked to long-term survival and post-LT complications, including renal dysfunction, PTDM, hyperlipidemia, and infections [70, 149, 150]. Thus, tacrolimus trough (C_0) levels should be kept between 6 and 10 ng/mL in the initial month after LT and thereafter between 5 and 8 ng/mL in patients who are receiving combination immunosuppression with mycophenolate or everolimus [151]. However, tacrolimus C_0 levels are variable, and monitoring area-under-curve (AUC) in the immediate post-LT period may be more useful in making treatment decisions regarding tacrolimus dose. C_0 levels and AUC have a poor correlation. This is important clinically, as patients with the same C_0 levels may have significantly different AUC [152]. AUC/C_0 ratio remains relatively stable in recipients over time and paints a better clinical picture of the overall immunosuppression [153]. However, this has not been studied prospectively post-LT. Tacrolimus levels 4 hours after dose (C4) have also been used previously to monitor for complications of over- or under-immunosuppression, but they did not fare superior to C_0 levels [154]. A personalized approach using weight-adjusted concentration/dose ratio in pediatric patients has been found useful in tacrolimus dose monitoring [155]. Tacrolimus C_0 variability within the individual patient correlates better with short-term and long-term complications post-LT [156, 157] and is emerging as a novel tool to guide therapeutic decisions.

38.9 Conclusion

Long-term graft survival has improved after LT due to better immunosuppression strategies after LT. This, in turn, has led to an increase in various complications linked to immunosuppression use. Better knowledge among clinicians and patients, along with frequent screening for these complications, is key to improve outcomes. Management focuses on minimization of immunosuppression, abstaining from smoking and alcohol consumption, regular exercise with maintenance of ideal body weight, and instituting cancer-specific screening programs. The role of novel modalities of therapeutic drug monitoring in addition to C_0 levels in minimizing immunosuppression-related complications after LT needs to be analyzed further in greater depth.

Conflict of Interest The authors declare no conflicts of interest.

Funding None.

References

1. Watt KDS, Pedersen RA, Kremers WK, Heimbach JK, Charlton MR. Evolution of causes and risk factors for mortality post-liver transplant: results of the NIDDK long-term follow-up study. Am J Transplant. 2010;10(6):1420–7.
2. Thaunat O. Finding the safe place between the hammer and the anvil: sounding the depth of therapeutic immunosuppression. Kidney Int. 2015;88(6):1226–8.
3. Wiesner RH, Fung JJ. Present state of immunosuppressive therapy in liver transplant recipients. Liver Transplant. 2011;17(Suppl3):S1–9.
4. Ojo AO, Held PJ, Port FK, Wolfe RA, Leichtman AB, Young EW, et al. Chronic renal failure after transplantation of a nonrenal organ. N Engl J Med. 2003;349(10):931–40.
5. Nevens F, Pirenne J. Renal disease in the allograft recipient. Best Pract Res Clin Gastroenterol. 2020;46–47:101690.
6. Allen AM, Kim WR, Therneau TM, Larson JJ, Heimbach JK, Rule AD. Chronic kidney disease and associated mortality after liver transplantation—a time-dependent analysis using measured glomerular filtration rate. J Hepatol. 2014;61(2):286–92.
7. Samstein B, Smith A, Freise C, Zimmerman M, Baker T, Olthoff K, et al. Complications and their resolution in recipients of deceased and living donor liver transplants: findings from the A2ALL cohort study. Am J Transplant. 2016;16(2):594–602.
8. Bahirwani R, Reddy KR. Outcomes after liver transplantation: chronic kidney disease. Liver Transplant. 2009;15(Suppl2):S70–4.

9. Charlton MR, Wall WJ, Ojo AO, Ginès P, Textor S, Shihab FS, et al. Report of the first international liver transplantation society expert panel consensus conference on renal insufficiency in liver transplantation. Liver Transplant. 2009;15(11):S1–34.
10. Stevens PE, Levin A, Kidney Disease: Improving Global Outcomes Chronic Kidney Disease Guideline Development Work Group Members. Evaluation and management of chronic kidney disease: synopsis of the kidney disease: improving global outcomes 2012 clinical practice guideline. Ann Intern Med. 2013;158(11):825–30.
11. Pacheco MP, Carneiro-D'Albuquerque LA, Mazo DF. Current aspects of renal dysfunction after liver transplantation. World J Hepatol. 2022;14(1):45–61.
12. Piano S, Gambino C, Vettore E, Calvino V, Tonon M, Boccagni P, et al. Response to terlipressin and albumin is associated with improved liver transplant outcomes in patients with hepatorenal syndrome. Hepatol Baltim Md. 2021;73(5):1909–19.
13. Fussner LA, Charlton MR, Heimbach JK, Fan C, Dierkhising R, Coss E, et al. The impact of gender and NASH on chronic kidney disease before and after liver transplantation. Liver Int. 2014;34(8):1259–66.
14. Wong RJ, Cheung R, Ahmed A. Nonalcoholic steatohepatitis is the most rapidly growing indication for liver transplantation in patients with hepatocellular carcinoma in the U.S. Hepatol Baltim Md. 2014;59(6):2188–95.
15. Sayiner M, Younossi ZM. Nonalcoholic steatohepatitis is becoming a top indication for liver transplantation worldwide. Liver Transplant. 2019;25(1):10–1.
16. Gonwa TA, Mai ML, Melton LB, Hays SR, Goldstein RM, Levy MF, et al. End-stage renal disease (ESRD) after orthotopic liver transplantation (OLTX) using calcineurin-based immunotherapy: risk of development and treatment. Transplantation. 2001;72(12):1934–9.
17. Duvoux C, Pageaux GP. Immunosuppression in liver transplant recipients with renal impairment. J Hepatol. 2011;54(5):1041–54.
18. Iglesias J, Frank E, Mehandru S, Davis JM, Levine JS. Predictors of renal recovery in patients with pre-orthotopic liver transplant (OLT) renal dysfunction. BMC Nephrol. 2013;14:147.
19. Lin YH, Lin CC, Wang CC, Wang SH, Liu YW, Yong CC, et al. The 4-week serum creatinine level predicts long-term renal dysfunction after adult living donor liver transplantation. Transplant Proc. 2012;44(3):772–5.
20. Gitto S, Falcini M, Marra F, MEDITRA Research Group. Metabolic disorders after liver transplantation. Metab Syndr Relat Disord. 2021;19(2):65–9.
21. Millson C, Considine A, Cramp ME, Holt A, Hubscher S, Hutchinson J, et al. Adult liver transplantation: UK clinical guideline – part 2: surgery and post-operation. Frontline Gastroenterol. 2020;11(5):385–96.
22. Utsumi M, Umeda Y, Sadamori H, Nagasaka T, Takaki A, Matsuda H, et al. Risk factors for acute renal injury in living donor liver transplantation: evaluation of the RIFLE criteria. Transpl Int. 2013;26(8):842–52.
23. Klintmalm GB, Feng S, Lake JR, Vargas HE, Wekerle T, Agnes S, et al. Belatacept-based immunosuppression in de novo liver transplant recipients: 1-year experience from a phase II randomized study. Am J Transplant. 2014;14(8):1817–27.
24. Yoshida EM, Marotta PJ, Greig PD, Kneteman NM, Marleau D, Cantarovich M, et al. Evaluation of renal function in liver transplant recipients receiving daclizumab (Zenapax), mycophenolate mofetil, and a delayed, low-dose tacrolimus regimen vs. a standard-dose tacrolimus and mycophenolate mofetil regimen: a multicenter randomized clinical trial. Liver Transplant. 2005;11(9):1064–72.
25. Boudjema K, Camus C, Saliba F, Calmus Y, Salamé E, Pageaux G, et al. Reduced-dose tacrolimus with mycophenolate mofetil vs. standard-dose tacrolimus in liver transplantation: a randomized study. Am J Transplant. 2011;11(5):965–76.
26. De Simone P, Fagiuoli S, Cescon M, De Carlis L, Tisone G, Volpes R, et al. Use of Everolimus in liver transplantation: recommendations from a working group. Transplantation. 2017;101(2):239–51.
27. Fischer L, Klempnauer J, Beckebaum S, Metselaar HJ, Neuhaus P, Schemmer P, et al. A randomized, controlled study to assess the conversion from calcineurin-inhibitors to everolimus after liver transplantation – PROTECT. Am J Transplant. 2012;12(7):1855–65.

28. Saliba F, De Simone P, Nevens F, De Carlis L, Metselaar HJ, Beckebaum S, et al. Renal function at two years in liver transplant patients receiving everolimus: results of a randomized, multicenter study. Am J Transplant. 2013;13(7):1734–45.
29. Sterneck M, Kaiser GM, Heyne N, Richter N, Rauchfuss F, Pascher A, et al. Long-term follow-up of five yr shows superior renal function with everolimus plus early calcineurin inhibitor withdrawal in the PROTECT randomized liver transplantation study. Clin Transpl. 2016;30(6):741–8.
30. Abdelmalek MF, Humar A, Stickel F, Andreone P, Pascher A, Barroso E, et al. Sirolimus conversion regimen versus continued calcineurin inhibitors in liver allograft recipients: a randomized trial. Am J Transplant. 2012;12(3):694–705.
31. Asrani SK, Wiesner RH, Trotter JF, Klintmalm G, Katz E, Maller E, et al. De novo sirolimus and reduced-dose tacrolimus versus standard-dose tacrolimus after liver transplantation: the 2000-2003 phase II prospective randomized trial. Am J Transplant. 2014;14(2):356–66.
32. Levitsky J, O'Leary JG, Asrani S, Sharma P, Fung J, Wiseman A, et al. Protecting the kidney in liver transplant recipients: practice-based recommendations from the American Society of Transplantation Liver and Intestine Community of Practice. Am J Transplant. 2016;16(9):2532–44.
33. Pageaux GP, Rostaing L, Calmus Y, Duvoux C, Vanlemmens C, Hardgwissen J, et al. Mycophenolate mofetil in combination with reduction of calcineurin inhibitors for chronic renal dysfunction after liver transplantation. Liver Transplant. 2006;12(12):1755–60.
34. Kornberg A, Küpper B, Thrum K, Krause B, Büchler P, Kornberg J, et al. Sustained renal response to mycophenolate mofetil and CNI taper promotes survival in liver transplant patients with CNI-related renal dysfunction. Dig Dis Sci. 2011;56(1):244–51.
35. Goralczyk AD, Bari N, Abu-Ajaj W, Lorf T, Ramadori G, Friede T, et al. Calcineurin inhibitor sparing with mycophenolate mofetil in liver transplantion: a systematic review of randomized controlled trials. Am J Transplant. 2012;12(10):2601–7.
36. Beckebaum S, Klein CG, Sotiropoulos GC, Saner FH, Gerken G, Paul A, et al. Combined mycophenolate mofetil and minimal dose calcineurin inhibitor therapy in liver transplant patients: clinical results of a prospective randomized study. Transplant Proc. 2009;41(6):2567–9.
37. De Simone P, Nevens F, De Carlis L, Metselaar HJ, Beckebaum S, Saliba F, et al. Everolimus with reduced tacrolimus improves renal function in de novo liver transplant recipients: a randomized controlled trial. Am J Transplant. 2012;12(11):3008–20.
38. Saliba F, Dharancy S, Salamé E, Conti F, Eyraud D, Radenne S, et al. Time to conversion to an Everolimus-based regimen: renal outcomes in liver transplant recipients from the EVEROLIVER registry. Liver Transplant. 2020;26(11):1465–76.
39. Lucey MR, Terrault N, Ojo L, Hay JE, Neuberger J, Blumberg E, et al. Long-term management of the successful adult liver transplant: 2012 practice guideline by the American Association for the Study of Liver Diseases and the American Society of Transplantation. Liver Transplant. 2013;19(1):3–26.
40. Fabrizi F, Dixit V, Martin P, Messa P. Chronic kidney disease after liver transplantation: recent evidence. Int J Artif Organs. 2010;33(11):803–11.
41. Demirci G, Becker T, Nyibata M, Lueck R, Bektas H, Lehner F, et al. Results of combined and sequential liver-kidney transplantation. Liver Transplant. 2003;9(10):1067–78.
42. Stone NJ, Bilek S, Rosenbaum S. Recent National Cholesterol Education Program Adult Treatment Panel III update: adjustments and options. Am J Cardiol. 2005;96(4A):53E–9E.
43. Laryea M, Watt KD, Molinari M, Walsh MJ, McAlister VC, Marotta PJ, et al. Metabolic syndrome in liver transplant recipients: prevalence and association with major vascular events. Liver Transplant. 2007;13(8):1109–14.
44. Anastácio LR, Diniz KG, Ribeiro HS, Ferreira LG, Lima AS, Correia MITD, et al. Prospective evaluation of metabolic syndrome and its components among long-term liver recipients. Liver Int. 2014;34(7):1094–101.

45. Madhwal S, Atreja A, Albeldawi M, Lopez R, Post A, Costa MA. Is liver transplantation a risk factor for cardiovascular disease? A meta-analysis of observational studies. Liver Transplant. 2012;18(10):1140–6.
46. Kardashian AA, Dodge JL, Roberts J, Brandman D. Weighing the risks: morbid obesity and diabetes are associated with increased risk of death on the liver transplant waiting list. Liver Int. 2018;38(3):553–63.
47. Nair S, Verma S, Thuluvath PJ. Obesity and its effect on survival in patients undergoing orthotopic liver transplantation in the United States. Hepatol Baltim Md. 2002;35(1):105–9.
48. Barone M, Viggiani MT, Losurdo G, Principi M, Leandro G, Di Leo A. Systematic review with meta-analysis: post-operative complications and mortality risk in liver transplant candidates with obesity. Aliment Pharmacol Ther. 2017;46(3):236–45.
49. Wong RJ, Cheung R, Perumpail RB, Holt EW, Ahmed A. Diabetes mellitus, and not obesity, is associated with lower survival following liver transplantation. Dig Dis Sci. 2015;60(4):1036–44.
50. Watt KDS, Charlton MR. Metabolic syndrome and liver transplantation: a review and guide to management. J Hepatol. 2010;53(1):199–206.
51. Luca LD, Westbrook R, Tsochatzis EA. Metabolic and cardiovascular complications in the liver transplant recipient. Ann Gastroenterol. 2015;28(2):183–92.
52. Krasnoff JB, Vintro AQ, Ascher NL, Bass NM, Paul SM, Dodd MJ, et al. A randomized trial of exercise and dietary counseling after liver transplantation. Am J Transplant. 2006;6(8):1896–905.
53. Cassiman D, Roelants M, Vandenplas G, Van der Merwe SW, Mertens A, Libbrecht L, et al. Orlistat treatment is safe in overweight and obese liver transplant recipients: a prospective, open label trial. Transpl Int. 2006;19(12):1000–5.
54. Wilding JPH, Batterham RL, Calanna S, Davies M, Van Gaal LF, Lingvay I, et al. Once-weekly semaglutide in adults with overweight or obesity. N Engl J Med. 2021;384(11):989–1002.
55. Newsome PN, Buchholtz K, Cusi K, Linder M, Okanoue T, Ratziu V, et al. A placebo-controlled trial of subcutaneous semaglutide in nonalcoholic steatohepatitis. N Engl J Med. 2021;384(12):1113–24.
56. Patton H, Heimbach J, McCullough A. AGA clinical practice update on bariatric surgery in cirrhosis: expert review. Clin Gastroenterol Hepatol. 2021;19(3):436–45.
57. Tsochatzis E, Coilly A, Nadalin S, Levistky J, Tokat Y, Ghobrial M, et al. International liver transplantation consensus statement on end-stage liver disease due to nonalcoholic steatohepatitis and liver transplantation. Transplantation. 2019;103(1):45–56.
58. Agarwal L, Sahu AK, Baksi A, Agarwal A, Aggarwal S. Safety of metabolic and bariatric surgery in obese patients with liver cirrhosis: a systematic review and meta-analysis. Surg Obes Relat Dis. 2021;17(3):525–37.
59. Mosko JD, Nguyen GC. Increased perioperative mortality following bariatric surgery among patients with cirrhosis. Clin Gastroenterol Hepatol. 2011;9(10):897–901.
60. Taneja S, Gupta S, Wadhawan M, Goyal N. Single-lobe living donor liver transplant in a morbidly obese cirrhotic patient preceded by laparoscopic sleeve gastrectomy. Case Rep Transplant. 2013;2013:e279651.
61. Mittal T, Ahuja A, Dey A, Malik VK, Sheikh MTM, Bansal NK, et al. Safety and efficacy of laparoscopic sleeve gastrectomy in patients with portal hypertension with liver function of Childs a. Surg Endosc. 2022;36(5):2942–8.
62. Diwan TS, Rice TC, Heimbach JK, Schauer DP. Liver transplantation and bariatric surgery: timing and outcomes. Liver Transplant. 2018;24(9):1280–7.
63. Zamora-Valdes D, Watt KD, Kellogg TA, Poterucha JJ, Di Cecco SR, Francisco-Ziller NM, et al. Long-term outcomes of patients undergoing simultaneous liver transplantation and sleeve gastrectomy. Hepatol Baltim Md. 2018;68(2):485–95.
64. Choudhary NS, Puri R, Saraf N, Saigal S, Kumar N, Rai R, et al. Intragastric balloon as a novel modality for weight loss in patients with cirrhosis and morbid obesity awaiting liver transplantation. Indian J Gastroenterol. 2016;35(2):113–6.

65. Singhal V, Dhampalwar S, Saigal S, Choudhary N, Saraf N, Chaudhary A, et al. Successful outcome of bariatric surgery in living donor liver transplant recipients with multidisciplinary approach: a preliminary experience. J Clin Exp Hepatol. 2021;11(1):144–8.
66. Lazzati A, Iannelli A, Schneck AS, Nelson AC, Katsahian S, Gugenheim J, et al. Bariatric surgery and liver transplantation: a systematic review a new frontier for bariatric surgery. Obes Surg. 2015;25(1):134–42.
67. Shivaswamy V, Boerner B, Larsen J. Post-transplant diabetes mellitus: causes, treatment, and impact on outcomes. Endocr Rev. 2016;37(1):37–61.
68. Sharif A, Hecking M, de Vries APJ, Porrini E, Hornum M, Rasoul-Rockenschaub S, et al. Proceedings from an international consensus meeting on posttransplantation diabetes mellitus: recommendations and future directions. Am J Transplant. 2014;14(9):1992–2000.
69. Grancini V, Resi V, Palmieri E, Pugliese G, Orsi E. Management of diabetes mellitus in patients undergoing liver transplantation. Pharmacol Res. 2019;141:556–73.
70. Song J, Li M, Yan LN, Yang JY, Yang J, Jiang L. Higher tacrolimus blood concentration is related to increased risk of post-transplantation diabetes mellitus after living donor liver transplantation. Int J Surg. 2018;51:17–23.
71. Younossi ZM, Stepanova M, Saab S, Kalwaney S, Clement S, Henry L, et al. The impact of type 2 diabetes and obesity on the long-term outcomes of more than 85 000 liver transplant recipients in the US. Aliment Pharmacol Ther. 2014;40(6):686–94.
72. Lv C, Zhang Y, Chen X, Huang X, Xue M, Sun Q, et al. New-onset diabetes after liver transplantation and its impact on complications and patient survival. J Diabetes. 2015;7(6):881–90.
73. Moon JI, Barbeito R, Faradji RN, Gaynor JJ, Tzakis AG. Negative impact of new-onset diabetes mellitus on patient and graft survival after liver transplantation: long-term follow up. Transplantation. 2006;82(12):1625–8.
74. John PR, Thuluvath PJ. Outcome of liver transplantation in patients with diabetes mellitus: a case-control study. Hepatol Baltim Md. 2001;34(5):889–95.
75. Alvarez-Sotomayor D, Satorres C, Rodríguez-Medina B, Herrero I, de la Mata M, Serrano T, et al. Controlling diabetes after liver transplantation: room for improvement. Transplantation. 2016;100(10):e66–73.
76. Charlton M, Levitsky J, Aqel B, O'Grady J, Hemibach J, Rinella M, et al. International liver transplantation society consensus statement on immunosuppression in liver transplant recipients. Transplantation. 2018;102(5):727–43.
77. Peláez-Jaramillo MJ, Cárdenas-Mojica AA, Gaete PV, Mendivil CO. Post-liver transplantation diabetes mellitus: a review of relevance and approach to treatment. Diabetes Ther Res Treat Educ Diabetes Relat Disord. 2018;9(2):521–43.
78. Halden TAS, Kvitne KE, Midtvedt K, Rajakumar L, Robertsen I, Brox J, et al. Efficacy and safety of Empagliflozin in renal transplant recipients with posttransplant diabetes mellitus. Diabetes Care. 2019;42(6):1067–74.
79. AlKindi F, Al-Omary HL, Hussain Q, Al Hakim M, Chaaban A, Boobes Y. Outcomes of SGLT2 inhibitors use in diabetic renal transplant patients. Transplant Proc. 2020;52(1):175–8.
80. Mahling M, Schork A, Nadalin S, Fritsche A, Heyne N, Guthoff M. Sodium-glucose cotransporter 2 (SGLT2) inhibition in kidney transplant recipients with diabetes mellitus. Kidney Blood Press Res. 2019;44(5):984–92.
81. Rajasekeran H, Kim SJ, Cardella CJ, Schiff J, Cattral M, Cherney DZI, et al. Use of canagliflozin in kidney transplant recipients for the treatment of type 2 diabetes: a case series. Diabetes Care. 2017;40(7):e75–6.
82. European Association for the Study of the Liver. Electronic address: easloffice@easloffice.eu. EASL clinical practice guidelines: liver transplantation. J Hepatol. 2016;64(2):433–85.
83. Reuben A. Long-term management of the liver transplant patient: diabetes, hyperlipidemia, and obesity. Liver Transplant. 2001;7(11 Suppl 1):S13–21.
84. Agarwal A, Prasad GVR. Post-transplant dyslipidemia: mechanisms, diagnosis and management. World J Transplant. 2016;6(1):125–34.

85. Overview | cardiovascular disease: risk assessment and reduction, including lipid modification | Guidance | NICE [Internet]. NICE; [cited 2023 Jan 24]. Available from: https://www.nice.org.uk/guidance/cg181.
86. Almutairi F, Peterson TC, Molinari M, Walsh MJ, Alwayn I, Peltekian KM. Safety and effectiveness of ezetimibe in liver transplant recipients with hypercholesterolemia. Liver Transplant. 2009;15(5):504–8.
87. Neal DA, Gimson AE, Gibbs P, Alexander GJ. Beneficial effects of converting liver transplant recipients from cyclosporine to tacrolimus on blood pressure, serum lipids, and weight. Liver Transplant. 2001;7(6):533–9.
88. McKenney JM, Sica D. Role of prescription omega-3 fatty acids in the treatment of hypertriglyceridemia. Pharmacotherapy. 2007;27(5):715–28.
89. Stegall MD, Everson G, Schroter G, Bilir B, Karrer F, Kam I. Metabolic complications after liver transplantation. Diabetes, hypercholesterolemia, hypertension, and obesity. Transplantation. 1995;60(9):1057–60.
90. Sheiner PA, Magliocca JF, Bodian CA, Kim-Schluger L, Altaca G, Guarrera JV, et al. Long-term medical complications in patients surviving > or = 5 years after liver transplant. Transplantation. 2000;69(5):781–9.
91. Canzanello VJ, Textor SC, Taler SJ, Schwartz LL, Porayko MK, Wiesner RH, et al. Late hypertension after liver transplantation: a comparison of cyclosporine and tacrolimus (FK 506). Liver Transplant Surg. 1998;4(4):328–34.
92. Martínez-Saldivar B, Prieto J, Berenguer M, de la Mata M, Pons JA, Serrano T, et al. Control of blood pressure in liver transplant recipients. Transplantation. 2012;93(10):1031–7.
93. VanWagner LB, Holl JL, Montag S, Gregory D, Connolly S, Kosirog M, et al. Blood pressure control according to clinical practice guidelines is associated with decreased mortality and cardiovascular events among liver transplant recipients. Am J Transplant. 2020;20(3):797–807.
94. Le MH, Yeo YH, Li X, Li J, Zou B, Wu Y, et al. 2019 global NAFLD prevalence: a systematic review and meta-analysis. Clin Gastroenterol Hepatol. 2021.
95. Shalimar EA, Bansal B, Gupta H, Anand A, Singh TP, et al. Prevalence of non-alcoholic fatty liver disease in India: a systematic review and meta-analysis. J Clin Exp Hepatol. 2022;12(3):818–29.
96. Patil DT, Yerian LM. Evolution of nonalcoholic fatty liver disease recurrence after liver transplantation. Liver Transpl. 2012;18:1147–53.
97. Malik SM, DeVera ME, Fontes P, Shaikh O, Sasatomi E, Ahmad J. Recurrent disease following liver transplantation for nonalcoholic steatohepatitis cirrhosis. Liver Transplant. 2009;15(12):1843–51.
98. Kakar S, Dugum M, Cabello R, Humar A, Ahmad J, Malik SM. Incidence of recurrent NASH-related allograft cirrhosis. Dig Dis Sci. 2019;64(5):1356–63.
99. Choudhary NS, Saraf N, Dhampalwar S, Mishra S, Gautam D, Lipi L, et al. Nonalcoholic fatty liver disease in living donor liver transplant recipients: a histology-based study. J Clin Exp Hepatol. 2022;12(5):1328–32.
100. Burke A, Lucey MR. Non-alcoholic fatty liver disease, non-alcoholic steatohepatitis and orthotopic liver transplantation. Am J Transplant. 2004;4(5):686–93.
101. Vallin M, Guillaud O, Boillot O, Hervieu V, Scoazec JY, Dumortier J. Recurrent or de novo nonalcoholic fatty liver disease after liver transplantation: natural history based on liver biopsy analysis. Liver Transplant. 2014;20(9):1064–71.
102. Finkenstedt A, Auer C, Glodny B, Posch U, Steitzer H, Lanzer G, et al. Patatin-like phospholipase domain-containing protein 3 rs738409-G in recipients of liver transplants is a risk factor for graft steatosis. Clin Gastroenterol Hepatol. 2013;11(12):1667–72.
103. Sprinzl MF, Weinmann A, Lohse N, Tönissen H, Koch S, Schattenberg J, et al. Metabolic syndrome and its association with fatty liver disease after orthotopic liver transplantation. Transpl Int. 2013;26(1):67–74.
104. Germani G, Laryea M, Rubbia-Brandt L, Egawa H, Burra P, O'Grady J, et al. Management of recurrent and De Novo NAFLD/NASH after liver transplantation. Transplantation. 2019;103(1):57–67.

105. Van Werven JR, Marsman HA, Nederveen AJ, Smits NJ, Ten Kate FJ, Van Gulik TM, et al. Assessment of hepatic steatosis in patients undergoing liver resection: comparison of US, CT, T1-weighted dual-echo MR imaging, and point-resolved 1H MR spectroscopy. Radiology. 2010;256(1):159–68.
106. Bhat M, Tazari M, Sebastiani G. Performance of transient elastography and serum fibrosis biomarkers for non-invasive evaluation of recurrent fibrosis after liver transplantation: a meta-analysis. PloS One [Internet]. 2017 Sep 1 [cited 2022 Sep 11];12(9). Available from: https://pubmed.ncbi.nlm.nih.gov/28953939/
107. Chalasani N, Younossi Z, Lavine JE, Charlton M, Cusi K, Rinella M, et al. The diagnosis and management of nonalcoholic fatty liver disease: practice guidance from the American Association for the Study of Liver Diseases. Hepatol Baltim Md. 2018;67(1):328–57.
108. Collett D, Mumford L, Banner NR, Neuberger J, Watson C. Comparison of the incidence of malignancy in recipients of different types of organ: a UK registry audit. Am J Transplant. 2010;10(8):1889–96.
109. Engels EA, Pfeiffer RM, Fraumeni JF, Kasiske BL, Israni AK, Snyder JJ, et al. Spectrum of cancer risk among US solid organ transplant recipients. JAMA. 2011;306(17):1891–901.
110. Saigal S, Norris S, Muiesan P, Rela M, Heaton N, O'Grady J. Evidence of differential risk for posttransplantation malignancy based on pretransplantation cause in patients undergoing liver transplantation. Liver Transplant. 2002;8(5):482–7.
111. Chandok N, Watt KD. Burden of de novo malignancy in the liver transplant recipient. Liver Transplant. 2012;18(11):1277–89.
112. Daniel KE, Eickhoff J, Lucey MR. Why do patients die after a liver transplantation? Clin Transplant. 2017;31(3).
113. Funk-Debleds P, Ducroux E, Guillaud O, Ursic-Bedoya J, Decullier E, Vallin M, et al. Subsequent nonmelanoma skin cancers and impact of immunosuppression in liver transplant recipients. J Am Acad Dermatol. 2018;79(1):84–91.
114. Tran M, Sander M, Ravani P, Mydlarski PR. Incidence of melanoma in organ transplant recipients in Alberta, Canada. Clin Transplant. 2016;30(10):1271–5.
115. Dierickx D, Habermann TM. Post-transplantation lymphoproliferative disorders in adults. N Engl J Med. 2018;378(6):549–62.
116. Tajima T, Hata K, Haga H, Nishikori M, Umeda K, Kusakabe J, et al. Post-transplant lymphoproliferative disorders after liver transplantation: a retrospective cohort study including 1954 transplants. Liver Transpl. 2021;27(8):1165–80.
117. Jiang Y, Villeneuve PJ, Fenton SSA, Schaubel DE, Lilly L, Mao Y. Liver transplantation and subsequent risk of cancer: findings from a Canadian cohort study. Liver Transplant. 2008;14(11):1588–97.
118. Sérée O, Altieri M, Guillaume E, De Mil R, Lobbedez T, Robinson P, et al. Longterm risk of solid organ De Novo alignancies after liver transplantation: a French National Study on 11,226 patients. Liver Transpl. 2018;24(10):1425–36.
119. Tiwari A, Saigal S, Choudhary NS, Saha S, Rastogi A, Bhangui P, et al. De Novo malignancy after living donor liver transplantation: a large volume experience. J Clin Exp Hepatol. 2020;10(5):448–52.
120. Na R, Grulich AE, Meagher NS, McCaughan GW, Keogh AM, Vajdic CM. De novo cancer-related death in Australian liver and cardiothoracic transplant recipients. Am J Transplant. 2013;13(5):1296–304.
121. Prenner S, Levitsky J. Comprehensive review on colorectal cancer and transplant. Am J Transplant. 2017;17(11):2761–74.
122. Ajithkumar TV, Parkinson CA, Butler A, Hatcher HM. Management of solid tumours in organ-transplant recipients. Lancet Oncol. 2007;8(10):921–32.
123. Chak E, Saab S. Risk factors and incidence of de novo malignancy in liver transplant recipients: a systematic review. Liver Int. 2010;30(9):1247–58.

124. van der Heide F, Dijkstra G, Porte RJ, Kleibeuker JH, Haagsma EB. Smoking behavior in liver transplant recipients. Liver Transplant. 2009;15(6):648–55.
125. Colmenero J, Tabrizian P, Bhangui P, Pinato DJ, Rodríguez-Perálvarez ML, Sapisochin G, et al. De Novo malignancy after liver transplantation: risk assessment, prevention, and management-guidelines from the ILTS-SETH consensus conference. Transplantation. 2022;106(1):e30–45.
126. Tjon ASW, Sint Nicolaas J, Kwekkeboom J, de Man RA, Kazemier G, Tilanus HW, et al. Increased incidence of early de novo cancer in liver graft recipients treated with cyclosporine: an association with C2 monitoring and recipient age. Liver Transplant. 2010;16(7):837–46.
127. Chakkera HA, Mandarino LJ. Calcineurin inhibition and new-onset diabetes mellitus after transplantation. Transplantation. 2013;95(5):647–52.
128. Dharnidharka VR, Lamb KE, Gregg JA, Meier-Kriesche HU. Associations between EBV serostatus and organ transplant type in PTLD risk: an analysis of the SRTR National Registry Data in the United States. Am J Transplant. 2012;12(4):976–83.
129. Carenco C, Assenat E, Faure S, Duny Y, Danan G, Bismuth M, et al. Tacrolimus and the risk of solid cancers after liver transplant: a dose effect relationship. Am J Transplant. 2015;15(3):678–86.
130. Kamdar KY, Rooney CM, Heslop HE. Post-transplant lymphoproliferative disease following liver transplantation. Curr Opin Organ Transplant. 2011;16(3):274–80.
131. Vera A, Contreras F, Guevara F. Incidence and risk factors for infections after liver transplant: single-center experience at the uUniversity Hospital Fundación Santa Fe de Bogotá. Colombia. Transpl Infect Dis. 2011;13(6):608–15.
132. Fishman JA, Issa NC. Infection in organ transplantation: risk factors and evolving patterns of infection. Infect Dis Clin N Am. 2010;24(2):273–83.
133. Pedersen M, Seetharam A. Infections after Orthotopic liver transplantation. J Clin Exp Hepatol. 2014;4(4):347–60.
134. Kawecki D, Pacholczyk M, Łagiewska B, Adadyński L, Lisik W, Sawicka-Grzelak A, et al. Urinary tract infections in the early posttransplant period after liver transplantation: etiologic agents and their susceptibility. Transplant Proc. 2011;43(8):3052–4.
135. Yadav SK, Saigal S, Choudhary NS, Saha S, Sah JK, Saraf N, et al. Cytomegalovirus infection in living donor liver transplant recipients significantly impacts the early post-transplant outcome: a single center experience. Transpl Infect Dis. 2018;20(4):e12905.
136. Fishman JA. Infection in solid-organ transplant recipients. N Engl J Med. 2007;357(25):2601–14.
137. Gandotra A, Mehtani R, Premkumar M, Duseja A, De A, Mallik N, et al. Invasive pulmonary Aspergillosis and tuberculosis complicated by Hemophagocytic Lymphohistiocytosis - sequelae of COVID-19 in a liver transplant recipient. J Clin Exp Hepatol. 2022;12(3):1007–11.
138. Lizaola-Mayo BC, Rodriguez EA. Cytomegalovirus infection after liver transplantation. World J Transplant. 2020;10(7):183–90.
139. Shibolet O, Ilan Y, Kalish Y, Safadi R, Ashur Y, Eid A, et al. Late cytomegalovirus disease following liver transplantation. Transpl Int. 2003;16(12):861–5.
140. Lee EC, Kim SH, Park SJ. Outcomes after liver transplantation in accordance with ABO compatibility: a systematic review and meta-analysis. World J Gastroenterol. 2017;23(35):6516–33.
141. Yadav SK, Saigal S, Choudhary NS, Saha S, Kumar N, Soin AS. Cytomegalovirus infection in liver transplant recipients: current approach to diagnosis and management. J Clin Exp Hepatol. 2017;7(2):144–51.
142. Fica A, Cervera C, Pérez N, Marcos MA, Ramírez J, Linares L, et al. Immunohistochemically proven cytomegalovirus end-organ disease in solid organ transplant patients: clinical features and usefulness of conventional diagnostic tests. Transpl Infect Dis. 2007;9(3):203–10.
143. Herrero JI, Quiroga J, Sangro B, Pardo F, Rotellar F, Alvarez-Cienfuegos J, et al. Herpes zoster after liver transplantation: incidence, risk factors, and complications. Liver Transplant. 2004;10(9):1140–3.

144. Levitsky J, Kalil A, Meza JL, Hurst GE, Freifeld A. Herpes zoster infection after liver transplantation: a case-control study. Liver Transpl. 2005;11(3):320–5.
145. De A, Ray D, Lamoria S, Sharma V, Khurana TR. Hepatic osteodystrophy and fracture risk prediction using FRAX tool in Indian patients with cirrhosis. J Gastroenterol Hepatol. 2020;4(5):945–9.
146. Leidig-Bruckner G, Hosch S, Dodidou P, Ritschel D, Conradt C, Klose C, et al. Frequency and predictors of osteoporotic fractures after cardiac or liver transplantation: a follow-up study. Lancet Lond Engl. 2001;357(9253):342–7.
147. Guichelaar MMJ, Schmoll J, Malinchoc M, Hay JE. Fractures and avascular necrosis before and after orthotopic liver transplantation: long-term follow-up and predictive factors. Hepatol Baltim Md. 2007;46(4):1198–207.
148. Kasturi KS, Chennareddygari S, Mummadi RR. Effect of bisphosphonates on bone mineral density in liver transplant patients: a meta-analysis and systematic review of randomized controlled trials. Transpl Int. 2010;23(2):200–7.
149. Hsiao CY, Ho MC, Ho CM, Wu YM, Lee PH, Hu RH. Long-term tacrolimus blood trough level and patient survival in adult liver transplantation. J Pers Med. 2021;11(2):90.
150. Song JL, Gao W, Zhong Y, Yan LN, Yang JY, Wen TF, et al. Minimizing tacrolimus decreases the risk of new-onset diabetes mellitus after liver transplantation. World J Gastroenterol. 2016;22(6):2133–41.
151. Brunet M, van Gelder T, Åsberg A, Haufroid V, Hesselink DA, Langman L, et al. Therapeutic drug monitoring of tacrolimus-personalized therapy: second consensus report. Ther Drug Monit. 2019;41(3):261–307.
152. Saint-Marcoux F, Woillard JB, Jurado C, Marquet P. Lessons from routine dose adjustment of tacrolimus in renal transplant patients based on global exposure. Ther Drug Monit. 2013;35(3):322–7.
153. Marquet P, Bedu A, Monchaud C, Saint-Marcoux F, Rérolle JP, Etienne I, et al. Pharmacokinetic therapeutic drug monitoring of Advagraf in more than 500 adult renal transplant patients, using an expert system online. Ther Drug Monit. 2018;40(3):285–91.
154. Ruijter BN, Tushuizen ME, Moes DJAR, de Klerk BM, van Hoek B. Tacrolimus 4-hour monitoring in liver transplant patients is non-inferior to trough monitoring: the randomized controlled FK04 trial. Clin Transpl. 2022;36(12):e14829.
155. Prusinskas B, Ohlsson S, Kathemann S, Pilic D, Kampmann K, Büscher R, et al. Role of Tacrolimus C/D ratio in the first year after pediatric liver transplantation. Front Pediatr [Internet]. 2021 [cited 2023 May 4];9. Available from: https://www.frontiersin.org/articles/10.3389/fped.2021.659608
156. Shemesh E, Bucuvalas JC, Anand R, Mazariegos GV, Alonso EM, Venick RS, et al. The medication level variability index (MLVI) predicts poor liver transplant outcomes: a prospective multi-site study. Am J Transplant. 2017;17(10):2668–78.
157. Rayar M, Tron C, Jézéquel C, Beaurepaire JM, Petitcollin A, Houssel-Debry P, et al. High Intrapatient variability of tacrolimus exposure in the early period after liver transplantation is associated with poorer outcomes. Transplantation. 2018;102(3):e108.

Chapter 39
Post-Transplant HCC: Recurrence, Surveillance and Management

Prashant Bhangui

Abstract Hepatocellular carcinoma (HCC) recurrence following liver transplantation (LT)—which remains the most definitive curative option for patients with cirrhosis and early-stage HCC—continues to pose a significant challenge for hepatologists and transplant surgeons. Despite the widespread use of selection criteria that now incorporate both tumor morphology and biological behavior, HCC recurrence remains a persistent issue and is a major determinant of long-term survival outcomes.

The therapeutic approach to recurrent HCC after LT depends on several key factors, including the time elapsed since transplantation, the pattern of recurrence (whether isolated or disseminated), graft function, and the recipient's overall performance status. This review outlines strategies for surveillance aimed at early detection of recurrence, assessment of tumor characteristics upon recurrence, and individualized treatment planning based on disease extent.

When recurrence is confined to a single organ—either within the graft or at an extrahepatic site—curative interventions such as surgical resection or local ablation (as opposed to systemic or palliative treatment alone) are associated with improved long-term survival. Core management principles include surgery, ablation, radiotherapy, systemic therapy, and modification of immunosuppression to incorporate mTOR inhibitors. Even in the context of recurrence, an aggressive, multimodal treatment strategy—when feasible—can significantly extend survival in selected patients.

Keywords Liver transplant for HCC · Post-transplant surveillance · Prognostication scores · Oligo-recurrence · Disseminated disease · Curative and palliative treatment

P. Bhangui (✉)
Institute of Liver Transplantation and Regenerative Medicine, Medanta – The Medicity, Gurgaon, Delhi NCR, India
e-mail: pbhangui@gmail.com

S. Saigal, D. Jothimani (eds.), *Fundamentals of Transplant Hepatology*,
https://doi.org/10.1007/978-981-95-2624-6_39

Key Highlights

- Post-transplant surveillance strategies should be individualized based on prognostication scores and recurrence risk calculations. In those with high recurrence risk, screening should involve cross-sectional imaging and AFP levels every 3–6 months.
- Once recurrence is detected, the immunosuppression regimen should be re-evaluated, and complete staging performed.
- The patient's functional status generally determines management of oligo-recurrence vs. disseminated disease, with curative or palliative treatment.
- Surgical resection or ablation of HCC recurrence (as opposed to systemic or palliative therapy alone) has been shown to be an independent predictor of long-term survival if recurrence is isolated to a single organ, whether it is in the liver or an extrahepatic site. Post-LT HCC recurrences develop in non-cirrhotic livers without portal hypertension, thus qualifying most patients for a safe surgery, which prolongs survival after HCC recurrence as compared to palliative treatment, whenever feasible. Ablative treatment modalities like RFA, MWA, and TACE are usually safe and well tolerated and may be repeated multiple times or combined in a multimodality approach.
- Use of non-invasive radiotherapy such as SBRT (focused ablation sparing adjacent normal liver parenchyma) is also effective for local control of pulmonary and skeletal oligo-recurrences, in addition to hepatic recurrences.
- Best results are usually obtained using multimodality treatment, including systemic therapy combined with surgery/ablation/radiotherapy. Systemic therapy with kinase inhibitors is advisable in all patients. Furthermore, combination therapy with mTOR inhibitors (sirolimus, everolimus) in order to reduce CNI doses may have some benefit over kinase inhibitors alone.

39.1 HCC Recurrence Post-LT

Liver transplantation (LT) is the best curative option for patients with hepatocellular carcinoma (HCC) with decompensated liver disease because it not only achieves oncological clearance but also treats the underlying chronic liver disease [1]. LT for patients with HCC should be guided primarily by the transplant benefit principle, that is, overall (OS) and recurrence-free survival (RFS) [2]. Several models have been proposed to predict recurrence in patients with HCC undergoing LT; however, a small proportion of patients do recur despite stringent selection criteria [3–5]. 10–20% of patients do have recurrence despite thorough preoperative evaluation to rule out extrahepatic disease and use of selection criteria based on tumor size and number, and recently, incorporating tumor biology too, when accepting patients with HCC for LT [6].

Tumor Recurrence: The Primary Determinant of Long-Term Outcomes Post-Liver Transplantation for HCC.

In patients undergoing liver transplantation (LT) for hepatocellular carcinoma (HCC), tumor recurrence remains the most critical factor influencing long-term outcomes. Despite LT being a potentially curative option, recurrence continues to be the "Achilles heel" of this approach. HCC recurrence is not only the leading cause of death post-transplant but also one of the most feared complications. Managing recurrent disease poses considerable challenges—particularly in cases with extrahepatic or multifocal recurrence—since no current treatment guarantees durable survival.

Recurrence rates differ depending on whether patients met conventional selection criteria, such as the widely adopted Milan criteria. For patients transplanted within the Milan criteria, recurrence ranges from 6% to 18%, while those beyond Milan experience recurrence rates between 20 and 30% [7]. Most studies report a median time to recurrence of about 13 months, with 80% occurring within the first 2 years post-transplant.

Regarding recurrence patterns [8]:

- 53% of cases involve only extrahepatic metastases (most commonly lungs \ [43%] and bones \[33%]).
- 31% have both intra- and extrahepatic involvement.
- 16% are confined to the graft liver.

Outcomes tend to be more favorable for liver-only recurrences, which are often amenable to locoregional therapies.

Several variables influence prognosis in recurrent HCC post-LT, including:

- Timing (early vs. late recurrence).
- Location (intrahepatic vs. systemic).
- Disease burden (oligo-metastatic vs. widespread dissemination).

This chapter will briefly review these prognostic indicators and provide a discussion of management strategies tailored to different clinical scenarios. We will also share our center's experience in treating HCC recurrence after LT.

39.2 Surveillance for HCC Recurrence Post-LT

Early detection, coupled with a prompt and multimodal treatment strategy, is essential for improving outcomes in post-transplant HCC recurrence [9]. Currently, no standardized global surveillance protocol exists, and strategies often vary by institution. Surveillance intensity may also differ depending on whether the patient underwent LT for HCC within conventional criteria or extended/locally advanced disease.

Given that most recurrences occur within the first 2 years after transplantation, close monitoring during this window is crucial for identifying treatable, potentially curable lesions—especially in cases of solitary, resectable metastases.

At our center, a study showed that 68% of recurrences occurred within the first 2 years, aligning with other reports, which document a median time to recurrence between 7 and 36 months [10–13]. Surveillance should target the most common sites of recurrence: lungs, bones, and the liver graft. Preferred imaging modalities include:

- Whole-body FDG-18 PET scans with triphasic CT angiography of the abdomen.
- Contrast-enhanced CT of the chest and abdomen with bone scans.

This imaging should be paired with tumor marker monitoring, particularly alpha-fetoprotein (AFP) and PIVKA-II (protein induced by vitamin K absence-II). It's important to note that not all HCCs secrete AFP. In non-AFP-secreting tumors, PIVKA-II often remains elevated and may serve as a more reliable marker.

39.2.1 Surveillance Frequency

- Every 3–6 months during the first 2 years post-transplant.
- Followed by every 6 months for at least 5 years thereafter [14].

This routine follow-up facilitates early identification of recurrence and timely initiation of therapy.

In a recent ILTS-ILCA Consensus Conference on LT for HCC (personal communication; the author participated as a working group member), it was recommended that individualized risk stratification be conducted using validated models, such as the RETREAT score [4]. For patients at intermediate to high risk, surveillance with contrast-enhanced cross-sectional imaging of the chest, abdomen, and pelvis should occur at least every 6 months. For high-risk patients with elevated pre-LT AFP, serum AFP monitoring is also advised, although the optimal testing interval remains to be defined.

39.3 Early vs. Late Recurrence

In patients undergoing LT for HCC, malignancy (mainly HCC recurrence) is an important medium-interval cause of death; it is responsible for 5.3% of deaths within the first year post-LT and increases to 20% in the 1- to 5-year interval and 14% after 5 years [15]. Early HCC recurrence (within the first year of LT) usually portends a worse prognosis [7, 16].

Early recurrence is defined as recurrence within 2 years of LT, and this is assumed to occur due to micro-metastases either before or at the time of hepatectomy or engraftment of circulating cancer cells. Late recurrence (beyond 2 years) occurs due to delayed engraftment of latent or indolent cancer cells.

Early recurrences are associated with worse and poor prognosis with median survival of 12 months, since there are few treatment options, whereas good outcomes have been noted with resection in late recurrences, especially when the recurrence is isolated and single.

One of the main reasons for limited treatment options is the fact that a majority of the recurrences present as widespread metastatic disease, which warrants the use of systemic therapy, but HCC is a chemotherapy-insensitive tumor. A recent study by Au et al. showed that early recurrences within one year of LT, liver recurrence, and AFP >200 ng/ml at recurrence predicted mortality following recurrence [17].

In patients with early recurrence, tyrosine kinase inhibitors (TKIs) like sorafenib or lenvatinib are first-line options, and regorafenib can be used as second-line. Use of TKIs has been shown to be safe and also associated with better outcomes compared to best supportive care alone. The use of immune checkpoint inhibitors (ICIs) has been associated with the risk of graft rejection with immune activation but may be cautiously considered within a clinical ICI/immunosuppression protocol or clinical trial. There is emerging evidence to show that ICIs may be safe when used for late recurrences, when the graft function is stable [18].

The role of reduced CNI exposure, especially in the early post-LT period, has been demonstrated in recent studies, and the use of mTOR inhibitors to maintain immunosuppression and their possible role in reducing recurrence per se has been proposed [19, 20].

39.4 Staging of HCC Recurrence

Management strategy as well as outcomes of HCC recurrence depend largely on whether the recurrences are isolated and single (oligo-recurrence) or disseminated. Once detected, a comprehensive staging is essential at recurrence, combining cross-sectional CT imaging with skeletal examination by a bone scan. Dual-tracer PET-CT has been shown to be effective for staging post-transplant HCC recurrence and also provides valuable information to guide clinical management [21].

Oligo-recurrence is further classified as intrahepatic and/or extrahepatic recurrence, and eligibility for treatment with curative intent is a key predictor of survival, compared to treatment with palliative intent or best supportive care. Rajendran L. et al. proposed an algorithm for the management of HCC recurrence based on the number of recurrences and site [22].

In general, there are no established consensus guidelines for management; it is best individualized. A multidisciplinary team approach, or tumor board, which includes transplant hepatology, surgery, diagnostic and interventional radiology, and oncology, should decide on what would be the best approach in an individual patient after a detailed evaluation and staging. A surveillance schedule has been proposed based on the RETREAT score— no surveillance for patients with RETREAT score of 0 (based on a 3% 5-year rate of recurrence), surveillance every 6 months for 2 years for patients with RETREAT score of 1–3, surveillance every 6 months for 5 years for patients with RETREAT score of 4, and surveillance every 3–4 months for 2 years followed by every 6 months for years 2–5 for patients with

RETREAT score of 5+ [23]. However, this protocol has yet to be prospectively validated. Treatment is either with a curative intent, surgical resection or ablation, or for palliation, which includes intra-arterial therapies (chemo- and radioembolization), and/or systemic therapy. Not being amenable to resection or ablation is in itself an independent predictor of poor prognosis in patients with HCC recurrence post-LT [10].

39.5 Management of Patients with Oligo-Recurrence

An algorithmic approach for managing oligo-recurrence is depicted in Fig. 39.1. Only a small subset (10–30%) of patients with recurrent hepatocellular carcinoma (HCC) present with isolated intrahepatic or extrahepatic metastases that are amenable to surgical resection. Surgical removal remains the preferred first-line therapy in such cases, particularly in patients with preserved allograft function and good performance status. Outcomes are most favorable in those with solitary tumors (<5 cm), well-differentiated histology, and no bone metastases [24]—showing a median survival of 20–27 months, compared to 9–10 months with non-surgical therapies and only 2.4–3.7 months with supportive care.

However, this improved survival may partly reflect selection bias, as resection is typically feasible in patients with later recurrences, fewer lesions, and better functional status. Surgical complexity increases in the setting of dense hilar adhesions, and successful resection demands a tumor-free residual liver of adequate volume. Immunosuppression further contributes to postoperative morbidity.

39.5.1 Ablation and Radiotherapy

For small, isolated liver recurrences not suitable for surgery, ablative techniques such as RFA (radiofrequency ablation), MWA (microwave ablation), or IRE (irreversible electroporation) are viable alternatives. These methods are most effective for tumors <3 cm situated deep within the liver parenchyma and away from vital structures. Tumor size, number, and limited extrahepatic spread are key predictors of treatment success [25].

Radiation therapy is also an option, particularly for larger lesions (2–7 cm). Image-guided stereotactic body radiotherapy (SBRT) offers precise targeting with minimal damage to surrounding tissue and may stimulate an anti-tumor immune response. Despite high local control rates (80–95% at 2 years), recurrence remains common.

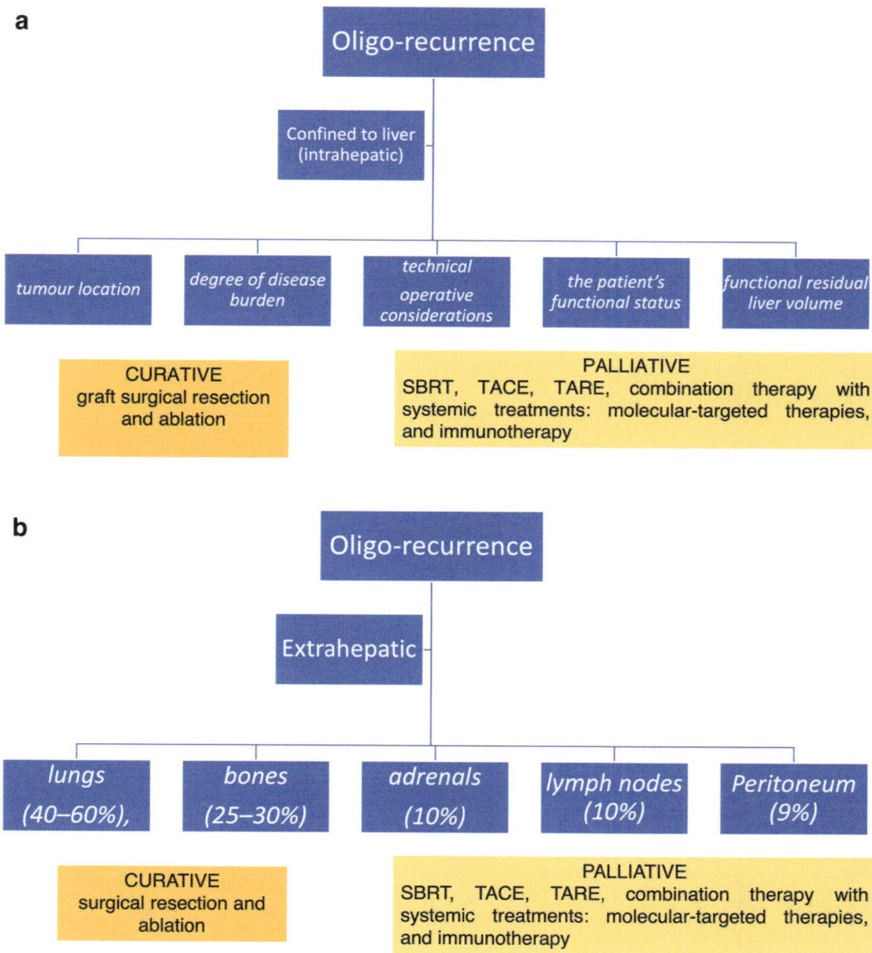

Fig. 39.1 (**a**) Management of intrahepatic oligo-recurrence. (**b**) Management of extrahepatic oligo-recurrence

39.5.2 Locoregional Therapies

For unresectable or multifocal intrahepatic recurrences, locoregional therapies such as TACE (transarterial chemoembolization) and TARE (transarterial radioembolization) are often utilized. TACE, however, can be technically challenging due to adhesions, altered vasculature, and risks of hepatic artery damage, which can impact graft survival [26]. In cases where TACE is not feasible, systemic therapies like sorafenib or lenvatinib offer comparable outcomes to TARE using Y90 microspheres [22].

39.5.3 *Management of Extrahepatic Oligo-Recurrence*

When recurrence is limited to extrahepatic sites, such as the lungs, local treatments like metastasectomy or ablation may be considered. In selected cases, even multiple pulmonary lesions can be resected, provided sufficient lung function remains. Reported median survival in such patients is 21–29 months, with 3-year survival rates ranging from 24% to 78%.

Other sites—such as vertebrae, adrenal glands, lymph nodes, and peritoneum—may also be treated with resection or ablation. SBRT has been proposed for bone and lung metastases. A combined strategy of surgery, local ablation, TKIs, and mTOR inhibitor-based immunosuppression has shown superior survival (1-year OS of 93.8% and 2-year OS of 52.6%) compared to systemic therapy alone (30.8% and 10.8%, respectively) [27].

39.5.4 *Post-LT HCC Recurrence: Prognosis and Immunosuppression*

Recurrence following LT is associated with worse survival compared to recurrence after surgical resection (median survival of 10–13 months vs. \~2 years). This poorer outcome is partly due to immunosuppression, which dampens immune surveillance and facilitates tumor progression. Elevated calcineurin inhibitor (CNI) levels early post-LT correlate with higher recurrence risk [28].

Recent studies (H2304 [19], H2307 [20]) suggest that switching early to mTOR inhibitors and reducing tacrolimus exposure may reduce recurrence rates. mTOR inhibitors (e.g., sirolimus, everolimus) not only reduce CNI toxicity but also suppress tumor growth by inhibiting cellular proliferation and angiogenesis. Their maximum benefit has been observed when recurrence occurs after 9 months post-LT, and mTORi is introduced within 3 months of recurrence [29].

Although clinical data are limited, combining mTORi with reduced-dose tacrolimus plus TKIs (sorafenib or lenvatinib) may offer a survival benefit in select patients.

39.6 Management of Disseminated Recurrence

Patients with disseminated HCC recurrence typically have a poor prognosis and are often managed with palliative intent (see Fig. 39.2). In some cases, based on individual assessments by a multidisciplinary team, a combination of locoregional therapies and systemic treatments may be attempted. Sorafenib alone provides a median survival of \~12 months but is often limited by side effects.

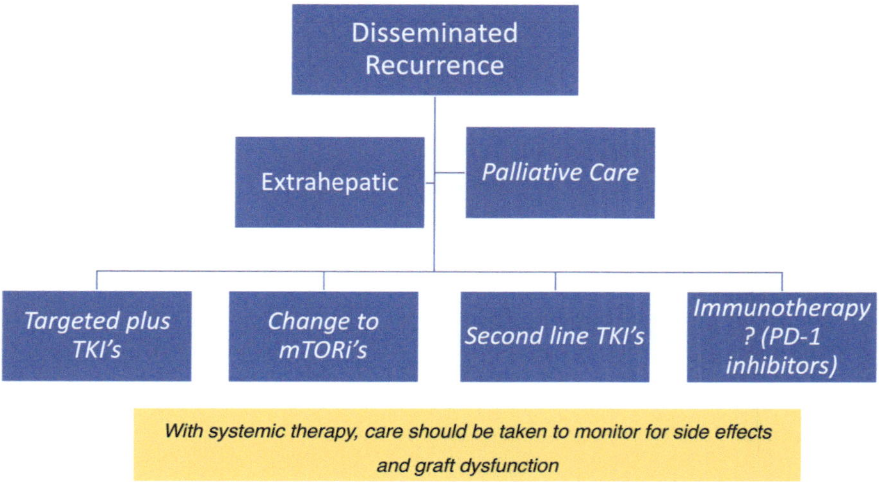

Fig. 39.2 Management of disseminated recurrence

Combining TKIs with mTOR inhibitors appears to improve tumor response in this setting [30–32]. The role of immunotherapy remains investigational, with ongoing trials evaluating anti-PD1 agents, TKIs, and other novel immune-based strategies [22].

39.7 Our Center's Experience

At our institution, living donor liver transplantation (LDLT) is offered to HCC patients without vascular invasion or extrahepatic disease, regardless of tumor size or number. Patients are stratified into low-, intermediate-, or high-risk categories based on morphologic and biological criteria and undergo either upfront LDLT or transplant after downstaging [6].

Pre-transplant evaluation includes:

- MDCT angiography.
- Whole-body FDG-18 PET scan.
- Bone scan.
- AFP and PIVKA-II levels.
- EUS-guided FNA of suspicious lymph nodes.

Post-transplant surveillance includes:

- CT scans every 6 months for 2 years, then annually.
- Ultrasound every 3 months for 2 years, then biannually.
- AFP monitoring every 3 months initially, later biannually.

In our analysis of 100 patients with post-LDLT HCC recurrence, the median time to recurrence was 16 months. Recurrence sites included lungs (53%), liver (37%), and bone (21%).

- 95 patients were treated with TKIs.
- 62 received mTOR inhibitors.
- 14 underwent surgical metastasectomy.
- 15 received SBRT.
- 18 were treated with ablation or locoregional techniques.

Survival outcomes:

- 1-year OS after recurrence: 57%
- 3-year OS: 24%
- Maximum survival: 7.5 years.

Poor prognostic factors included:

- Recurrence within 1 year of transplant.
- AFP >200 ng/mL at recurrence.
- Multiple sites of recurrence.

We found that multimodal therapy (surgery, ablation, TKIs, mTORi, and radiotherapy) significantly improved outcomes compared to TKI/mTORi alone. In patients unsuitable for directed therapy, we adopted a protocol of initiating mTOR inhibitors (everolimus 0.75 mg BID or sirolimus 1 mg OD), targeting trough levels of 3–5 ng/mL, while reducing and eventually stopping CNIs. Mycophenolate mofetil was added at low doses when required, titrated to maintain graft function.

39.8 Conclusion

In patients undergoing liver transplantation for HCC—especially beyond traditional criteria—post-recurrence survival can be significantly improved through aggressive, multimodal therapy. Careful surveillance, individualized treatment, and tailored immunosuppression adjustment are key to optimizing outcomes.

References

1. European Association for the Study of the Liver. Electronic address: easloffice@easloffice.eu; European Association for the Study of the Liver. EASL Clinical Practice Guidelines: management of hepatocellular carcinoma. J Hepatol. 2018;69:182–236.
2. Vitale A, Volk M, Cillo U. Transplant benefit for patients with hepatocellular carcinoma. World J Gastroenterol. 2013;19:9183–8.

3. Mazzaferro V, Sposito C, Zhou J, Pinna AD, De Carlis L, Fan J, et al. Metroticket 2.0 model for analysis of competing risks of death after liver transplantation for hepatocellular carcinoma. Gastroenterology. 2018;154:128–39.
4. Mehta N, Dodge JL, Roberts JP, Yao FY. Validation of the prognostic power of the RETREAT score for hepatocellular carcinoma recurrence using the UNOS database. Am J Transpl. 2018;18:1206–13.
5. Costentin C, Piñero F, Degroote H, Notarpaolo A, Boin IF, Boudjema K, et al. French-Italian-Belgium and Latin American collaborative group for HCC and liver transplantation. R3-AFP score is a new composite tool to refine prediction of hepatocellular carcinoma recurrence after liver transplantation. JHEP Rep. 2022;4:100445.
6. Bhangui P, Saigal S, Gautam D, Piplani T, Choudhary N, Chaudhary R, et al. Incorporating tumor biology to predict hepatocellular carcinoma recurrence in patients undergoing living donor liver transplantation using expanded selection criteria. Liver Transpl. 2021;27:209–21.
7. Fernandez-Sevilla E, Allard MA, Selten J, Golse N, Vibert E, Sa Cunha A, et al. Recurrence of hepatocellular carcinoma after liver transplantation: is there a place for resection? Liver Transpl. 2017;23:440–7.
8. de'Angelis N, Landi F, Carra MC, Azoulay D. Managements of recurrent hepatocellular carcinoma after liver transplantation: a systematic review. World J Gastroenterol. 2015;21:11185–98.
9. Bhangui P, Yadav S, Soin AS. Post liver transplant recurrence in patients with hepatocellular carcinoma: not necessarily the end of the road! Hepatoma Res. 2020;6:71–84.
10. Sapisochin G, Goldaracena N, Astete S, Laurence JM, Davidson D, Rafael E, et al. Benefit of treating hepatocellular carcinoma recurrence after liver transplantation and analysis of prognostic factors for survival in a large euro-American series. Ann Surg Oncol. 2015;22:2286–94.
11. Kornberg A, Küpper B, Tannapfel A, Katenkamp K, Thrum K, Habrecht O, et al. Long-term survival after recurrent hepatocellular carcinoma in liver transplant patients: clinical patterns and outcome variables. Eur J Surg Oncol. 2010;36:275–80.
12. Valdivieso A, Bustamante J, Gastaca M, Uriarte JG, Ventoso A, Ruiz P, et al. Management of hepatocellular carcinoma recurrence after liver transplantation. Transplant Proc. 2010;42:660–2.
13. Escartin A, Sapisochin G, Bilbao I, Vilallonga R, Bueno J, Castells L, et al. Recurrence of hepatocellular carcinoma after liver transplantation. Transplant Proc. 2007;39:2308–10.
14. European Association for the Study of the Liver. Electronic address: easloffice@easloffice.eu, European association for the study of the liver. EASL clinical practice guidelines: management of hepatocellular carcinoma. J Hepatol 2018;69:182–236.
15. Marrone G, Leone MS, Biolato M, Liguori A, Bianco G, Spoletini G, et al. Therapeutic approach to post-transplant recurrence of hepatocellular carcinoma: certainties and open issues. Cancers (Basel). 2023;15:5593.
16. Liang W, Wu L, Ling X, Schroder PM, Ju W, Wang D, et al. Living donor liver transplantation versus deceased donor liver transplantation for hepatocellular carcinoma: a meta-analysis. Liver Transpl. 2012;18:1226–36.
17. Au KP, Chok KSH. Multidisciplinary approach for post-liver transplant recurrence of hepatocellular carcinoma: a proposed management algorithm. World J Gastroenterol. 2018;24:5081–94.
18. Reig M, Forner A, Rimola J, Ferrer-Fàbrega J, Burrel M, Garcia-Criado Á, et al. BCLC strategy for prognosis prediction and treatment recommendation: the 2022 update. J Hepatol. 2022;76:681–93.
19. Fischer L, Saliba F, Kaiser GM, De Carlis L, Metselaar HJ, De Simone P, et al.; H2304 Study Group. Three-year Outcomes in De Novo Liver Transplant Patients Receiving Everolimus With Reduced Tacrolimus: Follow-Up Results From a Randomized, Multicenter Study. Transplantation. 2015;99:1455–1462.
20. Lee SG, Jeng LB, Saliba F, Singh Soin A, Lee WC, et al. Efficacy and safety of Everolimus with reduced tacrolimus in liver transplant recipients: 24-month results from the pooled analysis of 2 randomized controlled trials. Transplantation. 2021;105:1564–75.

21. Au KP, Dai WC, Chi-Yan Chan A, Cheung TT, Lo CM, Chok KS. Performance of dual-tracer PET-CT for staging post-liver transplant hepatocellular carcinoma recurrence. Transplant Direct. 2021;7:e769.
22. Rajendran L, Ivanics T, Claasen MP, Muaddi H, Sapisochin G. The management of post-transplantation recurrence of hepatocellular carcinoma. Clin Mol Hepatol. 2022;28:1–16.
23. Mehta N, Heimbach J, Harnois DM, et al. Validation of a risk estimation of tumor recurrence after transplant (RETREAT) score for hepatocellular carcinoma recurrence after liver transplant. JAMA Oncol. 2017;3:493–500.
24. Roayaie S, Schwartz JD, Sung MW, Emre SH, Miller CM, Gondolesi GE, et al. Recurrence of hepatocellular carcinoma after liver transplant: patterns and prognosis. Liver Transpl. 2004;10:534–40.
25. Huang J, Hernandez-Alejandro R, Croome KP, Yan L, Wu H, Chen Z, et al. Radiofrequency ablation versus surgical resection for hepatocellular carcinoma in Childs a cirrhotics-a retrospective study of 1,061 cases. J Gastrointest Surg. 2011;15:311–20.
26. Zhou B, Shan H, Zhu KS, Jiang ZB, Guan SH, Meng XC, et al. Chemoembolization with lobaplatin mixed with iodized oil for unresectable recurrent hepatocellular carcinoma after orthotopic liver transplantation. J Vasc Interv Radiol. 2010;21:333–8.
27. Yang Z, Wang S, Tian XY, Xie QF, Zhuang L, Li QY, et al. Impact of treatment modalities on patients with recurrent hepatocellular carcinoma after liver transplantation: preliminary experience. Hepatobiliary Pancreat Dis Int. 2020;19:365–70.
28. Pelizzaro F, Gambato M, Gringeri E, Vitale A, Cillo U, Farinati F, et al. Management of hepatocellular carcinoma recurrence after liver transplantation. Cancers (Basel). 2021;13:4882.
29. Kim M, Rhu J, Choi GS, Kim JM, Joh JW. Risk factors for poor survival after recurrence of hepatocellular carcinoma after liver transplantation. Ann Surg Treat Res. 2021;101:28–36.
30. Bhoori S, Toffanin S, Sposito C, Germini A, Pellegrinelli A, Lampis A, et al. Personalized molecular targeted therapy in advanced, recurrent hepatocellular carcinoma after liver transplantation: a proof of principle. J Hepatol. 2010;52:771–5.
31. Gomez-Martin C, Bustamante J, Castroagudin JF, Salcedo M, Garralda E, Testillano M, et al. Efficacy and safety of sorafenib in combination with mammalian target of rapamycin inhibitors for recurrent hepatocellular carcinoma after liver transplantation. Liver Transpl. 2012;18:45–52.
32. Sposito C, Mariani L, Germini A, Reyes MF, Bongini M, Grossi G, et al. Comparative efficacy of sorafenib versus best supportive care in recurrent hepatocellular carcinoma after liver transplantation: a case-control study. J Hepatol. 2013;59:59–66.

Chapter 40
De Novo Solid Organ Malignancy in Liver Transplant Recipients

Sanjay Kumar Yadav and Sanjiv Saigal

Abstract The liver transplant recipients are two to three times more likely to develop DNM as compared to the general population. The increased risk of DNM is mainly due to the additive effect of risk factors unrelated to transplant, like smoking, tobacco consumption, geography, age, and transplant-related risk factors like chronic exposure to immunosuppression and etiology of liver disease (PSC/alcohol). Skin cancer is the most common DNM, followed by post-transplant lymphoproliferative disease. The DNM in liver transplant recipients is biologically more aggressive and associated with shorter survival as compared to similarly staged matched cancer in the general population. It is one of the leading causes of death in liver transplant recipients on long-term follow-up. Abstinence from alcohol consumption and smoking is related to decreased risk of DNM in liver transplant recipients. The guidelines for screening of DNM are based on general population guidelines for specific cancers. The management of DNM is like the general population. CNI minimization or withdrawal with either addition or conversion to mTOR inhibitors is recommended in all patients after the diagnosis of the solid DNM.

Keywords De Novo Malignancy · Liver Transplant · Cancer · Immunosuppression · Tacrolimus

Key Highlights
- De Novo Malignancy (DNM) is one of the leading causes of death in long-term follow-up after liver transplant.
- Liver Transplant recipients are at high risk of developing DNM as compared to the general population.

S. K. Yadav
Narayana Health, Gurugram, Haryana, India

S. Saigal (✉)
Hepatology and Liver Transplant Medicine, Max Institute of Liver and Gastrointestinal Sciences, Max Super Specialty Hospital, Saket, New Delhi, India
e-mail: sanjivsaigal@hotmail.com

S. Saigal, D. Jothimani (eds.), *Fundamentals of Transplant Hepatology*,
https://doi.org/10.1007/978-981-95-2624-6_40

- The risk factors are similar to those in the general population, along with transplant-specific risk factors like chronic immunosuppression and infection with viruses with oncogenic potential.
- DNM is usually diagnosed in the advanced stage and is biologically more aggressive.
- Minimization of tacrolimus exposure should be considered in all patients to minimize the risk of DNM.
- Regular screening and surveillance should be done in all LT recipients.

40.1 Introduction

40.1.1 Epidemiology

Liver transplantation remains the gold standard treatment for patients with end-stage liver disease. Despite the challenges posed by the COVID-19 pandemic, over 8000 liver transplants were performed in the United States in 2020. Of these, 94.4% were adult recipients, 39.3% were classified as obese (BMI ≥30), and 28.9% had pre-existing diabetes. Alcoholic Liver Disease (ALD) was the leading indication for transplantation, accounting for 35.2% of cases. There has also been a steady increase in older recipients, with those aged 65 years and above comprising 22.4% of the total transplant population [1].

Advancements in surgical techniques, perioperative care, and immunosuppressive therapies have led to impressive short-term outcomes, with 1-year survival rates nearing 90% and 5-year survival rates around 75% at most transplant centers worldwide [1]. However, long-term survival has not seen a similar improvement, largely due to an increase in cardiovascular disease and malignancies following transplantation [2–4].

40.1.2 De Novo Malignancies (DNM)

De novo malignancies (DNMs) refer to new cancers that develop after solid organ transplantation. These include both solid tumors—such as hepatobiliary, aerodigestive (e.g., pancreatic, lung, colorectal), and skin cancers—as well as non-solid tumors like post-transplant lymphoproliferative disorders (PTLD) and non-Hodgkin lymphoma (NHL). This discussion focuses on solid tumors, as PTLD will not be covered in this chapter.

Data from large registries show that liver transplant recipients are 2–3 times more likely to develop DNMs compared to the general population [5, 6]. The reported overall incidence of DNM varies significantly, ranging from 3% to 16.5%, depending on the geographic location, patient risk factors, and length of follow-up

[5–10]. At 5 and 10 years post-transplant, the incidence of DNMs ranges between 10–14.5% and 20–32%, respectively [6, 11, 12] (Table 40.1).

A nationwide Japanese survey analyzing 9210 solid organ transplants (kidney 49.9%, liver 45.9%, heart 0.9%, lung 1.2%, pancreas 1.9%, small intestine 0.2%) reported an overall DNM incidence of 5.2%. Among these, kidney transplant recipients had the highest DNM rate (54.8%), followed by liver (38.8%), lung (3.8%), pancreas (1.9%), heart (0.1%), and small intestine (0.02%). The most frequently reported cancers was PTLD ($n = 87$), followed by kidney ($n = 43$), stomach ($n = 41$), colon ($n = 41$), and lung cancers ($n = 36$) [13].

Table 40.1 Incidence of DNM in studies with ≥1000 LT Recipients

Author, year, country	Number of LT recipients	Recipients with de novo malignancy	Common malignancies
Frezza et al.,1997, USA	1657	50 (3%)	Basal cell carcinoma, squamous cell carcinoma
Jain et al., 1998, USA	1000	57 (5.7%)	Skin, respiratory, oropharyngeal
Saigal et al., 2002, UK	1140	30 (2.6%)	Skin cancer, oropharyngeal, bladder, breast, leukemia
Sanchez et al., 2002, USA	1421	125 (8.8%)	Skin, lymphomas, lung
Oo et al., 2005, UK	1778	141 (7.9%)	Skin, large bowel and rectal, hematologic, lung, breast
Yao et al., 2006 USA	1043	50 (4.8%)	Skin, gastrointestinal
Jiang et al., 2008, Canada	2034	113 (5.5%)	Hematologic, colorectal, lung
Ettorre et al., 2013 Italy	1675	98 (5.9%)	PTLD, head and neck, lung, colorectal, Kaposi's sarcoma
Schrem et al.,2013, Germany	2000	115 (6%)	PTLD, lung, colorectal, gynecologic, breast, gastric/esophageal
Mangus et al.,2015, USA	1275	180 (14.1%)	Skin, gastrointestinal, hematologic, lung
Rademacher et al., 2017, Germany	1616	266 (16.5%)	Skin, hematologic
Sérée et al., 2018, France	11,226	1200 (10.7%)	Lung, esophagus, stomach, colorectal, larynx, oral/pharynx,
Studies from the east			
Park et al., 2012, Korea	1952	44 (2.3%)	Stomach, colorectal, breast, predominantly living donor series
Sanaei et al., 2015, Iran	1700	38 (2.2%)	PTLD, gastrointestinal, Kaposi's sarcoma, pancreatic
Tiwari et al., 2020, India	2100	21 (1%)	Oropharyngeal, lung, predominantly LDLT series
Yeh et al., 2020, Taiwan	2127	111 (5.2%)	Digestive most common

The geographical location influences the types of DNMs seen. For example, nonmelanoma skin cancers are most common in Western countries [14], while aerodigestive tract malignancies predominate in Asian populations[15–18]. Some studies suggest that living donor liver transplant (LDLT) recipients may have a lower DNM risk (1–2%) compared to deceased donor liver transplant (DDLT) recipients (6–14%), although these findings are limited by shorter follow-up periods [18].

40.1.3 Skin Cancers

Skin cancers represent the most frequent DNM in liver transplant recipients, accounting for up to 40% of all cases. Common types include cutaneous squamous cell carcinoma (cSCC), basal cell carcinoma (BCC), melanoma, and Kaposi's sarcoma (KS) [19]. Interestingly, around two-thirds of skin cancers in transplant recipients occur on partially sun-exposed or sun-protected sites, such as the genitals, especially in people of color.

There is a noted decline in skin cancer incidence, possibly due to the implementation of preventive strategies—including sun protection education, routine skin surveillance, and modification of immunosuppressive regimens [12, 20].

40.1.4 Post-Transplant Lymphoproliferative Disorder (PTLD)

PTLD is the second most common DNM in liver transplant recipients. Its reported incidence is 1–3% in adults and 6–10% in children, with a standardized incidence ratio (SIR) ranging from 3.9 to 21. While skin cancers typically do not impact overall survival, PTLD and solid organ cancers are linked to increased mortality in liver transplant recipients [21].

40.1.5 Colorectal Cancer (CRC)

Colorectal cancer is particularly common among liver transplant recipients with primary sclerosing cholangitis (PSC). Compared to the general population, liver transplant recipients face a 2.8-fold increased risk of developing de novo CRC. For those transplanted for non-PSC causes, the risk remains elevated at 1.8-fold. However, in patients with PSC-inflammatory bowel disease (IBD) and an intact colon, the risk is nearly 10 times higher compared to other liver transplant recipients [22, 23].

40.1.6 Lung, Head & Neck, and Genitourinary Cancers

Liver transplant recipients have a 2.3-fold higher risk of developing lung cancer compared to the general population. Similarly, the risk of head and neck cancers, including oropharyngeal cancers, is elevated. These cancers are typically diagnosed 34–61 months post-transplant [14, 24, 25]. Notably, oropharyngeal cancer is 25.5 times more common in patients transplanted due to alcohol-related cirrhosis than in those transplanted for other causes [26].

Among genitourinary cancers, the incidence of renal and prostate cancers is comparable to the general population. However, there is an increased risk of ovarian and cervical cancers in female liver transplant recipients [27, 28].

40.2 Survival After De Novo Malignancy

The de novo malignancy (DNM) in liver transplant recipients is biologically more aggressive and associated with shorter survival as compared to similarly staged matched cancer in the general population [29]. After the diagnosis of DNM, there is a 2- to 3-fold increase in the risk of death in transplant recipients as compared to age, cancer site, type, and cancer stage-matched general population cohort [30, 31]. After the diagnosis of de novo nonskin solid organ malignancy, the estimated 1- and 5-year patient survival was 62% and 47%, respectively, as compared to 79% one-year and 64% five-year patient survival in the general population [28]. The lymphoproliferative disorder is the most common cause of cancer-related death in transplant recipients. The use of alcohol and tobacco significantly increases the risk of and mortality related to these malignancies.

The possible reason for worse outcomes in transplant recipients with DNM includes a chronically immunosuppressed environment that predisposes them to biologically more aggressive tumors and less efficient cancer treatment in the transplant population as compared to the general population because of multiple comorbidities and rejection risks [32, 33]. Therefore, a multidisciplinary team approach with the involvement of the transplant team and transplant oncologist is essential to improve the efficacy of cancer treatment and improve survival [34].

40.3 Risk Factors for De Novo Malignancy

Liver transplant (LT) recipients are at a heightened risk for developing DNM due to a combination of transplant-related and non-transplant-related factors. Non-transplant-related risk factors include age, smoking, alcohol use, geographic region, and baseline disease etiology (such as primary sclerosing cholangitis or ALD). On the other hand, transplant-related factors—especially chronic exposure to immunosuppressive medications—also contribute significantly.

The type, dose, and duration of immunosuppressive therapy directly influence DNM risk. This risk typically begins to rise within the first year post-transplant and peaks between 6 and 10 years of follow-up. Mechanistically, this elevated cancer risk is attributed to oncogenic viral infections, chronic immune activation, cytokine-driven inflammation, insulin resistance, and impaired immune surveillance—all of which are worsened by long-term immunosuppression [35].

Chronic immunosuppression facilitates viral infections with oncogenic potential, such as:

- EBV (leading to PTLD/B-cell lymphoma).
- HHV-8 (Kaposi's sarcoma).
- HPV (anogenital cancers).
- HBV and HCV (linked to hepatocellular carcinoma).

40.3.1 Key Risk Factors (See Table 40.2 for Full List)

- Age: Older recipients, particularly those over 50 years, are at increased cancer risk.
- Cumulative Risk: A multicenter case-control study demonstrated a rising 5-year cancer incidence based on risk factors—0% in patients without any, 12.5% with 1–2, and 22.8% with 3–4 risk factors [36].

40.3.2 Alcohol and Smoking

Alcohol is a recognized carcinogen, particularly for aerodigestive tract and liver cancers. Its carcinogenic effects are mediated by acetaldehyde toxicity, DNA methylation interference, and disruption of retinoid metabolism. Alcohol's role in cancer may also be modulated by genetics, diet, and comorbidities [37]. Notably, combined exposure to alcohol and smoking significantly increases cancer risk and is associated with higher SIRs in transplant recipients.

Patients with ALD as the indication for transplantation have a higher DNM risk compared to those with other etiologies [24, 38, 39]. Additionally, current or former smokers face increased DNM incidence compared to non-smokers. Importantly, smoking cessation post-transplant may help reduce this risk [40].

Emerging data suggest that nonalcoholic steatohepatitis (NASH) is also an independent and growing risk factor for DNM after LT [41].

Table 40.2 Risk factors for solid organ DNM

Old age	
Male sex	
Geographical location of patients	
Light skin color	
Smoking	
Alcohol use	
Tobacco use	
The underlying cause of liver disease	PSC ALD NASH with HCC Metabolic syndrome Autoimmune live disease
Premalignant condition at the time of LT	Barret esophagus Colonic polyp Cervical dysplasia
Previous history of extrahepatic malignancy	Renal cell carcinoma
Prolong immunosuppression	Cyclosporin/tacrolimus Azathioprine
Oncogenic viral infection	Human papillomavirus Epstein-Barr virus H pylori
Sun exposer	

40.4 Immunosuppressive Agents and Oncogenesis

Experimental studies have shown that some immunosuppressants directly promote tumor development:

- Calcineurin inhibitors (CNIs) promote cancer via TGF-β signaling [42], reduced apoptosis, impaired DNA repair [43], and angiogenesis. CNIs also contribute to insulin resistance and beta-cell toxicity, increasing diabetes risk, which is itself a cancer risk factor.
- Azathioprine is associated with DNA repair impairment, further contributing to carcinogenesis [44].

A meta-analysis indicates that cyclosporine carries a higher DNM risk compared to tacrolimus or mycophenolate. This difference may stem from lower TGF-β induction and fewer tumor-promoting oxidative effects with tacrolimus [44].

A Spanish study further supported a dose-dependent oncogenic effect of tacrolimus, showing that high cumulative exposure (CET >10 ng/ml in the first month, >8 ng/ml thereafter) independently predicted cancer development. Therefore, dose moderation is especially important in high-risk individuals [36].

- Mycophenolate has not been linked to increased cancer risk. Some evidence suggests it may reduce DNM incidence, possibly due to CNI dose-sparing effects [44].
- mTOR inhibitors (sirolimus, everolimus) inhibit a pathway involved in cancer progression. While sirolimus may reduce tumor growth, its safety concerns (including increased mortality) limit use. Everolimus appears safer but has not demonstrated clear cancer-preventive benefits in LT recipients [36, 44].
- Induction therapies like anti-thymocyte globulin (ATG) have been linked to higher PTLD and DNM risks, whereas IL-2 receptor blockers do not appear to increase DNM risk [36, 44].

40.5 Prevention of De Novo Malignancy

Prevention strategies for post-transplant malignancies focus on modifying known risk factors. While age, sex, ethnicity, and underlying liver disease etiology are unchangeable, several lifestyle factors are modifiable and have proven significance in reducing DNM risk:

40.5.1 Key Preventive Measures

- Abstinence from alcohol and smoking is critical. Both habits increase DNM risk significantly. Structured addiction treatment and psychological support are recommended.
- Smoking cessation has been shown to reduce the risk of smoking-related cancers post-transplant.
- Obesity management is essential, as obesity is associated with various malignancies (breast, colon, endometrium, esophagus, gallbladder, and kidney). Bariatric surgery and exercise can reduce this risk.
- Metabolic syndrome should be proactively managed. This includes diabetes, hypertension, and dyslipidemia, all of which may influence cancer development.
- Medications like metformin, statins, and aspirin have shown potential protective effects against malignancies in some studies.

40.5.2 Counseling and Follow-Up

A comprehensive post-transplant care plan should include:

- Counseling on lifestyle modifications.
- Regular physical activity.

- A balanced diet.
- Emphasis on alcohol and tobacco abstinence.
- Ongoing evaluation and control of metabolic comorbidities.

These interventions should be integrated into routine follow-up visits and reinforced consistently to lower DNM risk over the long term.

40.6 Screening and Surveillance in Liver Transplant Recipients

The goal of cancer screening is to identify malignancies early, at a stage when curative treatment is still possible. Despite the higher incidence of DNMs in LT recipients, there are currently no transplant-specific, evidence-based screening guidelines. As a result, most screening practices are adapted from general population recommendations.

40.6.1 Skin Cancer

LT recipients are at significantly increased risk of developing skin cancers compared to the general population. Therefore, all patients should be educated on skin protection measures, including the use of sunscreen, protective clothing, hats, and sunglasses. An annual full-body skin examination by a dermatologist is recommended for all LT recipients [45].

40.6.2 Lung Cancer

Lung cancer is among the most common DNMs after transplantation. Chest X-rays are not reliable for screening, but low-dose CT (LDCT) scans have been shown to effectively detect early-stage lung cancer and reduce mortality in both the general population and LT recipients, particularly in smokers. LT recipients who are current smokers or quit within the last 15 years, with a smoking history exceeding 20 pack-years, should undergo annual LDCT chest imaging. Smoking cessation counseling and medical support should be offered to all smokers [45, 46].

40.6.3 Head, Neck, and Oropharyngeal Cancers

There are no formal screening recommendations for these cancers in the general population. However, LT recipients—especially those with PSC, alcohol-related liver disease, tobacco use, or HPV infection—are at increased risk. These individuals should undergo annual oral and ENT evaluations [45, 47, 48].

40.6.4 Colorectal Cancer (CRC)

General CRC screening begins at age 45–50 and continues to age 75, typically via full-length colonoscopy with multiple biopsies. LT recipients with PSC and IBD are at significantly higher risk for CRC and should undergo annual colonoscopies with random biopsies. In PSC-only patients (without IBD), colonoscopy is recommended 1 year after transplant, then every 3–5 years if no IBD is detected. For all other LT recipients, standard population-based screening guidelines apply.

Emerging data suggest that NASH patients over 50 with a history of HCC may also warrant earlier and more frequent CRC screening [49–51].

40.6.5 Prostate Cancer

LT recipients should follow general screening guidelines, including PSA testing and digital rectal exams as appropriate [45].

40.6.6 Urinary Tract and Renal Malignancies

Although bladder cancer appears more frequently in LT recipients, no standard screening is currently recommended. However, hematuria (blood in urine) should always prompt further investigation.

Renal cell carcinoma (RCC) is more prevalent among those with chronic kidney disease or those undergoing combined liver-kidney transplants. While no formal RCC screening guideline exists, annual abdominal ultrasonography is suggested in LT recipients to aid early detection [52].

40.6.7 Breast Cancer

The incidence of breast cancer in female LT recipients is comparable to the general population, so screening recommendations remain the same: mammography every 1–2 years for women aged 45–74, as long as their life expectancy is at least 10 years [45].

40.6.8 Cervical and HPV-Related Cancers

Due to impaired immune response, LT recipients are less effective at clearing HPV infections, which increases the risk for cervical cancer. Therefore, screening guidelines for immunocompromised populations—such as annual visual inspection, bimanual exams, Pap smears, and HPV testing—should be applied.

- All female LT recipients should undergo annual cervical cancer screening for three consecutive years.
- If HPV becomes negative, they can then follow general population screening protocols.
- If HPV remains positive, annual screening should continue.
- For recipients transplanted before age 21, screening should begin within a year of sexual debut and continue lifelong [45].

40.7 Current Gaps and Recommendations

Although the risk of DNM is well-established in LT recipients, current screening protocols remain largely based on general population data due to limited transplant-specific evidence. Moreover, many solid organ transplant (SOT) recipients are not even aware of standard screening guidelines [53].

Some cohort studies suggest that enhanced surveillance may improve survival, supporting the need for transplant centers to integrate DNM screening into routine follow-up protocols. Patient education on the importance of cancer screening should be part of post-transplant counseling.

Table 40.3 provides a summary of recommended cancer screening protocols tailored to LT recipients based on current evidence and should serve as a baseline reference for clinical practice.

Table 40.3 Screening Recommendation for DNM in LT Recipients

Malignancy type	Recommendations	Applicable transplant Recipients
Skin cancer	Annual dermatological examination Reduce sun exposure to skin-hats/long sleeves/pants Sunscreen application	All recipients
Colon cancer	Annual colonoscopy with random surveillance biopsy	IBD
Colon cancer	Colonoscopy with random surveillance biopsy every 3–5 years	PSC without IBD
Colon cancer	Colonoscopy with random surveillance biopsy every 5 years	NASH with HCC (>50 years of age)
Colon cancer	Adherence to guideline average risk population Screening age 45–75 years. FOBT yearly or CT colonoscopy every 5 years or colonoscopy every 10 years	All others
Lung cancer	Annual low-dose CT chest	ALD, smoker, ex-smoker
Oropharyngeal/ laryngeal cancer	Annual otolaryngology evaluation	ALD, smoker, ex-smoker, tobacco, oropharyngeal HPV
Cervical cancer, other gynecologic malignancy	Pelvic examination, PAP smear with HPV testing annually for 3 years HPV+ continue annually HPV negative: General population guideline	Female
Breast cancer	Annual mammography starting at the age of 40 years	Female
Prostate cancer	PSA annual starting at the age of 50 years	Male
Renal cancer	USG abdomen	Previous RCC, PCKD

40.8 Management of DNM after Liver Transplant

40.8.1 General Immunosuppression Management

There is growing evidence to suggest a potential link between chronic exposure to immunosuppressive drugs and oncogenesis [54]. Early minimization of tacrolimus using the CET tool should be considered to reduce the incidence of cancer in LT patients [36]. Concomitant immunosuppressive drugs such as mycophenolate may not increase the risk of cancer and could be useful if they allow for a safer and more effective tacrolimus minimization after LT. Despite the lack of randomized control trials showing the superiority of mTOR in reducing the risk of DNM and recurrent HCC after LT, several retrospective registry data have shown that the use of mTOR inhibitors is associated with a reduced incidence of de novo malignancies after kidney, heart, and LT [55–57]. Based on available evidence, international liver transplant society (ILTS). I guidelines have recommended the use of mTOR inhibitors for patients with DNM after LT [58].

40.8.2 Immunosuppression Adjustment in Liver Transplant Recipients with De Novo Malignancy

Modulating the immune response is an established therapeutic approach in cancer treatment. As such, reducing or discontinuing calcineurin inhibitors (CNIs) in LT recipients who develop DNM may offer clinical benefits. Another effective strategy involves the use of mTOR inhibitors, which are believed to lower cancer risk in post-transplant patients.

Studies in kidney transplant recipients have shown that reducing CNIs combined with either the addition of mTOR inhibitors (e.g., sirolimus) or complete conversion to mTOR-based regimens results in a 30–50% decrease in recurrence of nonmelanoma skin cancers (NMSC) [59, 60]. Based on this evidence, the 2018 ILTS consensus recommended the use of mTOR inhibitors for cutaneous squamous cell carcinoma in LT patients [61]. Similarly, for KS, immunosuppression should be minimized as much as possible, with conversion to an mTOR inhibitor being the preferred approach.

When it comes to solid organ DNMs, minimizing or withdrawing CNIs, alongside either adding or switching to an mTOR inhibitor, has been shown to reduce mortality by 55–75%, especially in patients with intermediate or advanced-stage cancers [62, 63]. Notably, none of these studies reported an increase in graft rejection or failure, suggesting that this immunosuppressive strategy is safe in the setting of DNM.

Therefore, CNI minimization and/or mTOR conversion are generally recommended for managing solid tumors in LT recipients, based on multiple nonrandomized studies.

40.8.3 ILTS 2022 Guidelines [45] on Immunosuppression in LT Patients with DNM

The International ILTS 2022 guideline on managing DNM after LT provides the following recommendations:

- CNIs should be reduced to the lowest effective dose to help lower the risk of developing or worsening DNM.
- Any adjustment in immunosuppression should aim to balance the risk of graft rejection with the need for optimal cancer therapy.
- mTOR inhibitors (sirolimus, everolimus) and mycophenolate mofetil (MMF) do not appear to increase cancer risk and are recommended components of CNI-sparing or minimization regimens for both prevention and management of cancer in LT recipients.
- When induction therapy is needed, IL-2 receptor antagonists are preferred.
- Lymphocyte-depleting agents should be avoided as induction agents due to their association with higher cancer risk [45].

40.8.4 Surgical Management and Other Modalities

The management of malignancy in LT recipients is the same as in the general population for surgery and chemoradiotherapy. In addition to this, the modification of immunosuppression medicine must be considered in LT patients with malignancy. However, the transplant surgical member/hepatologist should be part of the MDT for the management of DNM, given the complex nature of LT and the management of immunosuppression. Survival is highest among patients who underwent surgery with curative intent, followed by local ablative therapy or systemic or palliative therapy [36].

40.9 Conclusion

Liver transplant recipients carry a higher risk of developing de novo malignancies in the long term. Regular screening and surveillance protocols are of paramount importance for early detection and treatment.

References

1. Liver [Internet]. [cited 2023 Sep 4]. Available from: https://srtr.transplant.hrsa.gov/annual_reports/2020/Liver.aspx.
2. Durand F. How to improve long-term outcome after liver transplantation? Liver Int. 2018;38(S1):134–8.
3. Gelson W, Hoare M, Dawwas MF, Vowler S, Gibbs P, Alexander G. The pattern of late mortality in liver transplant recipients in the United Kingdom. Transplantation. 2011;91(11):1240–4.
4. Chandok N, Watt KD. Burden of de novo malignancy in the liver transplant recipient. Liver Transplant. 2012;18(11):1277–89.
5. Collett D, Mumford L, Banner NR, Neuberger J, Watson C. Comparison of the incidence of malignancy in recipients of different types of organ: a UK registry audit. Am J Transplant. 2010 Aug;10(8):1889–96.
6. Engels EA, Pfeiffer RM, Fraumeni JF, Kasiske BL, Israni AK, Snyder JJ, et al. Spectrum of cancer risk among U.S. solid organ transplant recipients: the transplant cancer match study. JAMA. 2011;306(17):1891–901.
7. Jiang Y, Villeneuve PJ, Fenton SSA, Schaubel DE, Lilly L, Mao Y. Liver transplantation and subsequent risk of cancer: findings from a Canadian cohort study. Liver Transplant. 2008;14(11):1588–97.
8. Sérée O, Altieri M, Guillaume E, De Mil R, Lobbedez T, Robinson P, et al. Longterm risk of solid organ de novo malignancies after liver transplantation: a French National Study on 11,226 patients. Liver Transplant. 2018;24(10):1425–36.
9. Zhou J, Hu Z, Zhang Q, Li Z, Xiang J, Yan S, et al. Spectrum of de novo cancers and predictors in liver transplantation: analysis of the scientific registry of transplant recipients database. PLoS One. 2016;11(5):e0155179.
10. Frezza EE, Fung JJ, van Thiel DH. Non-lymphoid cancer after liver transplantation. Hepato-Gastroenterology. 1997;44(16):1172–81.

11. Finkenstedt A, Graziadei IW, Oberaigner W, Hilbe W, Nachbaur K, Mark W, et al. Extensive surveillance promotes early diagnosis and improved survival of de novo malignancies in liver transplant recipients. Am J Transplant. 2009;9(10):2355–61.
12. Rademacher S, Seehofer D, Eurich D, Schoening W, Neuhaus R, Oellinger R, et al. The 28-year incidence of de novo malignancies after liver transplantation: a single-center analysis of risk factors and mortality in 1616 patients. Liver Transplant. 2017;23(11):1404–14.
13. Miyazaki T, Sato S, Kondo T, Kusaka M, Gotoh M, Saiki Y, et al. National survey of de novo malignancy after solid organ transplantation in Japan. Surg Today. 2018;48(6):618–24.
14. Piselli P, Verdirosi D, Cimaglia C, Busnach G, Fratino L, Ettorre GM, et al. Epidemiology of de novo malignancies after solid-organ transplantation: immunosuppression, infection and other risk factors. Best Pract Res Clin Obstet Gynaecol. 2014;28(8):1251–65.
15. Tsai HI, Lee CW, Kuo CF, See LC, Liu FC, Chiou MJ, et al. De novo malignancy in organ transplant recipients in Taiwan: a nationwide cohort population study. Oncotarget. 2017;8(22):36685–95.
16. Chen W, Zheng R, Zhang S, Zhao P, Li G, Wu L, et al. Report of incidence and mortality in China cancer registries, 2009. Chin J Cancer Res. 2013;25(1):10–21.
17. Park HW, Hwang S, Ahn CS, Kim KH, Moon DB, Ha TY, et al. De novo malignancies after liver transplantation: incidence comparison with the Korean cancer registry. Transplant Proc. 2012;44(3):802–5.
18. Tiwari A, Saigal S, Choudhary N, Saha S, Rastogi A, Bhangui P, et al. De novo malignancy after living donor liver transplantation: a large volume experience. J Clin Exp Hepatol. 2020;10:448–52.
19. Funk-Debleds P, Ducroux E, Guillaud O, Ursic-Bedoya J, Decullier E, Vallin M, et al. Subsequent nonmelanoma skin cancers and impact of immunosuppression in liver transplant recipients. J Am Acad Dermatol. 2018;79(1):84–91.
20. Menzies S, O'Leary E, Callaghan G, Galligan M, Deady S, Gadallah B, et al. Declining incidence of keratinocyte carcinoma in organ transplant recipients. Br J Dermatol. 2019;181(5):983–91.
21. Dierickx D, Habermann TM. Post-transplantation lymphoproliferative disorders in adults. N Engl J Med. 2018;378(6):549–62.
22. Singh S, Edakkanambeth Varayil J, Loftus EV, Talwalkar JA. Incidence of colorectal cancer after liver transplantation for primary sclerosing cholangitis: a systematic review and meta-analysis. Liver Transplant. 2013;19(12):1361–9.
23. Nicolaas JS, De Jonge V, Steyerberg EW, Kuipers EJ, Van Leerdam ME, Veldhuyzen-van Zanten SJO. Risk of colorectal carcinoma in post-liver transplant patients: a systematic review and meta-analysis. Am J Transplant. 2010;10(4):868–76.
24. Nure E, Frongillo F, Lirosi MC, Grossi U, Sganga G, Avolio AW, et al. Incidence of upper aerodigestive tract cancer after liver transplantation for alcoholic cirrhosis: a 10-year experience in an Italian center. Transplant Proc. 2013;45(7):2733–5.
25. Singh A, De A, Singh V. Post-transplant malignancies in alcoholic liver disease. Transl Gastroenterol Hepatol. 2020;5:30.
26. Jain A, DiMartini A, Kashyap R, Youk A, Rohal S, Fung J. Long-term follow-up after liver transplantation for alcoholic liver disease under tacrolimus. Transplantation. 2000;70(9):1335–42.
27. Engels EA. Epidemiologic perspectives on immunosuppressed populations and the immunosurveillance and immunocontainment of cancer. Am J Transplant. 2019;19(12):3223–32.
28. Watt KD, Pedersen RA, Kremers WK, Heimbach JK, Sanchez W, Gores GJ. Long-term probability of and mortality from De-novo malignancy after liver transplantation. Gastroenterology. 2009;137(6):2010–7.
29. Taborelli M, Piselli P, Ettorre GM, Baccarani U, Burra P, Lauro A, et al. Survival after the diagnosis of de novo malignancy in liver transplant recipients. Int J Cancer. 2019;144(2):232–9.
30. Acuna SA, Fernandes KA, Daly C, Hicks LK, Sutradhar R, Kim SJ, et al. Cancer mortality among recipients of solid-organ transplantation in Ontario, Canada. JAMA Oncol. 2016;2(4):463–9.

31. Na R, Grulich AE, Meagher NS, McCaughan GW, Keogh AM, Vajdic CM. De novo cancer-related death in Australian liver and cardiothoracic transplant recipients. Am J Transplant. 2013;13(5):1296–304.
32. Prenner S, Levitsky J. Comprehensive review on colorectal cancer and transplant. Am J Transplant. 2017;17(11):2761–74.
33. Ajithkumar TV, Parkinson CA, Butler A, Hatcher HM. Management of solid tumours in organ-transplant recipients. Lancet Oncol. 2007;8(10):921–32.
34. Rousseau B, Guillemin A, Tournigand C. Guidelines and tumor boards are required for solid organ recipients with de novo carcinoma. Oncotarget. 2019;10(29):2789–90.
35. Gutierrez-Dalmau A, Campistol JM. Immunosuppressive therapy and malignancy in organ transplant recipients: a systematic review. Drugs. 2007;67(8):1167–98.
36. Rodríguez-Perálvarez M, Colmenero J, González A, Gastaca M, Curell A, Caballero-Marcos A, et al. Cumulative exposure to tacrolimus and incidence of cancer after liver transplantation. Am J Transplant. 2022;22(6):1671–82.
37. Seitz HK, Stickel F. Molecular mechanisms of alcohol-mediated carcinogenesis. Nat Rev Cancer. 2007;7(8):599–612.
38. Saigal S, Norris S, Muiesan P, Rela M, Heaton N, O'Grady J. Evidence of differential risk for posttransplantation malignancy based on pretransplantation cause in patients undergoing liver transplantation. Liver Transplant. 2002;8(5):482–7.
39. Jiménez-Romero C, Justo-Alonso I, Cambra-Molero F, Calvo-Pulido J, García-Sesma Á, Abradelo-Usera M, et al. Incidence, risk factors and outcome of de novo tumors in liver transplant recipients focusing on alcoholic cirrhosis. World J Hepatol. 2015;7(7):942–53.
40. Mangus RS, Fridell JA, Kubal CA, Loeffler AL, Krause AA, Bell JA, et al. Worse long-term patient survival and higher cancer rates in liver transplant recipients with a history of smoking. Transplantation. 2015;99(9):1862–8.
41. Bhat M, Mara K, Dierkhising R, Watt KD. Gender, race and disease etiology predict de novo malignancy risk after liver transplantation: insights for future individualized cancer screening guidance. Transplantation. 2019;103(1):91–100.
42. Maluccio M, Sharma V, Lagman M, Vyas S, Yang H, Li B, et al. Tacrolimus enhances transforming growth factor-beta1 expression and promotes tumor progression. Transplantation. 2003;76(3):597–602.
43. Karran P, Attard N. Thiopurines in current medical practice: molecular mechanisms and contributions to therapy-related cancer. Nat Rev Cancer. 2008;8(1):24–36.
44. Zwart ES, Yüksel E, Pannekoek A, de Vries R, Mebius RE, Kazemier G. De novo carcinoma after solid organ transplantation to give insight into carcinogenesis in general—a systematic review and meta-analysis. Cancer. 2021;13(5):1122.
45. Colmenero J, Tabrizian P, Bhangui P, Pinato DJ, Rodríguez-Perálvarez ML, Sapisochin G, et al. De novo malignancy after liver transplantation: risk assessment, prevention, and management-guidelines from the ILTS-SETH consensus conference. Transplantation. 2022;106(1):e30–45.
46. Oudkerk M, Liu S, Heuvelmans MA, Walter JE, Field JK. Lung cancer LDCT screening and mortality reduction – evidence, pitfalls and future perspectives. Nat Rev Clin Oncol. 2021;18(3):135–51.
47. Liu Q, Yan L, Xu C, Gu A, Zhao P, Jiang ZY. Increased incidence of head and neck cancer in liver transplant recipients: a meta-analysis. BMC Cancer. 2014;14:776.
48. Chow LQM. Head and neck cancer. N Engl J Med. 2020;382(1):60–72.
49. Safaeian M, Robbins HA, Berndt SI, Lynch CF, Fraumeni JF, Engels EA. Risk of colorectal cancer after solid organ transplantation in the United States. Am J Transplant. 2016;16(3):960–7.
50. Razumilava N, Gores GJ, Lindor KD. Cancer surveillance in patients with primary sclerosing cholangitis. Hepatol Baltim Md. 2011;54(5):1842–52.
51. Nasser-Ghodsi N, Mara K, Watt KD. De novo colorectal and pancreatic cancer in liver-transplant recipients: identifying the higher-risk populations. Hepatol Baltim Md. 2021;74(2):1003–13.
52. Kälble T, Lucan M, Nicita G, Sells R, Burgos Revilla FJ, Wiesel M, et al. EAU guidelines on renal transplantation. Eur Urol. 2005;47(2):156–66.

53. Acuna SA, Huang JW, Scott AL, Micic S, Daly C, Brezden-Masley C, et al. Cancer screening recommendations for solid organ transplant recipients: a systematic review of clinical practice guidelines. Am J Transplant. 2017;17(1):103–14.
54. Rodríguez-Perálvarez M, De la Mata M, Burroughs AK. Liver transplantation: immunosuppression and oncology. Curr Opin Organ Transplant. 2014;19(3):253–60.
55. Kauffman HM, Cherikh WS, Cheng Y, Hanto DW, Kahan BD. Maintenance immunosuppression with target-of-rapamycin inhibitors is associated with a reduced incidence of de novo malignancies. Transplantation. 2005;80(7):883–9.
56. Cholongitas E, Mamou C, Rodríguez-Castro KI, Burra P. Mammalian target of rapamycin inhibitors are associated with lower rates of hepatocellular carcinoma recurrence after liver transplantation: a systematic review. Transpl Int. 2014;27(10):1039–49.
57. Jiménez-Romero C, Manrique A, Marqués E, Calvo J, Sesma AG, Cambra F, et al. Switching to sirolimus monotherapy for de novo tumors after liver transplantation. A preliminary experience. Hepatogastroenterology. 2011;58(105):115–21.
58. De Simone P, Fagiuoli S, Cescon M, De Carlis L, Tisone G, Volpes R, et al. Use of everolimus in liver transplantation: recommendations from a working group. Transplantation. 2017;101(2):239–51.
59. Dantal J, Morelon E, Rostaing L, Goffin E, Brocard A, Tromme I, et al. Sirolimus for secondary prevention of skin cancer in kidney transplant recipients: 5-year results. J Clin Oncol Off J Am Soc Clin Oncol. 2018;36(25):2612–20.
60. Campbell SB, Walker R, Tai SS, Jiang Q, Russ GR. Randomized controlled trial of sirolimus for renal transplant recipients at high risk for nonmelanoma skin cancer. Am J Transplant. 2012;12(5):1146–56.
61. Charlton M, Levitsky J, Aqel B, O'Grady J, Hemibach J, Rinella M, et al. International liver transplantation society consensus statement on immunosuppression in liver transplant recipients. Transplantation. 2018;102(5):727–43.
62. Rousseau B, Guillemin A, Duvoux C, Neuzillet C, Tlemsani C, Compagnon P, et al. Optimal oncologic management and mTOR inhibitor introduction are safe and improve survival in kidney and liver allograft recipients with de novo carcinoma. Int J Cancer. 2019;144(4):886–96.
63. Thimonier E, Guillaud O, Walter T, Decullier E, Vallin M, Boillot O, et al. Conversion to everolimus dramatically improves the prognosis of de novo malignancies after liver transplantation for alcoholic liver disease. Clin Transpl. 2014;28(12):1339–48.

Chapter 41
Monitoring of Immunosuppression and Drug Interactions in Liver Transplant Recipients

Anindita Phukan and Manav Wadhawan

Abstract Immunological interplay between donor cells and recipient immune system determines allograft function. Alloreactivity of recipient T-lymphocytes via activated dendritic cells against donor hepatocytes leads to liver rejection. Immunosuppressive drugs play a vital role in mitigating T-cell activation and proliferation, thus protecting the grafted liver. An ideal immunosuppressive drug should maintain normal liver allograft function, with minimal side effects. A detailed knowledge and understanding of immunosuppressive drugs and their interactions are essential for the effective management of liver transplant recipients. Drugs metabolized through cytochrome 3A4 may affect the therapeutic levels of calcineurin and mTOR inhibitors, increasing the risk of graft rejection or immunosuppressive drug toxicity. Several serum biomarkers focusing on T-cell function, cytokine release, and pharmacogenetics of immunosuppressive drug metabolism are in the pipeline, which may improve the clinical management of transplant recipients. Newer advancements in genomics, transcriptomics, and proteomics are likely to provide personalized immunosuppression, the way forward in the future.

Keywords Immunosuppression · Calcineurin inhibitors · Drug monitoring · Biomarkers · Drug interaction

Key Highlights

Given the narrow window, protocol-based therapeutic drug level monitoring is recommended in all liver transplant recipients.

Biomarkers based on immunophenotyping of blood samples are useful in predicting graft acceptance or rejection, thereby allowing clinicians to adjust the immunosuppression doses accordingly.

A. Phukan · M. Wadhawan (✉)
Institute of Digestive & Liver Diseases, BLK-Max Superspeciality Hospital, New Delhi, Delhi, India
e-mail: manavwadhawan@gmail.com

S. Saigal, D. Jothimani (eds.), *Fundamentals of Transplant Hepatology*,
https://doi.org/10.1007/978-981-95-2624-6_41

A thorough knowledge and understanding of immunosuppressive drugs and their interactions are essential in the effective management of liver transplant recipients.

41.1 Introduction

Alloreactivity refers to the immune response by the recipient upon identification of donor antigen as non-self and plays a key role in liver rejection. This alloantigen recognition occurs through binding of donor peptides to the host major histocompatibility complex (MHC) on the antigen-presenting cell (APC), leading to the cascade of activation and proliferation of host T-cells. Immunosuppressive drugs play a vital role in mitigating T-cell response, thus protecting the liver allograft from rejection. An ideal immunosuppressive drug should maintain normal liver allograft function, with minimal side effects. Therapeutic drug monitoring of immunosuppressive drugs in liver transplant recipients has a wider applicability, which helps to understand drug efficacy, compliance, drug toxicity, drug-drug interaction, and dose adjustments. Future management of liver transplant recipients may be guided by the use of serum biomarkers, including genomics, transcriptomics, and proteomics profiles, in order to provide personalized care.

Alloreactivity refers to the recipient's immune response upon recognizing donor antigens (alloantigens) as foreign. If not controlled, this immune reaction can result in organ rejection. The process begins when alloantigens are recognized and bind to major histocompatibility complex (MHC) peptides on the recipient's antigen-presenting cells (APCs). This MHC-alloantigen complex is then presented to the T-cell receptor (TCR) on the recipient's T-cells. Several other ligands on APCs—such as CD28, CD154, CD2, CD11a, and CD54—interact with corresponding receptors on T-cells, serving as co-stimulatory or inhibitory signals, which collectively lead to T-cell activation.

Once T-cells are activated, calcineurin is stimulated, which then activates NFAT (nuclear factor of activated T-cells). NFAT moves into the nucleus and promotes the transcription of interleukin-2 (IL-2). IL-2 is secreted by activated T-cells and binds to IL-2 receptors on neighboring T-cells, promoting cell cycle progression. This initiates clonal expansion of activated T-cells and drives cell-mediated cytotoxicity. The resulting release of cytokines and chemokines creates an inflammatory environment that contributes to graft failure. Immunosuppressive drugs work by targeting various stages of this immune cascade to prevent rejection and preserve graft function.

41.2 Targets of Immunosuppressive Agents in T-Cell Activation

Immunosuppressive drugs inhibit specific points in the T-cell activation pathway. These agents bind to receptors or signaling molecules in the cascade to block T-cell activation. For example, anti-thymocyte globulin (ATG) prevents TCR interaction with the MHC-alloantigen complex and inhibits T-cell proliferation, making it one of the most potent immunosuppressants. Calcineurin inhibitors, such as cyclosporine and tacrolimus, block calcineurin activation. Monoclonal antibodies like basiliximab and daclizumab target IL-2 receptors, thus inhibiting clonal T-cell expansion. Meanwhile, sirolimus and everolimus, which are mTOR (mammalian/mechanistic target of rapamycin) inhibitors, obstruct IL-2 receptor-mediated signal transduction. Immunosuppressants can also interfere with purine and pyrimidine synthesis (Fig. 41.1).

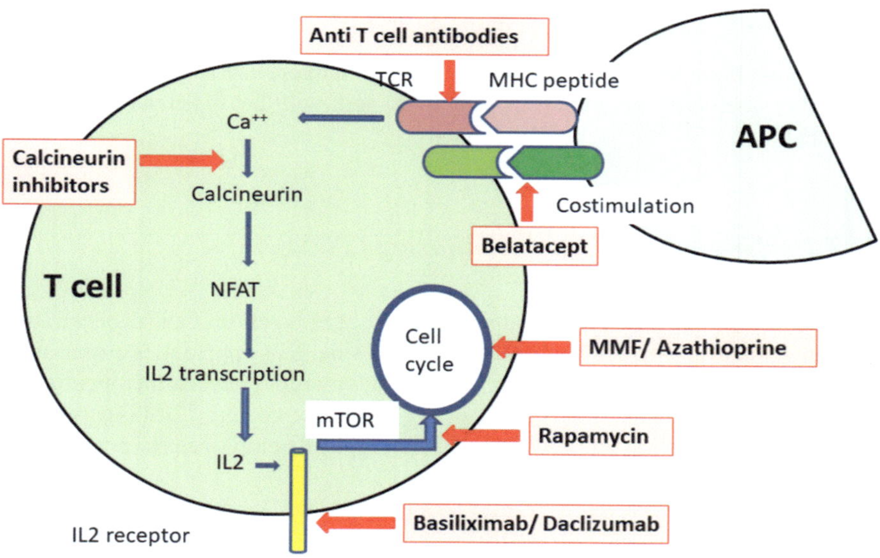

Fig. 41.1 T-cell cascade & targets for current immunosuppressive drugs

41.3 Monitoring Immunosuppression

Optimal immunosuppression is defined as achieving stable graft function with minimal systemic immune suppression. Currently, clinicians rely on judgment and immunosuppressant drug levels to monitor immune status. However, these are indirect markers and do not accurately reflect the real-time level of immunosuppression in an individual. Standard liver function tests are also limited, as they lack sensitivity and specificity for graft rejection and cannot reliably distinguish between acute rejection and other issues like infections. Additionally, these tests poorly correlate with histopathological severity.

Currently, immunosuppression monitoring involves two main methods:

1. Drug level monitoring.
2. Biomarker-based monitoring, which includes:
   - Markers of individual response to immunosuppressants.
   - Indicators of immune reactivity (e.g., tolerance or alloreactivity).
   - Markers of liver injury or graft dysfunction.

Although therapeutic drug monitoring (TDM) remains the standard, alternative biomarker methods are under investigation and will be discussed for better understanding.

41.3.1 Therapeutic Drug Monitoring (TDM)

TDM involves adjusting immunosuppressant dosages based on their concentration in biological fluids—typically whole blood or plasma. This approach is essential for drugs with a narrow therapeutic index, where the margin between therapeutic and toxic doses is small, increasing the risk of over- or under-dosing. TDM is commonly used for calcineurin inhibitors (CNIs) but is not typically employed for mycophenolate. Corticosteroids generally do not require TDM.

Tacrolimus (>90%), cyclosporine (>50%), and mTOR inhibitors (95%) accumulate primarily in red blood cells, so their trough levels are measured in whole blood. On the other hand, mycophenolic acid is found almost entirely in plasma (99.99%), with negligible amounts in cellular elements. Given its low variability and narrow dosing range, routine monitoring of mycophenolate levels is not generally deemed necessary.

While there is potential to monitor circulating free antibodies and antibody complexes (such as alemtuzumab), these tests are not yet available for clinical use.

41.3.2 Techniques for Drug Level Monitoring

TDM can be performed using either immunoassay-based or non-immunoassay methods. Non-immunoassay techniques include liquid chromatography (LC) and mass spectrometry (MS). Although immunoassays are user-friendly and provide quick results, LC-MS or tandem MS is considered the gold standard due to its higher precision and accuracy.

Immunoassays often suffer from cross-reactivity with drug metabolites, resulting in variable readings. In LC-MS, the sample is passed through a chromatographic column where components are separated based on their chemical and physical properties. These separated substances are then ionized and analyzed in a mass spectrometer. However, LC-MS is not without flaws—ions can remain in the collision cell, or matrix interference can affect ionic charge, potentially producing false-positive results. Despite these limitations, LC-MS remains the most reliable and accurate method available. Its use is particularly important in jaundiced patients, as bilirubin interferes with tacrolimus measurement in other methods.

41.3.2.1 Calcineurin Inhibitors (CNIs)

Tacrolimus shares immunosuppressive properties with cyclosporine but is more potent, requiring significantly lower blood concentrations to achieve a similar effect. In clinical settings, tacrolimus monitoring typically involves measuring the pre-dose or trough level (C0) due to its practicality, even though it doesn't always correlate perfectly with total drug exposure. Ideally, exposure should be assessed using the 12-hour area under the concentration—time–time curve (AUC), but this full AUC assessment is not feasible in routine practice.

To improve accuracy, limited sampling strategies (LSS) have been developed, showing a strong correlation with full AUC ($r > 0.9$). These abbreviated AUC methods can be especially helpful in patients who experience toxicity or rejection despite having a C0 within the target range. For example, a study by Capron et al., which included 90 liver transplant recipients on tacrolimus monotherapy, found no link between whole blood tacrolimus levels and histological rejection grade. However, a negative correlation was observed between tacrolimus concentration in peripheral blood mononuclear cells (PBMCs) and the degree of histological rejection. Moreover, intra-PBMC and whole blood tacrolimus levels showed poor correlation.

Dried blood spot (DBS) sampling is gaining interest as it allows easier, more frequent monitoring and the potential to calculate full AUCs. This method is less invasive, only requires a small blood volume (10–20 μL), and can be done at home, improving patient convenience.

Alongside traditional pharmacokinetic monitoring, pharmacodynamic biomarkers are being explored. These include markers within the CNI target pathway: calcineurin phosphatase activity, NFAT nuclear translocation (assessed via flow cytometry), NFAT-dependent gene expression, NFATc1 amplification, and IL-2 concentration or mRNA expression. However, these biomarkers have not yet entered routine clinical use due to their complexity, the need for specialized equipment, and a lack of proven clinical benefit.

41.3.2.2 Mycophenolic Acid (MPA)

MPA primarily distributes in plasma, with about 97% bound to albumin, making plasma or serum the most suitable matrices for measurement. MPA levels have been shown to correlate with clinical outcomes—higher plasma concentrations reduce the likelihood of acute rejection. Due to its low variability among individuals and narrow therapeutic window, routine therapeutic drug monitoring (TDM) is generally not required. However, similar to tacrolimus, DBS-based LSS methods for MPA monitoring are being investigated as promising alternatives for future use.

For pharmacodynamic monitoring, the most extensively studied biomarker is inosine monophosphate dehydrogenase (IMPDH) activity. IMPDH levels fluctuate in response to MPA concentrations. Low pre-transplant IMPDH activity or gene expression is associated with a greater risk of MPA-related adverse effects necessitating dose adjustments, while high pre-transplant IMPDH activity in PBMCs has been linked to increased risk of graft rejection.

41.3.2.3 mTOR Inhibitors

Once ingested, mTOR inhibitors—everolimus and sirolimus—are mainly distributed in red blood cells (75–80% for everolimus, 94% for sirolimus), so whole blood is used for concentration measurement. The key difference between the two lies in their half-lives: sirolimus has a longer half-life (~62 h), requiring once-daily dosing, whereas everolimus has a shorter half-life (~28 h), necessitating twice-daily dosing. Everolimus also reaches steady state more quickly.

There is a strong correlation between C0 and AUC for both drugs ($r \approx 0.9$), making C0 a reliable marker of exposure. As a result, limited sampling strategies are generally not needed. No current research links intracellular concentrations of mTOR inhibitors to transplant outcomes. However, given that these drugs are sequestered in erythrocytes—which lack immunologic function—measuring concentrations in PBMCs or graft tissue may offer better insights into therapeutic impact. Studies evaluating DBS-based monitoring for mTOR inhibitors are still lacking.

In terms of pharmacodynamic assessment, downstream targets of the mTOR pathway—such as phosphorylated 4E-BP1, S6 kinase β1, p70S6K1, and ribosomal S6 protein—have been proposed as drug-specific biomarkers. However, due to methodological complexity, long processing times, and a lack of standardization, these remain in the experimental stage and are not recommended for routine use.

41.3.2.4 Azathioprine

Azathioprine is the preferred immunosuppressant for pregnant transplant patients. It has a slower onset of action, taking 2–4 weeks to reach a steady state. Standard monitoring includes complete blood counts (CBC) and liver function tests to detect leukopenia or hepatotoxicity. According to recent British Society of Gastroenterology guidelines for inflammatory bowel disease, measurement of thiopurine metabolites (6-TGN and 6-MMP in erythrocytes) is recommended to avoid toxicity and under-dosing. However, there are no such recommendations for use in liver transplantation or autoimmune hepatitis (AIH).

41.4 Pharmacogenetics

Pharmacogenetics involves identifying inherent genetic markers within genes that influence drug responses. It holds promise in predicting drug dose requirements and monitoring potential adverse effects. Variations known as single-nucleotide polymorphisms (SNPs)—which are changes in a single base pair of DNA—have been identified in the CYP3A4 and CYP3A5 genes. These variations significantly impact drug metabolism and may allow for personalized medication dosing.

CYP3A4 is the primary enzyme responsible for metabolizing calcineurin inhibitors (CNIs) and mTOR inhibitors (mTORi). Among the most researched SNPs is **CYP3A5*1/*3. The CYP3A5*3 allele results in a non-functional protein due to alternative splicing, leading to reduced enzyme activity compared to the functional CYP3A5*1 allele. Individuals carrying **CYP3A5*1/*1 or *1/*3 genotypes are termed CYP3A5 expressors or rapid metabolizers and typically require 1.5 to 2 times higher doses of tacrolimus to reach the same therapeutic levels as non-expressors (those with the **CYP3A5*3/*3 genotype).

In liver transplantation, interpreting CYP3A5 genotypes is more complex than in other organ transplants, as both the recipient's intestinal and donor's hepatic CYP3A5 expression contribute to tacrolimus metabolism. As a result, both donor and recipient genotypes need to be considered. Two separate meta-analyses have shown that the recipient's CYP3A5 genotype predominantly affects tacrolimus dosing during the first month after transplant, while the donor's genotype becomes more influential thereafter as graft function improves.

The liver enzyme UGT1A9 is responsible for over half of mycophenolic acid (MPA) metabolism. Several SNPs in the UGT1A9 gene have been identified, including 275T > A, 2152C > T, 440C > T, and 331T > C. These genetic variants enhance MPA glucuronidation, thereby lowering systemic MPA exposure and necessitating higher doses to achieve the desired AUC (area under the curve).

However, clinical studies have not demonstrated any benefit of pharmacogenetics-guided MPA dosing when therapeutic drug monitoring (TDM) is already being employed. In addition, MPA pharmacodynamics is affected by genetic variations in the IMPDH1 and IMPDH2 genes.

The ABCB1 gene encodes an efflux transporter that removes xenobiotics into the bile. Polymorphisms in ABCB1 have been linked to changes in the bioavailability of tacrolimus, cyclosporine, and sirolimus. One study found a correlation between ABCB1 gene variations and tacrolimus-related nephrotoxicity in pediatric liver transplant recipients. Although ABCB1 influences the intestinal absorption and intracellular concentrations of CNIs and mTOR inhibitors, current evidence does not support its utility in improving therapy or transplantation outcomes.

Other genetic polymorphisms—such as those causing thiopurine S-methyltransferase (TPMT) deficiency and mutations in nudix hydrolase 15 (NUDT15)—are associated with myelotoxicity from drugs like azathioprine and 6-mercaptopurine, which are less commonly used in transplant medicine.

41.5 Biomarkers for Immune Response (Alloreactivity/Tolerance)

The availability of biomarkers identifying patients with a high risk of acute rejection (AR) could help to identify subjects who need an aggressive immunosuppressant therapy in the early post-transplant period. On the contrary, a biomarker to predict graft acceptance could allow using low doses of immunosuppressant drugs that could avoid or decrease the rate of adverse effects. The most commonly studied biomarkers, such as liver enzymes and pro-inflammatory cytokines, are non-specific and do not allow differentiation of graft dysfunction from other complications such as infections. Similarly, deranged liver functions can be secondary to biliary obstruction or disease recurrence (AIH, PBC, PSC). Biomarkers predicting graft acceptance are based on immunophenotyping of peripheral blood samples and non-specific genome analysis. Various biomarkers currently available & in development have been listed in Table 41.1 [1].

41.5.1 Cytokines/Chemokines

Cytokines are the mediators of the immune response and have been studied to understand the immune response post-transplant. Patients with the same drug levels are found to have different levels of cytokines, depicting a difference in immune response [2]. A study by Kim et al. has shown that combined detection of IL-10, IL-17, and CXCL10 at 1–2 weeks post-operation could predict acute rejection

Table 41.1 Summary of existing and promising Biomarkers of immunosuppression

Biomarkers	Clinical utility	Availability
Drug levels	Drug concentration levels as a marker of immunosuppression (e.g., tacrolimus, cyclosporine)	Commercially available
TPMT genotype/ phenotype	Useful to identify TPMT-deficient patients at risk for myelosuppression	Commercially available
Target enzyme: IMPDH	May predict risk for rejection or MPA-associated toxicity	Commercially available
Target enzyme: mTOR	May predict risk for rejection or mTOR inhibitor—associated toxicity	Research tool
NFAT	May assist to identify transplant recipients at higher risk for adverse effects and may be used to better guide CNI therapy	Research tool
CYP3A5 genotype	May assist in determining optimal tacrolimus starting dose	Commercially available
Total lymphocyte/ CD31 counts	Useful in ATG dose titration	Commercially available
IFN-g	Predictive of the risk for ACR Use for risk stratification and immunosuppression selection	Research tool
IL-2	Predictive of the risk for ACR	Research tool
CD154	Predictive of the risk for ACR after LT and assists immunosuppression minimization	Research tool
CD26 and CD28 T-cell surface antigens	Associated with ACR and/or malignancy after LT	Research tool
Tregs	Predictive of the risk for ACR, can be used to decide immunosuppression conversion	Research tool
Immune cell function assay	Measures intracellular ATP production marker of cell-mediated immune function	Commercially available
Liver function tests (AST, ALT, ALP, bilirubin)	Commonly used as a marker of liver injury and hence ACR; however, low sensitivity and specificity	Commercially available
Chemokines	May predict early allograft dysfunction	Research tool
GcfDNA	Early detection of transplant injury ("liquid biopsy"); guide changes in immunosuppression and minimization	Research tool

following adult liver transplantation [3]. Similarly, in other studies, IL-2 and its receptors (soluble IL-2 R) increased prior to rejection episodes [4].

IFN-γ could be used as a robust candidate biomarker in LT patients, as suggested by Milan et al. in their study, that showed an association between the percentage of IFN-γ CD8+ T-cells and soluble IFN-γ with the severity of AR [5]. Other cytokines that have shown promise include IL-4, IL-6, IL-15, IL-18, IL-23, and TNF-α. However, their utility is limited in clinical practice, as many of these cytokines cannot differentiate between ACR and infection. Membrane proteins like CD28 and Cd38 expressed on T-cells have also been seen in periods of acute rejection.

41.5.2 T-Cells

T-lymphocytes play a central role in the cell-mediated process of rejection. Certain donor-specific T-cells and T-regs (regulatory T-cells) have shown correlation with the risk of rejection[2] [6]. In a study, the correlation of donor-specific CD154 expression in T cytotoxic memory cells, as well as CD26- and CD28-expressing T-cells, has been shown with the risk for acute cellular rejection in transplant recipients [7].

Assessment of T-cell activation was proposed as the most appropriate method for assessing the state of immunosuppression in an individual. The immune cell function assays (ImmuKnow/Cylex) measure intracellular adenosine triphosphate (ATP) production in T-lymphocytes that correlates with T-cell activity. However, there is a lack of data on clinical usefulness [8]. Circulating CD4 + CD25highFoxP3+ regulatory T-cells have a negative correlation with RAI of acute rejection [9]. On the contrary, Th17 cells increase during rejection episodes, and thereby the T reg/Th17 ratio has been suggested as a candidate biomarker in the diagnosis of acute rejection.

41.5.3 Biomarkers for Chronic Rejection

Studies on biomarkers for chronic rejection are very limited, and all of them have been carried out on liver biopsies. C4d has been proposed as a marker of CR, which is seen in 100% of biopsies classified as CR [10]. Other markers like p21 WAF/Cip1 in biliary epithelial cells (percentage and number per portal tract) and their subsequent decrease on treatment of CR may prove to be valuable biomarker.

41.5.4 Donor-Specific Antibodies (DSAs)

Antibody-mediated rejection (AMR) mediated by the donor-specific antibodies can occur in the liver allograft, being involved in both acute and chronic rejections. Anti-HLA antibodies could also be suggested as potential biomarkers for managing immunosuppression after LT. De novo DSAs were almost exclusively against HLA class II antigens, and these patients had significantly lower patient and graft survival [11, 12].

To date, literature shows that high de novo DSAs, HLA class II DSAs, preformed DSA levels, IgG3 and are associated with allograft injury and AMR. These could be suggested as biomarkers of AMR in LTRs. However, more data and studies are required before DSAs are validated as a reliable biomarker of chronic rejection.

41.5.5 Biomarkers for Graft Acceptance (Immune Tolerance)

Operational tolerance is the absence of acute or chronic rejection with normal function and histology in immunocompetent recipients after discontinuing conventional immunosuppression for more than a year. Markers for immune tolerance include;

- NK cells: most robust markers of operational tolerance.
- gdTCR+ Cells: genes encoding for gamma-delta T-cells (γδTcell) are upregulated compared to the immunosuppression-dependent LT patients [13]. Moreover, Martinez et al. have also found a significant increase in the γδ1/γδ2 T-cell ratio in operationally tolerant patients.
- Regulatory T-cells: Increase in CD4+ CD25 T regulatory cells. Also, FoxP3 gene expression—mRNA on microarray studies—has been noted in blood samples as well as liver biopsies in tolerant patients [14].

All these markers are currently under further investigation as the science of immune tolerance is evolving.

41.5.6 Biomarkers Associated with Graft Dysfunction or Injury

Chemoattractant chemokines (CXC), such as CCL-2, CXCL-9, and CXCL-10, are small molecular weight proteins (8–14 kDa) that direct leukocyte migration. These are associated with inflammatory and immune responses after transplantation. High serum concentrations of these chemokines were associated with early allograft dysfunction [15].

Liquid biopsy is also emerging as a new tool in monitoring graft function post-organ transplant. Graft-derived circulating cell-free DNA (Gcf DNA), a marker of cell death released from necrotic or apoptotic cells in the transplanted organ, is another promising new biomarker of allograft dysfunction [16]. Quantitative measurement by ddPCR (droplet digital polymerase chain reaction) assay of donor-derived cell-free DNA (cfDNA) in plasma has been found to be more sensitive in detecting ACR than liver function tests [17, 18].

miRNAs are one class of small noncoding RNAs of 19–24 nucleotides that are important gene regulators at the post-transcriptional level. Many miRNAs seem to be associated with liver ischemia reperfusion injury and can predict ACR. miRNA-122, highly expressed in hepatocytes, shows considerable promise as a biomarker of hepatocyte injury [19]. The contribution of lymphocyte miRNA (such as miR-142-3p) during graft rejection has been studied, as lymphocyte infiltration into the liver is a major pathologic feature of rejection [20].

41.5.7 Future Biomarkers

There is ongoing advancement, especially in the fields of genomics, transcriptomics, and proteomics, in recent times. These have shown new perspectives for the panel of biomarkers. Whether these will simplify the monitoring of immunosuppression is the big question, which should be answered as more studies emerge on this.

41.6 Drug Interactions with Immunosuppressants

Immunosuppressive drugs used in liver transplantation have a narrow therapeutic index, meaning that small variations in drug concentration can significantly impact efficacy or toxicity. Therefore, factors such as individual metabolic capacity, genetic polymorphisms, and altered enzyme activity due to drug interactions can substantially affect the pharmacokinetics of these medications.

As noted earlier, both calcineurin inhibitors (CNIs) and mTOR inhibitors (mTORis) are primarily metabolized through the CYP3A4 and CYP3A5 pathways. Consequently, any medication that affects these enzyme systems can lead to clinically significant drug interactions involving CNIs and mTORis via the CYP3A enzyme family.

A detailed list of commonly encountered drug interactions is provided in Table 41.2, which should be readily accessible to all clinicians managing liver transplant patients. Familiarity with these interactions is essential for optimal patient care.

In addition, co-administration of nephrotoxic agents such as aminoglycosides, non-steroidal anti-inflammatory drugs (NSAIDs), and amphotericin B should be avoided when using CNIs, as these combinations can exacerbate renal impairment.

Potassium-sparing diuretics and antihypertensives—including amiloride, spironolactone, ACE inhibitors, and angiotensin receptor blockers (ARBs)—may increase the risk of severe hyperkalemia when used alongside CNIs.

Combining statins with cyclosporine can elevate statin levels, increasing the risk of myopathy or rhabdomyolysis, and should therefore be avoided. In patients requiring statin therapy, tacrolimus is generally preferred over cyclosporine due to a lower risk of interaction.

Azole antifungals and certain antibiotics like clarithromycin and azithromycin require caution when co-prescribed with CNIs or mTORis due to their potential to inhibit CYP3A metabolism and cause elevated immunosuppressant levels (refer to Table 41.2 for detailed interaction profiles).

Interactions between immunosuppressants themselves must also be considered (see Table 41.3). For instance, dose reduction of CNIs is advised during combination therapy with mTOR inhibitors, as both classes are CYP3A substrates and may mutually inhibit CYP3A enzyme activity, increasing drug levels.

Adjustments to immunosuppressive therapy—whether by initiating, withdrawing, or changing drug combinations—can alter blood drug concentrations,